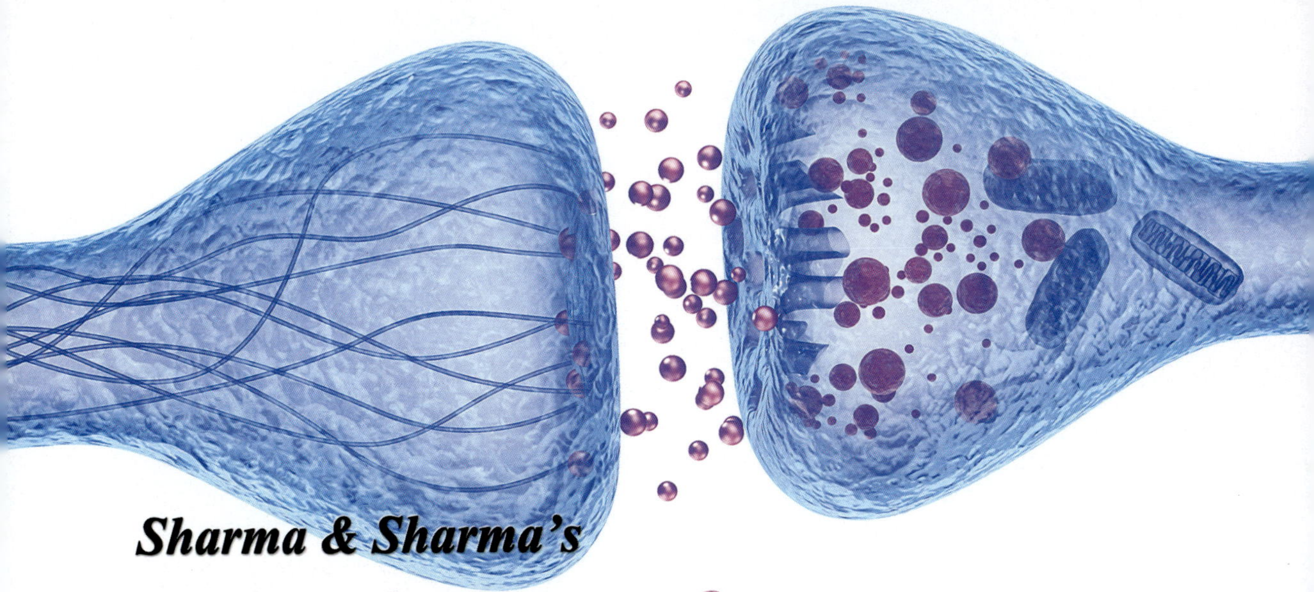

Sharma & Sharma's

Principles *of* PHARMACOLOGY

4th Edition

HL Sharma, PhD, MAMS

Formerly, Professor, Dept of Pharmacology, SMS Medical College, Jaipur;
Prof and Head, Dept of Pharmacology, Jaipur Dental College, Jaipur, Rajasthan, India;
Associate Prof, Dept of Pharmacology, Faculty of Medicine, Al-Fateh University, Libya;
Senior Research Fellow, Research Institute of Temple University, Philadelphia, on a National Institute of Mental Health Program, USA

KK Sharma (Late), MD, FAMS

National CME Coordinator cum Advisor, National Academy of Medical Sciences New Delhi, India; Formerly, Prof and Head, Dept of Pharmacology University College of Medical Sciences, Dilshad Garden, Delhi;
Prof and Head, Dept of Pharmacology, School of Medical Sciences & Research;
Dean, School of Allied Health Sciences, Sharda University, Greater Noida, UP, India

Revised by

Harsh M Joshi, MD

Faculty, Dept of Pharmacology, NHL Municipal Medical College
Gujarat University, Ahmedabad, Gujarat, India

Paras Medical Publisher

PRINCIPLES OF PHARMACOLOGY

PARAS

Paras Medical Publisher
5-1-475, First Floor, Putlibowli
Hyderabad–500095, India
parasmedpub@hotmail.com

Branch Office
2/25, Ground Flr., Arun House
Daryaganj, Ansari Road
New Delhi–100002, India

1st Edition 2007, Reprint 2008, 2010,
2nd Edition 2011, Rev. Reprint 2012,
Reprint 2013, 2nd Reprint 2013,
3rd Reprint 2015, 3rd Edition 2017
Rev. Reprint 2018, Rev. Reprint 2019,
1st Reprint 2020, 4th Edition 2023
1st Reprint, 2nd Reprint 2025

ISBN: 978-81-8191-550-4

To

Our Families

For their support, endurance and encouragement

PREFACE TO THE FOURTH EDITION

Dr KK Sharma (Late), with his vast knowledge and proficiency along with me, has laid the foundation and created this book through many years of involvement. Remembering his tireless hardwork, he has made endless contributions to this book. Lot of agonies on hearing the sudden demise of my friend. He was always with me, not only as a friend but also as a family member. In 25 years of our friendship, he always had a helping nature which kept our bond strong. My heartfelt condolences and I pray almighty God to give immense strength to his family to recover from the deepest sorrow. His contribution in the field of pharmacology was substantial and abundant. He was not only a good teacher, but also a renowned researcher for which he has received various awards. We as a reader of this book must remember such a great personality and feel privileged to learn from the legend.

Pharmacology as a medical discipline has the crucial aspects of drug details, which are constantly updating. The knowledge, attitude and practice owing to the approval of new drugs, discontinuation of drug and recent guidelines keep us dynamic. All who are involved in prescribing (medical doctors) and administration, evaluation and monitoring of drug responses (health professionals - pharmacists and nurses) must remember that in the era of internet, the expectation of patients are high and the community at large demand from them an up-to-date evidence-based knowledge about medicines with which they deal for their safe and effective use in their clinical practice.

The Competency Based Medical Education (CBME) provides an outcome-based strategy, which covers various aspects of teaching including different learning methods & assessment form the framework of competencies. This new edition covers all the elements of drug-related information, organised in the same format of sections, major topics and chapters on drug classes.

Further, I would like to express my gratitude to Dr Harsh M Joshi, Faculty, Department of Pharmacology, NHL Medical Collage, Ahmedabad who has revised the book by adding new chapters such as Dietary supplements, Nutraceuticals, National Health Programmes, Drugs used for skin and ocular disorders, Antibiotic Stewardship Programme, etc., according to the CBME curriculum, all the competencies are covered, which will strengthen the knowledge of medical undergraduates. For better understanding & correlation of undergraduate medical curriculum, a competency table with competency number along with corresponding chapter numbers & page numbers, is included; competency number is also mentioned under the particular chapter heading.

The recent US-FDA approved drugs are also emphasized in the pertinent chapters. The current guidelines of diseases are also updated which equips substantial information for undergraduates and postgraduate medical students. Advancement in molecular techniques, recent trends in development & understanding the pathophysiology of a disease and finding a newer target of drugs, as well as credible evidences focus on the impact of different treatment modalities of therapeutic outcomes.

The recently faced global pandemic of Novel Coronavirus Disease 2019 (COVID-19), caused by the Severe Acute Respiratory Syndrome Coronavirus-2 (SARS-CoV-2) has been associated with significant morbidity and mortality. Safe and effective COVID-19 vaccines are developed to reduce the spread of pandemic and to save millions of lives. An exclusive chapter is dedicated for vaccines including COVID-19 vaccines and all recently developed drugs have been added in the revised edition.

I would also thank Dr Vartika Srivastava, Faculty, Department of Pharmacology, Kalinga Institute of Medical Sciences, Bhubaneshwar for reviewing chapters and providing valuable suggestions.

To conclude, we all pray to God for happiness and healthy life

ॐ सर्वे भवन्तु सुखिनः, सर्वे सन्तु निरामयाः ।

The constructive critiques, comments and suggestions are always welcome. They can be sent to me through e-mail.

HL Sharma

drhl_sharma@yahoo.com

PREFACE TO THE FIRST EDITION

The book *'**Principles of Pharmacology**'* takes a refreshing and an innovative approach towards Pharmacology, which satisfies the requirements of the students. With a subject like pharmacology, which keeps on expanding so rapidly, the perennial problem in writing a textbook is how to present an updated and complicated matter in a simple and understandable language along with an interesting style. In the absence of such expertise, students get confronted with the dilemma of what to read from the book as self-study while teachers get vexed with a problem of what to teach in the classroom. Although the amount of information and method of presentation in the textbook differs from that of classroom, both are essential and interdependent. In a class, the teacher sows the seeds of knowledge in the minds of students but it is the books that provide water and manure to these seeds for sprouting and for blooming into flowers of knowledge.

Before the start of this venture, a majority of our students confessed that the subject matter of pharmacology was hardly accessible to them and that its understanding had always fallen short of what they longed for. They observed that textbooks are just stuffed with factual knowledge at the cost of building concepts and that they are always in a dire need of a self-explanatory book. We too, when we introspected our student life in retrospect, felt that their observations held solid ground. Hence, almost at the fag end of our professional life as a teacher, with enough experience at our command, we decided to write such a textbook that places high premium on basic understanding and building of concepts ignoring unnecessary details. We ourselves carry a heart of a dissatisfied student also which we kept on our desk while writing the chapters. If our heart beat normally after the end of the chapter, we considered our job done successfully. If there were arrhythmias, we explored for the reasons, rewrote the whole chapter, gave it to some students and our learned colleagues to have their feedback to ensure that the message was rightly conveyed.

Each chapter in this book starts with a summary of relevant anatomical, physiological and biochemical information so as to make subsequent pharmacological discussion comfortably comprehensible. To make the text more clear, concise and easy to recall at the time of examination, maximum use of innovative illustrations and tables has been made. To minimize the load of chemistry, the chemical structures of only those drugs have been incorporated, which help in explaining their mode of action or toxicity. Embedded in the text are some similies in the form of short stories, to conceptualise the more complicated aspects of the text easily. Every care has been taken to ensure that the book is free from errors but absolute perfection is usually unattainable. Hence, errors, if any, may please be communicated to us.

CONTENTS

SECTION 5—DRUG THERAPY OF INFLAMMATION & RELATED AUTACOIDS

SECTION 6—DRUGS AFFECTING GIT FUNCTIONS

SECTION 7—DRUGS ACTING ON CENTRAL NERVOUS SYSTEM

SECTION 8—HORMONES AND HORMONE ANTAGONISTS

SECTION 9—DRUGS ACTING ON RESPIRATORY SYSTEM

SECTION 10—DRUGS ACTING ON BLOOD & BLOOD FORMING ORGANS

SECTION 11—CHEMOTHERAPY OF MICROBIAL DISEASES

SECTION 12—CHEMOTHERAPY OF NEOPLASTIC DISEASES

SECTION 13—SPECIAL TOPICS

SECTION 14—APPENDICES

COMPETENCY TABLE

Code	Competency	Ch. No.	Page No.
PH1.1	Define and describe the principles of pharmacology and pharmacotherapeutics	1 2	1 7
PH1.2	Describe the basis of evidence-based medicine and therapeutic drug monitoring	80	972
PH1.3	Enumerate and identify drug formulations and drug delivery systems	3,4	10,17
PH1.4	Describe absorption, distribution, metabolism & excretion of drugs	5,6	27,21
PH1.5	Describe general principles and mechanism of drug action	7	59
PH1.6	Describe principles of pharmacovigilance & ADR reporting systems	8	107
PH1.7	Define, identify and describe the management of adverse drug reactions	7	72
PH1.8	Identify and describe the management of drug interactions	7	95
PH1.9	Describe nomenclature of drugs	1	1
PH1.10	Describe parts of a correct, complete and legible generic prescription. Identify errors in prescription and correct appropriately	73	929
PH1.11	Describe various routes of drug administration	4	17
PH1.12	Calculate the dosage of drugs using appropriate formulae for an individual patient, including children, elderly and patient with renal dysfunction	7	56, 940
PH1.13	Describe mechanism of action, types, doses, side effects, indications and contraindications of adrenergic and anti-adrenergic drugs	12 13	159 195
PH1.14	Describe mechanism of action, types, doses, side effects, indications and contraindications of cholinergic and anticholinergic drugs	10 11	111 132
PH1.15	Describe mechanism/s of action, types, doses, side effects, indications and contraindications of skeletal muscle relaxants	14	201
PH1.16	Describe mechanism/s of action, types, doses, side effects, indications and contraindications of the drugs which act by modulating autacoids, including: anti-histaminics, 5-HT modulating drugs, NSAIDs, drugs for gout, anti-rheumatic drugs, drugs for migraine	24 25 26	344 362 371
PH1.17	Describe the mechanism/s of action, types, doses, side effects, indications and contraindications of local anaesthetics	15	216

Code	Competency	Ch. No.	Page No.
PH1.18	Describe the mechanism/s of action, types, doses, side effects, indications and contraindications of general anaesthetics & preanesthetic medications	31	437
PH1.19	Describe the mechanism/s of action, types, doses, side effects, indications and contraindications of the drugs which act on CNS, (including anxiolytics, sedatives & hypnotics, anti-psychotic, antidepressant drugs, anti-maniacs, opioid agonists & antagonists, drugs used for neurodegenerative disorders, anti-epileptics drugs)	30 32–34 37 39 40	421 448 496 523 539
PH1.20	Describe the effects of acute and chronic ethanol intake	36	488
PH1.21	Describe symptoms & management of methanol & ethanol poisonings	36	488
PH1.22	Describe drugs of abuse (dependence, addiction, stimulants, depressants, psychedelics, drugs used for criminal offences)	35 38	479 514
PH1.23	Describe the process and mechanism of drug deaddiction	38	514
PH1.24	Describe the mechanism/s of action, types, doses, side effects, indications and contraindications of the drugs affecting renal systems including diuretics, antidiuretics–vasopressin & analogues	16 17	227 241
PH1.25	Describe the mechanism/s of action, types, doses, side effects, indications and contraindications of the drugs acting on blood, like anticoagulants, antiplatelets, fibrinolytics, plasma expanders	51	681
PH1.26	Describe mechanisms of action, types, doses, side effects, indications and contraindications of the drugs modulating renin-angiotensin and aldosterone system	18	254
PH1.27	Describe mechanisms of action, types, doses, side effects, indications & contraindications of antihypertensive drugs and drugs used in shock	19 71	262 919
PH1.28	Describe mechanisms of action, types, doses, side effects, indications & contraindications of drugs used in ischaemic heart disease (stable, unstable angina & myocardial infarction), peripheral vascular disease	20	282
PH1.29	Describe mechanisms of action, types, doses, side effects, indications and contraindications of the drugs used in congestive heart failure	22	315
PH1.30	Describe mechanisms of action, types, doses, side effects, indications and contraindications of the antiarrhythmics	21	296
PH1.31	Describe mechanisms of action, types, doses, side effects, indications & contraindications of the drugs used in management of dyslipidaemias	23	328
PH1.32	Describe mechanism/s of action, types, doses, side effects, indications and contraindications of drugs used in bronchial asthma and COPD	48 49	650 661

Code	Competency	Ch. No.	Page No.
PH1.33	Describe mechanism of action, types, doses, side effects, indications & contraindications of the drugs used in cough (antitussives, expectorants/mucolytics)	49	659
PH1.34	Describe the mechanism/s of action, types, doses, side effects, indications and contraindications of the drugs used as: (1) Acid-peptic disease and GERD; (2) Antiemetics and prokinetics; (3) Antidiarrhoeals; (4) Laxatives; (5) Inflammatory bowel disease; (6) Irritable bowel disorders, biliary and pancreatic diseases	27 28 29	390 402 411
PH1.35	Describe the mechanism/s of action, types, doses, side effects, indications & contraindications of drugs used in haematological disorders like: (1) Drugs used in anaemias; (2) Colony stimulating factors	50	663
PH1.36	Describe the mechanism of action, types, doses, side effects, indications and contraindications of drugs used in endocrine disorders (diabetes mellitus, thyroid disorders and osteoporosis)	45 46 47	613 624 633
PH1.37	Describe the mechanism of action, types, doses, side effects, indications and contraindications of the drugs used as sex hormones, their analogues and anterior pituitary hormones	41 43	550 584
PH1.38	Describe the mechanism of action, types, doses, side effects, indications and contraindications of corticosteroids	42	568
PH1.39	Describe the mechanism of action, types, doses, side effects, indications and contraindications of the drugs used for contraception	43	584
PH1.40	Describe the mechanism of action, types, doses, side effects, indications and contraindications of: (1) Drugs used in the treatment of infertility; (2) Drugs used in erectile dysfunction	41 44	560 610
PH1.41	Describe the mechanism of action, types, doses, side effects, indications and contraindications of uterine relaxants & stimulants	41	565
PH1.42	Describe general principles of chemotherapy	52	699
PH1.43	Describe and discuss the rational use of antimicrobials including Antibiotic Stewardship Programme	53–58 77	714 959
PH1.44	Describe the first-line antitubercular dugs, their mechanisms of action, side effects and doses	59	764
PH1.45	Describe the dugs used in MDR and XDR tuberculosis	59	764
PH1.46	Describe the mechanism of action, types, doses, side effects, indications and contraindications of antileprotic drugs	59	777

Code	Competency	Ch. No.	Page No.
PH1.47	Describe mechanisms of action, types, doses, side effects, indications and contraindications of the drugs used in malaria, Kala-Azar, amebiasis and intestinal helminthiasis	63 64 65	814 824 838
PH1.48	Describe mechanisms of action, types, doses, side effects, indications & contra. of drugs used in UTI/STD & viral diseases including HIV	61,62 83	789 801
PH1.49	Describe mechanisms of action, classes, side effects, indications and contraindications of anticancer drugs	67	853
PH1.50	Describe mechanisms of action, types, doses, side effects, indications and contraindications of immunomodulators and management of organ transplant rejection	69	891
PH1.51	Describe occupational and environmental pesticides, food adulterants, pollutants and insect repellents	89	1009
PH1.52	Describe management of common poisoning, insecticides, sting & bites	88	1005
PH1.53	Describe heavy metal poisoning and chelating agents	68	885
PH1.54	Describe vaccines and their uses	87	998
PH1.55	Describe & discuss following National Health Programmes including immunisation, tuberculosis, leprosy, malaria, HIV, filaria, kala azar, diarrhoeal diseases, anaemia & nutritional disorders, blindness, non-communicable diseases, cancer and Iodine deficiency	79	966
PH1.56	Describe basic aspects of geriatric and paediatric pharmacology	74	939
PH1.57	Describe drugs used in skin disorders	81	976
PH1.58	Describe drugs used in ocular disorders	82	981
PH1.59	Describe and discuss the following: Essential medicines; Fixed dose combinations; over the counter drugs; herbal medicines	6 9	57 110
PH1.60	Describe and discuss pharmacogenomics and pharmacoeconomics	78	963
PH1.61	Describe and discuss dietary supplements and nutraceuticals	84	989
PH1.62	Describe and discuss antiseptics and disinfectants	66	847
PH1.63	Describe drug regulations, acts and other legal aspects	76	955
PH1.64	Describe overview of drug development, phases of clinical trials and good clinical practice	8	97
PH3.5	To prepare and explain a list of P-drug for a given case/condition	9	111

CHAPTER 1

SECTION 1—GENERAL PRINCIPLES OF PHARMACOLOGY

Introduction

COMPETENCY PH1.1

WHAT IS PHARMACOLOGY

Whenever a study is made about a living organism, the first question which comes to our mind is, how does it work? In other words, what is the science of its normal vital processes? That is what we study in Physiology. The next question that follows is, what chemical reactions take place during its physiological functions? That is precisely what we study in Biochemistry. Then it automatically strikes us—can we alter its physiological or biochemical functions by means of some chemical agents? *Hence in Pharmacology we study as to how drugs can alter the physiological or biochemical functions of a living organism*. The term 'drug' is derived from the Greek word *"Pharmakon"* (English: *Pharmacon*) meaning a 'Drug' and *"Logos"* meaning a 'Science'. *Pharmacology can also be defined as a science which deals with the mechanism of action, therapeutic uses, adverse effects and fate of drugs in human beings or animals.*

WHAT IS A DRUG

Since Pharmacology, in a broader sense, covers all aspects of the knowledge about drugs, let us now define a drug: *A 'drug' is a chemical substance used for the treatment, cure, prevention or diagnosis of a disease in human beings or animals.*

This definition is, however, incomplete as it ignores the use of contraceptives which alter a physiological system to prevent pregnancy, which is not a disease. On the same analogy, the definition fails to recognize general anaesthetics as drugs as these are not used for any cure, diagnosis or prevention of a disease. Similarly, vaccines or antisera which alter the pathological state by formation of antibodies are also not properly covered by this definition.

World Health Organization (WHO) Scientific Group (in 1966) had to redefine the drug as *"any substance or product that is used or intended to be used to modify or explore physiological systems or pathological states for the benefit of the recipient."*

DRUG CATEGORIES

Drugs fall into two categories:

Non-prescription Drugs (OTC drugs)

These are safe drugs and can be sold **o**ver-**t**he-**c**ounter (OTC), by the chemist, without prescription, e.g., vitamins, antacids and paracetamol, etc.

Prescription Drugs

These are classified in various Schedules and Drug Acts. These drugs are used under medical supervision and dispensed by an order of a registered medical practitioner, e.g., antibiotics, anxiolytics, antidepressants and antihypertensive drugs, etc.

DRUG NOMENCLATURE

Every drug has three types of names.

Chemical Name

This is a name given according to the chemical constitution of a drug. These are very complex, hard to remember and difficult to use in a prescription (Table 1.1). Sometimes a code name, e.g., SKF-525-A (later named proadifen), may be given by the manufacturer for convenience before an approved name is allotted to the drug; but this is neither a chemical nor an official name. The vast majority of coded compounds never become drugs. The generic name is given only when such coded compound has the potential to be a useful drug.

Non-proprietary or Generic Name

These names are assigned by the United States Adopted Name (USAN) Council or by British Approved Name (BAN) Council, only when the drug has been found to be of potential therapeutic usefulness. These names are used uniformly all over the world by an international agreement through the WHO. When included in an official pharmacopoeia, the non-proprietary name becomes an *official name*. The non-proprietary/official name is frequently referred to as *generic name.* There may be variations in generic names given by USAN and BAN Councils, e.g., epinephrine and norepinephrine in USA are called adrenaline and noradrenaline, respectively in Europe and the UK; other examples include furosemide (in USA) versus frusemide (in UK) and cromolyn sodium (in USA) versus sodium cromoglycate (in UK). The allotment of generic names has some elements of drug categorization, because their common endings indicate their pharmacological classification. Examples include:

1. Drugs ending with "olol" belong to β-adrenergic receptor blockers, e.g., propranolol and atenolol (used to treat hypertension). Exception: Stanozolol which is an anabolic steroid.
2. Drugs ending with "caine" are usually local anaesthetics, e.g., lignocaine and prilocaine.
3. Drugs ending with 'dipine' are normally Ca^{2+} channel blockers used to treat hypertension, e.g., nifedipine and amlodipine.
4. Drugs ending with 'prazole' are grouped as proton pump inhibitors used to decrease gastric acid secretion, e.g., omeprazole and lansoprazole.
5. Drugs ending with 'cycline' are tetracycline group of antibiotics, e.g., doxycycline and minocycline.
6. Drugs ending with 'pril' are angiotensin converting enzyme inhibitors (ACE inhibitors) used to treat hypertension and heart failure, e.g., lisinopril, ramipril and enalapril.
7. Drugs ending with 'sartan' are angiotensin receptor antagonists used to treat hypertension, e.g., losartan, candisartan and telmisartan.
8. Oral hypoglycaemic agents (antidiabetic drugs) usually have "gli" in the middle or in the beginning of their spelling, e.g., glipizide, gliclazide, repaglinide, pioglitazone and sitagliptin.
9. Drugs ending with 'statin' are antihyperlipidaemic agents, e.g., atorvastatin and rosuvastatin.
10. Drugs ending with 'floxacin' are fluoroquinolone group of antibiotics, e.g., ciprofloxacin, ofloxacin.

Proprietary or Trade or Brand Name

Non-proprietary names, however, are sometimes difficult to pronounce or spell. The trade name selected by the pharmaceutical company to market the non-proprietary drug is usually small and easy to recall and therefore most widely used by the medical practitioners. This name is a copyright or registered name of the drug by which it is sold, by any drug company, in the market. Hence there may be several trade names, from different drug companies, for the same non-proprietary (generic) drug (see Table 1.1).

Prototype Drug

To permit an easy recognition of the drugs belonging to a particular group and to correlate their pharmacological effects, the attention is usually focussed on the original or the most commonly used drug belonging to a pharmacological group. Such a selected drug is called *prototype drug*, e.g., lignocaine is a prototype drug for local anaesthetics, while morphine is a prototype drug for narcotic analgesics. Prototype drug is usually the parental drug from which other drugs were developed.

SUBDIVISIONS OF PHARMACOLOGY

The broad science of pharmacology may be subdivided into the following categories listed below.

Pharmacokinetics

It deals with the **a**bsorption, **d**istribution, **m**etabolism and **e**xcretion (ADME studies) of the drugs. In short, it is a branch which deals with "what the body does to the drug".

Pharmacodynamics

It includes the study of (i) the biological effects produced by the drugs, (ii) the site at which and the mechanism by which it acts and (iii) the relationship of the plasma concentration of the drug with its response and duration of action. In short, it deals with "what a drug does to the body".

Pharmacotherapeutics

This deals with the clinical application of the pharmacodynamic and pharmacokinetic information about the drug in the prevention, treatment or diagnosis of a disease.

Table 1.1 Nomenclature of Drugs

Chemical name	Non-proprietary name	Proprietary name
Acetyl salicylic acid	Aspirin	**Ecospirin®** (USV, India) **Mejoral®** (CFL Pharma Ltd., India) **Loprin-DS®** (Unisearch, India) **Disprin®** (Rickett and Benckiser, India)
p-Acetamido phenol	Paracetamol	**Crocin®** (GSK, India) **Calpol®** (Burroughs Wellcome, India)
Aminobenzyl penicillin	Ampicillin	**Biocillin®** (Biochem Pharma, India) **Synthocillin®** (PCI, India) **Roscillin®** (Ranbaxy, India) **Albercillin®** (Aventis, India)

Trade names are usually suffixed by ® denoting registered name.

Clinical Pharmacology

It deals with the protocols of clinical evaluation of a new drug in healthy volunteers and patients. It devises scientific methodology for evaluating the therapeutic safety and efficacy of a drug by doing comparative clinical trials. It also includes the feedback monitoring of adverse effects of a drug, after its marketing.

Toxicology

It deals with the toxicity of drugs and poisonous effects of various chemicals in use (household, environmental, industrial or homicidal). It is also concerned with the symptoms and treatment of poisoning. Harm is the end point in toxicology while benefit is the end point of pharmacotherapeutics.

Chemotherapy

It deals with the treatment of systemic infections or malignancy with drugs that have selective toxicity for the infecting organism (living or multiplying) or malignant cell with minimal toxicity to host cells.

Pharmacogenetics

It is the study of inherited (single gene mediated) differences in drug metabolism or drug response in humans. For example, peripheral neuritis in slow acetylators while hepatotoxicity in fast acetylators of isoniazid (antitubercular drug).

Pharmacogenomics

This is a recent branch which overlaps pharmacogenetics. It makes the use of genetic make up (genome) of an individual so as to choose a particular drug therapy for the responders only and to avoid giving such drug to nonresponders (i.e., tailoring the drug therapy on the basis of an individual's genotype). For example, a recently introduced anticancer drug, *gefitinib*, is highly effective in curing lung cancer but only in those patients who have mutations in the tyrosine kinase receptor (10% of the cases), which is the target of action of this drug. Such individuals can be identified in advance by genotyping.

Pharmacoepidemiology

It is the study of the use of and effects of a drug in large population after its approval for clinical use. It is now well established that the *risk:benefit ratio* of the drug can be ascertained only after the drug is used widely by the general population.

Pharmacovigilance

Clinical trials conducted prior to drug approval cannot uncover every aspect of drug effect. Many are discovered later. The WHO suggests that every country should set up a pharmacovigilance center and the adverse drug reaction data of any new drug (even of an old drug) should be shared with global health care community through WHO-Uppsala monitoring center located in Sweden. *Pharmacovigilance* means continuous monitoring for unwanted effects and other safety related aspects of marketed drugs. It is the science related to the **D**etection, **A**ssessment, **U**nderstanding and **P**revention (DAUP) of adverse effects or any other drug-related problem.

Other allied fields of pharmacology are:

Pharmacy

Pharmacy differs from Pharmacology which is more of a profession that deals with the manufacture, compounding and dispensing of drugs for therapeutic use. With the rapid advancements of dosage forms of the drug, the pharmacist now is no longer required to prepare and dispense the drug since this is done for him by the pharmaceutical manufacturers. Hence with the changing trends, role of a pharmacy expert is of the community and hospital pharmacist, who has more specific knowledge about other properties of drugs such as stability, shelf life, preservation, handling of drug preparations and helping the patients in proper use of drugs.

Pharmacognosy

It is the study of the sources and identification of drugs from various sources such as plants, minerals, animals, etc.

Biopharmaceutics

The study of the effects of drug formulation on the therapeutic response.

SOURCES OF INFORMATION ABOUT DRUGS

Although textbooks, reviews and journals provide information about established drugs and furnish the ground for understanding newer ones, they obviously cannot include other details such as trade names, physical and chemical properties, identification, standards of purity and strength, methods of storage and dosage forms available for therapeutic use. These details are necessary from legal point of view for drug control. All such information about drugs is provided by Pharmacopoeias and Formulary (collectively known as Drug Compendia). ***Pharmacopoeias*** limit the drug information up to drug substances and dosage forms and its committee usually has predominance of physicians. ***Formulary*** on the other hand deals with pharmaceutical ingredients also and its committee has predominance of pharmacists (Table 1.2).

Table 1.2 Official Drug Compendia

Pharmacopoeias	Formulary
British Pharmacopoeia	Pharmaceutical Codex *(by Pharmaceutical Society of Great Britain)*
United States Pharmacopoeia	National Formulary *(by American Pharmaceutical Association)*
Indian Pharmacopoeia	National Formulary of India

Drug compendia could be *official* or *non-official.*

Official Compendia

Here information is provided by non-proprietary names of the drugs, not by trade names. It is a compilation of legally approved drugs for use in that country along with their legal standards of purity, quality and strength. Pharmacopoeias and formularies are official compendias.

Non-official Compendia

It serves as a secondary source of drug information. It provides very useful and miscellaneous information about drugs, both by trade names as well as by generic names for a medical practitioner or a pharmacist. This information is generalised and is not restricted to only those drugs which are approved for use by the legally constituted committee of that country.

For example:

1. *AMA Drug Evaluations*: by American Medical Association and Council on Drugs.
2. *Modern Drug Encyclopedia:* by Yorke Medical Books, New York, USA.
3. *Physicians' Desk Reference* (PDR): by Medical Economics Publications, USA.
4. *Martindale Extra Pharmacopoeia:* by Pharmaceutical Society of Great Britain.

LAWS GOVERNING DRUGS (DRUG SCHEDULES)

Definition of Controlled Substance Schedules

Drugs and other substances that are considered controlled substances under the Controlled Substances Act (CSA) are divided into five schedules. An updated and complete list of the schedules is published annually in ***Title 21 Code of Federal Regulations (C.F.R.) 1308.11 through 1308.15***. Substances are placed in their respective schedules based on whether they have a currently accepted medical use in treatment in the United States, their relative abuse potential and likelihood of causing dependence when abused. Some examples of the drugs in each schedule are listed below.

Schedule I

Substances in this schedule have no currently accepted medical use in the United States, a lack of accepted safety for use under medical supervision and a high potential for abuse. Some examples of substances listed in Schedule I are heroin, lysergic acid diethylamide (LSD), marijuana (cannabis), peyote, methaqualone and 3,4-methylenedioxy-methamphetamine ("Ecstasy").

Schedule II/IIN

Substances in this schedule have a high potential for abuse which may lead to severe psychological or physical dependence. Examples of Schedule II narcotics include hydromorphone, methadone, meperidine, oxycodone and fentanyl. Other Schedule II narcotics include morphine, opium, codeine, and hydrocodone. Examples of Schedule IIN stimulants include amphetamine, methamphetamine and methylphenidate. Other Schedule II substances include amobarbital, glutethimide and pentobarbital.

Schedule III/IIIN

Substances in this schedule have a potential for abuse less than substances in Schedules I or II and abuse may lead to moderate or low physical dependence or high psychological dependence. Examples of Schedule III narcotics include products containing not more than 90 mg of codeine per dosage unit and buprenorphine. Examples of Schedule IIIN non-narcotics include benzphetamine, phendimetrazine, ketamine and anabolic steroids such as testosterone.

Schedule IV

Substances in this schedule have a low potential for abuse relative to substances in Schedule III. Examples of Schedule IV substances include alprazolam carisoprodol clonazepam clorazepate, diazepam, lorazepam, midazolam, temazepam and triazolam.

Schedule V

Substances in this schedule have a low potential for abuse relative to substances listed in Schedule IV and consist primarily of preparations containing limited quantities of certain narcotics. Examples of Schedule V substances include cough preparations containing not more than 200 mg of codeine per 100 ml or per 100 g and ezogabine.

In India, the Legislative Laws related to drugs have a wider coverage. According to the Drugs and Cosmetics Act 1940 (along with the Drugs and Cosmetic Rules 1945) as amended by the Drugs and Cosmetic Rules 2001 (10th Amendment) the Schedules for the drugs are as under:

Schedule A gives the specimens of prescribed forms.

Schedule B states fees for test or analysis by the Central Drugs Laboratory or the Government Analyst.

Schedule C and C1 deals with biological and other special products.

Schedule D is devoted to exemption regarding import of drugs.

Schedule E1 gives a list of poisonous substances under Ayurvedic, Siddha and Unani systems of medicine.

***Schedule F and F(I)** give details of the standards of bacterial vaccines made from any microorganism pathogenic to man or other animals and also the vaccines made from other microorganisms which have any antigenic value.

Schedule FF gives details of the standards for ophthalmic preparations.

Schedule F (II) gives details of standards for surgical dressings and bandage cloth.

Schedule F (III) gives standards for umbilical tapes.

***Schedule G** details the drugs to be labelled with the words "Caution - it is dangerous to take this preparation except under medical supervision".

***Schedule H** deals with drugs and medicines which must be sold by retail only when a prescription by registered medical practitioner is produced. Most drugs fall under this schedule.

Schedule J gives the list of the ailments for which no drug should claim prevention or cure.

Schedule K lays down the condition under which certain cases are exempted from the provisions of Chapter IV of the Drugs Act.

***Schedule M** deals with Good Manufacturing Practices (GMP) and requirements of premises, plant and equipment (for allopathic medicines). Part I deals with good manufacturing practices and factory premises. Part II deals with plant and equipment.

Schedule M1 prescribes in detail requirements of factory premises for the manufacture of homeopathic drugs.

Schedule M-II prescribes requirements of factory premises for manufacture of cosmetics.

Schedule M-III prescribes requirements of factory premises for manufacture of medical devices.

Schedule N deals with the minimum equipment of a pharmacy and gives directions regarding: (a) entrance of a pharmacy, (b) premises, (c) furniture and apparatus, and (d) general provisions.

Schedule O deals with the provisions applicable to disinfectant fluids.

***Schedule P** deals with the 'expiry period' of and drug formulations. It gives period in months for which the drug is expected to retain its potency under the conditions of storage notified by licensing authority.

Schedule P-1 deals with pack sizes of drugs.

Schedule Q gives the list of dyes, colours and pigments permitted to be used in cosmetics and soaps.

Schedule R describes the standards for mechanical contraceptives.

Schedule R-1 prescribes standards of medical devices.

Schedule S prescribes standards for cosmetics.

Schedule T lays down the requirements of factory premises and hygienic conditions for ayurvedic and unani drugs.

Schedule U and U1 give the particulars to be shown in manufacturing records.

Schedule V gives details of standards for patent and proprietary medicines.

***Schedule W** gives the names of the drugs which shall be marketed under generic names only.

***Schedule X** gives the names of psychotropic drugs requiring special licenses for manufacture and sale.

***Schedule Y** specifies requirements and guidelines on clinical trials, import and manufacture of new drugs.

** Important schedules in common usage.*

CHAPTER 2

Nature and Sources of Drugs

COMPETENCY PH1.1

After knowing the drug definition, its categories, nomenclature and source of information, we must now discuss about various sources from which drugs are obtained and their chemical nature in a broader sense.

The drugs can be obtained from either of the following sources:

SYNTHETIC SOURCE

Presently, the majority of drugs are obtained synthetically or semi-synthetically. Some of the drugs which were earlier obtained from plant or animal source are today synthesized in the laboratories, the advantages being:

1. Their quality can be better controlled.
2. The process is easier and cheaper.
3. The chemical structure of the prototype drug can be modified in search of better, more potent and safer drug because the pharmacological activity of a drug is a function of its chemical structure and physical properties.

Numerous such examples would appear throughout the text in this book. Aspirin, paracetamol, phenytoin, chlorpromazine, amphetamine, chloroquine and various sulfa drugs belong to this class of drugs.

VEGETABLE SOURCE

Drugs belonging to the following categories are usually obtained from vegetable source.

Alkaloids

These are nitrogenous heterocyclic bases derived from plants. Alkaloids as such are insoluble in water but being alkali-like, they form salts with acids which are water soluble. Alkaloids are pharmacologically active principle of plants. Examples: atropine from *Atropa belladona*, quinine from *Cinchona* bark, morphine from *Papaverum somniferum* (poppy), reserpine from *Rauwolfia serpentina* and nicotine from tobacco leaves. The names of all alkaloids usually end with 'ne'.

Glycosides

Glycosides are those plant products, where a sugar moiety is joined to a nonsugar moiety with a ether linkage (-O-). However, if the sugar moiety is glucose, the glycoside is called a glucoside and if it is an aminosugar then it is called aminoglycoside.

Sugar	- O -	Non-sugar	—	Glycoside (e.g., digoxin)
Glucose	- O -	Non-sugar	—	Glucoside
Amino sugars	- O -	Non-sugar	—	Aminoglycosides (e.g., streptomycin)

On hydrolysis with mineral acids, all glycosides split up into the sugar and the non-sugar residues. The pharmacological activity of a glycoside resides in its non-sugar molecule which is called an 'aglycon' (or genin). The sugar portion, however, governs the pharmacokinetic characteristics of the glycoside. Some important examples of glycosides are cardiac glycosides used in the treatment of congestive heart failure, e.g., digitoxin, digoxin which are obtained from foxglove leaves (*Digitalis purpurea*) and ouabain obtained from *Stropanthus gratus*. Aminoglycosides are, rather, obtained from microorganisms (and not from plants source) and are used as antimicrobial agents.

Oils

The following three types of oils are generally used for various medical purposes.

i) Essential Oils (or volatile oils)

These are obtained from leaves or flower petals by steam distillation. These are steam volatile, have aroma, have no caloric or food value, do not form soaps with alkalis and do not become rancid (foul smell) on prolonged stay. These are mainly used as carminatives, astringents in mouth washes, or as flavouring agents, e.g., eucalyptus oil, clove oil, peppermint oil and ginger oil. Some of them may be solid at room temperature and sublimate on heating, e.g., menthol and camphor.

ii) Fixed Oils

These are non-volatile, have caloric or food value, form soaps with alkalis and become rancid after prolonged stay. These are obtained by solvent extraction of crushed seeds. Examples are groundnut oil, coconut oil and olive oil. Fixed oils have little pharmacological use except for castor oil (purgative) or arachis oil (demulcent).

Gums

These are the colloidal exudates of the plants. They either swell, or dissolve or form adhesive mucilage in water. These are used as emulsifying or suspending agents, e.g., gum acacia and gum tragacanth.

Tannins

These are non-nitrogenous phenolic derivatives from plant source and are soluble in water. They are mainly used as astringents, e.g., tinct. catechu and tinct. rhubarb.

Resins

These are polymers of volatile oil and are insoluble in water, e.g., benzoin (used as inhalation in common cold), tinct. benzoin (as antiseptic protective sealing over bruises), colophony (which is an oleoresin used as an ingredient in various plasters) and shellac (from *Lucifer lacca*, used for enteric coating of tablets). Balsams are also a type of resin (a mixture of resin, benzoic acid and volatile oil), e.g., Tolu balsam which is used as an expectorant in cough mixtures.

ANIMAL SOURCE

Many drugs are obtained from animal source and these comprise hormones, vitamins, vaccines and sera, e.g., insulin from pancreas, vitamin B_{12} from liver extract and thyroxine from thyroid; it also includes cholera, BCG, TAB, smallpox, polio and antirabies vaccines, antidiphtheria and antitetanus sera.

MICROBIOLOGICAL SOURCE

Some of the fungi, moulds and bacteria are important sources of many life-saving drugs, e.g., penicillin from *Penicilium notatum*, chloramphenicol from *Streptomyces venezuelae*, griseofulvin (an antifungal drug) from *Penicilium griseofulvum* and aminoglycoside group of antibiotics, like streptomycin from *Streptomyces griseus* and neomycin from *Streptomyces fradiae*.

MINERAL SOURCE

Many pharmacotherapeutic agents are obtained from the mineral source. These agents are solid or liquid and mineral preparations.

i) Solid/Powder and Liquid Preparations

The solid and powder preparations dispenced for medical use are: ferrous sulphate (in anaemia), magnesium sulphate (as purgative), aluminium hydroxide, calcium carbonate, sodium bicarbonate (as antacids) and kaolin (aluminium silicate) as adsorbent in antidiarrhoeal preparations. Tincture iodine and povidon iodine solutions used as antiseptics are some examples of liquid mineral preparations. Radioactive isotopes are a relatively newer source of mineral drugs, e.g., ^{131}I for the diagnosis and treatment of thyrotoxicosis and thyroid malignancy.

ii) Mineral Preparations

These are mostly petroleum products and are obtained by dry distillation of wood. These have no food value and do not become rancid. These are mainly used as vehicles for preparation of ointments, e.g., hard and soft paraffin and also as purgative-laxative, e.g., liquid paraffin.

GENETICALLY ENGINEERED/BIOTECHNOLOGY-BASED DRUGS/BIOPHARMACEUTICALS/ BIOLOGICAL AGENTS

Biotechnology-based drugs are prepared by genetic engineering which means the manipulation of genetic material using recombinant DNA technology. In this method a desired gene is inserted into a very fast multiplying non-pathogenic strain of some bacteria, e.g., *E. coli-K12*. This host cell will now produce large amounts of the gene-directed proteins which are required. *E. coli,* otherwise, does not synthesise these proteins. Examples: Humulin (human insulin by inserting proinsulin gene); Recombinax-HB (a hepatitis-B vaccine) and Human erythropoietin (a hormone that stimulates the production of RBC).

MONOCLONAL ANTIBODIES (MAbs) AS DRUG CARRIERS

Different antigens stimulate different B-cells to produce different antibodies. These antibodies, therefore, are called polyclonal antibodies. On the other hand, an antibody that recognizes and reacts only with a single and specific antigen is called a "**Monoclonal Antibody (MAb)**." These can be produced by the fusion of the B-cell (which produces an antibody against a desired antigen) with a cancer cell from mouse myeloma. The resulting hybrid cells (hybridoma) are then cloned to produce highly specific antibodies (MAbs) in larger amounts. These hybridomas now have an ability of B-lymphocyte to produce a single species of antibody and the capability of the cancer cell to grow endlessly. Cancer cells often have unique "tumour-associated antigens" expressed onto their surface. Therefore, MAbs can also be used to treat various cancers. For example, Rituximab is a MAb against "CD20 antigen" found on the surface of malignant B-lymphocytes of non-Hodgkin's lymphoma. It is given by slow IV infusion to such patients. If the spelling of a MAb ends up with "**omab**," it means it has been obtained from murine source (e.g., edricolomab); if it ends with "**zumab**," it is derived from human source (e.g., omalizumab), and if it ends with "**ximab**," it is a chimeric (part human-part murine) MAb (e.g., rituximab).

CHAPTER 3 Dosage Forms of the Drugs

COMPETENCY PH1.3, PH2.1

The pharmacist today is no longer called upon to prepare or to package the drugs at doctors' prescription, because this is now done for him by the pharmaceutical companies who prepare and supply the drugs in various dosage forms and formulations for administration to the patients. The drugs are not administered as such but are formulated as liquids, capsules, tablets or injections.

Formulation

It is a recipe by which a drug is prepared. It contains the list of active ingredients (the drug) and other substances, like excipients, vehicles, flavouring agents and preservatives, with the amounts contained therein.

Dosage Form

It is the form (e.g., as tablet or capsule or injection or oral liquid) in which the above formulation can be administered to a patient.

Excipients

These are pharmacologically inert substances which are added to the pharmaceutical preparation either to add bulk to the active drug (if it is used in extremely small quantities) or to mask (or lessen) the unpleasant taste, e.g., lactose, calcium lactate, starch, etc.

Vehicles

It is a broader term depicting the substances which are used to dissolve or suspend the drugs, in a pharmaceutical preparation, to make them better applicable (as in ointments) or more palatable (as in liquids), e.g., sugar syrups, cherry syrup, gum acacia and petroleum jelly, etc.

The dosage forms can be classified as:

SOLID DOSAGE FORMS

Powders

These may be simple (containing one drug) or mixture of drugs in a dried and finely pulverised form intended for internal or systemic use (e.g., aspirin powder, sodium bicarbonate powder). Some powders are used externally, e.g., dusting powder.

Effervescent Powders

These are powdered drugs mixed with sodium bicarbonate, critic acid or tartaric acid. When dissolved in water, they effervesce with evolution of carbon dioxide (e.g., Eno fruit salt) and thus make the mixture more palatable and tasty. The same formulation in tablet form (see below) is called dispersible tablet, e.g., Disprin (dispersible aspirin tablet).

Granules

These are small aggregates of powder held together by a binding agent (e.g., starch or alcoholic spray), e.g., vitamin D_3 granules. Some of these formulations can also be dissolved in a specified volume of water to make a suspension for immediate oral use in children, e.g., amoxycillin or ampicillin dry syrup.

Tablets

These are powdered or granulated form of drug compressed under heavy pressure into a round or disk-like shape suitable for swallowing.

i) Ordinary Tablets

These are uncoated compressed tablets, e.g., aspirin tablets, paracetamol tablets.

ii) Sugar-coated Tablets

These are tablets coated over by sugar to avoid bitter taste of ingredients, e.g., tab. chloroquine, tab. metronidazole.

iii) Film-coated Tablets

Transparent film coating is done by gelatin or cellulose derivatives so that tablet size or weight remains unaffected but its unpleasant taste is masked, e.g., Ceftum (cefuroxime film coated tab.); Dilgard (diltiazem film coated tab.).

iv) Enteric-coated Tablets

Coating is made of cellulose acid phthalate, shellac or keratin. This coating is resistant to gastric acid but dissolves at intestinal alkaline pH. The active drug is thus protected from destruction at acidic pH and incidence of gastric irritation is reduced, e.g., Diclofen-EC 50 mg (diclofenac enteric coated tab.), Enzar forte (enteric coated enzyme preparation), Dynasprin encotabs (enteric coated aspirin with dipyridamole) and Ecospirin- 75 (enteric coated aspirin tablets).

v) Long Tablets (retard tablets, sustained release tablets)

Aggregated drug particles have individual coating with different types of inert resins so that each type of coating dissolves at different time intervals. Such tablets provide a uniform and sustained release of the drug over a period of 10–12 hr and hence have a lower incidence of side effects, e.g., K Gard (pot. chloride retard tabs), Diclonac-SR (diclofenac sod. sustained release), Depin Retard (nifedipine retard tab.). Controlled release preparations are most appropriate for drugs of shorter half-life where poor compliance can lead to therapeutic failure.

vi) Pellets

These are sterile spheres (marketed in sterile vials) formed by compression of drug powder (particularly steroid hormones) which are implanted subcutaneously and form a depot, from which the drug is slowly released for a long duration of time, e.g., testosterone pellets.

vii) Lozenges

It is a tablet containing drug with sugar and a gum, and is meant for chewing or sucking for providing local effects in mouth or throat, e.g., various cough lozenges, like Strepsil.

Capsules

These are tasteless gelatin containers, of appropriate size, having powdered drug and excipients (if any) and are meant for swallowing, e.g., tetracycline cap., amoxycillin cap., chloramphenicol cap., etc. *Hard gelatin capsules* are used to enclose powdered drug (e.g., amoxycillin) while *soft gelatin capsules* are used to enclose oily drug (e.g., vit.E). The gelatin shell quickly dissolves in GIT fluid to release the drug for absorption into the circulation.

Spansules

These are longer acting capsules, practically same as described under Long Tablets (as above), but in capsule form, e.g., iron formulations, like Fefol, Isomack Retard (isosorbide dinitrate tab.), Angispan -TR. Spansules can be noticed as coloured beads of drug granules inside a capsule. These beads are coated with different resins which dissolve at different time intervals.

LIQUID DOSAGE FORMS FOR INTERNAL USE

Aqueous Solutions

These are subdivided into the following categories:

i) Syrups

These contain drug(s) in concentrated solution of sugar plus flavouring agents and permitted colours, e.g., various cough syrups, vitamin syrups.

ii) Liquors

These are aqueous solutions of medicinal substances which are either gases or are volatile or which sublimate, e.g., hydrogen peroxide solution, liquor ammonia and iodine solution. These are usually referred to as solutions.

iii) Linctus

These are viscous syrupy liquids containing the drug with some demulcent, like menthol. *These are to be sipped without dilution* to provide soothing effect in sore throat locally, e.g., cough linctus.

iv) Injections

These are sterile solutions or sterile suspensions of the drug in suitable solvent plus preservatives and are meant for parenteral use, e.g., injection digoxin, injection xylocaine. Some injections are supplied as dry solids in sterile vials. For these, aqueous vehicles like water for injection or Ringer solution for injection are used for preparing injection before use, e.g., procaine penicillin injection, chloramphenicol injection.

Depot Injection

It is a longer acting injectable preparation practically same as described under Long Tablets and Spansules (as above), but in injection form. The drug is dissolved in sterile oily base (e.g., fixed oil or oleic acid esters) from which it is slowly released for a prolonged duration, e.g., Testoviron depot (testosterone depot inj.); Anatensol (fluphenazine depot inj.)

Aqueous Suspensions

i) Mixtures

These are solid drugs dispersed homogeneously in water by means of some harmless suspending agent (agar agar), e.g., antidiarrhoeal mixtures and milk of magnesia etc.

ii) Emulsions

These are obtained when two or more immiscible liquid medicaments are dispersed together by means of some suspending agent (gum acacia). One of the liquids serves as continuous phase in which the other liquid is dispersed uniformly in fine droplet form, e.g., cod liver oil emulsion, liquid paraffin emulsion, castor oil emulsion. Milk is an example of a naturally occurring emulsion.

Alcoholic Solutions

i) Spirits

These are 10% v/v solution of volatile essential oils plus alcohol and are generally used as flavouring agents, masking agents and to some extent as preservatives, e.g., spirit chloroform, spirit ammonia aromaticus, peppermint spirit.

ii) Elixirs

These are pleasantly flavoured solutions of a drug in sugar syrup or glycerol *along with higher proportions of alcohol,* e.g., vitamin B-complex elixirs, cough elixirs; but these preparations are now on the decline. The very few that are left, are Lanoxin (digoxin) Elixir and Theophylline Elixir etc. Alcohol is used in elixirs as a solvent for drugs that are not sufficiently soluble in water alone. Alcohol in less than 10% concentration increases sweetness also.

iii) Tinctures

These are alcoholic extracts of plant drugs (drug contents 10–20% w/v), e.g., tinct. belladona, tinct. digitalis. Many tinctures are used as flavouring agents, e.g., tinct. cardamom Co. and tinct. Zingibaris (in such cases drug contents may range from 20% to 50%). Hydroalcoholic solutions of inorganic substances are also called tinctures, e.g., tinct. iodine which is used as an antiseptic.

Drops

These are mainly paediatric formulations which contain small amounts of highly concentrated solutions of drug(s), e.g., vitamin drops and enzyme drops. Eye/ear drops are also included in this category. These are sterile, isotonic buffered solutions of the drug. These are usually supplied in a vial with a dropper, e.g., sulfacetamide eye drops, gentamicin ear drops etc.

Enema

These are medicated liquid preparations for rectal administration and are used for evacuation of colon, e.g., soap water enema, procalys enema.

LIQUID DOSAGE FORMS FOR EXTERNAL USE

Liniments

These are liquid medicaments *to be rubbed on skin with friction.* It contains drug(s) in a liniment vehicle (fixed oil or soap) and water or alcohol. One ingredient is usually camphor which serves as counterirritant. These are mainly used as pain relievers or as rubefacient (making skin red), e.g., liniment camphor, and liniment turpentine. Such preparations are lesser in use.

Lotions

These are liquid medicaments *for local application but without rubbing*. They are generally used as antiseptics or for soothing, astringent and antipruritic effects, e.g., zinc calamine lotion, povidone iodine scrub lotion.

Tinctures and Solutions

These are hydroalcoholic solutions of inorganic substances (active drug contents 10–20% w/v), which depending on the methods of manufacturing are called tinctures, e.g., tincture iodine and tincture benzoin or solutions, e.g., povidone iodine solutlion which are used as antiseptics to sterlize the skin surfaces before surgery or to wash the wounds.

Ointments

These are soft, semi-solid masses containing the drug in a greasy base (like soft or hard paraffin or wool fat), e.g., soframycin skin ointment and silver sulfadiazine ointment. Some ointments are prepared in a water miscible base (vehicle). Ophthalmic ointments are sterile medicated ointments for eye ailments, e.g., chloramphenicol eye ointment, atropine eye ointment.

Cream

It is an emulsion, semisolid dosage form, usually containing > 20% water and volatile oil and/or < 50% hydrocarbons, waxes, or polyols as the vehicle. This dosage form is generally for external application to the skin or mucous membranes.

Gels

The active drug is dissolved in a liquid and then dispersed in some gelling agent (soft gelatin, etc.). These are usually transparent preparations, e.g., contraceptive gels. However, the term is also used for colloidal aqueous suspensions of hydrated inorganic substances, e.g., aluminium hydroxide gel.

Paste

It is like an ointment but it does not have a greasy base. Instead, they are prepared with some adhesive material (like starch) or a foaming agent (like carboxymethyl cellulose), e.g., zinc oxide paste, toothpastes, etc.

Plaster

It contains a drug mixed in a resinous base spread over a muslin cloth. Some plasters are coated with water repellent film also. The preparation remains hard at room temperature but becomes sticky at body temperature. These are meant for protective action and also for antiseptic action, e.g., zinc oxide plaster, belladona plaster and Band-Aid.

SPECIAL AND NOVEL DOSAGE FORMS

Inhalants

Liquid preparations containing a drug to be inhaled as vapour, e.g., tinct. benzoin inhalation and Karvol inhalant. The contents may be poured into a jug of boiling water and inhaled. Solid inhalants, like Fintal (sod. cromoglycate) are inhaled with the use of turbo spin inhaler.

Aerosols

These are devices in which therapeutically active ingredient(s) dissolved in a liquid is put inside a cylindrical container (nebulizer) and is then filled with a propellant gas (air or oxygen) under pressure. A push at the valve releases the drug through a microfined orifice in the form of liquid mist which is inhaled. If one push releases a measured dose of the drug, then these are called as "metered aerosols", e.g., salbutamol metered aerosol, terbutaline metered aerosol.

A spinhaler is an aerosol device in which therapeutically active ingredient(s) are packaged in the form of a powder, that are released upon activation of an appropriate valve system in the form of microfined powder mist, e.g., tiotropium metered spinhaler.

Suppositories (rectal), Pessaries (vaginal) and Bougies (urethral)

These contain the drug mixed with glycerine or gelatin or hard soap or coca butter. These remain solid at room temperature but become slippery and melt at body temperature. Suppositories are bullet shaped, pessaries are conical, while bougies are pencil shaped. For example: Dulcolax suppositories and Candizole-T (miconazole+ tinidazole) vaginal pessaries.

Transdermal Adhesive Patch

In these adhesive patches, the drug is incorporated into a polymer (usually polyisobutylene) which in turn is bonded to an adhesive plaster. The drug is delivered at the skin surface by diffusion, for percutaneous absorption into circulation. These preparations are designed to provide steady and smooth plasma concentration of the drug for a period ranging from 1–3 days from the site of their application (usually chest, abdomen, upper arm or mastoid region). Examples are transdermal patches of nitroglycerin (Nitroderm-TTS), nicotine (Nicotinell-TTS) and estradiol (Estraderm-TTS).

DRUG TARGETING: SPECIAL DRUG DELIVERY SYSTEMS

For better patient compliance and to improve the drug delivery, at the site where it is required, special drug delivery systems have recently been developed which have an added advantage of prolonged duration of drug action. Some of these systems are:

Ocuserts

These are thin elliptical microunits that contain the drug in a reservoir from which the drug is slowly released through a membrane by diffusion at a steady rate. For example: Pilocarpine ocusert used in glaucoma, which is placed under the lower eyelid to deliver pilocarpine for a period of 7 days, thus avoiding the need for instilling eye drops repeatedly every day.

Progestaserts

This is an intrauterine contraceptive device which is inserted into uterus where it delivers progesterone constantly at a specified rate for a period of one year.

Drug Encapsulated in Liposomes for Intravenous Infusion

Liposomes are minute vesicles produced by sonication of an aqueous suspension of certain phospholipids. They can be filled with non-lipid soluble drugs, which are retained until the liposome is disrupted. Amphotericin (an antifungal drug used to treat systemic mycoses) is available in a liposomal formulation for intravenous infusion; the preparation is less nephrotoxic and better tolerated than the conventional forms, albeit considerably more expensive.

Prodrugs

This is an inactive form of drug which gets metabolised in the body to an active drug. These are used to overcome the pharmacokinetic disadvantage of the useful drug. For example: Dopamine is very useful in treating parkinsonism, but it does not cross blood-brain barrier. Levodopa, its prodrug, can cross BBB, which is then converted to dopamine in the CNS. Prodrug may also be used to provide longer duration of drug action, e.g., esters of penicillins get slowly hydrolysed in the body to provide slow and sustained release of penicillins (e.g., Procaine Penicillin-G and Benzathine Penicillin-G).

Computerised Miniature Pumps

These are programmed to release drugs at a definite rate, either continuously as in the case of insulin or intermittently in pulses as in the case of GnRH (gonadotrophin-releasing hormone). These pumps may also be provided with glucose sensor devices which trigger the desired dose of insulin as per body's demand. Both invasive as well as non-invasive miniature pumps are now available.

Monoclonal Antibodies (MAbs) as Drug Carriers

Antibodies produced after immunisation are usually "polyclonal antibodies" because natural antigens have multiple epitopes (antigenic determinants) each of which generates separate clones of activated B-lymphocytes. On the contrary, those antibodies which are produced by a single clone and are directed against a single antigenic determinant (epitope), are called "monoclonal antibodies" (MAbs).

Large scale production of monoclonal antibodies against any specific antigen is now done by using "hybridoma technology". Hybridomas are somatic cell hybrids, obtained by fusing a specific B- lymphocyte (forming antibody against a specific antigen) with a mouse myeloma (tumour) cell. The resultant hybridoma, therefore, retains the antibody-forming capacity of the B-lymphocyte with an ability of the myeloma tumour cell to proliferate endlessly.

To generate these antibodies, the mouse myeloma cells are first grown in a culture deficient in hypoxanthine phosphoribosyl transferase (HPRT) enzyme so as to inactivate antigen and to prevent the subsequent formation of immunoglobulins (because a tumour cell itself has a specific antigen on its surface). These myeloma cells are then fused with B-lymphocytes, obtained from the spleen of mouse immunised with the desired antigen, in polyethylene glycol. The fused cells (hybridomas) are then placed in HAT medium and cloned. In HAT medium, only the hybridomas can survive and replicate. Such hybridomas can be maintained endlessly in this culture and can continue to produce monoclonal antibodies (MAbs) which can be eluted and purified for clinical use (Fig. 3.1).

Murine (rodents) MAbs are usually not prefe-rred these days, as they have a shorter half-life and induce a human antimouse antibody allergic reaction. Hence murine MAbs have now been partly humanised by genetic manipulation. These are called "Chimeric MAbs" in which murine variable region is coupled to the human constant region in the antibody structure (i.e., part human part mouse antibody).

However, totally humanised MAbs are the least antigenic. These are obtained either by recombinant DNA technology (by replacing a part of mouse gene sequence with human gene sequence) or by grafting of "complimentarity determining regions (CDRs)" of murine MAbs on human immunoglobulins framework *(For details see Fig. 69.5B)*.

Principle of naming the monoclonal antibodies: The name of any monoclonal antibody ends with a suffix "mab". The letter before "mab" indicates the source of the antibody, e.g., "o" for murine *(omab),* "xi" for chimeric, i.e. part human-part mouse *(ximab),* "zu" for humanized, i.e. more part human-less part mouse

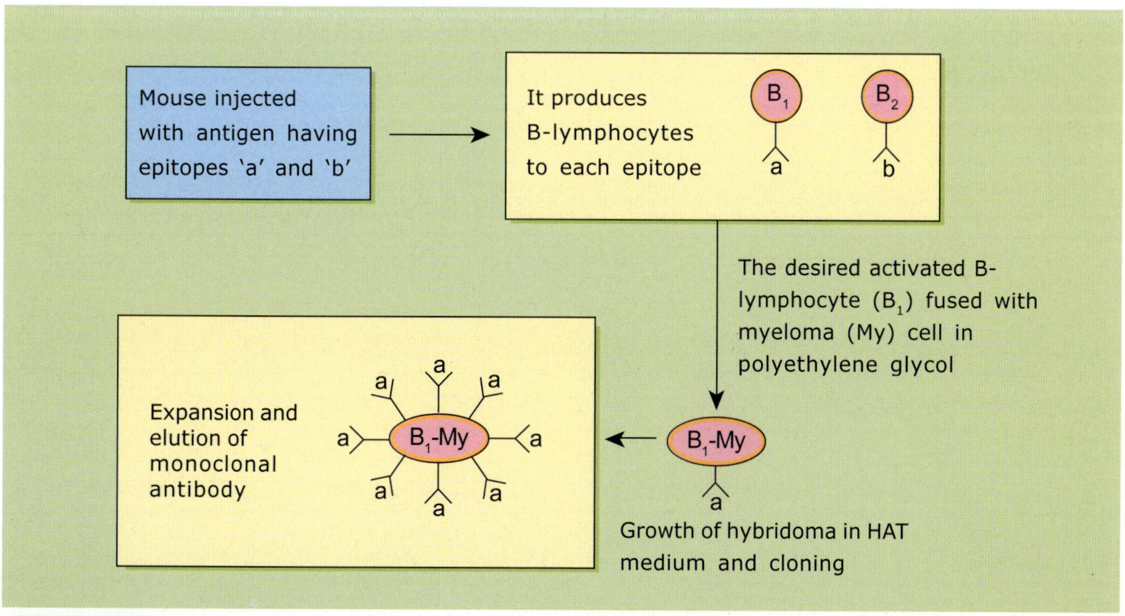

Fig 3.1 Synthesis of Monoclonal Antibodies (finer details have been ommited)

(zumab) and "u" for fully human. The letters appearing before these words denote their therapeutic use, e.g., "tu" for tumour, "vi" for virus and "ci" for circulation . If there is no such prefix then such a "MAb" is generally an immuno-modulator.

For example, *muromonab-CD3* is a murine anti-CD3 monoclonal antibody which is used to prevent transplant rejections (Ch. 69). *Rituximab* (Ch. 67) is a chimeric monoclonal antibody used to treat non-Hodgkin's lymphoma (tumour). *Palivizumab* (Ch. 61) is a humanised MAb that binds to fusion protein of respiratory syncytical virus (RSV) and thus prevents RS-viral infection in airways. *Abciximab* (Ch. 51) is a chimeric MAb which binds to GP IIb/IIIa receptors present on activated platelets to prevent their aggregation. *Edrecolomab* is a murine monoclonal antibody used to treat colorectal cancer (Ch. 67).

CHAPTER 4

How Drugs are Administered

COMPETENCY PH1.3, PH1.11

ROUTES OF DRUG ADMINISTRATION

For any drug to exert its pharmacological effects, it must reach its site of action. This usually necessitates its biotransportation across the cell membranes, which cannot be achieved unless the drug is purposely administered to produce its effects *systemically* or *locally*. Hence in this chapter the discussion will be centered around how drugs are administered, i.e., what are the different routes of their administration. The major routes of drug administration are:

I. Enteral Routes

i) Oral
ii) Sublingual
iii) Rectal

II. Parenteral Routes

A) Injections

i) Intravenous
ii) Intramuscular
iii) Intraperitoneal
iv) Intrathecal
v) Intramedullary
vi) Intra-arterial
vii) Intra-articular
viii) Subcutaneous
ix) Intracardiac
x) Epidural

B) Inhalational Administration

C) Transdermal Administration

III. Topical Routes

i) Conjunctival, Nasal and Auditory mucosal
ii) Vaginal and Urethral
iii) Inunction and Dermal

ENTERAL ROUTES

Placement of a drug directly into any part of the gastrointestinal tract is called an 'enteral' mode of administration (Gk. *enteron* = intestine).

i) Oral Administration

Site: Swallowing a drug through mouth.

Advantages: Most commonly used method as it is safe, convenient and painless procedure. Besides, it is economical as sterilization of drug is not essential.

Disadvantages: (i) Drugs have slower onset of action as their absorption is slow and erratic. Many drugs being highly polar (e.g., aminoglycoside group of antibiotics—streptomycin) or being quaternary salts (e.g., d-tubocurarine) are not absorbed and hence cannot be given orally to provide systemic effects, (ii) Drugs that are destroyed by digestive juices (e.g., penicillin-G, insulin, oxytocin and testosterone) cannot be administered by this route, (iii) Drugs having first-pass effect, i.e., those destroyed in liver before reaching systemic circulation (e.g., nitroglycerine morphine, isoprenaline) are not preferred to be given by this route, (iv) Palatability of drugs is essential and (v) Drugs cannot be given by this route to an unconscious and uncooperative patient or to a patient having nausea, vomiting and diarrhoea.

Examples with Dosage Forms: Majority of drugs in solid dosage forms (e.g., tablets, capsules and powders) or in liquid dosage forms (syrups, elixirs and mixtures) are usually given orally. Majority of drugs given orally provide *systemic effects,* excepting a few which are administered orally to provide *local effect,* e.g., antacids and antidiarrhoeal drugs, such as norfloxacin, neomycin, pectin and kaolin, etc.

ii) Sublingual (and buccal) Administration

Site: The drug is placed beneath the tongue or crushed in mouth and spread over the buccal mucosa.

Advantages: (i) Quick onset of action because of rapid absorption taking place through buccal or sublingual mucosal membrane, (ii) After absorption, the drug passes directly into the systemic circulation, bypassing the portal circulation, thus avoiding first-pass degradation and (iii) The drug can be spitted out if side effects are observed.

Disadvantages: (i) Distasteful, irritant drugs cannot be given; (ii) Unfortunately, drugs of higher molecular weights are not well absorbed by this route; otherwise, it could have been an extremely useful method for drugs like insulin or other peptides.

Examples with Dosage Forms: Isosorbide dinitrate and nitroglycerin tablets (for angina); and nifedipine in liquid form (after crushing the capsule, for hypertension). Drugs administered by this route mainly provide *systemic effects* except for the use of antiseptic lozenges which provide a *local effect* over buccal mucosa.

iii) Rectal Administration

Site: Through rectum.

Advantages: (i) Can be useful for patients having nausea and vomiting, (ii) First-pass degradation is relatively less, as a major portion of the drug is absorbed from external haemorrhoidal veins and (iii) Useful for gastric irritant drugs also.

Disadvantages: (i) Chances of rectal inflammation, (ii) Absorption is unreliable, (iii) Inconvenient and embarrassing to the patient.

Examples with Dosage Forms: (i) For *local effects*: bisacodyl and glycerine suppositories, enemas and ointments, (ii) For *systemic effects*: aminophylline (bronchodilator) and indomethacin (anti-inflammatory agent) suppositories.

PARENTERAL ROUTES

Routes other than "enteral" are called 'parenteral' routes of administration (Gk. *par* = aside from). Thus the administration of drugs by injection, by topical application to skin or by inhalation through the lungs are all parenteral. However, for convenience and better understanding, topical routes will be discussed separately.

A) Injections

Majority of them provide fast systemic effects bypassing first-pass inactivation.

i) Intravenous Administration

Site: Through lumen of the veins, mainly the antecubital vein.

Advantages: (i) The drug enters the systemic circulation directly, bypassing first-pass degradation (100% bioavailability). There is a quick onset of action and a lesser dose is required to achieve the desired plasma concentration (valuable in emergency), (ii) Can be employed even in unconscious, uncooperative patients and in those having nausea, vomiting and diarrhoea, (iii) Hypertonic solutions and GIT irritant drugs can also be infused by this route, (iv) Large volume of fluids can be infused at a uniform rate by this route, and (v) Amount of the drug can be controlled with an accuracy not possible by any other route.

Disadvantages: (i) Strict aseptic conditions are needed and the patient has to depend on somebody for giving an injection, (ii) Besides being painful, it is risky because once the drug is injected it cannot be recalled, (iii) Introduction of any particulate matter or air may produce embolism which may prove fatal, (iv) Drugs in suspension or oily drugs cannot be administered by this route, as a result there are no 'depot injections' available for this route and (v) Venous thrombosis, thrombophlebitis and necrosis around the site of injection can result if extravasation occurs.

Examples with Dosage Forms: Glucose (GDW), Glucose Normal Saline (GNS), dopamine and norepinephrine drips for I.V. infusion. Many antibiotics, barbiturate anaesthetics, diazepam, heparin, etc. are injected by this route. The route provides mainly *systemic effects* of drugs.

ii) Intramuscular Injection

Site: Deltoid muscle or gluteal mass of left or right buttock. Vastus muscle underlying the lateral surface of the thigh may also serve as an alternative area.

Advantages: (i) Absorption is more predictable, less variable and rapid compared to oral and subcutaneous route and (ii) Depot injections can also be given by this route, for obtaining sustained drug effects.

Disadvantages: (i) Perfect aseptic conditions are needed, (ii) Chances of abscess at the site of injection, (iii) Chances of nerve damage leading to paresis of muscle supplied by it and (iv) Large volumes cannot be administered (maximum of 5 ml).

Examples with Dosage Forms: Various antibiotics, antiemetics and depot injection of testosterone, and neuroleptics (haloperidol and perphenazine depot injection). The route provides mainly *systemic effects* of drugs.

iii) Intraperitoneal Administration

Site: Into the peritoneal space.

Advantages: Rapid absorption due to larger surface area.

Disadvantages: Painful, risky due to chances of adhesions and infections in peritoneal cavity (peritonitis). Aseptic conditions are needed.

Examples with Dosage Forms: Less in use except for administering dialysing fluids for peritoneal dialysis in cases of poisoning and renal failure. Most commonly used procedure for administering drugs in laboratory animals. The route provides mainly *systemic effects*.

iv) Intrathecal (intraspinal) Administration

Site: Into the subarachnoid space.

Advantages: The drug after diffusing from the lumbar sac passes into the the subarachnoid space, bypassing the blood-brain barrier and blood-CSF barrier. Thus, significant CSF levels are provided which otherwise are not possible by any other route. The drug acts directly on meninges and the spinal cord.

Disadvantages: Strict aseptic conditions and great expertise is needed to give such injections. Moreover, it is a painful and risky procedure.

Examples with Dosage Forms: (i) Many radiopaque contrast media for myelography (to visualise spinal cord), (ii) Xylocaine injection for providing spinal anaesthesia. Mainly provide *local effects* but certain antibiotics used to treat infectious meningitis do provide *systemic effects* when given by this route.

v) Intramedullary Administration

Site: Injection into the tibial or sternal bone marrow.

Advantages: Onset of action very fast as the vascular spaces of bone marrow communicate directly with the large veins.

Disadvantages: Risky, painful, strict aseptic conditions are needed and skill is also needed to give such injections.

Examples with Dosage Forms: Bone marrow transplantation. Sometimes (but rarely) blood is also transfused by this route, specially in children, if veins are not available. Mainly provide *systemic effects.*

vi) Intra-arterial Administration

Site: Into the lumen of the desired artery.

Advantages: Greater concentration of the drug can be delivered at the desired site of action.

Disadvantages: Great expertise and aseptic conditions are required.

Examples with Dosage Forms: Radiopaque contrast media for coronary angiography and cerebral angiography, and many anticancer drugs, are perfused through the artery to treat malignancy involving limbs. The route mainly provides *local effects, in the areas supplied by the injected artery.*

vii) Intra-articular Administration

Site: Injection directly into the joint space.

Advantages: Ensures higher concentration of drug in a localised area.

Disadvantages: (i) Strict aseptic conditions are needed, (ii) Repeated administration into the joint space may further damage the joint and (iii) Painful procedure.

Examples with Dosage Forms: Hydrocortisone or gold chloride injection for the treatment of rheumatoid arthritis. The route provides *local effects* of the drug.

viii) Subcutaneous Administration

Site: Injection into the subcutaneous tissue under the skin.

Advantages: (i) Smooth but slower absorption for a longer period compared to intravenous or intramuscular route, (ii) Depot injections or implants can also be made.

Disadvantages: (i) Suitable for only small volumes of drugs (maximum 1 ml), (ii) Irritant drugs cannot be administered as sloughing and necrosis may result, (iii) Not suitable in the states of shock as reduced peripheral circulation decreases the rate of absorption.

Examples with Dosage Forms: Subcutaneous injection of local anaesthetics (for *local effects*) and of insulin (for *systemic effects*). Vaccines are administered preferably by this route as the active protein reaches the lymphoid tissue directly, through lymphatics, without getting destroyed elsewhere in the body (e.g., by peptidases and esterases in the muscle mass).

Other related (cutaneous) routes are as follows:

a) Intradermal (intracutaneous) Route

The drug is injected into the outer layers of skin.

The amount of drug given is small and absorption is slow. A tuberculin syringe is used to give such an injection. Example: Injection of BCG vaccine, diagnostic tests and allergic sensitisation testing in patients.

b) Dermojet Injections

It is a subcutaneous needleless injection of a drug by means of a high-velocity jet projected through a microfined orifice. It is a painless procedure, useful for mass inoculation.

c) Pellet and Biodegradable Implants

The drug as a solid pellet or packed in biodegradable tubes is implanted under the skin to provide a uniform but a slow release of the drug lasting over months, e.g., testosterone and contraceptive implants (for systemic effects).

ix) Epidural Injection

The drug is injected through a vertebral interspace between the dura of the spinal cord and the lining of the spinal canal, e.g., lidocaine injection to provide the epidural nerve block (*local effect*).

x) Intracardiac Injection

This injection is given by a long needle into the heart muscle through the left fourth intercostal space close to the sternum, e.g., injection of adrenaline to restart the heart beat in cases of sudden cardiac arrest (*local effect*).

B) Inhalational Administration

Site: Inspiration through nose or mouth.
Advantages: (i) Faster absorption and hence quick onset of action due to larger surface area of alveoli and (ii) Self administration is also possible.
Disadvantages: Bronchial irritation leading to increased bronchial and salivary secretions.
Examples with Dosage Forms: Oxygen and general anaesthetics inhalation (for *systemic effects*); metered aerosol preparations of salbutamol and isoprenaline for treatment of bronchial asthma and inhalation of sodium cromoglycate through spin inhaler as prophylaxis for bronchial asthma (*local effect*).

C) Transdermal Administration

Transdermal administration is considered under parenteral route because the patches, though applied topically, provide the systemic effects.

Site: Adhesive matrix (patch) containing drug is applied to chest, upper abdomen, or mastoid region.
Advantages: Slow but sustained release of the drug for several days; bypasses first-pass hepatic inactivation.
Disadvantages: Nil; however, if irritation results, the site of application can be changed.
Examples with Dosage Forms: Nitroglycerin (for angina), scopolamine (for motion sickness) and nicotine (for smoking cessation) transdermal patches for *systemic effects.*

TOPICAL ROUTES

i) Conjunctival, Nasal and Auditory Mucosal

Ointments or isotonic aqueous solutions of drugs, like sulfacetamide, chloramphenicol, gentamicin and ciprofloxacin are applied or instilled onto the conjunctiva for *local effects*. Drugs can also be administered as nasal drops, nasal sprays and as ear drops. However, absorption through mucous membrane can lead to *systemic effects* also.

ii) Vaginal and Urethral

Solutions, ointments, emulsion, foams, tablets, suppositories and pessaries of various sulfa drugs, antifungal agents and metronidazole are used for *local application* into the vagina while various drug solutions and pencil-shaped bougies are available for urethral use.

iii) Inunction and Dermal

Site: Rubbing the drug preparation onto the skin (Inunction) or can be dusted or sprayed over the surface of the skin (Dermal).
Advantages: Safe and convenient.
Disadvantages: (i) Difficulty in ascertaining the amount of the drug absorbed, (ii) Systemic absorption may take place if the skin has abrasions.
Examples with Dosage Forms: Various antibiotic--antifungal ointments, powders and solutions, various lotions, liniments, creams and ointments for their antiseptic, antipruritic and analgesic *effects locally.* Similarly, antiseptic powders are dusted while analgesic preparations are sprayed to provide local effects.

CHAPTER 5 How Drugs are Biotransported

COMPETENCY PH1.4

Once the drug is administered, it must move, from where it was administered, to the tissues or cells where it will act. This movement or translocation of drug from one side of the biological barrier to the other is called biotransport and the mechanisms underlying the transfer of a drug across the biological barriers are called the transport mechanisms. At all levels, whether a drug is absorbed, distributed, metabolized or excreted, it (or its metabolite) has to pass across the cell membrane. Hence, before we discuss its pharmacokinetics (i.e., what the body does to the drug) we should first study as to how the drugs are biotransported across the cell membranes and how their physico-chemical characteristics (and of the environment too) influence their biotransportation.

The major transport mechanisms are as under:

I. Passive Diffusion (Non-ionic or simple diffusion)
II. Carrier Mediated Transport
   1) Facilitated Diffusion
   2) Active Transport
III. Pinocytosis/Phagocytosis
IV. Filtration

PASSIVE DIFFUSION

It is a transfer process in which the drug molecules pass through a biological barrier from the phase of higher concentration to the phase of lower concentration (i.e., along the concentration gradient) without requiring any expenditure of energy by the biological system (Fig. 5.1).

Nonelectrolytes (i.e., nonionised drugs) can diffuse passively across the biological barriers at a rate proportional to their lipid:water partition coefficient. That means, drugs that are highly lipid soluble can diffuse rapidly, whereas those that are less lipid soluble will diffuse more slowly. For weak electrolytes (i.e., partly ionised drugs), the diffusion would depend upon the degree of ionisation of the drug, the pH of the surrounding environment and the lipid:water partition coefficient of their undissociated form. The weak electrolytes are either weakly acidic drugs (i.e., which form salts with bases, e.g., phenytoin *sodium*, phenobarbitone *sodium*, *sodium* salicylate, *sodium* sulfadiazine and *potassium* penicillin-V. Such drugs are available as their sodium or potassium salts) or weakly basic drugs (i.e., which form salts with acids and are available as hydrochlorides or sulphates etc., e.g., morphine *hydrochloride*, amphetamine *sulphate*, atropine *sulphate*, ephedrine *hydrochloride*, and chloroquine *phosphate*).

Since the rate of passive diffusion of any weak acid or a weak base depends on its degree of ionisation which in turn depends upon the pH of the surrounding medium, a relationship exists between its dissociation constant (pKa of the drug), the pH of the environment (in which it is placed) and the extent of its ionisation. This relationship is expressed by Henderson–Hasselbalch equation given below.

$$\text{pKa (Acid)} = \text{pH} + \log \frac{[\text{Conc. of Nonionised Acid}]}{[\text{Conc. of Ionised Acid}]} \quad \textbf{(1)}$$

$$\text{pKa (Base)} = \text{pH} + \log \frac{[\text{Conc. of Ionised Base}]}{[\text{Conc. of Nonionised Base}]} \quad \textbf{(2)}$$

The implications of Henderson–Hasselbalch equations **(1)** and **(2)** vis-a-vis passive diffusion (absorption) are as follows:

1. The stronger the acid (or weaker the base), the lower will be its pKa value. On the contrary, stronger the base (or weaker the acid), the higher will be its pKa.

2. Weakly acidic drugs, like aspirin, phenytoin and barbiturates, remain predominantly nonionised in acidic media and are better absorbed from places like stomach; while weakly basic drugs, like morphine, diazepam and amphetamine remain predominantly nonionised at alkaline pH and thus are better absorbed from intestine.
   This situation is reversed for acidic drugs at alkaline pH and for basic drugs at acidic pH. However, the shorter stay of the drug in stomach with its limited surface area, compared with that of intestine, outbalances the importance of this pH factor. Accordingly, the net absorption from intestine usually exceeds that from stomach.
3. If pKa of the drug is equal to the pH of the medium (in which it has been placed), it would remain 50% ionised and 50% nonionised.
4. For every upward or downward shift of one unit in pH (of the environment) there is 10-fold increase or decrease in the ratio of the ionised and nonionised fraction of the drug, depending upon whether the drug was a weak acid or a weak base.
5. Strongly acidic or strongly basic drugs and quaternary ammonium compounds remain predominantly ionised at all pH and are, therefore, poorly absorbed.

Explanation for 2, 3 and 4

Suppose a weakly acidic drug (pKa = 3) is placed at different acidic pH (2 or 3). Then

$$\text{pKa (acid)} = \text{pH} + \log \frac{[\text{Nonionised fraction}]}{[\text{Ionised fraction}]} \quad \textbf{(1)}$$

OR

$$3 = 3 + \log \frac{[\text{Nonionised fraction}]}{[\text{Ionised fraction}]}$$

OR

$$0 = \log \frac{[\text{Nonionised fraction}]}{[\text{Ionised fraction}]} \quad \textbf{(1a)}$$

Taking antilog of both sides, the above equation (1a) becomes

$$1 = \frac{[\text{Nonionised fraction of acid}]}{[\text{Ionised fraction of acid}]}$$

That means if pKa of the drug is equal to the pH of the environment the ratio of its nonionised:ionised fraction is 1:1 (or 50:50).

If the same drug is placed at pH = 2, then after substituting the values of pKa and pH in equation **(1)** we get

$$3 = 2 + \log \frac{[\text{Nonionised fraction}]}{[\text{Ionised fraction}]}$$

OR

$$1 = \log \frac{[\text{Nonionised fraction}]}{[\text{Ionised fraction}]} \quad \textbf{(1b)}$$

Taking antilog of both sides of equation **(1b)** we get

$$10 = \frac{[\text{Nonionised fraction}]}{[\text{Ionised fraction}]}$$

That means, by just a downward shift of one unit in pH (from 3 to 2) the resultant ratio of the nonionised:ionised fraction of the same drug becomes 10:1 (i.e., ten-fold increase in nonionised fraction—hence better absorption). All the above situations would be reversed for the basic drugs and one can derive all the stipulated rules cited above just by substituting the appropriate values of pKa and pH in equation **(2)**.

Further, it may be emphasised that, conditions which favour the neutral (nonionised) form of the drug will enhance the drug permeation (absorption). Contrarily, conditions that favour ionisation will restrict the translocation of weak electrolytes, since the proportion existing as the diffusible (nonionised) form is low. This leads to a phenomenon called as "ion trapping". For example, the nonionised form of weakly acidic drug (e.g., aspirin; pKa 3.5) which crosses the gastric mucosa (pH 2), reverts to the ionised form within the cell (pH 7) and hence slowly passes to the extracellular fluid. This type of *"ion trapping"* possibly also contributes to gastric mucosal cell damage caused by aspirin.

CARRIER-MEDIATED TRANSPORT

Polar compounds such as sugars and amino acids and certain drugs of therapeutic interest cannot penetrate membranes by passive diffusion but are moved by carrier systems present on the membrane surface. These carrier molecules, which are usually proteins, combine with the drug substrate in question and form a complex. This drug-carrier complex exhibits better permeability than the drug alone. After the complex crosses the membrane, the carrier dissociates from the drug. The carrier then either returns to the original side of the membrane for reuse or is essentially produced on one side and eliminated at the other side. The carrier-mediated transports are of two types:

Facilitated Diffusion

The characteristic features of this process are:

a) Carrier can move a drug substrate along its concentration gradient only (down-hill diffusion, Fig. 5.1)

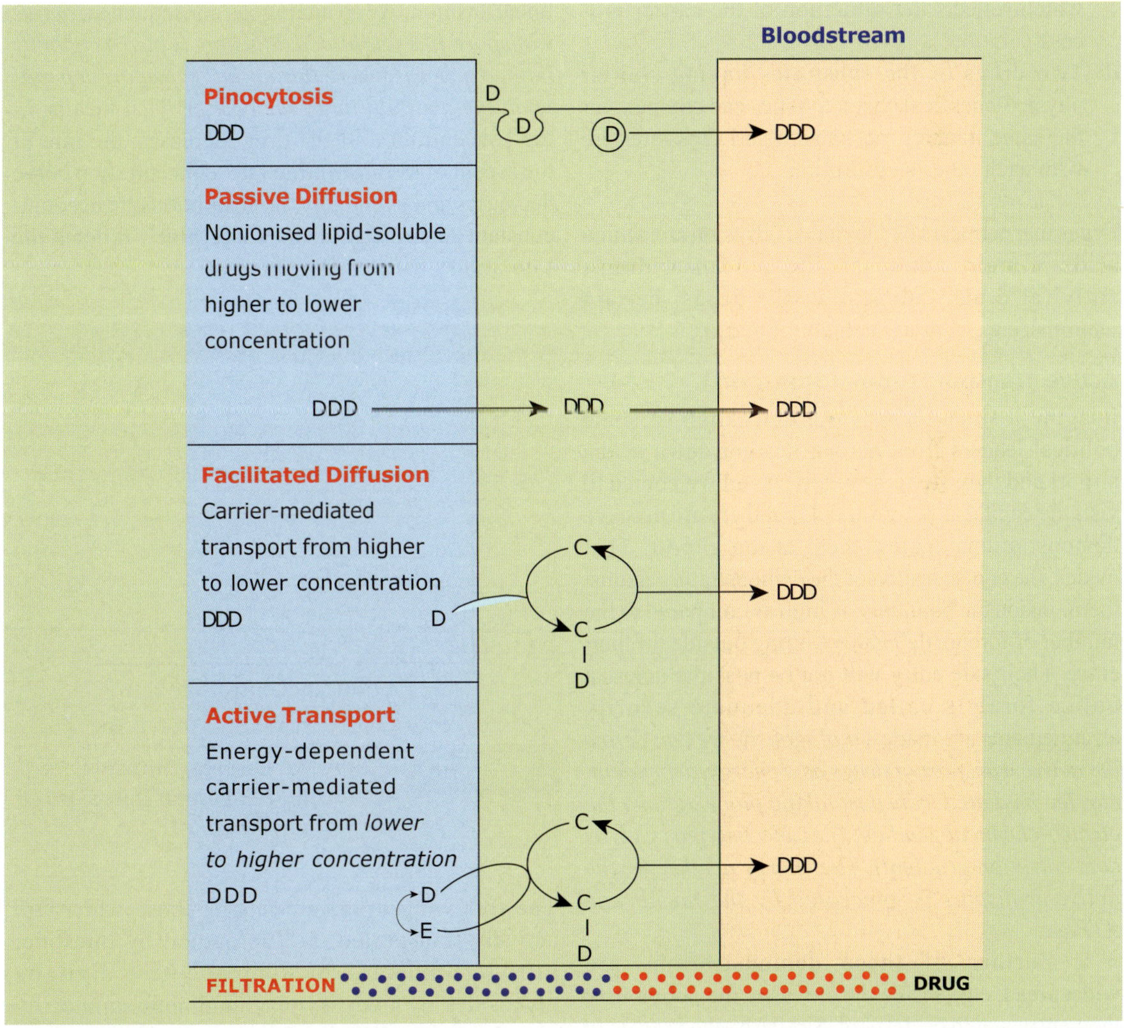

Fig 5.1 Processes of Biotransportation. D = drug; E = energy; C = carrier.

b) As in passive diffusion, no extracellular energy is required for translocation of drugs and
c) It is a capacity limited process, i.e., the rate of diffusion depends upon the binding ability of the drug to its carrier and is limited by the availability of carrier. The plot describing the absorption rate-concentration relationships for the passive diffusion is linear over the entire concentration range while that of facilitated diffusion shows linear relationship at concentrations only at lower range. As the concentration increases, the rate of ascent of the curve decreases and eventually the absorption rate becomes constant regardless of the dose, which reflects the saturation of the carrier process (Fig. 5.2).
d) Two drugs or the substrates having similar physico-chemical characteristics can compete for the same transfer mechanism and thus interfere with each other's absorption.

Drugs that permeate by facilitated diffusion are: amino acids in brain; antimetabolite-anticancer drugs; antiviral drugs; adenosine-like drugs; certain vitamins, e.g., riboflavin, thiamine and B_{12}.

Active Transport (up-hill transport)

Imagine a situation where a delegation of some political leaders from abroad has got down at the airport and they are to be received and welcomed to visit the capital as per protocol; but there are massive demonstrations against them at the airport. That means, the concentration of the demonstrators against them, inside the boundary, is high as compared to the number of foreign delegates waiting outside for their entry. Their safe entry will not be possible unless a police force is called and adequate security arrangements are made. *Analogously, we can define the active transport of drugs as a energy-dependent, carrier-mediated transport taking place against the electro-chemical gradient (i.e., electrical as well as concentration gradient). The energy needed for the active transport is generated by the membrane ATPase.*

Further, if these demonstrations are widespread, e.g., inside the city also, then obviously their entry would be delayed. Similarly, *the process of active transport can be blocked by inhibiting cell metabolism or by reducing the ATP levels by giving agents like sodium cyanide, sodium fluoride or 2,4-dinitrophenol.* Moving the story a step further, as the entry of the Head of the delegation is taking place under police cover, other members of the delegation would also be seeking their entry under the same security cover. *In a similar manner, the drugs or substrate, having similar physico-chemical characteristics can also compete for the same carrier-mediated active transport process.* A step further, if the number of delegates is large, while the police force is meagre to control the massive demonstrations, their entry cannot take place in a linear fashion. As an analogous consequence, *active transport, like facilitated diffusion, is also a capacity limited process where this up-hill transport depends upon the availability of the carrier.* That means, as the concentration of the drug increases, the rate of the ascent of the absorption rate–concentration curve decreases and eventually the absorption rate becomes constant regardless of the dose, which reflects the saturation of the carrier process (Fig. 5.2).

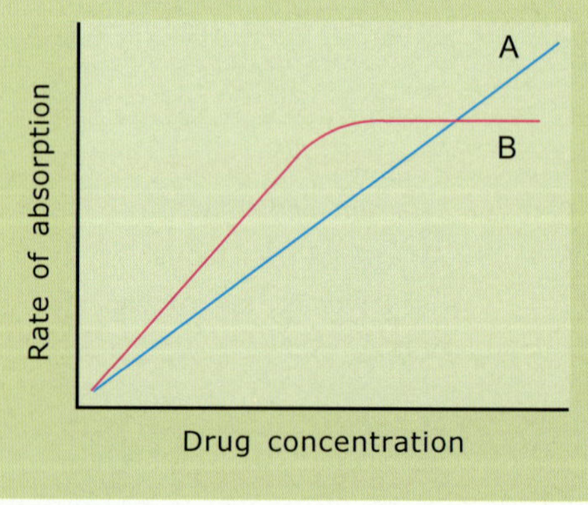

Fig 5.2 Curve A: Passive Diffusion. Curve B: Facilitated Diffusion or Active Transport.

The following drugs are among those which are actively transported: 5-Fluorouracil by intestine; nitrogen mustard by lymphocytes; digitalis glycosides by liver; sympathomimetic amines by neural tissue and choline by cholinergic neuron.

Depending upon the driving force, the active transport can be subdivided into *primary or secondary active transport* (Fig. 5.3).

In ***primary active transport,*** the bio-transportation of drugs is directly coupled with ATP hydrolysis for deriving the energy (i.e., energy-dependent) and is usually carried by ABC (**A**TP **B**inding **C**assette) group of biotransporters (e.g., P-glycoprotein). ABC transporters work like "evacuators" and mediate the unidirectional efflux of many drugs like antibiotics, anticancer drugs, HIV protease inhibitors, digoxin and anticonvulsants.

In ***secondary active transport,*** one ion or the solute (X) supplies the driving force for the transport of other ion/solute (Y). Depending on the direction of flux of X and Y, the transporters can be called either a *symporter* or an *antiporter.* A *symporter (or cotransporter)* transports X and Y in the same direction (e.g., $Na^+/K^+/2Cl^-$ symporter, Ch.16). An *antiporter (*or *exchanger* or *counter-transporter),* on the contrary, transports X and Y in the opposite directions (e.g., Na^+ and H^+ exchanger, Ch. 16). These transport mechanisms are not directly linked to ATP hydrolysis (as discussed above). The transportation here is driven by a difference in electrochemical gradient established by the active transport (or even by facilitated diffusion) of X and Y.

Membrane Transporters

Membrane transporters are usually the proteins that control the therapeutic response or toxicity of a drug through their ability to influx or efflux the drug from a cell. These are located in intestine, kidney, lung, liver and BBB, etc., and control absorption, tissue distribution and elimination of a drug. There are two superfamilies of drug transporters.

ATP Binding Cassette (ABC) Superfamily of Transporters

These are involved in primary active transport and are coupled to ATP hydrolysis and energy generation out of the hydrolysis. There are 7 subclasses of this group (ABC-A to ABC-G) which are encoded by 49 genes. The most important example is P-glycoprotein (also called $ABCB_1$ or MDR-1). The multi-drug resistance (MDR) gene is a member of the functionally

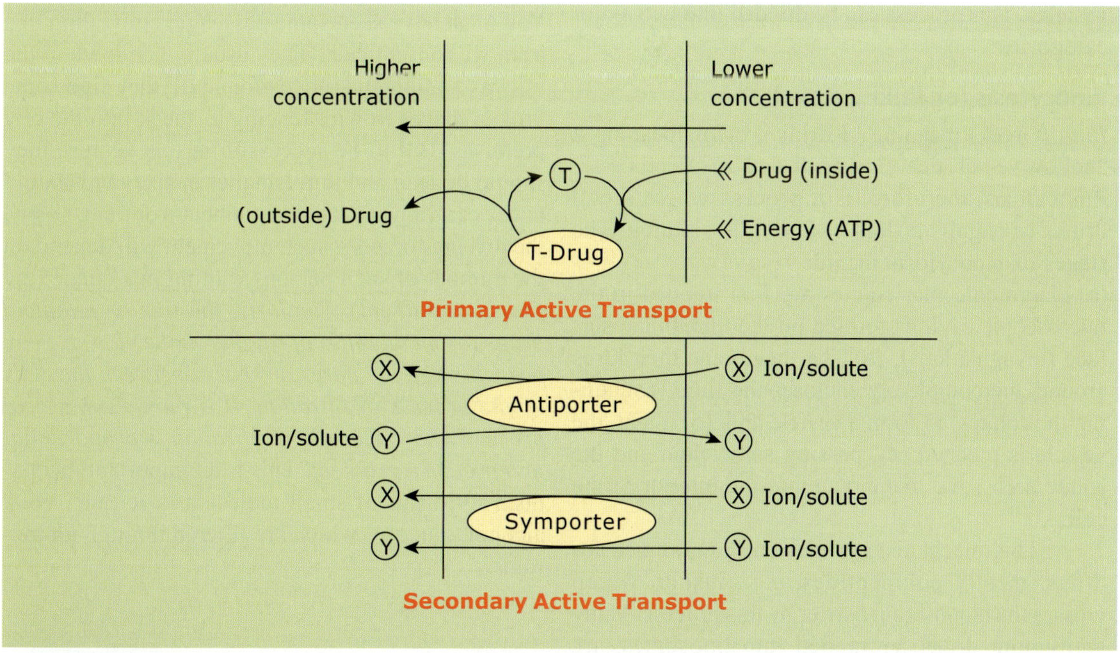

Fig 5.3 Classification of Membrane Transport Mechanisms. T = ATP Binding Cassette (ABC) Group of Transporters (e.g., P-glycoprotein)

diverse ABC transmembrane superfamily of transport proteins and the multiple drug resistance occurs from a single mutation of *MDR1* gene. Hence the name MDR1 for the P-glycoprotein. MDR1 inducers or inhibitors can lead to serious drug-drug interactions (Ch. 22, Ch. 62).

Solute- Linked Carrier (SLC) Group of Transporters

The SLC superfamily of transporters are involved in facilitated diffusion or secondary active transport. 43 SLC families, encoded by different genes, are known till date. Prominent SLC transporters are various neurotransmitter transporters (Ch. 10) like for serotonin, norepinephrine and dopamine. SLC transporters that are non-neuronal include glucose transporters (GLUT, Ch.47), cholesterol transporters (Ch. 23), and a variety of renal symporters and antiporters (Ch. 16) etc.

PINOCYTOSIS/PHAGOCYTOSIS (ENDOCYTOSIS)

The mechanism of transport by endocytosis involves the cellular uptake of exogenous molecules or complexes, inside plasma membrane-derived vesicles. This process can be divided into two major categories:

Pinocytosis (or fluid uptake)

Pino (Greek) meaning "I drink", *cytos* meaning a "hollow vessel" denoting a cell, and *osis* "a process". Pinocytosis, therefore, is a process where a cell drinks or engulfs a fluid or a drug in solution. The stages of pinocytosis include (Fig. 5.1):

(a) Macromolecular solutes are first trapped in the microscopic cavities formed on the membrane surface (invaginations). (b) The membrane then fuses around and completely encloses the fluid (containing the solutes) to form a vesicle and (c) Later, the vesicle is pinched off, passing some fluid and the solute across the membrane into the interior of the cell.

This mechanism is of some importance for drugs, mostly polypeptides, e.g., insulin which crosses the blood-brain barrier by this process. Many antitumour drugs, entrapped into liposomes, are biotransported by this method. Receptor mediated absorption of LDL in liver also takes place through pinocytosis.

Pinocytotic activity is rather marked at the alveoli of the lungs and at the walls of blood vessles but this process does not represent the transfer mechanism for large quantities of materials, since the number of vesicles that would have to be formed is beyond the capacity.

Phagocytosis (uptake of particles)

In some cases, the particulate matter can also be transferred by local invagination of the cell membrane. Such a process is termed as phagocytosis (*phago* meaning "to eat"). The process is rare but certainly poisoning by botulinum toxin and allergic reactions occurring after ingestion of offending proteins (antigens) are well-known examples for this type of absorptive process. Both these processes require an expenditure of cellular energy, but the translocation of the drug does not require its combination with any carrier as is seen in active transport or facilitated diffusion.

FILTRATION

You must have seen some passengers travelling in a train without a ticket. They usually get down at the railway station and move around till they find some broken places in wire fencing to sneak into the city premises. But to be successful in this venture they should be lean and thin (smaller in size) and should not be carrying any luggage (unbound or free). Lastly, the driving force for such movement will depend on the number of such persons waiting in a queue (the pressure gradient). *Similarly, the free or unbound drugs (or metabolite) of smaller molecular size can pass through the pores or spaces between the cells by the process of filtration. It is purely a physical process where the rate of filtration is proportional to a pressure gradient.* This is an important mechanism for drugs of small molecular size (e.g., urea, alcohol, glucose) which are filtered through glomerulus.

CHAPTER 6 Pharmacokinetics

COMPETENCY PH1.4, PH1.59

HOW DRUGS ARE ABSORBED

Although the transport processes described in *Chapter 5* can adequately account for the passage of drugs across any biological membrane, they can hardly explain their movement over any great distance. How then is the movement of drugs over greater distances accomplished? The circulatory system, then, serves as a common pathway for carrying drugs from the inner side of the biological barrier to any tissue or organ. Hence, unless the drug is purposely injected directly into the blood stream (where absorption is completely bypassed), getting to its site of action involves two separate processes. The first of these is *absorption,* i.e., the movement of drug into the blood stream from its site of administration. The second process then is *distribution*, i.e., movement of drug molecules from the blood into the tissues (to be discussed later). We shall here discuss only some important sites from where the drug enters into the systemic circulation. The factors affecting absorption shall be discussed along with bioavailability of drugs (see following text).

ABSORPTION VIA GASTROINTESTINAL TRACT

Some aspects about the absorption of drugs through GIT have already been discussed earlier (refer Ch. 4 and Ch. 5), and shall be discussed again in factors affecting absorption and bioavailability. Briefly speaking, the absorption of drugs from GIT is mainly by passive diffusion through the lipid sheath. Few drugs, however, are small enough to diffuse through the pores in the cell membrane; while uptake of sugar and other nutrients is by active transport. The gut is more permeable to nonionised lipid-soluble form of drugs and less permeable to the ionised form. The ability of a drug to be absorbed via GIT and to reach the systemic circulation is compromised as a result of drug loss due to: (i) its efflux by the P-glycoprotein localised in the enterocytes, (ii) its metabolism in these cells and liver, (iii) by vomiting or (iv) by disease that may affect drug absorption. The whole process of absorption through GIT is summarised below.

From mouth: Saliva pH is slightly acidic, but the pH of stimulated saliva (as with sublingual drugs) reaches 7.4 (alkaline). Hence, lipid-soluble (non-ionised) basic or neutral drugs can be absorbed form this site. After the sublingual absorption, the drug directly goes into systemic circulation, bypassing first-pass metabolism (i.e., metabolism of a drug taking place in liver/intestine/lungs before it reaches systemic circulation). For example: isosorbide dinitrate given sublingually for angina.

From stomach: pH acidic. Hence, lipid-soluble (unionised) acidic or neutral drugs are absorbed from this site. After absorption they pass through hepatic portal system before going to systemic circulation – hence chances of *first-pass* metabolism are increased.

From intestine: pH alkaline. Hence, lipid-soluble (unionised) basic or neutral drugs are absorbed from here, e.g., morphine. Because of the larger surface area, it is the major site of absorption for most of the drugs. However, the drugs have to pass through hepatic portal system before going to systemic circulation: hence, there are chances of *first-pass effect.* From liver, some drugs may be secreted into intestine through bile and are reabsorbed back (*enterohepatic circulation,* see following text).

From large intestine or colon: pH alkaline. Hence, unionised (lipid soluble) basic or neutral drugs are absorbed from this site. From external haemorrhoidal vein, the major amount of the drug goes directly to systemic circulation, hence minimal first-pass effect.

The rate of absorption from fastest to lowest is: sublingual → rectal → oral.

ABSORPTION VIA PARENTERAL SITES

Drugs when injected intravenously are completely absorbed and rapidly distributed, as they reach the bloodstream directly without crossing any membrane. Absorption following intramuscular and subcutaneous injections usually occurs by *passive diffusion* from the injection site to the plasma or lymph. *Filtration* through channels in the endothelial capillary membrane is also very efficient (Ch. 5). Absorption of drugs from intramuscular injection is usually more rapid than from subcutaneous sites, because of the higher vascularity of the muscle compared to the subcutaneous tissue but the difference is not large. The extent of absorption from highest to lowest is: intravenous → intramuscular → subcutaneous. However, the absorption from S.C. and I.M. route is reduced in patients with circulatory failure (e.g., shock) in whom the tissue perfusion gets decreased.

ABSORPTION VIA LUNGS

Lipid-soluble drugs when given in a vapourised form (general anaesthetics), or as aqueous solution spray (salbutamol) or as spray of suspended microfined particles (disodium cromoglycate) are absorbed by simple diffusion from the pulmonary epithelium and mucous membrane of trachea and lungs. Absorption is rapid because of the large surface area and high vascularity. First-pass metabolism is avoided.

ABSORPTION VIA TOPICAL SITES

Absorption of most drugs through the intact skin is of course poor as the keratinised epidermis behaves like a barrier to permeability. However, the underlying dermis is quite permeable to many lipid-soluble drugs and therefore significant absorption can occur if the skin is abraded. As discussed above, a transdermal application of some drugs (nitroglycerin, scopolamine and clonidine) and application of some drugs on mucous membranes (e.g., oxytocin and vasopressin as nasal spray) enhances the systemic absorption mainly because of the thin and highly vascular absorbing surface. Ophthalmic drugs in the form of eye drops or ointment are absorbed through the cornea.

METHODS FOR DELAYING ABSORPTION

Using an Appropriate Dosage Form

The "slow release" dosage forms, like retard tablets (e.g., potassium chloride retard tabs. and diclofenac sodium sustained release tabs.), spansules (e.g., iron formulations, like Fefol® and isosorbide dinitrate spansule), depot injections (e.g., testosterone depot inj. and fluphenazine depot inj.) and subcutaneous implants (e.g., testosterone pellets) are some ways to obtain a slow but sustained absorption of drugs (refer Ch. 3).

Changing the Physical Characteristics of the Drug

Physical characteristics of some drugs may also be changed to retard their rate of absorption, e.g., insulin zinc suspension. Depending upon the pH of the reaction, insulin can form a fine amorphous zinc suspension (semilente) which is relatively rapidly absorbed or a cloudy zinc suspension (ultralente) which is slowly absorbed. Each can be used separately depending upon the effect desired or can also be mixed together (lente) to produce an immediate but sustained effect. Similarly, procaine penicillin-G is such a salt of penicillin which is only slightly water souble. When injected as an aqueous suspension it is slowly absorbed and exerts a prolonged action.

Adding a Vasoconstrictor Drug or Applying a Tourniquet

The addition of a vasoconstricting drug, like noradrenaline or adrenaline to a solution of a local anaesthetic, e.g., xylocaine, reduces the absorption of the local anaesthetic into the general circulation. This usefully prolongs the local anaesthetic effect and reduces the chances of systemic toxicity.

Application of a tourniquet to arrest the blood flow, followed by the I.V. injection of local anaesthetic below the tourniquet (e.g., in whole limb) delays the systemic absorption but prolongs the local anaesthetic effect. Decreased peripheral blood flow in conditions of "shock" significantly reduces the rate of absorption of injected drugs.

METHODS TO FACILITATE ABSORPTION

The rate limiting factors in absorption from the injection site are: (a) diffusion through the tissue and (b) removal by local blood flow. The importance of the former is shown by the powerful effect of hyaluronidase, an enzyme which breaks down the intercellular matrix. Adding hyaluronidase to the injection fluid increases the rate of diffusion through the interstitial spaces and greatly speeds up the drug absorption. Similarly the absorption from the site of injection may be increased by increasing the local blood flow by applying hot fomentation or doing massage.

BIOAVAILABILITY OF DRUGS

In case you hire a set of persons (i.e., men of same age, height, weight and strength) from different nationalities to complete a desired task in stipulated time, you will notice that the rate at which these persons appear at the desired site of work and the extent to which they perform their job differ from persons of one nationality to another. In other words, their availability at the desired site and their work output is not identical. The same holds true with the drugs also. Different brands of the same generic drug can be *chemically equivalent* (i.e., they may satisfy all the chemical and physical standards as laid down in the pharmacopoeia), yet may not be *biologically* or *therapeutically equivalent* (i.e., may not yield similar concentration of drug in bloodstream at the same time and may not provide the same therapeutic effect) if given by any route other than intravenous.

BIOAVAILABILITY is defined as per US Food and Drugs Administration as "*the rate at which and the extent to which the active concentration of the drug is available at the desired site of action* (or practically speaking in the bloodstream)". Probably the term bioavailability came into existence through an unusual incidence of phenytoin toxicity in epileptic patients which occurred in the year 1968 in Australia and due to the differences in the bioavailability observed with different digoxin formulations in the year 1971.

In Australia, in the year 1968, there was a sudden outbreak of phenytoin toxicity in epileptic patients. The pharmaceutical firm which was marketing "Dilantin Sodium Capsules" was using calcium sulphate as inert excipient. Since stocks of calcium sulphate got exhausted, they substituted it with lactose thinking that this minor change in inert excipient should be immaterial. But with this "reformulated product" the plasma concentration of phenytoin reached around 30 μg/ml leading to phenytoin toxicity. The reason was that lactose gets more easily wetted. This resulted in faster dissolution with implied quicker absorption and consequently higher plasma concentration, leading to toxicity.

BIOAVAILABILITY is an *absolute term* which requires measurement of both the true rate and total amount (extent) of drug that reaches the general circulation from an administered dosage form.

EQUIVALENCE is a *relative term* which means a comparison of two different brand products of the same drug with a set of established standards.

Equivalence could be of several types:

BIOEQUIVALENCE

If two or more similar dosage forms of the same drug reach the blood circulation at the same relative rate and to the same relative extent, these are called bioequivalent preparations (brands) of the generic drug. In other words, the two similar dosage forms of one drug entity can be called bioequivalent if their plasma level profiles are comparable and superimposable or fall within specific (and regulated) limits. For example, two brand preparations of phenytoin like Dilantin (Parke Davis) and Eptoin (Boots) may or may not be bioequivalent.

Differences in bioavailability are primarily seen with oral dosage forms because bioavailability of any drug after I.V. administration is 100 percent and is sometimes assumed to be close with I.M. or S.C. route also. The latter may not always be true because some drugs, like phenytoin, digoxin, diazepam and chlordiazepoxide partly get precipitated at the site of injection and hence their bioavailability gets reduced, if given by S.C. or I.M. route.

Differences of less than 25% in bioavailability among several formulations of one drug will usually have no significant effect on clinical outcome, hence such formulations can be called as bioequivalent. Thus measurements of bioavailability are immaterial for drugs having higher margin of safety, e.g., with water-soluble vitamins, antacids and some antimicrobials having large therapeutic index. *But the differences in bioavailability assume a much greater concern with drugs that show a steep dose-response relationship, i.e., with drugs which obey zero-order or mixed-order elimination kinetics* (e.g., phenytoin, warfarin and other oral anticoagulants, digoxin and aspirin in high doses) *and with drugs having a narrow margin of safety* (e.g., theophylline, cyclosporine, antiarrhythmics, antidiabetics like insulin and first generation of oral hypoglycaemic drugs and adrenal steroids). In such cases, the patient should be stabilised with one brand formulation only and that brand should never be changed (unless the changed brand is bioequivalent to the one that was being used). Because, if a patient who is stabilised on one brand product is switched over to another brand of the same drug, there could be either a therapeutic failure (due to decreased bioavailability) or drug intoxication (due to increased bioavailability). For these reasons, before issuing the license for marketing, the "generic equivalent" of the branded drug, the drug regulatory authorities (like DCGI in India and FDA in USA), lay stress on evidence of their bioequivalence so that the generic drug can be substituted for its branded product without affecting the clinical outcome.

CHEMICAL EQUIVALENCE

If two or more dosage forms of the same drug contain the same labeled quantities of the drug as specified in pharmacopoeia, these are called chemically equivalent drugs. For example, Dilantin® and Eptoin® may be *chemically equivalent* if they contain same quantity of phenytoin on chemical assay. The two brands of a drug may be chemically equivalent but may not be bioequivalent.

PHARMACEUTICAL EQUIVALENCE

In the above example of chemical equivalence, if the two drug formulations or dosage forms of the same active drug entity also contain other similar ingredients, e.g., exipicients (binders or dispersing agents, etc), these two dosage forms are considered to be pharmaceutically equivalent. Such two pharmaceutically equivalent formulations if are administered by the same route (e.g., oral or parenteral) at the same time in different subjects, these would show a pharmacokinetic bioequivalence.

THERAPEUTIC EQUIVALENCE

The two brand products of one drug can be considered as therapeutically equivalent, if they provide an "identical *in vivo* pharmacological response" as measured by control of symptoms or a disease and safety profile. For example, Dilantin® and Eptoin® may or may not be pharmocokinetically bioequivalent but show *therapeutic equivalence* if both provide same pharmacological response qualitatively.

CLINICAL EQUIVALENCE

If one structurally different drug can provide the same clinical response as another mechanistically related drug, these are then considered to exhibit clinical equivalence. For example, trifluperazine (belonging to phenothiazine group) may be *clinically equivalent* to haloperidol (belonging to butyrophenone group) if both provide equivalent therapeutic results in the treatment of schizophrenia.

MEASUREMENT OF BIOAVAILABILITY

To compare the bioavailability, the absorption pattern of two brand products of the same drug is studied after oral administration. Thereafter, the plasma concentration of the drug, from both the formulations, is plotted against time (till plasma concentration has fallen to a predetermined end point: say, 10 percent of the peak value). From the plasma concentration – time curves, thus obtained, three important characteristics are noted and compared (Fig. 6.1).

a) Peak plasma concentration (Cmax),
b) Time to attain the peak plasma concentration (tmax),
c) The area under the curve (AUC) of plasma concentration versus time curve (till plasma concentration has fallen to 10% of the peak value).

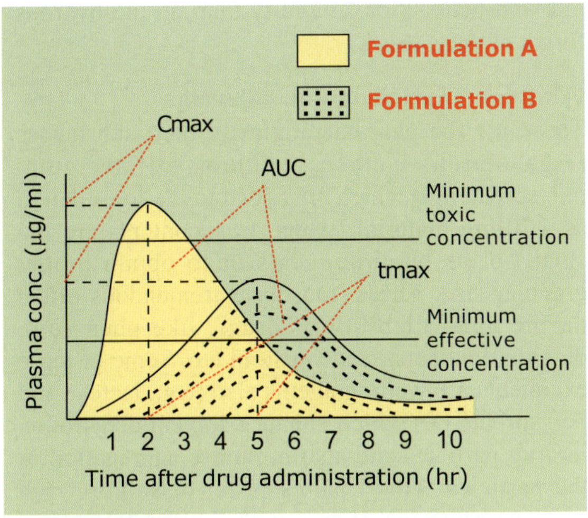

Fig 6.1 Parameters of Bioavailability

The first two parameters are simple indicators for the rate of absorption. An increased rate means a higher peak at a shorter time. In contrast, the third parameter, i.e., AUC reflects the extent of absorption. It denotes the total amount of drug absorbed into the circulation during a specified period. Ideally speaking, for the product to be considered bioequivalent, the peak plasma concentration (Cmax), time to reach peak plasma concentration (tmax) and the areas under the curves should not be significantly different. The AUC is expressed in the units of mg-hr/ml and can be calculated by several methods. One method is to use a planimeter: an instrument for mechanically measuring the area of plane figures. Another proce - dure is "cut and weigh" method, that means to cut out the area under the entire curve on rectilinear graph paper and to weigh it on an analytical balance. The third method is mathematical, using trapezoidal rule.

However, the measurement of AUC is a better index of bioavailability for drugs to be given for a longer period because here the total drug absorbed becomes more crucial than the peak concentration achieved or the time required to achieve the peak concentration.

The quantitative evaluation of the bioavailability of any oral dosage form can be done by comparing the AUC obtained after oral administration of a single dose with that obtained when the same drug, in the same dose, is given intravenously (100 percent absorption).

$$\text{Drug Bioavailability (\%)} = \frac{\text{AUC (oral)}}{\text{AUC (IV)}} \times 100$$

FACTORS INFLUENCING ABSORPTION AND BIOAVAILABILITY

These can be broadly classified as follows:

A. Pharmaceutical factors
B. Pharmacological factors

Pharmaceutical Factors

The first thing to happen to a drug, administered by any route (other than I.V.), is that it must dissolve and become available for absorption. Therefore, the first important influence upon bioavailability is the formulation of the drug in the form of tablet, capsule, suspension or solution that can be taken by the patient. Generally, one would expect the bioavailability of a drug to decrease in the following order: solution > suspension > capsule > tablet > coated tablet. Although this ranking is not universal, it nevertheless provides a useful guideline. On oral administration, two processes precede the actual absorption process and these are summarised in Fig. 6.2.

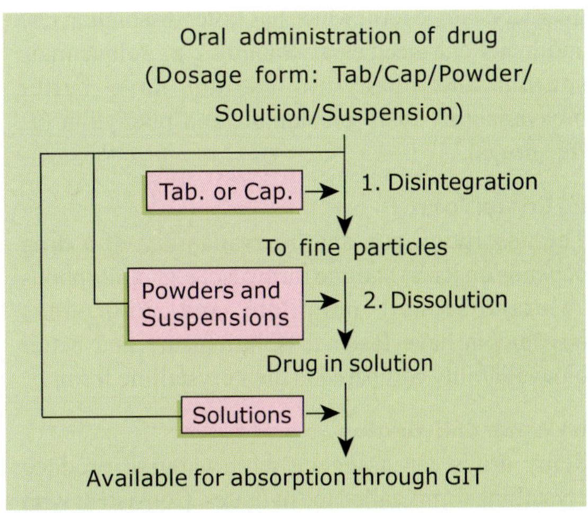

Fig 6.2 Pharmaceutical Factors of Bioavailability

The first step, i.e., the *disintegration* of the solid dosage form into fine particles depends on the type of the dosage form. Hard tablets and coated tablets take greater time to disintegrate as compared to ordinary tablets and capsules. The time required for disintegration is saved in powders and suspensions.

The second step is the *dissolution* of the active drug from fine particles to solution. Obviously, both the rate and extent to which the drug is absorbed are more when the drug is administered in solution form (saves time from disintegration and dissolution). Both are rate-limiting steps in the process of absorption and bioavailability. Various pharmaceutical or formulation factors which can affect disintegration and dissolution are discussed below.

i) Particle Size

A drug usually dissolves more rapidly when its surface area is increased by decreasing its particle size. For this reason poorly soluble, slowly dissolving drugs are often marketed in microfined or finely particled form to facilitate their absorption and to enhance the bioavailability, e.g., microfined aspirin, spironolactone, griseofulvin and digoxin.

ii) Salt Form

The dissolution rate of a particular salt is usually different from that of the parent compound. Salts of weakly acidic drugs as a rule, are highly water soluble. Free acidic drug is precipitated from these salts in a microcrystalline form which has faster dissolution rate and hence enhanced bioavailability, e.g., tolbutamide sodium and phenytoin sodium have better bioavailability than tolbutamide and phenytoin (as free drugs).

iii) Crystal Form

The absorption rate and bioavailability of a drug depends on its crystalline form also, e.g., amorphous chloramphenicol palmitate and amorphous novobiocin have faster dissolution rate and better bioavailability compared to their crystalline forms.

iv) Water of Hydration

Many drugs can associate with water to produce crystalline forms called the hydrates. Consistent with the theory, the anhydrous forms of caffeine, theophylline and ampicillin have faster dissolution rate and better bioavailability than do the hydrous forms of these drugs.

v) Nature of Excipients and Adjuvants

These are the pharmacologically inert substances (e.g., starch, lactose, calcium sulfate, gum, polysorbate-80) which are added to the formulation as a filling material (when drug contents are too small) or as binding agents or to obtain proper granular size. These, too, have tremendous effect on the bioavailability of drugs, like phenytoin, digoxin, levodopa, and warfarin etc. Some of these excipients are wetting agents also (e.g., lactose and polysorbate-80) which enhance solvent penetration in drug particles and also minimise aggregation of the particles. This ensures faster dissolution and quicker absorption. Hence, with a drug which obeys zero-order or mixed-order elimination kinetics or with a drug which has a low margin of safety, change from one brand formulation to another could lead to either therapeutic failure or intoxication due to different excipients/adjuvants used which can affect the bioavailability.

vi) Degree of Ionisation

Nonionised lipid-soluble drugs are better absorbed whereas strongly acidic or basic drugs or highly ionised drugs show reduced bioavailability from GIT, e.g., streptomycin, neostigmine, acetylcholine and its analogues and d-tubocurarine.

Pharmacological Factors

In addition to the pharmaceutical factors described above, other pharmacological and physiological factors also affect the absorption and bioavailability and these are discussed below:

i) Gastric Emptying and Gastrointestinal Motility

In general, factors that accelerate gastric emptying, permit drugs to reach the large absorptive surface area of small intestine sooner, and increase the bioavailability unless the drug is slow to dissolve. The converse is equally true and important. Gastric emptying is promoted by fasting, anxiety, lying on right side, hyperthyroidism and with gastrokinetic drugs like metoclopramide. Gastric emptying is retarded by fatty diet, endogenous depression, lying on left side, pyloric stenosis, hypothyroidism and with drugs like atropine, propantheline, imipramine and chlorpromazine.

ii) Gastrointestinal Disease

There are several pathophysiological factors that affect drug absorption. The outcome of coeliac disease (malabsorption of fats) is complex. Some drugs, like amoxycillin and pivampicillin show decreased absorption; others, like cephalexin show increased absorption, while some show no change, e.g., ampicillin. In chronic inflammation of ileum (Crohn's disease), however, there is a disproportionate absorption of individual components from tablets of cotrimoxazole: the absorption of trimethoprim is decreased while that of sulfamethoxazole is increased. In gastroenteritis, there is a decreased absorption of drugs if given orally.

iii) Food and Other Substances

In general, gastrointestinal absorption is favoured by an empty stomach while the absorption rate (not the extent) is reduced after the ingestion of food. However, both the rate and extent of absorption of certain antibiotics (e.g., rifampicin) is reduced after meals. Absorption of tetracyclines is also markedly reduced if taken with milk or milk products (forms poorly absorbed complex with calcium ions). Absorption of certain antifungal drugs (e.g., griseofulvin) is enhanced by administering the drug with a fatty diet. Vitamin C keeps iron in its ferrous form and therefore increases its bioavailability.

iv) First-Pass Effect

All drugs taken orally, first of all pass through GIT wall and then through portal system before reaching systemic circulation. First-pass effect means the drug degradation occurring before the drug enters the systemic circulation. The net result is the decreased bioavailability and diminished therapeutic response. Thus, bioavailability of l-dopa, morphine, nitroglycerin, isosorbide dinitrate and propranolol/labetalol is less, if given orally, due to significant first- pass effect.

v) Drug-Drug Interactions

Differences in bioavailability can also be observed due to drug-drug interactions. For example, liquid paraffin decreases the bioavailability of fat-soluble vitamins as it emulsifies fats and therefore causes deficiency of fat-soluble vitamins like A, D, K and E. Antacids containing aluminium, calcium and magnesium and haematinics containing iron cause reduced bioavailability of tetracyclines (because the resultant chelated complex is poorly absorbed). Barbiturates reduce the bioavailability of several drugs due to enzymatic induction. Probenecid blocks penicillin excretion and thus enhances its bioavailability (refer following text).

vi) Pharmacogenetic Factors

Large differences in bioavailability often exist among humans due to pharmacogenetic reasons. Obviously, slow acetylators of isoniazid show increased bioavailability and therefore are more subject to isoniazid-induced neurotoxicity (e.g., American Whites, Israelis and Scandinavians). Contrarily, fast acetylators, like Eskimos, Japanese and Chinese show reduced bioavailability. Some persons have atypical plasma pseudocholinesterase which has a very low hydrolysing capacity for succinylcholine. In such cases even 1/6th of the dose of succinylcholine provides the same effect as the therapeutic dose in normal cases. For details refer the relevant portions in Chapter 7.

vii) Miscellaneous Factors

Besides these factors, multiple other factors like (a) route of administration, (b) area of absorbing surface and (c) state of circulation at the site of absorption (as in shock, where tissue perfusion gets decreased), also affect the bioavailability and these have been appropriately discussed earlier.

HOW DRUGS ARE DISTRIBUTED

If you sprinkle salt all over your plate, which has different eatable items, it is not necessary that the salt will land only on the potatoes. Most of it will land on the other parts of the meal as well. Thus, *drug distribution* means the pattern of "scattering" of the specified amount of drug among the various locations within the body. Once absorbed into the bloodstream, a drug is distributed to all organs including those not relevant to its pharmacological or therapeutic effect. Thus, after absorption the drug may not only get reversibly associated with its site of action (receptor) but may get bound to plasma proteins or may accumulate in various storage sites or may enter into the tissues which are not involved in its primary action (though may be involved in metabolism and excretion). This part of pharmacokinetics which deals with *distribution, metabolism* and *excretion* is termed as *drug disposition*, because these three phases precisely decide the fate of the drug after absorption.

The drugs may be evenly, or unevenly or selectively distributed in different body compartments, which are physiological in character rather than anatomical entities (Fig. 6.3).

PHYSIOLOGICAL BARRIERS TO DRUG DISTRIBUTION

Blood-Brain Barrier

Endothelial cells of brain capillaries differ from peripheral capillaries of the body, as they are very tightly joined and lack intercellular pores. In addition, these brain capillaries are also enveloped by less permeable cells known as the glial cells. Morphologically this constitutes the "Blood-Brain Barrier" (BBB; Fig. 6.4). Anatomically, there exists a dual barrier in the CNS: *the blood-brain barrier* and *the blood-CSF barrier* (located in the choroid plexus). The BBB places certain constraints on the passage of drugs from the blood to the brain and the CSF. In fact, there are a number of efflux transporters also, located at the BBB (like p-glycoprotein and $ABCC_1$), which act as molecular barrier to complement this morphological barrier. As a result it protects the brain tissue, both from toxic substances that circulate in the blood and from neurotransmitters like epinephrine, norepinephrine and dopamine etc., which have systemic peripheral effects but could bind to CNS receptors to cause adverse effects if their access were permitted. As a rule, only lipid-soluble, nonionised form of drugs penetrate more easily to brain as compared to water-soluble ionised form of the drug. Thus volatile anaesthetics like ether and chloroform, ultrashort-acting barbiturate like thiopental, narcotic analgesics like morphine and heroin, dopamine precursor like l-dopa, sympathomimetics like amphetamine and ephedrine and drugs like diazepam and propranolol can pass through BBB; while polar compounds like dopamine, serotonin and streptomycin and quaternary substances like d-tubocurarine, hexamethonium, neostigmine and acetylcholine fail to penetrate the BBB. Inflammatory conditions as in cerebral meningitis, or viral infections of brain or heat stress usually alter the permeability characteristics of BBB and as a result drugs like penicillins and chloramphenicol which otherwise have a poor penetration through BBB, exhibit increased permeability in these disease states. There

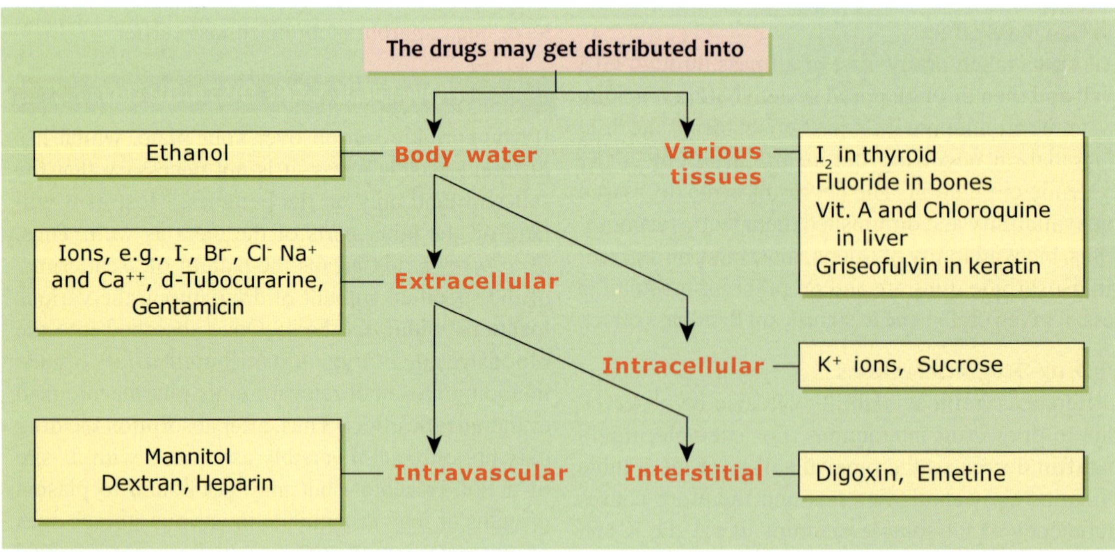

Fig 6.3 Possible Pathways of Drug Distribution in Various Physiological Compartments

are five regions of the brain which are relatively permeable or leaky (because of no occluding zonulae) and thus do not constitute part of BBB. These are: pituitary gland, pineal body, median eminence, choroid plexus capillaries and area prostema near the floor of fourth ventricle which includes chemoreceptor trigger zone and vomiting centre (Fig. 6.4).

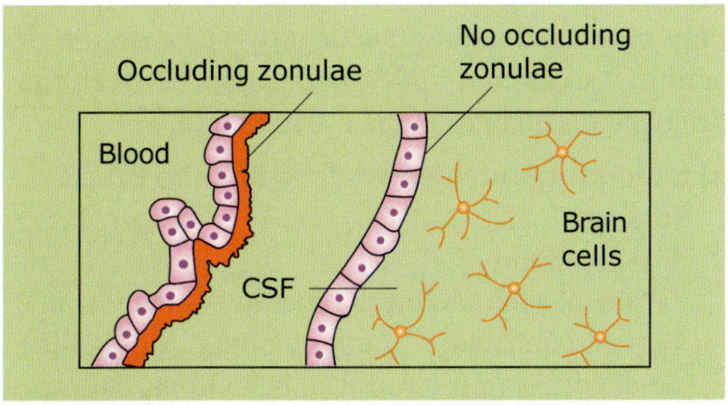

Fig 6.4 Blood-Brain & CSF-Brain Barriers

Blood-CSF and CSF-Brain Barrier

Cerebrospinal fluid is secreted by the epithelial cells of the choroid plexus and these are lined by occluding zonulae (Fig. 6.4). That means (as in the case of BBB) only nonionisable lipid-soluble drugs can pass from blood to the CSF. On the contrary, the CSF-brain barrier is composed of the epithelial cells lining the ventricles, but these are not connected by occluding zonulae. Hence the CSF-brain barrier is extremely permeable to drug molecules from CSF to brain cells. Clinical advantage may be taken of this fact for the proper distribution of drugs, like penicillins into brain. Penicillin being less lipid soluble has poor penetration through BBB but if given by intrathecal route it can cross CSF-brain barrier and reach the brain in sufficient concentration to treat conditions like brain abscess.

Placental Barrier

The placental membrane, like any other cell membrane is lipid in nature and readily allows the transfer of non-polar lipid-soluble substances mainly by a process of passive diffusion. However, other transport mechanisms, like active transport (e.g., for amino acids and glucose) and pinocytosis (e.g., for maternal immunoglobulins) are also operative. Even some influx transporters are reported to be present on placental membrane. Thus, lipid-soluble nonionisable drugs, like hypnotics, narcotics, general anaesthetics, cardiac glycosides, alcohol, neuroleptics and certain antibiotics can readily cross placental barrier; while polar substances and quaternary ammonium compounds, like d-tubocurarine, and substances with very high molecular weight, e.g., dextran and insulin, cannot cross placental barrier.

Since some degree of foetal exposure is likely to occur with virtually all drugs, and since consequences of such exposure are usually not known, it is normally advised that the drug administration during pregnancy should be severely restricted. For example, certain drugs when given in first trimester may lead to congenital abnormality in the foetus (teratogenic effects), e.g., thalidomide, phenytoin, trimethadione, streptomycin, and methotrexate. Similarly, the drugs administered during the last trimester may affect the vital functions of the foetus, e.g., administration of morphine during labour can lead to foetal asphyxia while the use of antithyroid drugs (like carbimazole) can cause neonatal goitre.The foetal plasma is slightly more acidic than that of the mother (7.0 *vs* 7.4). Hence ion trapping of basic drugs (like morphine) occurs in foetal plasma; because once inside, a basic drug would get ionised and cannot be diffused out. Certain physiological variations (as seen with BBB) can also alter the permeability characteristics of placental barrier, e.g., hypoxia increases permeability of drugs through placental barrier.

SPECIAL COMPARTMENTS FOR DRUG DISTRIBUTION (SANCTUARY COMPARTMENTS)

Besides plasma proteins, other tissues of the body can also act as reservoirs for drugs, but usually the sites where drugs get accumulated are not those where they exert their pharmacological effects. The classical examples of drugs getting distributed in such reservoirs are given below:

Cellular Reservoir

A drug may have a great affinity for plasma proteins, yet be primarily distributed in tissues. This situation would occur if the tissue has an even higher affinity for the drug. This affinity could be due to several reasons, e.g., binding to tissue proteins (lipoproteins) or to nucleoproteins. Examples are digoxin and emetine in skeletal muscles, heart, liver and kidney (bound to muscle proteins); iodine in thyroid; chloroquine in liver (tissue proteins) and retina (nucleoproteins); cadmium, lead and mercury in kidney (muscle protein, metallothionein) and chlorpromazine in eye (affinity to retinal pigment melanin).

Fat as Reservoir

Highly lipid-soluble drugs, like thiopentone and DDT, get selectively accumulated in fat and adipose tissue. The fat is, however, a sluggish reservoir due to lesser blood flow but, if the body fats start depleting, as occurs during starvation, the stored drug may be mobilised and toxicity may ensue.

Transcellular Reservoir

Aqueous humour (e.g., chloramphenicol and prednisolone), CSF (e.g., aminosugars and sucrose), endolymph, joint fluid (e.g., ampicillin), pleural (e.g., imipramine and methadone), pericardial and peritoneal sacs can also serve as drug reservoirs.

Bones and Connective Tissue as Reservoirs

Many drugs, like tetracyclines, cisplatin, lead, arsenic and fluorides, form a complex with bone salts and get deposited in nails, bones and teeth. Antifungal drug griseofulvin has an affinity for keratin precursor cells and is selectively accumulated in the skin and finger nails.

Plasma Protein Binding as Drug Reservoir

Drugs usually bind to plasma and cellular proteins in a reversible manner and in dynamic equilibrium, as shown by the following equation:

$$\text{Free drug} + \text{Protein} \Leftrightarrow \text{Drug-Protein complex}$$

Thus, extensive protein binding results in the blood which serves as a circulating drug reservoir. But, it is only the free fraction of the drug which is pharmacologically active while the protein bound component is inert. Similarly, it is the free fraction of the drug which can diffuse through the capillary wall (and also through-blood-brain barrier), be metabolised and be excreted through glomerulus, saliva, CSF and milk. The protein bound component is not accessible to capillary diffusion, metabolism or excretion. As the free or unbound drug is eliminated from the body, more drug dissociates from the drug–plasma protein complex to replace the free drug that was lost. Thus, extensive protein binding does not prevent the drug from reaching its site of action but only prolongs the drug availability and duration of action. Association and dissociation between the drug and plasma protein is usually rapid.

a) Important Proteins that Contribute to Drug Binding

1. **Plasma Albumin**
   Of the plasma proteins, albumin is the most important contributor to drug binding. Most of the acidic drugs (e.g., warfarin, penicillins, sulfonamides, tolbutamide and salicylic acid) in principle bind to albumin.
2. **α_1-Acid Glycoproteins (α_1-AGP)**
   While acidic drugs primarily bind to albumin, many lipophilic basic drugs, like quinidine, imipramine, lidocaine, chlorpromazine, propranolol and analogues, and spiroperidol, bind avidly to α_1-acid glycoproteins. The plasma α_1-AGP is an acute-phase reactant protein, i.e., its plasma concentration increases in physiological stress and pathological states (e.g., in myocardial infarction, arthritis, cancer and in Crohn's disease).
3. **Tissue Proteins and Nucleoproteins**
   Some drugs, particularly those having high apparent volume of distribution, specifically bind to tissue proteins, e.g., digoxin, emetine and chloroquine.
4. **Miscellaneous Binding Proteins**
   Only a few drugs are appreciably bound to other proteins, e.g., steroids are bound to corticosteriod binding globulin—transcortin; thyroxine to α-globulins, and antigens to gamma globulins.

b) Clinically Important Aspects of Plasma Protein Binding

1. Highly plasma protein bound drugs remain largely restricted to the vascular compartment and tend to have lower volumes of distribution (cf following text).

2. Highly protein bound drugs are difficult to be removed by dialysis and need special techniques for treatment of their poisoning.
3. The binding of drugs to plasma proteins is a capacity-limited and saturable process. In liver disease, uraemia and in all disease states causing hypoalbuminaemia, even the therapeutic dose of the drug can lead to higher concentration of the free drug because of reduced protein binding. However, in certain conditions like physiological stress, myocardial infarction, Crohn's disease and inflammation, plasma concentration of acute-phase reactant protein (e.g., α_1-acid glycoprotein) increases. Therefore, binding of some basic drugs, like propranolol and quinidine, increases in such pathological states.
4. More than one drug can bind to the same site of albumin. This can give rise to displacement interactions wherein a drug bound with higher affinity will displace the one having lower affinity. Theoretically, the increased free drug concentration (of the displaced drug) could have the potential to cause greater adverse effects. But practically, the consequences are not that serious (for exceptions, see below) because most of the drugs obey first-order elimination kinetics and hence, the clearance of the free drug (after displacement) also increases proportionately. However, acidic drugs (as they are bound to albumin) do not generally displace basic drugs (because these are bound to α_1-acid glycoproteins) and vice versa.

c) Some Clinically Important Displacement Reactions

1. Phenylbutazone, salicylates and some sulfonamides displace tolbutamide from its binding sites leading to hypoglycaemia.
2. Salicylates, indomethacin, phenytoin and tolbutamide displace warfarin resulting in increased risk of haemorrhage.
3. Sulfonamides and vitamin K can displace endogenous ligands, like bilirubin from the protein binding sites leading to kernicterus in neonates.
4. Salicylates displace methotrexate.

Yet, it is also true that the importance of drug interactions, purely due to displacement from protein binding sites, has been over-emphasised. Due significance should only be given when:

a) The displaced drug is more than 95% protein bound. Suppose a drug is 99% protein bound, i.e., it has 1% free drug component which is active. Now, even if just 1% is displaced, then the bound form becomes 98.01% while the concentration of the free active form increases from 1% to 1.99% which is almost double of the earlier value and is thus liable to cause toxicity.

b) The displaced drug is not only extensively protein bound but has a smaller apparent volume of distribution also (see following text). Under this criterion, drugs like warfarin (99% bound, aVd 9.8 L/70 kg), tolbutamide (98% bound, aVd 8 L/70 kg) and phenytoin (90% bound, aVd 40 L/70 kg) are the most potential candidates to cause toxicity after getting displaced from plasma protein binding sites. Because of their low aVd, these drugs remain primarily in plasma and that too in their free form to produce toxicity.

Lastly, displacement interactions are rare with basic drugs presumably because (a) they bind to different loci than do the acidic drugs, and (b) because most of them have large aVd values.

APPARENT VOLUME OF DISTRIBUTION (aVd)

To grasp the concept of aVd let us explain it with an example: 500 μg of digoxin provides a plasma concentration of 0.78 μg/L in a 70 kg adult person. From this it follows that if 0.78 μg of digoxin is contained in one litre of plasma, 500 μg of digoxin (present in the body) would require 641 L of plasma, to reach the same concentration. Neither there is so much plasma nor is so much body volume available for distribution. The intracellular volume is 28 L, interstitial volume is 10 L and plasma volume is 4 L. This makes the total distribution volume equal to 42 L. Digoxin, therefore, exhibits volume of distribution far in excess (approx. 16 times higher) of the total body water (42 L), which is seemingly impossible to explain. This serves to emphasise two points that:

1. Volume of distribution does not represent a real volume but must be regarded as the size of the pool of the body or fluids (available space) that would be theoretically required if the drug was distributed equally throughout all portions of the body.

2. Digoxin is widely distributed in the body including muscles and adipose tissue, leaving a small fraction to be distributed in plasma.

Apparent volume of distribution, therefore, means the total space which should apparently be available in the body to contain the known amount of the drug.

$$\text{aVd} = \frac{\text{Total amount of drug in body (mg/kg)}}{\text{Conc. of the drug in the plasma (mg/L)}}$$

aVd is expressed in the units of L/70 kg body weight or in L/kg. From the ongoing discussion, the following generalisations can be made:

a) If the drug does not cross capillary walls (high molecular weight, e.g., heparin and insulin or lesser lipid-soluble drugs) and is given by intravenous route, its aVd is equal to plasma water, i.e., 3 L.
b) Drugs highly bound to plasma proteins (less bound to tissue proteins) have a low aVd value (e.g., tolbutamide, furosemide and warfarin). Conversly, lesser the plasma protein binding (higher tissue binding) greater is the aVd for the drug (e.g., chloroquine and metoprolol).
c) aVd for many drugs may be much more than the actual body volume (e.g., digoxin, imipramine and analogues, phenobarbitone and analogues and morphine). It means that such drugs are widely distributed in body including muscles and adipose tissue. Such drugs are difficult to be removed by haemodialysis if toxicity appears. Dialysis is fruitful only for those drugs which have smaller aVd (e.g., for warfarin, aspirin, tolbutamide and sulfonamides). If a drug having smaller aVd has lesser protein binding also, it is easier to remove by haemodialysis.
d) Generally speaking, a value of aVd < 5 L implies that the drug is retained within the vascular compartment (e.g., heparin, insulin, warfarin and furosemide). A value of aVd approximating 15 L suggests that the drug is restricted to the extracellular fluid (e.g., aspirin, tolbutamide, gentamicin, d-tubocurarine and amoxycillin) while large volume of distribution (aVd > 20 L) indicates distribution throughout the total body water (e.g., ethanol, phenytoin, methyldopa and theophylline) or penetration in various tissues (e.g., digoxin, imipramine, phenobarbitone, morphine and chloroquine). Pathological states, like congestive heart failure, uraemia and cirrhosis of liver, however, can alter aVd of many drugs by altering distribution of body water and protein binding.

REDISTRIBUTION OF DRUGS

This is a typical mode of drug distribution observed particularly with highly lipid-soluble drugs. Sometimes the drug action is terminated after its withdrawal because of its redistribution in viscera, muscle mass, lean tissue and fat, e.g., after giving IV injection of ultrashort-acting barbiturates (thiopentone). These drugs, being highly lipid soluble, enter the brain very rapidly (in one circulation time, i.e., one minute after their I.V. injection) causing general anaesthesia. But being highly lipid soluble they also diffuse out of the brain through blood circulation and are then redistributed in the muscle, lean tissues and fat. As a result their action gets terminated. It is because of this rapid removal from brain and redistribution to other tissues that single dose of ultrashort-acting barbiturate is very short acting. In short, the general anaesthetic effect after giving one I.V. injection of thiopentone occurred due to its rapid distribution in the brain but its effects were terminated due to its redistribution in the muscle mass and fat in the periphery.

HOW DRUGS ARE BIOTRANSFORMED

The processes of absorption and distribution, as discussed earlier, summarily determine the speed of onset of drug effect. In order that the drug action may not continue indefinitely, body mechanisms, like biotransformation, excretion and tissue redistribution (though in limited cases) start acting on the drug to terminate its actions. The net result of these processes contributes to the duration of the drug action. We shall first start our discussion as to how the drug action is terminated by the process of biotransformation. Detoxification and drug metabolism are the other two loosely referred terms which are used interchangeably, but not correctly, with biotransformation.

BIOTRANSFORMATION means enzyme-catalysed biochemical transformation of drugs within the living organism. The metabolites thus formed are much less lipid soluble, hence not reabsorbed from the renal tubules and thus are finally excreted. The biotransformation of drugs, which is the more preferred term, occurs mainly in liver, although kidney, intestine, adrenal cortex, lungs, placenta and skin may also be involved to some extent. The dead tissues, like nails and hair, *per se*, are not involved in drug biotransformation.

The biotransformation reaction of any drug may have three different consequences with respect to pharmacological activity of its metabolite:

1. ***Formation of an inactive metabolite from the pharmacologically active drug:*** This is the usual case, e.g., phenobarbitone (active drug) is converted to hydroxyphenobarbitone (inactive metabolite).
2. ***Formation of an active metabolite from an inactive (prodrug) or a lesser active drug.***

For example:

L-Dopa (inactive) PRODRUG → Dopamine (active) in basal ganglia

Parathion (inactive) PRODRUG → Paraoxon (active) in liver

Talampicillin (inactive) PRODRUG → Ampicillin (active)

The term PRODRUG refers to a precursor drug that in itself has little or no biological activity but is metabolised to a pharmacologically active metabolite.

3. ***Formation of an active metabolite from an equally active drug:***

Diazepam (active) → Oxazepam (active)

Amitriptyline (active) → Nortriptyline (active)

Imipramine (active) → Des-imipramine (active)

Codeine (active) → Morphine (active)

FIRST-PASS METABOLISM

All drugs taken orally, first of all, pass through GIT wall and then through portal system, before reaching the systemic circulation. *First-Pass Metabolism* or the *pre-systemic metabolism* or the *First-Pass Effect* means the drug metabolism occurring before the drug enters the systemic circulation (Table 6.1). The net result is the decreased bioavailability of the drug and consequently a diminished therapeutic response, because a significant amount of the drug is inactivated before reaching the systemic circulation. The first-pass effect may be bypassed if the drug is administered parenterally (e.g., I.V. infusion of xylocaine in combating arrhythmias) or sublingually (e.g., isosorbide dinitrate in antagonising

Table 6.1 Examples of the Drugs Undergoing First-Pass Effect

First-Pass Metabolism Occurring in		
Liver	**Intestinal Mucosa**	**Bronchial Mucosa**
Isosorbide dinitrate	l - Dopa	Nicotine
Glyceryl trinitrate	α-Methyldopa	Isoprenaline
Morphine	Tyramine	
Pethidine	Testosterone	
Xylocaine	Progesterone	
Imipramine	Chlorpromazine	
Amitriptyline		
Propranolol		

anginal pain). If a drug, after oral administration, furnishes metabolites which are active, the significance of first pass decreases (e.g., propranolol); but in liver disease it acquires greater significance as the oral bioavailability of the drug might go much higher.

CHEMICAL PATHWAYS OF DRUG BIOTRANSFORMATION

Drug biotransformation reactions are commonly grouped into two types:

A) Phase I Reactions

These are degradative reactions. The drug is diminished to a smaller polar/non-polar metabolite by introduction of a new group. These reactions are mainly microsomal, except a few which are non-microsomal, and include oxidation, reduction or hydrolysis reactions. *The metabolite formed may be active or inactive.*

B) Phase II Reactions

These are synthetic reactions and are also called as conjugation reactions. These reactions may be catalysed by microsomal, mitochondrial or cytoplasmic enzymes. *The metabolite formed is usually polar, water soluble and is mostly inactive.*

Some drugs originally contain reactive groups (e.g., NH_2, OH or COOH) capable of being conjugated and may therefore undergo phase II reactions immediately without having to go through phase I; while in others, the metabolites, formed after phase I reactions, may undergo phase II process, if they acquire these reactive groups in their molecules during metabolism.

THE DRUG METABOLISING ENZYMES

i) Microsomal Enzymes

These are the drug metabolising enzymes which are located primarily on the *smooth-surfaced endoplasmic reticulum* of the liver. However, these are present in intestinal mucosa, lungs and in kidney also. The principal enzymes are mixed function oxidases (MFOs) or cytochrome P-450 (these are haemoproteins and are so-named because, in their reduced form they can combine with carbon monoxide giving a product whose absorption peak is at 450 cm^{-1}). Glucuronyl transferase is also a microsomal enzyme. *The rough-surfaced endoplasmic reticulum* contains ribosomes which are involved in protein synthesis. The microsomal enzymes are non-specific in action, can be induced or activated and can metabolise only lipid-soluble drugs. Microsomal enzymes are concerned primarily with phase I reaction—oxidation, reduction and hydrolysis—and also phase II glucuronyl conjugations.

Specific forms of cytochrome P-450 (CYP) enzymes have been classified into families designated by numbers 1,2,3,4 etc., and subfamilies designated by letters A, B, C, D etc., on the basis of amino acid sequence and cDNA cloning studies; another number is added to indicate the specific isoenzyme, e.g., CYP2D6 is the cytochrome P-450 enzyme belonging to family 2, subfamily D with gene number 6. In humans, 12 CYPs from three families (1 to 3) are responsible for drug metabolism. These are : CYP1A1, 1A2, 1B1, 2B1, 2A6, 2B6, 2C8, 2C9, 2C19, 2D6, 2E1, 3A4 and 3A5. The most important CYPs for drug metabolism belong to three subfamilies, viz, CYP3A, CYP2D and CYP2C (also CYP2E to some extent). These exhibit genetic polymorphism (existence of different forms in gene regulation). The characteristic features of these CYPs are noted below;

CYP3A4 and CYP3A5: Nearly 50% of xenobiotics (drugs and other chemical substances) are metabolised by these CYPs because these are present not only in liver but also in intestine (first-pass) and kidney. Barbiturates (sedative-hypnotics), carbamazepine and phenytoin (anticonvulsants) and rifampicin (antitubercular drug) are their *inducers.* While erythromycin and clarithromycin (macrolide group of antibiotics), ketoconazole and fluconazole (antifungal drugs), verapamil and diltiazem (Ca^{2+} channel blockers) as well as ritonavir (antiretroviral drug against AIDS), act as their *inhibitors*. CYP3A5 is usually less active than CYP3A4.

CYP2D6: This CYP subfamily metabolises about 25–30% of the commonly used drugs. Its important *inhibitors* are quinidine and fluoxetine. *Inducers* are less common, rather unknown. However, there are greater incidences of genetic polymorphism with this CYP. Some persons may be genetically deficient in CYP2D6 or may have an altered activity of this enzyme due to genetic polymorphism. Such persons will be poor responders to analgesic actions of codeine because these are unable to metabolise codeine to morphine.

CYP2C8 and CYP2C9: These CYPs metabolise about 15–18 (10%) commonly used drugs, some of which have a low margin of safety (e.g., phenytoin and warfarin). Barbiturates and rifampicin are its *inducers. Inhibitors* are less known (except for fluconazole and fluvastatin).

CYP2C19: It metabolises about 12–15 frequently used drugs including diazepam (antianxiety) and omeprazole (proton-pump inhibitor) group. As above it is *induced* by barbiturates and rifampicin. Inhibitors are less known.

CYP1A1 and CYP1A2: Only a few drugs are metabolised by this subfamily. These include theophylline (bronchodilator), warfarin (anticoagulant), clomipramine (antidepressant) and paracetamol (minor pathway). However, this subfamily is *induced* by several drugs and other polltuants (procarcinogens), e.g., barbiturates, rifampicin, carbamazepine, smoking and charcoal-broiled meat.

CYP2E1: It metabolises very few drugs like general anaesthetics (halothane and enflurane etc), alcohol (minor pathway) and paracetamol (minor pathway but forming a hepatotoxic metabolite). Chronic consumption of alcohol *induces* this enzyme; disulfiram (antabuse) *inhibits* this enzyme also (besides inhibiting aldehyde dehydrogenase).

ii) Non-microsomal Enzymes

Enzymes of non-microsomal origin are present in cytoplasm, mitochondria of hepatic cells (and other tissues) and in plasma. Examples of such enzymes are monoamine oxidase, esterases, amidases, transferases and conjugages. Reactions catalysed by them are all phase II reactions (except glucuronide conjugation), certain oxidations, reductions and hydrolytic reactions. These are non-inducible but can be inhibited and usually show genetic variation (e.g., pseudocholine esterase and acetyl transferase etc.).

PHASE I REACTIONS

A) Oxidations

1. Microsomal Oxidations (CYP dependent)

The oxidative processes catalysed by the microsomal enzymes are as follows:

- ***Aromatic Hydroxylations***

As with phenobarbitone to p-hydroxyphenobarbitone. Other examples include phenytoin, propranolol, amphetamine, and warfarin.

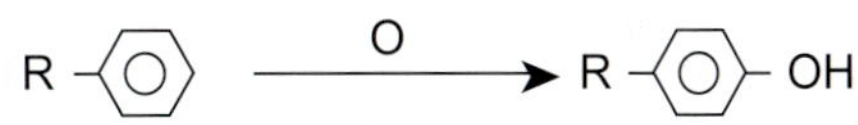

- ***Aliphatic Hydroxylations*** (side chain hydroxylation)

$$R.CH_2.CH_3 \xrightarrow{O} R.CHOH.CH_3$$

As with pentobarbitone to hydroxypentobarbitone. Other examples: digitoxin and ibuprofen.

- ***N-, O- and S-Dealkylation***

$$R.NHCH_3 \xrightarrow{O} R.NH_2 + HCHO$$

$$R.N\,(CH_3)_2 \xrightarrow{O} R.NHCH_3 + CH_3CHO$$

As with mephobarbitone to phenobarbitone; morphine to normorphine and amitriptyline to nortriptyline; *nor* means removal of one alkyl group from amino nitrogen (N-dealkylation).

$$R\text{-}OCH_3 \xrightarrow{O} R\text{-}OH + HCHO$$

As with phenacetin to paracetamol. A similar metabolic pathway of codeine to morphine is also through O-dealkylation.

$$R\text{-}SCH_3 \xrightarrow{O} RSH + HCHO$$

Example: 6-methylthiopurine to mercaptopurine.

- ***N- and S-Oxidation***

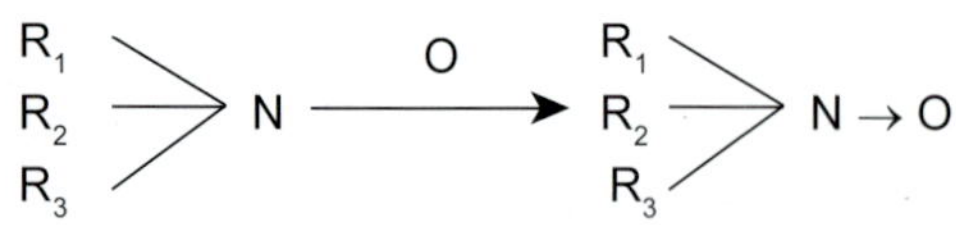

Example: Trimethylamine to trimethylamine N-oxide; also N-oxidation of chlorpheniramine, quinidine and dapsone.

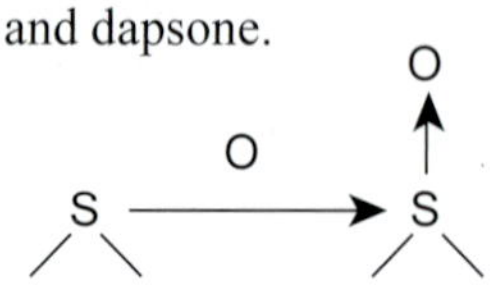

Example: Chlorpromazine to chlorpromazine sulfoxide and cimetidine to cimetidine sulfoxide.

- ***Deamination***

$$R\text{-}CHNH_2\text{-}R \xrightarrow{O} R.COR + NH_3$$

Example: Amphetamine to phenylacetone derivative.

- ***Desulfurisation***

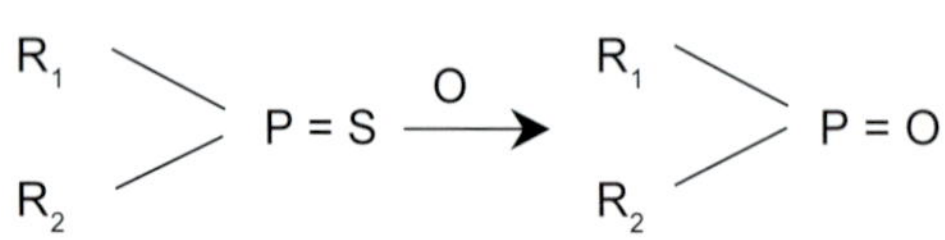

Example: Parathion to paraoxon.

2. Non-microsomal Oxidations (cytochrome P-450 independent)

- ***Mitochondrial Oxidations***

$$R\text{-}CH(OH).CH_2NH_2 \xrightarrow{O} R.CH(OH).COOH + NH_3$$

Example: Oxidation of catecholamines, like epinephrine by monoamine oxidase to vinyl-mandelic acid.

- ***Cytoplasmic Oxidation (dehydrogenation)***

$$C_2H_5OH \xrightarrow{O} CH_3CHO \xrightarrow{O} CH_3COOH$$

Example: Oxidation of alcohol by alcohol dehydrogenase to acetaldehyde and then by aldehyde dehydrogenase to acetic acid.

- ***Plasma Oxidative Processes (oxidative deamination)***

$$\text{Histamine} \xrightarrow[\text{Histaminase}]{O} \text{Imidazole acetic acid}$$

$$\text{Xanthine} \xrightarrow[\text{Xanthine oxidase}]{O} \text{Uric acid}$$

Example: oxidative deamination of histamine and xanthine

B) Reductions

1. Microsomal Reductions

The reductive processes catalysed by microsomal enzymes are:

- ***Nitro Reduction***

$$R\text{-}NO_2 \xrightarrow[\text{Hepatic nitro reductase + FADH}]{} R.NH_2$$

Example:Chloramphenicol to its arylamine metabolite.

- ***Azo Reduction***

Example: Prontosil (prodrug) to sulfanilamide; reduction of sulfasalzine.

$$R\text{-}N = N\text{-}R_1 \xrightarrow[\text{Hepatic azo reductase + FADH}]{O} RNH_2 + R_1NH_2$$

- ***Keto Reduction***

$$R\text{-}\overset{\overset{\Large O}{\|}}{C}\text{-}R_1 \longrightarrow R\text{-}\overset{\overset{\Large OH}{|}}{CH}\text{-}R_1$$

Example: Cortisone to hydroxycortisone and reduction of methadone and naloxone to their corresponding hydroxylated metabolites.

2. Non-microsomal Reductions

$C(Cl)_3CH(OH)_2 \longrightarrow C(Cl)_3\text{-}CH_2OH$

Chloral hydrate → Trichloroethanol

C) Hydrolysis

1. Microsomal Hydrolysis

Hydrolytic reactions are rarely microsomal, except for the hydrolysis of pethidine to pethidinic (meperidinic) acid and hydrolysis of lidocaine by hepatic membrane bound esterase.

2. Non-microsomal Hydrolysis

Mainly for esters and amides. Enzymes involved are primarily the esterases and amidases but also peptidases, proteases and phosphatases. *Examples:* Procaine to PABA by plasma choline esterase; atropine to tropic acid; hydrolysis of β-lactam ring of penicillin-G and hydrolysis of procainamide by amidases.

PHASE II REACTIONS

Conjugations

1. Microsomal Conjugations

- ***Glucuronide Conjugation***

This is the sole example of microsomal conjugation. Other conjugations are non-microsomal. Parent drugs or their phase I metabolites that contain phenolic, alcoholic, carboxylic, amino or mercapto groups can undergo conjugation reaction with uridine diphosphate glucuronic acid (UDPGA) catalysed by microsomal UDP-glucuronyl transferase enzymes to yield drug-glucuronide conjugates which are polar, readily excreted and often inactive (except morphine glucuronide which is active).

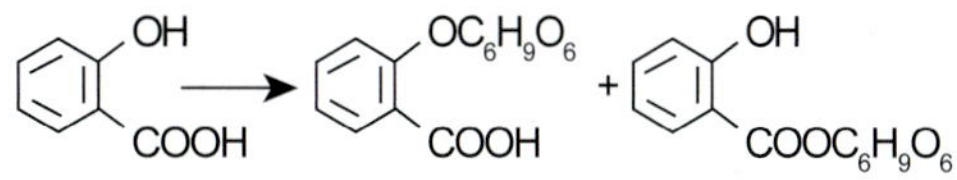

Salicylic acid — Ether glucuronide — Ester glucuronide

In general:

$$\text{Drug + UDPGA} \xrightarrow[\text{Glucuronyl transferase}]{\text{Microsomal}} \text{Drug glucuronide + UDP}$$

Examples: Drugs like morphine, paracetamol, aspirin, chloramphenicol, diazepam and sulfonamides. Natural endogenous substance like bilirubin is also conjugated as glucuronide by this process.

2. Non-microsomal Conjugation

- ***N-Acetyl Conjugation (in cytosol)***

This reaction is catalysed by *N*-acetyltransferase which utilises acetyl coenzyme-*A* as a cofactor and takes place in cell cytoplasm of various organs. A number of aromatic amines, like isoniazid, PAS, dapsone, sulfonamides, procainamide and histamine undergo N-acetylation.

$$R\text{-}NH_2 \xrightarrow[\text{Acetyl CoA}]{\text{N-acetyl transferase}} R.NH.COCH_3$$

- ***Sulfate Conjugation (in cytosol)***

This reaction is catalysed by a family of enzymes called sulfotransferases that are present in the cell cytoplasm of various organs. The essential cofactor (sulfate donor) for this enzyme is 3' phosphoadenosine-5-phosphosulfate (PAPS). Sulfate conjugates being highly polar compounds are readily excreted in the urine. Many phenolic, alcoholic and aromatic amine drugs undergo sulfate conjugation and these include aspirin, methyldopa, paracetamol, hydroxycoumarins, corticosteroids and chloramphenicol.

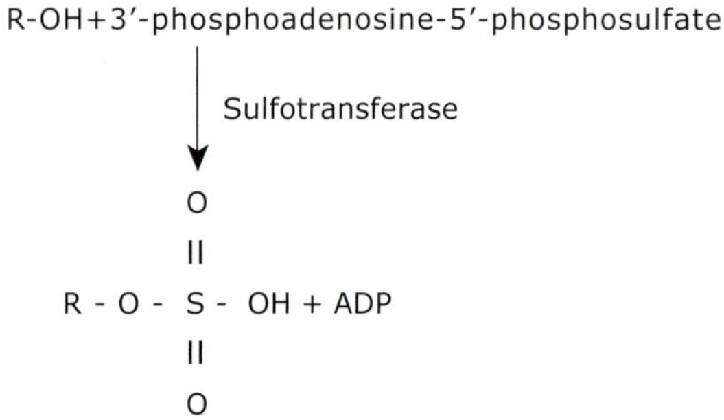

- ***Amino Acid Conjugation (in mitochondria)***

Acyl-coenzyme-A derivatives of carboxylic acid drugs (e.g., aspirin, benzoic acid, nicotinic acid and deoxycholic acid) can couple with glycine or glutamine in presence of AcCoA-glycine transferase enzymes in mitochondria; *but it is a minor metabolic pathway.*

- ***Methyl Conjugation (in cytosol)***

Many catecholamines (e.g., dopamine and epinephrine) are O-methylated, while amines (like histamine) are N-methylated in this way. The catalysing enzyme is transmethylase while cofactor (methyl donor) is S-adenosine methionine. *However, this is again a minor metabolic pathway.*

- ***Glutathione Conjugation (in cytoplasm)***

Many epoxides, NO_2 group containing drugs and hydroxylamines (e.g., ethacrynic acid and sulfobromophthalein) undergo glutathione conjugation in the presence of glutathione-S-transferase enzyme present in cytosol (or in microsomes). *This is also a minor metabolic pathway.*

- ***Ribosides and Riboside Phosphates***

Many purines and pyrimidines, used as antimetabolites in cancer chemotherapy, form their active metabolites by forming ribonucleosides and ribonucleotides. *This is again a minor metabolic pathway.*

NON-ENZYMATIC BIOTRANSFORMATION (HOFMANN ELIMINATION)

Some drugs like atracurium (skeletal muscle relaxant) are metabolised in the plasma spontaneously through molecular rearrangement without involvement of any enzyme action. Such non-enzymatic biotrans-formation of drugs is called Hofmann elimination.

Table 6.2 Enzyme Inducers, Enzyme Induced and Consequential Increase in Drug Metabolism

Enzyme Inducer	Enzyme Induced	Drugs whose metabolism is enhanced and clinical effect reduced
Phenobarbitone, Phenytoin Carbamazepine, Efavirenz Glucocorticoids, Pioglitazone	CYP3A4	Midazolam, Alprazolam, Barbiturates themselves, Ritonavir, Ca^{2+} channel blockers, Vit. D_3, Theophylline, Macrolide
Rifampicin, Phenobarbitone	CYP3A4 & CYP2C9	Oral contraceptives, Warfarin, Ibuprofen, Tamoxifen, Tolbutamide, Losartan
Smoking, Charcoal-broiled meat	CYP1A2	Theophylline, Warfarin, Imipramine, Paracetamol, neuroleptics
Chronic ethanol intake, Isoniazid	CYP2E1	Ethanol itself, General anaesthetics (e.g., halothane), Paracetamol

ENZYME INDUCTION

Several drugs, on repeated administration, stimulate or induce the growth of smooth endoplasmic reticulum. This stimulation/induction, *although reversible*, usually leads to an enhanced microsomal enzyme activity. The induction results in an accelerated metabolism and consequently in a decreased pharmacological response of not only the inducer itself but also of the co-administered drugs utilizing same enzymatic pathway.

Enzyme induction, although most prominent in liver, can also occur to some extent in the intestine, lung, placenta and kidney, e.g., CYP1A1 isoenzyme is induced in the lungs of cigarette smokers. Since enzyme induction requires the synthesis of proteins, it *occurs gradually* over a period of 1–2 weeks to attain its maximal effect and requires an equal time to dissipate after the enzyme inducer is stopped. Some of the common enzyme inducers, specific forms of cytochrome P-450 which they induce and the drugs whose metabolism they enhance are listed in Table 6.2.

Clinical Relevance of Enzyme Induction

A) Clinical consequences of increased drug metabolism include: (1) decreased plasma levels and decreased therapeutic effect of the co-administered drug, (2) decreased drug effect if its metabolite is inactive, and (3) increased drug activity if its metabolite is active. The following examples would illustrate this:

i) Unwanted pregnancy can result, even in the users of oral contraceptive pills, if potent enzyme inducers, like phenytoin or rifampicin, are used concomitantly.
ii) Patients on enzyme-inducing drugs, like barbiturates, would need higher doses of oral anticoagulants, like warfarin. Conversely, if barbiturates are suddenly withdrawn but the doses of anticoagulants are not proportionately reduced, the bleeding from an injury may be enhanced.
iii) Enzyme inducers, like phenytoin, accelerate the metabolism of vitamin D_3 leading to osteomalacia (side effect).
iv) Enzyme inducers, like barbiturates, usually enhance their own metabolism leading to the development of pharmacokinetic (metabolic) tolerance (adverse effect).

B) Enzyme induction can even lead to drug toxicity, e.g., ethanol drinkers have more probabilities of developing hepatotoxicity from paracetamol overdose or even with therapeutic doses due to increased production of *N*-acetyl-P-benzoquinoneimine, a hepatotoxic metabolite of paracetamol.

C) The knowledge of enzyme induction can also be used for therapeutic benefits, e.g., to treat neonatal jaundice. Phenobarbitone can be given to the pregnant mother, 7–14 days prior to labour or to the infant soon after birth to induce the foetal hepatic glucuronyl transferase enzyme which catalyses the conjugation of bilirubin to glucuronic acid. Hence, bilirubin gets conjugated (metabolised) faster and excreted through bile.

ENZYME INHIBITION

One drug may inhibit the metabolism of another drug with resultant increase in the circulating levels of the slowly metabolised drug and prolongation or potentiation of its pharmacological effects. The enzyme inhibition can either be of hepatic microsomal mixed function oxidase (MFOs) or of enzymes having specific functions, e.g., xanthine oxidase, monoamine oxidase and aldehyde dehydrogenase etc. Enzyme inhibition, unlike induction, is a *rapid process* but is *usually reversible*. However, it could also be irreversible as in the case of *secobarbital overdoses*. Secobarbital, in the course of its metabolism by cytochrome P-450, inactivates the enzyme and ends up in an impairment of its own metabolism.

Some of the common enzyme inhibitors, the enzymes which they inhibit and the drugs whose metabolism they retard are listed in Table 6.3.

Clinical Relevance of Enzyme Inhibition

a) Potentially Adverse Consequences

1. Unexpected nausea/vomiting and tremors due to theophylline with concomitantly administered chloramphenicol or erythromycin (enzyme inhibitor).

Table 6.3 Enzyme Inhibitors, Enzyme Inhibited and Consequential Retardation of Drug Metabolism

Inhibitors	Enzymes inhibited	Drugs whose metabolism is inhibited
Cimetidine	Hepatic microsomal MFOs	Phenytoin, warfarin, antidepressants, theophylline, diazepam, quinidine, testosterone
Sod. valproate	Hepatic microsomal MFOs	Phenytoin, phenobarbital, primidone
Erythromycin	Hepatic microsomal MFOs	Theophylline, warfarin, carbamazepine, cyclosporine
Ciprofloxacin group (except ofloxacin)	Hepatic microsomal MFOs	Theophylline
Chloramphenicol	Hepatic microsomal MFOs	Terfenadine, tolbutamide, phenytoin, warfarin
Verapamil and diltiazem	Hepatic microsomal MFOs	Theophylline, carbamazepine, cyclosporine
Allopurinol	Xanthine oxidase	6-Mercaptopurine, azathioprine
MAO inhibitors	Monoamine oxidase	Morphine, pethidine, tricyclic antidepressants
Disulfiram, tolbutamide, metronidazole	Aldehyde dehydrogenase	Alcohol, phenytoin and warfarin
Ecothiophate	Acetylcholine esterase	Suxamethonium, propanidid
Captopril, enalapril	Angiotensin-converting enzyme	Angiotensin I
Carbidopa	L-Aromatic aminoacid decarboxylase	l-Dopa

2. Enhanced bleeding tendency with dicumarol when administered with cimetidine (enzyme inhibitor).
3. Severe respiratory depression with morphine when given with MAOIs (monoamine oxidase inhibitors).
4. Severe ataxia and drowsiness with phenytoin in combination with dicumarol or chloramphenicol.
5. Precipitation of cardiac arrhythmias with terfenadine when given in combination with chloramphenicol or ketoconazole (enzyme inhibitor).

b) Therapeutically Beneficial Consequences

1. Increased accessibility of l-dopa in brain when given along with carbidopa (l-aminoacid decarboxylase inhibitor). Carbidopa prevents peripheral decarboxylation of l-dopa. More l-dopa is now available to pass through BBB.
2. Aversion to alcohol after prior administration of disulfiram (aldehyde dehydrogenase inhibitor). Further conversion of acetaldehyde to acetic acid is thus prevented which leads to nausea, vomiting and headache (aversion to alcohol).

Table 6.4 Some Examples of Genetic Polymorphism in Drug Metabolism

Genetic defect	Drug	Therapeutic use	Clinical consequences
Atypical pseudocholinesterase (inherited as autosomal recessive trait)	Succinyl choline	Neuromuscular blocker	Prolonged aponea due to retarded metabolism
Slow N-acetylation Rapid N-acetylation (inherited as an auto-somal recessive trait)	Isoniazid Isoniazid	Antitubercular Antitubercular	Peripheral neuropathy; Hepatotoxicity
Faulty expression of CYP2D6 (autosomal recessive trait)	Codeine	Opioid analgesic	Reduced analgesia

3. Reversal of skeletal muscle paralysis due to d-tubocurarine by neostigmine (acetylcholinesterase reversible inhibitor).

FACTORS AFFECTING DRUG METABOLISM

Age

Neonates have low microsomal enzyme and glucuronyl transferase enzyme activity and these attain full functional capacity several weeks after the birth. Thus neonates are potentially predisposed to the life-threatening cyanotic condition, called 'grey baby syndrome' after administration of chloramphenicol, which is primarily metabolised by glucuronyl conjugation. Similarly, elderly persons, above the age of 60, have a reduced hepatic blood flow. Hence metabolism of drugs, like propranolol and pethidine (whose rate of metabolism is governed by hepatic blood flow) exhibit slow metabolism and increased incidence of toxicity.

Sex

The differences in the rate of metabolism due to sex are important in various animal species *but are seldom important in human beings*. Male rats sleep for a shorter duration than females, after receiving hexobarbital, as their microsomal enzyme activity is higher than in females.

Species

Examples of species-dependant variations in drug metabolism are few. However, some of these can be cited. Rabbits metabolise atropine faster than man as they have high atropine esterase activity in the liver and plasma.

Race

Racial differences in metabolism are less, although important. Chinese have a high alcohol dehydrogenase but a low aldehyde dehydrogenase activity. Hence they exhibit higher plasma concentration of aldehyde (and therefore headache, palpitation, etc.) after consuming alcohol.

Genetic Variation

Some well-studied examples of genetic variation in the rate of drug metabolism are given in Table 6.4.

Nutrition and Diet

The diet rich in protein and low in carbohydrate enhances the rate of metabolism of many drugs. Rich protein diet supplies glycine and cysteine which are essential to form conjugated metabolites of the drug. On the other hand, diets very poor in protein and rich in carbohydrate slow down the rate of drug metabolism (e.g., starvation leads to enzyme inhibition).

Disease

The activity of hepatic cytochrome P-450 enzymes are impaired to varying degrees in a number of pathological states, like viral hepatitis, alcoholic hepatitis, active or inactive liver cirrhosis, hepatocellular carcinoma and heavy metal poisoning. Similarly, hypothyroidism decreases the metabolism of digoxin, methimazole and practolol while hyperthyroidism enhances the rate of metabolism of various drugs.

Drug-drug Interactions

Many drugs affect the rate of metabolism of other drugs. This happens due to either *enzyme induction* or *enzyme inhibition* as discussed above.

HOW DRUGS ARE ELIMINATED

ROUTES OF DRUG ELIMINATION

Drugs are eliminated from the body either unchanged or as water-soluble metabolites. Both the processes of metabolism and excretion are essential for the elimination of drugs from the body. The major routes of drug excretion are: (a) Renal, (b) Biliary, (c) Faecal and (d) Alveolar.

Other minor routes of drug excretion include: (a) Milk, (b) Skin, (c) Hair, (d) Sweat and (e) Saliva.

Renal Excretion

Kidney is the most important organ for elimination of free drugs (e.g., frusemide, gentamicin, d-tubocurarine and digoxin) and their metabolites. The three key processes that determine the renal excretion of drugs are: (i) Glomerular filtration, (ii) Active tubular secretion, and (iii) Passive tubular reabsorption (Fig. 6.5).

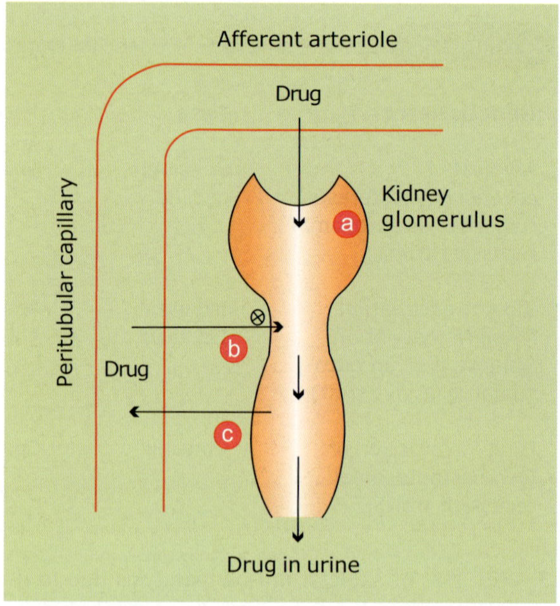

Fig 6.5 a) Glomerular Filtration, b) Active Tubular Secretion, c) Passive Tubular Reabsorption

i) Glomerular Filtration

Several factors influence the renal excretion by glomerular filtration: (i) *Molecular size:* drugs having small molecular size are more readily filtered. Usually the drugs having molecular weight above 20,000 are unable to be filtered. Thus macro-molecular substances like heparin, dextran and insulin (irrespective of their protein binding) are unable to pass through glomerulus, (ii) *Plasma protein binding:* only the free drugs can be filtered through glomerulus, while protein binding decreases the renal excretion. For example, a drug like wafarin which is 98% bound to albumin, is excreted to an extent of only 2% through glomerulus, (iii) *Renal blood flow*: greater the glomerular perfusion, faster is the drug removal from the plasma.

ii) Tubular Secretion

Glomerular filtration removes at the most 20% of the drug from the blood reaching the kidney. The rest 80% of the drug passes on to the proximal tubule from where it is secreted into the tubular lumen. Tubular secretion is an energy-requiring carrier-mediated active transport and hence protein binding, which is a hindrance for glomerular filtration, does not interfere with the tubular secretion primarily because the carrier itself is a protein and also because the resultant decrease in the plasma concentration of the free drug subsequently promotes the dissociation of the protein-bound drug. *There are two independent carrier systems operating at this level: one is for acidic drugs*, like penicillins, salicylic acid, thiazide diuretics, probenecid, indomethacin, methotrexate, sulfonamides, glucuronide metabolites of these drugs and for some endogenous substances, like uric acid; *another is for basic drugs*, like morphine, quinidine, procaine, quinine, neostigmine, quaternary ammonium compounds and for some endogenous substances, like dopamine, choline, histamine and serotonin. Each carrier system is relatively nonselective and therefore the drugs having similar physico-chemical characteristics compete for the same carrier system. For example, probenecid (a weak acid) competitively inhibits the tubular secretion of penicillins and amoxycillin, thereby increasing the plasma half-life and effectiveness of penicillins in the treatment of certain infective diseases. Similarly, weakly acidic drugs (e.g., lactic acid, salicylic acid and thiazide diuretics) interfere with the secretion of an endogenous substance, uric acid, with resultant rise in plasma uric acid levels sufficient to precipitate the attack of gout in predisposed individuals. However, there are no drugs which can be used clinically to block the active secretion of basic drugs and such drug interactions have little clinical significance.

iii) Tubular Reabsorption

The renal tubule behaves like a typical lipid barrier especially in the distal region. Hence the reabsorption of drugs through the distal tubule predominantly takes place by passive diffusion, and its extent is dependent upon the (i) lipid solubility, (ii) ionisation constant (pKa) of the drug and (iii) pH of the urine. Hence as a rule, since the pH of the urine is acidic, all acidic drugs (e.g., salicylates, barbiturates and sulfonamides) remain predominantly nonionised and have more chances of their reabsorption than excretion. On the contrary, if the pH of the urine is made alkaline by giving sodium bicarbonate or sodium citrate, the ionisation of acidic drugs would increase. As a result, their reabsorption would be retarded while excretion would be facilitated. Alkalisation of urine, therefore, is a part of the therapeutic regimen in the cases of salicylate or barbiturate poisoning.

Weakly basic drugs, like morphine or amphetamine, are predominantly excreted in acidic urine (due to their high ionisation). Their excretion can further be hastened by making urine more acidic by giving ascorbic acid (or ammonium chloride). On the contrary, if the pH of the urine is made alkaline, their reabsorption would increase while excretion would be retarded. Strongly acidic or basic drugs remain ionised at all pH ranges and hence are not reabsorbed (rather excreted). Quaternary ammonium compounds and aminoglycoside antibiotics being highly polar drugs are not reabsorbed (rather primarily excreted).To sum up, the amount of drug excreted is the sum of the total amount filtered and secreted minus the amount reabsorbed.

Biliary Excretion and Enterohepatic Circulation

Liver cells transfer various drugs and endogenous substance like bilirubin, from plasma to bile, by means of a transport system similar to that of the renal tubule. *Drugs that show significant elimination through bile include:* quinine, colchicine, d-tubocurarine, corticosteroids and erythromycin. These are then subsequently eliminated through faeces. *Some drugs are secreted through bile, but after being delivered to intestine, are reabsorbed back and the cycle is repeated (enterohepatic circulation).* Typical such example is of digitoxin, which after being partly converted into an active metabolite, digoxin, is excreted through bile and then reabsorbed back from the gut (enterohepatic circulation). Vitamin D_3 and indomethacin are also excreted in the bile, in partly free form, and undergo enterohepatic circulation. *On the other hand, certain drug metabolites (particularly the glucuronides) are excreted through bile and delivered to the intestine where these metabolites are deconjugated or hydrolysed (by gut enzymes) releasing the parent active drug again. This free drug is then reabsorbed and the cycle is repeated (enterohepatic circulation).* Such examples include: thyroxine, morphine, chloramphenicol, tetracycline, phenolphthalein and ethinyl estradiol. Sometimes the drugs, particularly the basic drugs, like morphine, have to be removed by gastric lavage in order to prevent their enterohepatic circulation. In case of morphine poisoning, morphine that diffuses into stomach would be predominantly ionised due to acidic pH of the gastric juice; and would therefore be poorly absorbed. If it is not removed by gastric lavage at this stage, it would reach intestine and will get significantly reabsorbed (enterohepatic circulation) because of its poor ionisation at alkaline pH. *The net result of enterohepatic circulation is the prolongation of drug action as the drug serves as a small circulating reservoir.*

Faecal Elimination

Substances excreted in faeces are mainly (i) orally ingested drugs which are not absorbed through the gut, e.g., magnesium sulfate, streptomycin, neomycin, bacitracin, cholestyramine and certain purgatives, and (ii) certain drugs (or their metabolites) which are excreted through bile but are not reabsorbed from the intestinal tract as described earlier, e.g., erythromycin and corticosteroids.

Alveolar Excretion

Gases and volatile liquids, e.g., general anaesthetics, nitrous oxide, ether and alcohol are eliminated through breath, irrespective of their lipid solubility, because the excretion of drugs here depends on their partial pressure in the blood. Certain essential oils like eucalyptus oil and garlic oil are eliminated through expectoration.

Excretion Through Breast Milk

Excretion of drugs in the breast milk is important, not because of the amount excreted but because of the unwanted pharmacological effects in the nursing infant. Drugs are transferred to the breast milk according to pH partition principle. Therefore, the basic drugs, being predominantly nonionised at plasma alkaline pH can diffuse through the mammary epithelium and get accumulated in the milk. Once diffused into milk, these drugs cannot be reabsorbed back to plasma, because at relatively acidic pH of milk they get substantially ionised (ion trapping; Fig. 6.6).

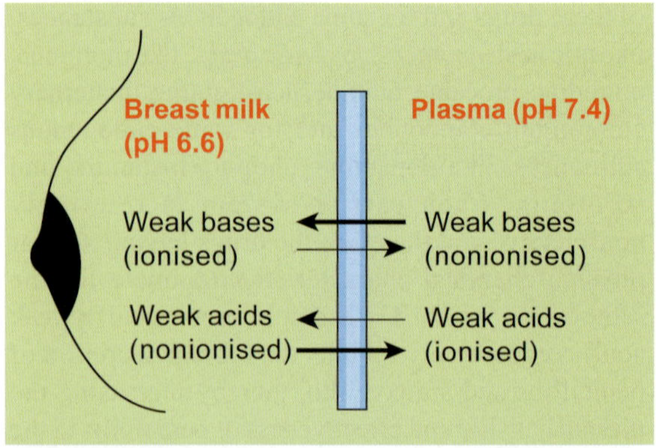

Fig 6.6 Drug Secretion in Breast Milk

Hence, as a rule, basic drugs, e.g., chloramphenicol, tetracyclines, ergotamine, morphine, metronidazole, carbimazole, certain immunosuppressive/cytotoxic drugs, bromocriptine, estrogen/progesterone, oral contraceptives, diazepam, antihistamines and senna alkaloids (purgatives) are excreted more through milk as compared to acidic drugs. Certain non-electrolytes like ethanol and urea readily enter the breast milk, independent of the milk pH. Certain acidic drugs, although being less secreted, can cause serious side effects in infants, e.g., sulfonamides (kernicterus and allergy), penicillins (allergy), ampicillin (diarrhoea), dapsone (haemolytic anaemia), phenindione (bleeding), phenobarbitone (drowsi-ness), phenytoin (methaemoglobinaemia) and theophylline (restlessness). Infants are particularly sensitive to drug-induced haemolysis during neonatal period (some infants may also have G6PD deficiency). Hence, the following drugs should also be avoided (or be administered with caution) in breast-feeding mother, e.g., chloramphenicol, chloroquine, primaquine, quinine, quinidine, procainamide, nitrofurantion, nalidixic acid, dapsone, isoniazid, probe-necid and cotrimoxazole (sulfonamides in general).

Excretion Through Skin, Hair, Sweat and Saliva

Elimination of drugs through these routes is quantitatively unimportant. To cite a few examples, griseofulvin is secreted *through keratin precursor cells*; arsenic, mercury salts and iodides are secreted *through hair follicles;* iodine, potassium iodide, lithium and phenytoin are secreted *through saliva*, while certain amines and urea derivatives are secreted *through sweat.*

KINETICS OF DRUG ELIMINATION

Once the drug is administered intravenously, it enters the blood and is rapidly distributed to various tissues. By taking repeated blood samples, the fall in the plasma concentration of the drug, as related to the time, can be plotted on a graph and from such plots the plasma half-life ($t_{1/2}$) of a drug can be measured.

The PLASMA HALF-LIFE ($t_{1/2}$) means the time duration in which the plasma concentration of the drug falls by 50% of the earlier value. Obviously, $t_{1/2}$ does not reflect on absorption kinetics of the drug, but reflects on its elimination (clearance) kinetics.

The BIOLOGICAL EFFECT HALF-LIFE is the time duration in which the principal pharmacological effect of the drug declines by half.

The plasma half-life of a drug is one of the important pharmacokinetic parameters to be considered (along with 'apparent volume of distribution') while preparing the dose schedule of any drug. The rate and the pattern of drug elimination (and also of absorption for that matter) follows either First-Order or Zero-Order or Mixed- Order Kinetics.

First-Order Kinetics

Majority of the drugs obey first-order kinetics of elimination. The characteristic features of first-order elimination are as follows:

i) *A constant fraction* of the drug is eliminated at a *constant interval of time*. For example, plasma concentration declining *at a rate of 50% per two hours*:

100 (μg/ml) —50%, 2 hrs→ 50 (μg/ml) —50%, 2 hrs→ 25 (μg/ml) → and so on

ii) The rate of drug elimination is directly proportional to the plasma concentration. That means, if the plasma concentration is increased (by increasing the dose), the rate of elimination also increases proportionately.

For example, higher plasma concentrations would also decline at the rate of 50% per two hours (in the above example).

200 (μg/ml) —50%, 2 hr→ 100 (μg/ml) —50%, 2 hr→ 50 (μg/ml) —50%, 2 hr→ 25 (μg/ml)

iii) In other words, the $t_{1/2}$ of any drug, following first-order kinetics, would always remain constant irrespective of the dose (Fig.6.7 a,b).

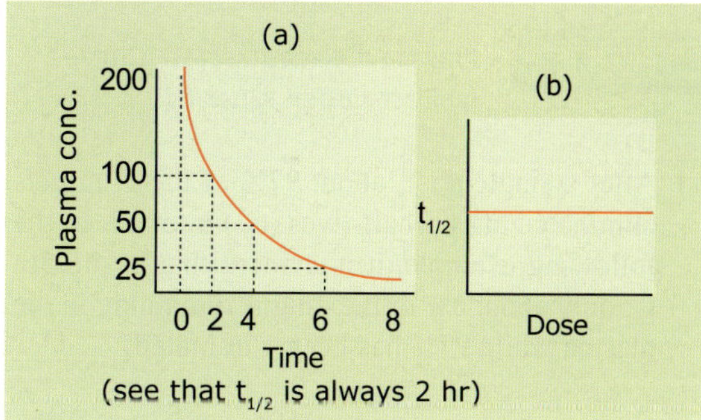

Fig 6.7 Constant $t_{1/2}$ in First-Order Kinetics

It can be noted from the above examples that the $t_{1/2}$ is still 2 hours even when the plasma concentrations were doubled.

iv) If the fall in plasma concentration (on arithmetic scale) is plotted against time, the resultant "plasma fall-out curve" would be curvilinear; but if the logarithms of plasma concentrations are plotted against time, the resultant "plasma fall-out curve" would be linear (Fig. 6.8 a,b).

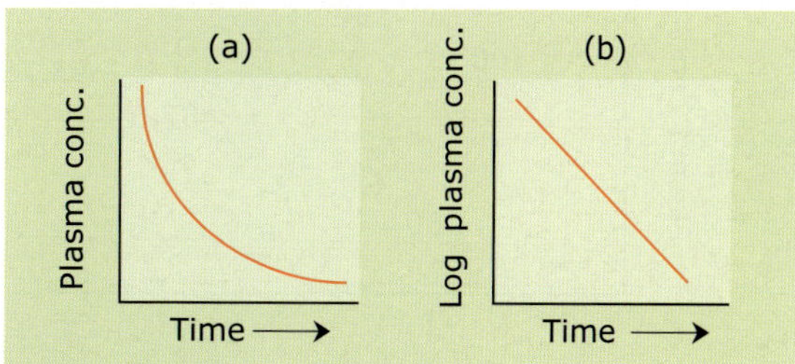

Fig 6.8 Plasma Fall-Out Curve in First-Order Kinetics

The same holds true when we talk of absorption, following first-order kinetics, and the related plasma concentration curves versus dose (Fig. 6.9 a,b).

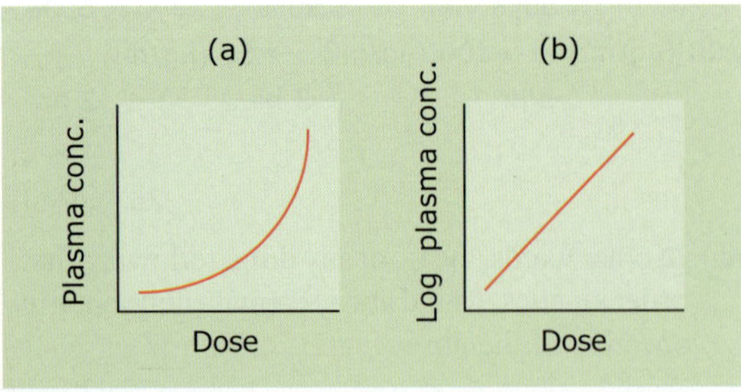

Fig 6.9 Plasma Concentration Curve in First-Order Kinetics

v) After a single dose, about 97% of the drug gets eliminated after 5 half-lives ($t_{1/2}$) interval. In the following example, it is evident that at the 5th $t_{1/2}$ only about 3% of the drug is remaining in the plasma while 97% has been eliminated.

100 (µg/ml) —50%, I $t_{1/2}$→ 50 (µg/ml) —50%, II $t_{1/2}$→ 25 (µg/ml) —50%, III $t_{1/2}$→ 12.5 (µg/ml) —50%, IV $t_{1/2}$→ 6.25 (µg/ml) —50%, V $t_{1/2}$→ 3.125 (µg/ml)

vi) On the contrary, if a fixed dose of the drug is administered at every half-life, five half-lives would be needed for 97% achievement of its steady state level in the body. Up to 5th half-life, the plasma concentration keeps on increasing but thereafter it reaches a *steady state level* (or *plateau level*) where the rate of absorption equals the rate of elimination and thus subsequent administration of same doses thereafter, have hardly any effect on plasma concentration. Ideally, during drug treatment, a steady state plasma concentration is maintained within a known effective therapeutic range; because at a lower level than this, the drug would be ineffective and at high levels it would lead to overdosage toxicity (Fig. 6.10).

vii) If the dose of the drug (obeying first-order kinetics of elimination) is doubled, its duration of action is prolonged for one more half-life.

100 (µg/ml) —2 hr, I $t_{1/2}$→ 50 (µg/ml) —2 hr, II $t_{1/2}$→ 25 (µg/ml)

Effect starts (at 100 µg/ml); *Effect vanishes* (at 25 µg/ml)

Duration of effect is 4 hr, i.e., two $t_{1/2}$

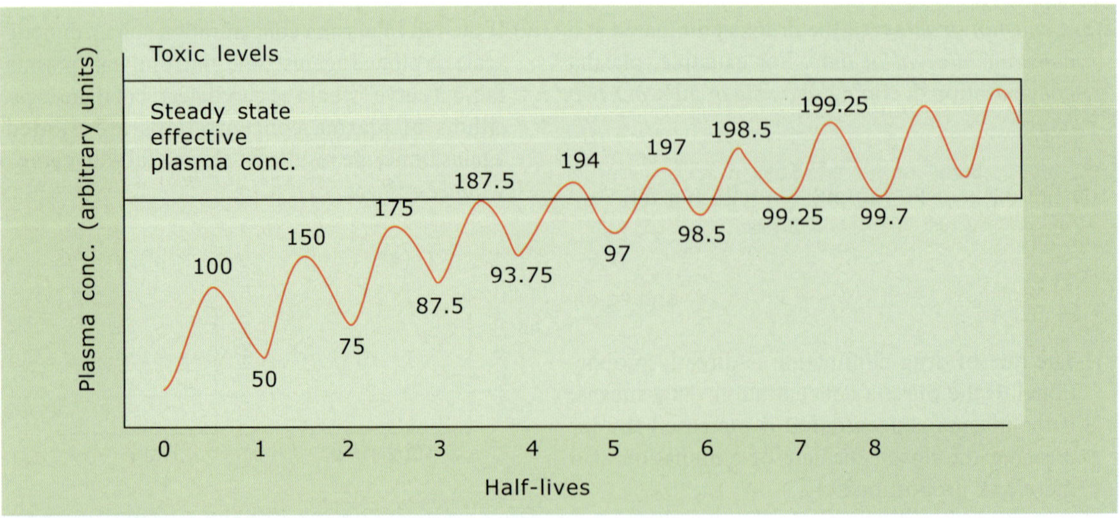

Fig 6.10 Steady State Concentration in Five Half-Lives

$$200(\mu g/ml) \xrightarrow{2\text{ hr}} 100(\mu g/ml) \xrightarrow{2\text{ hr}} 50(\mu g/ml) \xrightarrow{2\text{ hr}} 25(\mu g/ml)$$

I $t_{1/2}$ II $t_{1/2}$ III $t_{1/2}$

After doubling the dose

Effect vanishes
Duration of effect is 6 hr, i.e., three $t_{1/2}$

viii) The "log plasma concentration fall-out curve" of a drug having high 'apparent volume of distribution' (but obeying first-order kinetics of elimination), exhibits two slopes (Fig. 6.11). An initial rapidly declining phase due to distribution (called as α-phase) and later linearly declining phase due to elimination (called as β-phase). Hence, at least two half-lives (i.e., distribution $t_{1/2}$ and elimination $t_{1/2}$) can be calculated from these two slopes.

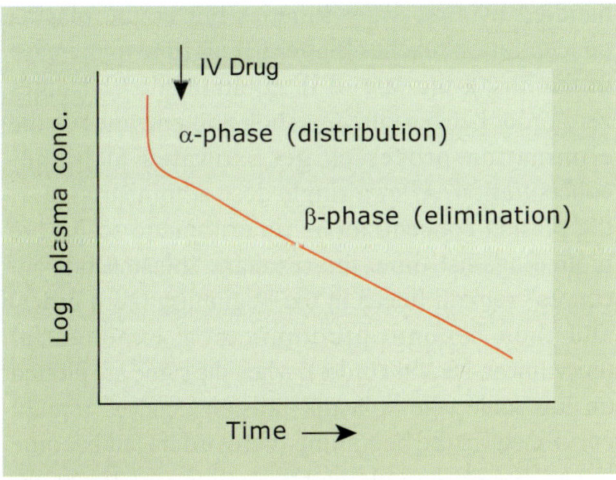

Fig 6.11 α- & β-Phase of Drug Clearance

In practice, usually the elimination half-life derived from the β slope is called the $t_{1/2}$ of such a drug; although the total half-life of this drug is usually longer than its elimination $t_{1/2}$.

ix) Mathematically, the half-life of elimination ($t_{1/2}$) can be calculated from the following formula:

$$t_{1/2} = \frac{0.693}{K}$$

where K is the elimination rate constant and 0.693 is the natural log of 2. The value of K can be calculated from the "slope" of the straight line obtained by plotting the log of plasma concentration against the time of observation. Thus:

$$\text{Slope} = -\frac{K}{2.303}$$

where the negative sign merely signifies that the plasma concentrations are declining after single dose drug administration. Slope is called tan Θ which is equal to - (k/2.303).

Zero-Order Kinetics

Hardly a few drugs obey *zero-order kinetics* in true sense. However, an example can be cited of ethyl alcohol whose metabolism is of zero order at virtually all plasma concentrations. The characteristic features of *zero-order kinetics* are:

i) *A constant or a fixed quantity of the drug is eliminated (or absorbed) per unit time.* For example, plasma concentrations declining at a rate of 25 μg per hour (instead of 25%; a constant fraction as discussed in first-order kinetics).

$$50\ (\mu g/ml) \xrightarrow[1\text{ hr}]{25\ \mu g} 25\ (\mu g/ml) \xrightarrow[1\text{ hr}]{25\ \mu g} \text{Nil}$$

ii) This means that the rate of elimination (or of absorption for that matter) is proceeding at a fixed rate, independent of the concentration of the drug in the plasma. In other words, increasing the dose does not result in a proportionate rise in the extent of elimination.

For example, higher plasma concentrations would also decline at the rate of 25 μg per hour in the case cited above.

$$100\ (\mu g/ml) \xrightarrow[1\text{ hr}]{25\ \mu g} 75\ (\mu g/ml) \xrightarrow[1\text{ hr}]{25\ \mu g} 50\ (\mu g/ml) \xrightarrow[1\text{ hr}]{25\ \mu g} 25(\mu g/ml)$$

iii) Hence $t_{1/2}$ of a drug following zero-order elimination kinetics is never constant (Fig. 6.12).

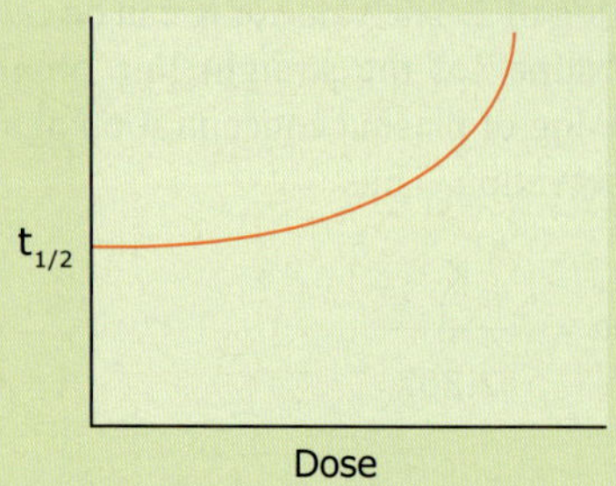

Fig 6.12 Variable $t_{1/2}$ in Zero-Order Kinetics

Note that 50 μg/ml plasma conc. fell to 25 μg/ml in 1 hr (i.e., $t_{1/2}$ = 1 hr); while 100 μg/ml plasma concentration fell to 50 μg/ml in 2 hr (i.e., $t_{1/2}$ = 2 hr).

iv) If such a fall in plasma concentration (in arithmetic scale) is plotted against time, the resultant "plasma fall-out curve" is steeply linear; but if logarithms of plasma concentrations are plotted against time, these "plasma fall-out curves" become curvilinear,

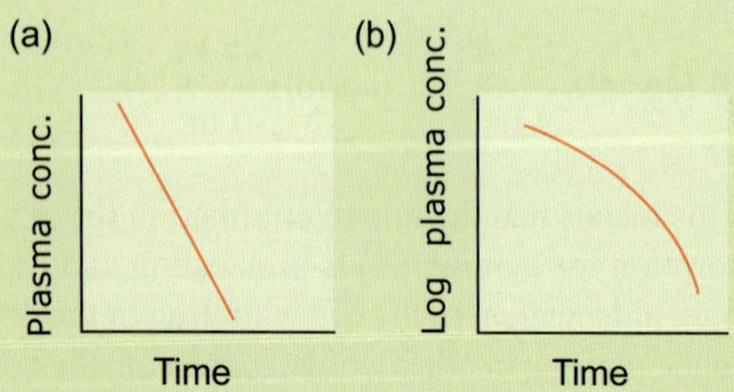

Fig 6.13 Plasma Fall-Out Curves in Zero-Order Kinetics

because here the plasma concentrations are falling at a constant rate, unaffected by the plasma levels existing in the body (Fig. 6.13 a,b). The same holds true when we talk of absorption and the related plasma concentration curves *versus dose* (Fig. 6.14 a,b).

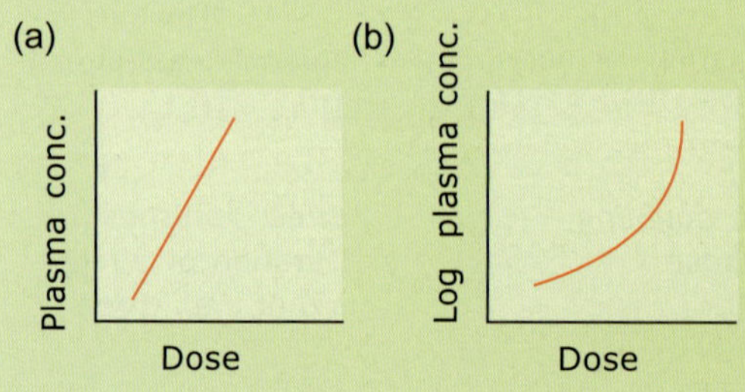

Fig 6.14 Plasma Conc. Curve in Zero-Order Kinetics

Michaelis-Menten Kinetics (or Mixed-order Kinetics or Saturation Kinetics)

Some important drugs, like phenytoin, digoxin, warfarin, dicumarol, tolbutamide and aspirin (higher doses) obey mixed-order elimination kinetics. It is a dose-dependent kinetics where smaller doses are handled by first-order kinetics but as the plasma concentration reaches higher values (due to increase in the dose), the rate of drug elimination becomes zero order because the metabolising enzymes or the elimination processes get saturated at higher concentration. After a single dose administration, if the plasma concentrations (in arithmetic scale) are plotted against time, the resultant "plasma fall-out curves" remain linear in the beginning (zero order) and then become predominantly exponential (curvilinear, i.e., first order); when the same are plotted on log scale, the "plasma fall-out" curves remain curvilinear in the beginning (zero order) but become linear (first-order kinetics) thereafter (Fig. 6.15 a,b).

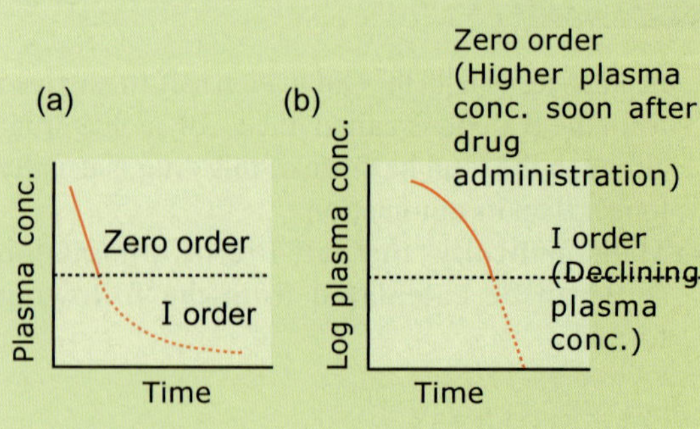

Fig 6.15 Plasma Concentration Fall-Out Curve in Mixed-Order Kinetics

If we talk of this type of kinetics for absorption, the "plasma concentration curves" (in arithmetic scale) *versus dose* would remain curvilinear in the beginning (i.e., first order) and then becoming linear (i.e., zero order) later after the saturation of enzymatic processes. The "plasma concentration (log scale) versus dose curve" however, remains linear in the beginning (first order) but becomes curvilinear later (zero order) (Fig. 6.16 a,b).

The changes from primarily first-order to predominantly zero-order kinetics with an increase in the dose, produces a risky and unpredictable

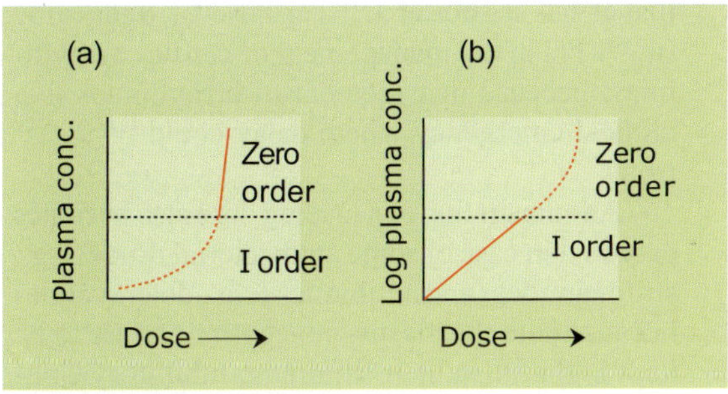

Fig 6.16 Plasma Concentration Curve in Mixed-Order Kinetics

pharmacokinetic state because with such drugs $t_{1/2}$ changes with the dose. It may remain constant at the maintenance dose but would increase if the dose is further increased. The clinical use of such drugs, therefore, needs proper monitoring and the maintenance of their plasma concentration because a small increase in the dose would shoot up the plasma concentration resulting in drug toxicity.

DOSING SCHEDULES

Given below are some basic concepts, regarding dose schedules of drugs, which are primarily based on the pharmacokinetic principles detailed so far.

a) The drugs having very short half-life (e.g., norepinephrine—1 to 2 min; dopamine—5 min; dobutamine—2 min; and oxytocin —3 to 5 min) are usually given by a constant I.V. infusion to maintain their steady state plasma concentration.
b) For the drugs having a short $t_{1/2}$, i.e., between 30 min to 2 hr (e.g., cephalexin < 1 hr; benzylpenicillin < 1 hr; and paracetamol 2 hr), it becomes very inconvenient to administer them at every half-life. In such cases, provided the drug is having a high margin of safety and is obeying first-order elimination kinetics, the dose can be so increased that the drug can be administered at every 6 to 8 hourly interval (refer foregoing discussion, because for such drugs doubling the dose increases the duration of their effect by one $t_{1/2}$).
c) The drugs having $t_{1/2}$ between 4 to 12 hr, are usually administered at every half-life interval.
d) The drugs having medium half life (12–24 hr) are usually given at 12 hourly interval. For drugs having half-life of 24 hr, half of the therapeutic dose is given at "every half of the half life"; e.g., if the therapeutic dose is 50 mg and the $t_{1/2}$ of the drug is 24 hr, then the dose is scaled down to 12 hr by simple proportion as follows and is administered at 12 hourly interval:

$$\frac{50 \times 12}{24} = \text{25 mg to be given at 12 hourly interval.}$$

e) For drugs having longer $t_{1/2}$, the situation is different; because such drugs usually have a high volume of distribution, slow rate of clearance and are cumulative in nature, e.g., digoxin ~40 hr (640 L), desipramine 20–60 hr (30–60 L), diazepam ~40 hr (50–70 L), digitoxin ~168 hr (38 L) and chloroquine ~40 hr (130 L). Since five half-lives are needed to reach the steady state plasma concentration, several days would be wasted in obtaining the desired therapeutic effect. If there is no clinical emergency (e.g., anxiety neurosis to be treated with diazepam or moderate depression to be treated with desipramine), it matters little if the steady state levels are reached after a few days. Contrarily, if there is a clinical emergency, like congestive heart failure with atrial fibrillation (where digoxin is to be used), or hyperpyrexia due to malaria (where chloroquine is to be used) such a delay is bound to be fatal for the patient. In such cases, an initial *loading dose* (or priming dose) is given to reduce the time needed to reach the steady state plasma concentration (Fig. 6.17). The *loading dose* is then followed by a *maintenance dose* to maintain the already attained steady state plasma concentration.

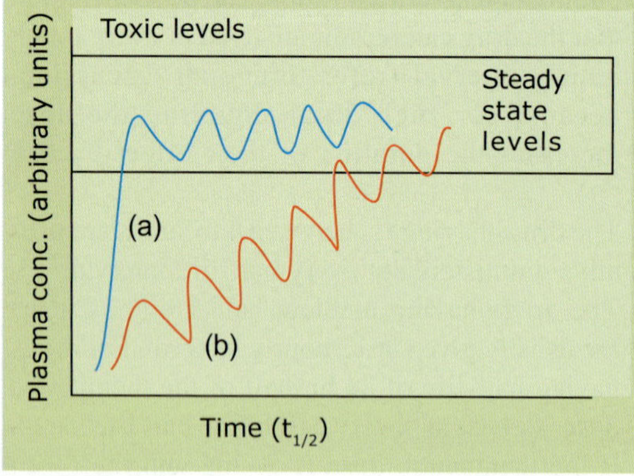

Fig 6.17 (a) Steady State Plasma Concentrations, Rapidly Attained after a Loading Dose and then Main-tained by Administering Main-tenance Doses. (b) Steady State Levels Being Achieved in a Regular Course after Repetitive Dosage.

The loading dose can be calculated by the following formula:

Loading dose = Desired plasma conc (mg/L) x aVd (L/kg body weight)

For example: If the desired plasma concentration of digoxin for therapeutic effect is 1–2 µg/L and its aVd is 640 L then its loading dose should be 640 to 1280 µg (or 0.64 to 1.28 µg). In practice an average, i.e., 0.9 mg is administered. The maintenance dose is usually half of the loading dose to be administered at every half-life. In the above example it comes to 0.45 mg every 40 hours. But it is very inconvenient to give this maintenance dose every 40 hours. Hence the dose is scaled down to every 24 hours by simple proportion as follows:

$$\frac{0.45 \times 24}{40} = 0.27 \text{ mg}$$

In practice, however, a maintenance dose of 0.25 mg of digoxin is administered every 24 hr and considering its nature of accumulation, it is given only 5 days a week.

In the case of chloroquine (for the treatment of malaria), the loading dose is essential on two counts; firstly, because it has a longer $t_{1/2}$ and secondly, because it has a tendency to selectively accumulate in the liver which further delays the attainment of the desired steady state plasma concentration.

Sometimes, it may be necessary to give the loading dose of the drug irrespective of the fact that it has a shorter $t_{1/2}$, e.g., use of lignocaine ($t_{1/2}$=1 hr) in the management of cardiac arrhythmias; because management of arrhythmias is a clinical emergency where delay could be disastrous.

Administration of a loading dose also becomes essential in case of some antibacterial drugs (e.g., sulfonamides) and antibiotics (e.g., doxycycline) because here the plasma concentrations are to be kept higher than their Minimum Inhibitory Concentration (MIC) to avoid the danger of the development of bacterial resistance.

f) All these rules apply to the normal healthy persons because $t_{1/2}$ is dramatically altered in renal/liver disease and due to pharmacogenetic variations. Adjustment in doses and dose intervals will therefore be needed in such diseased states.

Renal disease (or reduced cardiac output) often reduces the clearance of drugs, if their elimination depends on renal function. The suitable dose for a patient with renal disease may be calculated by multiplying the normal therapeutic dose with the ratio of the patient's creatinine clearance to normal creatinine clearance value (approximately 100 ml/min), as expressed below:

$$\text{Corrected dose} = \text{Normal dose} \times \frac{\text{Patient's creatinine clearance}}{\text{Normal creatinine clearance (100 ml/min)}}$$

Problem: The normal therapeutic adult dose of a drug is 100 mg (I.V.) two times a day. Its clearance is almost entirely by glomerular filtration. A patient with renal disease shows creatinine clearance of 33 ml/min. What shall be the corrected dose regimen of this drug for this patient in such a situation?

Answer:

$$\text{Corrected dose} = 100\ \text{mg} \times \frac{33\ \text{ml/min}}{100\ \text{ml/min}}$$

$$= 33\ \text{mg (I.V) twice a day}$$

There are several drugs which are excreted not only by renal but through non-renal routes as well. In such a case, the above equation should be applied to that percentage of the dose which is eliminated by the kidney.

Example: If a drug is cleared 70% by kidney and 30% by liver and its normal therapeutic dose is 100 mg/day, the corrected dose in a patient with creatinine clearance of 50 ml/min will be:

$$\text{Corrected dose} = (30) + (70 \times \frac{50}{100})$$

$$= (30) + (35)$$

$$= 65\ \text{mg/day}$$

Because of the difficulties in obtaining accurate 24 hr urine collections to measure creatinine clearance directly, it is usually estimated using the following equation:

$$(CL)_{cr}\ \text{Men} = \frac{(140 - \text{Age in yr})\ (\text{Weight in kg})}{72 \times \text{Scr}}$$

where $(CL)_{cr}$ is creatinine clearance in ml/min, while Scr is serum creatinine concentration in mg/100 ml. This formula is scaled down to 85% for females.

$$(CL)_{cr}\ \text{Women} = \text{Male value} \times 0.85$$

Evaluation of renal function, on the basis of serum creatinine concentration, in the elderly can be misleading because creatinine is a product of muscle metabolism and its production is reduced as the muscle mass declines with age. Thus, seemingly normal serum creatinine values in ICU patients may at times be associated with significant impairment of renal function. For example, with the same serum creatinine values of 1 mg/100 ml, a 80-yr-old man will have creatinine clearance of 60 ml/min (approx.) while a 40-yr-old person (of same weight) will have $(CL)_{cr}$ value of 100 ml/min approximately.

FIXED-DOSE DRUG COMBINATIONS

The fixed-dose drug combination means the combination of two different drugs in a single pharmaceutical formulation. It never means a concomitant drug therapy, wherein two (or more) drugs are given separately for treatment of a disease. Rational fixed-dose formulation of two drugs can be advantageous, but illogical or inappropriate combination could be dangerous.

As a rule, if two drugs are to be combined in a single pharmaceutical formulation, these should have approximately equal $t_{1/2}$; e.g., cotrimoxazole (antibacterial drug) is a combination of sulfamethoxazole ($t_{1/2}$ 11 hr) and trimethoprim ($t_{1/2}$ 10 hr); sulfadoxin ($t_{1/2}$ 160 hr) is combined with pyrimethamine ($t_{1/2}$ 112 hr) for treatment of malaria; clavulanic acid ($t_{1/2}$ 1–1.5 hr) is combined with ampicillin ($t_{1/2}$ 1–1.5 hr) or with amoxycillin ($t_{1/2}$ 1–1.5 hr) for treatment of various infections, and carbidopa ($t_{1/2}$ 2 hr) is combined with levo dopa ($t_{1/2}$ 1.7 hr) for the treatment of parkinsonism.

The ratio of the doses of each component in such a formulation would, however, depend on their apparent volume of distribution and peak plasma concentration (at steady state) of individual drug.

For example: since $t_{1/2}$ as well as aVd of amoxycillin (1–2 hr; 0.21 L/kg) matches to the $t_{1/2}$ and aVd of clavulanic acid ($t_{1/2}$ 1–1.5 hr, 0.20 L/kg), these can be combined in their standard dose regimen, i.e., amoxicillin 500 mg + clavulanic acid 125 mg and this fixed-dose formulation could be administered as 1 to 2 tab 8 hourly, as usual.

In the case of cotrimoxazole (trimethoprim + sulfamethoxazole), the $t_{1/2}$ of trimethoprim (10 hr) and of sulfamethoxazole (11 hr) are almost identical. For synergism, the optimal ratio of the **M**inimum **I**nhibitory **C**oncentration (MIC) is 1:20 (if these drugs are acting independently *in vitro*). But the aVd of trimethoprim (1 to 2 L/kg) is 5 to 6 times greater than that of sulfamethoxazole (0.2 L/kg), i.e., it is widely distributed and attains lower plasma concentration than sulfamethoxazole. Hence if trimethoprim is mixed with sulfamethoxazole in a ratio of 5:20 (or 1:4), the peak plasma concentrations should mimic the ratio of 1:20 which is optimal for synergism *in vitro*. However, to avoid development of resistance, the ratio of trimethoprim:sulfamethoxazole is kept slightly higher (1:5) than the theoretical ratio of 1:4.

Advantages of Fixed-dose Formulation

i) Convenience in dose schedule and better patient compliance.
ii) Enhanced effect of the combination, e.g., both trimethoprim and sulfamethoxazole, individually are bacteriostatic but the combination, called cotrimoxazole, is bactericidal.
iii) Minimisation of side effects, e.g., combining carbidopa with levodopa not only reduces the doses required for levodopa but minimises peripheral side effects due to dopamine by preventing the metabolic degradation of levodopa (to dopamine) peripherally by l-aminoacid decarboxylase enzyme.

Disadvantages of Fixed-dose Combinations

i) The dose of any component drug cannot be adjusted independently if desired.
ii) If the pharmacokinetic characteristics of two drugs do not match, there would be unacceptable range of fluctuations in the plasma concentration of the component drugs at steady state (since fixed-dose combinations are given at a fixed interval).
iii) It becomes difficult to identify one particular drug which is causing harmful/beneficial effects. For example, the patient's positive response to a particular anaemia (iron deficiency anaemia or megaloblastic anaemia with neurological deficits due to B_{12} deficiency or megaloblastic anaemia due to folate deficiency) cannot be ascertained from a fixed-dose combination of iron, vit. B_{12} and folic acid.

Thus, the therapeutic aims should be clear and the fixed-dose combinations should not be prescribed unless: (i) there is a good reason to believe that the patient needs all the drugs in the formulation and (ii) the pharmacokinetic parameters of the component drugs match with each other.

CHAPTER 7 Pharmacodynamics

COMPETENCY PH1.5, PH1.7, PH1.56, PH1.8

PHARMACODYNAMICS

Pharmacodynamics (*pharmakon* = drug, *dynamics* = action or activity) is the study of the biochemical and physiological effects of drugs and their mode of action. It deals with the relationship between the plasma concentration of the drug and its response as well as its duration of action. In short, it covers all aspects relating to "what a drug does to the body". Effects of drugs are only *quantitative*, but never *qualitative*. That means, the drugs can accelerate or depress the normal physiological or biochemical functions of an organ but cannot confer entirely a new activity on it. The type of response produced by the drug is called its *effect*, but how and where the effect is produced is called its *action*. Therefore, *effects* are measured and quantified while *actions* are identified. In other words, drug action always precedes the drug effect. For example, miosis produced by pilocarpine is its effect. However, it results due to parasympathetic stimulation of the circular muscles of iris, which is its action (or say, the effect of this action is miosis).

HOW DRUGS ACT ON LIVING ORGANISM

(The Site and Mechanism of Drug Action)

Prior to understanding this, we must know where the drugs can act, i.e., their probable site of action. Knowing only about the effects of drug signifies little about its site of action, because two drugs may exhibit the same effect but their site of action may differ. To exemplify: the site of action of pilocarpine, for producing miosis, is the circular muscle of iris; however, morphine also produces miosis but its site of action is the 3rd cranial nerve nucleus (stimulation).

The Site of Drug Action

The drugs may act at *extracellular, cellular* or *intracellular* sites.

Extracellular Site of Action

For example, antacids neutralising gastric acidity; chelating agents forming complexes with heavy metals; or magnesium sulfate acting as osmotic purgative by retaining the fluid inside the lumen of intestine and thus increasing the faecal bulk.

Cellular Site of Action

For example, action of acetylcholine on nicotinic receptors of motor end plate, leading to contraction of skeletal muscle; or inhibition of membrane-bound ATPase by cardiac glycosides; or effect of sympathomimetics on heart muscle and blood vessels.

Intracellular Site of Action

For example, trimethoprim or sulfa drugs act by interfering with the synthesis of folic acid which is an intracellular component; or incorporation of 5-fluorouracil (an anticancer drug) into messenger RNA in place of uracil.

Mechanism of Action of Drugs

Drugs act by *receptor mediated* or by *non-receptor mediated mechanisms* or by *targeting specific genetic changes*.

Receptor Mediated Mechanisms

Majority of drugs produce their effects through an interaction with some chemical component of the living cell called as *receptor*. It is a specific macromolecular protein (membrane bound or intracellular) which is capable of binding with the specific functional groups of the drug or endogenous substance. Its structure resembles the 3-dimensional configuration of the drug in the same way as the levers of a lock are the 3-dimensional mirror image of the grooves of the key with which it opens. Binding of a drug with its receptor results in the formation of *drug-receptor complex* (DR) which is responsible for triggering the biological response.

$$D + R \rightleftharpoons [DR] \rightsquigarrow \text{Response}$$

This binding is usually *specific* and *reversible* (when there is formation of hydrogen bonds, van der Waals bonds or electrostatic bonds) but in certain cases *irreversible* also (e.g., organophosphorous insecticides which bind *irreversibly* to acetylcholinesterase by forming a covalent bond). At times the binding may be *stereoselective* also, i.e., if the drug has optical isomers, then usually it is *levo* or *dextro* form which is active, e.g., l-epinephrine, l-morphine, d-amphetamine are active while their opposite optical isomers are not.

Since receptors are, broadly speaking, macromolecular proteins with which the drug is presumed to interact, there may be several types of receptors, e.g., receptor for hormones, autacoids, growth factors and neurotransmitters. Thus the term 'receptor' has been used operationally to denote any cellular macromolecule to which a drug binds to imitate its effects. If the binding of the drug to some chemical components of the cell does not lead to any pharmacological effect (as in the case of drug binding to plasma proteins), then the component is not called as the receptor but is merely referred to as '*acceptor site*' or '*non-specific binding site*'.

The overall drug effect is attributed to the following two factors:

Affinity: Which means the capability of a drug to form the complex with its receptor (DR complex), e.g. the key entering the key hole of the lock has got an affinity to its levers.

Intrinsic Activity or Efficacy (E): Which means the ability of a drug to trigger the pharmacological response after making the drug-receptor complex (to exemplify: if the same key after entering into the key hole of the lock opens it too, it has got intrinsic activity also; otherwise, only affinity).

On the basis of affinity and efficacy, the drugs can be broadly classified as:

Agonists: Which have both the high affinity as well as high intrinsic activity (E = 1) and therefore can trigger the maximal biological response or mimic the effects of the endogenous substance after combining with the receptor, e.g., methacholine is a cholinomimetic drug (agonist) which mimics the effect of acetylcholine on cholinergic receptors.

Antagonists: Which have only the affinity but no intrinsic activity (E = 0). These drugs bind to the receptor but do not mimic, rather block or interfere with, the binding of an endogenous agonist. For example, atropine blocks the effects of acetylcholine on the cholinergic-muscarinic receptors (for details of the types of antagonism see following text). When two drugs are binding to the same receptor and at the same site, why is it that one is acting as an agonist while another is serving as an antagonist? This central question in pharmacodynamics is answered by considering "*the concept of dual nature of the receptors*", wherein the molecular forces during drug-receptor interaction, with the agonist only, alter the receptor conformation (antagonists are unable to activate the inactive receptor conformation).

Receptor usually exists in at least two conformations—the active (Ra) and inactive (Ri) (Fig. 7.1).

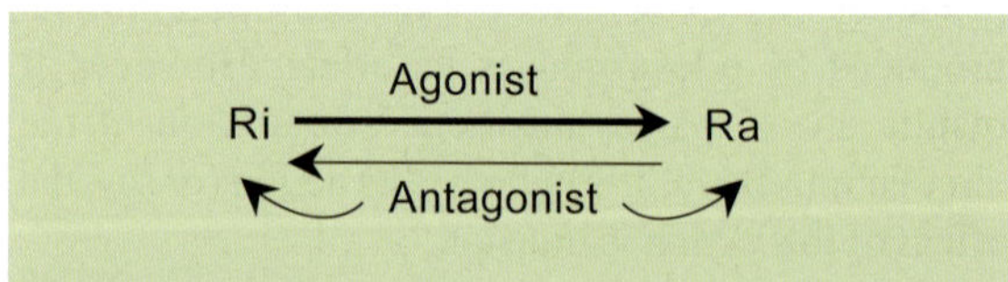

Fig 7.1 The Drug Action Viewed in Terms of Two-State Model of Receptor Activation.

These Ra and Ri conformations might relate to: (i) the open or the closed state of any ion channel or (ii) the active or inactive states of protein tyrosine kinase, or (iii) the productive or non-productive G-proteins (for details refer the latter part of this chapter). If Ra and Ri conformations are in equilibrium, the extent to which this equilibrium will be perturbed shall be determined by the relative affinity of the drug for these two conformations.

In such a situation, the following features may be manifested (Fig. 7.2):

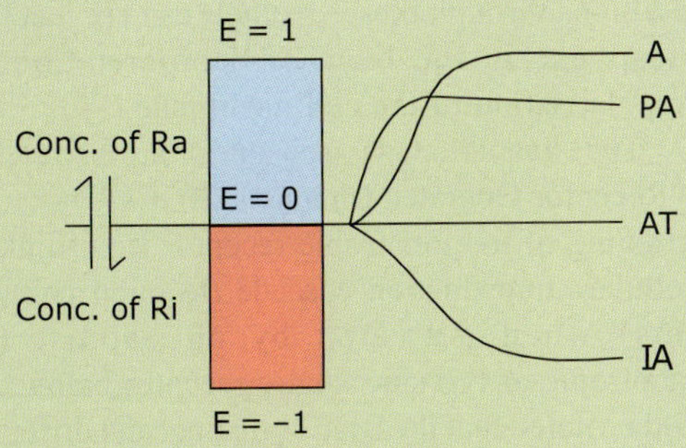

Fig 7.2 The Differential Influence of Agonist (A), Partial Agonist (PA), Antagonist (AT) and Inverse Agonist (IA) on Relative Distribution of Active (Ra) and Inactive (Ri) States of Receptors.

1. *When the drug has a very high affinity for the active conformation (Ra) than for inactive (Ri):* Such a drug will be an agoinst as it will shift the equilibrium towards the active state (Ra), i.e., it will activate the receptor (Fig. 7.2; see curve 'A').
2. *When the drug binds to both of these conformations (Ra and Ri) with equal affinity:* Such a drug would serve as an antagonist, as it will not perturb the equilibrium, i.e., it would neither activate the receptor nor will it shift the equilibrium towards any side (Fig. 7.2; curve 'AT').

There are some additional subtypes besides these two categories of the drugs:

Partial Agonists: These have full affinity to the receptor but with low intrinsic activity (E = zero to one) and hence these are only partly as effective as agonists. For example, pentazocine (a narcotic analgesic) is a partial agonist at the μ receptor subtype of opioid receptor.

Partial agonists influence the relative distribution of Ra and Ri in a slightly different manner. These have slightly higher affinity for Ra than for Ri (Fig. 7.3) and hence shift the equilibrium toward Ra to a lesser extent than true agonist (Fig. 7.2; curve 'PA'). Such drugs therefore display an intermediate effectiveness between the agonist and the antagonist.

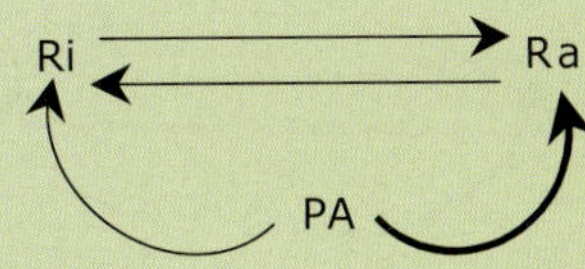

Fig 7.3 Partial Agonist (PA) has Slightly Higher Affinity for Ra (active state of the receptor), Although Lesser in Comparison to Agonist.

Inverse Agonist (IA): There are certain receptors like $GABA_A$ receptors which remain inherently in the Ra (active) state even in the absence of an endogenous ligand or an exogenously administered agonist. It is this inherent or basal activity of the $GABA_A$ receptor that protects a normal person from undue anxiety. Benzodiazepines (Ch.32) simply facilitate GABA binding to the $GABA_A$ receptor. Inverse agonists inactivate such constitutively active receptors and therefore prevent even its basal activity. As a result, inverse agonists produce an effect opposite to that of an agonist/drug even in its absence. They have full affinity but the efficacy (E) ranges between zero to minus one (Fig. 7.2, curve IA). For example: β-carbolines act as inverse agonists at benzodiazepine receptor and produce effects like anxiety, insomnia and seizures which are just the opposite of the therapeutic effects of benzodiazepines (antianxiety, sedation, anti-epileptic).

Inverse agonist differs from a competitive antagonist in the sense that while a competitive antagonist has no effect in the absence of agonist, the inverse agonist shows opposite effects by deactivating the receptor (which has a basal activity) even in the absence of agonist. Hence, these are also called *negative antagonists*. It is also implied that if the pre-existing equilibrium lies more towards Ri (inactivated state), the negative antagonism may not be evident and will be difficult to be distinguished from competitive antagonism (Fig 7.4 b).

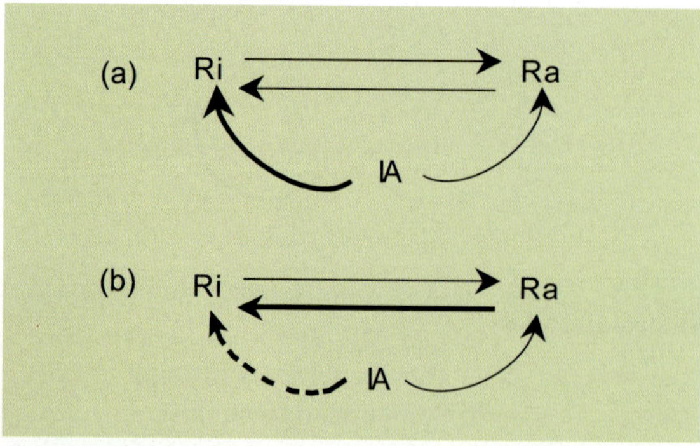

Fig 7.4 (a) Inverse Agonist (IA) has Preferential Affinity for Ri (Inactive State of The Receptor). (b) if Pre-existing Equilibrium Lies More Towards Ri, Inverse Agonism may not be seen.

Receptor Types & Signal Transduction Mechanisms

In terms of both molecular structure and the nature of transduction mechanisms, we can distinguish six receptor types.

1. Ion-channel Coupled Receptors (Ionotropic Receptors): These receptors are localised on cell membrane and are coupled directly to an ion channel. These "agonist regulated ion channels" (also known as ligandgated ion channels) open only when the receptor is occupied by an agonist. The subsequent flow of ions through these channels can elicit cellular response in the form of depolarisation or hyperpolarisation of the cell membrane (Fig. 7.5).

The "ligand-gated ion channels" are also called the "Receptor Operated Channels (ROCs)" because functioning of the ionotropic receptor is not linked to cellular transduction cascade (to elicit cellular events) when activated by an agonist (cf metabotropic or tyrosine kinase receptor below). It should be noted that the ROC is distinct and different than "Voltage Operated (or gated) ion Channel (VOC). In ROC the ion conductance through the channel is regulated by a drug or a neurotransmitter binding to a specific " ligand binding site". On the contrary, in the VOC the ion conductance is modulated through alterations in the voltage gradient across the plasma membrane (sec Ch. 15 & 19 and the following text). Further, in ROC, the ligand binding site and the channel are functionally distinct ; but in VOC there is no ligand binding site, rather its "gating" is controlled by changes in membrane potential. The ROC is conventionally described as a "channel with a receptor site" where an agonist opens the channel, the antagonist prevents the agonist from opening the channel (Fig 7.5b), while an inverse agonist closes the open channel.

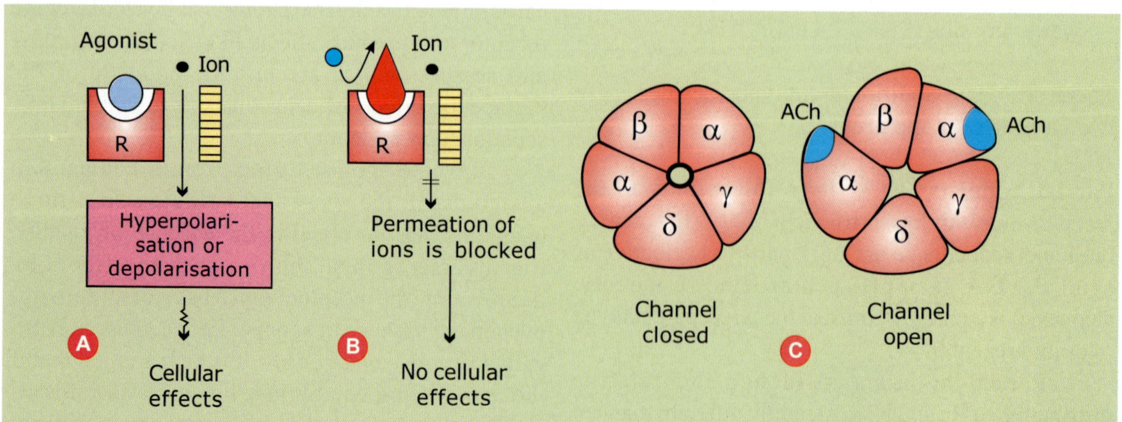

Fig 7.5 (a) Agonist Regulated Ion Channel. (b) Blockade of Ion Channel by an Antagonist which Lacks Intrinsic Activity (c) Two ACh molecules bind to two α subunits to open the channel of nicotinic-cholinergic receptor.

Examples include: nicotinic-cholinergic receptor; $GABA_A$ receptor; glutamate receptor and the glycine receptor. Some drugs are the allosteric modifiers of channel gating, e.g., benzodiazepines allosterically enhance the chloride transport through the $GABA_A$ chloride channel.

The best exemplified nicotinic-acetylcholine receptor operated channel consists of 5 protein subunits (2α+β+γ+ δ). All of them pass across the cell membrane and surround a central pore. In order to activate the receptor and open the channel one molecule of ACh should bind to each of the α subunits. The ROC then comes in "open state", otherwise remains in "closed state" (Fig. 7.5 c). ROC transductions are very rapid (milliseconds).

2. G-Protein Coupled Receptors (Metabotropic Receptors): These are membrane bound receptors which are coupled to the effector system (enzyme/ channel) through ***guanosine diphosphate (GDP)/ guanosine triphosphate (GTP) binding proteins*** called *G-proteins*. Examples include: muscarinic-cholinergic receptors, adrenoceptors, dopaminergic receptors, 5HT receptors, opiate receptors and purine receptors.

G-Protein Coupled Receptors (GPCRs) are composed of 7 transmembrane helices which have an extracellular domain as drug or neurotransmitter binding site and an intracellular domain that couples to G-protein. G-proteins are heterotrimeric molecules, i.e., having 3 subunits designated as α, β and γ subunits (these three α, β and γ subunits are so tightly bound together that they did not dissociate from each other and therefore written as αβγ subunit,not as plural). Their further classification is based on the identity of their distinct α-subunits. Thus, it is believed that there are 3 main varieties of Gα-proteins (Gs, Gi and Gq; although 17 variants are known). Among these, Gs and Gi produce stimulation or inhibition of adenyl cyclase, respectively; while Gq stimulates phospholipase-C activity.

In the "resting state", the αβγ subunit of G-protein is linked with one another and GDP is bound to the α subunit. Binding of an agonist (e.g., epinephrine) to a G-protein coupled receptor (e.g., β_1 adrenoceptor) causes the exchange of GTP for

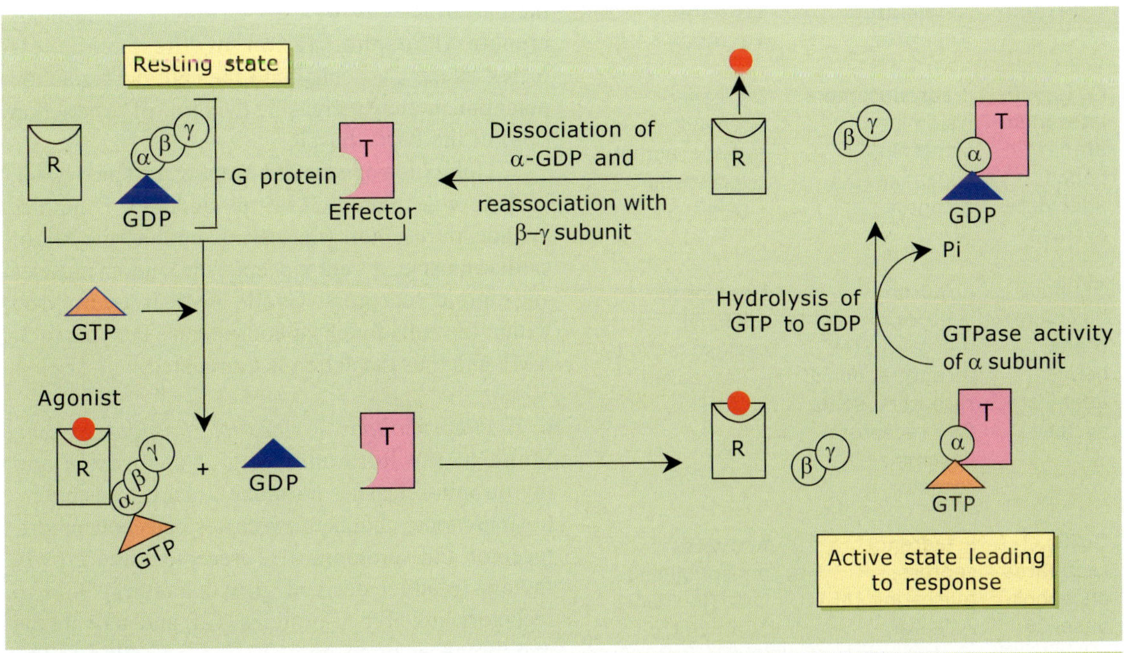

Fig 7.6 Mechanism of Activation and Action of G-Proteins.

GDP on the α-subunit. The β-γ subunit then dissociates from α-GTP complex which now interacts with target protein (T; in this case adenylyl cyclase) and activates it.The activated effector then propagates transduction mechanisms through second messengers to produce effects. The first messenger is the agonist itself. Stimulation of these receptors provides responses that lasts several seconds or minutes. When the agonist is no longer present (or dissociates) the receptor reverts to its resting state. In this process, the GTP on the α-subunit is hydrolysed to GDP and the effector protein (e.g., adenylate cyclase) is deactivated (Fig. 7.6).

The α-subunit possesses an intrinsic GTPase activity, which leads to hydrolysis of GTP to GDP. The α-subunit bound to GDP then reunites with β-γ subunit so that the cycle can continue. Depending upon the receptor subtype (e.g., α_2 adrenoceptors) and the specific G-protein isoform (e.g., Gi), the activity of the effector protein (e.g., in this case adenylate cyclase) can also be inhibited. Major G proteins and their receptors and effectors are summarised in Table 7.1.

Table 7.1 G-Proteins and their Receptors and Effectors

G-Protein	Associated Receptor	Effector Pathway
Gs (stimulates membrane-bound adenylate cyclase)	β-adrenoceptors, histamine, serotonin, dopamine (D_1) receptor	Increased adenylyl cyclase activity →increased cAMP
Gi (inhibits membrane-bound adenylate cyclase)	α_2-adrenoceptors, muscarinic (M_2) receptors, opioid receptors, some 5HT receptors; dopamine (D_2) receptor	Decreased adenylyl cyclase activity →decreased cAMP
$Gq/G_{12/13}$ (activates phospholipase-C)	α_1-adrenoceptors, muscarinic (M_1) receptor, angiotensin receptor (AT_1)	Activates phospholipase-C →↑IP_3, ↑DAG, ↑Ca^{2+} entry

Primarily there are 3 G-protein coupled effector systems: **(a)** *Adenylate cyclase-cAMP system,* **(b)** *Phospholipase-C-inositol phosphate system* and **(c)** *Ion channels.*

a) *Adenylate cyclase:cAMP System:* Cyclic AMP is a prototype second messenger and is synthesised by adenylyl cyclase under the influence of different G-proteins coupled to their respective receptors. Stimulation of adenylyl cyclase (and hence ↑ cAMP) is mediated by Gs while inhibition (and hence ↓ cAMP) by Gi. Fig. 7.7 shows, as an example, the ways in which increased cAMP production in response to β-adrenergic activation (by Gs) affects the glycogen and fat metabolism in liver and muscles. The result is a coordinated response in which stored energy, in the form of glycogen or fat, is made available as glucose to fuel the muscle contraction. Other examples of regulation by cAMP-dependent protein kinase include the increased activity of Ca^{2+} channels in the heart muscle. Phosphorylation of these channels increases the Ca^{2+} entry into the cell, during action potential, thereby increasing the force of contraction (FC) of the heart muscle.

Inhibition of adenylyl cyclase, mediated by Gi, leads to a decreased cAMP production. Examples include M_2 receptors (muscarinic-cholinergic-M_2) of cardiac muscle, α_2- adrenoceptors in smooth muscles and opioid receptors. Cyclic AMP is hydrolysed within the cells by phosphodiesterase enzyme to 5-AMP and thus the action is terminated.

b) *The Phospholipase-C:Inositol Phosphate System*: Some of the hormones (e.g., vasopressin and thyrotropin-releasing hormone), neuro-transmitters (on muscarinic-cholinergic receptor, catecholamine α_1 receptor and serotonin $5HT_2$ receptor) and growth factors (platelet derived growth factors) bind to receptors linked to G-proteins (Gq) and activate the membrane enzyme phospholipase-C (PLC). The stimulation of PLC leads to the hydrolysis of phosphotidyl inositol 4,5-diphosphate (PIP_2) which

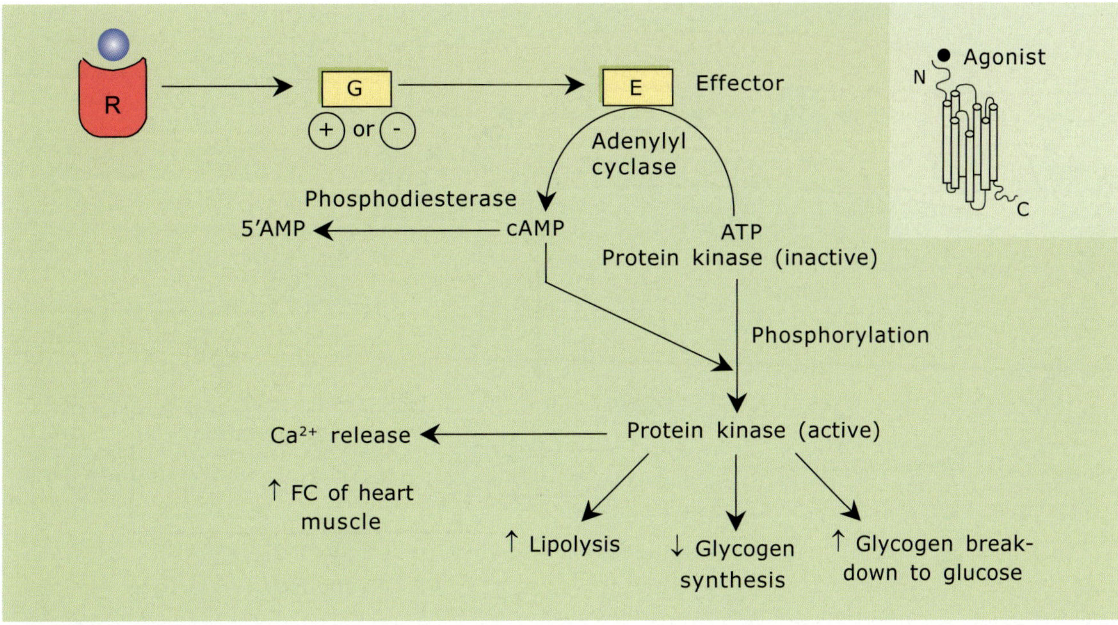

Fig 7.7 Regulation of Energy Metabolism and Contractility of the Heart by cAMP Dependent Protein Kinases. Inset. 7-transmembrane helical topology of G-protein coupled receptor (R). N terminal: Agonist binding domain; C terminal: G-protein coupling domain.

is the phospholipid component of plasma membrane. On hydrolysis, PIP_2 splits into two second messengers: diacylglycerol (DAG) and inositol-1,4,5-triphosphate (IP_3). DAG remains confined to the membrane, while IP_3, being water soluble, diffuses through cytoplasm where it triggers the release of Ca^{2+} from storage vesicles. The raised cytoplasmic concentration of Ca^{2+} promotes the binding of Ca^{2+} to calmodulin (Cam)—a Ca^{2+} binding protein which regulates the activities of various enzymes (responses like contraction, secretion and enzyme activation etc.). DAG activates a phospholipid and the calcium sensitive protein kinase-C (PKC) which then phosphorylates specific protein (enzymes) substrates (S) leading to the response (e.g., release of hormones, increase or decrease in neurotransmitter release and inflammatory responses etc.) (Fig. 7.8).

As in the cAMP system, multiple mechanisms exist to damp or terminate signaling by phosphoinositide pathway. IP_3 is inactivated by dephosphorylation to inositol and then to phosphotidyl inositol monophosphate (PIP, a precursor of PIP_2). DAG, on the other hand, is either phosphorylated to phosphatidic acid and finally converted back to phospholipids or it is deacetylated to arachidonic acid (a precursor of prostaglandins). Ca^{2+} is removed from the cytoplasm by calcium pump through active transport.

c) *Ion Channel Regulation*: G-protein coupled receptors can control the functioning of ion channels (e.g., K^+ and Ca^{2+} channels) by mechanisms that do not involve any role of second messengers (e.g., cAMP or inositol phosphate). For example, in cardiac muscle, muscarinic ACh receptors (M_2) are known to enhance K^+ permeability (thus hyperpolarising the cells and inhibiting electrical activity). Opioid analgesics also reduce neuronal excitability by opening K^+ channels by this mechanism.

d) *Guanylate cyclase:cGMP System*: Though of lesser significance, GPCRs also activate guanylate

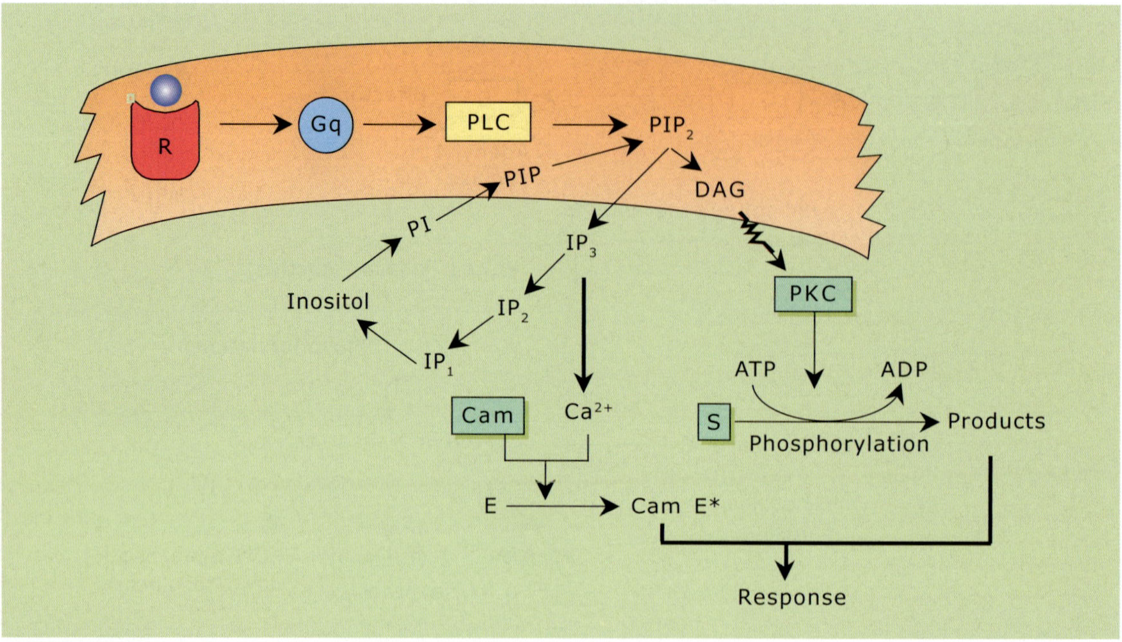

Fig 7.8 The Ca^{2+}-Phosphoinositide Signaling Pathway.

cyclase which converts GTP to cGMP (a 4th second messenger), which stimulate cGMP-dependent protein kinase. It causes dilatation of vascular smooth muscle by dephosphorylation of myosin light chains. Some drugs like sildenafil (used to treat erectile dysfunction) produce vasodilatation by interfering with the enzyme that metabolises cGMP.

3. **Kinase-linked Receptors**: These receptors are directly linked to tyrosine kinase (e.g., receptors for insulin and various growth factors) or to guanylate cyclase (e.g., receptors for atrial natriuretic peptide). *These are the receptors that are ligand (agonist) activated transmembrane enzymes having catalytic activity.* The agonist binding to the extracellular domain of these receptors produces a conformational change that results in dimerisation followed by autophosphorylation of the tyrosine residues in the intracellular tyrosine binding domain. These phosphorylated tyrosine residues then couple with SH_2 domain of Grb_2 protein which results in a series of events, culminating in the responses like mediating the actions of a variety of growth factors, peptide mediators (which stimulate mitogenesis) and of insulin (Fig. 7.9a). Other related receptors are *cytokine receptors* which controls the synthesis and release of many inflammatory mediators.

A few hormones (e.g., atrial natriuretic peptide) also have a similar architecture but the intracellular domain here is not tyrosine kinase but is guanylyl cyclase (GC) which after synthesising a second messenger (cyclic GMP), provides cellular responses (Fig. 7.9b).

4. **Intracellular Receptors (Cytosolic Recep-tors)**: This nuclear receptor family senses signals from the lipid-soluble substances (e.g., vit.A and D) and other hormonal substances (such as corticosteroids, sex hormones and thyroid hormone) to influence the gene expression. This family consists of 3 categories. The main category of nuclear receptors belongs to steroidal hormones (glucocorticoid, mineralocorticoid, estrogen, progestogen and androgens). Their receptors are located in the cytoplasm, in an inactive state, complexed with heat shock protein-90 (hsp-90) and some other proteins. Glucocorticoids have a very high affinity to this receptor. When they cross the cell membrane, the glucocorticoid receptor dissociates from hsp-90 and forms a homodimer (GR+GR) complex with glucocorticoids which then translocates into the

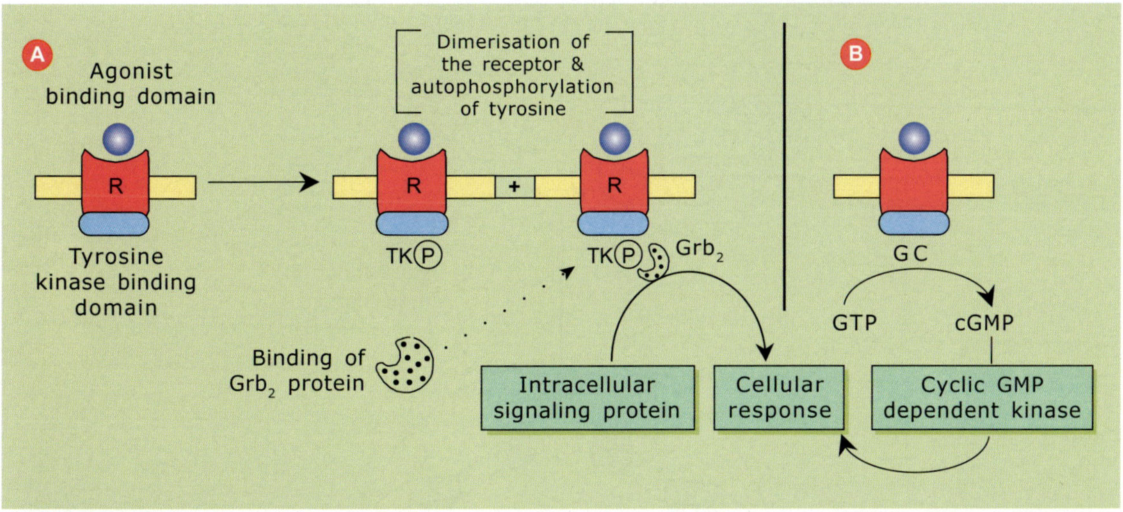

Fig 7.9 Transmembrane Signaling by Ligand (agonist) Activated Receptor Linked to (a) Tyrosine Kinase, (b) Guanylyl Cyclase.

cell nucleus. Once inside the nucleus, these dimers *transactivate* or *transrepress* the genes by binding to the positive or negative *Glucocorticoid Responsive Elements* (GRE; Fig. 7.10). This they do by recruiting some *coactivators* or *corepressors* (not shown). Alterations in gene transcription leads to a change (either up or down) in the desired protein expression.

Other categories of nuclear receptors include receptors for thyroid hormone (TR), receptors for vit A and D, and **P**eroxisome **P**roliferator **A**ctivated **R**eceptor (PPAR) which acts as a lipid sensor and modulates lipid metabolism (Ch. 23) within the cell. While steroid receptors are present in the cytoplasm and translocate, after forming dimers, into the nucleus to initiate gene transcription, the other 2 categories of nuclear receptor are present mainly within the nucleus and act after forming heterodimers with **R**etinoid **X**-**R**eceptor (RXR), i.e., in these dimers RXR is an obligate dimer (e.g., TR+RXR or PPAR+RXR).

Because gene transcription is a relatively slow (min to hrs) and a long-lasting process, drugs that target these receptors often require a longer period of time for the onset of action and show longer lasting effects than do drugs that act through ion-channels (milli seconds) or through GPCRs (few sec to min) or through tyrosine-kinase receptor (min).

5. **Enzymes as Receptors**: A large variety of enzymes (both intra- or extra-cellular) also serve as potential molecular targets for the drugs.

Drugs can either mimic the enzyme's substrate (after binding with its 'active' site) or may bind to its allosteric site to produce the effect. One example of this class of receptors is *angiotensin-converting enzyme* (ACE) which converts angiotensin I to the vasoconstrictor angiotensin II. ACE enzyme is therefore a receptor for ACE inhibiting drugs which lower blood pressure by inhibiting the enzymatic conversion from angiotensin I to angiotensin II. Another example is of a*cetylcholinesterase* (AChE) *enzyme* which degrades the neurotransmitter acetylcholine. AChE inhibitors prevent degradation of acetylcholine and thus enhance cholinergic activity in the cholinergic synapse. AChE, therefore, serves as a receptor for AChE inhibitors. Similarly, the dihydrofolate reductase (an intracellular enzyme) serves as a receptor for an antibacterial drug trimethoprim and for an anticancer drug methotrexate. These drugs act by inhibiting this enzyme.

6. **Drugs Which Act Through Modulation of Voltage-Gated Ion Channels (Voltage-Operated Channels, VOCs)**: Voltage-operated channels (VOCs) like ROCs (discussed above) are ion channels that are gated only by voltage. That means, the gating (or opening

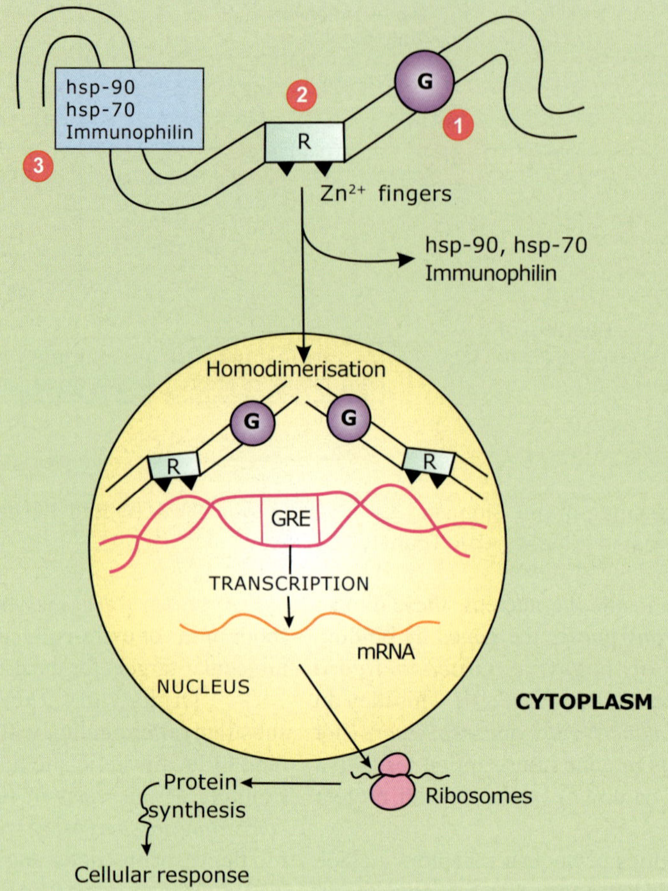

Fig 7.10 Cytosolic Receptor Mediated DNA Transcription (Exemplified by Glucocorticoid Receptor Functioning). Key—R = Receptor; G = Glucocorticoid drug; GRE = Glucocorticoid responsive element; 1 = Agonist binding site; 2 = DNA binding site; 3 = Transcription activating domain (this site becomes active only after dissociation of inhibitory proteins, e.g hsp-90, hsp-70 and immunophilin; hsp = heat shock protein)

or conductance) of the ion channel is controlled by changes in membrane potential. These are typed as voltage-gated Na-channels (Ch. 15&21), K-channels (Ch. 19 & 21) and Ca-channels (Ch. 19, 20 & 21) which are discussed in details in the relevant chapters.

ROCs (e.g., nicotinic ACH receptors) appear to assume only 2 states, 'open' or ' closed', while VOCs undergo a third state also, called ' refractory' (or 'inactivated') state. In this state the channel is unable to 'open' (or reactivate) for a certain period of time even when the membrane potential returns to a voltage that normally opens or activates the channel. Unlike ROCs, voltage-gated channels have no major endogenous modulator (like a acetylcholine). However, certain drugs can prolong or shorten the duration of different states of the same ion channel. This`state-dependent binding' is important for the mechanism of local anaesthetics, antianginal and antiarrhythmic drugs.

Receptor Desensitisation

Receptor-mediated responses to drugs and hormones often 'desensitise' with time. After reaching an initial high level, the response gradually diminishes over seconds or minutes even in the continuing presence of the agonist. This desensitisation is usually reversible (Fig. 7.11), which distinguishes it from the "down-regulation" of receptors as described below. It is a self-defence mechanism provided by nature to protect our cells from excessive stimulation.

Many kinds of receptors undergo desensitisation, e.g., at the neuromuscular junction there is evidence that the desensitisation is caused by a slow conformational change in the receptor resulting in the tight binding of the agonist molecule without opening of the ion channel. Similarly, GPCRs, e.g., β-adrenoceptors, on desensitisation become unable to activate adenylate cyclase, though they can still bind to the agonist molecule.

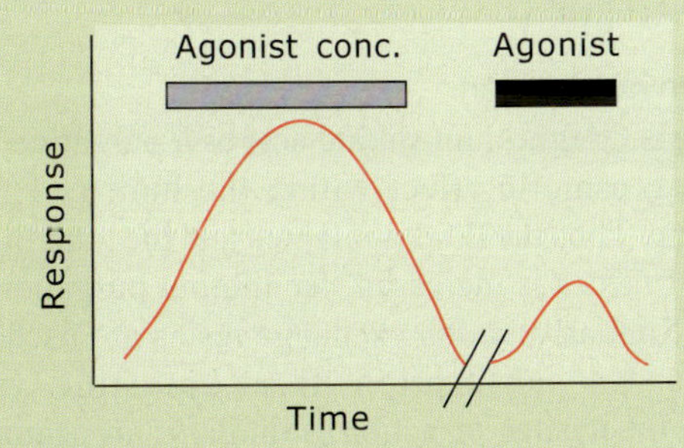

Fig 7.11 The Response to an Agonist Versus Time During the Phase of Desensitisation.

Up- and Down-regulation of Receptors

Prolonged exposure to high concentration of agonist (whether administered as a drug or overproduced as a neurotransmitter) causes a reduction in the number of receptors available for activation (down-regulation of receptors). This results due to endocytosis or internalisation of the receptors from the cell surface.

On the other hand, prolonged occupation of receptors by a blocker (antagonist) leads to an increase in the number of receptors (up-regulation) with subsequent increase in receptor sensitivity. This probably results due to externalisation of the receptors out again from inside of the cell surface. Sometimes, other hormones can also bring about up-regulation of certain receptors. For example, in thyrotoxicosis, the thyroid hormones bring about up-regulation of $\beta_1$receptors of cardiac muscle which increases cardiac sensitivity to catecholamines leading to tachycardia.

Down-regulation of receptors may be responsible for diminished effects seen in severe asthmatics who no longer respond to β_2 adrenoceptor agonist, like salbutamol. In endogenous depression there is down-regulation of α-adrenoceptors (with concomitant up-regulation of β-adrenoceptors); and the prolonged use of tricyclic antidepressants results in down-regulation of β-receptors (with relatively up-regulation of α-receptors).

Spare Receptors (receptor reserve)

Maximal efficacy means a state at which receptor - mediated signaling is maximal and that, further increase in the drug dose does not produce any additional response. Theoretically, it should happen when all the receptors get occupied by the drug. Normally, the drugs can produce the maximal response when even less than 100% of receptors are occupied. The remaining unoccupied receptors are just serving as receptor reserve and are called *spare receptors*. Experimentally, spare receptors can be demonstrated by using irreversible antagonist (to prevent binding of an agonist to available receptors) and showing that by using higher concentration of agonist, the maximal response can still be produced. About 90% of insulin receptors are just serving as spare receptors. Thus there is an immense functional reserve to make sure that adequate amount of glucose enters into the cell. On the contrary, a human heart has only 5–10% of β-adrenoceptor spare receptor reserve. Hence a little functional reserve exists in the failing heart and to obtain maximum contractility most receptors must be occupied. This surplus of receptors, over the number actually needed, is not just a wasteful biological management. It is the economy of hormone or neurotransmitter secretion and utilisation which we achieve at the expense of some additional receptors.

Denervation Supersensitivity of Receptors

In denervated muscles, the new receptors are synthesised (fast up-regulation) and these then proliferate all along the cell surface or membrane surface. A similar proliferation of new receptors can occur if these are subjected to prolonged blockade by any antagonist. Such receptors show supersensitivity to even small amounts of the neurotransmitter being made available despite receptor blockade or due to some active collateral innervation. The pharmacological basis of tardive dyskinesia (excessive involuntary oro-buccal-lingual motions; a side effect of neuroleptics after prolonged use) is explained on the basis of supersensitivity of dopamine receptors. Due to long-term dopamine receptor blockade by a neuroleptic drug, the striatal nerve cells start synthesising new dopamine receptors which are supersensitive to even small amounts of dopamine still coming through the neurons after neuroleptic blockade. This supersenstitive response causes the dopaminergic inputs to outweigh the cholinergic inputs and thus the patient exhibits the afore-mentioned excessive movements which are diametrically opposite to parkinsonism.

Receptor Related Diseases

There is now a considerable interest in the role of receptor changes in the aetiology of certain diseases. Practically all patients with myasthenia gravis have antibodies developed against the cholinergic nicotinic receptors at motor end plate. In some forms of insulin resistant diabetes, antibodies develop against insulin receptors. Other interesting examples of receptor related diseases are testicular feminisation (male pseudohermaphroditism) due to androgen receptor insensitivity and the familial hypercholesterolaemia due to decrease in the receptors for the low-density lipoproteins (LDL receptors).

Non-receptor Mediated Mechanisms

Not all drug actions are mediated by receptors. They may act by a chemical action or by physical action or through other modes as discussed below:

1. By Chemical Action

Neutralisation. For example, antacids act by neutralising gastric hyperacidity. The anticoagulant action of heparin constitutes another example. It is a strongly acidic mucopolysaccharide and acts by neutralising the basic groups of various clotting factors and thus prevents the action of thrombin (extracellular site of action).

Chelation. Some drugs (the chelating agents) trap the heavy metals (Pb, Hg, Ca, Cu and Fe) in their ring structure, and form water-soluble complexes which are then finally excreted. For example, EDTA (chelates Ca^{2+}), calcium disodium edetate (chelates Pb^{2+}), dimercaprol (chelates Hg^{2+}), penicillamine (chelates Cu^{2+}) and deferoxamine (chelates iron). All these drugs are used to treat heavy-metal poisoning (an extracellular site of action).

Ion Exchangers. For example, anion exchange resin like cholestyramine exchanges Cl^- ions from the bile salts. The resultant complex is not absorbed and is excreted out. The drug is thus used as a cholesterol lowering agent.

2. By Physical Action

Osmosis. Magnesium sulfate acts as a purgative by exerting osmotic effect within the lumen of the intestine. Thus the fluid is retained and the total fluid bulk of faeces is increased, facilitating purgation.

Similarly, cation exchange resins are used to reduce Na^+ absorption from intestine (all extracellular sites of action). Similary, an osmotic diuretic, mannitol acts nonspecifically by changing the osmolarity in the nephron directly.

Adsorption. Kaolin adsorbs bacterial toxins and thus acts as an antidiarrhoeal agent. Methylpolysiloxane and simethicone adsorb gases and are used as antiflatulent.

Protectives. For example, various dusting powders to provide local effects.

Demulcents. These drugs coat the inflamed mucous membrane and provide a soothing effect, e.g., pectin (in antidiarrhoeal preparations); menthol and syrup vasaka (in cough linctus).

Astringents. They precipitate and denature the mucosal proteins and thus protect the mucosa by firming up the mucosal surface, e.g., tannic acid in gum paints.

Saturation in the Biophase. For example, general anaesthetics simply saturate the cellular sites (called the biophase) of central nervous system. They get packed in between the membrane lipids and thus hinder some metabolic functions or disrupt the membrane organisation.

3. By Counterfeit or False Incorporation Mechanisms

For example, sulfa drugs and antineoplastic drug like methotrexate, act by this mechanism. Bacteria synthesise their own folic acid from PABA, for their growth and development. Sulfa drugs resemble PABA in their chemical configuration and therefore falsely enter into the synthetic process in place of PABA. The folic acid derivative now formed contains a sulfa drug moiety in place of PABA and is therefore, nonfunctional and is of no utility for bacterial growth and development. As a result, the bacteria get deprived of the required folate and their growth ceases (bacteriostatic action). Similarly, methotrexate resembles folic acid and irreversibly binds to the dihydrofolate reductase enzyme responsible for folic acid synthesis. Hence the production of the active form of folic acid (folinic acid) is prevented. Consequently, the synthesis of purine nucleotides and ultimately the DNA production is hindered leading to the death of cancerous cells (cytotoxic action).

4. By Virtue of Being Protoplasmic Poisons

Certain drugs like germicides, and antiseptics like phenol and formaldehyde act non-specifically as protoplasmic poisons causing the death of bacteria.

5. Through Formation of Antibodies

Some drugs like vaccines produce their effects by inducing the formation of antibodies and thus stimulate the defence mechanisms of the body, e.g., vaccines against smallpox and cholera (providing active immunity) and antisera against tetanus and diphtheria (providing passive immunity).

6. Through Placebo Action

The placebo (*I please*) is a pharmacodynamically inert and harmless substance which is sometimes given to the patient in dosage form which resembles the actual medicament exactly in size, shape, colour, smell and weight. If the physician commands a good confidence of the patient, even a pharmacologically inert substance (the placebo) given by him to his patient can bring dramatic relief in the subjective symptoms associated with his psychological problems (e.g., anxiety, headache, pain, insomnia, tremors and lack of appetite etc.). Such a patient is called as placebo reactor and the drug is called *placebo*. Usually starch or lactose are used as placebo in solid dosage forms. The placebo effect is not mediated through any receptor action. It is simply the faith in the treating physician which is providing the clinical benefits. Placebo can bring relief in subjective symptoms only (mainly psychogenic manifestations) but not in objective responses, i.e., it cannot increase or decrease neutrophils, eosinophils or total leucocyte count of the patient suffering from leukaemia. Apart from this compassionate use in therapy, placebos are also used in double-blind clinical trials of a new drug to distinguish the real pharmacodynamic effect of a drug from the personal bias of the investigator and to avoid false positive or negative conclusions (refer Ch.8).

7. By Targeting Specific Genetic Changes

The knowledge of altered gene function in cancer cells has allowed the dream-designing of novel anticancer drugs that specifically target these genetic changes. These include: (i) the inhibitors of *ras*-modifying-enzyme farnesyl transferase that reverses the malignant transformation in cancer cells containing the *ras* oncogene and (ii) the inhibitors of specific tyrosine kinase that block the activity of oncogenic kinases. Other promising approaches include: delivering a gene to cancer cells rendering them sensitive to drugs or delivering a gene to healthy host cells to protect them from chemotherapy or tagging of cancer cells with genes that make them immunogenic.

WHAT DRUGS DO TO A LIVING ORGANISM

(The Qualitative Aspects of Drug Effects)

After dealing with how drugs act (i.e., their site of action and their mechanism of action) we must now see what they do to the body, i.e., the qualitative aspects of their pharmacodynamic effects. The drugs, besides producing the desirable or beneficial effects, can also cause undersirable adverse effects due to drug factors or by some non-drug factors (see text below). The aim of pharmacotherapy is to provide maxium benefits with minimal risk due to adverse effects. Here, we first discuss the adverse drug reactions (ADRs) from the view point of their types and the basis of their occurence and then proceed to discuss how the drug effects could be measured quantitatively to assess their margin of safety. The pharmacodynamic effects of the drug could be classified as shown in Fig. 7.12.

ADVERSE DRUG REACTIONS

Expected Undesirable Effects (Type-A ADRs)

Type A adverse effects are called *augmented effects*. These are largely predictable and are dose depenedent. Their incidence rate is high but mortality is rare or very low. Reduction in dose can minimise these adverse effects. These are manifested as:

1. Side Effects

These are undesirable effects which are observed even with the therapeutic doses of the drug and are usually mild and manageable.

For example. Dicyclomine (an anticholinergic drug) relieves pain of intestinal colic due to its antispasmodic action (desirable effect) but side-by-side also causes dryness of mouth even in its therapeutic doses (side effect). Similarly, promethazine (an antihistaminic drug) has antiallergic action (desirable effect), but it also produces sedation in therapeutic doses (side effect). Several drugs produce epigastric distress as their side effect. However, proper adjustment of the dose (in previous cases) or use of countermeasures, like antacids (in epigastric distress) usually minimises the symptoms of side effects.

2. Secondary Effects

These are indirect consequences of the main pharmacodynamic action of the drug.

For example. Development of superinfection after suppression of bacterial flora by antibiotics and weakening of host defenses after the use of corticosteroids. As above, these effects may occur even when the drug is used in therapeutic dose but can be predicted from the pharmacological profile of the drug.

3. Toxicity

These are exaggerated form of side effects which occur predictably either due to overdoses or after prolonged use of the drug. The reason could be pharmacodynamic (e.g., bleeding due to high doses of heparin, or coma due to high doses of barbiturates) or pharmacokinetic (e.g., crystaluria

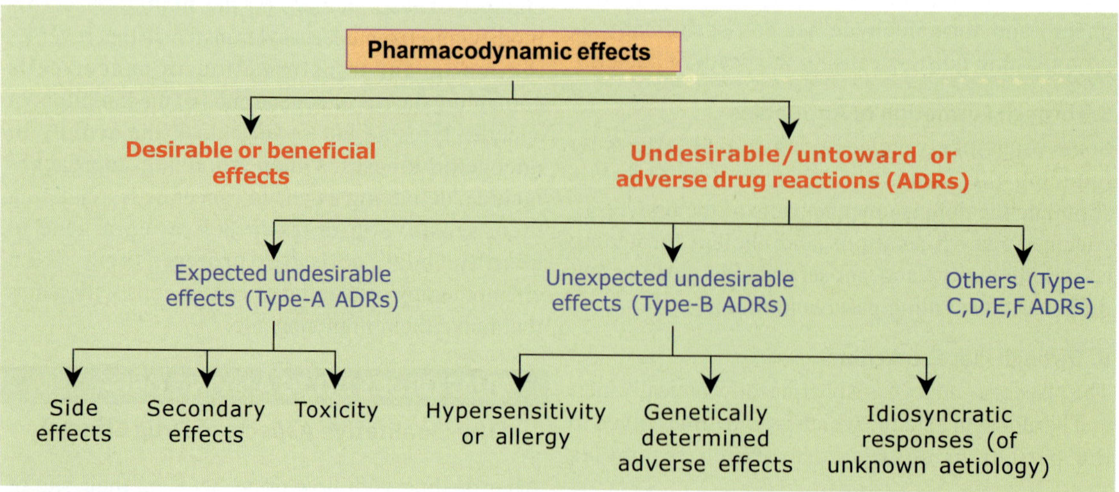

Fig 7.12 The Pharmacodynamic Effects of a Drug.

or glomerular nephritis due to precipitation of sulfonamides in acidic urine, or nephrotoxicity due to gentamicin in cases having renal insufficiency). Certain drugs in high doses may cause poisoning, e.g., delirium, hyperpyrexia, and hallucinations with overdoses of atropine (atropine poisoning; a pharmacodynamic reason).

Unexpected Undesirable Effects (Type-B ADRs or Bizarre effects)

These arise unexpectedly, even when the drug is used in therapeutic doses, by a mechanism unrelated to the main pharmacological effect of the drug. These include, either immunologically mediated reaction to the drug, or pharmacogenetically mediated adverse response or idiosyncratic reaction due to peculiarities of an individual for which no definite genotype has been described. These are grouped as unpredictable responses because firstly, there is no linear relationship with drug doses, and secondly, the predictive tests, if any, are uncertain, expensive and unpracticable. These are relatively uncommon but, if occur, mortality rates are high. Reduction in the dose does not reduce the risk for type-B ADR. These include:

1. Drug Allergy (hypersensitivity reactions)

Allergic responses to drug occur when there has been previous exposure to drug (or its metabolites) and when this sensitised individual is re-exposed to the same drug again. It is loosely termed also as hypersensitivity.

During the first uneventful exposure, the drug (or its metabolite) acts as hapten, which after combining with host proteins, becomes antigenic. Specific antibodies are formed against this antigen which keep on circulating. On re-exposure there is then antigen-antibody response which results in the release of the chemical mediators of allergy (histamine, 5HT, leukotrienes, SRS-A and PAF, etc.) causing effects like urticaria, rhinitis, pruritus, asthma, and anaphylactic shock (exaggerated and immediate type of hypersensitivity characterised by hypotensive shock, bronchoconstriction, angioneurotic oedema, laryngospasm followed by death) (Fig. 7.13 a,b).

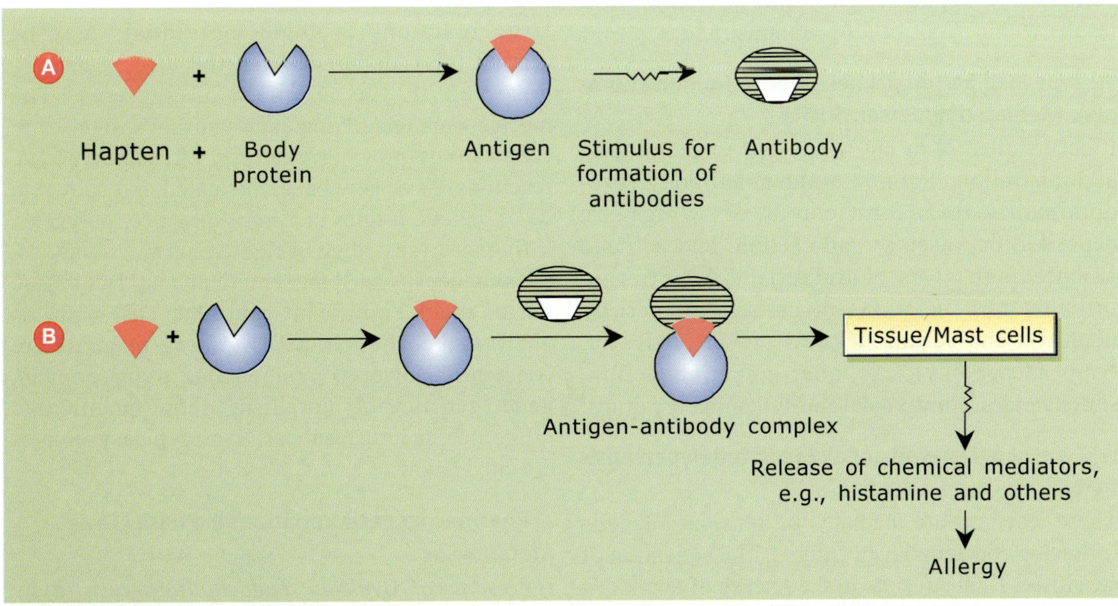

Fig 7.13 Mechanism of the Allergic Response. (a) After Initial or First Exposure to the Drug. (b) After Subsequent or Second Exposure to the Same Drug.

Drugs may elicit following types of allergy:

i) Type I or Immediate Type (Humoural Antibodies)

Allergy develops within minutes and lasts for 2–3 hr. The drug causes formation of tissue-sensitising IgE antibodies that are fixed to mast cells or leucocytes. The subsequent exposure to drug, degranulates mast cells or activates leucocytes with release of chemical mediators (histamine, serotonin etc.) of allergy. The patient, if untreated, suddenly passes into anaphylactic shock. For example anaphylaxis after parenteral administration of penicillins, or streptokinase or radiocontrast media.

ii) Type II or Accelerated Allergy or Antibody-dependent Cytotoxic Hypersensitivity (Humoural Antibodies)

It results when a drug (antigen) binds to RBC and is recognised by IgG antibody. The antigen-antibody reaction then triggers the lysis of RBC either by activating complement system or by the action of cytotoxic T cells or by phagocytosis by macrophages. For example: thrombocytopenia, agranulocytosis, haemolysis, fever and systemic lupus erythematosus after the use of quinidine, cefotetan (a cephalosporin) and penicillin-G. It results within 72 hr of drug administration.

iii) Type III or Serum sickness type or Immune Complex Mediated Hypersensitivity

It occurs after 72 hr but within 1–2 weeks of drug administration. Soluble antigen–antibody (predominantly IgG) form complexes which are deposited on vascular endothelium and activate complement. It is characterised by allergic inflammatory reactions in tissues, glomerular nephritis and serum sickness (fever, urticaria, lymphadenopathy), e.g., after giving ampicillin, sulfonamides, nonsteroidal anti-inflammatory drugs.

iv) Type IV or Delayed or Cell Mediated Hypersensitivity

These reactions are mediated by sensitised T cells following contact with an antigen. The activation of sensitised T cells results in the release of cytokines which activate macrophages, granulocytes and natural killer cells to generate an inflammatory response, e.g., hypersensitivity pneumonitis, contact dermatitis, photosensitivity and rashes with fever.

Type II, III and IV hypersensitivity reactions are treated by giving glucocorticoids (hydrocortisone I.V. or prednisolone I.V.). Anaphylactic shock following Type I hypersensitivity reaction should be treated promptly with: inj adrenaline (1:1000) 0.3–0.5 ml I.M + inj hydrocortisone 100–200 mg I.V. + inj diphenhydramine (an antihistamine) 25–50 mg I.M. or I.V.

Cross Allergy: The cross allergy within the members of the same group of drugs is most common. Why allergy is very common with some drugs like penicillins and why the same drug does not cause allergy in all individuals is not exactly clear. Desensitisation can be attempted in some limited cases only (e.g., in patients allergic to antitubercular drug). In this procedure, a very small amount of allergen is administered, which is then gradually increased until a therapeutic dose is tolerated. This procedure is usually done under the cover of a corticosteroid, a β-adrenoceptor blocker and an antihistamine which inhibit chemical mediator release and action.

2. Genetically Determined Abnormal Responses of a Drug

Drug reactions in some individuals may be qualitatively different from the effects usually observed in the majority of subjects. The mechanisms underlying such unusual responses to certain drugs (previously categorised as idiosyncratic reactions) have now been elucidated and shown to be of genetic origin. In clinical practice, polygenic influences (sex, diet, weight, pharmacokinetics, receptor density and other environmental factors) are not of much significant consequences so far as pharmacogenetic variations in drug response are concerned. However, variations due to single mutant gene (genetic polymorphism) show quantitative differences in drug response. Some typical examples are cited below.

a) Pharmacogenetic Variations in Phase I Drug Metabolism

i) ***Presence of Atypical Pseudocholinesterase (faulty hydrolysis):*** Incidence of the presence of atypical pseudocholinesterase in the population is 1:2500. The inheritance of this trait is autosomal recessive. The neuromuscular blocking action of succinylcholine is terminated within 5 min by the hydrolysis due to normal pseudocholinesterase in plasma. However, the genotype atypical pseudocholinesterase cannot hydrolyse succinylcholine (may take 1–2 hr). In such cases, even the therapeutic dose of succinylcholine leads to a prolonged respiratory failure. The atypical pseudocholinesterase can easily be detected by measuring its inhibition by dibucaine (a local anaesthetic drug). Normal pseudocholinesterase is inhibited 80% by dibucaine while atypical pseudocholinesterase is inhibited only to the extent of 20%. Thus "dibucaine number" is the measure of the percentage inhibition of plasma cholinesterase. The atypical plasma cholinesterase has a low dibucaine number. Normal "dibucaine number" is 80.

ii) ***Hydroxylase Polymorphism (faulty oxidation)***: Normally, phenytoin (an anticonvulsant drug) is hydroxylated and thus oxidised by mixed function oxidases. In slow hydroxylators, phenytoin toxicity increases. The defect is transmitted as autosomal recessive trait.

b) Pharmacogenetic Variations in Phase II Drug Metabolism

i) ***Acetylator Status***: Many drugs are metabolised by hepatic N-acetylase enzyme. This enzyme is non-inducible, i.e., variations in drug response are not due to the concomitant use of enzyme inducers; rather, the differences are due to the presence of higher or lower amounts of N-acetylase in the liver. Thus there are two phenotypes in the population: the *rapid acetylators* (like Eskimos and Japanese) or *slow acetylators* (like Egyptians, Mediterranean Jews and Swedes). It is inherited as an autosomal recessive trait. The acetylator status of an individual significantly affects the nature of adverse effects with drugs which are mainly metabolised through N-acetylation (e.g., isoniazid and dapsone). In *slow acetylators*, isoniazid gets accumulated after repeated doses leading to neurotoxicity (peripheral neuritis) because isoniazid inhibits pyridoxine kinase which converts pyridoxine to its active form pyridoxyl phosphate. Addition of vitamin B_6 (pyridoxine), therefore, controls the side effects. In *fast acetylators,* isoniazid is metabolised faster providing higher concentrations of a metabolic product, acetyl hydrazine, causing hepatotoxicity. Dapsone therapy also, in slow acetylators, may lead to haemolysis.

c) Pharmacogenetic Variation in Drug Response due to Enzyme Deficiency

i) ***Glucose-6-phosphate Dehydrogenase (G6PD) Deficiency*** in RBCs is inherited as a sex-linked recessive trait. It is common amongst Africans and American Negros (incidence is 5–10%) but about 10 million people belonging to other races (Mediterranean Jews, Middle East and South East races) are supposed to be deficient in G6PD enzyme.

Certain drugs which have oxidising properties, like primaquine (antimalarial), sulfonamides, sulfones and nitrofurantoin (all antibacterials) cause haemolytic anaemia in cases having G6PD deficiency; because, in absence of G6PD, NADPH is not regenerated and consequently glutathione reduction is prevented. Due to deficiency of reduced glutathione, methaemoglobin (Fe^{3+}) is not converted to haemoglobin (Fe^{2+}) and thus haemolytic anaemia results. Other oxidising drugs, like quinine, chloroquine (all antimalarials) and quinidine (antiarrhythmic drug) may also cause haemolysis in G6PD deficient individuals but have a lesser risk.

ii) ***Uroporphyrinogen Synthetase Enzyme Deficiency***: Another clinically important example in this category is the effect of many drugs (e.g., barbiturates, carbamazepine, phenytoin, chloramphenicol and oral contraceptives) in precipitating attacks of intermittent porphyria in susceptible individuals who are *deficient in uroporphyrinogen synthetase,* an enzyme required for haem synthesis. Thus porphyrin-containing haem precursors accumulate giving rise to acute intermittent porphyria characterised by gastrointestinal, neurological and behavioural disturbances. It is inherited as an autosomal dominant trait, which is more common in Swedes and in North European races.

3. Idiosyncratic Drug Responses

These are harmful and sometimes fatal reactions that occur in a small minority of individuals, for which the cause is yet poorly understood. A few examples can be cited:

i) A condition of malignant hyperpyrexia, a dangerous idiosyncratic reaction to drugs like halothane, succinylcholine and neuroleptic drugs, like chlorpromazine and haloperidol. It is supposed to be an inherited trait, though the exact basis is not yet known.

ii) Occurrence of aplastic anaemia with a single dose or with low doses of chloramphenicol is in approximately 1:50,000 patients. The cause is not yet clear.

iii) Aspirin-induced late-onset asthma or chronic renal failure and thiazide diuretics induced erectile impotence are some other examples of idiosyncratic reaction due to drugs.

Majority of idiosyncratic reactions have now been found to have a genetic basis and therefore are classified under genetically determined Type -B ADRs.

Other Types of Adverse Drug Effects

Type A (augmented) and Type B (bizarre) are most important and fundamental type of adverse drug effects. Other types of ADRs include:

Type C (Chronic effects) ADRs: These are the adverse effects that are associated with prolonged use of the drug. For example, orofacial dyskinesia after prolonged use of phenothiazine neuroleptics and Cushing syndrome after chronic use of prednisolone, analgesic nephropathy with aspirin and colonic dysfunctions after prolonged use of laxatives.

Type D (Delayed effects) ADRs: These are the adverse effects that occur remotely from the treatment, i.e., delayed adverse effects occurring in patients years after the treatment, or effects appearing in their children who did not receive that treatment, e.g., secondary cancers in patients treated with alkylating agents for Hodgkin's disease or clear-cell carcinoma of vagina in the daughters of women who took diethylstilbestrol during pregnancy. Teratogenic effects (impaired foetal developments) are also covered under type-D ADRs.

Type E (End-of-treatment effects) ADRs: These ADRs occur when a drug is suddenly discontinued, e.g., rebound hypertension after abrupt withdrawal of propranolol (β-adrenoceptor blocker); withdrawal seizures after suddenly stopping phenytoin (anti-epileptic drug) and adrenocortical insufficiency after sudden stopping of prednisolone (a glucocorticoid).

Type F (Failure of a drug to produce the desired effect) ADRs: In some people administration of a drug does not produce therapeupic effect due to genetic variability, i.e., polymorphism of the drug torget protein or as a result of some unknown reasons. Such a failure of the drug to producethe desired effect is considered Type F ADR.

Type C, D, E and F ADRs are not properly covered under type A and B ADRs. Adverse drug effects are the most common cause for ***iatrogenic diseases*** (i.e., diseases induced by drug therapy). Iatrogenic disease may persist even after the offending drug has been withdrawn. For example: reserpine leads to endogenous depression; glucocorticoids precipitate diabetes and hypertension; aspirin causes peptic ulcer; chlorpromazine produces parkinsonism and hydralazine causes systemic lupus erythematosus.

Specific Toxicity of Some Particular Drugs

Toxic effects of drugs can be: (a) related to their principal pharmacological action, e.g., hypoglycaemic coma with insulin, bleeding with anticoagulant drugs, and arrhythmias with cardiac glycosides or (b) unrelated to their principal pharmacological action. The latter are specific toxicities with some particular drugs.

Such toxicities often involve a chemically reactive metabolite (rather than the parent drug) and are at times immunological in nature also. Examples include liver or kidney damage, bone marrow suppression, carcinogenesis and teratogenesis (impaired foetal development). Such effects, which are liable to occur with any kind of chemical or a drug, fall conventionally into the area of toxicology rather than pharmacology. Example of drugs causing organ toxicities and teratogenicity are listed in Table 7.2.

Table 7.2 Specific Toxicities Due to Drugs, Unrelated to their Principal Pharmacological Action

Type of toxicity	Drug
Carcinogenicity	Tobacco, estrogens, progestogens, radio-isotopes
Endocrinal	
Hyperglycaemia	Thiazide diuretics
Thyroid dysfunction	Amiodarone
Haemopoietic toxicity	
Haemolytic anaemia	Sulfonamides, methyldopa
Agranulocytosis	Carbimazole, phenylbutazone
Aplastic anaemia	Clozapine, cytotoxic drugs
Megaloblastic anaemia	Chloramphenicol, phenytoin, methotrexate
Heart	
Heart failure	Doxorubicin (anticancer drug)
Arrhythmias	Astemizole and terfenadine (antihistamines), emetin
Hepatotoxicity	
Hepatic cell injury *Cholestatic jaundice*	Paracetamol, phenytoin, chlorpromazine, rifampicin, erythromycin, androgens
Hepatitis	Isoniazid (fast acetylators)
Cirrhosis liver	Alcohol, methotrexate
Immunologically induced hepatitis	Halothane, enflurane
Neurotoxicity	
Peripheral neuropathy	Isoniazid
Subacute myelo-optic neuropathy (SMON)	Iodochloro hydroxy quinoline (amoebicidal drug)
Ocular toxicity	
Cataract	Glucocorticoids
Pigmented retinopathy	Chloroquine, chlorpromazine
Optic neuritis	Ethambutol (antitubercular drug)
Ototoxicity	Aminoglycoside group of antibiotics, salicylates (high doses), chloroquine, ethacrynic acid (diuretic)
Renal toxicity	
Allergic-type interstitial nephritis and nephropathy	Nonsteroidal anti-inflammatory agents
Nephrotic syndrome	ACE inhibitors, penicillamine
Glomerular nephritis	Sulfonamides
Tubular necrosis	Aminoglycoside group of antibiotics
Teratogenicity *(foetal abnormalities)*	Thalidomide, penicillamine, warfarin, phenytoin, valproate, trimethadone, folate antagonists (e.g., methotrexate), antithyroid drugs, androgens, progestogens, tetracyclines and retinoids (Vit. A derivatives)
Miscellaneous	
Influenza like syndrome	Rifampicin
Distortion of taste	Metronidazole, captopril
Pancreatitis	Asparaginase (anticancer drug)
Gingival hyperplasia	Phenytoin
Lupus erythematosus	Hydralazine, procainamide
Gout	Loop diuretics
Osteomalacia	Phenytoin
Haematuria	Cyclophosphamide
Staining of teeth and bone deformities	Teracyclines and fluorides

HOW DRUG EFFECTS CAN BE MEASURED

(The Quantitative Aspects of Drug Effects)

Up to this point we have considered some of the fundamental principles of pharmacodynamics on rather a qualitative basis. These principles must also find expression in quantitative terms as well; only then they can provide the basis for evaluation and comparison of drug effectiveness and safety. One of the basic principles of Pharmacology states that the degree of effect produced by a drug depends on the quantity of the drug administered, i.e., the dose.

WHAT IS A DOSE

It is the required amount of drug in weight, volume, moles or International Units, that is necessary to provide a desired effect. In clinical practice it is called as a *therapeutic dose*, while for experimental purposes (in animals) it is called as an *effective dose*. The therapeutic dose varies from person to person and from one clinical situation to the other and hence is indicated by a range. For example: the dose of aspirin to provide relief from pain is 300 mg to 1 g wherein 300 mg is the minimum dose while 1 g is the maximum dose which can be given to an individual for different analgesic purposes. The drugs can be administered as:

Single Dose

For example, a single oral dose of albendazole (400 mg) is sufficient to eradicate roundworms or a single I.M. dose of 250 mg of ceftriaxone can be given to treat gonorrhoea.

Daily Dose

It is the quantity of a drug to be administered in 24 hr, either all at once or in equally divided doses (the dose interval is decided on the basis of the plasma half-life along with other parameters, like aVd as discussed earlier). For example, 10 mg daily dose (all at once) of cetrizine is sufficient to relieve allergic manifestations; while a daily dose of erythromycin (an antibiotic) is 1 g per day to be given in 4 equally divided doses (i.e., 250 mg every 6 hr).

Total Dose

It is the maximum quantity of the drug that is needed during the complete course of the therapy. For example, the total dose of procaine penicillin-G for the treatment of early syphilis is 6 million units and this is given as 0.6 million units per day for 10 days.

Loading Dose (priming dose)

It is the large dose of the drug to be given initially to provide the effective plasma concentration rapidly. The clinical situations, where the administration of the loading dose is essential, have already been discussed earlier (Ch. 6).

Maintenance Dose

The loading dose is normally followed by a maintenance dose which is usually half of the loading dose. This is needed to maintain the steady state plasma concentration attained after giving the loading dose. The pharmacokinetic basis of giving a maintenance dose has already been discussed earlier (Ch. 6).

MEASUREMENT OF DRUG EFFECTS

(Quantitative Aspects of Drug Effects)

After giving a dose, the drug effects can be measured for quantitative assessment of its safety and efficacy. Before discussing the quantitative aspects of drug action, we must realise the complexity of the problem in the sense that we are now dealing with so many variables like *the dose, the plasma concentration, the isolated tissue or the whole subject or the population on which the response is to be measured and, of course, the response itself*. For plotting any curve and to derive quantitative information, we must have three variables: *One independent variable* to be plotted on X-axis (abscissa), the *other dependent variable* to be plotted on Y-axis (ordinate) and *the third, a constant variable,* which being common, can be eliminated and therefore not shown on the graph.

Thus we can draw the *dose–plasma concentration curve* by plotting doses on abscissa (independent variable) versus plasma concentration on ordinate (dependent variable), eliminating the subject to whom the doses were administered (constant variable). Alternatively, we can plot a *time–*

plasma concentration curve by plotting time on abscissa (independent variable) versus plasma concentration on ordinate (dependent variable), ignoring the subject in whom plasma concentrations were measured at different time intervals after giving a particular dose (constant variable). In this chapter we shall examine the magnitude of drug effect as a function of the dose administered. In other words, we are restricting our discussions to three variables, i.e., *the dose, the response and the tissue or the subject or group of population on which the response is to be measured.*

Two situations can now result: (a) we can depict the relationship between different doses (graded doses) and their relative response by plotting the graded doses (independent variable) on abscissa versus the relative response (dependent variable) on the ordinate, eliminating the isolated tissue or the single subject (constant factor) to whom the doses were administered. The graphic curve thus obtained is called as the *graded dose–response curve*; (b) alternatively, we can eliminate the response either by quantifying it or by prefixing its criteria on "all or none" basis (i.e., death or no death, anaesthesia or no anaesthesia, or by quantification like "25% rise in pulse rate from the basal value"). Thereafter, we can obtain a curve by plotting doses (independent variable) on abscissa versus the number of subjects providing this "prefixed" response (dependent variable) on ordinate. Obviously, the response, being quantified or prefixed on "all or none" basis, is a constant factor common to all subjects and can be eliminated. The curve, so obtained, is classified as "*quantal dose–response curve*". All these relationships are merely the graphic representations of mathe-matical expressions.

GRADED DOSE–RESPONSE CURVES

The graded dose-response curves are obtained by administering increasing doses of the drug to a single subject or to an isolated tissue. When the doses (in arithmetic scale) are plotted on abscissa, against the percent response, it will be noted that as the dose is increased, the magnitude of response also increases until a stage comes when a further increase in the dose elicits no further increase in the effect. The response at this stage is called as the "*maximal response (MR)*" or the ceiling response while the corresponding dose is called as the "*maximal dose (MD)*" or the ceiling dose. The graphic representation of such simple graded dose-response curve takes the form of a hyperbola (Fig. 7.14).

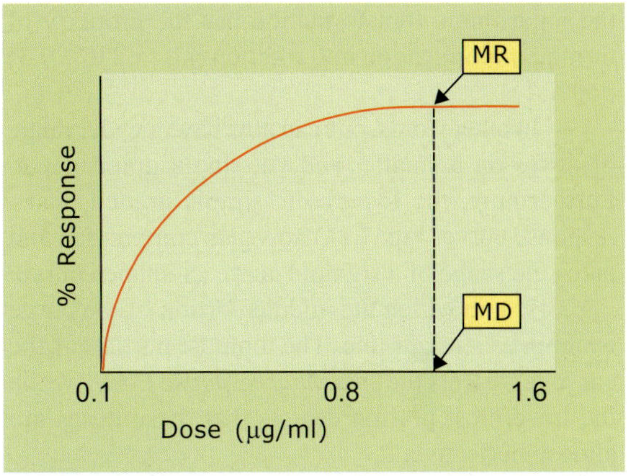

Fig 7.14 Simple Graded Dose-Response Curve

Limitations of a Simple Graded Dose–Response Curve

The initial portion of the curve (Fig. 7.14) is so steep that it is virtually impossible to guage the magnitude of increase in the response corresponding to the small increase in the doses. Precisely speaking, when the effect is approaching a maximum, large increments in dose (0.8 to 1.6 mg/ml) produce such changes in response which are actually too small to be evaluated with accuracy. On arithmetic scale, it is extremely difficult to display a dose range in which the largest dose (1.6 mg/ml) is several times that of the smallest (0.1 mg/ml). As a result, the huddling together of so many doses is inevitable or else an unusually wider graph paper would be needed to accommodate all these doses.

What we need is to have such an abscissa scale which can accommodate wider dose range on a smaller graph paper. It can be achieved if the doses are converted to their logarithms, i.e., when the doses are plotted on log scale.

LOG DOSE–RESPONSE CURVES

On the logarithmic scale, it may be noted that although each selected dose (0.1, 0.2, 0.4, 0.8 and 1.6 µg/ml) is just the double of its preceding dose, the interval between their log values is equal (1·0, 1·3, 1·6, 1·9 and 0·2, i.e., having a constant interval of 0.3) because the logarithmic transformation has the property of turning multiplication into addition (i.e., x 2 to + 0.3) (Fig. 7.15).

In other words, one can now have a wider range of doses on a smaller and yet single graph paper. Furthermore, the hyperbolic simple graded dose–response curve (Fig. 7.14) now gets compressed and takes the shape of a sigmoid curve (S-shaped curve, Fig. 7.15), in which the middle portion of the curve is almost a straight line. The topmost portion of the curve represents the "*maximal response (MR)*" while the lowermost portion depicts that these doses are almost ineffective.

The effect of increasing doses of histamine causing muscle contraction of guinea pig ileum and of acetylcholine causing contraction of frog rectus muscle are some examples where such *log dose–response relationships could be obtained.*

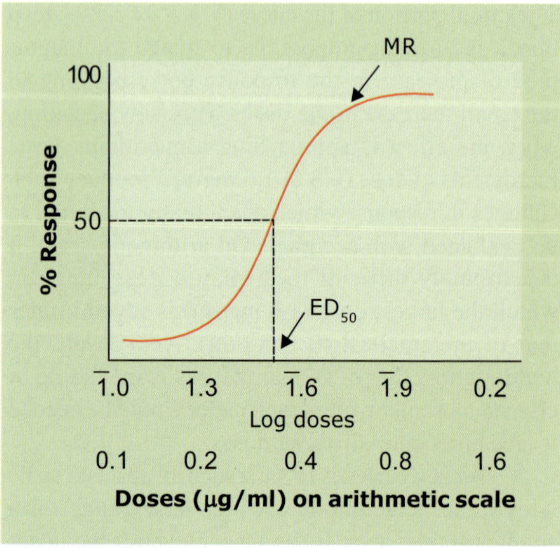

Fig 7.15 Calculation of ED_{50} from LDR Curve

Information Derived From Log Dose–Response Curves

i) From the middle porition of the curve (i.e., the linear segment) one can find out the ED_{50} of a drug. The ED_{50} here means *effective dose* which can provide 50% of the maximal response (because in this type of study, the isolated tissue is a constant factor which have been eliminated; obviously, since the study has been made on a single isolated tissue/subject, one cannot have 50% of the subject). Smaller the ED_{50}, more potent is the drug (Fig. 7.15).

ii) Frequently, two drugs produce the same effect by the same mechanism. In such cases the LDR curves of both the drugs run parallel to each other and among them the LDR curve of the less potent drug would be located on the right side, on the dose axis (Fig. 7.16).

For example, let us assume that drug A and drug B are producing the same effect by the same mechanism and drug B is half as potent as drug A. Then, in comparison, the response obtained by any dose of drug A would match with the response obtained with twice the dose of drug B. Therefore, all the corresponding points on the LDR curves of both the drugs will remain equally spaced, while the points on the curve of weaker drug B, will always lie equally spaced towards the right side of the curve for drug A. Converse is also true, i.e., two drugs that have non-parallel LDR curves, although may elicit qualitatively similar response, act by different mechanisms.

iii) Further, it also follows that the location of the LDR curve on the abscissa reflects the *affinity* of the drug with its receptor. The curve for the drug with greater affinity (i.e., acting at the lower concentration), will lie close to the ordinate (drug A, Fig. 7.16), while the curve for the drug with lesser affinity will lie farther towards right (drug B, Fig. 7.16).

iv) The LDR curves also help to differentiate between the *relative potency* and the *relative efficacy* of the drug. Hence the positioning of LDR curves of two drugs along the abscissa (the dose axis) provides an expression of their relative potencies. ***Potency*** means the dose of a drug required to

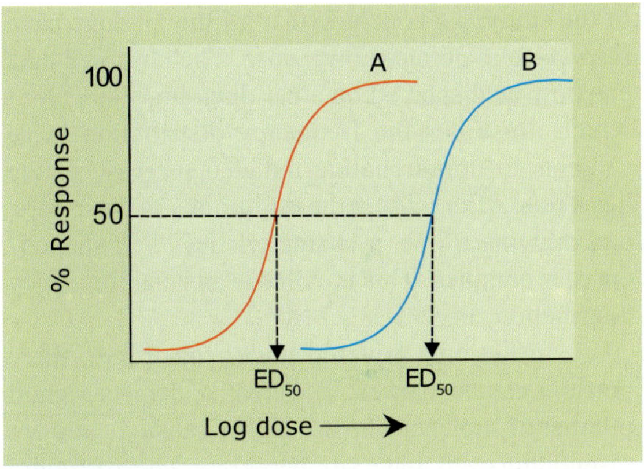

Fig 7.16 LDR Curves of Two Drugs With Different Potency

produce a standard effect. The closer the LDR curve is towards the ordinate, smaller is the dose required to produce the given effect and hence greater the potency. ***Efficacy***, on the other hand, denotes the maximal response as reflected by the height of the LDR curve on its ordinate (i.e., the response axis). In Fig. 7.17, the drug A is more potent than B or C but is less efficacious; the drug B is less potent but more efficacious than A, while more potent and equally efficacious than C.

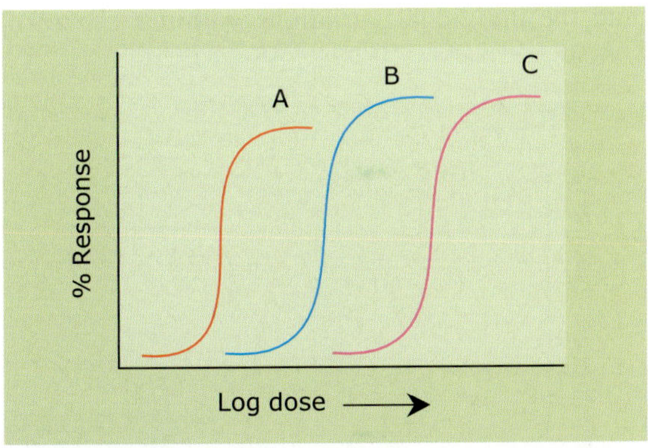

Fig 7.17 Difference Between Efficacy and Potency

Similarly, the drug C is less potent but more efficacious than A while less potent but equally efficacious to B. The potency of a drug tells us nothing about its efficacy and safety and is, therefore, a relatively unimportant characteristic for therapeutic purposes. Low potency becomes disadvantageous only when the size of the therapeutic dose is too awkward to administer, otherwise what really matters in therapeutics is that the dose should be both effective and safe, whatever be its magnitude.

QUANTAL DOSE–RESPONSE CURVES

So far, we have seen that the graded dose–response relationship is obtained in a single biological unit such as the isolated tissue or a single subject. The response elicited, e.g., contraction of smooth muscle, was measurable on a continuous scale. However, there are many pharmacological effects which cannot be measured as graded response on a continuous scale. For example, if you have to measure the acute toxicity of a drug, your criteria of response would be either death of an experimental animal or no death (there cannot be a go between like 'half dead' by the particular dose of the drug). Similarly, if you are studying the effect of barbiturates (thiopental) to induce anaesthesia, the response could be measured only on "all or none" basis, i.e., either anaesthesia or no-anaesthesia by a particular dose. One can prefix other responses as well, on "all or none" basis, e.g. 25% rise in heart rate from the base line (thus eliminating those subjects showing less than 25% rise, with a particular dose, as non-responders). Such predetermined responses on "all or none" basis are called as "quantal responses". Hence, when you keep the response as fixed it becomes a constant factor which can be eliminated as it is common to all subjects in a population. You can, now, derive another valuable relationship between the doses and the number of subjects exhibiting a "particular response" with these doses. A graphic curve can thus be obtained by plotting different doses on the abscissa (independent variable) versus the number of subjects providing a prefixed response, on the ordinate (dependent variable). The quantal dose–response curve, unlike graded dose–response curves, does not relate the dose of the drug to its magnitude of response, rather it relates the dose to the frequency with which it produces a predetermined response in a group of subjects or a population. By the term *frequency*, we mean the number of subjects exhibiting the 'stated response' to a certain dose of the drug. In a population, one would expect individuals to range from *very sensitive* (responding to unexpectedly low doses) to *sensitive* (responding to usual doses) and *least sensitive* (responding to uncommonly high doses).

To illustrate how a quantal dose–response curve is plotted between the subjects responding to the dose of a drug, the following example can be cited.

Suppose, we have to study the effect of I.V. infusion of noradrenaline on the enchancement of heart rate in dogs. The criterion of response has been fixed as "25% enhancement in the heart rate" and the test group consists of 50 dogs. When we have an infusion of 10 ng/kg/min, this end point was observed in 2 dogs only. Now these 2 dogs have to be eliminated from further experiments because once they have responded to 10 ng/kg/min dose these would respond to higher dose as well. When the dose was increased to 15 ng/kg/min, 4 more dogs elicited 25% rise in heart rate (in other words till now a total of 4+2 = 6 dogs have responded to a dose up to 15 ng/kg/min). Further, with 20 ng/kg/min infusion, another 6 dogs responded (i.e., by now 2+4+6 = 12 dogs in all, have responded to 20 ng/kg/min) and so on (Fig.7.18 a,b). After completion of the study, we conclude that all the 50 dogs have responded to 50 ng/kg/min dose. The observed data can now be displayed on a bar diagram (Fig. 7.18a) which illustrates the frequency distribution these subjects to noradrenaline-induced increase in the heart rate. After joining the mid-points of these bars, and drawing a line, a characteristics "bell shaped" curve is obtained. This is called a "normal frequency distribution curve" (Fig. 7.18 b).

In the area covered under this curve, three portions can be marked. The area 'A' depicts a small number of subjects who are highly sensitive and are responding even to the smaller doses. The maximum number of responders are found in the middle portion of the dose range (area 'B') while again a smaller number of subjects are least sensitive (or hyporeactive) because these have responded only to higher doses (area 'C'). The curve is called as "normal" because the quantitatively identical response in a population, produced by different doses, is distributed in a normal manner and can be expected in almost all types of such studies (e.g., while finding out IQs of thousands of people).

Limitations of Normal Frequency Distribution Curve

Although the bell-shaped curve provides adequate information concerning the average dose of a drug and the individual variations within a group of

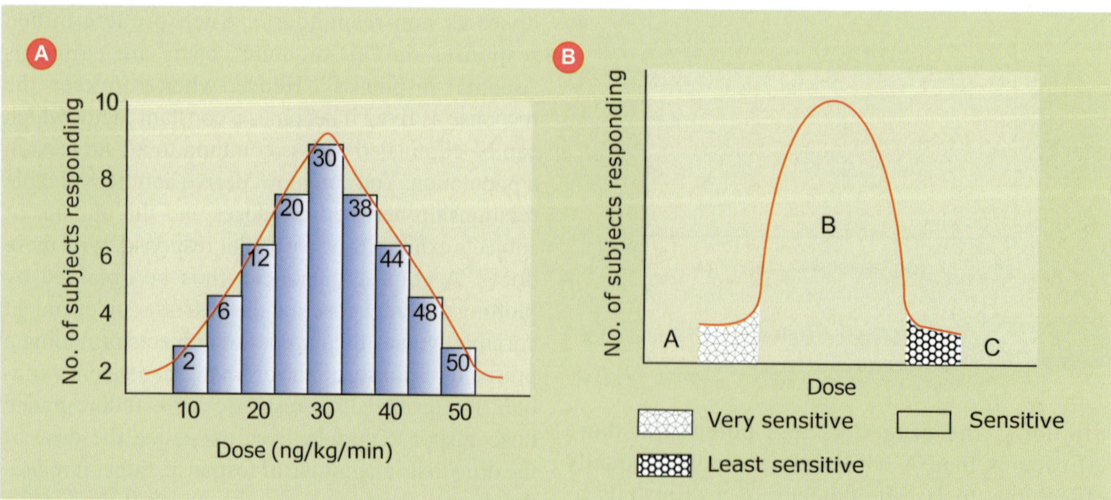

Fig 7.18 (a), (b) Frequency Distribution Curves

subjects, one cannot handle the data for calculation of ED_{50} or LD_{50} (see below), in the way these were handled with S-shaped LDR curves.

Summation of the Frequency Histogram

A convenient method of overcoming this shortcoming is to replot the data between the doses of the drug (in the log scale) on the abscissa and the cumulative percentage of animals responding, on the ordinate.

For example, as before, 2 out of 50 dogs responded to 10 ng/kg/min dose, i.e., the cumulative percent of animals responding is 4%. Similarly, when a total of 6 dogs out of 50 responded to 15 ng/kg/min dose, the cumulative percentage would be 12% and so on, till 50 out of 50 dogs have responded (100%). By doing such type of summation for every dose, one can obtain a sigmoid curve as shown in Fig. 7.19. This curve resembles the log dose-response curve with the difference that now it is plotted between the doses of the drug and cumulative percentage of subjects providing an "all or none" response (Fig. 7.19).

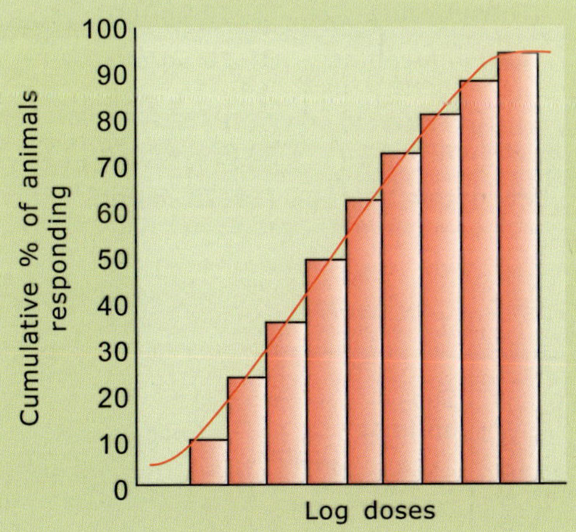

Fig 7.19 Summation of Frequency Histogram

Information Derived From Quantal Dose–Response Curves

i) As with LDR curves, from the middle linear segment of the curve, one can find out ED_{50} of the drug. ED_{50} here means a dose which provides a predetermined response in 50% of the subjects (Fig. 7.20).

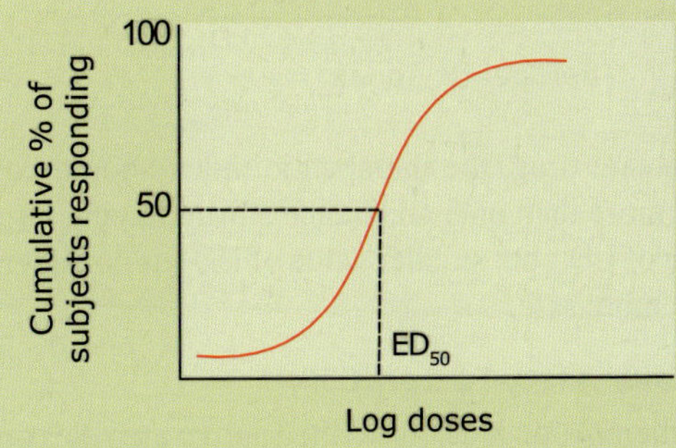

Fig 7.20 Calculation of ED_{50} from Quantal LDR

ii) Similarly, if mortality studies are made, we can find LD_{50} of the drug, which means a dose which is lethal to 50% of the subjects (Fig. 7.21). Mortality (and hence LD_{50}), is always a quantal response, as the criteria of death is an "all or none" phenomenon (Fig. 7.21).

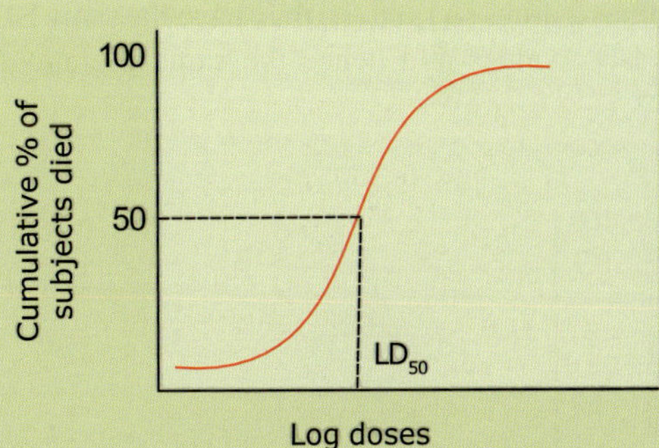

Fig 7.21 Calculation of LD_{50} from Quantal LDR

EVALUATION OF DRUG SAFETY

Therapeutic Index (margin of safety)

The safety of a drug depends on by what factor the dose producing a desirable effect is separated from the dose eliciting toxic effects. For finding out the margin of safety, we must calculate the *median lethal dose (LD_{50})* and *the median effective dose (ED_{50})* of the drug and then express their ratio. Such an expression is called as "therapeutic ratio" or the *therapeutic index*. Hence the

$$\text{Therapeutic Index} = \frac{LD_{50}}{ED_{50}}$$

For a safe drug, the therapeutic index should be at least more than one, and hence a drug having larger value of LD_{50} but smaller value of ED_{50} is considered to be more safe.

Certain Safety Factor (CSF)

The therapeutic index described above provides only an approximation of the relative safety of a drug. The drug safety, however, can be better assessed by having the ratio derived from the extremes of the respective quantal response curves, i.e., by finding out the ratio between the dose effective in 99% of the subjects (ED_{99}) and the dose which is lethal to 1% of the subjects (LD_1). This ratio is called *Certain Safety Factor (CSF)*

$$\text{Certain Safety Factor} = \frac{LD_1}{ED_{99}}$$

At times 2 drugs (A) and (B) may have the same ED_{50} and LD_{50} values and hence the same therapeutic index (Fig 7.22).

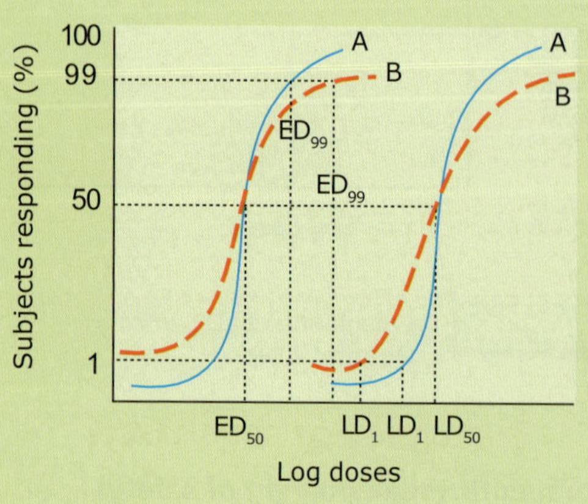

Fig 7.22 Calculation of Standard Safety Margin

An entirely different picture of their relative safety would emerge if we compare their certain safety factor. Obviously, drug (A) is more safe as its certain safety factor is more than one (because of higher LD_1 and lower ED_{99} values) as compared to drug (B). Hence, better judgement of relative safety can be made by utilising the extremes of LDR curves (ED_{99} & LD_1) of any drug.

Therapeutic Window

The frequency distribution diagram (Fig. 7.23) reveals that the same dose regimen produces a high plasma concentration and toxicity in some patients while a low plasma concentration or insufficient response in others. In between, there is an optimal therapeutic range of plasma concentrations at which most of the patients experience the desired effects. This optimal therapeutic range of plasma concentrations of the drug is called its *therapeutic window*. The plasma concentrations of some drugs (characterised by their low therapeutic index) that fall within the therapeutic window are given below:

Theophylline	(5–10 μg/ml)
Carbamazepine	(4–10 μg/ml)
Digoxin	(0.5–1.4 ng/ml)
Lithium	(0.8–1.4 mEq/L)
Phenytoin	(10–20 μg/ml)

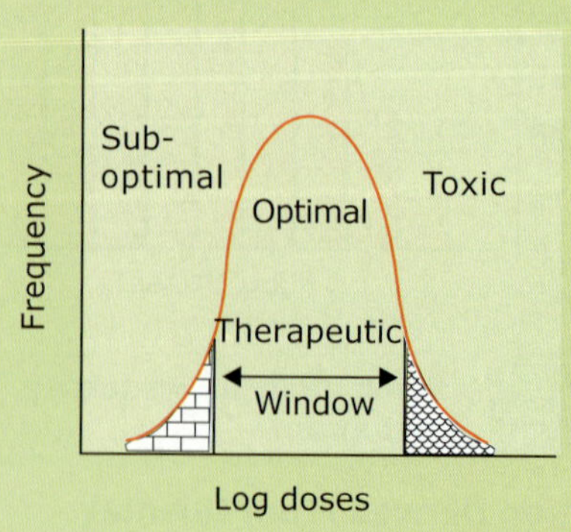

Fig 7.23 Therapeutic Window

FACTORS INFLUENCING DOSAGE AND DRUG RESPONSE

We have already defined the DOSE earlier. DOSES is its plural. However, there is another term called DOSAGE which literally means "the method of dosing" and represents a decision about four variables:

A. The dosage form and the amount of the drug to be administered at one time
B. The route of administration
C. The interval between doses, and
D. The duration for which the drug administration is to be continued.

For example: Cap Amoxycillin 500 mg, to be taken at 8 hourly interval, for 5 days is the usual *dosage* of this drug for a case of upper respiratory tract infection.

Here we deal with the following basic question: If an accepted normal dose of a drug is prescribed, why do some patients show either too much or too little response and what are the factors which influence the dosage of the drug and its response? A multitude of factors which influence the drug response in an individual and which necessitate an adjustment in drug dosage are discussed below.

BIOLOGICAL FACTORS

Various biological factors, account for the differences in drug response in individuals, e.g., difference in body weight, size, age, sex, inherited characteristics and the general state of health. It also includes variability in drug response attributable to conditions of drug administration *excluding those factors where drug effects are dependent on the previous administration of the same or concurrent administration of other drugs.*

Age, Body Weight and Body Surface Area

An average adult dose of a drug is calculated on the basis of the quantity that will produce a desired effect in 50% of population between 18 to 65 years of age and weighing about 70 kg (or 150 lb). Since the dose required is roughly proportional to body size and body build, the variation in effects produced by a drug can be minimised when the dose is determined on the basis of amount per kilogram of body weight. A special case of pharmacokinetic variation, leading to variations in drug response, is encountered in relation to dosage in children of different ages.

Many formulae are available for calculating the dose for a child who, obviously, requires a lesser dose than an adult. These formulae are based on age, weight or body surface area of a child.

i) Young's Formula

This is applicable for children up to 12 yr of age, and makes the assumption that a 12yr-old-should receive one-half of the adult dose.

$$\text{Child's Dose} = \frac{\text{Age in years}}{\text{Age} + 12} \times \text{Adult Dose}$$

ii) Dilling's Formula

It makes an assumption that a 20-yr-old should receive an adult dose.

$$\text{Child's Dose} = \frac{\text{Age in years}}{20} \times \text{Adult Dose}$$

iii) Clark's Formula

This is based simply on proportional body weight as related to an average adult weighing about 70 kg (150 lb).

$$\text{Child's Dose} = \frac{\text{Wt. of child (lb)}}{150} \times \text{Adult Dose}$$

However, for children, ***body surface area***, which is based on both height and weight, is a more precise index than body weight alone for adjustment of drug doses. Hence a more accurate method for calculating a dose for a child should be on the basis of his Body Surface Area (BSA). On obtaining the BSA, the child's dose can be calculated by the following formula:

$$\text{Child's Dose} = \frac{\text{BSA (m}^2\text{)}}{1.8} \times \text{Adult Dose}$$

The surface area rule is based on the assumption that the average adult weighing about 70 kg has a corresponding surface area of about 1.8 (approximately).

Nomograms are available which are generally used for finding out BSA from height and weight. In case, nomograms are not available readily with the physician, the following formula can also be used for a simplified approximation.

(1.5 x wt in kg) + 10 = Percentage of adult dose to be given to the child

OR

(0.7 x wt in lb) + 10 = Percentage of adult dose to be given to the child

Medicaments for topical use are usually not governed by these rules. Similarly, doses of antisera used for passive immunization (e.g., ADS and ATS) are not modified by age.

Sex

Drug responses in men and women are not always the same for which there may not be a satisfactory answer. Some paradoxical drug responses in women can, however, be cited. Morphine and barbiturates may produce excitation prior to sedation in women. Ephedrine may produce more excitation and tremors in women than in men. On the contrary, a number of drugs, like clonidine, α-methyldopa, β-blockers, diuretics and ketoconazole can cause loss of libido only in men but not in women.

Environment and Time of Drug Administration

The subjective effects of a drug may be markedly affected by the setup in which the drug has been taken. For example, slightly higher doses of sedative-hypnotics are needed to induce sleep in day light than at night. It has been noticed that glucocorticoids taken as single morning dose, minimise the risk of pituitary-adrenal suppression which is a serious hazard of long-term steroid therapy.

Psychological and Emotional Factors

Non-pharmacological factors also influence the drug response in certain individuals. Some patients even respond to the administration of pharmacologically inert material called the PLACEBO (Latin word meaning "I will please"). For details refer earlier discussion.

Derived from Latin, a NOCEBO ("I will harm") is the opposite of a PLACEBO ("I will please"). While the ***placebo*** relieves the symptoms of illness by creating expectations for the good, a ***nocebo*** harms by creating a panic or fear for nothing. ***Nocebo reactors*** are usually pessimistic persons whose symptoms of illness do not respond to medication. The harm of pessimism may be transient, chronic or even fatal. For example, patients are reported to die on the operation table because before entering the operation theatre, they were thinking that their death was imminent. Nocebo reactors usually prefer to consult a "Tantrik" (a witch doctor) or a soothsayer instead of a doctor, as they believe that some "black art" is responsible for their ailment. In such cases medicine hardly works unless it is profoundly supported by psychotherapy.

Genetic Factors and Idiosyncrasies

A small cross-section of a supposedly homogeneous population respond to drugs in an entirely unusual and highly unpredictable fashion. Some of these are genetically determined abnormal responses to drugs (pharmacogenetic reason). Others are idiosyncrasies, for which a satisfactory answer is still obscure. For details refer earlier discussion.

Metabolic Disturbances and Pathological State

Almost all the principles of pharmacokinetics have been developed from the data collected in normal healthy subjects. Drugs, however, are usually administered to people in whom the physiological, metabolic or biochemical processes are functioning at an abnormal level. It is, therefore, expected that a disease-induced abnormality may also modify a drug effect. A few examples can be cited:

i) Low acidity decreases iron (Fe^{2+}) absorption and results in a decreased response to iron therapy.

It also decreases aspirin absorption by favouring its ionisation;

ii) Bioavailability of drugs having first-pass metabolism is increased in patients having liver disease;

iii) In patients with impaired renal functions, drugs like streptomycin, gentamicin and kanamycin may accumulate to toxic levels causing nephrotoxicity and ototoxicity as these are not adequately excreted via kidneys;

iv) Patients with hyperthyroidism are very sensitive to sympathomimetics and are relatively resistant to digitalis or morphine. On the other hand, patients with hypothyroidism respond to these drugs in the opposite manner;

v) Drugs given orally in diarrhoea and vomiting may prove to be ineffective.

The Route and Frequency of Drug Administration

The route of administration governs the speed and intensity of drug response (refer Ch. 4). Drugs are usually administered according to their half-lives. But, at times, their administration has no bearing on their $t_{1/2}$. For example, the half-life of streptomycin is 2–4 hr, yet for the treatment of tuberculosis it is given in a dose of 15 mg/kg/day as a single I.M. injection for 2 to 3 months and then twice a week thereafter. It is because the *Mycobacterium tuberculosis* is a slow multiplying bacteria and once these are exposed to the antimicrobial action of streptomycin they remain inhibited for about 48–72 hr (post-antibiotic effect).

Sometimes a drug may exhibit an entirely diffe-rent response when administered by different routes. For example, magnesium sulfate causes purgation when given orally, reduces swelling when applied locally, but causes CNS depression and hypotension when given intravenously. At times, different mode of administration of the same drug is preferred for different therapeutic purposes. For example, oxytocin is infused slowly by I.V. route for induction of labour; it is given by I.M. injection to check postpartum haemorrhage while for let-down of milk from engorged breasts it is administered by intranasal spray.

MODIFIED DRUG EFFECTS AFTER REPEATED ADMINISTRATION OF A SINGLE DRUG

Drug Tolerance

Tolerance is characterised by the need to increase the dose in order to produce the pharmacological response of equal magnitude and duration. In other words, it is an inability of the subsequent administration of the same dose, of the same drug, to be as effective as its initial dose. Graphically, the log dose–response curve of a tolerant person shows a shift towards right side because higher than initial doses are required to achieve the same effect (Fig. 7.24).

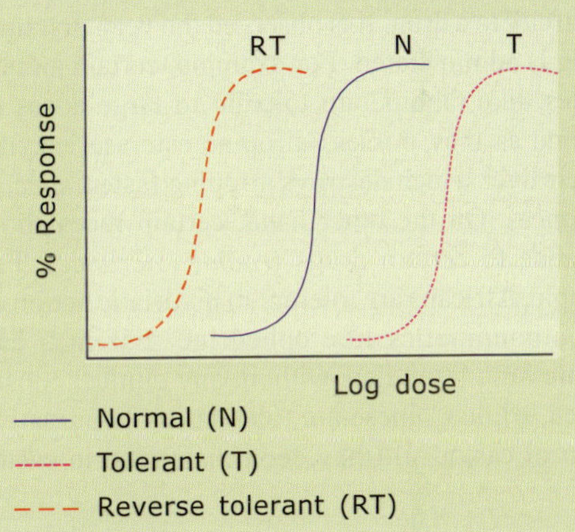

Fig 7.24 Development of Tolerance and Reverse Tolerance

Tolerance is a common phenomenon seen usually with CNS active drugs, like morphine, alcohol, barbiturates, LSD and amphetamine etc. It is not necessary that tolerance would develop uniformly to all pharmacological effects of a drug. For example, tolerance develops to all pharmacological effects of morphine (to varying degrees) except for miosis and constipation. The tolerance developed to CNS active drugs is frequently associated with either psychological or physical dependence. In the present discussion, however, we are concerned with the general aspects of this phenomenon and the mechanism involved for its development.

There is another term called as "reverse tolerance" (or sensitisation) which is also observed with an intermittent dosing schedule but is opposite to the phenomenon of tolerance. With reverse tolerance there is a leftward shift of the log dose–response curve, such that for a given dose there is a greater response than seen after the initial dose (Fig. 7.24). For example, after repeated daily administration of a dose of cocaine or amphetamine in rats, there is a gradual increase in their motor activity even though the dose remains constant.

Drug tolerance may be of the following types:

i) Innate (natural or congenital) Tolerance

This refers to the genetically determined lack of sensitivity to a drug. It is observed the very first time a drug is administered. For example, certain animal species, like rabbits, are tolerant to large doses of atropine as they possess atropine esterase enzyme in their liver which destroys atropine faster (*species tolerance*). On the other hand, certain races show tolerance to certain drugs (*racial tolerance*). For example, Africans are tolerant to mydriatic action of sympathomimetics like ephedrine. Eskimos can tolerate high fatty diets without any clinical consequence, while Chinese are tolerant to the purgative action of castor oil (they cook their food in castor oil).

ii) Acquired Tolerance

This is seen by repeated use of a drug in an individual who was initially responsive. This type of tolerance is not inherent, rather is acquired at a later stage after repeated administration of the drug. The acquired tolerance can result due to either pharmacokinetic or pharmacodynamic reasons. The tolerance developing through the first mechanism is called as *drug disposition (*or *metabolic) tolerance,* and that by second mechanism is called as *cellular adaptive* or *target tissue* or *pharmacodynamic tolerance*.

1. Drug Disposition or Metabolic Tolerance

This type of tolerance may occur when a drug reduces its own absorption or increases its own metabolism through microsomal enzyme induction. The net result is the decrease in the effective concentration of the drug at the site of action. The higher doses taken by the tolerant person are simply compensating for the losses incurred due to faster drug disposition.

The example for the pharmacokinetic tolerance resulting due to poor absorption is that of alcohol. Chronic alcoholics can tolerate large amounts of alcohol because of their thickened (indurated) gastric mucosa which reduces the extent of alcohol absorption. The examples of pharmacokinetic tolerance resulting due to increase in the rate of biotransformation through enzyme induction are barbiturates (see earlier text). An example of pharmacokinetic tolerance resulting due to faster excretion is that of amphetamine. This drug suppresses appetite and when the person continues taking the drug in preference to food, ketosis results. Ketosis acidifies the urine and promotes ionisation of this basic drug, leading to its faster excretion. As a result more dose is needed to produce the same euphoric effects.

2. Cellular Adaptive (target tissue or pharmacodynamic) Tolerance

This type of tolerance may be attributed to some kind of adaptive changes that have taken place within the system after repeated drug administration. This may result due to either (1) drug-induced changes in the receptor density (down-regulation) or (2) impairment in receptor coupling to signal transduction pathways (see earlier discussion). Examples include drugs like morphine and its congeners, caffeine, nicotine and LSD.

3. Acute Tolerance (Tachyphylaxis)

This term is used to describe the acute development of tolerance after a rapid and repeated administration of a drug at shorter intervals.

Tachyphylaxis may result primarily due to any of the following reasons:

a) Gradual depletion of the agonist from the storage vesicles with no chances of its replenishment because of the repeated administration of the drug at short intervals. For example, tachyphylaxis seen with indirectly acting sympathomimetics like ephedrine, amphetamine and tyramine. These drugs act by releasing catecholamines (from the storage sites), the synthesis of which is unable to match its release. Hence, further response decreases due to nonavailability of adequate stores of catecholamines.

b) Tachyphylaxis may also occur as a result of a change in the sensitivity of target cells (pharmacodynamic reason). For example, tachyphylaxis to nitroglycerin is observed among workers exposed to this drug in its manufacturing industry. On Monday or Tuesday, these workers suffer severe headache (vasodilatory effects of nitroglycerin) which gradually disappears by Friday due to the development of tachyphylaxis. After enjoying their weekend on Saturday and Sunday when they return to their job on Monday, the headache reappears (and hence the term called "Monday disease" to describe the return of symptoms after a weekend away from work).

Difference between tachyphylaxis and tolerance

1. Tachyphylaxis is rarely seen in clinical practice since repeated administration of drugs at short intervals is not customary in therapy. However, it can be demonstrated experimentally on isolated tissues etc. Tolerance, on the other hand, is observed clinically.

2. Tachyphylaxis develops faster due to repetition of doses in quick succession. Tolerance develops slowly and is observed with intermittent dosing schedules (e.g., after every 2nd or 3rd day).

3. In tolerance, the original effect of the drug can still be obtained by increasing the dose, which is not possible in tachyphylaxis, either due to exhaustion of mediators or due to faster desensitisation of target cells (with no chances of recovery due to repeated dosing in quick succession).

iii) Cross Tolerance

Another characteristic feature of tolerance is that of cross tolerance among drugs belonging to the same category. For instance, individuals tolerant to morphine are also tolerant to heroin and other narcotic analgesics.

Drug Resistance

It refers to unresponsiveness of microorganisms to an antimicrobial agent after its repeated use and is akin to the phenomenon of tolerance seen in higher organisms. The drug resistance could be of three types:

i) Natural Resistance

Some microorganisms have always been resistant to certain antibiotics, e.g., Gram-negative bacilli are normally unaffected by penicillin-G; *Mycobacterium tuberculosis* is insensitive to tetracyclines or cephalosporins etc. This type of resistance poses no significant clinical problem as only the proper drugs which are effective against the particular microorganisms are to be selected.

ii) Acquired Resistance

It is the subsequently developed resistance by a microorganism (which was initially sensitive) due to the use of an antimicrobial agent over a period of time. For example, some bacteria like staphylococci, coliform or tubercle bacilli quickly and most commonly develop resistance to the antimicrobial agents used. In the past 20 years, highly penicillin resistant gonococci have emerged. This type of resistance develops either by gene transfer (conjugation, transduction or transformation) or by mutation.

iii) Cross Resistance

If a microorganism resistant to one antimicrobial agent exhibits resistance to another antimicrobial drug belonging to the same category (to which the organism was not exposed earlier), it is called as cross resistance. For example, a microorganism becoming resistant to one sulfa drug exhibits resistance to all sulfonamides. Sometimes, unrelated drugs also exhibit partial cross resistance, e.g., a microorganism resistant to erythromycin exhibits resistance to lincomycin.

Drug Allergy

Allergy is an adverse, unexpected response to the usual therapeutic doses of a drug resulting from a previous exposure to the same substance (refer earlier discussion). If such an unusual response occurs, the physician has to not only take care of the toxicity but also seek an alternative drug for the therapy.

Cumulation

Cumulation occurs when the rate of removal or inactivation of a drug is slower than the rate of its administration. Such a phenomenon can lead to dangerous overdosage and toxicity. Cumulation is more likely when the drug has a long half-life (e.g., digoxin, emetine, chloroquine and heavy metals like lead) but may also be associated with certain highly lipid-soluble drugs having shorter half-lives, e.g., thiopental, where considerable quantities of the drug still remain in the body due to its redistribution to tissues and fat. For drugs like digoxin, a loading dose is given initially to achieve the desired level of the drug in the body and the therapy is continued with such smaller doses that the drug input into the body equals the drug removed from the body in the interval between the doses. These are called as maintenance doses. This practice is followed to avoid accumulation. If care is not taken in selecting the proper maintenance dose and its dosage schedule, the toxicity may result due to cumulation. That is why, the maintenance dose of digoxin is given 5 days a week to avoid the risk of cumulation after long-term therapy. The retinal toxicity resulting after prolonged use of chloroquine is a result of its cumulative toxicity.

MODIFIED DRUG EFFECTS AFTER CONCURRENT ADMINISTRATION OF TWO DIFFERENT DRUGS

Summation

When two drugs elicit the same response, *but with different mechanism,* and their combined effect is equal to the algebraic sum of their individual effects, the drugs are said to exhibit summation of effects (Fig. 7.25).

Thus a tablet containing aspirin and codeine is providing analgesic effect due to summation as these work by different mechanisms.

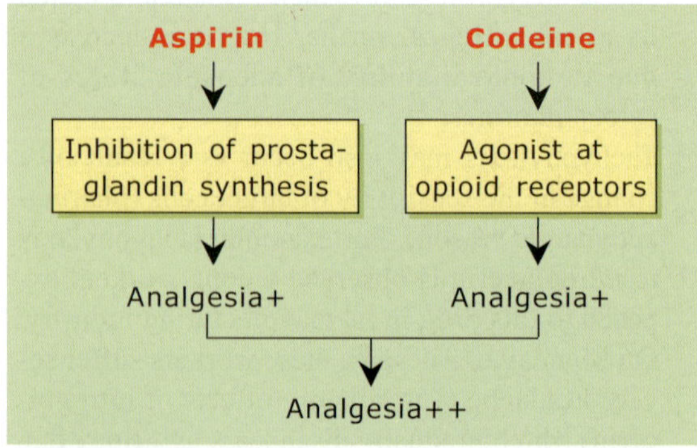

Fig 7.25 Summation of Drug Effects

Additive Effects

This term is usually used in those cases in which the combined effect of two drugs, *acting by the same mechanism,* is equal to that expected by simple addition. For example, ibuprofen and paracetamol apparently act by the same mechanism and hence their combined analgesic effect is an additive effect (Fig. 7.26).

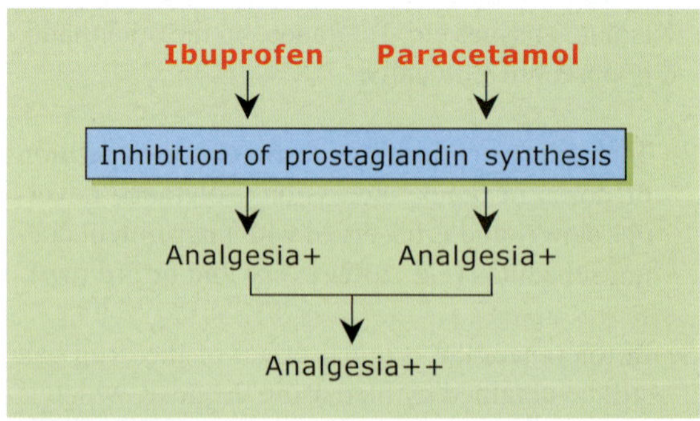

Fig 7.26 Addition of Drug Effects

Synergism

When the combined effect of two drugs is greater than the algebraic sum of their individual effects, the phenomenon is called as synergism. The net outcome of synergism is either the potentiation or prolongation of effects. This may result when two drugs act at different sites or when one drug alters the pharmacokinetics of the other drug. The best example of synergistic action of two drugs acting at different sites is that of sulfamethoxazole combined with trimethoprim. Individually, each drug is bacteriostatic but the combination (cotrimoxazole) becomes bactericidal. In this combination, sulfamethoxazole inhibits the folic acid synthesis in the bacteria by competing with PABA for the enzyme dihydropteroic acid synthetase while trimethoprim sequentially blocks folic acid synthesis by inhibiting dihydrofolate reductase (Fig. 7.27). Other such examples where two drugs show synergistic action by acting through different sites is the synergistic action of antihypertensive drugs (e.g. β-blockers) with diuretics (frusemide).

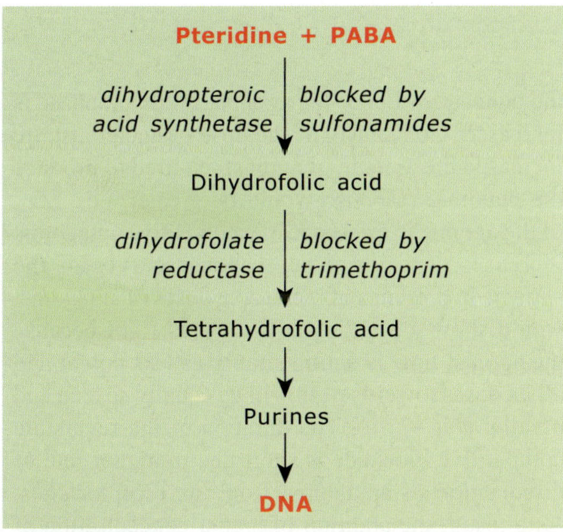

Fig 7.27 Synergistic Effect of Drugs

An example of synergism where one drug alters the pharmacokinetics of the other is: Levodopa + Carbiodopa (for the treatment of parkinsonism). Carbidopa prevents the peripheral metabolic degradation of levodopa, thus favouring greater amounts of levodopa to reach the brain (Fig. 7.28).

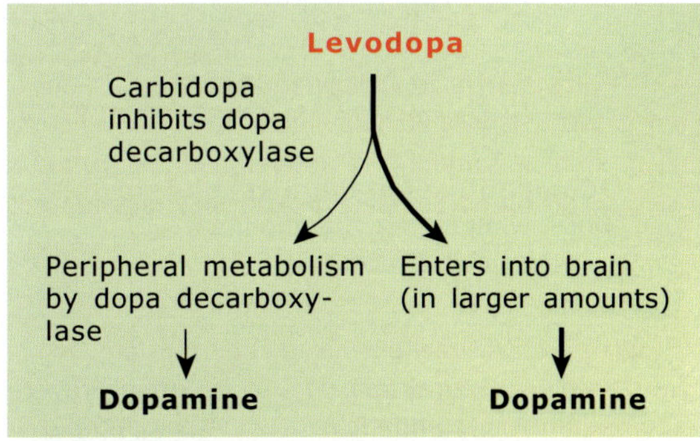

Fig 7.28 Synergistic Effect of Drugs

Drug Antagonism

Any time when the combined effect of two drugs is less than the sum of the effects of the individual drugs, the phenomenon is called as drug antagonism. There are four mechanisms by which one drug may oppose the action of another, and these are:

i) Chemical Antagonism

This is when the drugs act merely as chemical antidotes to each other; for instance, the anticoagulant effect of the strong negatively charged macromolecule heparin is antagonised by protamine which is a highly positively charged protein. This is analogous to the neutralization of excess gastric acid by any of the antacids like aluminium hydroxide, magnesium hydroxide or sodium bicarbonate; or to the chelating action of drugs, like BAL or calcium sodium edetate, which form inactive soluble complexes with heavy metals like arsenic or lead.

ii) Physiological or Functional Antagonism

This is when two agonists, acting at different receptors, counterbalance each other by producing opposite effects on the same physiological system. For example, CNS stimulants antagonise the effects of CNS depressants, or the effects of histamine on blood pressure (vasodilatation) can be cancelled out by norepinephrine (vasoconstriction). The essential point about physiological antagonism is that the effects produced by the two drugs counteract each other, but each drug is unhindered in its ability to elicit its own response (unlike pharmacological antagonism; see below).

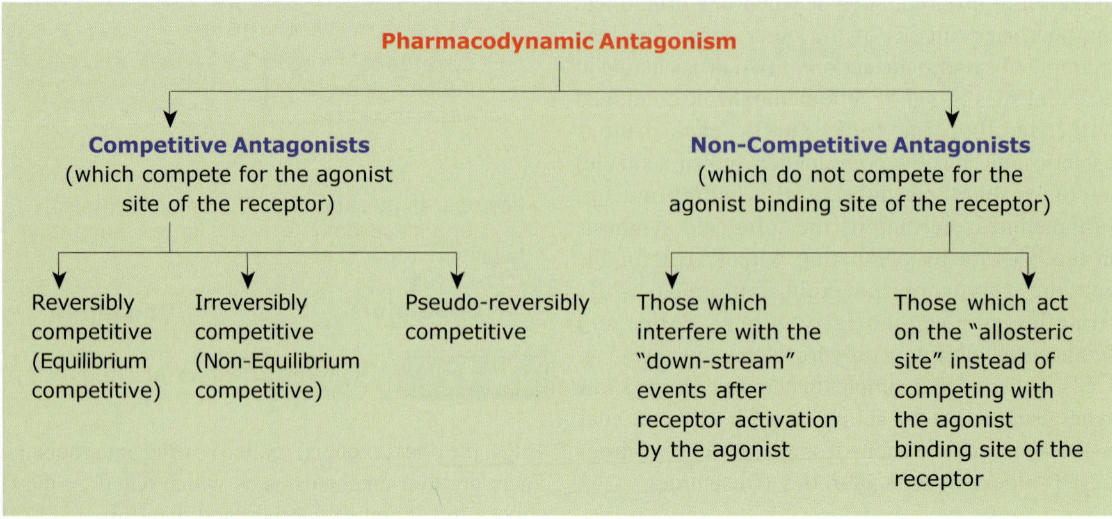

Fig 7.29 Classification of Pharmacodynamic Antagonism

iii) Pharmacological (Pharmacodynamic) Antagonism

It is a pharmacodynamic antagonism (for classification see Fig. 7.29) wherein the antagonist *either* competes with the agonist for its binding sites on the receptor *(competitive antagonism) or* may antagonise the effects of agonist by acting at a site different from the agonist receptor site *(non-competitive antagonism).*

a) Competitive Antagonism

This is the most commonly observed pharmacological antagonism. Here, the antagonist combines and competes with the same receptor sites as does the agonist but does not induce its own response (i.e., has no intrinsic activity). These are classified into 3 subtypes depending on the type of the bonding formed between the antagonist and the receptor.

i) *Reversibly Competitive or Equilibrium Competitive Antagonism*: This type of antagonism is frequently observed with antagonists that bind reversibly (by forming weak bonds) to the same receptor sites as that of agonists. Hence, the antagonism can be overcome (surmounted), and the maximal response of the agonist can be attained if the concen-tration of the agonist, in the biophase is increased. Conversely, if the dose of antagonist are increased the amount of agonist required to produce the maximal response would be greater, i.e., ED_{50} of the agonist in presence of a competive antagonist increases. The log dose–response curves of the agonist, in presence of increasing doses of antagonist would show a parallel shift towards right because the agonist now is acting simply as less potent and all its doses towards right will be equally spaced and parallel (Fig. 7.30). The duration of the reversible competitive blockade is short due to higher rate of dissociation of antagonist from the receptor sites. As a result, the addition of higher concentration of agonist reduces the overall receptor occupancy of the antagonist and a new competitive equilibrium is rapidly established between the agonist and the antagonist (hence the term 'equilibrium competitive antagonism').

Examples: Atropine is a reversibly competitive antagonist of acetylcholine or bethanechol at various muscarinic receptors; naloxone is a similar antagonist of morphine at different opioid receptors while propranolol is a similar antagonist of norepinephrine at β_1 adrenoceptor.

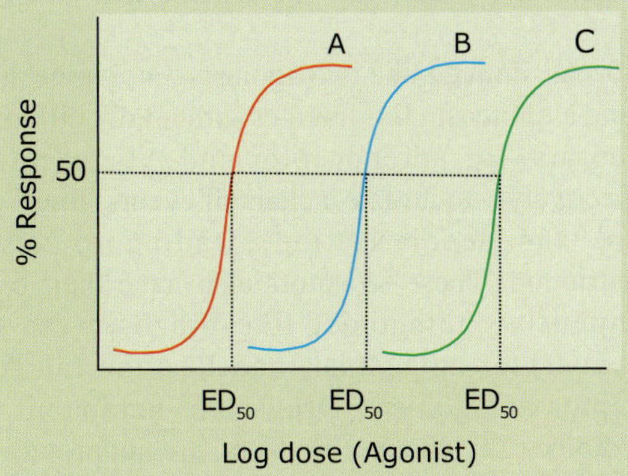

A: LDR curve for agonist alone.
B: LDR curve for agonist in presence of competitive antagonist.
C: LDR curve for the agonist plus increasing concentration of competitive antagonist.

Fig 7.30 Competitive Antagonism

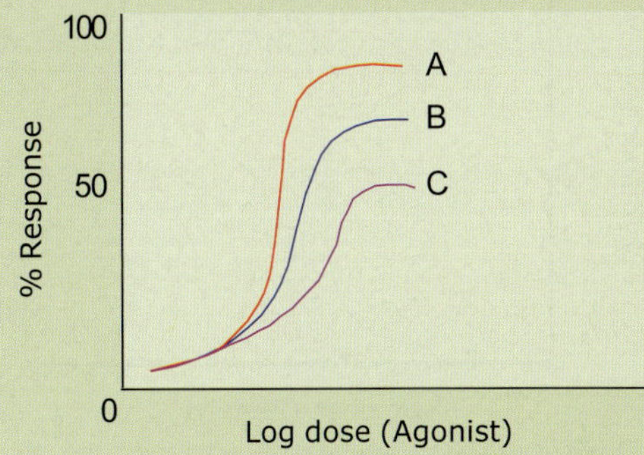

A: LDR curve for agonist alone.
B: LDR curve for agonist in presence of irreversible antagonist.
C: LDR curve for the agonist plus increasing concentration of irreversible antagonist.

Fig 7.31 Irreversibly Competitive Antagonism

ii) *Irreversibly Competitive or Non-Equilibrium Competitive Antagonism*: Such antagonists also have only the affinity for the same receptor sites (as of the agonists) but bind to it in an irreversible manner by forming a stable covalent bond. Here the antagonist dissociates very slowly or not at all from the receptors and its effects cannot be overcome even by increasing the concentration of the agonist (i.e., unsurmountable). Characteristically, the LDR curves of the agonist (in presence of this antagonist) would show reduced efficacy (i.e., reduced maximal response of the agonist) but unaltered potency (i.e., no change in the location of the curve at dose axis; see Fig. 7.31). The duration of action of the irreversible antagonist is longer as its rate of dissociation from the receptor is very slow. As a result an equilibrium between the antagonist and the agonist cannot be established even after increasing the doses of agonist (hence the term 'non-equilibrium competitive antagonism').

Example: Dibenamine (a haloalkylamine) is an irreversible competitive antagonist of norepinephrine at α_1 adrenoceptor.

iii) *Pseudo-reversible Antagonism*: In few cases (e.g., phenoxybenzamine, a pseudo reversible α_1 adrenoceptor blocker or methysergide, a pseudoreversible 5HT receptor blocker) the classical irreversible antagonism, described above, may not be that obvious. This happens due to a lesser degree of receptor occupancy by pseudoreversible type of antagonist, and also due to availability of spare receptors. As a result, increasing concentrations of the agonist, in presence of such antagonist will initially shift the LDR curves to the right showing the maximal response (because of the response from spare receptors), but eventually if the concentration of this antagonist is increased there will be reduction in the maximal response (Fig.7.32). Hence the term: 'pseudo-reversible competitive antagonism'.

b) Non-Competitive Antagonism

Some texts refer the "irreversible antagonism" as "non-competitive antagonism". It is now clear that the term "non-competitive" should be reserved for antagonism that does not involve occupation of same receptor sites. It is of 2 subtypes: the antagonist may interfere with the down-stream events after receptor activation by the agonist *or* a drug may antagonise

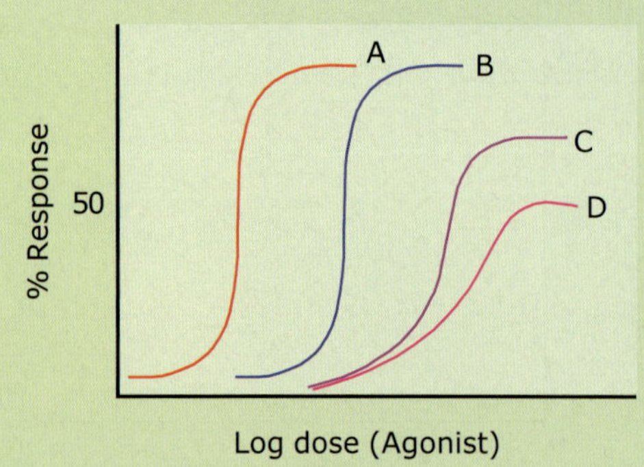

A: LDR curve for agonist alone.
B: LDR curve for agonist in presence of pseudo-reversible antagonist.
C & D: LDR curve for the agonist plus increasing concentration of pseudo-reversible antagonist.

Fig 7.32 Pseudo-reversible Antagonism

the effects of other drug by acting at a modulatory site (or allosteric site) of the receptor beyond the binding site for the agonist.

i) *Non-competitive Antagonism Through Interference in the Down-stream Events of Receptor Activation*: To understand this type of antagonism let us follow the scheme laid down in Fig. 7.33.

As noticed, the two agonists—norepinephrine and angiotensin II—interact with totally different receptors—α_1 adrenoceptor and AT_1 receptor, respectively—to initiate a chain of events (free Ca^{2+} entry and depolarisation) leading to vasoconstriction. These receptors also have their own competitive antagonist like prazosin (an α_1 adrenoceptor antagonist) and losartan (an AT_1 receptor antagonist). Drugs like verapamil or nifedipine (Ca^{2+} channel blockers) are not providing antihypertensive effects by virtue of being α_1 or AT_1 receptor antagonist but by preventing the opening of voltage-gated Ca^{2+} channel. Thus, they inhibit the Ca^{2+} entry associated with depolarisation which leads to vasodilatation. Calcium channel blocking drugs are therefore non-competitive antagonist of both norepinephrine and angiotensin II because instead **of blocking α_1 or AT_1** receptors, they have blocked the down-stream chain of events due to receptor activation by both these agonists.

The non-competitive antagonism as well as the irreversible competitive antagonism exhibit the same pattern of log dose–response curve as shown in Fig. 7.31. But the irreversible competitive

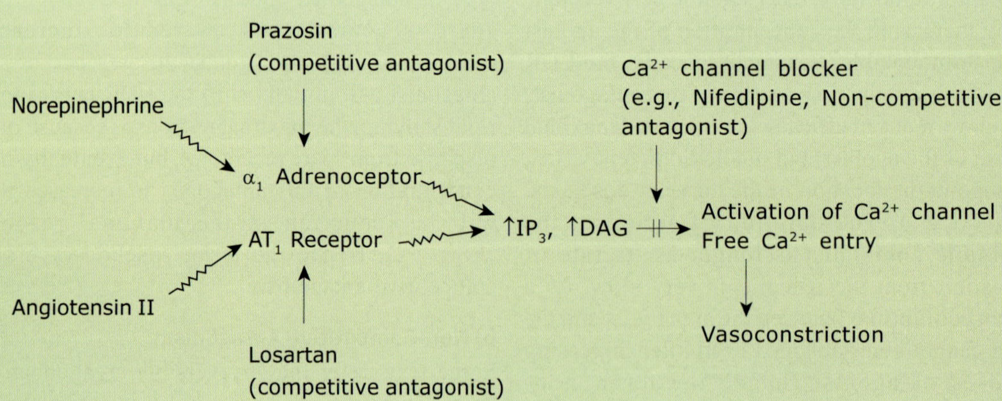

Fig 7.33 Difference Between Competitive and Non-competitive Antagonist. A single example can be cited to distinguish these antagonisms: NE actions on α_1 adrenoceptors can be blocked by a competitive antagonist—prazosin; a pseudo-reversible antagonist—phenoxybenzamine; an irreversible antagonist—dibenamine; and a non-competitive antagonist—nifedipine.

antagonists are specific against one type of agonists, while the non-competitive antagonists are non-specific in action as they can antagonise different agonists acting through more than one receptor system, provided their final down-stream events are same.

ii) *Antagonism Through Allosteric Receptor Site Binding*: Allosteric receptor antagonists bind to the receptor at a site other than the agonist site. They do not compete directly with agonist for receptor binding but rather prevent the receptor activation by the agonist. Example: Flumazenil (by binding to benzodiazepine site) antagonises the effects of benzodiazepines by preventing the binding of GABA to $GABA_A$ receptor. Hence flumazenil does not compete directly with the agonist (GABA) for its binding site at $GABA_A$ receptor but rather prevents its activation by modulation through allosteric (Fig. 7.34) binding. Such antagonists do not affect the inherent basal receptor activity (as of $GABA_A$ receptor, cf inverse agonists).

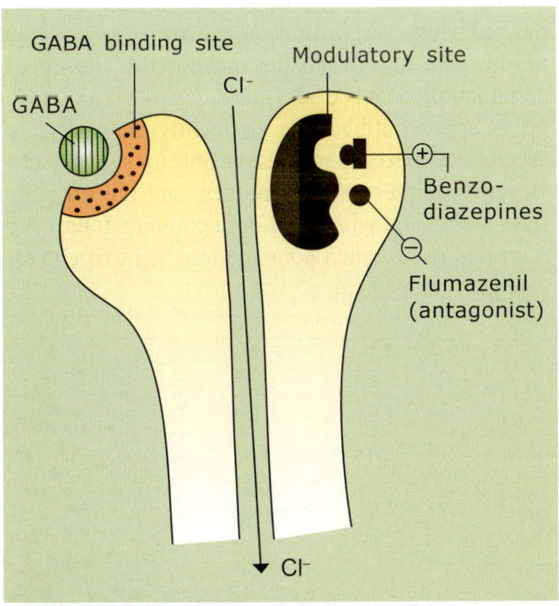

Fig 7.34 Non-competitive Antagonism Through Allosteric Receptor Binding Site

Similarly, bicuculline which is a competitive antagonist of binding of GABA to its receptor sites, indirectly blocks the effects of benzodiazepines (BZDs) like diazepam non-competitively; becuase BZDs facilitate GABA-ergic activity by binding at the modulatory site of GABA receptor (i.e., binding sites of both the drugs are different).

Drug Combinations

Multiple drug therapy involves either (a) the concurrent administration of more than one drug (leading to drug-drug interactions) or (b) simultaneous administration of two drugs mixed in a single dosage form (the fixed-dose formulations).

i) Drug-Drug Interactions

An alteration in the effectiveness or toxicity of one drug due to another simultaneously administered drug is known as drug-drug interaction. Drug interactions may result in: (a) adverse effects wherein there is a decrease in the effectiveness or an increase in the toxicity of one drug in the presence of other drug or (b) biological interference with laboratory tests which may mislead the diagnosis or (c) beneficial effects, wherein there is an increase in the effectiveness or a decrease in the toxicity of one drug in the presence of another.

Adverse drug interaction can happen either (a) *in vitro*, for example penicillins and amino-glycoside group of antibiotics inactivate each other if mixed in the same syringe; thiopentone and suxamethonium, in the same syringe culminate precipitation; or (b) *in vivo,* where drug interactions occur either due to *pharmacokinetic reasons* or due to *pharmacodynamic reasons.*

Pharmacokinetic reasons include:

1. *Alteration in absorption* e.g., antacids of Ca^{2+}, Mg^{2+}, Al^{3+} group, or milk or iron decrease the effect of tetracyclines by hindering its absorption; and liquid paraffin decreases the absorption of fat-soluble vitamins A, D and E;
2. *Alteration in distribution,* e.g., salicylates and sulfonamides displace tolbutamide and warfarin from their protein binding sites leading to hypoglycaemia and haemorrhage, respectively;
3. *Alteration in metabolism,* e.g., enzyme inducers like barbiturates decrease the anticoagulant

effect of warfarin while rifampicin blunts the effects of oral contraceptives. Conversely, enzyme inhibitors like tolbutamide or metronidazole produce antabuse type of effects after alcohol consumption; and MAOIs potentiate respiratory depression due to morphine because of enzymatic inhibition;

4. *Alteration in excretion,* e.g., acidification of urine increases excretion of basic drugs like amphetamine and morphine; while alkalinisation of urine accelerates excretion of acidic drugs, like phenobarbitone and salicylates.

Drug interactions of pharmacodynamic nature result due to:

(a) *Different types of pharmacological antagonism as discussed above* or (b) *interference with neuronal uptake or neurotransmitter release* (e.g., tricyclic antidepressants, like imipramine blunt the antihypertensive effect of clonidine) or (c) *additive or summative action* (e.g., aminoglycosides + d-tubocurarine lead to respiratory paralysis; aminoglycosides + ethacrynic acid increase ototoxicity and digitalis + propranolol lead to brady-cardia due to unopposed vagal effects of digitalis) or (d) *changes in ionic balance* (e.g., digitalis + loop diuretics increase digitalis toxicity due to hypokalaemia; corticosteroids decrease the effects of antihypertensive drugs due to Na^+ retention).

Examples of drug interactions which interfere with diagnostic tests (and thus mislead the diagnosis) include:

(a) Nalidixic acid, salicylate and vitamin C which provide a false-positive test of urine sugar with Benedict's solution or with Clintest (as these are reducing agents by themselves) and (b) estrogens exhibit false-positive rise in the values of serum thyroxine (as they cause hyperproteinaemia).

Drug interactions can lead to beneficial effects either (a) in therapeutics (e.g., a combination of sulfamethoxazole + trimethoprim called cotrimoxazole, has synergistic antibacterial activity; combination of carbidopa + levodopa, in the treatment of parkinsonism, provides enhanced levels of levodopa in brain as carbidopa prevents peripheral degradation of levodopa by dopamine decarboxylase) or (b) in the management of poisoning (e.g., use of naloxone in morphine poisoning and use of atropine + pralidoxime in the treatment of organophosphorous poisoning).

ii) Fixed-dose Drug Combinations

Concurrent but separate administration of drugs permits proper manipulation of the dosage of individual drugs so that the maximum benefits can be achieved with minimum undersirable effects. The timing of administration can also be adjusted if desired. However, in a *fixed-dose drug combination* neither the individual dosage nor the timing of administration can be adjusted if desired. If any toxic effect appears it becomes frequently impossible to ascertain which drug was responsible for such effects. Because of these disadvantages, and the possible risks associated with fixed-dose combinations, only a limited use of such combinations is justified (for examples refer Ch. 6).

CHAPTER 8 Drug Discovery and Clinical Evaluation of New Drugs

COMPETENCY PH1.6, PH1.64

Until the end of nineteenth century, the useful life of a drug was considered to be 30 to 50 years but by the end of twentieth century it came down to one or two decades. This has resulted because of the strict regulations governing the development of new drugs that have evolved over the last three decades, to assure their safety and efficacy. In this chapter we shall trace the development of a new drug from its genesis in the chemical laboratory, to its final acceptance as a safe and useful therapeutic agent, under Schedule Y of Drugs and Cosmetics Act (10th Amendment) 2001, which were amended later in 2005.

Broadly speaking the *drug development* process can be divided into 3 main phases, namely:

1. ***Drug discovery phase,*** during which the candidate molecules are chosen on the basis of their pharmacological properties.
2. ***Preclinical phase,*** during which a wide range of animal studies are performed, e.g., pharmacokinetic, pharmacodynamic and toxicity studies.
3. ***Clinical trial phase,*** during which the *lead compound* is evaluated for efficacy, safety, and adverse effects in human volunteers and patients.

DRUG DISCOVERY PHASE

Most new drugs are discovered and identified through one of the following approaches:

1. Random Screening

It is a sort of blind hitting procedure where new chemical entities (natural or synthetic) are subjected to a battery of pharmacological screening procedures designed to explore different types of biological activity. Such tests include studies on animal behaviour, animal models of the disease and on isolated tissues as well. Although such approaches are cumbersome, time consuming, expensive and seemingly inefficient in providing fruitful results, nonetheless, these are at times valuable, since many drugs like morphine, atropine, digitalis and quinidine were derived this way from folklore medicinals. Cyclosporine, an immunosuppressant drug which was discovered during the course of routine screening of fungal products, constitutes another such example.

2. Serendipity (happy observation, by chance)

Sometimes, a new use is discovered for an old drug or its side effects find a new therapeutic application. For example, lignocaine (local anaesthetic) and phenytoin (antiepileptic) were later used as antiarrhythmics. Methotrexate, an anticancer drug, is also used for psoriasis, while cyclophosphamide and azathioprine (both cytotoxic drugs) are also used to prevent tissue rejection in kidney transplant. Penicillin was also discovered this way, which heralded the beginning of antibiotic therapy.

3. Rational Drug Designing

Two basic strategies are used in rational drug designing. First is the *compound-centered approach*, another is *target-centered approach.*

Promising agents, through *compound-centered approach,* could be obtained from *natural products,* e.g., penicillin from the mold *penicillum notatum*; paclitaxel—an anticancer drug—derived from Pacific yew tree; and cyclosporine—an immunosuppressive drug—obtained from fungus. The main disadvantage in obtaining lead products from natural source is that these are often complex molecules which are difficult to be synthesised. It is ultimately difficult to synthesise their modified analogues also. Hence *lead optimisation* becomes difficult (see below). Compound centered drug designing can be followed for *synthetic products* also. Drugs, this way, can be developed from the pharmacological data obtained from structure activity relationship of an established drug, e.g., a dozen or so β-adrenoceptor blocking drugs available today are based on propranolol structure; or plethora of "triptans" are based on sumatriptan introduced to treat migraine; or 6 to 7 H_2-receptor antagonists (cimetidine, ranitidine etc.) are available after modifying the structure of histamine. Although it is a more logical approach, yet due to the pressure from the drug industry and their marketing promotion strategies, the "molecular modification" has ended up in "molecular manipulation". As a result, the so-called "new drugs" are virtually serving as only "me-too drugs" with no added advantage over the already existing drugs. This has rather resulted in drug explosion.

The second is the *target-centered approach* where valid biochemical or molecular targets are used to search for promising compounds. For example, it was known that inhibition of angiotensin-converting enzyme (ACE) blocks conversion of angiotensin I to angiotensin II and hence lowers the blood pressure. Hence it made sense to look for ACE inhibitors (lisinopril, ramipril and fosinopril etc) or for vascular angiotensin II receptor antagonists (losartan, candesartan and telmisartan etc) as useful antihypertensive drugs. A large number of drugs which are now available were developed following the target-centered approach. With this approach their is high likelihood of getting useful promising agents for *lead optimisation.*

4. Designing of a Prodrug or an Active Metabolite as a Drug

Prodrug is an agent that is administered as the precursor of a drug and is converted into active therapeutic agent inside the body. Sometimes, an effective drug is tailored to fit such predetermined specifications. For example, the unquestioned success of levodopa, as a prodrug of the neurotransmitter dopamine, in the treatment of parkinsonism. Besides prodrugs, active metabolites of certain drugs are also found to possess therapeutic advantages over the parent drug. For example, paracetamol, an active metabolite of phenacetin, was introduced as a safe analgesic this way. Similarly, the active metabolite of procainamide, *N*-acetyl procainamide, is an effective antiarrhythmic drug which does not cause lupus-like syndrome that occurs with procainamide.

After the synthesis or isolation of compounds, their purity is ascertained by physico-chemical and analytical studies. These are then subjected to biological screening. The desired aim of this screening procedure is to find LEAD COMPOUNDS which have a potential of becoming a new drug. Next comes the stage of LEAD OPTIMISATION where the aim is to identify one or two drug canditates suitable for further investigation. Attempts are made to increase its potency on its targets and to optimise it with other properties like pharmacokineties and adverse effects. Three to five years may be spent to come to this stage. The promising LEAD COMPOUND selected this way is then subjected to preclinical evaluation. The clinical trials follow only when the results of preclinical evaluations are encouraging.

PRECLINICAL EVALUATION PHASE (ANIMAL STUDIES)

Initially, animal studies are performed to define the pharmacological profile of the lead compound. The aim during preclinical phase of development is to satisfy all the requirements that are needed before a compound is considered fit to be tested for first time in humans. Much of this work, especially the toxicological studies, is done according to the standards laid down in a formal operating code known as *"Good Laboratory Practices"*. This ensures reliability and reproducibility of laboratory data and minimises human errors. Figure 8.1 shows various stages in drug development right from finding and optimisation of the lead compound, to the development of a "typically new drug" for clinical use. Out of the 10000 compounds screened during drug discovery phase, only 10 qualify the phase of preclinical evaluation which are then subjected to clinical trials in humans. Studies during the preclinical phase usually require 1.5 to 2 yr for completion.

The major areas of preclinical evaluations are:

Pharmacodynamic Studies

Here actions relevant to the proposed therapeutic use (and other effects) are studied on animals. For example, in search for an antihypertensive activity of the lead compound, the study can be undertaken on

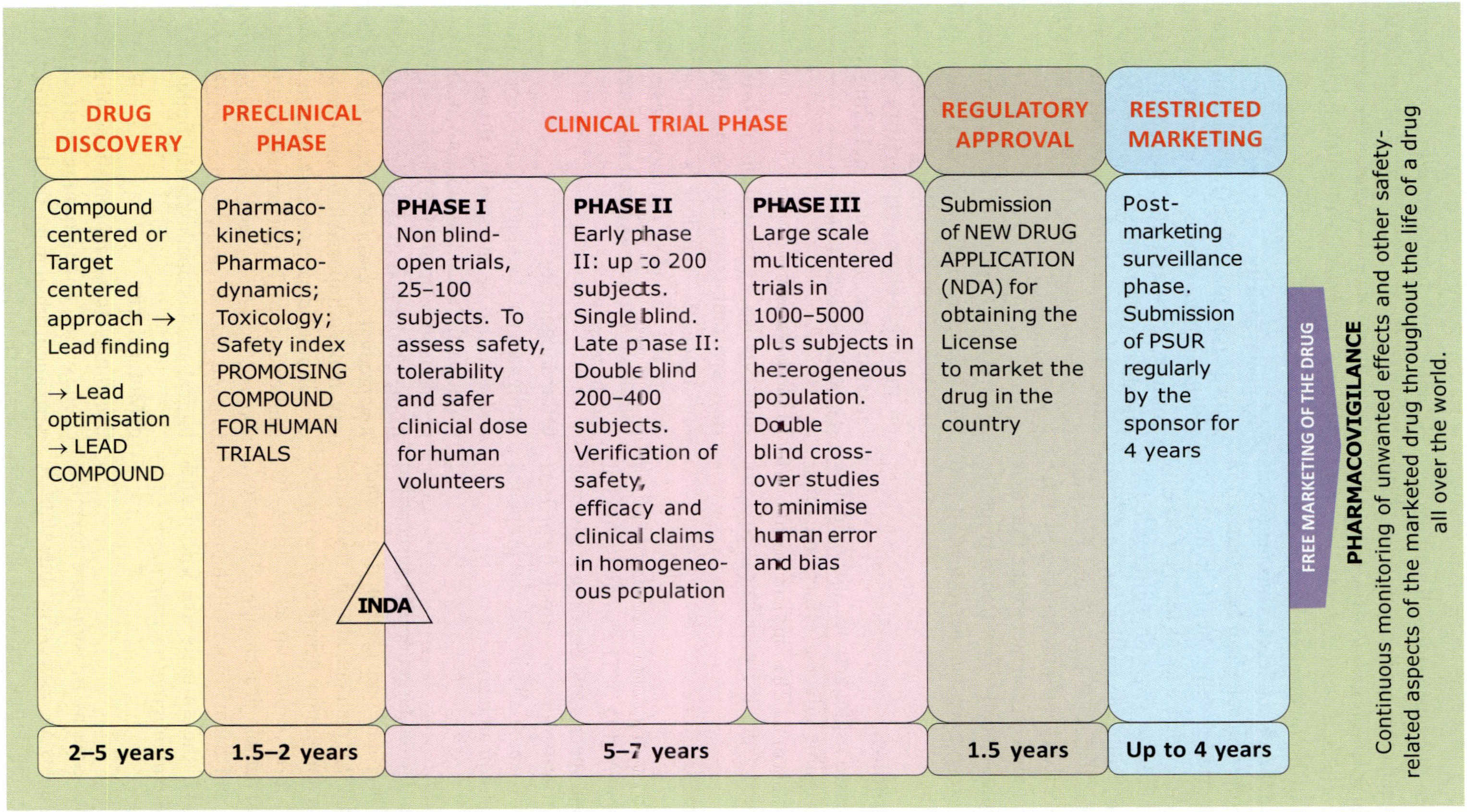

Fig 8.1 Stages Involved During Development of a 'New Drug'. PSUR = Periodic Safety Update Report; INDA = Investigational New Drug Application.

dogs, cats or rats to find out systolic-diastolic blood pressure changes and other cardiac effects like ECG changes, ionotropic-chronotropic effects, cardiac output and total peripheral resistance. Once the lead compound exhibits promising results, the studies can be further made at cellular level. Thus the effects on vascular and other muscles can be evaluated *in vitro* on isolated arteries/veins, heart or ileum of rat or guinea pig. An evidence for its receptor activity can also be gathered *in vitro* on cultured cells. Depending on the results, the studies can be further extended to molecular level to find out receptor affinity and selectivity by performing *in vitro* receptor binding studies on cell membrane fractions from organs or cultured cells. The graded response assays or quantal assays are then performed to find out ED_{50} of the drug.

Toxicological Studies

If the agent possessed useful activity, it should now be studied for possible adverse effects on other major organ systems. The major kinds of information needed from the preclinical toxicity studies are:

1) Acute Toxicity

The aim is to find out the *acute dose that is lethal to 50% of the animals* (LD_{50}). The study is done at least on two animal species and the drug is given in graded doses to several groups of animals by *at least two routes,* one of which should be the proposed route to be used in human beings.

2) Subacute Toxicity

The aim is to identify the target organs susceptible to drug toxicity. *Three doses* are used on *two animal species*. The animals are maintained at the maximum tolerated doses for a minimum period of *four weeks to a maximum of three months* so as to allow for the development of pathological changes. Thereafter, the biochemical and haematological changes are evaluated. Finally, the animals are killed and subjected to *histopathological examination.*

3) Chronic Toxicity

The goals are the same as for subacute toxicity. However, such studies are especially important if the drug is intended for chronic use in human beings. Usually *two animal species (one rodent and one non-rodent)* are used. The duration of study may range from *one to two years.* These studies may also run simultaneously with clinical trials, to cut short the time factor.

4) Special Toxicity

Nowadays, toxicological data on teratogenicity (including the effects on reproductive functions), mutagenicity and carcinogenicity have become mandatory after the unfortunate episode of thalido-mide disaster in 1961 which left more than 10,000 newborns congenitally deformed and crippled due to phocomelia.

a) Effect on Reproductive Performance

Studies are carried out on rats treated with the test drug before and after mating period. Effects of drugs on mating behaviour, fertility, parturition and lactation are noticed, including perinatal and postnatal effects if any.

b) Teratogenicity

Such studies are carried out in *two animal species* (rats and rabbits) to assess the effect of drugs on organogenesis. The drug is given, after the mating, during the period of organogenesis. Foetus is then examined for any skeletal or visceral abnormality (birth defects).

c) Carcinogenicity

Malignant and benign tumours occur spontaneously and can also be induced by drugs sometimes as a result of mutation. The unknown aetiology of most spontaneous cancers, the long latent period involved in the production of drug-induced tumours and the low predictive power of animal tests for carcinogeni-city, make it impossible to say that a compound will or will not be carcinogenic in man. However, such studies can still be performed on at least *two animal species, by giving same doses as used for chronic toxicity, for two years* with assessment of haemato-logical and histopathological findings.

d) Mutagenicity

Drugs may cause abnormalities of genetic material (genes and chromosomes) of cells so that a permanent change in the hereditary constitution occurs (muta-tion). When a mutation occurs in reproductive cells (spermatozoa or ova), then a hereditary defect occurs which may appear in the first generation progeny of the individual. However, if it is a recessive kind of trait, it may become evident only when two individuals affected by the chemical mutagen mate. This type of the toxicity is studied on the genetic stability of the bacteria (AMES TEST): For example, *Salmonella typhi* cannot grow (or dies) in a histidine-deficient culture medium. However, if a drug is a mutagen, it will induce mutation of *S. typhi*. As a result the mutant strains of *S. typhi* can still grow even in the histidine-deficient medium.

Mutagenicity can also be studied on mammalian cell cultures but are very difficult to be performed. However, there is an increasing interest in this problem. Where a mutation occurs in somatic cells (non-reproductive cells), these tissues (e.g., bone marrow cells), may develop abnormal characteristics and become malignant (leukaemia). However, genotoxicity data for anticancer drugs (because of shorter life expectancy of cancer patients) is not required unless phase II trials are completed.

e) Local Toxicity

These studies are required when the drug is used topically. These may include: (a) dermal toxicity studies, (b) dermal photo-toxicity studies, (c) vaginal toxicity tests, (d) ocular toxicity studies, (e) inhalational studies and (f) allergy studies. If the drug is given per rectal route, then rectal tolerance tests (e.g., rectal inflammation etc.) are to be performed. If a drug is to be given parenterally, then the inflammatory reactions at the site of injection are to be examined.

Pharmacokinetic Studies

After performing toxicological studies, the promising test compound is subjected to pharmacokinetic studies in several species of animals, like rats, dogs and sometimes monkeys. Besides studying its absorption, distribution, metabolism and excretion, these studies also establish its relative bioavailability after its oral or parenteral administration. Its elimination half life ($t_{½}$) is also estimated from the pharmacokinetic data.

Assessment of Safety Index

From the toxicological and pharmacodynamic data, the LD_{50} and ED_{50} of the test compound are found, respectively. From these data, its *therapeutic index* and *certain safety factor* is also calculated (refer Ch. 7). Besides Safety Index, other safety parameters like Maximum Tolerated Dose (MTD), No Adverse Effect Level (NoAEL) dose, and Human Equivalent Dose (HED) are determined in species akin to humans (like monkeys), ultimately to calculate First in Human (FIH) dose which will later be used in Phase I clinical trials.

When the preclinical studies predict that the test drug holds promise, the time comes to put it to human trials and to launch a program for clinical trials that will decide whether the test drug is only a drug or it can acquire the status of a medicine. A suitable formulation of this lead compound, for intended clinical route of administration, is then developed and its stability is ascertained.

CLINICAL TRIAL PHASE (HUMAN TRIALS)

CLINICAL TRIALS mean a systematic study of a new drug in human subjects to generate data for discovering or verifying the *clinical claims* or *pharmacological* and *adverse effects* with an aim to determine the safety and efficacy of the drug in question.

The procedure followed during the trials should comply with an elaborate code known as "*Good Clinical Practice* (GCP)" prescribed by the International Conference on Harmonization (ICH) and Declaration of Helsinki. The GCPs provide details about designing the trial, collection of the data, recording of information, statistical analysis, documentation and reporting the results of clinical trials.

When the new compound passes the preclinical pharmacological screening, the manufacturer may file a "Preclinical New Drug" or "Investigational New Drug" application (IND application) to an authorized Drug Control body of the respective country. In UK it is to be submitted to the Committee on Safety of Medicine (CSM); in USA, to the Food and Drug Administration (FDA), while in India, to the Drugs Controller General, Govt. of India, New

Delhi. The IND application must contain the following information about the test drug in question:

a) The chemical structure, its source, its manufacturing data with details of its purity.
b) The preclinical data about pharmacodynamics, pharmacokinetics and toxicological studies with ED_{50} and LD_{50} data.
c) Specification of dosage forms in which it has to be administered to human beings.
d) A detailed description of the investigational protocol to be undertaken (including the dose and route of administration).
e) The names and qualifications of each investigator and the facilities available to them.
f) An agreement from the sponsors to submit annual progress report regularly.
g) A certification that "informed consent" will be obtained from human volunteers and that "ethics of research in human beings" will be strictly followed. The sponsors have to also ensure that copies of all informational material have been supplied to each investigator (through Investigator`s Brochure).

Only when the approval is given by the regulatory body, the drug can be administered to the men for clinical trials.

Ethics Committee and Its Responsibilities

At the Institutional level (where the trials are conducted) the regulatory bodies rely on an Independent Ethics Committee (IEC) to ensure the rights and welfare of the participants in the clinical trials. The responsibilities of Ethics Committee are:

a) To review and accord its approval to a clinical trial according to the protocol. The clearance report should be enclosed along with IND application.
b) To safeguard the rights, safety and well-being of the trial subjects who have given their consent including those who are homeless or refugees or minors or others who are incapable of giving personal consent.
c) To make a periodical review of the ongoing trial and to ensure that the standard operation procedures (SOPs) and the protocols are being followed. For this, they may visit the study site or can review the periodic study-progress reports furnished by the investigator or may examine the internal audit reports, provided by the sponsor.

In case, the IEC revokes its approval accorded to a trial protocol, it must record its reason for doing so and must communicate this decision to the investigator, to the sponsor and to the licensing authority as well. The IEC should keep a copy of SOPs being followed and should maintain a record of its proceedings.

The IEC should have at least 7 members. They should appoint among themselves a Member Secretary and a Chairperson (who should be from outside the Institution). Other 5 members should be a mix of medical/nonmedical persons with one layperson from the community. For review of each protocol, the quorum of IEC should have at least 5 members preferably: one clinician, one medical scientist (preferably a Pharmacologist), one legal expert, one non-medical or a social scientist and one lay person from the community. Proper gender representation in the IEC is also advisable. The subject experts also be invited from time to time to offer their views. Only those IEC members who are not connected to the clinical trial or to the sponsor of the trial can vote or express their opinion officially in the matters of trial.

Informed Consent from Human Volunteers and Ethics of Research In Human Volunteers

The law requires that the investigator should obtain the written informed consent from every human volunteer on the format prescribed by the regulatory authority. The investigator must provide the information about the study verbally as well as by providing a "patient information sheet" in a language that is understandable by the subjects participating in the trial. Both the "**p**atient **i**nformation **s**heet (PIS)" as well as the "**i**nformed **c**onsent **f**orm (ICF)", are known as ICF Document and should be approved by the IEC before submitting to the licensing authority. Any change in the ICF Document due to any reason later should be first approved by the IEC and submitted to the Licensing Authority prior to its implementation. If a subject is not able to give an informed consent (e.g., disabled person, unable to read or write, or mentally ill person), the same may be obtained from a legally authorized acceptable representative who must append his/her signature in the ICF. The human volunteers or the patient volunteers should have the right to choose whether or not they should participate in the proposed trial, i.e., they have the "right to autonomy". The investigator or the sponsor has no right to select "martyrs for the society through persuasion or lure".

The basic elements of such informed consent are:

1. The statement that the study involves research and an explanation of the purpose of the research.
2. Expected duration of the subject's participation.
3. Description of the procedures to be followed (including all invasive procedures if used).
4. An explanation of the possible discomforts and risks to the participant.
5. A description of the anticipated benefits to the subject, expected from the trial (e.g., when the volunteers are like cancer patients).
6. A disclosure of alternative therapies or procedures available currently to the subject.
7. An assurance that the subject's medical records would be maintained confidentially and about the person who will have access to these records.
8. Trial treatment schedules and the probability for random assignment of the subject for each treatment.
9. A disclosure about whom to contact for trial-related queries and in the event of trial-related injury.
10. The anticipated payment, if any, to the subject for participating in the trial.
11. An explanation about the compensation and/or treatment available to the subject in the event of trial-related adverse effects.
12. An assurance that his/her participation in the trial is voluntary and that the subject is free to withdraw from the study at any time without paying any penalty.

Additional elements, which may be explained while filling the Informed Consent Form (ICF):

1. Total number of subjects enrolled for the trial.
2. A statement that depending upon the circumstances the subjects's participation can be terminated by the investigator without the subject's consent.
3. A statement that the subject or his/her representative will be notified timely if new findings appear during the trial which may affect the subject's willingness to continue his participation.
4. A statement that the particular treatment may involve risk to the female subjects or to the foetus if the subject is or may become pregnant. As a rule, women with child-bearing potential are not included in clinical trials unless rigorous teratological studies in animals reveal that the drug is safe. Even for clinical trials with new contraceptive drugs, no women should be used as subjects if they are willing to bear the child either during the trial period or immediately after the end of clinical trial.

Thus, although a large number of subjects participate in the clinical trials, almost every subject is fully informed about the action of the drug, the purpose of study and the benefits to be derived out of the trial.

Use of "Placebo" during the Trials

A new drug is frequently compared with a "placebo" to nullify the subject bias. The placebo is an inert substance having the same appearance as the drug under investigation.

- The "placebo controls" are necessary when the trials are to be conducted on healthy volunteers, in whom the therapeutic benefits of the new drug are difficult to be ascertained, e.g., when a new drug is claimed to be an appetite stimulant or a suppressant; that means, when the subjective effects of the drug are under study. These are equally appropriate in the clinical trial of an absolutely new drug for which there are no existing counterparts to compare with, e.g., the evaluation of the clinical efficacy of an entirely new vaccine.
- Placebo controls are not permissible when to give a placebo means withholding a drug from a group

of patients who could have been benefited by its use. That means, placebo has no place in the trials of a new drug in the patients suffering from a disease for which an effective drug is already available for comparison, e.g., a new antiarrhythmic drug to be evaluated in the patients suffering from ventricular arrhythmias. Hence in such situations, the new drug should properly be compared with the existing established drug by randomly assigning the patients in 2 or 3 experimental groups.

- However, for the sake of human ethics, consent should also be obtained from the subjects for the use of the placebo. He/she should be explained that an "inert preparation" may be used and why it will be used during the trial. That means, the investigator should make the volunteer understand the basic concept of distinguishing between the "imaginary benefits" and the "actual therapeutic benefits" of the new drug.
- Allocation of patient volunteers in different experimental groups poses another ethical problem. In most cases, a comparison has to made between the new drug and the standard drug, which is already available for a particular disease. Hence, it also becomes necessary to eliminate the "observer's bias" that may develop during the investigation. If it is not known whether one treatment is better than the other, the best way of getting equivalent groups is by allocating the patients by "random allocation" to each group. The function of randomization is basically to eliminate the observer's bias, known or unknown, that could affect assignment of the volunteers to a particular treatment.

PHASES OF CLINICAL TRIALS

1. Phase I

It is the phase of clinical pharmacological evaluation of the new drug and is performed on a small number (25–100) of healthy volunteers. If the drug is expected to have significant toxicity (as in the case of anticancer drugs or drugs to be used in AIDS therapy), the volunteers with the particular disease are used rather than healthy volunteers. The objectives of this necessary but cautious phase of investigation are:

i) to check for *safety* (i.e., whether the drug affects any cardiovascular, hepatic or renal functions adversely) and to check its *tolerability* (i.e., does the drug produce any unpleasant symptom like headache, nausea and vomiting).
ii) to determine whether humans and animals show significant pharmacokinetic differences.
iii) to determine a *safe clinical dosage range in humans*. The selection of an initial human dose is difficult because the toxicological data on animals are of limited usefulness (quantitatively) for selecting such a dose. The common rule is to begin with 1/5th or 1/10th of the maximum tolerated dose (mg/kg) in animals and calculating it for an average human body weight of 70 kg. The drug is then given in small increments till the therapeutically effective dose is attained by clinical observation.
iv) to determine the pharmacokinetics of the drug in humans so as to decide whether the deficiency in drug effects, if any, is a result of its lack of absorption or its faster elimination.
v) to detect any predictable toxicity.

These trials are NON-BLIND or OPEN LABEL; that means both the investigator and the subjects know what is being given. Phase I trials are usually performed by clinical pharmacologists in a research centre especially equipped for pharmacokinetic studies.

2. Phase II

In this phase, the drug is studied for the first time in patients with target disease, to determine its efficacy (i.e., proof of claims). The main purpose of phase II trial is to gather evidence that the drug has the effects as suggested by preclinical trials. Hence an end point is decided. It may be *definitive end point* (which measures the drug effect directly, e.g., pain relief is the end point for testing an analgesic) or a *surrogate end point* (which is predictive of the definitive end point, e.g., reduction in the tumour size is the surrogate end point for survival by anticancer drugs). These trials are divided into EARLY and LATE PHASES.

In the EARLY PHASE II, a small number of patients (up to 200) are studied in detail to observe the potential therapeutic benefits and side effects. The idea is to establish a dose range for more definitive therapeutic trials to be undertaken in the late phase. It is usually a SINGLE BLIND design where only the subject does not know whether he is taking an inert placebo (if used) or a positive control drug (i.e., an established standard medicine) or the new drug (under trial).

The LATE PHASE II trials are conducted on a larger number of patients (200–400) in a controlled DOUBLE BLIND manner, where the investigator is also ignorant (besides the subject) whether he is prescribing a placebo, or a positive control medicine or the new drug under trial. This is done to rule out the influence of preconvinced notion or of benign communication by the investigator to his subjects.

In such a design, a third party holds the code identifying each medication and this code is not deciphered until all the clinical data have been collected.

In short, the phase II trials are carefully controlled blind studies (single as well as double) in a homogeneous population to ensure safety and efficacy of the new drug in a specific disease.

3. Phase III

These are large-scale multicentered (heterogeneous population) randomized double-blind trials in patients (1000–5000 plus) to further establish the safety and efficacy. These are designed to minimise errors in the information gathered in Phase I and II trials. Therefore these trials are made using DOUBLE-BLIND CROSS-OVER designs like those set out in Table 8.1.

The term *cross-over design* means that the standard drug, the placebo and the new drug are given in alternating periods and the sequence is systematically varied (as per Latin square rule) so that different subsets of patients receive each of the possible sequences of the treatment (see Table 8.1). All the three phases of clinical trial usually take 5–6 years for completion.

At the end of this trial, statistical analysis of the data is performed. Initially, relatively simple tests, like the student t-test or the chi-square tests are applied to determine the significance of results. However, complex statistical methods may also be needed like non-parametric tests, analysis of variance with confidence limits and covariance etc. Providing details of these methods is beyond the scope of this text.

Table 8.1 Double-Blind Cross-Over Design of Phase III Trial

Patient groups (randomised)	Medication given*		
	Week 1	Week 2	Week 3
I	Standard drug	Placebo	New drug
II	Placebo	New drug	Standard drug
III	New drug	Standard drug	Placebo

**Each therapeutic period arbitrarily lasts for 7 days with an interval of one week, in between, for wash out of preceding medicament.*

New Drug Application. Once the phase III trials are completed satisfactorily the sponsors can file a "New Drug Application" with the Drug Control authorities of that country. The new drug application usually contains thousands of pages and includes complete detailed monograph of the product, the results of the trials, the proposed registered name of this product and the package insert. The data are reviewed by the Drug Control authorities and even by outside consultants who may require further information or clarification. If the documentation is acceptable and is in compliance with the regulations, the drug control authorities can allow the drug to enter the market with "New Drug Status".

4. Phase IV

Once approval is obtained to market the drug, phase IV of the trials begins. It is the post-licensing phase—field trials. The phase IV has no fixed duration as it is the surveillance phase during the post-marketing clinical use of the drug. The performance of the drug is monitored for several years, immediately after marketing, to discover relatively rare side effects (e.g., congenital effects) or previously unknown drug interaction or even a previously unknown therapeutic use detected by a chance discovery. During the "New Drug Status" period, the manufacturer is expected to report any new information about the drug concerning its safety. Such *Periodic Safety Update Report* (PSUR) is to be submitted every six months for first 2 years and then annually for the next 2 years. The drug may remain in "New Drug Status" (i.e., in controlled marketing) for several years until the Drug Control authorities are confident about its release to unrestricted marketing.

ORPHAN DRUGS

At times, the drug is not developed into a usable medicine, because the costs incurred will not be recovered by the developer. As a result the free market economy is liable to leave some rare disease as untreated (for example: some uncommon cancers and rare parasitic infections). Such a disease is called as *orphan disease*, the drug as *orphan drug*, and the sufferer as *orphan patient*. Such drugs are, however, developed by government-offered incentives, like tax relief and by providing exclusive marketing rights to the pharmaceutical company. More than 300 drugs are having orphan status. However, some examples of these drugs with their proposed use are listed in Table 8.2.

The "New Drug Application" for orphan drugs receives highest priority at all stages of the drug review process. For example, the treatment of New Drug Application enables the patients, not qualified for participation in ongoing studies, to be treated with investigational drugs outside controlled clinical trials. Such priorities in processing the application are given when: (i) the drug is intended to treat a rare or a serious life-threatening disease for which no satisfactory alternative drug is available and (ii) the drug is under investigation in a controlled clinical trial and the sponsor is also actively pursuing the marketing approval of such investigational drug.

When no priority treatment of investigational new drug is in effect but the drug is under trial (for some orphan disease), a physician may also obtain the drug for "compassionate use" in orphan patient. In such a situation he may submit an application to Drug Control authorities requesting them to

Table 8.2 Orphan Drugs and Orphan Diseases

Orphan drug	Orphan disease
Acetyl cysteine	For paracetamol overdose toxicity
Miltefosine	For kala azar
Anagrelide	For polycythaemia vera
Antithrombin III (human)	For hereditary anti-thrombin III deficiency
Arginine butyrate	For sickle cell disease and β-thalassemia
Atovaquone	For AIDS associated *Pneumocystis carinii* pneumonia
Betaine	For homocystinuria
2-Chlorodeoxy-adenosine	For acute myeloid leukaemia
Fomepizole	Methylalcohol poisoning
Erythropoietin	For anaemia of end-stage renal disease and anaemia associated with cancers
Factor XIII (plasma)	For congenital factor XIII deficiency
Relaxin (human)	For progressive systemic sclerosis
Denileukin diftitox	For cutaneous T-cell lymphoma refractory to other drugs

authorise him to use an investigational new drug for such a use. According to Orphan Drug Act of FDA an orphan disease is the one which affects less than 200,000 persons in USA.

PHARMACOVIGILANCE

Not all hazards can be known before a drug is marketed and used widely by the general population. Many additional risks or additional benefits are only identified after the drug is widely used by a large community of the people. Clinical trials conducted prior to drug approval cannot uncover every aspect of health of the approved drug. For example, teratogenic effects of thalidomide and more recently of isotretinoin were identified through observational method but not through experimental methods. Similarly, the association between certain appetite suppressant drugs (e.g., fenfluramine and phentermine) and pulmonary hypertension as well as valvular heart disease is an example where serious adverse effects of these drugs were discovered only when they came into widespread use. Liver toxicity and the subsequent withdrawal of troglitazone (an antidiabetic drug) from the market is another example to the valuable contribution of **p**ost-**m**arketing **s**urveillance (PMS). These are also called post-licensing phase trials or phase IV trials or **p**ost-**a**pproval **s**urveillance **s**tudies (PASS). It is the surveillance phase during the post- marketing clinical use of the drug which is important in determining the real safety issues and status of a drug. During the new drug marketing period of 4-year, the manufacturer is expected to report any new information about the drug like a rare side effect observed, a new drug interaction revealed or even a new clinical use (off-level use) detected by a chance discovery. Hence during the first 4-year of marketing a new drug, the manufacturer has to submit the **P**eriodic **S**afety **U**pdate **R**eports (PSURs) every six months for first 2-year and then once annually for the next 2-year. Lately WHO had suggested that every country should generate broad-based ADR data about the drugs already in clinical use or for those licensed for marketing all through the life of a drug. WHO prepared a document on " Safety Monitoring of Medicinal Products" and suggested guidelines for "setting up and running a pharmacovigilance centre" in every country. In this effort not only pharmaceutical industries but practising doctors, nursing staff, hospital pharmacists, clinical research organisations and clinical pharmacologists should participate in their national pharmacovigilance program and the ADR data of a new drug (even of an old drug) should be shared with global health care community through WHO Uppsala Monitoring Centre located in Sweden.

PHARMACOVIGILANCE (Greek: *Pharmakon* = a drug, *vigilare* = to be observant) means to remain vigilant and observe the adverse effects of drugs by continuously monitoring for unwanted effects and other safety related aspects of marketed drugs.

WHO defines "pharmacovigilance as the science and activities relating to the **D**etection, **A**ssessment, **U**nderstanding and **P**revention (DAUP) of adverse effects or any other drug-related problems and generally referes to the continuous monitoring of unwanted effects and other safety related aspects of marketed drugs."

PHARMACOVIGILANCE PROGRAMME OF INDIA (PvPI): A NATION-WIDE PHARMACOVIGILANCE PROGRAMME

In the year 2010, the Ministry of Health & Family Welfare (MoHFW), Government of India through its two inter-collabrative Departments- the Central Drugs Standard Control Organization (CDSCO), New Delhi and the Indian Pharmocopoeia Commission (IPC), Ghaziabad started a Nation-wide Pharmacovigilance Programme by the name of Pharmacovigilance Programme of India (PvPI). The CDSCO is an Organization which is involved in giving marketing authorization/licence for new drugs and control of standard of drugs imported or manufactured in the country. In the latter process, the IPC assists the CDSCO by expermenting and testing of drugs to maintain the standards of medicinal products marketed in India and by publishing, Indian Pharmacopoeia (IP), and National Formulary of India (NFI) time to time. Since, administratively both the CDSCO and the IPC are headed by the Drugs Controller General of India (DCGI), the regulatory authority of medicinal products in the country, it was thought that the (PvPI) will be fine-tuned by the two departments of the MoHFW.

The objective of PvPI are:

1. to monitor ADRs in Indian population,
2. to create awareness amongst health professionals about the importance of ADR reporting in India,
3. to monitor benefit-risk profile of medicines approved, marketed and used in the country,
4. generate independent evidence-based recommendations on the safety of medicines,
5. communicate safety-related findings of medicines to all stakeholders,
6. support the CDSCO in formulating safety-related regulatory decisions for medicines,
7. create a national centre of excellance at par with global drug safety monitoring standards.

It was decided that the PvPI shall be coordinated by the IPC, Ghaziabad as a National Coordinating Centre (NCC) for the PvPI (NCC-PvPI). The operation of the PvPI will be overseen and guided by a Steering Committee at the level of CDSCO and a Strategic Advisory Committee at the level of IPC/NCC.

The PvPI was envisaged to work through the inclusion of MCI recognized Medical Colleges & Hospitals, Private and Corporate Hospitals, Public Health Programmes and Autonomous medical Institutes like AIIMS, New Delhi and other States and Indian Council of Medical Research (ICMR), etc. as ADR Monitory Centres (AMCs) (A list of nationwide AMCs is available at: *http://cdsco.nic.in/pharmacovigilance.htm)*. All ADRs are reported through filling an uniform ADR Form, called "Suspected Adverse Reaction Reporting Form" designed by the CDSCO/ICC and available at all AMCs all over the country. The pharmacovigilance staff at the AMCs will check the validity of the report and if possible conduct causality assessment. The ADR or ICSR (Individual Case Safety Report) forms will then be dispatched to the NCC-PvPI as per the standard operating practices (SOPs).

The NCC-PvPI is mandated to conduct a final causality assessment and upload the reports into the National Pharmacovigilance Database. The NCC is also responsible to prepare a consolidated report of ADRs collected at defined time intervals. All the ADRs from all other sources (Industry, Health care professionals, National Immunization Programmes, etc.) will also be databased at the NCC.

The NCC will also implement and integrate pharmacovigilance activities into public health programmes involving mass usage of drugs, such as for anti-malarial, anti-tubercular and anti-retroviral medications. Lastly, the integrated ADR data will be transmitted through *vigiflow* interface into the WHO-Uppsala Monitoring Centre (UMC) ADR Database (called *vigibase*) located in Sweden, where ***signal*** processing can be carried out under the safety data exchange agreements.

CAUSALITY ASSESSMENT

The causality assessment is the structured and standardized assessment of ADRs as reported through the ICSR for the likelihood of involvement of suspected drug in causing particular event in a given patient. Basically it is an exercise to assess whether there is a reasonable possibility that the adverse event associated with the suspected product or study medication. After the causality between the noted adverse event and suspected drugs is established, it is called ADR, until then it is known as adverse drug event only.

SIGNAL means the first alert about the problem and hazard with a drug. It can be generated at the level of doctors, nursing staff, pharmacist or a dentist in the field. It is the reported information on a possible causal relationship between an adverse event and a drug (the relationship being unknown or incompletely documented previously). Usually, more than a single report is required to generate a "***signal***" and it depends on the seriousness of the event and the quality of the information. The reporting of the suspected drug related adverse event can include: (a) any suspected drug interaction, (b) any reaction causing death, (c) any life-threatening reaction, (d) any reaction which required hospitalisation, (e) any reaction which caused disability (significant or permanent), (f) any reaction that required intervention to permanent impairment or damage, and (g) possible causal relationship with an observed congenital abnormality.

The signal or the data on the uses and risks of the new or old drug can also be generated from pharmacoepidemiological studies which can be classified as *experimental* (e.g., clinical trials) or *observational* (e.g., case reports, case-control studies, cohort studies and quasi-experimental study designs).

Pharmacoepidemiology means a study of the effects of drug when used in general population or in specific group types. The observational pharmacoepidemiological studies are hypothesis-testing studies regarding a drug and its adverse effect. *Case-control studies* are undertaken if there are only a few cases of adverse effects. The results of this study compare or relate the risk of adverse effect/toxicity in the cases being treated, with the controls which are either free of the disease or susceptible to the disease. *Cohort* means a group of patients with a common demographic (like Tamils living in Tamil Nadu) or statistical characteristics, e.g., born at about the same time, sharing common historical or cultural background. These studies follow-up a large group of patients for long time to assess the outcome of an exposure common to cohort. *Quasi-experimental study* is like an experimental study (e.g., clinical trials) except that it lacks random assignments of subjects to treatment groups.

CHAPTER 9

Concept of Essential Medicines and Rational Use of Drugs

COMPETENCY PH1.59, PH3.5

CONCEPT OF ESSENTIAL MEDICINES

Truly speaking, only a handful of drugs are required to treat most of the diseases, in most of the people, for most of the times. As per the WHO Directives (1975), such essential drugs should remain available in all hospitals at all times. As per WHO definition (1975) "*the Essential Drugs are those drugs that satisfy healthcare needs of the majority of population and which should, therefore, be available at all times, in adequate amounts and in appropriate dosage forms*." With this aim, the WHO published its first model of Essential Drug List (EDL) in 1977. Later, in 2003, the WHO introduced a new term "Essential Medicines" in place of "Essential Drugs" because at times the term "drug" may give a wrong impression as "drugs of abuse (addiction)". *The WHO in 2002, defined Essential Medicines as those that satisfy the priority healthcare needs of the population.* They are selected with due regard to public healthcare relevance. *These medicines are supposed to be available for proper functioning of the basic healthcare system at all times, in adequate amounts, in appropriate dosage forms, with assured quality, with adequate information and at a price the individual and the community can afford.* With these aims in view, now the WHO has published its 20th model of "Essential Medicines List (EML)" in 2017; WHO model of Essential Medicines 22nd List (2021) – 479 drugs; WHO model of Essential Medicines for children 8th List (2021) – 350 drugs. These essential lists are published every 2 years. The next list will be in 2023. The WHO, however, suggested that their model EML is only a guideline. It is expected that other countries should prepare their own EML according to their own requirement; because a particular drug may be essential for one country but may not be essential for another country. For example: New zealand is a snake free country. Hence antisnake venom serum may not be an essential medicine for this country. But this could be officially an Essential Medicine for India, Pakistan, Bangladesh and other African countries. It is expected that every country should have its own EML which should be updated after every 2–3 years according to changing medical needs and availability of new and better drugs. It was also recommended that the cost of the total treatment should also be considered as a major criterion for including any medicine in such EML. That means, the clinical benefits from the drug should be more but the treatment cost should be low (i.e., better cost: benefit ratio).

In India, the National List of Essential Drugs was released by the Directorate General of Health Services, MoHFW, for the first time in 1996. This National List of Essential Medicines (NLEM) was later revised in 2003, 2011, 2015 and the latest in 2022. The first State level EML in India was prepared by Ministry of Health, Government of National Capital Territory of Delhi in 1994. These EMLs are available with respective State hospitals and are published in many textbooks of pharmacology for the benefit of medical students.

Currently, National List of Essential Medicines (NLEM) was revised which plays an important role in ensuring accessibility of affordable quality medicines. Total 384 Drugs are included in NLEM 2022; 34 new drugs added while 26 from the previous list have been dropped. The medicines have been categorized into 27 therapeutic categories.

RATIONAL USE OF DRUGS

In 1985 WHO, for the first time defined the rational use of medicines as "*patients receive medications appropriate to their clinical needs, in doses that meet their own requirements, for an adequate period of time, and at lowest cost to them and their community*." The rational use of drugs is based on the rule of Right: that means the *Right drug,* to the *Right patient,* in *Right dosage,* at a *Right cost* with *the Right documentation*. It should also fulfil the

SANE criteria. Which means that the **S**afety, **A**ffordability, **N**eed and **E**fficacy of the drug should always be considered before prescribing it to the patient.

THE CONCEPT OF P-DRUGS

It is expected that every doctor should select his **P-drug** (preferred or personal drug) to treat a particular disease. He may choose his P-drug by comparing the efficacy, safety, suitability and the total cost of treatment with this drug vis-a-vis other drugs used to treat the same disease.

Steps in Choosing the P-drug (Table 9.1)

1. **Define the Diagnosis**
   Let us follow an example of choosing a P-drug for patient of angina pectoris. Suppose you have specified the final diagnosis as "stable angina pectoris" caused by a partial occlusion of the coronary arteries.
2. **Specify the Therapeutic Objective**
   Since the patient is having an acute attack of angina, the immediate requirement is to provide quick relief from pain. This can be achieved by increasing the oxygen supply to or by reducing the oxygen demand of the cardiac muscle.

   It is difficult to increase the oxygen supply in the case of arteriosclecrotic occlusion in the coronary artery, because such stenosis cannot be dilated with drugs. This leaves only one option and that is to reduce the oxygen demand of the cardiac muscle.

   Now this is your therapeutic objective which can be achieved in four ways: (a) by decreasing the preload, (b) by decreasing the contractility, (c) by decreasing the heart rate or (d) by decreasing the afterload of the cardiac muscle.
3. **Make a List of Effective Group of Drugs**
   There are three groups of drugs with such an effect: The nitrates, the β-blockers and the calcium channel blockers.
4. **Choose an Effective Group by Comparing Efficacy, Safety, Suitability and Cost of Treatment**
   a) ***Efficacy***
   The therapeutic objective is that the drug should work as soon as possible. Hence not only pharmacodynamics but pharmacokinetics is important as well. Nitrates cause peripheral vasodilatation and thus decrease oxygen demand by decreasing preload and afterload of the cardiac muscle. β-blockers and the calcium channel blockers decrease preload, contractility, heart rate and afterload. All groups contain drugs or their dosage forms with a rapid effect. Nitrates have high first-pass metabolism but their sublingual tablets with rapid effect are available, while for β-blockers or calcium channel blockers injectable forms are available (cost factor will be considered later).

   b) ***Safety***
   In all the three groups, the side effects are more or less equal. With nitrates there is headache, tachycardia and flushings; with beta-blockers there is hypotension, bradycardia and chances of AV block, provocation of asthma and impotence (on prolonged use); with calcium channel blockers there is tachycardia, hypotension, dizziness and AV block. However, side effects with nitrates are milder.

   c) ***Suitability***
   For a patient of angina pectoris, the dosage form of the drug should be such that it can be administered by himself during the attack and which should guarantee a rapid effect. Here again the nitrates have an edge over β-blockers and calcium channel blockers as these are available as sublingual tablets; other group of drugs are available as injectables (for faster relief).

   d) ***Cost of treatment***
   Nitrates are usually inexpensive drugs as compared to other group of drugs.
   Hence it can be concluded that among the three groups of drugs, nitrates are the group of first choice considering efficacy, safety, suitability and the cost.
5. **Choose a P-drug from the Effective Group of Drugs**:
   In general, three types of nitrates are available for the treatment of an acute attack: glyceryl trinitrate (nitroglycerin), isosorbide mononitrate

and isosorbide dinitrate. All the three are available as sublingual tablets with a rapid effect. Transdermal patches, sprays and ointments are also available but these are very costly besides having slow onset of action (except spray). There is no difference in safety, efficacy and suitability between these three types of nitrates.

Hence, the ultimate choice between the three types of nitrates depends on the cost. Usually, the sublingual tablets of glyceryl trinitrate are the cheapest. Hence the P-drug of choice for an attack of angina pectoris for such patient would be sublingual tablet of nitroglycerin 1 mg for an acute attack. If an attack persists, a second tablet can be taken after 15 min. However, since the active drug here is volatile, the tablets become ineffective after sometime. Hence the patient should be advised not to buy these tablets in bulk. Isosorbide dinitrate sublingual tablets could serve as second alternative for 'P drug' (Table 9.1).

Table 9.1 Summary of Criteria for Selecting a P-Drug

1. Define the diagnosis.
2. Specify the therapeutic objective.
3. Make a list of effective group of drugs.
4. Choose the effective group of drugs.

	Efficacy	**Safety**	**Suitability**	**Cost**
Group A				
Group B				
Group C				

5. Choose a P-drug from this group

	Efficacy	**Safety**	**Suitability**	**Cost**
Drug 1				
Drug 2				
Drug 3				

6. Finalise the drug, dosage form, dose schedule and duration of treatment.
7. Monitor the treatment through follow-ups.

General Introduction

COMPETENCY PH1.14

The human nervous system is composed of two main divisions: the ***Central Nervous System*** consisting of the brain and the spinal cord, and the ***Peripheral Nervous System*** consisting of all afferent (sensory) neurons carrying nerve impulses from sensory organs in the periphery to the CNS, and all efferent (motor) neurons which carry nerve impulses from the CNS to the effector cells in the peripheral tissues. Based primarily on the part of the body that responds, the *peripheral nervous system* is subdivided into *Somatic Nervous System* and *Autonomic Nervous System (ANS)*. Traditionally, the ANS and the somatic nervous system are usually described as an output or efferent portion of peripheral nervous system. Hence, mainly the efferent pathways (which convey the output messages) of ANS and somatic nervous system shall be dealt in this chapter.

SOMATIC NERVOUS SYSTEM

The somatic nervous system consists of two types of neurons: the *sensory neurons* that carry information from cutaneous and special sensory receptors in the peripheral organs to the CNS, and the *motor neurons* which conduct impulses from the CNS to skeletal muscles only. Since the effect of motor neurons can be consciously controlled, the efferent (motor) part of the somatic nervous system is concerned primarily with the voluntary functions, like locomotion, respiration, posture and deep tendon reflexes.

The axons of somatic motor neurons extend from the CNS and are myelinated. These emerge from the ventral horn of the grey matter of the spinal cord and run uninterrupted, without any ganglia or synapse in between, straight up to Neuromuscular Junction (NMJ), which is also called myoneural junction.

The neurotransmitter released by somatic nerves at the neuromuscular junction (NMJ) is acetylcholine (ACh), which then stimulates the cholinergic nicotinic receptors present on the motor end plate (see following text for details). The somatic motor neurons are therefore cholinergic in character. The stimulation of these neuromuscular nicotinic receptors (N_M receptors) by ACh produces contraction of the skeletal muscle (Fig. 10.1). However, an excessive stimulation of N_M receptors by ACh (cholinergic crisis) leads to initial fasciculations or jerks (due to persistent depolarisation) which is followed by flaccid paralysis (ultimately desensitisation of N_M receptor with loss of muscle tone). Blockade of N_M receptors by drugs leads to progressive flaccid paralysis (but without fasciculations). Similarly, the section of the somatic nerve (or its complete degeneration) leads to paralysis or atrophy of the skeletal muscle supplied by that nerve.

AUTONOMIC NERVOUS SYSTEM (ANS)

The ANS consists of the afferent neurons that convey information from the receptors located primarily in the viscera to the CNS, and the efferent neurons which conduct impulses from the CNS to the effector organs. Since the efferent responses of the ANS are not under conscious control, they are autoregulatory or involuntary in nature. As the term ANS suggests, the activities of this system are maintained autonomically and no atrophy of organs occurs even after section of an autonomic nerve. On the contrary, the section of the autonomic nerve or its complete degeneration rather produces a denervation supersensitivity of autonomic receptors of the organ supplied by that nerve. The main physiological processes which ANS regulates are: contraction and relaxation of smooth muscles, all exocrine and some endocrine secretions, the heart beat, the blood pressure and certain metabolic functions.

The ANS consists of three main anatomical divisions:

- Parasympathetic Nervous System (or cholinergic division)
- Sympathetic Nervous System (or adrenergic division)
- Enteric Nervous System (ENS).

Almost all autonomic nerves (whether sympathetic or parasympathetic) have a relay center in between, called ganglion, which lies outside the CNS. In other words the autonomic nerves are actually composed of a set of two neurons termed as *preganglionic neuron* and the *postganglionic neuron,* named after their location relative to the ganglia. Thus, the ganglion is actually a region of synaptic contact between the preganglionic and the postganglionic neurons. The intervening space of this junctional region is called as the ganglionic synapse. The ganglia in between the preganglionic and the postganglionic parasympathetic fibres are called *parasympathetic ganglia*, while those connecting preganglionic and postganglionic sympathetic fibres are called *sympathetic ganglia* (Fig. 10.1).

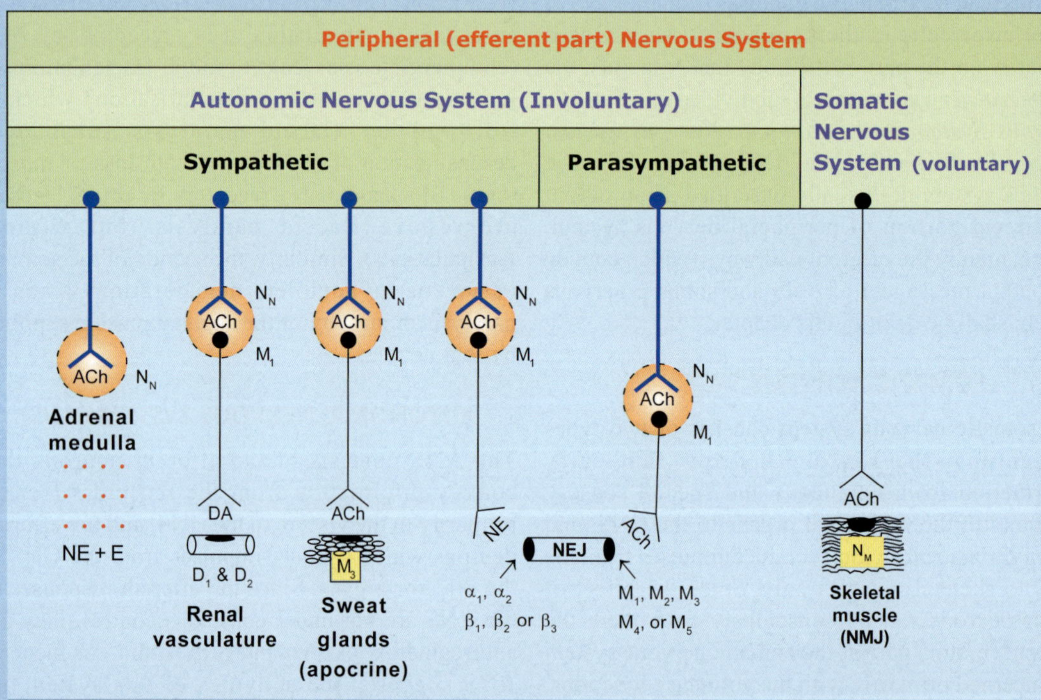

Key: Preganglionic fibres; Postganglionic fibres

ACh—Acetylcholine; NE—Norepinephrine, E—Epinephrine, DA—Dopamine;

N_M—Nicotinic cholinergic receptor (muscular type) at neuromuscular junction (NMJ);

N_N—Nicotinic cholinergic receptor at ganglia (neuronal type); α_1, α_2, β_1, β_2, β_3—Alpha and beta adrenergic receptor subtypes; M_1 to M_5—Muscarinic cholinergic receptor subtypes; D_1 & D_2—Dopamine receptor subtypes at renal vasculature;

NEJ—Neuroeffector junction at the smooth muscle of the effector organ.

Fig 10.1 Distribution of Cholinergic and Adrenergic Neurons in Peripheral Nervous System

The division of ANS into the *parasympathetic* and *sympathetic* components depends upon the emergence of their preganglionic fibres from the CNS. The parasympathetic preganglionic fibres are myelinated and emerge from the cranial and the sacral regions of the CNS. Hence, it is analogously designated as *cranio-sacral outflow.* The cranial outflow is carried out by the III (oculomotor), VII (facial), IX (glossopharyngeal) and X (vagus) nerves. The sacral outflow is carried out by 2nd, 3rd, and 4th sacral segments of the spinal cord. The cell bodies of the sympathetic preganglionic neurons are located within the lateral horns of the first thoracic to the third lumbar segments of the spinal cord (both inclusive). Hence, the sympathetic outflow is also termed as *thoraco-lumbar outflow.*

Parasympathetic Nervous System

Parasympathetic Innervation of Peripheral Effector Organs

The basic plan of the parasympathetic innervation of peripheral organs is depicted in Figure 10.2. The oculomotor nerve (III cranial nerve) carries parasympathetic fibres to ciliary muscle of eye and circular muscle of iris. The facial nerve (VII cranial nerve) carries fibres to salivary glands, lacrimal glands and submaxillary glands. The glossopharyngeal nerve (IX cranial nerve) carries fibres to parotid gland and nasopharynx, while the vagus nerve (X cranial nerve) carries fibres to heart, lung and gastrointestinal tract. The sacral outflow carries parasympathetic fibres destined to pelvic organs and genitourinary tract. The sacral fibres emerge from the spinal cord in a bundle of nerves known as *nervi erigentes* (because stimulation of these nerves evokes genital erection). The parasympathetic ganglia related to oculomotor (ciliary ganglia), facial (sphenopalatine and submandibular ganglia), glossopharyngeal nerve (otic ganglia) and that related to sacral nerves (pelvic ganglia) lie close to the wall of the effector organ supplied by them. On the other hand, those related to vagus nerve lie within the wall of the effector organs (heart, lungs, intestine) (Fig. 10.2).

Parasympathetic ganglia are therefore also referred to as terminal ganglia. The parasympathetic postganglionic fibres are therefore shorter in length as compared to their preganglionic fibres. The parasympathetic preganglionic fibres are usually myelinated while the postganglionic fibres are non-myelinated (except for the ciliary parasympathetic postganglionic fibres which are myelinated).

The parasympathetic preganglionic fibres tend to synapse with only a very little number of postganglionic parasympathetic fibres. Further, the ramification of postganglionic parasympathetic fibres at the neuroeffector junction (NEJ) is least diffused. Hence, the area covered may be less, but the intensity of parasympathetic effect is more. The only exception to this is in the Auerbach and Meissner plexuses where the ratio of pre:postganglionic vagal fibres is 1:8000.

Parasympathetic Neurotransmitters (Fig. 10.1)

- Acetylcholine (ACh) is the neurotransmitter at all the autonomic (sympathetic or parasympathetic) ganglionic synapses.
- All postganglionic parasympathetic fibres release ACh at Neuroeffector Junction (NEJ).
- As an exception, the postganglionic sympathetic fibres to apocrine sweat glands, although sympathetic in origin, are cholinergic in character (as the neurotransmitter released at the sweat glands is acetylcholine). That is why during stress, anxiety or apprehensions there is increased sweating (adrenergic sweat).
- The term "cholinergic fibres" means all such fibres which release ACh as a neurotransmitter. Thus, (i) all somatic motor neurons to skeletal muscles (NMJ), (ii) all preganglionic parasympathetic or sympathetic fibres (including adrenal medulla), (iii) all postganglionic parasympathetic fibres to neuroeffector junction (NEJ) and (iv) postganglionic sympathetic fibres to sweat glands of palm and sole are cholinergic fibres in character.

Acetylcholine Receptors (Fig. 10.1)

The acetylcholine receptors are subdivided into NICOTINIC and MUSCARINIC receptor subtypes. These are named after the alkaloids (nicotine and muscarine) originally used for their identification. The term cholinoceptor means the receptors (nicotinic or muscarinic) which respond to ACh.

Nicotinic Receptors

The receptors located on neuromuscular junction (NMJ) and at all autonomic ganglia (including adrenal

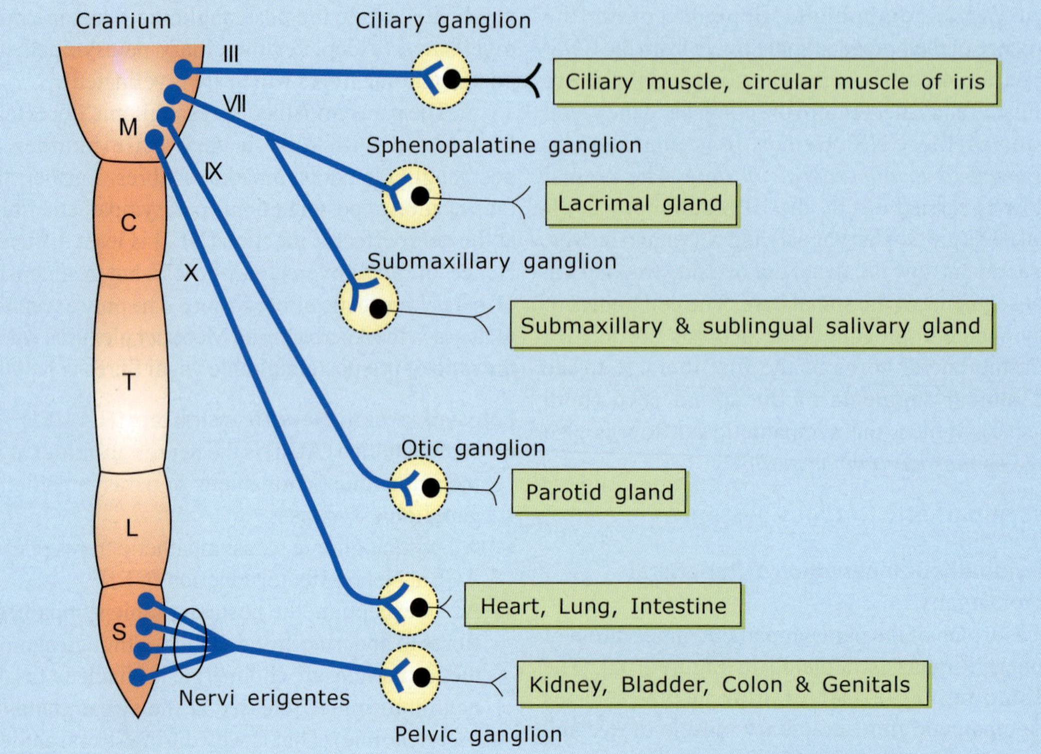

Key: M—Medullary; C—Cervical; T—Thoracic; L—Lumbar; S—Sacral
myelinated preganglionic parasympathetic fibres. myelinated postganglionic parasympathetic fibres (to ciliary muscle). non-myelinated postganglionic parasympathetic fibres (see text). Note that preganglionic parasympathetic fibres are long while postganglionic parasympathetic fibres are short. Also, the parasympathetic ganglia related to III, VII, IX and pelvic nerves are lying close to while that related to X (vagus) nerves are embedded within the wall of the effector organ.

Fig 10.2 The Parasympathetic Nervous System and its Effector Organs. (The Cranio-sacral Outflow is Bilaterally Paired But Only One Side Has Been Illustrated.)

medulla) are *nicotinic receptors.* These receptors are also present in the brain and appear to be located presynaptically where they play a facilitatory role in the release of other transmitters like dopamine and glutamate. However, the nicotinic receptors present at the neuromuscular junction (NMJ), at the autonomic ganglia and in the CNS are not identical and show molecular heterogeneity.

The nicotinic receptor subtypes are classified as *muscle type* (N_M), *neuronal type* (N_N) and *central nicotinic receptors.* This classification is based on the existence of selective agonists and antagonists which can distinguish these receptors (Table 10.1).

The selective agonists at the nicotinic receptors present at autonomic ganglia (N_N) are: DMPP (dimethyl phenyl piperazinium) and epibatidine (obtained from the skin of South American frog); while the selective antagonists at these receptors are: hexamethonium and trimethaphan. Similarly, the selective agonist of the nicotinic receptors at the neuromuscular junction (N_M) is PTMA (phenyltrimethyl-ammonium), while the selective antagonists are d-tubocurarine and α-bungarotoxin. Both these nicotinic receptors are the members of the "ligand gated ion channel" family of the receptors. The five protein subunits of the receptor are arranged around a central core forming a channel. This channel is normally closed but opens upon the binding of ACh (or any agonist). As the channel opens, Na^+ ions are permitted to flow down their concentration gradient to cause depolarisation (Fig. 10.3) (for details, refer to Ch.7).

Muscarinic Receptors

The receptors present at the parasympathetic neuroeffector junction (NEJ) at all smooth muscles and glands are muscarinic cholinergic receptors. These receptors are currently divided into five

Table 10.1 Comparison of the Nicotinic Receptor Subtypes

NICOTINIC RECEPTORS			
Characteristics	**Muscle type (N_M)**	**Neuronal type (N_N)**	**In CNS**
1. Location	At skeletal neuromuscular junction (NMJ); Postsynaptic	At all autonomic ganglia and at adrenal medulla; Postsynaptic	At sensory nerve terminals and in other parts of brain but mostly located presynaptically
2. Function	Contraction of skeletal muscle	Transmission of impulse through autonomic ganglia and firing of postganglionic neuron, and secretion of NE & E from adrenal medulla	Presynaptic facilitation of the release of dopamine and glutamate
3. Mechanism	Ligand gated ion channel family of receptors - opening of cation (Na^+) channel (end plate depolarisation)	Same as for N_M receptors	—
4. Agonists	ACh, Succinyl choline, PTMA*, Nicotine	Nicotine, DMPP* Epibatidine*	—
5. Antagonists	d-Tubocurarine α-Bungarotoxin*	Hexamethonium Trimethaphan*	—

Key: DMPP—Dimethylphenyl piperazinium
PTMA—Phenyltrimethyl ammonium
* More specific action

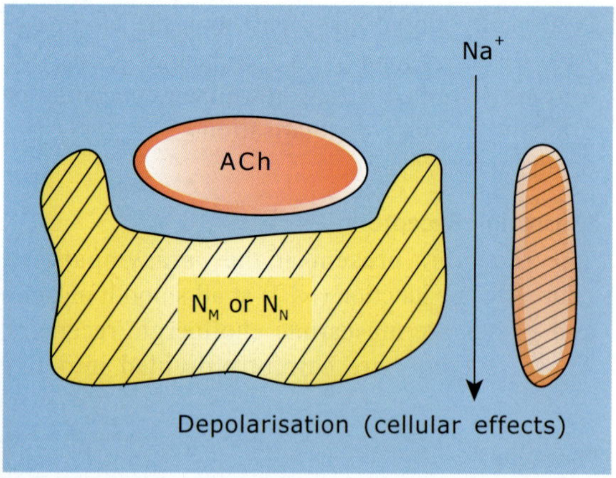

Fig 10.3 Functioning of Nicotinic Receptors.

subtypes (M_1 to M_5) depending upon (i) the pharmacological specificities of their agonists and antagonists and (ii) the findings from the molecular cloning of the human genes for these receptors. Three of these (M_1,M_2 & M_3) are well characterised while characteristics of the remaining two (M_4 & M_5) are less certain (Table 10.2).

M_1 receptors (neuronal and gastric) are found on the autonomic ganglia, in the CNS (cerebral cortex) and on gastric paracrine cells. The latter are also known as gastric muscarinic receptors. They mediate excitatory effects, e.g., increase in gastric acid secretion following vagal stimulation. These are also involved in slow excitation of sympathetic ganglia and central neurons by ACh. Two experimental drugs McNA-343 and oxotremorine are fairly selective agonists at M_1 receptor, while pirenzepine and telenzepine are selective antagonists at this receptor.

M_2 Receptors (cardiac): These are mainly located on myocardium, on smooth muscles and also on the presynaptic terminals of the peripheral and central neurons. *These exert mainly inhibitory effects,* e.g., their activation results in vagal inhibition of the heart (decrease in heart rate and conductivity).

Available agonists are non-selective; however, methacholine has prominent M_2 agonistic action, while antagonists like AF-DX 116 and tripitramine exhibit fairly selective antagonistic actions on M_2 receptor.

M_3 Receptors (glandular): These are located mainly on the glandular and visceral smooth muscles. *Their activation results in mainly excitatory effects,* e.g., increase in sweating, bronchial and salivary secretions and the contraction of visceral smooth muscles. However, their activation stimulates the release of nitric oxide from neighbouring endothelial cells causing relaxation of vascular smooth muscle. No selective agonist is available at present except bethanechol which has prominent agonist action on these receptors. However, selective M_3 receptor antagonists like darifenacin and tolterodine are available.

M_4 and M_5 receptors are largely confined to CNS but their functional role is poorly understood. The characteristics of muscarinic receptor subtypes are summarised in Table 10.2.

All muscarinic receptors (M_1 to M_5) belong to the family of G-protein coupled receptors. *The odd numbered members of this group* (M_1, M_3 & M_5) act through a common mechanism, i.e., through inositol phosphate pathway. The ACh (or any agonist) binds to these receptors, which are linked to Gq proteins, and activates the membrane enzyme phospholipase-C (PLC), which in turn hydrolyses phosphatidyl inositol-4,5–diphosphate (PIP_2) into diacylglycerol (DAG) and inositol-1,4,5,-triphosphate (IP_3) (second messengers). DAG activates a phospholipid and the Ca^{2+} sensitive protein kinase-C (PKC) which then phosphorylates specific enzyme substrate(s) leading to the response. IP_3 diffuses out of the cytoplasm where it triggers the release of Ca^{2+} from storage vesicles. The raised cytoplasmic Ca^{2+} concentration promotes the binding of Ca^{2+} to calmodulin (Cam) leading to the responses like depolarisation and increased secretions etc. (refer Fig. 7.8, Ch.7 where R is M_1, M_3 or M_5 while agonist is ACh).

The evenly numbered receptors (M_2 & M_4) are linked to Gi proteins. Their activation inhibits adenylate cyclase and thus reduces the intracellular cAMP concentration (Fig. 10.4). This opposes the response due to activation of the β_1 adrenergic receptor (which stimulates the Gs linked adenylate cyclase). In the myocardium cAMP increases the force of contraction, whereas, in intestines it causes relaxation. Consequently, an activation of M_2

Table 10.2 Comparison of Muscarinic Receptor Subtypes

MUSCARINIC RECEPTORS			
Characteristics	**M_1 (neuronal)**	**M_2 (cardiac)**	**M_3 (glandular)**
1. Location	Neural: Ganglia (autonomic and enteric), gastric paracrine cells, CNS (cortex and hippocampus)	Cardiac: SA node, AV node, atrium, ventricle; neural: presynaptic terminals	Exocrine glands, smooth muscles, vascular endothelium
2. Function	Gastric acid secretion, GI motility, CNS excitation	SA node: ↓ rate of impulse generation. AV node: ↓ velocity of conduction ↓ contractility: vagal bradycardia	↑ exocrine secretions, smooth muscle contraction[1]
3. Mechanism[2]	↑ IP_3, ↑ DAG, ↑ cytoplasmic Ca^{++}, depolarisation	Inhibition of adenylate cyclase (↓ cAMP) and opening of K^+ channels Inhibits neuronal Ca^{++} channels (presynaptic inhibition of ACh release)	Same as for M_1 receptors
4. Agonists	M_cNA-343*, oxotremorine	Methacholine	Bethanechol
5. Antagonists	Pirenzepine* Telenzepine*	AF-Dx 116* Tripitramine*	4-DAMP Tolterodine Darifenacin*

[1] Relaxation occurs at urinary and intestinal sphincters, which results due to release of peptides from parasympathetic nerves. Blood vessels also relax as a consequence of the release of nitric oxide (other smooth muscles contract).
[2] All muscarinic receptors belong to the family of G-protein coupled receptors.
* More selective agonist or antagonist.

receptors opposes these effects in heart and intestine by decreasing cAMP levels. M_2 receptors in pacemaker cells of the heart, however, act by activating K^+ channels through Gi proteins resulting in hyperpolarisation and a decrease in the heart rate (Fig. 10.4).

Presynaptic Cholinergic Receptors and Their Role in Cholinergic Transmission

The nicotinic or muscarinic receptors present on the effector organs (NEJ) are usually located postsynaptically (as discussed above). Hence these are termed as postsynaptic or postjunctional receptors. On activation, these receptors produce or mimick the responses of the neurotransmitter

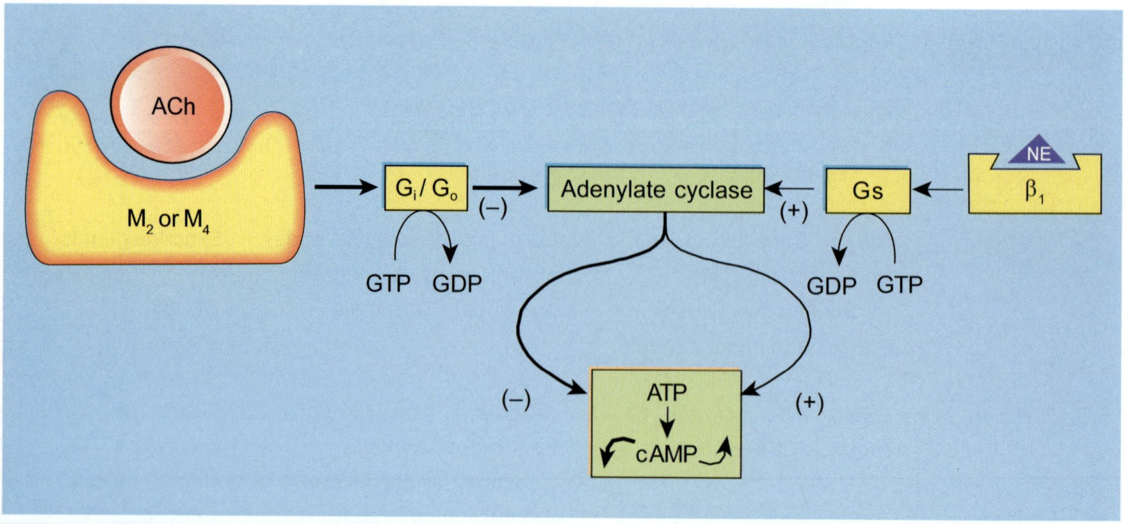

Fig 10.4 Functioning of M_2 and M_4 Receptors Through Inhibition of Adenylate Cyclase (bold face arrows). Interactions with Beta Adrenergic Receptor (lighter arrows). *Key*: ACh—Acetylcholine, NE—Norepinephrine.

(ACh). However, there exists an additional class of receptors which regulate the release of ACh at the effector site. These receptors are located on the cholinergic axon terminals (i.e., presynaptic or prejunctional). *Activation of these presynaptic receptors usually inhibits the ACh release from the axon terminals, through negative feedback mechanism*. Contrarily, the blockade of these receptors, by antagonists, rather facilitates the release of ACh. In all automobiles, there is an accelerator and a brake. The activation of the accelerator, enhances the speed while activation of the brake slows down the speed of the vehicle. Analogously, the postsynaptic receptors are like accelerator whose activation leads to an enhanced response; while presynaptic receptors act like brakes, whose activation decreases the release of the neurotransmitter and thus diminishes the response (Fig. 10.5).

The presynaptic release of the neurotransmitter (ACh) is regulated by the following mechanisms:

1. ***By Homotropic Receptor Interaction***. Where ACh released from its nerve terminal acts on its presynaptic autoreceptor and inhibits its own release (Fig. 10.5A).
2. ***By Heterotropic Receptor Interaction***. Where one neuron (e.g., sympathetic neuron) may control the neurotransmitter release of the other neuron, e.g., a parasympathetic neuron (Fig. 10.5B). In intestine, there is an anatomical proximity of the sympathetic and the parasympathetic postganglionic neuron; and the α_2 adrenergic receptors are located on these cholinergic nerve terminals. Hence these α_2 receptors (although being postsynaptic to sympathetic neuron) are located presynaptically on the cholinergic neuron. Now, the norepinephrine released from the adrenergic neuron is virtually activating α_2 receptors which are located presynaptically on the cholinergic neuron. Such presynaptic activation of α_2 receptors on cholinergic neuron would ultimately inhibit the release of ACh from these neurons. This explains the observed intestinal relaxant effects of norepinephrine (Fig. 10.5B).

The functioning of the presynaptic nicotinic receptor is rather an exception to the rule, as paradoxically the activation of the presynaptic nicotinic receptor, however, facilitates the release of ACh.

The presynaptic receptors regulate transmitter release mainly by inhibiting Ca^{2+} entry into the nerve terminal

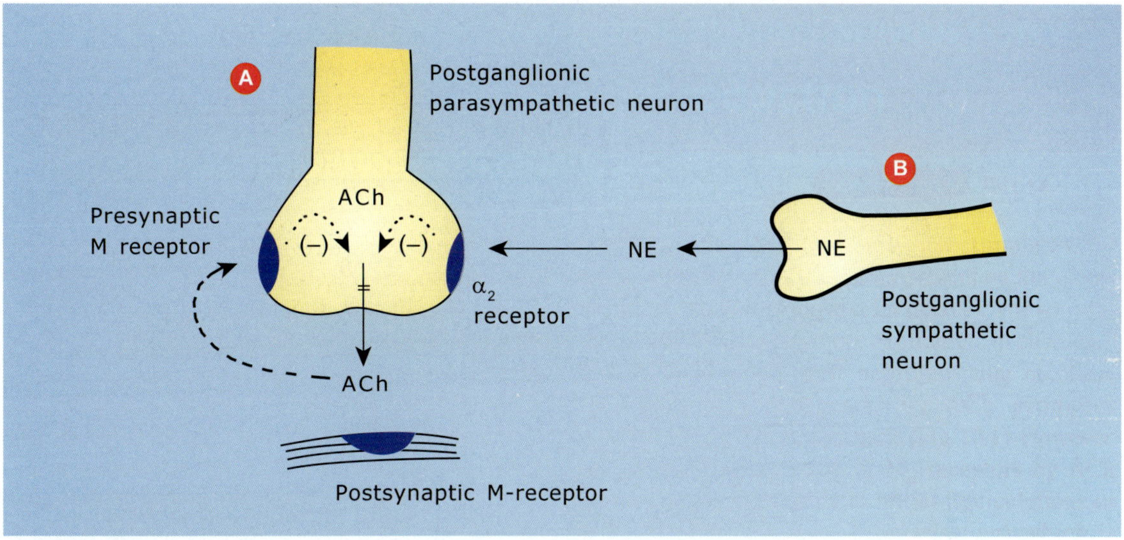

Fig 10.5 (A) Homotropic Presynaptic Receptor Interaction.
(B) Heterotropic Presynaptic Receptor Interaction.

or by increasing K^+ permeability (leading to hyperpolarisation) or by impairment of the coupling between increased $[Ca^{2+}]$ i and vesicle discharge.

Sympathetic Nervous System

Sympathetic Innervation of Peripheral Effector Organs

The sympathetic preganglionic neurons have their cell bodies in the lateral horn of the grey matter of the thoracic and lumbar segments of the spinal cord. These neurons leave the spinal cord through the ventral root of the spinal nerves from the first thoracic to the third lumbar segments (both inclusive). Hence, the sympathetic outflow is also termed as the *"thoraco-lumbar outflow"*.

Just outside the spinal cord, these neurons leave the spinal nerve and communicate with the *paravertebral chain of 22 sympathetic ganglia,* which lie bilaterally on either side of the spinal column. Each ganglia is connected to each other (above and below) by the nerve trunk (Fig. 10.6).

Although these 22 ganglia are placed bilaterally from cervical to sacral vertebra, the white rami communicates with them only in T_1–T_{12} and L_1–L_3 region (i.e., in only 15 ganglia) and it is from here the sympathetic outflow takes place. The three cervical ganglia at the top and the four sacral ganglia at the bottom are not communicated with white rami. The preganglionic fibres to these ganglia run directly upward (to 3 cervical ganglia) or downward (to 4 sacral ganglia), making no synapse in between. These finally make synapse with their postganglionic neurons at superior cervical or sacral ganglia. Through superior cervical ganglia, the sympathetic innervation goes to radial muscle of iris, smooth muscles of eyelids, salivary glands and blood vessels of head and neck. Through sacral ganglia, the sympathetic innervation goes to sex organs and bladder etc (Fig. 10.6).

Between T_1 and T_4, the preganglionic fibres originating from white ramus make a synapse with postganglionic fibres in paravertebral ganglia. The name ("white") indicates that they contain myelinated fibres. The postganglionic neurons (non-myelinated) then pass through the gray ramus communicantes to most of the major organs like heart, thorax and respiratory tract. Between T_5–L_3, however, some preganglionic fibres, after entering the chain of paravertebral ganglia, pass straight without making any synapse. These fibres, later synapse with the postganglionic neurons in another set of ganglia called as the *prevertebral ganglia.*

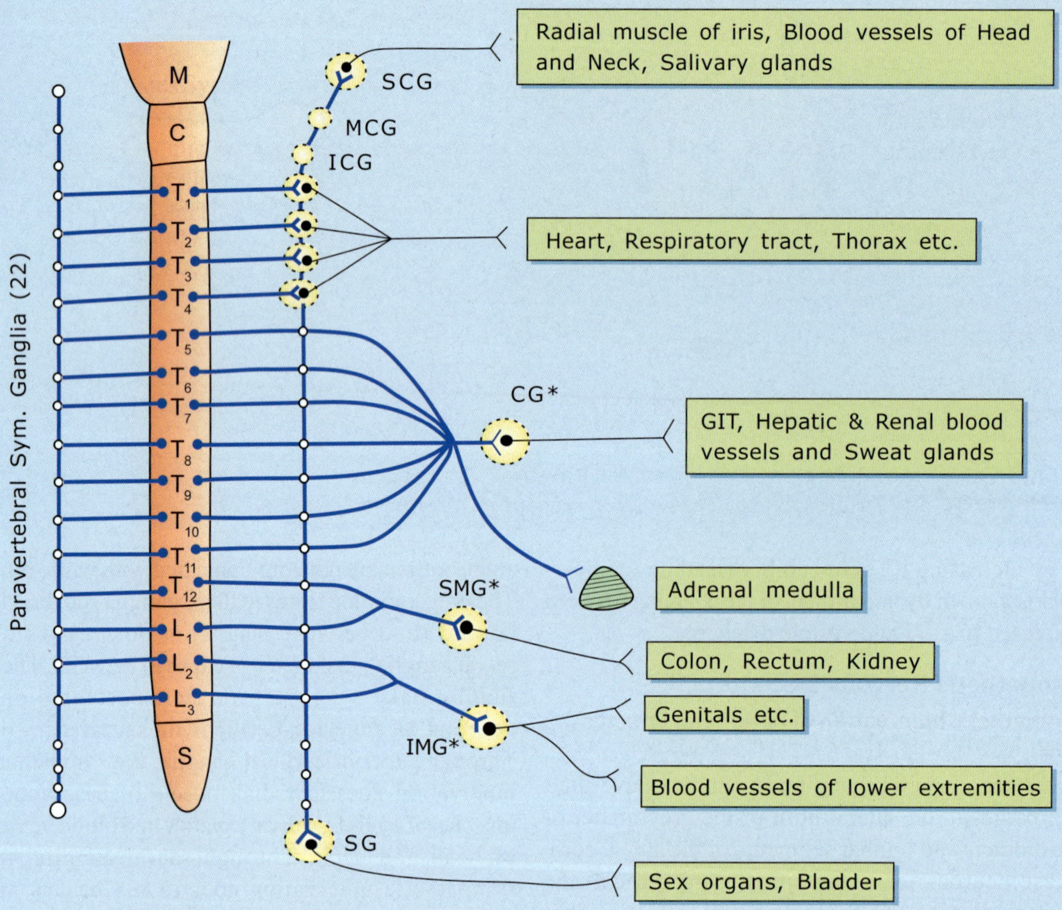

Key: preganglionic neuron; postganglionic neuron; * - prevertebral ganglia (not bilaterally paired); SCG—Superior cervical ganglia; MCG—Middle cervical ganglia; ICG—Inferior cervical ganglia; CG—Coeliac ganglia; SMG—Superior mesenteric ganglia; IMG—Inferior mesenteric ganglia; SG—Sacral ganglia; M—Medulla; C—Cervical; T—Thoracic; L—Lumbar; S—Sacral. Although paravertebral sympathetic ganglia (22) chain is bilaterally paired, yet for convenience, the innervation has been shown only on the right side of the figure.

Fig 10.6 Sympathetic Nervous System and its Effector Organs.

These ganglia, however, are not bilaterally paired and lie in front of vertebrae, on the ventral surface of aorta. There are three main prevertebral ganglia:

1. ***Coeliac Ganglia (or coeliac plexus)***. Preganglionic nerves from T_5–T_{11} form this ganglion. It lies near the junction of coeliac artery and aorta. The postganglionic neurons from this ganglion innervate stomach, liver, spleen, small intestine, proximal colon and renal blood vessels.
2. ***Superior Mesenteric Ganglia (or plexus)***. Preganglionic nerves from T_{12}–L_1 form this ganglion. It lies near the junction of the superior mesenteric artery and the aorta and innervates colon, rectum and kidneys, through postganglionic fibres.
3. ***Inferior Mesenteric Ganglia (or plexus)***. Preganglionic fibres from L_2–L_3 form this ganglion. This lies adjacent to the inferior mesenteric artery and supplies to distal colon, rectum, bladder and genitalia, through postganglionic fibres.

Some preganglionic fibres (from T_{10}–T_{11}) terminate into chromaffin cells of adrenal medulla, i.e., there are no further postganglionic fibres thereafter. The adrenal medulla is considered, embryologically and functionally, equivalent to sympathetic prevertebral ganglia. Sympathetic preganglionic fibres (related to paravertebral ganglia) are either shorter or are equal in length to the postganglionic fibres. On the contrary the preganglionic fibres (related to prevertebral ganglia) are long compared to their respective postganglionic fibers. Preganglionic sympathetic fibres tend to synapse with a large number of postganglionic fibres which in turn have a more diffused ramification (Fig. 10.6 obviously is an oversimplification) at neuroeffector junction (NEJ). Hence, the effects of sympathetic neurotransmission are more widespread as compared to parasympathetic neurotransmission.

Sympathetic Neurotransmitters (Fig. 10.1)

- As discussed above, the neurotransmitter at the sympathetic ganglia is acetylcholine (ACh)
- In general, all postganglionic sympathetic fibres (with few exceptions) release norepinephrine (NE) at the neuroeffector junction (NEJ) (in UK, norepinephrine and epinephrine are named as noradrenaline and adrenaline respectively).

  The exception are (a) the postganglionic sympathetic fibres to sweat glands. These fibres are sympathetic in origin but are cholinergic in character, because the neurotransmitter released here is acetylcholine (ACh); (b) some postganglionic fibres supplying to the arterioles of skeletal muscle. As discussed above, these fibres are also sympathetic in origin but cholinergic in character. When activated (particularly during exercise) these show vasodilatation instead of constriction; (c) some postganglionic sympathetic neurons (particularly at splanchnic and renal blood vessels). These fibres are sympathetic in origin but dopaminergic in character, as the neurotransmitter released here is dopamine (DA). Although dopamine is a major neurotransmitter in brain, it also plays an important role in the periphery in these blood vessels (see following text—dopamine receptors).
- The chromaffin cells of adrenal medulla are innervated by the preganglionic sympathetic nerve fibres where the neurotransmitter is ACh. On stimulation these cells secrete epinephrine (E) directly into the bloodstream along with small amounts of norepinephrine (NE).

Adrenergic Receptors

A diagramatic representation of the currently known adrenergic receptor subtypes along with examples of agonists (agents that stimulate) and the antagonists (agents that block) is presented in Fig. 10.7.

Among dopamine receptor subtypes, only D_1 and D_2 have some limited peripheral role as discussed above. However, classically these should not be considered as adrenergic receptors.

α-Adrenergic Receptors

These are of two types: α_1 and α_2, both of which are G-protein coupled receptors (metabotropic receptors)

i) **α_1 Adrenergic Receptors**: Although the tissue distribution and functional role of different subtypes of α_1 receptors is not clear, yet *as a rule these α_1 receptors are present postsynaptically and when activated by an agonist these produce excitatory effects in most of the organs (e.g., vascular smooth muscle, salivary glands, bronchi, uterus, radial muscle of iris, urinary bladder neck, liver cells) EXCEPT in intestines*

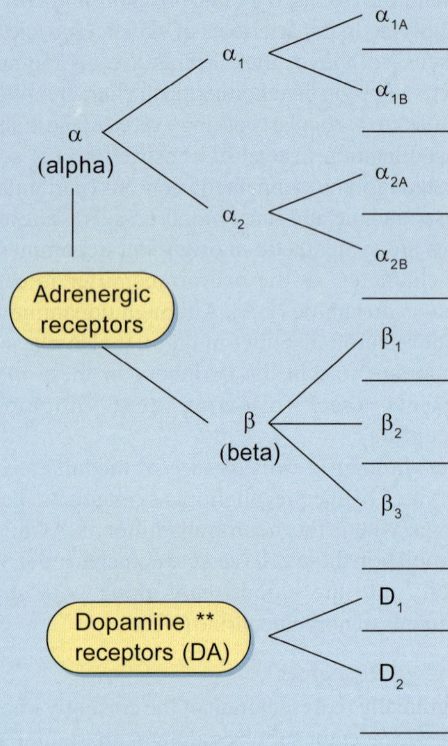

Receptor	AGONISTS	ANTAGONISTS
$α_{1A}$	A61603* Phenylephrine Methoxamine	5-methylurapidil* Tamsulosin* Prazosin, Terazosin
$α_{1B}$	Phenylephrine Methoxamine	CEC*, Prazosin, Terazosin
$α_{2A}$	Oxymetazoline* Clonidine	Yohimbine
$α_{2B}$	Oxymetazoline Clonidine	ARC-239* Yohimbine
$β_1$	Dobutamine* Xamoterol*	Atenolol* Acebutolol
$β_2$	Terbutaline Salbutamol*	ICI-118551 Butoxamine
$β_3$	BRL-37344* AD-9677* Mirabegron	Cyanopindalol CGP-20712A
D_1	Fenoldopam*	SCH-23390*
D_2	Bromocriptine	Sulpiride

Key: * – more specific action. ** – classically not an adrenergic receptor. Only those DA receptor subtypes have been shown which have some peripheral role.

Fig 10.7 Adrenergic Receptor Subtypes and their Agonists and Antagonists.

where they produce inhibitory effects (relaxation).

All $α_1$ receptors are activated by agonists like phenylephrine and methoxamine and blocked by prazosin and terazosin. $α_1$ receptor has further subtypes as $α_{1A}$, $α_{1B}$, $α_{1C}$, $α_{1D}$ and $α_{1L}$. Although the location of these subtypes is known, the differences in their mechanism of action are not clearly defined. Even their *selective* agonists and antagonists are not available, except for *tamsulosin* which is a selective antagonist of $α_{1A}$ receptor which is located at the urinary bladder neck, urinary sphincter and prostate. Tamsulosin is therefore used to treat benign prostate hyperplasia.

The excitatory responses of $α_1$ *receptor activation* are mediated through inositol phosphate pathway (as described in Ch. 7, Fig. 7.8 where R is $α_1$ receptor and agonist is phenylephrine). *The inhibitory (relaxant) effects of* $α_1$ *receptor activation* in the gut result due to different mechanism. Here these G-protein coupled receptors are acting through an increase in the ionic permeability of K^+ ions leading to hyperpolarisation (relaxation), without involving any role of second messenger (like IP_3 and DAG as discussed above).

ii) **α_2 Adrenergic Receptors**: These are located mainly presynaptically on the sympathetic postganglionic neuron. Stimulation of these receptors by the released neurotransmitter (NE) or by any exogenously administered agonist (like *clonidine*) decreases the release of the neurotransmitter NE. (Fig 10.8A, presynaptic homotropic receptor activation). The neurotransmitter potency order is E =NE.

Presynaptic α_2 receptors are also located on the cholinergic nerve terminals of the gut. When these receptors are activated, the release of ACh is decreased from the cholinergic neuron leading to relaxation (Fig. 10.8B, heterotropic presynaptic receptor interaction. See Fig. 10.5 for details). On the other hand, the blockade of this presynaptic α_2 receptor by α_2 receptor antagonist (like *yohimbine*) would provide an enhanced flow of NE.

Although α_2 receptor is considered to exist mainly presynaptically, yet the radioligand binding studies have shown it to be present postsynaptically as well, e.g., in brain (decrease in sympathetic outflow), in platelets (causing aggregation) and on β-pancreatic cells (inhibiting insulin release).

Three subtypes of α_2 receptors, α_{2A}, α_{2B} and α_{2C}, have been identified but the difference in their mechanism of action and their characteristic agonist and antagonist are not known. *Thus, in brain, the α_2 receptors whether present postsynaptically or presynaptically, decrease the sympathetic outflow* (in the periphery) *upon their activation* (*leading to hypotension*). The vascular smooth muscle possesses postsynaptic α_1 as well as α_{2B} adrenergic receptors, both of which mediate contraction of blood vessels. In higher doses, clonidine may activate these α_{2B} receptor which may lead to even hypertension due to initial vasoconstriction. However, clonidine has higher affinity for α_{2A} than α_{2B}.

The α_2 receptor agonists inhibit adenylate cyclase through an inhibitory G-protein (Gi) and reduce the intracellular cAMP concentration. The reduced cAMP concentration results in a decreased activation of cAMP dependent protein kinase and consequently in a diminished response (i.e., hypotension, Fig. 10.9).

β-Adrenergic Receptors

β-adrenergic receptors are subdivided into β_1, β_2 and β_3 subtypes. The availability of β-receptor antagonists with high selectivity for either β_1, β_2 or β_3 subtypes has led to this classification. None of the typical β_1 or β_2 antagonists can potentially inhibit β_3 receptor (Fig. 10.7).

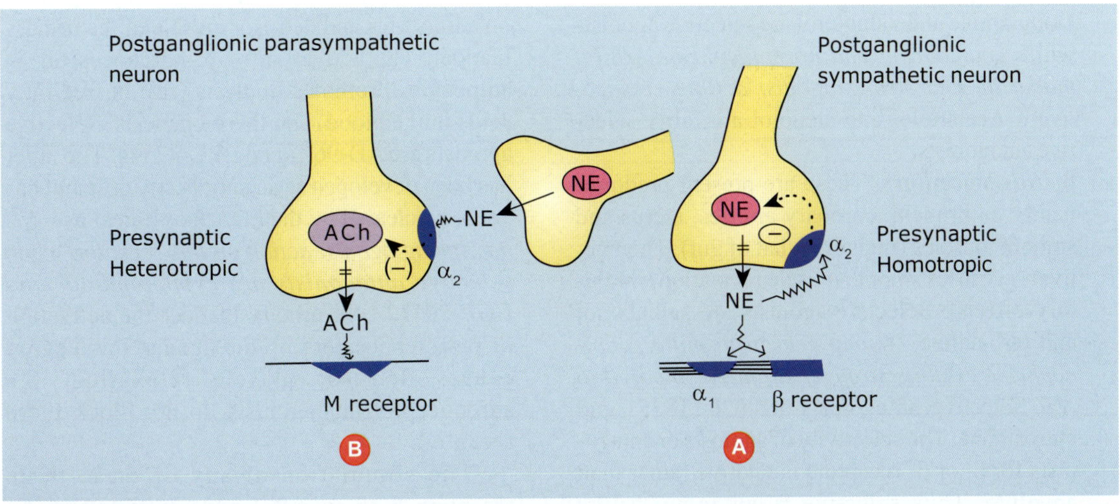

Fig 10.8 Presynaptic α_2 Receptor and the Regulation of NE (A) or ACh (B) Release From the Adrenergic or Cholinergic Neuron.

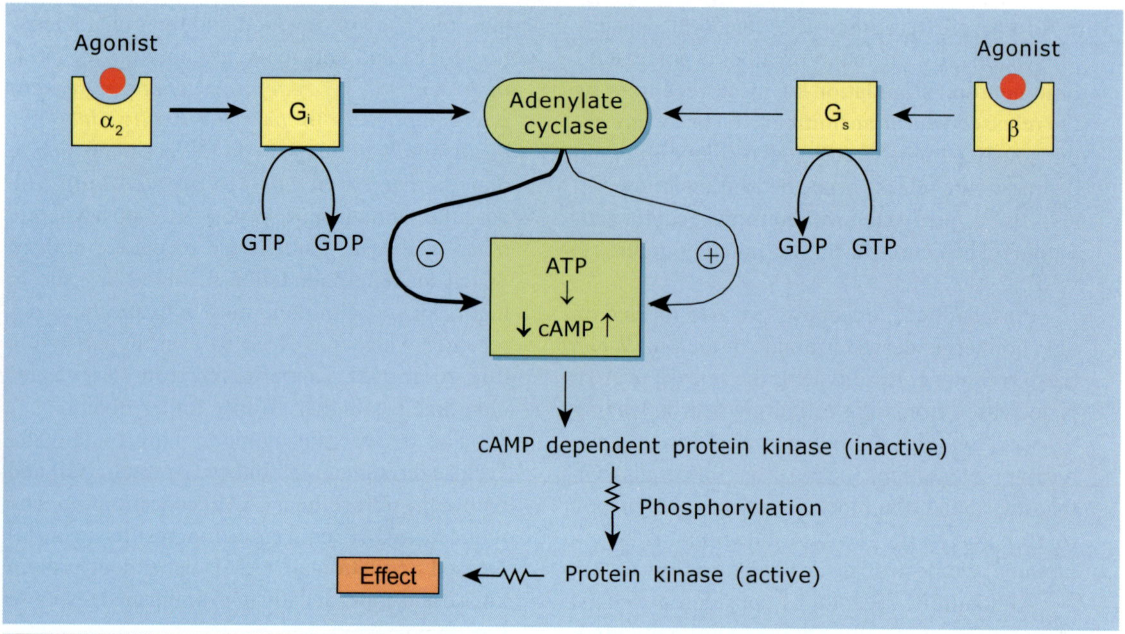

Fig 10.9 Activation (+) and Inhibition (-) of Adenylate Cyclase by β-Receptor Agonists (thin arrows) and α_2-Receptor Agonists (thick arrows) respectively.

i) **β_1-Adrenoceptors**: These are found mainly in the heart where these produce positive inotropic and positive chronotropic effects (i.e., excitatory effects) upon activation by agonists (e.g., NE). They are also present on the juxta-glomerular cells of the kidney where these promote renin release. Dobutamine and xamoterol are selective agonists while *epinephrine and norepinephrine exhibit moderate and strong agonist actions, respectively.* Acebutolol and atenolol are fairly selective antagonists.

ii) **β_2-Adrenoceptors**: These are present predominantly on bronchi, coronary arteries, uterus and smooth muscles (including that of gut). Their activation causes smooth muscle relaxation (inhibitory effects). Selective agonists are salbutamol and terbutaline. *Among neurotransmitters, epinephrine exhibits stronger affinity compared to NE.* Selective antagonists are ICI-118551 and butoxamine. The selectivity of agonists or antagonists for β_1 or β_2 receptors is relative rather than absolute. Thus selective β_1 antagonists like atenolol and metoprolol invariably have some β_2 receptor antagonist action also, which may cause some unwanted effects like bronchoconstriction, whereas selective β_2 agonists like salbutamol which causes bronchodilatation can also exhibit excitatory effects (β_1 effects) on heart (tachycardia).

iii) **β_3-Adrenoceptors**: These *receptors* are present on adipocytes and detrusor muscle of the urinary bladder. The activation of β_3-adrenoceptors in adipocytes promotes lipolysis (rise in free fatty acids in the blood) and thermogenesis. Selective agonists are AD-9677 and BRL-37344. The latter has been developed as an antiobesity drug but has yet to be cleared by the FDA for clinical use. *NE has strong agonist action on this receptor, while selective antagonists are cyanopindalol and CGP-20712A.* In urinary bladder the activation of β_3-adrenoceptors by the agonist mirabegron causes detrusor muscle relaxation. β_2-adrenoceptor anatagonists do not block these receptors.

The stimulation of any of these three receptors, β_1, β_2, and β_3 leads to an activation of membrane bound enzyme adenylate cyclase which catalyses the conversion of ATP to cAMP.

Table 10.3 Characteristics of Adrenoceptors

Receptor	Location	G-Protein	Second messenger	Function
α_1	Postsynaptic, most smooth muscles, salivary glands, liver cells	G_q	↑ IP_3 ↑ DAG	↑ Ca^{++} conc., contraction of smooth muscle, ↑ secretions
α_2	Presynaptic on adrenergic or cholinergic nerve terminals; Postsynaptic in brain; β-Pancreatic cells Vascular smooth muscle (α_{2B})	G_i	↓ cAMP	↓ NE release ↓ Central sympathetic outflow ↓ Insulin release Vasoconstriction
β_1	Postsynaptic at cardiac muscle, Juxtaglomerular apparatus; also presynaptic at adrenergic and cholinergic nerve terminal (but mainly postsynaptic)	G_s	↑ cAMP	↑ In heart rate ↑ Force of contraction ↑ In renin release
β_2	Post- as well as presynaptic in bronchi, coronary arteries, uterus and smooth muscles; also in myocardium	G_s	↑ cAMP	↑ NE and E release, Relaxation of smooth muscle ↑ Glycogenolysis ↑ Heart rate ↑ Force of contraction
β_3	Postsynaptic at adipocytes	G_s	↑ cAMP	↑ Lipolysis, ↑ Thermogenesis
	Postsynaptic at urinary bladder detrusor muscle	G_s	↑ cAMP	Bladder detrusor muscles relaxation (increased bladder capacity to retain urine)

The cyclic AMP then activates an intracellular enzyme (cAMP-dependent protein kinase) which phosphorylates various intracellular proteins leading to the biological effects (Fig. 10.9). The pharmacological characteristics of adrenoceptors are summarized in Table 10.3.

iv) **Presynaptic β Receptors**. These belong to β_1/β_2 receptor subtypes and have been identified on adrenergic nerve terminals. Activation of these receptors by any agonist (or NE), facilitates the neurotransmitter release; an effect which is opposite to that usually observed after presynaptic α_2 adrenergic receptor activation as discussed earlier (Fig. 10.10).

The reason as to why the presynaptic α-receptor (α_2) activation retards the release of NE whereas an activation of presynaptic β-receptor (β_2) rather faciltates the NE release is not yet clear. It seems that this strange type of combined positive and negative feedback mechanisms have been provided by the nature to manage the "need based" release of NE. It is well known that the circulating epinephrine

(E) can be accumulated by the sympathetic varicosities and is subsequently coreleased with NE. Epinephrine having higher affinity for β_2 receptor can activate presynaptic β_2 receptor to facilitate NE release from the adrenergic neuron. The presynaptic β-receptors in our body are just serving as a "*choke*" which is provided in petrol driven vehicles. If we are at rest and are faced with a sudden unexpected emergency, there should be an immediate release of sufficient NE. Activation of β_2 receptor , by coreleased E, would provide a positive feedback for instant NE release (in the same way as activation of choke provides instant petrol to the engine). Thereafter, if the optimal concentration of NE is surpassed in the synaptic cleft, the presynaptic α_2 receptors get activated which slow down or terminate the further release of NE by negative feedback mechanism.

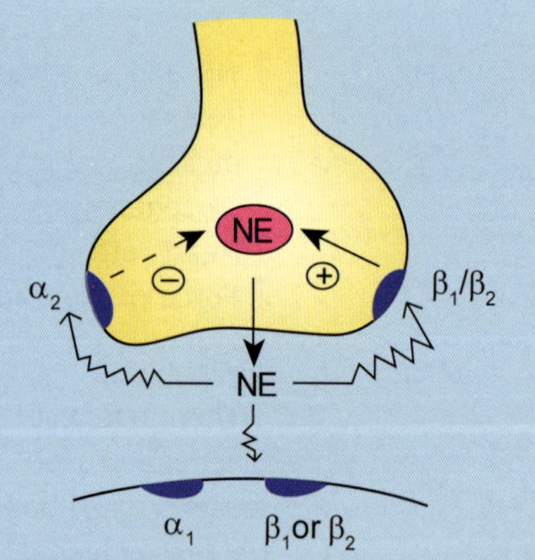

Fig 10.10 Presynaptic Autoreceptors that Regulate the Release of Neurotransmitter (NE) from Adrenergic Neuron: Activation of Presynaptic β_1/β_2 Receptor Facilitates (+), While that of Presynaptic α_2 Receptor Inhibits (-) the NE Release.

Dopamine Receptors

Dopamine (DA) is an endogenous catecholamine neurotransmitter, like NE and E, which produces a variety of biological effects that are mediated by interactions with specific DA receptors. Although DA serves as a precursor of NE and E, this endogenous amine does not have noticeable sympathomimetic action. At higher doses it, however, activates β_1 receptors. At still higher doses it can activate α_1 receptors as well. Although DA receptors are distinct from α and β receptors and are particularly important in CNS, yet these have some valuable role to play in the splanchnic and renal vasculature.

Although at least five subtypes of DA receptors exist, the D_1 *subtype* appears to be more important in the periphery (renal, mesenteric and coronary vascular beds). The D_2 *subtype* is pharmacologically more important in the CNS but it is found presynaptic as well. The original D_1 receptor family now includes D_1 and D_5 and is associated with stimulation of adenylate cyclase (i.e., ↑ cAMP), while D_2 receptor family consists of D_2, D_3 and D_4. Their activation inhibits adenylate cyclase activity (i.e., ↓ in cAMP), opens K^+ channels and blocks Ca^{2+} channels. Dopamine through D_1 receptor activation (which has more pharmacological role to play in the periphery) causes vasodilatation in the renal and mesenteric arteries; and increases myocardial contractility by direct stimulation of β_1 receptor (to save us from renal failure and shock in E-situations like blood loss during fighting). The pharmacological characteristics of DA receptors are presented in Table 10.4, while agonists and antagonists at D_1 and D_2 receptors are listed in Fig. 10.7.

Autonomic Innervations: Exceptions and Rules

Most body organs receive dual innervation, i.e., fibres from both parasympathetic as well as sympathetic divisions. These two divisions usually have opposing effects on a given organ (one causing inhibition while the other causing excitation). However, it is an over-simplified statement and not a rule.

Parasympathetic is an energy saving and a restorative system. Thus the food is digested and absorbed to provide energy, while the wastes are eliminated. ***The sympathetic division***, on the other hand, prepares the body for emergency situations which of course involve expenditure of energy. In

Table 10.4 Characteristics of D_1 and D_2 Receptors

Receptor	Location	G-Protein	Second messenger	Function
D_1	Postsynaptic, brain, renal, mesenteric, coronary vascular bed and myocardium	G_s	↑ cAMP and/or PIP_2 hydrolysis	Vasodilatation of renal vasculature
D_2	Mainly in the CNS; also presynaptically at nerve terminals, also in renal vascular bed	G_i	↓ cAMP ↑ K^+ conductance; Blocks Ca^{++} channels	↓ NE release; Modulates DA release

the normal situations, the sympathetic division counteracts the parasympathetic effects to a certain degree only, so as to provide the desired energy to the body. But in the "E-situations" (Emergency, Exercise and Embarrassment), the sympathetic system sets in motion a series of physiological responses either to fight the crisis or to fly for safety. However, the following are some exceptions to the basic rule of dual innervation.

i) ***Only sympathetic (no parasympathetic) innervation:*** Radial muscle of iris, smooth muscles of eyelids, nictitating membrane, pilomotor muscle, ventricular myocardium, bladder neck (trigone), seminal vesicle and vas deferens.

ii) ***Only parasympathetic (no sympathetic) innervation:*** Circular muscle of iris, ciliary muscle, larcrimal glands, mucous membrane of GIT and bronchial tree, pancreatic exocrine glands, detrusor muscle of bladder and erectile tissue of penis.

iii) ***Only adrenergic receptors (but no sympathetic innervation):*** Adipocytes (lipolysis), liver cells (gluconeogenesis), skeletal muscle cells (glycolysis) do have β-receptors but no sympathetic innervation.

iv) ***Only cholinergic receptors (but no parasympathetic innervation):*** Blood vessels have muscarinic receptors but have no parasympathetic innervation. Hence they respond only to exogenously given ACh (I.V.).

v) Usually, sympathetic system is antagonist to the parasympathetic, ***yet at salivary glands the effect of both the systems is complementary to each other,*** as stimulation of both promotes salivary secretions. However, parasympathetic stimulation makes saliva more watery (due to vasodilatation) while sympathetic stimulation makes the saliva more viscid (due to vasoconstriction). This system has been provided by nature to save us from embarrassment. Needless-to-say, the dripping saliva along the chin, would look very awful in the situations when you are fighting.

vi) ***Fibres which are sympathetic in origin but cholinergic in character*** : The postganglionic sympathetic fibres to sweat glands, arterioles of skeletal muscles and external genitalia are cholinergic in character, although sympathetic in origin. At these sites, the neurotransmitter released is ACh (not NE); otherwise, at all postganglionic sympathetic fibres and at effector organs the neurotransmitter released is NE.

Cotransmission in the ANS

Had ACh and NE been the only neurotransmitters in the ANS, the neurotransmission in different organs should have been completely blocked by anticholinergic or noradrenergic blocking drugs. However, this is not true. That shows that autonomic neurons also contain some other substances as well, which have potential activity at the relevant postsynaptic sites. This means that autonomic neurotransmission also encompasses other chemical substances which function as

COTRANSMITTERS. We would restrict our discussion to ATP, VIP and NPY (neuropeptide Y) only, because evidence for their function as contransmitters in ANS is quite substantial.

Both ATP and NE are found within the same storage granule in the sympathetic neuron. Both NE and ATP elicit excitation (contraction) after their release from adrenergic nerve terminal such as those in vas deferens and the vasculature but the response to ATP is rapid (and is blocked by ATP antagonist, *suramine*), while that of NE is slow (and is blocked by α-adrenoceptor blocker, *prazosin*). Drugs like *isoprenaline* (a β-receptor agonist) may provide a differential release of contransmitter and the neurotransmitter (inhibits ATP release while enhances NE release) from the sympathetic nerve terminal.

Similarly, the Vasoactive Intestinal Peptide (VIP) regulates the secretions of saliva during cholinergic stimulation. Here, the secretory responses are produced by ACh while the vasodilatation is partly contributed by VIP. It has been revealed that in GIT, sphincter relaxation is partly facilitated by synergistic action of VIP to ACh response.

At sympathetic nerve terminals, NE and NPY (neuropeptide Y) are stored in separate vesicles. As compared to NE, NPY is released at a higher frequency. This maintains a balanced release of neurotransmitters under varying impulse patterns. In the periphery, NPY action is synergistic to NE (vasoconstriction).

Recently, attention has been focused on the rapidly growing list of peptide group of cotransmitters that are found in the organs innervated by ANS. This list includes enkephalins, substance-P, thyrotropin releasing hormone (TRH), gonadotropin releasing hormone (GnRH), somatostatin and calcitonin gene related peptide (CGRP).

Nonadrenergic–Noncholinergic (NANC) Transmission in ANS

The smooth muscles of many tissues, which are innervated by ANS, get relaxed following stimulation by external electrodes even when there was a total adrenergic and cholinergic blockade. This suggests some existence of non-adrenergic-noncholinergic (NANC) transmission in ANS.

Some of the NANC fibres are motor fibres that cause the release of purines (ATP, adenosine etc.). Purine, especially adenosine, is produced in the cells mainly as a by-product of ATP-breakdown. The main effects of adenosine are: vasodilatation, inhibition of platelet aggregation, bronchoconstriction and neuroprotection during ischaemia. Other NANC fibres are some sensory fibres because when activated by sensory inputs these are capable of releasing peptide transmitters from the sensory nerve ending itself. These peptides (e.g., VIP, CGRP and NPY) are potent agonists at many autonomic effector tissues.

Many nonpeptides, e.g., nitric oxide (NO) and endothelins have also been identified as potentially important NANC transmitters in vascular responses.

In response to a variety of vasoactive agents and even physical stimuli, the endothelial cells release a short lived vasodilator called *endothelium derived releasing factor* (EDRF) which has now been identified as nitric oxide (NO). The latter has also been shown to be released from certain nerves, which innervate blood vessels. All blood vessels have muscarinic receptors located on endothelial cells (with no cholinergic innervation). Activation of these receptors by exogenously administered ACh releases EDRF (i.e., NO) which diffuses to the smooth muscle to cause relaxation. It has a negative inotropic action on the heart as well. In contrast, the endothelin peptides (which are stored and released by vascular endothelial cells and act as NANC transmitter) contribute to the maintenance of vascular homeostasis by reversing (i.e., contraction) the response of nitric oxide (i.e., relaxation).

ENTERIC NERVOUS SYSTEM (ENS)

Although semi-autonomous part of ANS, some prefer to classify it as a third division of ANS. The Enteric Nervous System (ENS) is a well organised collection of different neurons located in the wall of GIT with a specific purpose of controlling its functions. While the parasympathetic and the sympathetic nervous system are essentially linked with CNS and cannot function without it, the ENS has sufficient integrative capability to function

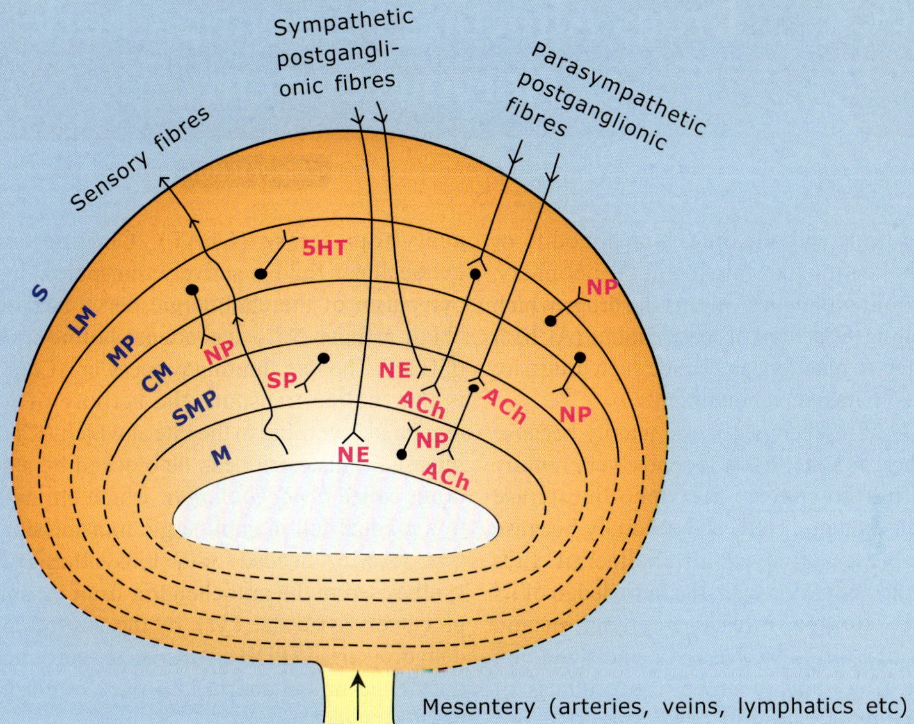

Key: LM—longitudinal muscle; MP—myenteric plexus (Auerbach's); CM—circular muscle: SMP—submucosal plexus (Meissner's); M—mucosa; S—serosa; NE—norepinephrine; ACh—acetylcholine; 5HT—serotonin; SP—substance-P; NP—neuropeptide

Fig 10.11 A Simplified Representation of the Layers of the Wall of Stomach/Small Intestine/Colon.

independently of the CNS (hence called 'brain of the gut'). ENS controls the motility, exocrine and endocrine secretions and the microcirculation of GI tract. It is modulated by both the parasympathetic and sympathetic nervous system.

The intestine receives a dual innervation from the ANS, with parasympathetic cholinergic activity generally increasing the motility of intestine (while relaxing the sphincters) and sympathetic noradrenergic activity usually decreasing the motility of the gut (while causing sphincters to contract). The preganglionic parasympathetic fibres consist of vagal and sacral efferents. These generally make a contact at the ENS ganglia present in the myenteric (MP) and submucosal plexus (SMP). The sympathetic fibres are postganglionic, but some of them end upon the postganglionic cholinergic neurons (heterotropic interaction) where they inhibit ACh release (relaxation) as discussed earlier; while others end directly at intestinal smooth muscles (β_2 effect—relaxation).

Besides ACh and NE, many other neurotransmitters or neuromodulators have been identified in the ENS and these include neuropeptide (NP), substance P (SP), serotonin (5HT), dopamine (DA) and cholecystokinin (CCK) (Fig. 10.11). Under the influence of these neurotransmitters and neuromodulators, the plexus perform their peristaltic and other functions and also coordinate motor activity in the total absence of CNS control.

CHAPTER 11

Drugs Affecting Parasympathetic Nervous System

COMPETENCY PH1.14, PH1.58, PH1.52

This chapter deals with the drugs which modify or affect the cholinergic transmission in the periphery. The term "cholinomimetics" means the drugs which imitate or mimic the actions of acetylcholine (ACh) at the neuroeffector junction, and hence such drugs are also called as "parasympathomimetics".

ACh is of no therapeutic use mainly because of its ultrashort action (t½ few seconds; very rapidly hydrolysed by the enzyme acetylcho-linesterase present in the synaptic cleft) and secondly because of its widespread activity at all cholinergic sites throughout the body. However, the knowledge of its biosynthesis, storage, release, degradation and receptor actions forms the basis for understanding the pharmacology and therapeutic usefulness of other cholinomimetic drugs. Considering ACh as a prototype drug, its pharmacology will be discussed prior to the pharmacology of other cholinomimetics.

ACETYLCHOLINE (PROTOTYPE DRUG)

Chemically, ACh is the acetic acid ester of choline (Fig. 11.1).

$$CH_3.\overset{\overset{\displaystyle O}{\|}}{C}.O.CH_2CH_2N^+(CH_3)_3Cl^-$$

Fig 11.1 Chemical structure of Acetylcholine

Biosynthesis

The neurochemical events inside and outside the cholinergic nerve terminal are summarised in Fig. 11.2.

ACh is synthesised in the axon terminal by acetylation of choline with acetylcoenzyme-A (AcCoA). The reaction is catalysed by the cytosolic enzyme choline acetyltransferase (ChAT). Choline from the extracellular fluid is actively transported inside the cytoplasm of the cholinergic nerve terminal by a "high affinity Na^+- dependent-choline transporter (CHT)". The rate limiting process in ACh synthesis is the choline transport, the activity of which is regulated according to the rate at which ACh is being released. This carrier can be blocked by a group of drugs called *hemicholiniums*, which ultimately lead to a gradual fall in cholinergic transmission.

AcCoA needed for the biosynthesis of ACh is synthesised in the mitochondria from its immediate precursor, pyruvate (Pyr), by the enzyme pyruvate dehydrogenase (PDH). AcCoA is then transported out of the mitochondria into the cytoplasm by an unknown mechanism.

Storage

Once formed in the axon cytosol, ACh is actively transported into vesicles by another carrier called vesicle associated transporter (VAT). This active vesicular uptake of ACh is selectively blocked by *vesamicol* (resulting in a slowly developing neuromuscular block). ATP and certain Peptides (P) are also stored in the vesicles as cotransmitters (Fig. 11.2).

Release

The arrival of an action potential at the nerve terminal causes an influx of Ca^{2+} ions, thereby triggering the release of ACh by exocytosis. The exocytosis mechanism involves an interaction between the proteins associated with vesicles *(synaptobrevin)* and the nerve ending membrane (*syntaxin*). This interaction results in the fusion of the vesicle and nerve ending membrane, opening of a pore toward extracellular space and the release of ACh. *Botulinum toxin* (a bacterial toxin from *Clostridium botulinum)* enzymatically alters synaptobrevin to prevent the release of ACh from all cholinergic fibres. The death

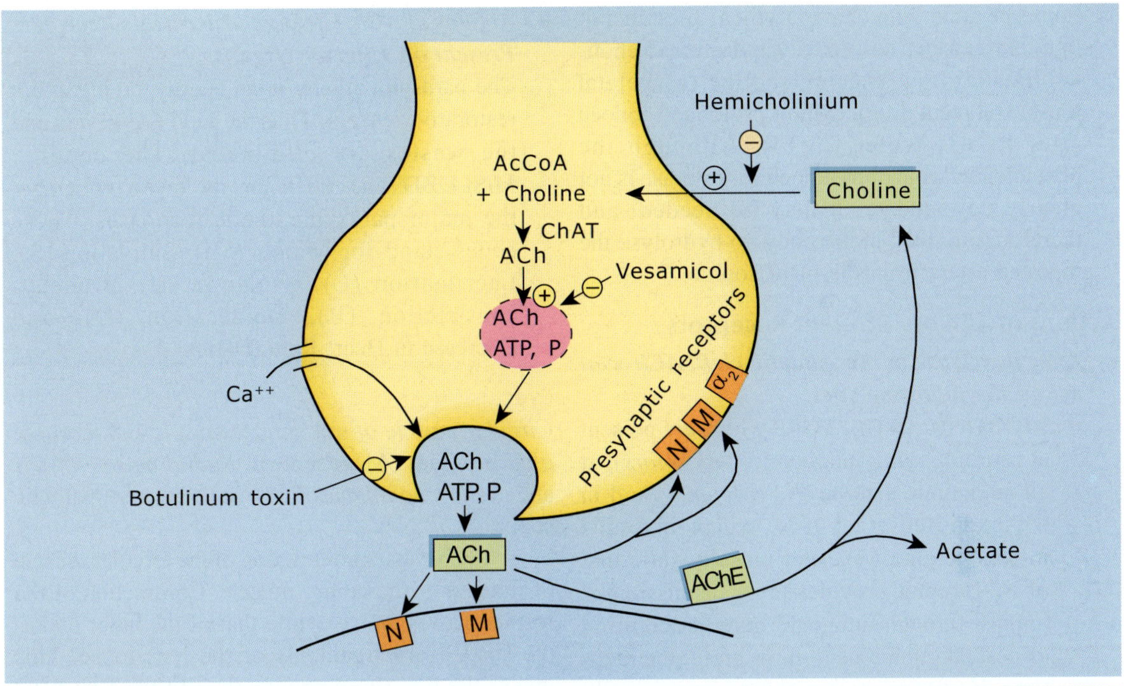

Fig 11.2 Neurochemical Events During the Synthesis, Storage, Release, Degradation and Actions of ACh on Postsynaptic and Presynaptic Receptor Sites.

in botulism occurs due to respiratory paralysis. The transmitter release, which requires nerve action potential through Ca^{2+} entry, is prevented by *local anaesthetics* and *tetrodotoxin.*

Metabolism (termination of action)

Acetylcholine is hydrolysed by an enzyme called *acetylcholinesterase* to choline and acetic acid and thus its actions are terminated. CHOLINE is then recycled in acetylcholine biosynthesis. The cholinergic synapse is very rich in acetylcholinesterase (AChE) and therefore the $t_{1/2}$ of ACh is very short (few seconds). Cholinesterase (ChE) is of two types:

1. **True Acetylcholine Esterase**
   It is a membrane bound enzyme present in the cholinergic synaptic cleft. It is highly specific in hydrolysing ACh and other acetylesters (e.g., methacholine) but does not hydrolyse benzoylcholine, butyrylcholine and succinylcholine. It is mainly localised in neuronal membrane, cholinergic synaptic cleft and to a small extent in RBC and placenta.

   In RBC, the AChE is possibly connected with some ion transport mechanism. In placenta it acts independently of nervous system, and works probably as an autacoid. Placenta has no parasympathetic innervation but it is, however, rich in ACh, choline acetylase, AcCoA, choline and AChE. Here ACh causes vasodilatation and thus facilitates the nutrition of the embryo. AChE, therefore, is needed there to terminate the action of ACh.

2. **Plasma Cholinesterase (pseudocholine esterase or butyrylcholine esterase)**
   It is synthesised in liver and found predominantly in plasma and also in intestine. Its actions are nonspecific as it hydrolyses succcinylcholine, benzoylcholine and butyrylcholine esters more easily than ACh and acetylcholine esters. Genetic variations are commonly seen with this enzyme.

Some persons who have atypical pseudocholinesterase, which only slowly hydrolyses a cholinomimetic drug, succinylcholine (a skeletal muscle relaxant drug), exhibit prolonged apnoea after its use (refer Ch.14). Although the physiological role of pseudocholinesterase is not clearly defined, yet it may be needed, and therefore provided in the body, to hydrolyse the ingested esters from the plant source.

Actions of ACh on Different Receptors

- ***After its release in the synaptic cleft, ACh can act on the following sites:***
  i) **NICOTINIC RECEPTORS** which are present at neuromuscular junction (*N_M receptors*), at all autonomic ganglia (*N_N receptors*) and in the brain. Activation of N_M receptors results in contraction of skeletal muscle while that of N_N receptor provides the transmission of impulse through autonomic ganglia and firing of postganglionic neuron. In brain, the nicotinic receptors are located presynaptically and facilitate the release of dopamine and glutamate.
  ii) **MUSCARINIC RECEPTORS** which are present at the parasympathetic neuroeffector junction at all smooth muscles and glands. Three subtypes—M_1, M_2 and M_3 are well characterised. *M_1 receptors* are found on sympathetic ganglia, on gastric parietal cells and in cerebral cortex. These mediate excitatory effects. Another odd numbered member of this group *(M_3 receptors)* are located mainly on glandular and visceral smooth muscles. Their activation also results in excitatory effects (except for vasodilatation due to release of nitric oxide from neighbouring endothelial cells). *M_2 receptors* are mainly located on myocardium, on some smooth muscles and also on presynaptic terminals of peripheral and central neurons. These exert mainly inhibitory effects. Activation of presynaptic M_2 receptor, inhibits ACh release (refer Ch.10 and Fig. 10.5 for details).

- ***Actions of ACh Through Muscarinic Receptors Present on Effector Organs:***
  The parasympathetic is an energy saving and a restorative system. Thus the food is digested and the wastes are eliminated. The codes "MiSLUBD" and "DHR" are the keys to remember the major parasympathetic responses. These codes stand for Miosis (Mi), Salivation (S), Lacrimation (L), Urination (U), Bronchoconstriction (B), Defaecation (D), and Decrease in Heart Rate (DHR).

Eye

Circular muscle of iris, *ciliary muscle* and *lacrimal glands* possess M_3 receptors. *Radial muscle of iris* and *eyelid smooth muscles* have no parasympathetic supply.

ACh causes contraction of the circular muscle of iris and of the ciliary muscle. Contraction of the former causes *miosis* while that of the latter makes the suspensory ligaments of the lens loose. This makes the lens more convex (by reducing its focal length) and thus the eye's focus is *accommodated for near vision*. The ciliary muscle contraction (aided by stretching of pupil due to miosis) also opens the pores of the canal of Schlemm which facilitates drainage of aqueous humour (Fig. 11.3B), and *reduces intraocular pressure* (more particularly in the patients suffering from glaucoma). Stimulation of M_3 receptors at lacrimal glands produces *lacrimation* (due to vasodilatation).

Salivary Glands

Salivary glands have M_3 receptors, stimulation of which produces *watery saliva* (partly due to vasodilatation resulting from the release of bradykinin).

Lungs

Smooth muscle of bronchi as well as *mucous glands* possess M_3 receptors.The stimulation of the former causes *bronchoconstriction* while that of latter causes increased *bronchial secretions.*

Gastrointestinal System

GIT smooth muscles, sphincters and gastric glands all have M_3 receptors. *The gastric parietal cells,* however, possess M_1 receptor. As a result of M_3

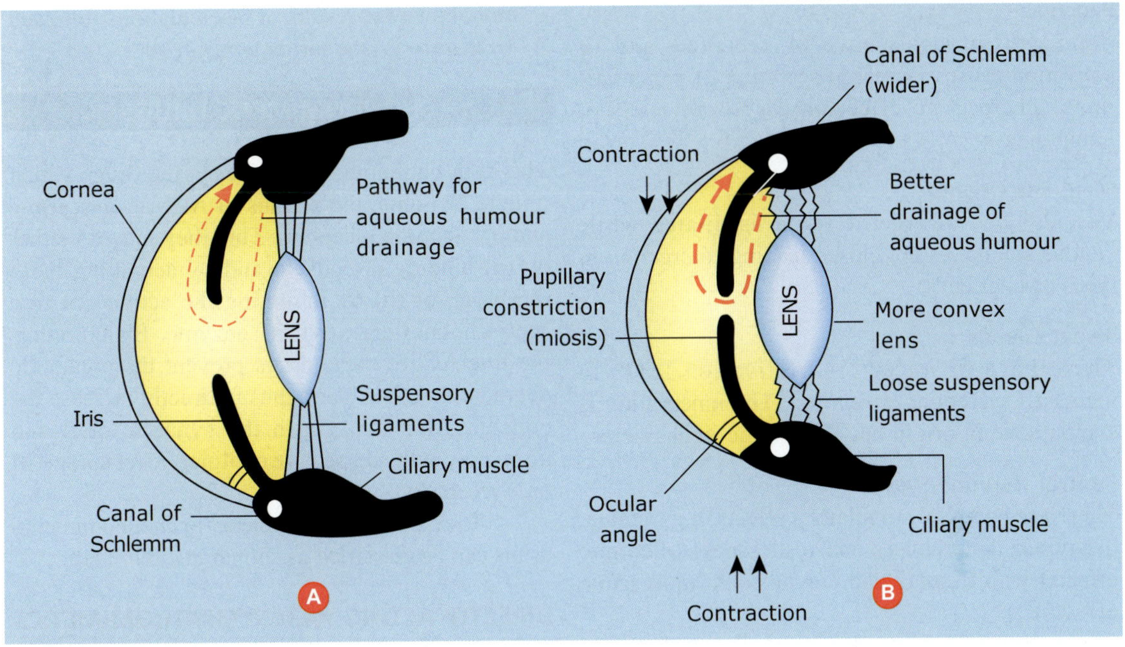

Fig 11.3 Effect of Released Acetylcholine on Eye: A) Normal Eye; B) After the Effect of ACh.

activation, there is an *increase in the motility* and tone of GIT smooth muscle, *relaxation of sphincters* and increased secretions from the gastric glands (defaecation). Stimulation of M_1 receptors *promotes gastric acid secretions.*

Heart

Parasympathetic supply is only up to SA node, atria, and AV node but not below. *The ventricular myocardium* has muscarinic receptors but no innervation, hence can exhibit a decrease in contractile strength (but only in response to exogenously administered ACh). At *SA node, atria and AV node* there are M_2 receptors. Effect of M_2 receptor activation at SA node and atria provides a *decrease in the heart rate* (negative chronotropy) and decrease in the force of contraction (negative inotropy), respectively. M_2 receptor activation at AV node causes *decrease in the conduction velocity* and increase in the refractory period.

Blood Vessels

Arteries have no parasympathetic innervation, but have M_3 receptors. Hence, if a cholinomimetic is given exogenously, a transient but a marked fall in blood pressure (due to vasodilatation) can be observed which, however, cannot occur after parasympathetic nerve stimulation. The endothelium of most blood vessels releases EDRF (endothelium derived relaxing factors, e.g., nitric oxide and other cotransmitters) which causes vasodilatation due to M_3 receptor activation by exogenously administered cholinomimetics. The fall in blood pressure evokes baroreceptor reflex, resulting in equivalent compensatory sympathetic discharge at the heart. As a result, ACh administration (I.V.) initially causes *bradycardia*, but after a brief spell, it is followed by tachycardia. *Systemic veins* have neither parasympathetic innervation nor M-receptors.

Liver and Kidney

Have no parasympathetic innervation.

Urinary Bladder

Both the *detrusor muscle* and the *sphincter* have M_3 receptors. Stimulation causes contraction of detrusor muscle and relaxation of sphincter, leading to voiding of urinary bladder (urination).

Pancreas

Acini cells probably have M_3 receptors and its activation causes increased secretion of pancreatic juice. There is no effect on β-cells of islets of Langerhans.

Male Sex Organs

Vascular bed of erectile tissue is dilated while venous sphincters are closed leading to *erection of penis* (M_3 effect).

Sweat Glands

These have M_3 receptors. Activation leads to increased secretions (*sweating*). The innervation is sympathetic in origin but cholinergic in character.

Central Nervous System

There are complex stimulatory effects, e.g., ataxia, behaviour disturbances and restlessness (nicotinic effects) with tremors and convulsions (muscarinic effects).

- ***Actions of ACh Through Nicotinic Receptors***

The nicotinic actions of ACh include:

i) Stimulation of sympathetic as well as parasympathetic ganglia (N_N receptors), which ultimately results in discharge of either ACh or NE from the respective postganglionic neurons. Since most organs have a dual innervation, the net result of discharge would promote the dominant tone of that particular organ. For example, blood vessels are dominated by sympathetic tone, therefore the nicotinic receptor activation at the ganglia would cause vasoconstriction through sympathetic postganglionic nerve discharge. Similarly, the gut is dominated by parasympathetic tone, hence ACh would increase the motility and secretions because of parasympathetic postganglionic nerve discharge.

ii) Stimulation of adrenal medulla to discharge epinephrine (adrenaline), because the adrenal medulla is a sort of modified ganglion where ACh serves as a neurotransmitter stimulating N_N receptors present on it.

iii) Stimulation of nicotinic receptors at the neuromuscular junction (N_M receptor) resulting in the spasm of the skeletal muscle. Prolonged activation, however, results in fasciculations followed by paralysis (see earlier text; Ch.10).

CHOLINOMIMETIC DRUGS

The term cholinomimetics means the drugs which imitate or mimic the actions of ACh at muscarinic and/or nicotinic receptors. This they may do either by (a) binding directly to and by activating these receptors, or (b) by inhibiting the activity of true acetylcholinesterase (AChE) enzyme. By inhibiting the true AChE, these drugs prevent the metabolic degradation of ACh and thus indirectly increase the concentration of ACh in the synaptic cleft and ultimately at the respective cholinergic receptors (M or N receptors).

The parasympathomimetic (or cholinomimetic) drugs can be classified as shown in Table 11.1.

DIRECTLY ACTING PARASYMPATHOMIMETICS

As discussed earlier, these drugs directly activate cholinergic receptors and therefore can elicit ACh like action even after denervation. The prototype agent is acetylcholine.

Synthetic Cholinesters

These include methacholine, carbachol and bethanechol. Among these, methacholine and carbachol are obsolete.

BETHANECHOL is totally resistant to hydrolysis by true AChE as well by pseudocholinesterase and hence its t½ is sufficiently long. It has mainly muscarinic actions (particularly at urinary bladder and GIT) but is devoid of nicotinic effects.

Its main uses are (i) to reverse post-operative and post-partum atony of bladder and to combat urinary retention as it occurs in neurogenic bladder. α_1-Adrenoceptor blockers, e.g., terazosin, usually serve as an useful adjunct in reducing the resistance to the urine outflow (see following text). For acute retention, 2.5 mg of bethanechol can be injected (S.C). In chronic cases 10–15 mg of the drug can be given orally daily with meals until automatic voiding starts; its administration then, is slowly withdrawn; (ii) to treat GIT atony (without obstruction), e.g., to expel gases from intestines prior to radiological

Table 11.1 Classification of Parasympathomimetic Drugs

PARASYMPATHOMIMETICS		
DIRECTLY ACTING	**INDIRECTLY ACTING (anticholinesterases)**	
	REVERSIBLE*	**IRREVERSIBLE****
1. **Acetylcholine (prototype)** 2. **Synthetic Choline Esters** i) Methacholine ii) Carbachol iii) Bethanechol 3. **Natural Alkaloids** i) Muscarine ii) Nicotine iii) Pilocarpine iv) Arecoline 4. **Miscellaneous** i) Tremorine ii) Oxotremorine iii) Cevimeline	1. **Natural Alkaloids** Physostigmine 2. **Quaternary Compounds** i) Edrophonium ii) Neostigmine iii) Pyridostigmine iv) Ambenonium v) Demecarium vi) Rivastigmine	1. **Organophosphates** i) Isoflurophate (DFP) ii) Ecothiophate iii) Paraoxon iv) Parathion v) Malathion vi) Diazinon 2. **Carbamates** Propoxur

* These drugs have short to intermediate duration of action.
** These drugs usually have a longer duration of action.

examination or to revert post-operative and post-partum paralytic ileus of the gut. For this, the drug can be given orally in a dose of 10–20 mg three times a day, and (iii) to treat salivary gland malfunction (xerostomia; as an alternative to pilocarpine).

***Precautions**:* It should not be given by I.V. route because the sudden rise in its plasma concentration may lead to cardiovascular collapse. It can be administered orally or subcutaneously for systemic effects.

***Contraindications and Undesirable Effects**:* The signs and symptoms of overdosage can be readily predicted from the pharmacological profile of ACh. These include CNS stimulation, miosis, spasm of accommodation for distant vision, broncho-constriction, abdominal cramps, flushing, sweating and salivation. The *major contraindications* to its use are:

- ***Hyperthyroidism*** (because the patient may develop atrial fibrillation and cardiac arrhythmias)
- ***Bronchial asthma*** (because bronchoconstriction may aggravate asthma)
- ***Peptic ulcer*** (as these drugs promote gastric acid secretion)
- ***Myocardial infarction*** (because of the danger of developing conduction block—AV dissociation).

Natural Alkaloids

There are three major alkaloids in this group—muscarine, arecoline and pilocarpine.

MUSCARINE is obtained from poisonous mushroom *Amanita muscaria* and has mainly muscarinic effects. It is not used therapeutically. However, toxicity can result by consuming mushrooms of the genus *Inocybe or Clitocybe.*

Treatment of its poisoning consists of parenteral administration of atropine (1 to 2 mg I.M., every 30 min) with adequate supportive measures for respiration, circulation and pulmonary oedema. Mushroom poisoning is also called as *mycetism.*

ARECOLINE is the chief alkaloid of areca or betel nuts. It has no therapeutic use.

PILOCARPINE is the chief alkaloid obtained from the leaves of the shrub *Pilocarpus jaborandi.* It is a tertiary amine and hence crosses blood-brain barrier. It has a dominant muscarinic action (mainly through M_3 receptor agonist action) but also has mild nicotinic actions at the ganglia (N_N receptors). Pilocarpine is too toxic for systemic use. Besides usual side effects of bethanechol, pulmonary oedema is the major hazard of the systemic pilocarpine therapy. However, main therapeutic uses include:

a) **Ophthalmic Use**: (i) For the initial treatment of open angle glaucoma where it is instilled into the eye as 0.5% to 4% solution. Reduction in intraocular pressure occurs within few minutes and lasts for 4 to 8 hrs, (ii) To counteract the mydrasis produced by atropine (as pilocarpine produces miosis), (iii) To break adhesions between the iris and the lens (as in iridocyclitis) where it is instilled alternately with homatropine (a mydriatic).
b) **As Sialagogue**. Pilocarpine (5 to 10 mg orally) can also be used to stimulate salivary secretions in patients after largyngeal surgery and to treat xerostomia resulting after radiotherapy.

CEVIMELINE (30 mg, orally TDS) is also used to treat xerostomia in patients undergoing cancer chemotherapy or suffering from Sjogren syndrome. Side effects include decreased visual acuity in central field and diarrhoea.

Miscellaneous Agents

TREMORINE and OXOTREMORINE are synthetic tertiary amines. Oxotremorine is an active metabolite of tremorine. These are not used therapeutically but used only as investigative research tools, to simulate Parkinsonism-like symptoms in animal models.

INDIRECTLY ACTING PARASYMPATHOMIMETICS (AChE INHIBITORS OR ANTICHOLINESTERASES)

These agents inhibit acetylcholinesterase (AChE) enzyme, which is present in synaptic cleft and is responsible for rapid hydrolysis of acetylcholine (ACh). As a result, these drugs prolong the action as well as increase the indirect availability of ACh at the muscarinic and/or nicotinic receptors after its release from postganglionic parasympathetic neurons. Unlike directly acting parasympathomimetics (discussed above), these drugs do not show any activity on denervated organs (because these drugs act by protecting ACh from its degradation, after its release, while in denervated organ there is no ACh release from the cholinergic neuron).

Reversible (Competitive) Inhibitors of AChE

To this category belong: Physostigmine, neostigmine, pyridostigmine, edrophonium, ambenonium, demecarium, and rivastigmine.

During the process of its degradation, ACh combines with AChE through electrostatic attraction at two points, i.e., between quaternary nitrogen of ACh and anionic (negative) site of AChE; and between carbon of the acetoxy group of ACh and the –OH group of the serine residue of AChE. The enzyme substrate complex (AChE-ACh) is thus formed (step I) which is followed by cleavage of the ester linkage (O-CO-CH_3) with regeneration of choline (step II). The remaining acetylated enzyme (acetylated AChE) then reacts with water to regenerate the active enzyme AChE (step III) (Fig. 11.4).

The reversible anticholinesterase drugs bear a structural resemblance to ACh. They combine with the anionic and the esteratic sites of AChE. This complex is less readily hydrolysed than AChE-ACh complex. It results in a temporary inhibition of the enzyme (because AChE regeneration is now taking a longer time). This inhibition prolongs the duration of action of ACh released in the synaptic cleft. Among these drugs, only edrophonium has a shorter duration of action (10 min). This is so because, edrophonium forms the complex only at the anionic (negative) site, thereby reversibly preventing the binding of ACh with AChE. The reactivation of

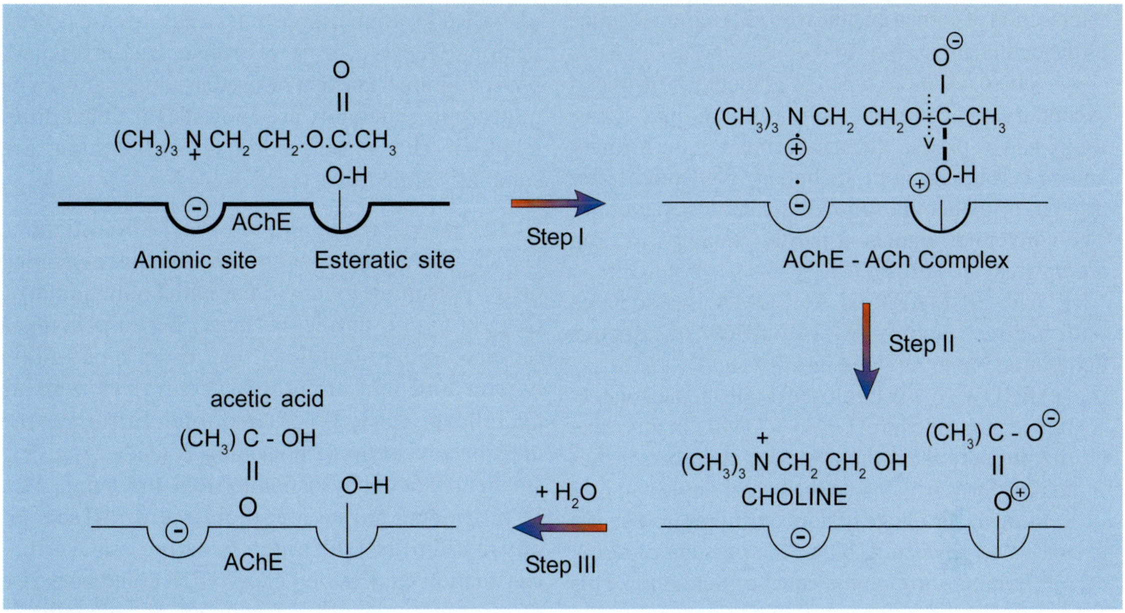

Fig 11.4 Mechanism of Acetylcholine Hydrolysis by Acetylcholinesterase

edrophonium-bound AChE complex does not require the hydrolysis of edrophonium (like that of ACh); rather, soon after its detachment from AChE, it gets rapidly eliminated through kidney. Hence, the reversibility of its binding to AChE and its subsequent rapid renal elimination (after its detachment from AChE) accounts for its short duration of action.

Among anticholinesterase drugs, IT IS ONLY PHYSOSTIGMINE which is a naturally occurring alkaloid, a tertiary amine and being lipid soluble can cross blood- brain barrier. REST OF THE DRUGS are synthetic quaternary ammonium compounds and being ionised cannot cross blood-brain barrier.

Natural Alkaloids

PHYSOSTIGMINE (ESERINE) is an alkaloid obtained from the dried ripe seeds of *Physostigma venenosum*. Being a tertiary amine, it is highly lipid soluble and shows better absorption in all body compartments including CNS. It has marked muscarinic effects (M_1 to M_3) and also stimulates ganglia; but its nicotinic effects at motor end plate (neuromuscular junction) are negligible. Being highly toxic, it has only limited use.

Therapeutic Uses

A) ***Ophthalmic Use:*** Ophthalmic uses of physostigmine resemble those of the pilocarpine, i.e., (a) for reversal of mydriasis, (b) to prevent adhesions between pupil and the lens and (c) for the treatment of open angle glaucoma. Physostigmine, though more potent than pilocarpine, is highly lipid soluble, very toxic and poorly tolerated and hence is rarely used; rather has become obsolete. Its ophthalmic preparations are not available in India and in several countries. However, it is available in USA as ESERINE (generic): 0.25 and 0.5% eye drops.

Management of Glaucoma: Glaucoma is characterised by an increase in intraocular pressure (IOP) which, if persistent, can lead to damage to optic disc resulting in blindness. Usually, glaucoma is caused by the impaired drainage of aqueous humour which is produced by the ciliary epithelium in the posterior chamber of the eye. Normally, aqueous humour flows into the anterior chamber by passing between the lens and the iris and then out through the pupil. Finally, it leaves the anterior chamber by flowing through the trabecular mesh work and into the canal of Schlemm, which lies at the base of an angle formed at the intersection of cornea and the iris. This region is called as the ocular angle (Fig. 11.3).

There are three types of glaucoma—primary, secondary and congenital. Out of these three types, drugs can be used in the management of the primary and in certain types of secondary glaucoma (after trauma, or glaucoma following cataract operation). The congenital glaucoma hardly responds to drug therapy, except surgery.

The PRIMARY GLAUCOMA is associated with a direct disturbance in outflow of aqueous humour and is subdivided into:

i) NARROW ANGLE (closed angle, acute congestive or angle closure) GLAUCOMA: In this case, the pressure from the posterior chamber pushes the iris forward, closing the ocular angle and preventing the drainage of aqueous humour. The iris may also physically block the passage of aqueous humour through the canal of Schlemm. This is a medical emergency. Patients present with a painful red eye, sweating, headache with nausea and vomiting as a result of rapid rise in IOP. The drugs may control the acute attack but the long term management is often surgical (partial iridectomy or placement of hole in the peripheral iris by laser).
ii) WIDE ANGLE (open angle, chronic simple) GLAUCOMA: Here the ocular angle remains wide but the trabecular meshwork starts losing patency due to progressive degeneration. Consequently, the outflow of aqueous humour gets impeded. In this type the surgical intervention is not much useful and the control of IOP is usually dependent upon long range drug therapy.

The cholinomimetic drugs decrease the IOP in both the types of glaucoma, yet the mechanism by which the IOP is lowered is different. In closed angle glaucoma, the pupillary constriction lowers the IOP by pulling the iris away from the trabecular meshwork with consequent opening of the ocular angle. In wide angle glaucoma, it is the contraction of the longitudinal ciliary muscle which stretches the trabecular meshwork and opens the tubules to facilitate the drainage of aqueous humour (decrease in IOP). The treatment is started with an instillation of 0.5% pilocarpine, three times a day. In case it alone is not effective or if response is diminished, physostigmine can also be used in combination with pilocarpine (but rarely used nowadays). Other drugs used in the management of glaucoma are summarised in Table 11.2.

B) ***Belladona (atropine) Poisoning:*** Physostigmine is a specific antidote for atropine (datura) poisoning or for poisoning by any other anticholinergic drug (e.g., tricyclic antidepressants) because being a tertiary amine alkaloid, it can cross blood-brain barrier and can antagonise central as well as peripheral toxicity of atropine. Initially, the diagnosis of atropine poisoning is made by giving smaller doses of physostigmine (0.5. to 1.0 mg I.M.). If the usual parasympathomimetic effects of physostigmine (flushing, sweating, salivation, lacrimation etc.) are not observed, it could be a case of atropine poisoning. Treatment of poisoning is then made by giving 2 mg I.V. or I.M. of physostigmine initially, or additional doses thereafter if necessary. Parenteral preparation of physostigmine is not available in India. In USA it is available as 1 mg/ml injection for I.M./I.V use in the name of ESERINE (generic).

Synthetic Quaternary Compounds

These include edrophonium, neostigmine, pyridostigmine, distigmine, ambenonium and demecarium.

Being quaternary compounds, these drugs are least absorbed and do not cross blood-brain barrier. However, these drugs have important therapeutic (as well as toxic) effects on skeletal muscle neuromuscular junction. Low (therapeutic) doses moderately prolong and intensify the actions of physiologically released ACh at motor end plate. This results in strengthening of muscles weakened by curare-like drugs or by the disease called myasthenia gravis. In addition, these drugs also possess direct agonist action at nicotinic receptors of neuromuscular junctions (N_M) which also contributes to their effectiveness in the therapy of myasthenia gravis. These drugs differ in their duration of action. An approximate duration of action of these drugs are as under:

Table 11.2 Drugs Used in the Treatment of Glaucoma*

Group/Drugs	Mechanism	Dose regimen
1. **Directly acting cholinomimetics** PILOCARPINE	Ciliary muscle contraction, pupillary constriction, pulling of iris, opening of trabecular meshwork, increased drainage of aqueous humour, decrease in IOP.	0.5–4% eyedrops topically TDS; or as sustained release ocular inserts. Also as adjuvant in ACG.
2. **Reversible Anti-AChE**		
PHYSOSTIGMINE[1]	– do –	0.25–5% eyedrops topically TDS
DEMECARIUM[2]	– do –	0.25–5% topically twice/week.
3. **Irreversible Anti-AChE**		
ECOTHIOPHATE[2]	– do –	0.05–0.25% eyedrops topically once in two weeks.
ISOFLUROPHATE[2]	– do –	0.03% eyedrops topically once in two weeks.
4. **Beta blockers**[3]	These drugs reduce the aqueous humour formation by blocking β_2 receptors present on ciliary epithelium.	Also as adjuvants in ACG.
TIMOLOL		0.25%–0.5% BD a day.
BETAXOLOL		– do –
LEVOBUNOLOL		0.25%–0.5% eyedrops OD.
CARTEOLOL		1% eyedrops.
5. **Nonselective alpha agonists**[4]	Facilitate outflow of aqueous humour ***via*** the uveoscleral veins.	
EPINEPHRINE	Dipivefrine is a prodrug of epinephrine. It has a better penetration through cornea, better ocular tolerance and longer duration of action.	0.5–2% eyedrops topically.
DIPIVEFRINE		0.1% eyedrops BD or TDS
6. **Selective Alpha$_2$ agonists**[5]	Reduce the formation of aqueous humour by α_2 receptor agonist action present on ciliary epithelium. These are potent ocular hypotensives which do not cross blood-brain barrier, hence no systemic effects (like clonidine).	Also as adjuvants in ACG.
APRACLONIDINE		0.5–1% eyedrops topically.
BRIMONIDINE		0.2% eyedrops BD. Use of both selective α_2 agonists is restricted for acute rise in IOP after laser trabeculoplasty.
7. **Carbonic anhydrase inhibitors**[6]	Reduce aqueous humour formation by decreasing the secretion of HCO_3^- ions from ciliary body epithelium.	Orally can be used in ACG.
ACETAZOLAMIDE		250–500 mg, 3 times a day orally.
DORZOLAMIDE		2% eyedrops BD
BRINZOLAMIDE		1% eyedrops TDS

contd.

Group/Drugs	Mechanism	Dose regimen
8. **Hypertonic solutions** MANNITOL (20%) GLYCEROL	Reduce IOP by inducing intraocular dehydration by osmotic action.	Mainly used to terminate the acute attack of ACG. Infused intravenously. Glycerol given orally
9. **Prostaglandins**[7] LATANOPROST BIMATOPROST TRAVOPROST TAFLUPROST	Reduce IOP by increasing uveoscleral outflow.	Also as adjuvants in ACG. 0.005% eyedrops once daily 0.03% eyedrops once daily 0.004% eyedrops once daily 0.0015% (15microgram/mL) eyedrops once daily

1 Produces systemic side effects on prolonged use. Not well tolerated. Produces follicular conjunctivitis, retinal detachment and hypersensitivity reactions. Not available in India. Rarely used - obsolete.

2 Longer acting, can cause muscle spasm, and systemic side effects. Can induce cataract formation and retinal detachment on long-term use. Reduces plasma cholinesterase levels, potentiates succinylcholine action and causes death due to prolonged apnoea. Rarely used.

3 Mild systemic side effects associated with systemic beta blockers (e.g., bradycardia, bronchoconstriction etc.) *Topical side effects*—dryness of eye. *Advantages*—no change in pupil size, hence no diminution of vision in the dim light and in the patients of cataract; convenient dosing schedule with no fluctuations in IOP. *Betaxolol* is less potent than *timolol*. Although its β_2 blocking actions are negligible, its more selective and potent β_1 blocking actions cause negligible bronchoconstriction. *Carteolol* facilitates ocular perfusion and retinal blood flow, besides decreasing the formation of aqueous humour. Hence it also protects the optic nerve from damage which is a consequence of glaucoma. It is better tolerated than betaxolol or timolol. *Levobunolol* is longer acting. Usually once daily instillation is sufficient.

4 Ocular allergic reactions are common; systemic side effects are possible; redness in eye (due to rebound vasodilatation after vasoconstriction).

5 Tachyphylaxis and ocular irritation may limit their long-term use.

6 Used as an adjuvant with either β-blockers or with miotics. Side effects include paraesthesia, hypokalaemia and anorexia. *Dorzolamide* and *Brinzolamide* are topical carbonic anhydrase inhibitors.

7 Preferred drugs nowadays. Well tolerated. Do not affect pupil size or accommodation. Benign brown pigmentation of iris on long-term use.

* Drug treatment is helpful manily in open angle glaucoma. Drugs can be used to terminate the acute attack of angle closure glaucoma (ACG), but definitive treatment is surgical.

Edrophonium 5–15 min; Neostigmine 0.5–2 hrs; Pyridostigmine 3–6 hrs; Ambenonium 4–8 hrs.

Efgartigimod Alfa

Efgartigimod alfa is an approved drug for the treatment of myasthenia gravis (MG). IgG autoantibodies are responsible for MG. This drug is antagonist of the Fc receptors (FcRn), preventing IgG recycling and subsequently reducing autoantibodies responsible for myasthenia. It is given subcutaneously or via i.v. infusion. It is used for the treatment of generalized myasthenia gravis in adult patients. Adverse effects: Stuffy nose, sore throat, headache and allergic reactions.

Therapeutic Uses

A) *Treatment of Myasthenia Gravis*

Aetiology: It is an acquired autoimmune disorder causing skeletal muscle fatiguability and weakness. It is associated with the production of IgG antibody that binds to ACh receptors (N_M) at the post-junctional motor end plate. Anti-ACh receptor antibody titre is raised in 90% of patients of myasthenia gravis. The reduction in the number of receptors (N_M) results in the reduction of the amplitude of the end plate potential which in turn fails to trigger an action potential. The characteristic symptoms of the disease thus involve weakness of the muscle and fatigue which worsens after the exercise but goes off after the rest. In contrast to "physiological fatigue" the skeletal muscle weakness in such patients is not associated with muscle pain. In early stages of the disease, the fast moving muscles are affected first. Thus, symptoms start with ptosis, diplopia, slurring of speech, difficulty in swallowing and weakness of extremities. Thereafter, all muscles get progressively involved including respiratory muscles. The thymus shows pathological abnormality in about 75% cases of myasthenia gravis (which substantiates the immunological aetiology of this disease).

Diagnosis: **(i)** By measuring anti-ACh receptor titre by immuno-precipitation assay; **(ii)** By EMG recording of the response to the nerve stimulation at frequency of 3 per second (but prior to giving any medication); **(iii)** ***By Edrophonium test:*** This test is useful if the anti-ACh receptor antibody titre measurement is not available, or is negative but the patient clinically shows the signs of muscular weakness. The muscular paralysis could either be a consequence of myasthenic disease or could be due to an excessive cholinergic activity (cholinergic crisis) at the motor end plate (a physiology which is just the opposite of myasthenia gravis). The cholinergic crisis at motor end plate would lead to persistent depolarisation of the motor end plate with no chances of repolarisation. Hence a new action potential is neither generated nor can it be triggered in the adjacent membrane. As the action potential fails, the contraction cannot be elicited and hence the muscle fibre remains in a relaxed state (muscle paralysis). To start with, 1–2 mg I.V. test dose of edrophonium chloride is injected (the drug, being very short acting, carries least risk). If the muscle weakness is due to cholinergic overactivity at the motor end plate, the patient's condition will worsen further; but if no cholinergic side effects develop, a further 5–8 mg I.V. dose of the drug is injected. The patient of myasthenia gravis will now show an obvious improvement in muscle strength, abolition of ptosis and an increase in vital capacity. Edrophonium, being short acting, the response usually lasts for about 5 min; **(iv)** By detection of antistriated muscle antibody and **(v)** By thymoma identification and CT scanning of the thymus.

Treatment: Once the diagnosis of myasthenia gravis is established, treatment is started with any reversible anti-AChE agent of intermediate duration of action.

Initially, the doses are given on an empirical basis as follows, but later titrated for prolonged therapy:

Neostigmine 15–30 mg, per day, orally in divided doses or 0.5–2.5 mg IM/SC with gradual increment till therapeutic goals are achieved.

Pyridostigmine 60 mg, three times a day, orally; gradually increased till satisfactory response.

Ambenonium 2.5–5 mg, 6 hrly, orally.

- ***Titration of doses during prolonged therapy with reversible anti-AChE drugs***

After the prolonged treatment or with overtreatment with anti-AChE drugs, the patient's condition may swing between myasthenic crisis (due to therapeutic failure as a consequence of low doses) or cholinergic crisis (a toxicity due to overtreatment by higher doses). Both the conditions would end up in muscular weakness. In such a situation, the doses of anti-AChE drug (e.g., neostigmine) have to be adjusted. Prior to such dose adjustments, a differentiation has to be made between these two conditions by giving edrophonium (2 mg, I.V). If the condition worsens, the muscular weakness is due to overdosing with neostigmine (i.e., cholinergic crisis). Obviously, the doses of neostigmine have to be reduced. On the contrary if the condition of the patient improves, the muscle weakness is due to myasthenic crisis (due to underdosing of neostigmine). Consequently, the doses of neostigmine, in such a case, have to be increased.

- ***Toxicity of reversible anti-AChE drugs***

i) *Muscarinic side effects:* Flushing of face, salivation, sweating, lacrimation, nausea, vomiting, abdominal cramps and bronchoconstriction.
ii) *Nicotinic side effects:* Muscle fasciculations and twitching, muscular weakness and tremors.

- ***Treatment of toxic effects***

If muscarinic side effects become prominent (during therapy with neostigmine), treatment can be done with atropine (0.5 mg, S.C.). However, it must be remembered that neostigmine toxicity itself is identified by its muscarinic manifestations. Hence, the nonjudicious use of atropine may mask its muscarinic side effects and the patient may suddenly pass into the state of cholinergic crisis. Moreover, tolerance to muscarinic side effects (due to anti-AChE drugs) eventually develops at a later stage. Hence, atropine treatment for the management of neostigmine toxicity may not even be necessary.

- ***Drugs which aggravate myasthenia gravis***

Antibiotics	: Aminoglycosides (e.g., streptomycin and gentamicin etc.), polymixins and colistin
Antiarrhythmics	: Procainamide, quinidine and propranolol
CNS depressants	: Morphine (profound respiratory depression)
Miscellaneous	: d-tubocurarine, quinine, methoxyflurane and lithium.

- *Other therapeutic measures which can be considered for the management of myasthenia gravis have been summarised in Table 11.3.*

B) ***Paralytic Ileus and Atony of Urinary Bladder***

This can be relieved by using 0.5–1 mg S.C. dose of neostigmine. A longer acting drug, *distigmine,* can also be used in a dose of 5 mg orally every second day.

C) ***Glaucoma***

0.25 to 0.5% solution of *demecarium* is applied topically, in the eye, twice a week. Demecarium can also be used in the management of accommodative convergent strabismus affecting children. Demecarium is a longer acting congener of neostigmine

D) ***Postoperative Decurarization (treatment of curare poisoning and cobra bite)***

Neostigmine (0.5–1 mg, I.V.) or edrophonium (10 mg, I.V.) along with atropine, rapidly reverses muscle paralysis induced by d-tubocurarine given during anaesthesia or by poisoning due to snake venom neurotoxin (cobra bite).

E) ***Paroxysmal Atrial and Supraventricular Tachycardia***

Edrophonium is preferred but it is not commonly used as Ca^{2+} channel blockers are now preferred over edrophonium.

Irreversible Inhibitors of AChE

This group consists of organophosphorous compounds, e.g., diflos (DFP), ecothiophate, parathion, malathion, diazinon, and carbamate derivatives, e.g., propoxur and carbaryl.

Irreversible AChE blockers are usually pentavalent organophosphorous compounds containing a labile fluoride group (as in DFP) or a labile organic group (as in ecothiophate and parathion etc.). These drugs are called as irreversible blockers because they phosphorylate the esteratic site of AChE irreversibly by forming a covalent bond. During this process, the labile group is released leaving the remaining part of the drug molecule attached covalently with the esteratic site of AChE through its phosphorous atom (Fig. 11.5).

After phosphorylation, the AChE becomes inactive and is usually very stable (resistant to hydrolysis) due to covalent bonding. The recovery of AChE therefore depends on its new synthesis which may take few weeks.

Ecothiophate, however, is an exception. It has a quaternary nitrogen which can bind also to the anionic site of the enzyme. Hence, slow hydrolysis can still occur, over the course of few days, so that its action is not strictly irreversible (although the drug is longer acting).

The phosphorylated AChE enzyme can undergo a fairly rapid process of "ageing" which means that within a period of 1–2 hrs, the AChE-drug complex undergoes molecular rearrangement and becomes completely resistant to hydrolysis (i.e., no reactivation of AChE). The "ageing of the complex" is probably due to the loss of one alkyl or one alkoxy group, leaving a much more stable monoalkyl or monoalkoxy-phosphoryl-AChE complex. Organophosphates having diisopropyl group (e.g., DFP) are more prone for "ageing" as compared to

Table 11.3 Other Therapeutic Measures for the Treatment of Myasthenia Gravis

Drug/Procedure	Dose	Remarks
1. **Glucocorticoids** Prednisolone	10 mg once a day or on alternate day, to be increased slowly to a maximum of 100 mg once a day or on alternate day	In the patients receiving high doses of prednisolone, it is advisable to prescribe additional potassium. When an acceptable improvement is obtained with steroid treatment, the doses can be reduced slowly (5–10 mg every month). As the patient improves with glucocorticoids, the doses of anti-AChE drugs can be reduced.
2. **Immunosuppressants**		
Azathioprine	2.5 mg/kg per day	Complete blood count and liver function tests should be performed every week for the first two months and then every month thereafter. Improvement is slow and often takes 6–12 months
Cyclosporine	2–5 mg / kg per day orally	May be beneficial in advanced cases.
3. **Thymectomy**	—	Advisable when myasthenia is associated with thymoma or when the disease is not controlled with a combination of prednisolone and anti-AChE drug or with prednisolone and azathioprine. Anti-AChE drugs should be withheld for 24 hrs post-operatively and readministered after doing edrophonium test.
4. **Plasmapheresis**	—	Advisable in non-responders to thymectomy and treatment with steroids and anti-AChE agents. Improvement correlates with the reduction of the titre of anti-N_M receptor antibodies.

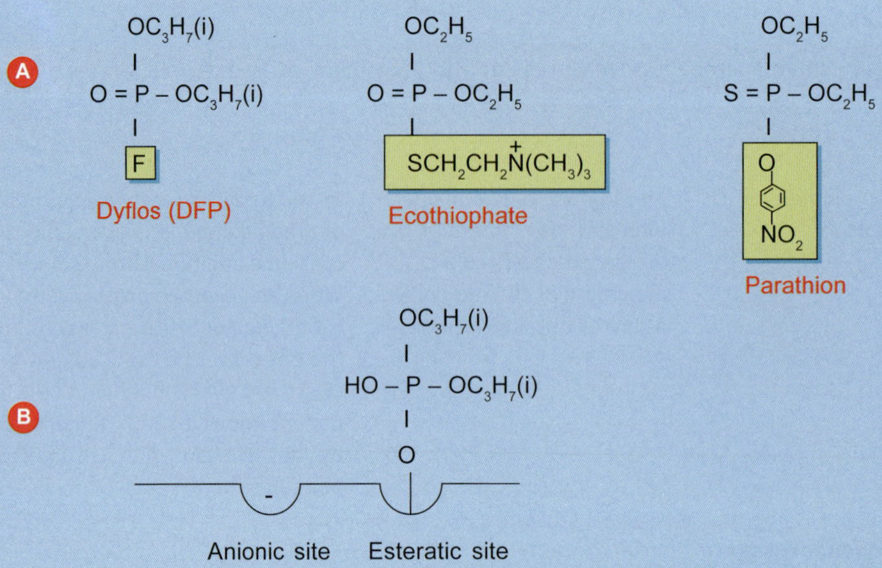

Fig 11.5 (A) Structural Formulae of Some Organophosphorous Compounds; [box] Labile Portion of the Molecule. (B) Phosphorylated Acetylcholine Esterase Enzyme.

those having diethyl (e.g., parathion) or dimethyl groups (as in malathion).

Pharmacological Effects

These drugs are volatile non-polar substances of very high lipid solubility. As a result, these are rapidly absorbed through mucous membranes and even through unbroken skin. These are mainly used as insecticides or pesticides and are better known for their toxicity, which is manifested as combination of muscarinic, nicotinic and CNS side effects.

i) *Muscarinic toxic manifestations*: Diarrhoea, urination, miosis, bronchoconstriction, lacrimation, salivation, sweating, bradycardia, and hypotension.
ii) *Nicotinic toxic manifestations*: Fasciculations of skeletal muscles leading to paralysis.
iii) *CNS toxic manifestations*: Restlessness, tremors, convulsions, ataxia and respiratory arrest.

Treatment of Organophosphorous Poisoning

Poisoning with organophosphorous compounds (organophosphorous poisoning) can occur due to occupational or accidental or suicidal reasons. The treatment is done by using acetylcholinesterase enzyme reactivating drugs along with atropine (to counteract muscarinic and central side effects). The AChE reactivating drugs are *pralidoxime* (2-PAM, i.e., pyridine-2-aldoxime methyl chloride), *obidoxime* and *diacetylmono-oxime* (DAM).

Pralidoxime (Fig. 11.6 and 11.7) reactivates the enzyme AChE by attaching with the anionic site which lies vacant in the phosphorylated enzyme (2-PAM has a quaternary nitrogen akin to ACh). Its oxime group, which is now in the close proximity with the phosphorylated esteratic site, attracts the phosphate group (phosphate transfer to –NOH group of 2-PAM). The oxime-phosphonate complex diffuses out, leaving the regenerated AChE enzyme in an active form (Fig. 11.6, 11.7).

The shortcomings in the use of oximes as antidotes to organophosphorous poisoning are as under:

i) Reactivation of the phosphorylated AChE is no longer possible if it has undergone the process of "ageing". This holds true for all the oxime reactivators.

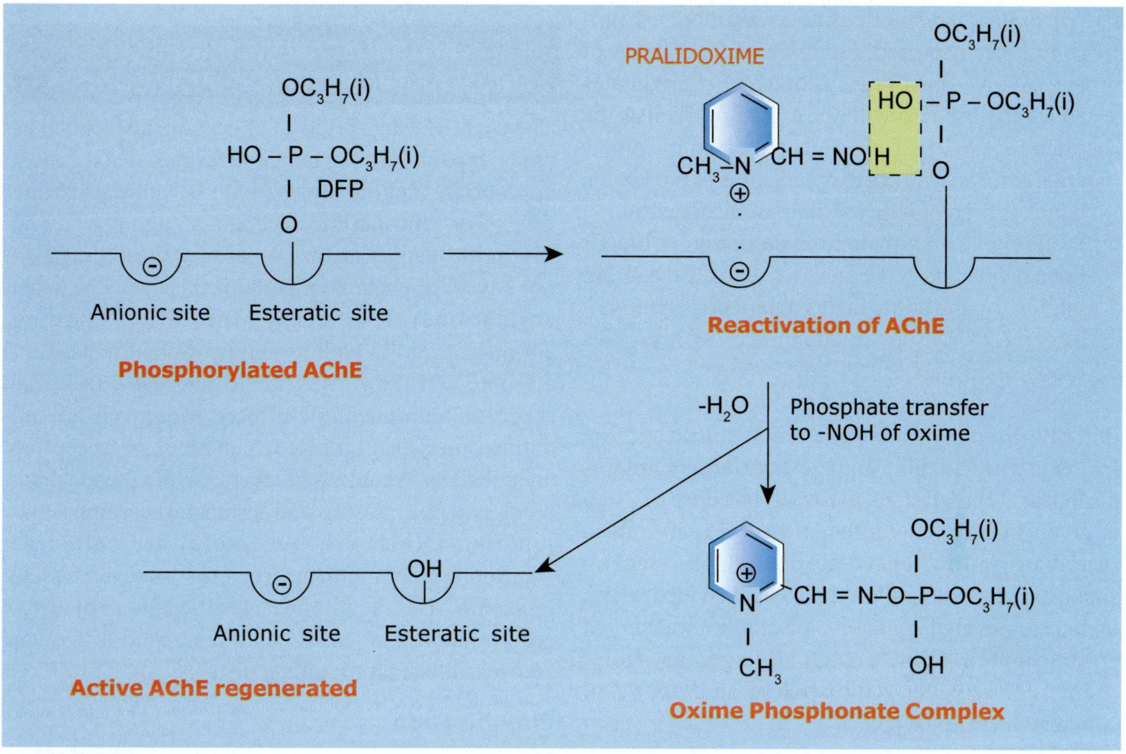

Fig 11.6 Reactivation of Phosphorylated AChE by Oxime Reactivators

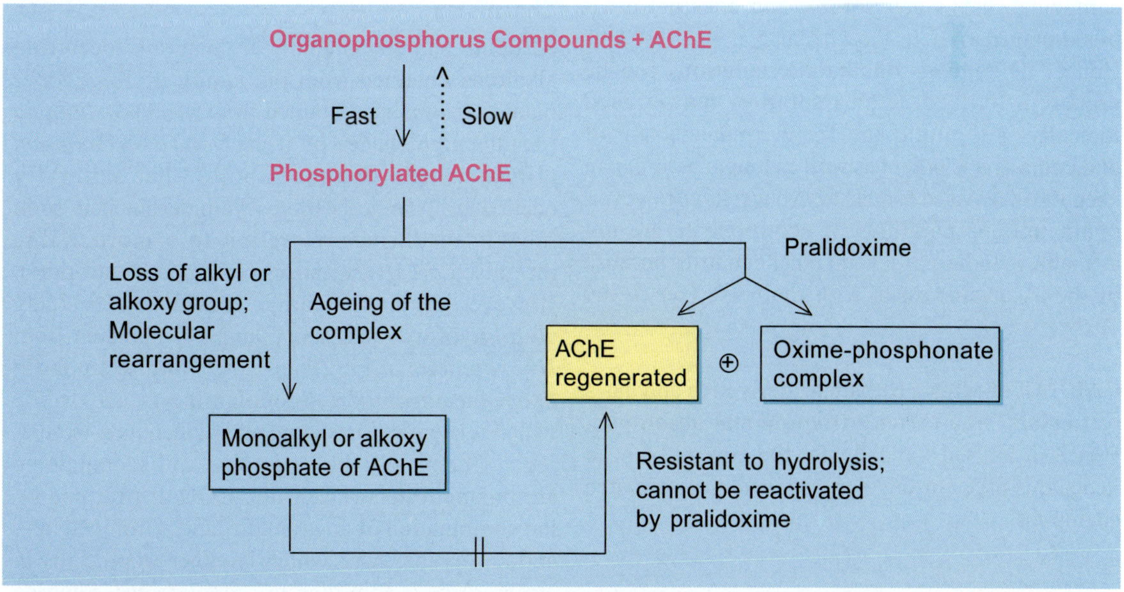

Fig 11.7 Schematic Representation of the Treatment of Organophosphorous Poisoning by Pralidoxime

ii) All oximes are ineffective as antidotes if poisoning has occurred due to carbamate group of anti-AChE drugs (e.g., propoxur). Carbamates attach themselves with the anionic as well as the esteratic site of AChE. Hence the anionic site is not free for attachment to pralidoxime or obidoxime which is prerequisite for their mode of action.
iii) Pralidoxime and obidoxime do not cross blood-brain barrier and hence cannot reactivate the AChE inhibited in the brain. In this regard diacetylmonooxime (DAM) has an advantage, as it crosses blood-brain barrier.

Initially, *atropine* is administered in a dose of 2 mg I.V. every 10–15 min until muscarinic symptoms disappear. Thereafter, *pralidoxime* in a dose of 1–2 g is given by slow I.V. infusion over 15–30 min to reactivate and to regenerate the AChE. General supportive measures should also be provided which include removal of contaminated clothes, washing of contaminated skin, gastric lavage, artificial respiration, oxygen administration and control of convulsions by diazepam.

Therapeutic Uses of Irreversible AChE Inhibitors

ECOTHIOPHATE: Being a quaternary ammonium compound, it is water soluble and does not cross blood-brain barrier. Its local irritancy is also very low. Hence, its aqueous ophthalmic solutions can be prepared. Its 0.05–0.25% solution can be used topically as a miotic and for the management of glaucoma as it is potent as well as longer acting (can keep IOP decreased for one to two weeks). However, ophthalmic preparations of ecothiophate are not available in India and several other countries because of the associated risks with their use (see Table 11.2).

CARBARYL: It is a carbamate derivative and has a particularly low toxicity from dermal absorption. Hence, it is used topically for the control of head lice and is used for this purpose in some medicated shampoos.

ANTIMUSCARINIC DRUGS OR MUSCARINIC RECEPTOR ANTAGONISTS

The class of drugs referred to here are also called as parasympatholytics or anticholinergics. But the most appropriate and the precise term is "antimuscarinic drugs" or "muscarinic receptor antagonists". The first term seems incorrect because these drugs do not "lyse" the parasympathetic nerves. The term anticholinergics means the drugs having antimuscarinic as well as antinicotinic effects. But, atropine and the related drugs dealt here lack any cognizable antinicotinic effects. Moreover, among antinicotinic drugs, those which block N_N receptors are called as "ganglion blockers" while those which block synaptic transmission at somatic neuromuscular junction (NMJ) (N_M receptors) are called as "neuromuscular blocking drugs" or "skeletal muscle relaxants". Hence, atropine and allied group of drugs are preferably called as "antimuscarinic drugs" or "muscarinic receptor antagonists".

Classification

Muscarinic receptor antagonists are classified as shown in Table 11.4.

Chemistry

Atropine and scopolamine are naturally occurring alkaloids obtained from the family of *Solanaceae* plants. *Atropine* is obtained from *Atropa belladona* (deadly nightshade) or from *Datura stramonium* (Jimson weed or thorn-apple). The naturally occurring atropine is l-hyoscyamine but it is soon racemised during extraction to a more stable racemised *dl- Hyoscyamine* (commercial atropine). However, the antimuscarinic activity resides solely with *l*-hyoscyamine. *Scopolamine* is obtained from *Hyoscyamus niger* (henbane) and also from *Scopolia carniolica*. Scopolamine is *l-hyoscine* which is several times more potent than its *d*-isomer.

Chemically, both atropine and scopolamine are organic esters (i.e., with –COO-gr.) formed by the combination of an aromatic acid—tropic acid—and an organic base which is either tropine (as in atropine) or scopine (as in scopolamine). Scopine

Table 11.4 Classification of Muscarinic Receptor Antagonists.

ANTIMUSCARINIC DRUGS*			
Natural alkaloids	**Semisynthetic derivatives**	**Synthetic derivatives**	
ATROPINE (dl-hyoscyamine)	HOMATROPINE and its salts ATROPINE methionitrate HYOSCINE methylbromide BENZTROPINE IPRATROPIUM bromide TIOTROPIUM bromide	EUCATROPINE CYCLOPENTOLATE TROPICAMIDE FLAVOXATE OXYBUTININ PIRENZEPINE TELENZEPINE TRIHEXYPHENIDYL PROCYCLIDINE	PROPANTHELINE OXYPHENONIUM GLYCOPYRROLATE DICYCLOMINE CLIDINIUM TOLTERODINE FESOTERODINE PIPENZOLATE VALETHAMATE DROTAVERINE
SCOPOLAMINE (l-hyoscine)			

Miscellaneous group of drugs possessing significant antimuscarinic effects are: Antihistamines (DIPHENHYDRAMINE, PROMETHAZINE, ORPHENADRINE); phenothiazine group of antipsychotics (CHLORPROMAZINE, THIORIDAZINE); butyrophenone group of antipsychotics (HALOPERIDOL); tricyclic antidepressants (AMITRIPTYLINE, IMIPRAMINE)

differs from tropine in having an epoxide group (i.e., oxygen bridge) between C6 and C7 (Fig. 11.8).

Semisynthetic derivatives are obtained by combining the natural organic base (tropine or scopine) with any organic acid (e.g., with mandelic acid as in *homatropine*). *Synthetic derivatives* do not have tropine or scopine portion in their chemical structure. Both the semisynthetic or synthetic derivative could be *tertiary amines* (where the amine nitrogen is trivalent) or *quaternary amine salts* where the tertiary amino nitrogen is loaded with an additional alkyl group, making this nitrogen as tetravalent with a positive charge on it (Fig. 11.8).

Pharmacokinetics

- **Absorption**: Atropine, scopolamine and the tertiary amine antimuscarinic drugs are well absorbed from the gut and across the conjunctival membrane. If prepared in a suitable vehicle, these can be absorbed by transdermal route (e.g., scopolamine transdermal patch). Quaternary compounds, in contrast, are poorly absorbed and do not cross blood-brain barrier because of their poor lipid solubility.
- **Distribution**: Except for quaternary compounds, rest of the antimuscarinic drugs get widely distributed in all body compartments. Scopolamine in particular is rapidly and fully distributed in CNS and has greater effects there than most other antimuscarinic drugs.
- **Metabolism**: About 50% of atropine and 80% of scopolamine is metabolised by liver as conjugates (phase II). Some animal species (e.g., black rabbits) are resistant to atropine actions because they possess specific enzyme, atropine esterase, which degrades atropine at a faster rate than humans.
- **Excretion**: About 50% of atropine is excreted unchanged through urine. Half-life (t½) is about 3 hrs. Atropine effects decline rapidly in all organs except the eye, where the effects last for about 72 hrs or even longer.

Pharmacodynamics

Mechanism of Action

Atropine and related drugs compete with ACh or other muscarinic agonists for the common binding site on the muscarinic receptor (M_1 to M_5). Hence, these

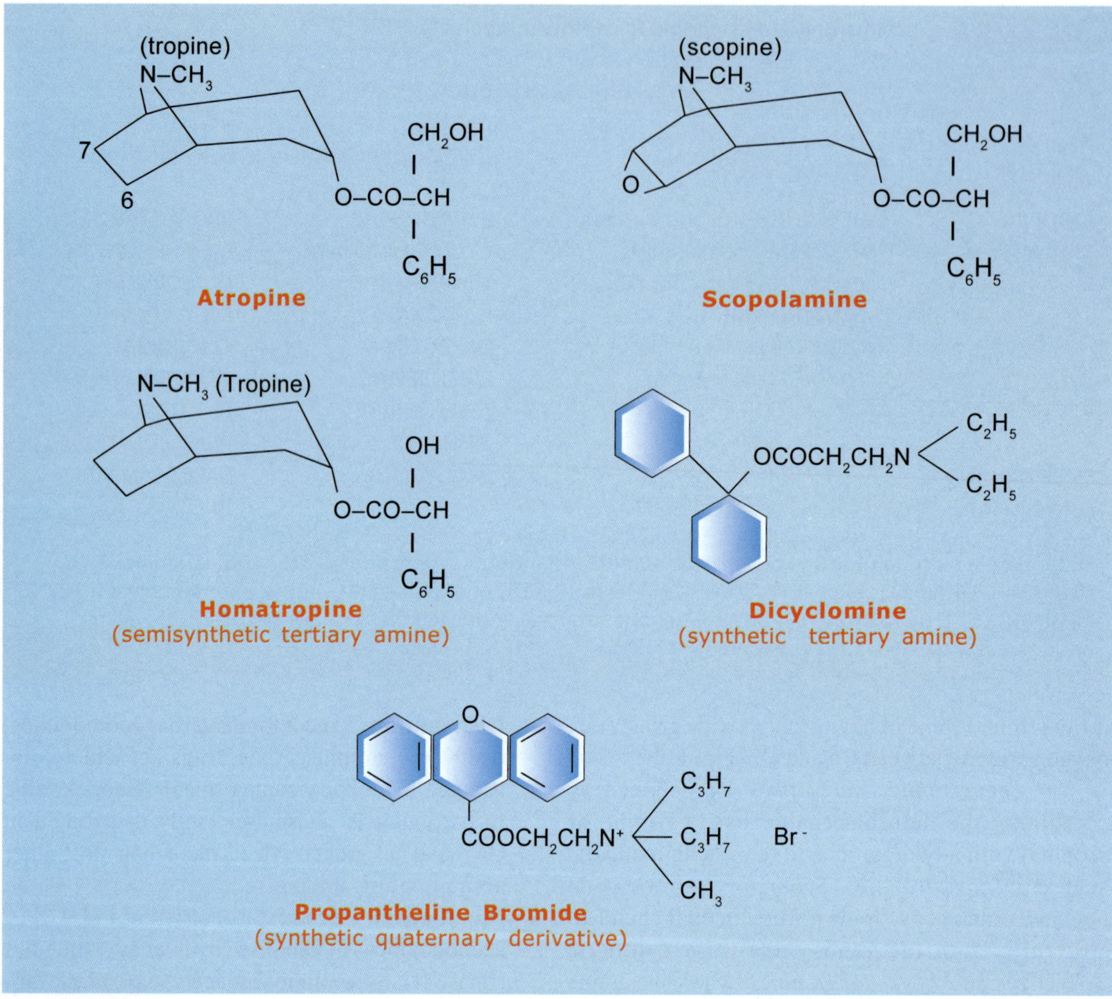

Fig 11.8 Chemical Structures of Some Representative Antimuscarinic Drugs.

drugs are competitive antagonists of the action of ACh and other muscarinic agonists. This antagonism is reversible (or surmountable) and therefore the blockade by smaller doses of atropine can be overcome by the larger concentration of ACh or muscarinic agonists. When atropine binds to M-receptors it blocks all actions that are brought about by ACh or muscarinic agonist (e.g., release of IP_3 from M_1 and M_3 activation and inhibition of adenylate cyclase from M_2 receptor activation; see Ch.10 also). The M-receptor antagonists are more efficacious in antagonising the effects of exogenously administered choline esters than antagonising the responses obtained after parasympathetic postganglionic nerve stimulation. This is because, ACh during nerve stimulation is released so close to the M-receptor that the atropine molecule, being bulky, cannot effectively intercept between ACh and the M-receptor.

Both atropine and scopolamine are non-selective antagonists and hence block all (M_1 to M_3) muscarinic receptors. However, more selective antagonists for M_1, M_2 and M_3 receptors are now available (refer Table 10.2).

Effects on Different Organ Systems and Therapeutic Applications

The effectiveness of antimuscarinic drugs varies according to the tissue. The following is the sequence of sensitiveness of different smooth muscles and glands toward atropine action.

Sweat, Bronchial and Salivary glands >> Heart and Eye >> Bladder and GIT >> Gastric glands

This order of relative sensitivities is not a consequence of differences in the affinity of atropine for different M-receptors at these sites, because atropine does not show selectivity toward different M-receptors (M_1 to M_5). The most likely determinant seems to be the extent of the parasympathetic tone by which the particular organ is governed. The higher the tone, the more shall be the sensitivity of the organ toward the drug.

Central Nervous System

Effect: Atropine has almost no detectable CNS effects in low doses. In therapeutic doses it has only mild stimulant effect on medullary centres. In higher doses it stimulates higher cerebral centres and in toxic doses the central excitation becomes still more prominent leading to restlessness, irritability, disorientation, hallucinations and delirium. With still larger doses, the stimulation is followed by depression leading to circulatory collapse, paralysis, coma and respiratory failure leading to death.

Scopolamine has a greater permeability through blood-brain barrier. In contrast to atropine, *scopolamine in low as well as in therapeutic doses normally causes CNS depression.* In therapeutic doses, it produces drowsiness, amnesia, fatigue, dreamless sleep (with a reduction in REM sleep) and depression of vomiting centre (antiemetic effect) by suppressing vestibular excitation (see below). However, in toxic doses, scopolamine causes agitation, excitement and hallucinations (like atropine). With still larger doses, like atropine, the stimulation is followed by depression leading to coma and respiratory failure.

Therapeutic Uses

a) **Motion Sickness**: Whenever the body is rotated or its equilibrium is disturbed (e.g., during landing and take off by an aeroplane or while travelling on a ship) the vestibular apparatus sends nauseating signals to vomiting centre. ACh serves as an excitatory neurotransmitter in such emesis of labyrinthine origin (i.e., motion sickness). *Scopolamine* (0.6–1.0 mg, S.C.) is often effective in preventing motion sickness. Besides blocking muscarinic receptors in labyrinths and in vestibular pathways, it possesses CNS depressant actions also. Transdermal patches of scopolamine are also available. When applied on to the skin behind the ear, it provides a steady state release of scopolamine (0.5 mg over a period of 3 days) with minimal side effects. The drug, however, should be given prophylactically as it is much less effective once the nausea or vomiting has developed.

b) **Parkinson's Disease**: Tremors and rigidity associated with Parkinson's disease seem to result from the relative dominance of cholinergic activity (over the dopaminergic) in the basal ganglia. Hence the combination of antimuscarinic drug with a dopaminergic drug usually provides more effective results than either drug alone. Muscarinic receptor antagonists are also used to treat the extrapyramidal side effects that commonly occur with antipsychotic drug therapy. The centrally acting anticholinergic drugs (mostly synthetic tertiary amines) like *benztropine* (1–5 mg per day orally) or *benzhexol (trihexyphenidyl*, 2–10 mg per day orally) or *procyclidine* (5–15 mg per day orally) or *biperiden* (2–10 mg per day orally) can be given for this purpose.

c) **Diagnosis of Alzheimer's Disease**: Instilling a low dose of short acting antimuscarinic drug tropicamide in the eyes of a patient with a suspected diagnosis of Alzheimer's disease has been found to exhibit unexpectedly marked dilatation of the pupil (due to changes in receptor sensitivity associated with the disease).

Eye

Effects: Circular muscle of iris, ciliary muscle and lacrimal glands possess M_3 receptors. When instilled in eye, atropine or other tertiary amine antimuscarinic drugs, block M_3 receptors present in pupillary constrictor muscle and produce mydriasis, which is a consequence of unopposed sympathetic dilator activity (radial muscle of iris possesses α_1 adrenoceptors). Thus, in true sense, this type of mydriasis is a passive (indirect) mydriasis* because the normal pupillary responses being blocked, the eyes become unresponsive to light (loss of light reflex). The wide pupillary dilatation results in photophobia. The blockade of M_3 receptors at the ciliary muscle of lens abolishes all responses to cholinergic stimulation. Consequently, the suspensory ligaments get tightened resulting in flattening of the lens (i.e., it becomes less convex) and the eyes get set for distant vision. This effect is termed as paralysis of accommodation or cycloplegia. Both mydriasis and cycloplegia can be the precipitating factor for the rise in intraocular pressure particularly in elderly persons or in individuals with shallow anterior chambers or with narrow angle glaucoma. This effect is due to falling of iris back over the canal of Schlemm (due to mydriasis) which obstructs the drainage of aqueous humour (Fig. 11.9). The fourth ocular effect of antimuscarinic drugs is decrease in lacrimation due to blockade of M_3 receptors at lacrimal glands. As a result, patients receiving large doses of atropine or tertiary amine antimuscarinic drugs often complain of "dry or sandy eyes".

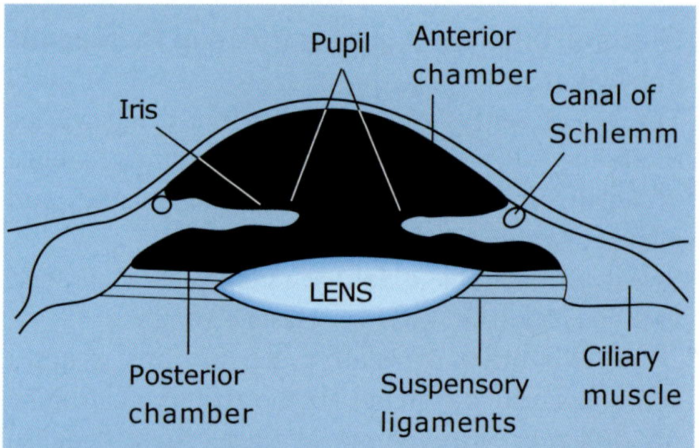

Note: (i) The flattening of lens (less convex) due to stretching of the ligaments (loss of accommodation for near vision) and (ii) obstruction in the flow of aqueous humor due to crowding of iris over the canal of Schlemm (because of mydriasis).

Fig 11.9 Effect of Atropine on Eye.

Note: *In active mydriasis by sympathomimetics, the pupillary dilatation is not accompanied with loss of accommodation or with loss of light reflex because sympathomimetics neither affect ciliary muscle nor circular muscle of iris (no sympathetic innervation).

Therapeutic Uses

a) **As mydriatic**: Ophthalmoscopic examination of the retina is greatly facilitated by mydriasis while accurate measurement of refractive error needs ciliary paralysis. Therefore, antimuscarinic drugs, administered topically as eyedrops are extremely useful in doing a complete eye examination. Instead of atropine, semisynthetic or synthetic substitutes like *tropicamide, eucatropine* or *cyclopentolate* are now preferred for this purpose as their duration of action is shorter while side effects are minimal (lesser risk of precipitating glaucoma). The relative potency and duration of action of these drugs (as compared with atropine) are summarised in Table 11.5. Antimuscarinic drugs are preferred when mydriasis along with cycloplegia is required, otherwise α-adrenoreceptor agonists, e.g., phenylephrine which produce a short-lasting mydriasis is sufficient for fundoscopic examinations (Table 11.5).

b) **To prevent adhesions in inflammatory conditions of the eye**: Antimuscarinic mydriatics may be alternated with miotics (e.g., pilocarpine) to prevent adhesions between the iris and the anterior surface of the lens, as in iridocyclitis, iritis or uveitis. A longer acting preparation like *homatropine* (alternated with pilocarpine) is more valuable for this indication.

Cardiovascular System

Effects: With usual clinical doses 0.4 to 0.6 mg, I.M. or S.C., atropine causes a transient bradycardia initially. There are no accompanying changes in blood pressure or cardiac output. Since this bradycardia is also seen with muscarinic M_1 receptor antagonists that do not cross blood-brain barrier (e.g., pirenzepine) it seems to result due to blockade of presynaptic M_1 receptors on vagal postganglionic

Table 11.5 Characteristics of Antimuscarinic Drugs for Ophthalmic Use.

Drug	Conc. %	Mydriasis duration	Cycloplegia duration	Comments
Atropine	1	7–10 days	7–12 days	May produce systemic effects
Scopolamine	0.5	3–7 days	3–7 days	- do -
Homatropine	1–2	1–3 days	1–3 days	Unsatisfactory cycloplegia in children[1]
Eucatropine	2–5	12–24 hrs	—	Least cycloplegia, less rise in IOP
Cyclopentolate	0.5–1	24 hrs	6–18 hrs	Not suitable for children[2]
Tropicamide	0.5–1	6–8 hrs	6–8 hrs	Less cycloplegia, less rise in IOP; commonly used

1 Due to their high ciliary muscle tone
2 Absorbed through nasolacrimal duct and causes transient behavioural abnormalities like restlessness, disorientation, ataxia, amnesia and hallucinations.

parasympathetic neurons. Blockade of presynaptic M_1 receptors facilitates the release of ACh on SA node and hence the bradycardia. However, further doses of atropine cause progressive tachycardia by blocking vagal effects on M_2 receptors on the SA node. The tachycardia is modest by about 18–20 beats per minute (with 1 mg I.M. dose of atropine). This is because there is no direct effect on sympathetic system (only the existing parasympathetic tone is getting inhibited). The atropine-induced tachycardia is most noticeable in teenagers because their vagal tone is high (i.e., they have low pulse rate); but in infants and elderly, one fails to distinguish the atropine-induced acceleration in the heart rate because their vagal tone is low (i.e., they already have a higher pulse rate).

The ventricles, because of a lesser degree of parasympathetic control, are less affected by atropine-like drugs given in therapeutic doses. The inhibition of vagal activity at heart, by atropine, may facilitate AV conduction, may shorten the functional refractory period of the AV node and may increase the ventricular rate in the patients who have atrial flutter or fibrillation.

Although all blood vessels contain muscarinic receptors, these are devoid of parasympathetic innervation. Hence there is hardly any effect of atropine on blood pressure. However, the transient fall in blood pressure due to exogenously administered cholinomimetics is easily blocked by pretreatment with atropine. Higher doses of atropine dilate cutaneous blood vessels, especially of the face (atropine flush). The mechanism of this anomalous response is not known. However, this could happen either due to histamine release or due to a direct compensatory vasodilator activity of atropine to permit the radiation of heat to offset the atropine-induced fever (because atropine fever is not associated with sweating).

Therapeutic Uses: The cardiovascular uses of muscarinic antagonists are of limited nature. Adequate doses of atropine can abolish reflex vagal cardiac slowing or asystole, e.g., while injecting contrast media during cardiac catheterisation. In certain cases of second degree heart block, in which vagal activity is a contributory factor (such as digitalis toxicity), atropine may lessen the degree of heart block. Atropine (I.V.) can be very cautiously given to treat sinus bradycardia occurring with myocardial infarction; because too low doses will aggravate bradycardia (which may end up in AV block and severe hypotension) while higher doses will cause tachycardia which may extend the infarct by increasing the oxygen demand.

Respiratory System

Effects: Both smooth muscle and secretory glands of the pulmonary airway receive vagal para-sympathetic innervation and have predominantly M_3 receptors. Atropine-like drugs inhibit secretions of nose, mouth, pharynx and bronchi and thus dry the mucous membrane of the respiratory tract. These drugs also reduce the laryngospasm during general anaesthesia. However, drying of mucous secretions and suppression of mucociliary clearance are undesirable side effects of atropine in patients with airway disease as this leads to the formation of mucous plugs which can dangerously obstruct the air flow and predispose the patient to infection. However, owing to the introduction of ipratropium bromide, anticholinergic therapy of respiratory disease has been revived. Ipratropium and similar agents like tiotropium and oxitropium antagonise bronchoconstriction induced by histamine, bradykinin and $PGF_{2\alpha}$. They also block the indirect effects of inflammatory mediators that are released during the attacks of asthma. Besides, these drugs have lesser drying effect on sputum (no risk of forming mucous plugs) and do not inhibit mucociliary movements.

Therapeutic Uses

a) ***Bronchial asthma and chronic obstructive pulmonary disease (COPD)***: Since *ipratropium* and its congeners reduce bronchial secretions, have least drying effect on sputum, do not interfere with mucociliary clearance and cause bronchodilatation, these are the preferred drugs for the treatment of COPD (where cholinergic tone is the most important contributory factor). *Ipratropium* can be given as a nebulised bronchodilator in an acute attack of asthma along with a β_2 adrenoceptor agonist, e.g., salbutamol. *Tiotropium*, a new drug, has a longer duration of bronchodilator activity and can be given once daily.

b) ***Preanaesthetic medication***: To reduce bronchial secretions (which is a contributory factor in producing laryngospasm) and to prevent excessive vagal effect on heart, drugs like *atropine*, *scopolamine* and *glycopyrrolate* are sometimes used as preanaesthetic agents; but after the advent of non-irritating anaesthetic agents (like halothane and enflurane etc.), the use of muscarinic receptor antagonists is nowadays declining. However, *scopolamine* has an advantage because of its CNS depressant effects (amnesia and tranquillisation) while *glycopyrrolate* (0.1 to 0.3 mg, I.M.) causes less tachycardia and reduces bronchial and salivary secretions more effectively and hence the latter drug is at times preferred for preanaesthetic medication.

Gastrointestinal Tract

Effects

a) ***Gastric Secretions***: Antimuscarinic drugs can reduce the basal secretions of gastric acid by 40 to 50%. Vagal stimulated secretions are inhibited to a lesser extent by these drugs. Basal secretions (fasting phase) are blocked more effectively than that stimulated by food, alcohol or nicotine (i.e., of intestinal phase). The concentration of the acid is not necessarily lowered as secretion of HCO_3^- is also blocked along with H^+. Not only the volume of secretion, but the total amount of H^+, HCO_3^- pepsin and mucin, are all reduced. The effect of antimuscarinic drugs on salivary secretions is more marked. The mouth becomes dry and thus swallowing as well as talking become difficult.

b) ***Motility***: Antimuscarinic drugs are very effective in reducing the tone and the motility of the gut, right from stomach to colon. This results in prolongation of gastric emptying time, closure of sphincters, decrease in tone, amplitude and frequency of peristaltic movements (i.e., intestinal transit time is lengthened). As in other tissues, the effect of exogenously administered cholinomimetics is more effectively blocked than the effects of parasympathetic nerve stimulation. Since local hormones and noncholinergic neurons in the enteric nervous system also modulate the GIT functions, even the potent antimuscarinic drugs cannot totally block the GIT functions. Serveral of the synthetic antimuscarinic drugs also possess some inherent "spasmolytic" activity in addition to their antimuscarinic effects. Such drugs (see below) can relax the gut in absence as well as in the presence of cholinoceptor stimulants. These drugs also relax the bile duct and gall bladder.

Therapeutic Uses

a) ***Peptic Ulcer***: Until the introduction of H_2 histamine receptor blockers (e.g., *ranitidine* and *famotidine*) and proton pump inhibitors (*omeprazole* and *lansoprazole*), the antimuscarinic drugs were mainly used to treat peptic ulcer. For this purpose, the classical quaternary antimuscarinic drugs like *propantheline* and *glycopyrrolate* were more preferred because they do not cross blood-brain barrier and therefore produce less side effects. Yet, these drugs being non-selective muscarinic receptor blockers, exhibit uncomfortable side effects like blurred vision, dry mouth, constipation and urinary retention which limits their clinical utility. Moreover, these drugs are not useful for the management of gastric ulcers as they increase the gastric emptying time and thus prolong the exposure of the ulcer bed to gastric acid. Similarly, these drugs were not preferred in cases suffering from reflux esophagitis as they delay the gastric emptying and relax the lower esophageal sphincter (LES) and thus exacerbate the condition due to the reflux of gastric acid mixed food contents into the esophagus.

However, with the development of selective M_1 blockers such as *pirenzepine* and *telenzepine*, an interest in the use of antimuscarinic drugs for the management of peptic ulcers has been revived. *Pirenzepine* (50 mg thrice a day, orally) or the more potent ***telenzepine*** (3 mg per day, orally) provide the same rate of healing of duodenal ulcers as the H_2 receptor blocker ranitidine provides. These drugs were also found to be equally effective in preventing the recurrence of duodenal ulcers. At therapeutic doses, the usual side effects like dry mouth, blurred vision, constipation and urinary retention were relatively low with these drugs. The CNS side effects are not observed as these drugs do not cross blood-brain barrier. These drugs probably act by blocking of M_1 receptors at paracrine cells in gastric mucosa that release histamine when activated by neurally secreted ACh (i.e., by activation of cholinergic fibres in vagus pathway, arising from sight, smell and taste of food, etc). Pirenzepine and telenzepine are not available in India.

b) ***As antispasmodics***: Semisynthetic drugs like *methylatropine* and *hyoscine methylbromide*, tertiary amine derivatives like *dicyclomine*, and quaternary compounds like *propantheline, oxyphenonium, glycopyrrolate, clidinium bromide* and *pipenzolate methylbromide* are used in the conditions of hypermotility of the gut as in intestinal colic, traveller's diarrhoea, irritable bowel syndrome, mild dysentery and diarrhoea associated with diverticulitis. For symptomatic relief from diarrhoea, these drugs are often combined with an opioid antidiarrhoeal like diphenoxylate (a nonanalgesic from opioid group with least addicting liability). These drugs can also be used for the treatment of biliary colic. Newer antispasmodics have been dealt under the section of genitourinary tract (see following text).

c) ***To reduce excessive salivation***: Belladona alkaloids and the synthetic tertiary amine derivatives, like *dicyclomine* are very effective in reducing excessive salivation associated with heavy metal poisoning or parkinsonism. However, the doses must be adjusted properly so that secretions are not reduced to a point where dryness of mouth becomes troublesome for eating food.

Genitourinary Tract

Effects: The smooth muscle of ureters and urinary bladder wall is relaxed by antimuscarinic drugs and hence the voiding is slowed (urinary retention). The antimuscarinic drugs have no significant effect on uterus. Although these drugs cross placental barrier, the foetus is apparently not affected.

Therapeutic Uses: ***Dicyclomine*** (10–20 mg BD oral) and ***oxybutinin*** (5 mg BD oral) are used in the treatment of renal colic and to relieve ureteral smooth muscle spasm. The latter drug has M_3 selective action and is used to relieve bladder spasm after urologic surgery. It is also valuable in reducing involuntary voiding in patients with neurologic disorders. When given orally or when instilled by catheter into the bladder, ***oxybutinin*** improves the bladder capacity.

Solifenacin (5–10 mg BD oral), ***tolterodine*** (2 mg BD oral) and ***fesoterodine*** are the latest addition for treating urinary urge incontinence in adults through their M_3 selective antimuscarinic action. All these three drugs have the least anticholinergic side effects.

Propaverine is a newer addition in this series with negligible CNS side effects. The use of antimuscarinic drugs to relieve bladder spasm may prove hazardous in patients having prostatic hyperplasia because in such elderly patients, the urinary retention may be very painful.

Flavoxate (200 mg TDS oral), a directly acting smooth muscle relaxant, having anticholinergic-antispasmodic activity is another drug which is useful in urinary urge incontinence and for suprapubic pain in cystitis and urethritis.

Valethamate (10 mg BD oral), is another anticholinergic-antispasmodic drug which is very useful especially in delayed dilatation of cervix during delivery.

Drotaverine (40–80 mg BD or TDS orally), an effective spasmolytic drug, has slightly different mode of action. It acts on spastic sites by inhibiting phosphodiesterase-IV enzyme and thus corrects cAMP and Ca^{2+} imbalance to relieve smooth muscle spasm, including uterine spasms in early pregnancy as well as in dysmemorrhoea.

Sweat Glands

Effects: Thermoregulatory sweating is suppressed by atropine. Sweat glands have M_3 receptors and are innervated by cholinergic nerves which are sympathetic in origin. In adults, the skin may become dry and hot but the rise in body temperature (atropine fever) results only in toxic doses; while in infants and children (below 5 yrs) even therapeutic doses may cause "atropine fever".

Therapeutic Uses: Hyperhydrosis is sometimes treated with antimuscarinic drugs (like darifenacin, a selective M_3 receptor blocker) but these are rarely effective because apocrine (rather than eccrine) glands are involved in sweating. A summary of the therapeutic uses of antimuscarinic drugs has been provided in Table 11.6.

Miscellaneous Uses

As discussed earlier, atropine is also used for:

a) Treatment of mushroom poisoning.
b) Treatment of muscarinic side effects of neostigmine (used for the management of myasthenia gravis).
c) Treatment of organophosphorous poisoning where atropine is used as an adjuvant drug (to control muscarinic side effects) along with AChE reactivating drug, pralidoxime.

Adverse Effects and Toxicity

Because of the broad range of pharmacological actions, the desirable effects of antimuscarinic drugs at one organ may be considered as an adverse effect on the other. For example, mydriasis and cycloplegia are considered as therapeutic effects when examining the fundus of an eye, the same become adverse effects when you use an antimuscarinic drug to relieve intestinal colic. However, the most common side effects are (a) dryness of mouth, (b) blurred vision and photophobia, (c) constipation, (d) urinary retention, (e) decreased sweating and (f) precipitation of glaucoma.

Atropine toxicity or poisoning usually results because of accidental reasons or suicidal intentions. The toxicity occurs due to overdosing in adults (above 80 mg orally). Infants and young children are usually very susceptible to atropine toxicity. At times even a dose of 10 mg orally could be lethal to them.

Atropine intoxication in children could even result from its absorption through conjunctiva or after giving an antidiarrhoeal drug containing atropine.

Symptoms of poisoning include dry skin (*as dry as bone)*, hyperpyrexia, flushing of face (*as red as beet)*, mydriasis, photophobia (*as blind as bat)*,

Table 11.6 A Summary of the Therapeutic Uses of Antimuscarinic Drugs*

Clinical condition	System	Drugs used
a) Motion sickness b) Parkinson's disease c) Diagnosis of Alzheimer's disease d) Amnesia with twilight sleep	**CNS**	a) Scopolamine (SC or transdermal) b) Trihexyphenidyl (Benzhexol), Benztropine, Procyclidine c) Tropicamide (as eye drops in low doses) d) Scopolamine (with morphine) (rare use)
a) As mydriatic b) Iridocyclitis, Iritis, Uveitis	**EYE**	a) Tropicamide, Eucatropine, Cyclopentolate, and Homatropine b) Homatropine (alternated with pilocarpine)
a) To abolish reflex vagal cardiac slowing or asystole b) Second degree heart block as with digitalis toxicity	**CVS** (limited use)	a) Atropine (rare use) b) Atropine (rare use)
a) Bronchial asthma and chronic obstructive disease b) Preanaesthetic medication	**RESPIRATORY SYSTEM**	a) Ipratropium (in a nebulised form along with salbutamol), Oxitropium, Aclidinium (both short acting), Tiotropium (long acting) b) Glycopyrrolate, Atropine, Scopolamine
a) Peptic ulcer b) Antispasmodics To relieve excessive salivation	**GIT**	a) Pirenzepine, Telenzepine, Propantheline b) Dicyclomine, Clidinium bromide, Pipenzolate methyl bromide, Oxyphenonium, and Glycopyrrolate c) Dicyclomine
a) Renal colic b) Urinary urge incontinence c) Nocturnal enuresis d) Delayed dilatation of cervix during delivery e) Uterine spasm in dysmenorrhoea and during early pregnancy (I & II trimester)	**GENITO-URINARY TRACT**	a) Dicyclomine, Oxybutinin b) Flavoxate, Solifenacin, Darifenacin, Imidafenacin,Tolterodine, Fesoterodine (Uroselective antimuscrinic drugs) c) Propaverine d) Valethamate e) Drotaverine
a) Hyperhydrosis	**SWEAT GLANDS**	a) Darifenacin**, Dicyclomine (rare use)

* For details refer text; ** Investigational drug

dry mouth, slurred speech, difficulty in micturition, confusion, delirium, restlessness, hallucinations (*as mad as hen)* and tachycardia. It is followed by coma, cardiovascular collapse and respiratory paralysis. Scopolamine is more toxic than atropine.

For diagnosis of atropine poisoning, *physostigmine* (1 mg I.M.) may be used. If the typical salivation, sweating and lacrimation do not occur, intoxication with atropine is almost certain. **Treatment of poisoning** is then made by giving 2 mg I.V. or I.M of physostigmine initially, or additional doses, thereafter, if necessary (physostigmine is metabolised rapidly, hence repeated doses may be needed). Physostigmine, being tertiary alkaloid, crosses blood-brain barrier and thus can counteract peripheral as well as central toxicity of atropine or scopolamine. To prevent convulsions and delirium, small doses of *diazepam* may also be given (I.M.). Supportive measures like gastric lavage, artificial respiration, ice bags sponging to reduce fever are also necessary. For young children 0.5 mg physostigmine may be given by slow I.V injection.

CHAPTER 12 Drugs Affecting Sympathetic Nervous System

COMPETENCY PH1.13

Norepinephrine (NE) is the major neurotransmitter in the peripheral sympathetic nervous system, whereas epinephrine (E) is the primary hormone secreted by adrenal medulla (epinephrine functions as hormone as, after its release, it acts at different sites during circulation). Dopamine (DA), the metabolic precursor of NE and E, is the third neurotransmitter in sympathetic nervous system. Although it is found predominantly in basal ganglia, limbic system, CTZ and in anterior pituitary, specific receptors for this neurotransmitter have been identified on splanchnic and renal blood vessels. All the three neurotransmitters chemically belong to catecholamine group (Fig. 12.1).

The physiological and metabolic responses that follow after stimulation of sympathetic nervous system are usually mediated by the major neurotransmitter NE, although cotransmitters like peptides also contribute to sympathetic effects on effector organs. However, during stress, adrenal medulla is also stimulated and releases E in the circulation. This chapter deals with the aspects of how the drugs modify and influence the noradrenergic neurotransmission in the periphery.

ADRENOCEPTOR AGONISTS

The term adrenoceptor agonist means a drug which stimulates any (or most) of the adrenoceptors (α and/or β). Synonymously, these drugs are also called as sympathomimetics which means the drugs which mimic the actions of catecholamines at the neuroeffector sites. Many of the actions of agonists that activate the adrenergic receptors can be understood from the known physiological effects of natural catecholamines. Most of the available agonists are structural analogues of NE or E and bear a catecholamine nucleus. However, some are non-catecholamine derivatives also. These synthetic drugs have a variety of advantages such as oral bioavailability, crossing of blood-brain barrier, longer duration of action and receptor specific action. Such increased receptor specificity improves their safety profile. Looking to the multiplicity of available adrenoceptor agonists, it is impossible to select and discuss a single prototype sympathomimetic drug. The text below describes the prototypic actions of E and NE rather than prototype drug in order to explain the varied actions, uses and adverse effects of different sympathomimetics. Prior to this, a summary has been provided about the biosynthesis, storage, release, degradation and receptor action of NE and E (also of DA) which forms the basis for understanding the pharmacology and therapeutic usefulness of different sympathomimetic drugs.

ADRENERGIC NEUROTRANSMITTERS (NE, E AND DA)

The chemical structures of all the three adrenergic neurotransmitters have been shown in Fig. 12.1. The steps in the biosynthesis of DA, NE and E are summarised in Fig. 12.2, while the proposed sites of action of different drugs on the synthesis, storage, release, action and fate of NE at neuroeffector junction is shown in Fig. 12.3.

Biosynthesis

The starting material for the biosynthesis of NE is L-phenylalanine (a dietary amino acid) which is absorbed from the gut and oxidised in the liver by phenylalanine hydroxylase (conventionally called hepatic hydroxylase) to form L-tyrosine. The circulating L-tyrosine is then actively transported into the cytoplasm of the noradrenergic neuron. Within the neuronal cytoplasm, L-tyrosine is then hydroxylated by tyrosine hydroxylase to l-dopa (dihydroxyphenylalanine). *This is the rate limiting step in the synthesis of NE* (i.e., increase in the neuronal cytoplasmic NE concentration inhibits the

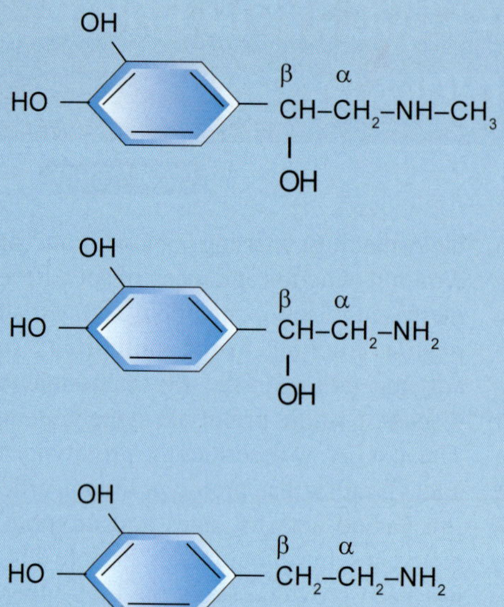

Fig 12.1 Chemical Structures of Major Catecholamines. All catecholamines have two features in common, i.e., a benzene ring with two adjacent -OH group, called a CATECHOL NUCLEUS and an AMINE containing side chain (with either a primary amine $-NH_2$ group or a secondary amino -NH- group). In norepinephrine, *nor* means removal of one alkylgroup (e.g $-CH_3$ gr.) from the amino nitrogen (i.e., from $-NHCH_3$ of epinephrine). Dopamine differs from NE and E as it does not have a -OH group at β-carbon atom of the side chain.

activity of tyrosine hydroxylase enzyme through the negative feedback mechanism and will inhibit the further conversion of L-tyrosine to L-dopa). *2-methyl-p-tyrosine* is a drug which inhibits tyrosine hydroxylase enzyme. Hence it is used to control the discharge of NE and E during surgical removal of the adrenal tumour in the cases of phaeochromocytoma. The drug is especially useful in the patients who respond poorly with phenoxybenzamine and/or propranolol.

Thereafter, L-dopa is converted to dopamine by cytoplasmic L-amino acid decarboxylase (usually called dopa decarboxylase in the context of L- dopa). In the dopaminergic neurons, within the CNS, this is the last step in the biosynthetic process, because DA serves as a main neurotransmitter in the CNS. *Carbidopa* is the drug which inhibits dopa decarboxylase enzyme in the periphery and thus saves L-dopa from its peripheral metabolic degradation. Carbidopa with L-dopa, is therefore a synergistic combination for the treatment of parkinsonism because it increases the availability of L-dopa in the brain where it is converted to DA.

Dopamine synthesised in the neuronal cytoplasm is then actively transported to storage vesicles of axon terminals (or varicosities) where it is oxidised to norephinephrine by dopamine-β-hydroxylase located in synaptic vesicles. The affinity carrier for DA, located in the wall of storage vesicle, can be inhibited by the drug *reserpine*. This results in the disruption of vesicular storage of NE (i.e., depletion of NE stores).

The adrenal medulla has two distinct types of catecholamine containing cells—those with NE and those with E. The latter type of the cells contain an enzyme called phenylethanolamine-*N*-methyltrans-

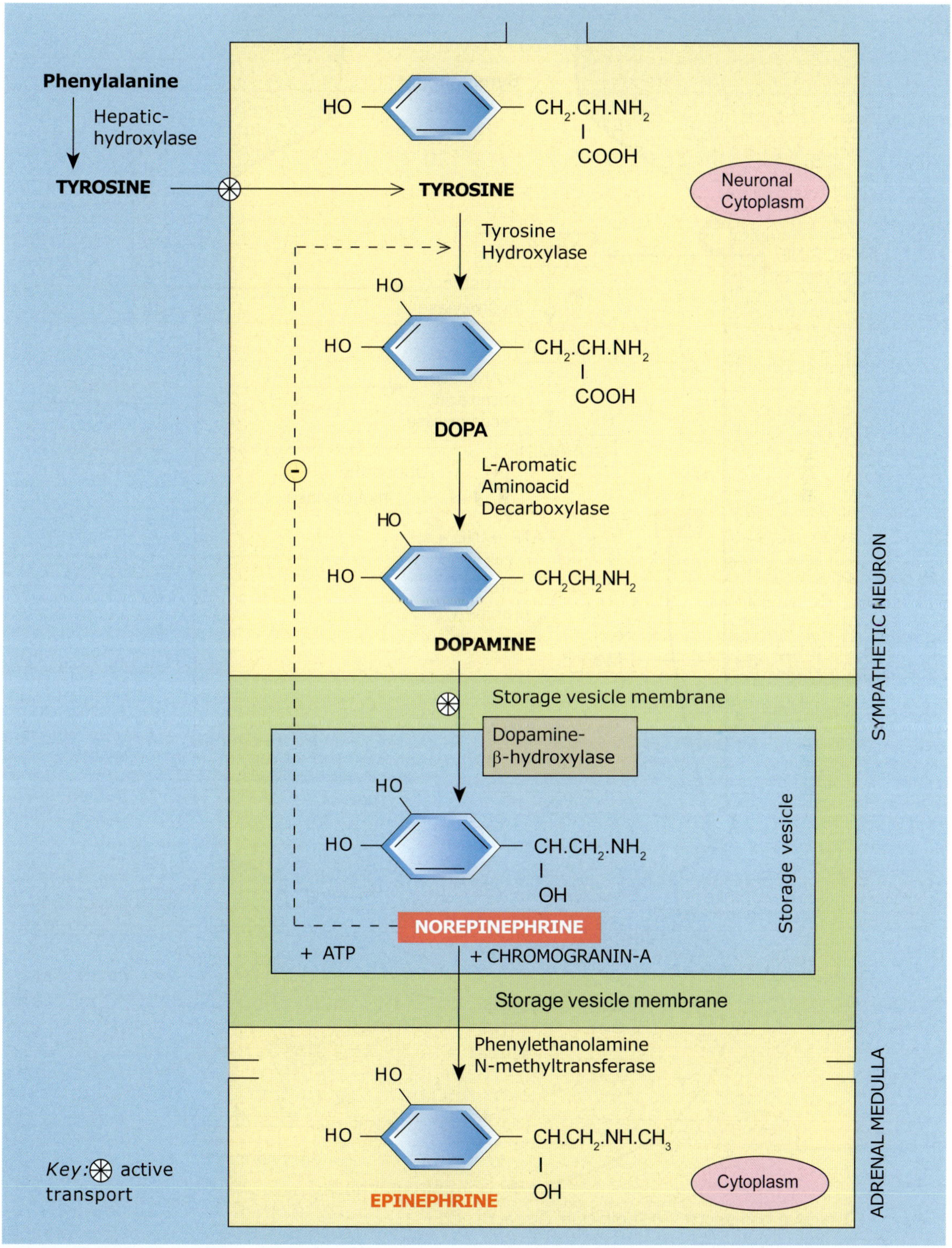

Fig 12.2 Schematic Version of the Synthesis of Dopamine, Norepinephrine and Epinephrine.

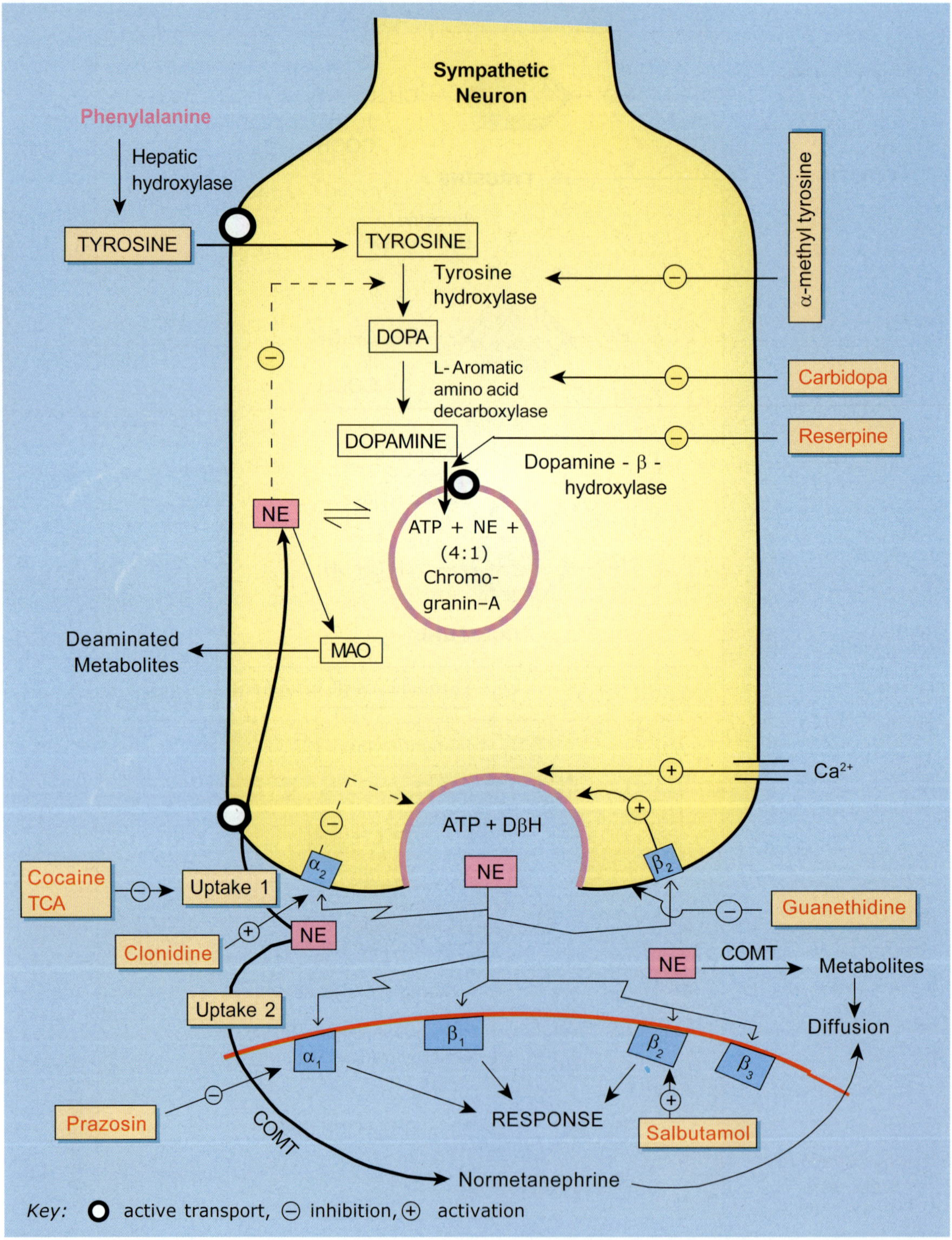

Fig 12.3 Sites of Action of Drugs on Synthesis, Storage, Release, Action and Fate of Norepinephrine.

ferase. In these cells, the NE formed in the granules leaves these structures by a process of diffusion and is methylated in the cytoplasm of adrenal medulla to epinephrine. Probably certain amount of intra-adrenal glucocorticoids is required for catalysing the methylating enzyme. After its synthesis, E then reenters the chromaffin granules where it is stored, until released. In adults, about 80% of catecholamines is present as E in adrenal medulla, while NE makes up for the remaining 20%.

Storage

The endogenous NE, in the nerve terminal, is then stored in the synaptic vesicles as a complex with ATP (4 molecules of ATP per molecule of NE) with the help of a soluble binding protein called chromogranin-A. ATP itself has a transmitter function at adrenergic synapse (see cotransmitters, Chapter 10). Inside the storage vesicle, there is acidic pH which confers a positive charge (protonation) on the amino group of NE. This prevents its outside diffusion (leakage) through the vesicle membrane. Complexation with ATP prevents excessive osmotic pressure inside the vesicle which also helps to prevent leakage of NE.

Release

Action Potential Induced Release

An action potential along the terminal axon brings about the membrane permeability changes. Thus, Na^+, Ca^{2+} and Cl^- enter while K^+ comes out. The influx of Ca^{2+} disrupts the storage vesicle to release NE, ATP, chromogranin along with small amounts of dopamine-β-hydroxylase enzyme into the synaptic cleft by exocytotic process. In this process, the storage vesicle membrane fuses with the neuronal membrane, allowing the storage vesicles to release its contents into the synaptic cleft. The storage vesicles are retained within the nerve terminal and thereafter refilled with NE. This release process may be inhibited by drugs like *bretylium* and *guanethidine* (refer Ch.13).

It is possible to promote the release of NE from the postganglionic sympathetic nerve terminals by two ways. One is by activating N_N receptors of the autonomic ganglia by nicotine or by DMPP. The action potential thus generated is propagated to the axon terminal to activate the Ca^{2+} dependent exocytotic release of NE from the storage vesicles of the postganglionic sympathetic neuron into the synaptic cleft. Another way to evoke the release of NE from the storage vesicles is by using indirectly acting sympathomimetic amines like *amphetamine* and *tyramine*. These drugs are transported into the postganglionic nerve terminal by the active uptake process (see below) and displace NE from the storage vesicles, and then liberate it into the synaptic cleft by a process which neither requires vesicle exocytosis nor is Ca^{2+} - dependent.

Spontaneous Release

This process is of lesser importance. The random migration of storage vesicles towards the end of neuron varicosity can result in the spontaneous discharge of NE. This release is very small and simply modifies the ongoing activity of the effector cell.

Inactivation of NE and E (Termination of effect) by Reuptake and Metabolism

Metabolism is not the main mechanism for the termination of effect of NE and E. Infact the effects of NE and E are terminated by: (1) active reuptake into nerve terminal (uptake-1; 80% by *catecholamine transporter*) and subsequent reuptake into storage vesicle (vesicular reuptake by *vesicular monoamine transporter*); (2) uptake into postsynaptic non-neuronal cell membrane (uptake-2; 20%); and (3) metabolic degradation by the enzymes: **m**ono**a**mine **o**xidase (MAO) located intraneuronally (also intracellularly, e.g., in the cells of effector organs like heart, smooth muscles of blood vessels, bronchi, etc) and by **c**atecholamine-**O**-**m**ethyl**t**ransferase (COMT) located intracellularly. However, the reuptake of released/administered NE/E as described in (1) and (2) above not only the primary mechanism of termination of their effect but also enables these monoamines to be used again for neurotransmission. Since MAO and COMT enzymes are located intraneuronally/intracellularly, reuptake of NE or E into the cells necessarily precedes metabolic degradation. Neuronal reuptake (uptake-1) is inhibited by drugs like *cocaine* and *tricyclic antidepressants*. Inhibition of the uptake-1 leads to potentiation of the effects of NE and E. Vesicular reuptake is blocked by *reserpine* (Fig. 12.3).

The transmitter that is released and that enters into the nerve terminal after uptake-1, can be metabolised by MAO. The COMT and MAO, present particularly in liver, play a major role in degrading endogenously circulating as well as exogenously administered catecholamines. Both MAO and COMT are widely distributed throughout the body (intestines, liver, kidney and brain) but it is only MAO which is found in adrenergic neuron (not COMT).

COMT is, rather, located mainly in the cytoplasm. Two different isozymes of MAO (MAO-A and MAO-B) are found in varying proportions in periphery and in the CNS. Their characteristics are listed in Table 12.1. MAO converts catecholamines (NE, E and DA) ultimately to the corresponding carboxylic acids by oxidative deamination. COMT converts catecholamines to their O-methyl derivatives by O-methylation of one of the catechol-OH groups. MAO can further degrade the O-methyl metabolite produced by COMT. Analogously, COMT O-methylate the carboxylic acid metabolite produced by MAO. Thus, both NE and E when acted upon by MAO produce 3,4-dihydroxy-mandelic acid which when O-methylated by COMT produces 3-methoxy-4-hydroxymandelic acid or vanillyl-mandelic acid (VMA). Similary, E and NE when acted upon by COMT provide metanephrine and normetanephrine, respectively, which when acted upon by MAO provide 3-methoxy-4-hydro-xymandelic acid (VMA). *The final metabolite of NE and E is vanillyl mandelic acid (VMA).*

These metabolites are excreted through urine as their sulphate or glucuronide water-soluble conjugates. Estimation of VMA in 24-hr urine sample provides an estimate of NE and E turnover in an individual (normal values for VMA are 2–4 mg in 24-hr urine sample). Such an estimation is useful in the diagnosis of phaeochromocytoma, an adrenaline secreting tumour.

Dopamine, in the peripheral tissue, gets converted to 3,4-dihydroxyphenyl acetic acid (DOPAC) by MAO which when acted upon in sequence by COMT provides homovanillic acid (HVA). Similarly dopamine, if first acted upon by COMT, provides 3-methoxytyramine which then undergoes oxidative deamination by MAO *to provide the final metabolite HVA*. The pathways of the metabolism of NE, E and DA are depicted in Fig. 12.4.

Action on Different Receptors

The liberated NE, then stimulates the postsynaptic adrenoceptors (α_1, β_1, β_2 and β_3 as the case may be) and elicits the end organ response. Epinephrine (E) activates all the known adrenoceptor subtypes while NE primarily activates α_1, α_2, β_1 and β_3 subtypes and has relatively weak activity at β_2 receptors. Neurotansmitters (NE and E) released into the neuroeffector junction can also activate presynaptic adrenoceptors (α_2 and β_2) on sympathetic nerve terminals. Activation of these receptors plays an important role in the modulation of vesicular neurotransmitter release (see below). After their release in the synaptic cleft, NE/E can act on the following receptor sites (for adrenoceptor details, refer Chapter 10).

Table 12.1 Distinictive Properties of Different MAO Enzymes

Characteristics	MAO–A	MAO–B
1. Distribution	Adrenergic neuron, intestine, liver, kidney placenta	Dopaminergic neuron, brain, platelets, liver
2. Specific substrate	NE, 5HT	DA, phenylethylamine
3. Specific inhibitor*	Clorgyline, Moclobemide	Selegiline (Deprenyl)

* Tyramine is a nonspecific substrate while tranylcypromine is a nonspecific inhibitor for both MAO isozymes.

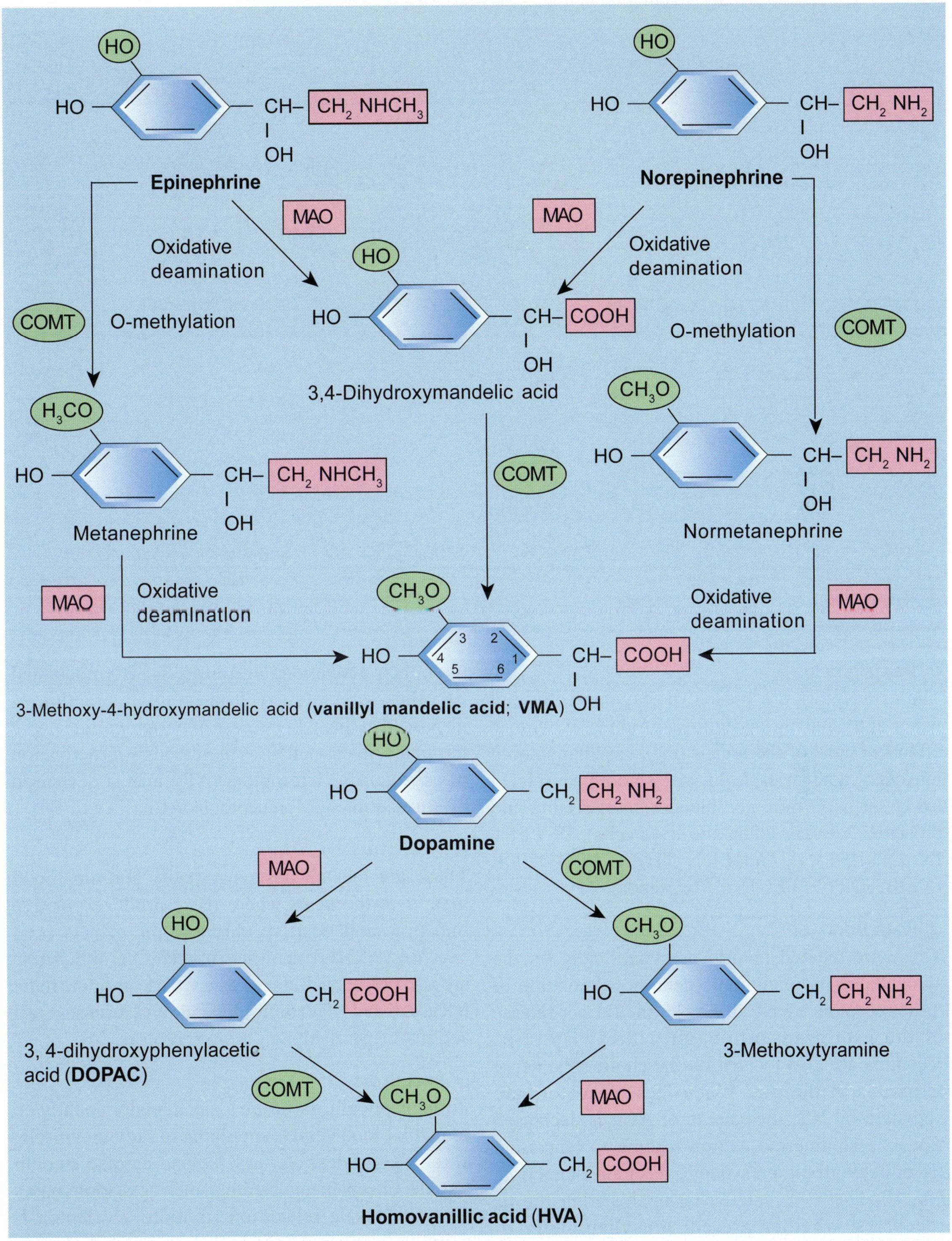

Fig 12.4 Metabolism of Catecholamines by COMT (catechol-o-methyl transferase) and MAO

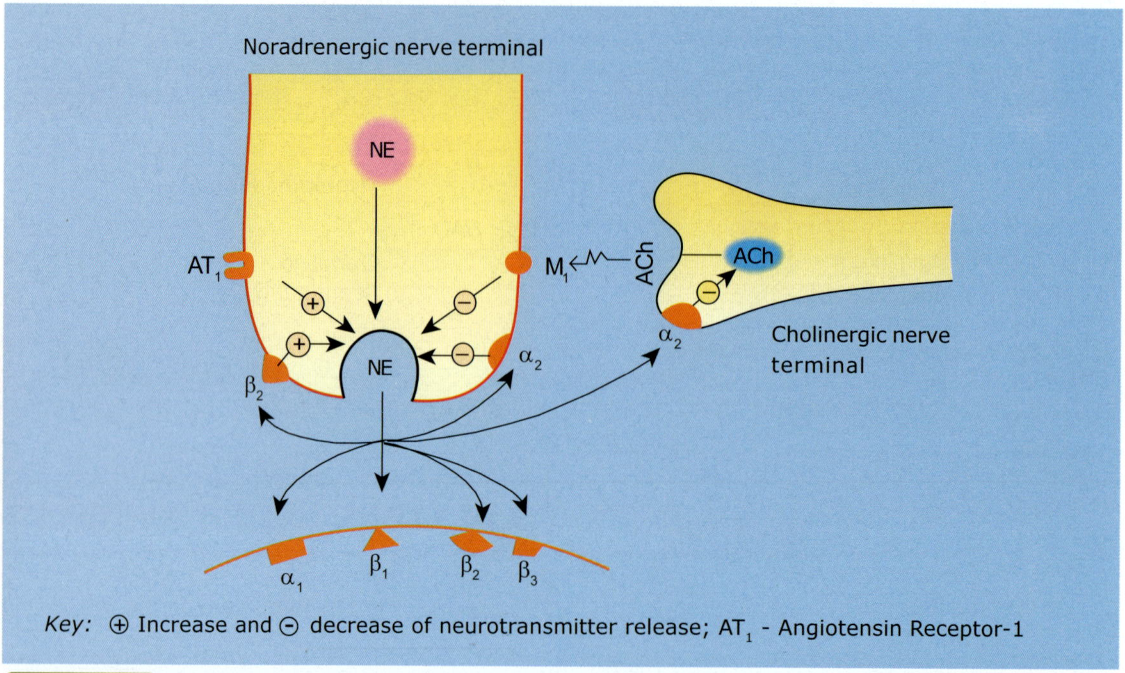

Fig 12.5 Modulation of NE Release.

α_1 Receptors

These receptors are present postsynaptically and when activated by an agonist produce excitatory effects in most of the organs (e.g., vascular smooth muscles; radial muscle of iris; smooth muscle in lower urinary tract, i.e., bladder base, urethra and prostate; salivary gland and liver cells), EXCEPT IN INTESTINE WHERE THEY PRODUCE INHIBITORY EFFECTS, i.e. relaxation.

α_2 Receptors

These are located mainly presynaptically on the sympathetic postganglionic neuron. Stimulation of these receptors by NE decreases the further release of the neurotransmitter (NE). Presynaptic α_2 receptors are also located on the cholinergic nerve terminals of the gut. When these receptors are activated by NE, the release of ACh is decreased from the cholinergic neuron leading to relaxation (refer heterotropic presynaptic receptor interaction, Ch. 10, Fig. 10.5 and 10.8). In the brain the α_2 receptors, whether present presynaptically or postsynaptically, decrease the sympathetic outflow upon their activation. NE release is also modulated by other receptors (heteroreceptor interaction as discussed earlier). In the case of noradrenergic nerve terminals, release of NE is increased by an activation of angiotensin-II receptors (AT_1) and is decreased by stimulation of M_1 receptor by ACh (Fig. 12.5).

β_1 Receptors

These are located postsynaptically and are found mainly in the heart where these produce positive inotropic and positive chronotropic effects (i.e., excitatory effects), upon activation by NE or E. These are also present in kidneys where these promote renin release. E and NE exhibit moderate and strong agonist actions respectively, on these receptors.

β_2 Receptors

Postsynaptically, these are located predominantly on bronchi, blood vessels supplying to skeletal muscle, coronary arteries, uterus, GIT and cardiac smooth muscle. Except in myocardium, their activation causes smooth muscle relaxation (inhibitory effects). E exhibits stronger affinity to β_2 receptor compared to NE (very little affinity).

β_2 receptors have also been identified *pre-synaptically* on adrenergic nerve terminals. Activation of presynaptic β_2 receptors by NE or E facilitates the neurotransmitter release (an effect which is opposite to that observed with activation of α_2 receptor as discussed above; Fig. 10.8, 12.3 & 12.5).

β_3 Receptors

These are present on adipocytes. Their activation promotes lipolysis (rise in blood free fatty acids) and thermogenesis. NE has 10-fold stronger agonist action on β_3 receptors compared to E.

For further details about adrenoceptors and their subtypes refer Chapter 10, and Fig. 10.7.

Receptor Regulation

The responses mediated by adrenoceptors are not constantly same. Their density and efficacy is subject to regulation by the level of ongoing activity and other physiopathological influences. Three processes have considerable clinical significance: (a) desensitisation, (b) up- and down-regulation of receptors and (c) denervation supersensitivity.

Continued receptor stimulation by an agonist causes ***desensitisation*** of the receptor, i.e., it becomes less responsive to the agonist. Tolerance, refractoriness and tachyphylaxis are some loose terms which are also used as synonyms to desensitisation. This process usually develops rapidly which distinguishes it from the process of "down-regulation" discussed below. The mechanism in desensitisation of effector cells to responses mediated by β-receptor has been extensively studied. Desensitisation of β-receptor occurs due to phosphorylation of its serine residue by an enzyme *β-adrenergic receptor kinase* (β-ARK). The phosphorylation of β receptor by β-ARK, facilitates its association with a protein *β arrestin* which disrupts its coupling to Gs-protein (i.e., receptor transduction is hindered). If the β agonist is removed, the serine residues are dephosphorylated and the β receptor mediated activation of Gs-protein is restored. Clinical examples include desensitisation of β_2 receptors in bronchial asthma patients treated with β_2 agonists.

Down-regulation of receptors is a phenomenon more commonly seen with tyrosine-protein kinase receptors, e.g., with insulin receptors while both up- and down-regulation is observed with G-protein coupled receptors, e.g., α and β-receptors. Prolonged exposure to high concentration of agonist causes a reduction in the number of receptors available for activation (down-regulation). This results due to endocytosis or internalisation of the receptors from the cell surface. On the other hand, prolonged occupation of the receptors by an antagonist leads to an increase in the number of receptors (***up-regulation***) with subsequent increase in receptor sensitivity. This probably results due to externalisation of the receptors out again from inside of the cell surface. Sometimes, other hormones can also bring about up-regulation of certain receptors. For example, in thyrotoxicosis, the thyroid hormones bring about up-regulation of β_1 receptors of cardiac muscle which increases cardiac sensitivity to catecholamines, leading to tachycardia. The process of up- or down-regulation of receptors takes several days and takes equally long time for restoration to normalcy.

An "extreme form of up-regulation" occurs if the receptors/effector organs are deprived of an agonist over a prolonged period. This results in ***supersensitivity*** of the receptor as well as of the effector organ. *Supersensitivity* can also result after denervation, or after continued blockade of the receptor by an antagonist or by administering a drug which depletes the neurotransmitter. In these situations, the new receptors are synthesised which then proliferate all along the cell surface. Such receptors are hyper-reactive to even small amounts of the neurotransmitter being made available despite receptor blockade. Examples include, rebound hypertension observed after sudden withdrawal of clonidine or β_1 receptor blockers (also refer Chapter 7).

Responses of Effector Organs to Sympathetic Stimulation

Eye

The radial pupillary dilator muscle of iris contains α_1 receptors. Sympathetic stimulation or activation by sympathomimetic drugs like phenylephrine causes mydriasis (NE, if instilled topically, does not produce mydriasis as it does not cross conjunctival membrane). In contrast to atropine, it produces an active mydriasis (refer Chapter 11). The ciliary muscle possesses β_2 receptors but, because of parasympathetic predominance, there is insignificant effect on accommodation. However, there is decrease in intraocular pressure as α_1 agonists increase the outflow of aqueous humour. Smooth muscles of eyelid have α_1 receptors, hence get constricted. Active mydriasis (more light) with no cycloplegia (no blurred vision) is one of the desired physiological responses set by sympathetic nervous system to prepare the body to fight or to run away from emergency situations.

Circular muscle of iris and lacrimal glands have no sympathetic innervation (no need of tears if you are fighting).

Salivary Glands

Sympathetic activation produces *thick* salivary secretions. The reduced salivary secretions is a consequence of reduced blood flow caused by vasoconstriction (watery saliva dripping along the chin would have looked very ridiculous and embarrassing during fight or flight).

Lungs

Bronchial smooth muscle possesses β_2 receptors which cause relaxation (bronchodilation). The blood vessels of the mucous membrane of upper respiratory tract (nasal and bronchial mucosa) get constricted by adrenaline (circulating or administered) and hence sympathetic stimulation causes decongestion. Both bronchodilatation (β_2 effect) and mucosal vasoconstriction (α_1 effect) increase the diameter of lumen and decrease bronchial resistance. Epinephrine also inhibits the release of allergic mediators from the mast cells (β_2 effect) and thus reduces congestion by this mechanism also (both bronchodilatation and decongestion help the body to meet the emergency situations of fight or flight).

Heart

Direct effects on the heart result mainly by β_1 receptors, though α_1 and β_2 receptors are also involved. The sympathetic activation increases the heart rate (activation of β_1 receptors at SA node), enhances conduction and decreases effective refractory period (AV node- β_1 receptor activation), increases automaticity by activating β_1 receptors at Purkinje fibres and increases the force of contraction (β_1 receptor stimulation of ventricular myocardium). All these accelerating effects on heart help the body to prepare itself for fight or flight.

Blood Vessels

Vascular smooth muscle tone is governed by the presence of α_1 and β_2 receptors. Alpha$_1$ receptors increase arterial resistance, whereas β_2 receptors promote smooth muscle relaxation. There are major differences in the types of receptors (α_1 or β_2) present in different vascular beds. *The skin, mucosal, splanchnic and renal blood vessels* have predominantly α_1 receptors and therefore constrict during sympathetic stimulation ($\alpha_1 > \beta_2$). However, D_1 receptors promote vasodilatation of renal arteries, hence renal vascular resistance does not increase as appreciably as of skin, mucosal and splanchnic blood vessels. *Coronaries* have predominantly β_2, α_2 and D_1 receptors and therefore exhibit vasodilatation.

Sympathetic stimulation also increases myocardial contractility and increases its oxygen demand producing local hypoxia. This local hypoxia in turn dilates the coronaries (over-riding α_1 stimulated coronary vasoconstriction if any). Recently α_2 receptors have been found located on the endothelial cells of coronary arteries, stimulation of which results in the release of nitric oxide causing vasodilatation. *The innervation to some skeletal muscle blood vessels* is sympathetic in origin but cholinergic in character. Nevertheless, since the postsynaptic receptors on smooth muscles being predominantly β_2 (role of α_1 receptor is only marginal), the overall effect of sympathetic stimulation is vasodilatation (or reduced peripheral vascular resistance). The *pulmonary blood vessels* have both α_1 and β_2 receptors. Since the α_1 effect slightly dominates over β_2 effect, the net result is mild pulmonary vasoconstriction (decongestion). There is no change in *cerebral vascular resistance* ($\alpha_1 = \beta_2$). There is hardly any change in the tone

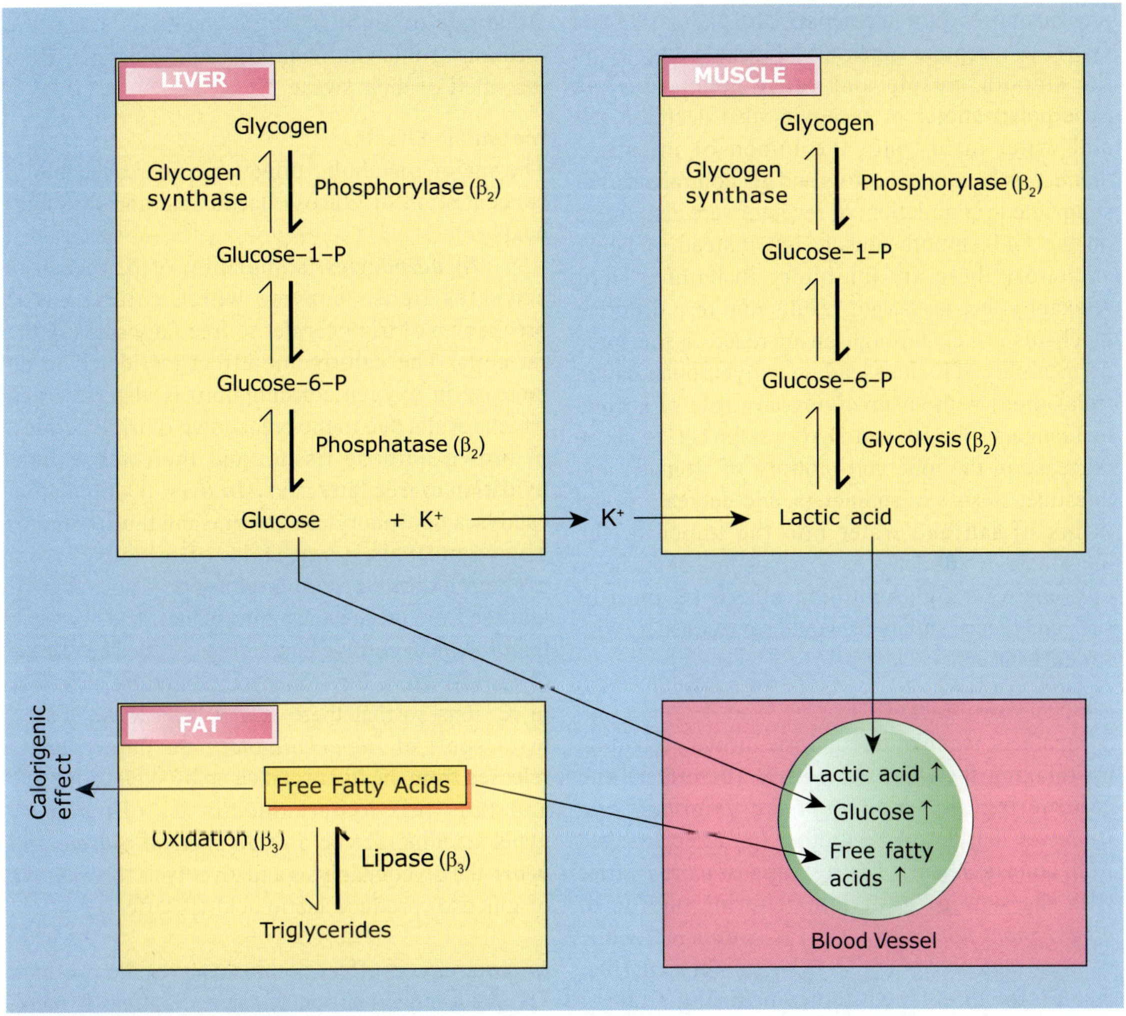

Fig 12.6 Metabolic effects of catecholamines

(resistance) of *systemic veins* as α_1 receptor effect is antagonised by β_2 effect ($\alpha_1 = \beta_2$).

Hence to meet out the demands of the body during fight of flight, the coronaries get dilated to maintain enough blood supply to the heart; skeletal muscle blood vessels get dilated to meet the demand of exercising muscle; blood supply to the brain is not disturbed; veins which have to return blood to heart are not affected; renal perfusion is not compromised but the demands of coronaries and skeletal blood vessels are compensated by drifting some blood from skin, pulmonary mucosa and splanchnic blood vessels. Pulmonary vasoconstriction would lead to decongestion which would further help lungs to cope with the situations like flight or fight (an added advantage to bronchodilatation).

Gastrointestinal System

Smooth muscles of stomach and intestines have α_2 and β_2 receptors. α_2 receptors are located presynaptically at the cholinergic neuron and their stimulation reduces the tone as well as the motility indirectly by reducing the release of ACh through presynaptic activation (refer heterotropic presynaptic receptor interaction, Ch.10, Fig. 10.5 and 10.8). β_2 receptors appear to be located directly on the smooth muscle and cause relaxation via hyperpolarisation. α_2 receptors also decrease salt and water influx into the lumen of intestine. *Sphincters* have α_1 receptors and get contracted after sympathetic stimulation. α_1 receptors are also found on the GIT smooth muscle but instead of being excitatory these are inhibitory in nature. Their relaxant effect in the gut results due to a different mechanism, i.e., through an increase in the ionic permeability of K^+ ions leading to hyperpolarisation (relaxation) without involving any role of second messengers (like IP_3 and DAG , refer Ch. 11). The decrease in the tone and motility of stomach and intestine, closure of sphincters, and decrease in the influx of salt and water into the lumen of the intestines, are all such effects, which favour the body to prepare for fight or flight; otherwise, most of such emergency situations would have ended up with soiled trousers.

Genitourinary Tract

Sympathetic stimulation can foster urinary retention by relaxing the *detrusor muscle* (β_3 effect) and contracting the *bladder base trigonal and sphincter* muscle of the urethra (α_1 effect) (saved from embarassment). The response of *uterus* varies with the state of gestation. Uterine muscle of *nonpregnant uterus* ($\alpha_1 > \beta_2$) is contracted, while of *pregnant uterus* ($\beta_2 > \alpha_1$) gets relaxed (less chance for threatened abortion during fight or flight). In men ejaculation is facilitated by activation of α_1 receptors in *vas deferens, seminal vesicles* and *prostate.*

Skin

Secretion of sweat from sweat glands located on the palms, sole, and forehead is increased during psychologic stress due to sympathetic stimulation (adrenergic sweat). Sweat glands in these areas are regulated by sympathetic-cholinergic post-ganglionic fibres that activate M_3 receptors (refer Ch.10). Pilomotor muscles are contracted (α_1 effect) leading to piloerection (raising of hair). Piloerection increases the perception to the surroundings, and helps the body to cope with the situations of fight or flight. Animals sense the location of their kith and kin, during danger, from the smell of their sweat.

Metabolic Effects

The major metabolic effects are increased blood concentration of glucose, lactic acid and free fatty acids (Fig. 12.6).

In adipocytes, stimulation of β_3 receptors activates lipase enzyme which catalyses the breakdown of triglycerides to free fatty acids in the fat cells. The calorigenic effect (reflected in an increase in oxygen consumption) is also observed which results due to the breakdown of triglycerides, in brown adipose tissue, and their subsequent oxidation to free fatty acids. ***In liver***, β_2 stimulation catalyses phosphorylase enzyme and thus promotes glycogenolysis (synthesis of glucose from glycogen) and gluconeogenesis (synthesis of glucose from lactate and amino acids). The net result therefore is hyperglycaemia. (Fig. 12.6). The release of glucose from liver is accompanied by an efflux of K^+ ions so that there is *hyperglycaemia* with a brief spell of *hyperkalaemia*; but later the K^+ released from the liver is taken up by skeletal muscle and thus this hyperkalaemia is followed by hypokalaemia (see below). ***In skeletal muscle and heart,*** the glycogenolysis and glycolysis (breakdown of glucose) produce lactic acid (β_2 effect).

In pancreas, α-effect dominates over the β-effect. The predominant action of catecholamines is on α_2 receptors of the pancreatic-B-islet cells which leads to diminution in insulin secretion. There is also increase in glucagon secretion from the pancreatic-A-islet cells through activation of β_2 receptors. These effects further contribute to hyperglycaemia (Fig. 12.7).

Skeletal Muscle

There is facilitation of neuromuscular transmission by a presynaptic α-receptor action which increases the amount of ACh release at the neuromuscular junction. Usually a heterotropic presynaptic receptor interaction in ANS decreases the release

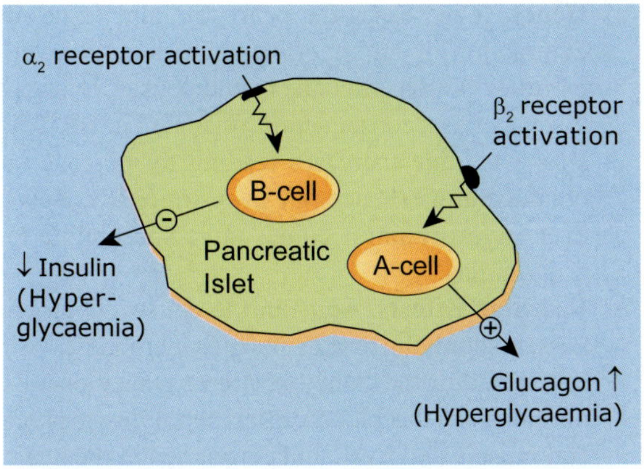

Fig 12.7 Regulation of Insulin and Glucagon Secretion by A and B cells of the Islets of Langerhans.

of the neurotransmitter (in this case, of ACh as discussed in Ch.10). However, in apparent contrast to ANS, stimulation of α-receptor at cholinergic neuron of somatic motor system, increases ACh release perhaps as a result of enhanced influx of Ca^{2+}. Since distribution of β_2 receptors predominates over α_1 receptors in skeletal muscle blood vessels, the relaxation produced by β_2 receptor activation improves the blood flow to skeletal muscle (it is only partly counteracted by vasoconstrictor action of meagre number of α_1 receptors). The net result is "antifatigue effect" during stressful situations, e.g., fight and flight situations.

Central Nervous System

These effects are not that important. But during stress there may be anxiety, apprehension, arousal, restlessness and in extreme situations tremors.

Kidney

There is renin release from the juxtaglomerular apparatus in the kidney (β_1 effect). There is increase in the motility and tone of ureter (α_1 effect).

Other Effects

(a) Inhibition of histamine release through mast cell membrane stabilisation (low incidence of itching if you are hiding behind or under the shrub); (b) inhibition of lymphocytic activity; (c) more uptake of K^+ from ECF to ICF which results in the fall of plasma K^+ levels (β_2 effect). Decrease in serum K^+ levels can precipitate cardiac arrhythmias due to stress.

SYMPATHOMIMETICS

These drugs mimic the actions of endogenous catecholamines. Sympathomimetic drugs can be classified into three groups on the basis of their mode of action:

Directly Acting Sympathomimetics

- These drugs act directly on pre- and/or postsynaptic α and β-adrenergic receptors and produce expected pharmacological effects.
- These can exhibit effects even after the denervation of postganglionic adrenergic neuron.
- Repeated dosing with these drugs, unlike indirectly acting sympathomimetics, does not lead to tachyphylaxis.

Indirectly Acting Sympathomimetics

- These do not have a direct stimulant action on adrenoceptors. Rather, these are taken up by neuronal membrane (uptake-1) and, once inside the neuronal cytoplasm, enter into the storage vesicle from where they displace NE from its stores. The displaced/released NE then activates the adrenoceptors.
- Denervation of postganglionic adrenergic neuron prevents their action (as they have no direct action on postsynaptic receptors).
- Repeated dosing, at short intervals, leads to tachyphylaxis, as neuronal NE stores get depleted after repeated dosing and no more NE is available now for release, unless the NE stores are replenished.
- These drugs, usually, are more lipid soluble than NE or E. Hence they have better penetration through blood-brain barrier and are better absorbed through the gut.

Mixed Action Sympathomimetics

These drugs act indirectly through displacement (release) of NE from its stores as discussed above (major mode of action). Also, these have a direct action on α and β receptors (like NE and E).

Individual groups of sympathomimetics have been discussed, in detail, as below.

DIRECTLY ACTING SYMPATHOMIMETICS

On the basis of their mode of action, these drugs can be classified as in Fig. 12.8.

Endogenous Catecholamines

These are sympathomimetic amines that contain two adjacent OH groups in the benzene nucleus (see earlier text). These drugs share the following characteristics:

a) High potency in activating α and/or β receptors
b) Rapid inactivation (very short t½): These have only a brief spell of action when given parenterally (hence usually given by I.V. infusion). These are ineffective when given orally, because of being polar and partly because of their inactivation by COMT present in gut wall and by MAO present in liver and gut wall.
c) Poor penetration into the CNS (being polar). However, they do produce anxiety, tremors and headaches (in high doses) which probably represent enhancement of DA-mediated processes in CNS.

Epinephrine (Adrenaline)

It is primarily secreted from adrenal medulla (80–90%) along with NE (10–20%). Naturally occurring epinephrine is optically active and the levoform is more potent than the dextro form. It is unstable, rapidly oxidised by light and air and is converted to an inactive coloured toxic substance called adrenochrome. Solutions are, therefore, kept in amber coloured bottles with reducing agents like sodium metabisulphite or ascorbic acid.

The relative receptor affinity epinephrine is: $\beta_2 > \beta_1 = \alpha_1 = \alpha_2$. As a result at low doses β_2 effects predominate over α and β_1 effects. However, the latter effects (α & β_1) are stronger at high doses due to fewer blood vessels being endowed with β_2 receptors, i.e., skeletal muscle blood vessels only. It also has weak β_3 agonist activity.

Cardiovascular Effects

Epinephrine is a very potent vasoconstrictor and cardiac stimulant.

a) **Heart**. It increases the heart rate and force of contraction (β_1 and β_2 effects) which is followed by reflex bradycardia due to compensatory vagal discharge as a consequence of the rise in BP. The stroke volume increases leading to increase in cardiac output (hence rise in systolic BP). However, myocardium becomes more susceptible to arrhythmias.
b) **Vascular Effects**. Epinephrine constricts blood vessels supplying to skin, mucous membrane, viscera including the kidney (α effect). Dilatation predominates in the blood vessels supplying to skeletal muscle and liver, and coronaries in the heart (β_2 effect). Total peripheral resistance decreases because vascular β_2 receptors are more sensitive than α-receptors. The cumulative effect therefore is an increase in the systolic BP coupled with slight decrease in diastolic BP.
c) **Blood Pressure**. Moderate dose produces a biphasic response, i.e., a rise in BP due to α_1 and β_1 actions, resulting into more rise in systolic than diastolic. Subsequently, as the plasma concentration of E declines, the β_2 effects get unmasked (β_2 receptors, being more sensitive than α_1 respond even with lower doses of E). As a result, mean BP falls below normal before returning to control values (Fig.12.9A) This fall in BP (due to β_2 action), becomes more apparent after pretreatment with an α-blocking drug (Dale's vasomotor reversal phenomenon, Fig. 12.9B). However, if pretreatment is done with a β-blocker then mainly the hypertensive effect is noted (called blockade of Dale's vasomotor reversal phenomenon: Fig.12.9C).

Effects on Smooth Muscles

a) **Bronchial Smooth Muscle**. Epinephrine causes powerful bronchodilatation (β_2 effect) and decrease in bronchial secretions (α_1 effect due to decrease in bronchial microcirculation). Hence cumulatively, there is decrease in bronchial resistance.
b) **GIT**. Gut relaxation (α_2 and β effect) occurs with constriction of sphincters (α_1 effect) but these effects are of no clinical significance.
c) **Urinary Tract**. There is relaxation of detrusor muscle (β_3 effect) with contraction of smooth

DIRECTLY ACTING SYMPATHOMIMETICS

CATECHOLAMINES

Endogenous

- EPINEPHRINE (Adrenaline)
  Has $\alpha_1 + \alpha_2 + \beta_1 + \beta_2$ and weak β_3 action
- NOREPINEPHRINE (Noradrenaline)
  Has $\alpha_1 + \alpha_2 + \beta_1 + \beta_3$ action with poor β_2 receptor action
- DOPAMINE
  Mainly $D_1 + D_2 + \beta_1$ effects with little α, (α action is seen only in high doses) but no β_2 or β_3 action

Synthetic

- ISOPRENALINE (Isoproterenol)
  $\beta_1 + \beta_2 + \beta_3$ action
  No α-action
- DIPIVEFRINE
  Prodrug of epinephrine
- DOBUTAMINE
  Mainly β_1 action.
  Little α_1 effect. No DA receptor or β_2 or β_3 action
- DOPEXAMINE
  $D_1 + D_2 + \beta_2$ receptor action
- FENOLDOPAM
  Selective D_1 agonist

NON-CATECHOLAMINES

- **α_1 Selective agonists**
  PHENYLEPHRINE
  METHOXAMINE
  NAPHAZOLINE
  OXYMETAZOLINE
  XYLOMETAZOLINE
  MIDODRINE
- **α_2 Selective agonists**
  CLONIDINE
  APRACLONIDINE
  BRIMONIDINE
  α-METHYLDOPA
- **β_1 Selective agonists**
  PRENALTEROL, but seldom used. However in catecholamine-synthetic group-dobutamine is used
- **β_2 Selective agonists**
  Short acting β_2 agonists (SABA)
  SALBUTAMOL (albuterol)
  ORCIPRENALINE (metaproterenol)
  TERBUTALINE, PIRBUTEROL, CLENBUTEROL
  Long acting β_2 agonists (LABA)
  BAMBUTEROL, SALMETEROL
  FORMOTEROL, EFORMOTEROL
  INDACATEROL, OLODETEROL, VILANTEROL
- **β_3 Selective agonists**
  MIRABEGRON
  BRL-37344

Fig 12.8 Directly Acting Sympathomimetics

muscle of trigone and urethral sphincter (α_1 effect). Micturition is therefore hindered.

d) **Uterus**. Nonpregnant human uterus constricts ($\alpha_1 > \beta_2$), otherwise relaxation (pregnant uterus $\beta_2 > \alpha_1$). However, effects vary with species and gestational status.

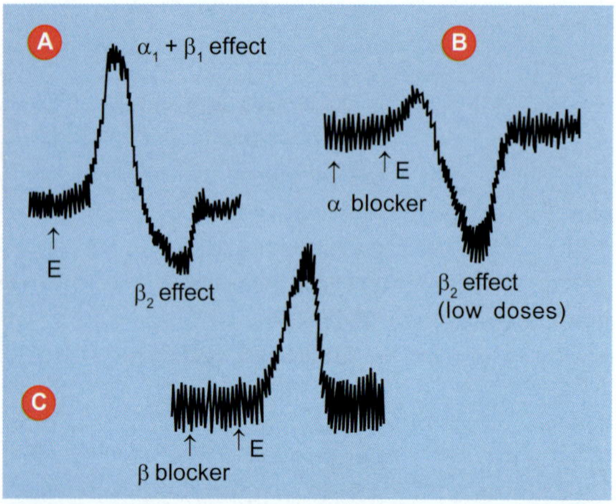

Fig 12.9 (A) Normal Effect of Epinephrine on BP; (B) Dale's Vasomotor Reversal Phenomenon; (C) α Effect (↑BP) Seen after β-blockade

Metabolic Effects

a) Hyperglycaemia due to glycogenolysis in liver (β_2) and skeletal muscle (α_1 and β_2).
b) Increase in free fatty acids due to lipolysis in adipose tissue (α and β_3).
c) Inhibition of insulin release (α_2).
d) Calorigenic effects (rise in BMR and CVS effects cause rise in body temperature; β_3).

Miscellaneous Effects (for details, refer earlier text)

a) Active mydriasis in eye due to contraction of radial muscle of iris (α_1).
b) Thick salivary secretions (α_1).
c) Piloerection and sweating of palms and soles (α_1).
d) Inhibition of histamine release through mast cell membrane stabilisation.
e) Anxiety and tremors (CNS effects).

Therapeutic Uses (remember ABCDE)

a) **Allergy (Anaphylactic shock)**: It is the drug of first choice in acute hypersensitivity reactions (type 1), like acute anaphylactic shock, because it relieves bronchospasm, angioneurotic oedema of larynx, prevents release of histamine from mast cells and maintains BP in anaphylactic shock (given intramuscularly ; 0.3–0.5 ml 1:1000 solution). In anaphylactic shock the absorption of adrenaline, if given S.C., is very poor. Hence, preferred route is I.M.
b) **Bronchial Asthma**: Because it causes bronchodilatation and decongestion of bronchial mucosa (given S.C. 0.3–0.5 ml of 1:1000 solution or as aerosol).
c) **Cardiac Resuscitation**: Intracardiac injection of epinephrine (0.1 mg/ml) can be used to reverse sudden cardiac arrest like with drowning and electrocution (contraindication: ventricular fibrillation).
d) **To prolong the Duration of Local Anaesthetic Action**: Epinephrine because of its vasoconstricting effect antagonises the vasodilating effects of LA and also retards their systemic absorption from their desired site of action. Hence, not only the duration of LA action is prolonged but their systemic toxicity also decreases (given S.C. or intradermal in combination with any LA).
e) **To control Epistaxis (as a local haemostatic)**: To control bleeding as in epistaxis and in ENT surgery (used as a spray to have clear vision).

Adverse Effects

a) Increase in BP may lead to cerebral haemorrhage.
b) Increase in cardiac work and contractility may lead to coronary insufficiency—hence may precipitate angina, palpitation, and even arrhythmias (specifically if the patient is receiving digitalis). Epinephrine may induce pulmonary oedema.
c) CNS side effects may include tremors, anxiety and headaches.

Contraindications & Interactions

- **Hyperthyroidism.** Due to up-regulation of α receptors on the vasculature and of β-receptors in the heart, a hyperthyroid individual may become hyper-responsive to epinephrine. In such cases the dose must be reduced.
- **Angina and hypertension** (as discussed earlier).

- Tricyclic antidepressants, as these drugs prevent the reuptake of E into the adrenergic neuron (thus availability of E at receptor site increases).
- Halothane group of general anaesthetics, as they increase the sensitivity of myocardium towards catecholamines.
- MAOIs (as the metabolism of E is hampered; hence availability of E increases).

Norepinephrine (noradrenaline; levarterenol)

Endogenous norepinephrine (NE) is the l-isomer which is more potent than the d-isomer. Chemically NE differs from E in having "amino nitrogen devoid of $-CH_3$ substitution" (i.e., it has a $-NH_2$ group in place of $-NHCH_3$; Fig. 12.1). It is a chemical mediator liberated from the postganglionic sympathetic nerve endings, adrenal medulla (10–20%) and constitutes 97% of the secretions from the tumour phaeochromocytoma. It is predominantly an α-agonist with relative receptor affinity as $\alpha_1 = \alpha_2 > \beta_1 >> \beta_2$. It also possesses significant β_3 agonist action.

Features Distinguishable from Epinephrine

Cardiovascular Actions. NE raises both systolic as well as diastolic BP, mainly due to cardiac stimulation (β_1) and rise in total peripheral vascular resistance (α_1). Cardiac output, however, is unchanged. Reflex bradycardia (due to compensatory increase in vagal discharge) is evident secondary to hypertension produced by NE. If atropine (which blocks the transmission of vagal effects) is given prior to NE, this hypertension is followed with tachycardia. The coronary blood flow increases (due to rise in mean arterial pressure and also due to production of adenosine—a vasodilator metabolite of myocardial metabolism). As NE has a predominant α-action, it does not exhibit Dale's vasomotor reversal phenomenon (very little β_2 action, unlike E).

Other Sympathomimetic Actions. These are minimal and clinically unimportant in therapeutic doses.

Therapeutic Uses. Injection of NE (4 mg or 2 ampoules) is dissolved in one litre of 5% glucose solution prior to I.V. infusion (0.5 to 1.0 ml/min). It may be carefully used to treat cardiogenic shock (hypotensive state as a consequence of surgical shock or MI) as it increases vascular resistance and decreases blood flow to vital organs. However, dopamine is preferred as it does not reduce blood flow to kidney (with NE there is associated risk for renal shutdown). It is not suitable for S.C., I.M. or undiluted direct I.V. injection because of the danger of necrosis at the site of injection (powerful vasoconstrictor).

Adverse Effects, Precautions and Contraindications. These are similar to that of E. However, its infusions should be tapered off gradually to avoid sudden fall in BP. Extravasation into the subcutaneous tissue should be carefully watched to avoid tissue necrosis at the site of infusion (powerful vasoconstriction).

Dopamine (DA)

DA is an endogenous catecholamine which is the immediate precursor of NE and E. Chemically it differs from NE and E by an absence of a –OH group at the β-carbon atom of the side chain (Fig.12.1). Additionally, it also has an important neurotransmitter role in CNS. The metabolism of DA is shown in Fig. 12.4. When given parenterally it does not cross BBB and exhibits no central effects.

Features Distinguishable from NE and E

When given I.V. in therapeutic doses (up to 2–5 μg/kg/min, I.V.) it acts on D_1 receptors and causes dilatation of renal vessels resulting in increased glomerular filtration rate, renal blood flow and excretion of sodium. Around 5–10 μg/kg/min, I.V., it also stimulates β_1 receptors resulting in an increase in cardiac output but the total peripheral resistance and mean blood pressure are unchanged due to simultaneous renal and splanchnic vasodilatation through D_1 receptor. However, in higher doses (above 10 μg/kg/min, I.V.), it can cause vasoconstriction by activating α_1-receptor nullifying the beneficial effects of low doses of DA.

Therapeutic Uses. It is used in conditions of low cardiac output with compromised renal functions (advantage of increased cardiac output with renal vasodilatation), such as *cardiogenic shock resulting from MI, trauma or surgery. Also used in the treatment of congestive heart failure, renal and liver failure.* Before administering DA to the patients of shock, hypovolaemia, if present, must be corrected. The contents of ampoule (40 mg/ml) are diluted in 100 ml of 5% dextrose solution or in 0.9% normal saline so as to give a final concentration of 400 µg/ml. This is given as an infusion at a rate of 5 to 10 µg/kg/min. The BP, HR and urine flow should be continuously monitored not only to adjust the dose but to obtain beneficial effects.

Adverse Effects. These include nausea, vomiting, tachycardia, ectopic beats, hypertension (in high doses) and cardiac arrhythmias (although incidence is lower).

Synthetic Catecholamines

These are synthetic catecholamines containing two adjacent OH groups in the benzene nucleus.

Isoprenaline (isoproterenol)

Isoprenaline predominantly stimulates β_1 and β_2 adrenergic receptors. Its action on β_3 receptors can also be demonstrated (e.g., increased lipolysis) but these are not clinically significant. It has negligible α-receptor action ($\beta_1 = \beta_2 >> \beta_3 >>>> \alpha$). Its chemical structure is given in Fig. 12.10.

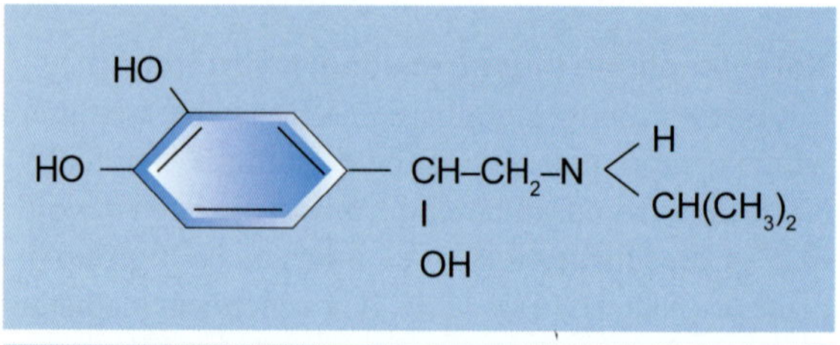

Fig 12.10 Chemical Structure of Isoprenaline.

Features Distinguishable from E and NE

Cardiovascular Effects (Fig. 12.11). It exerts a positive inotropic and chronotropic effect on heart causing an increase in cardiac output (β_1 effect). Because of its cardiac stimulant action it may

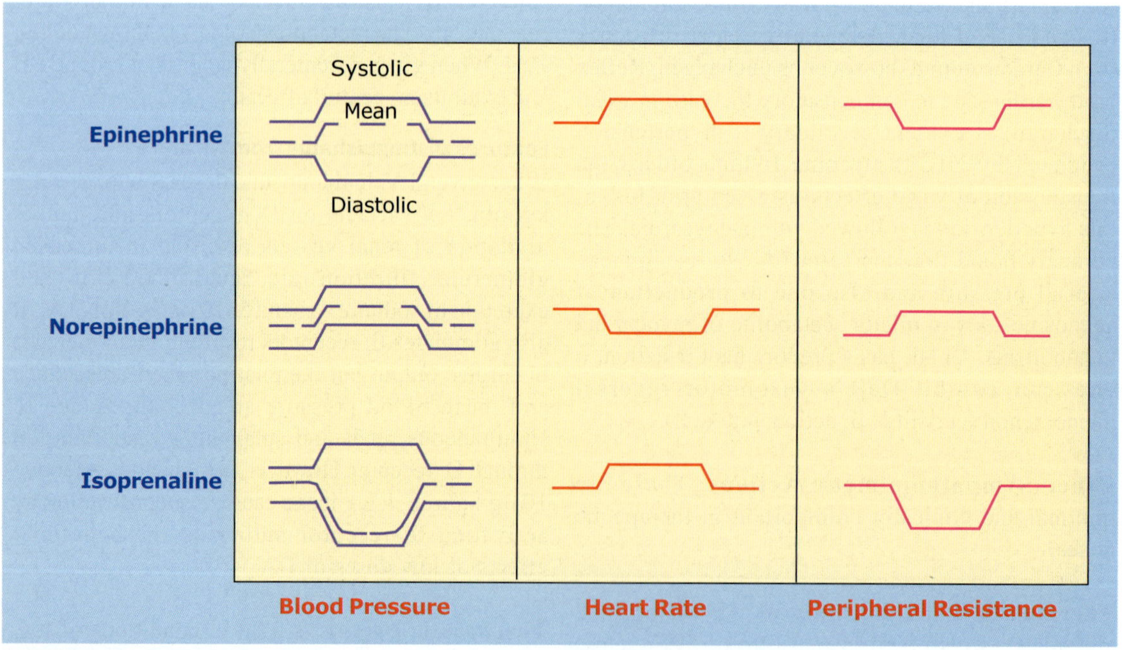

Fig 12.11 Comparative Cardiovascular Effects of Epinephrine, Norepinephrine and Isoprenaline (refer text).

slightly increase systolic BP but the mean arterial and diastolic BP are greatly reduced. It dilates the arterioles of skeletal muscle (β_2 effect) resulting in decreased peripheral resistance.

Effects on Smooth Muscles. Isoprenaline relaxes bronchial as well as gastrointestinal smooth muscles. It relieves bronchoconstriction mainly due to its β_2 agonist action and partly due to inhibition of antigen-induced histamine release (Fig. 12.11).

Pharmacokinetics. It is readily absorbed when given parenterally or as an aerosol. Compared to E and NE it is taken up by the sympathetic neurons to a much lesser extent and hence it is stable to MAO degradation but is metabolised by COMT present in liver and other tissues.

Therapeutic Uses. It is rarely used, but can be employed in emergency situations to increase heart rate in patients with bradycardia or heart block (prior to insertion of an artificial cardiac pacemaker). Availability of selective β_2 agonist drugs has made its use in bronchial asthma almost obsolete.

Adverse Effects. Its cardiac stimulant effects may lead to palpitations, sinus tachycardia and at times serious arrhythmias.

Dipivefrine

It is a prodrug for epinephrine with enhanced corneal permeability. Its 0.1% solution is used for the treatment of glaucoma. Ocular side effects may include photosensitivity and conjunctival hyperaemia.

Dobutamine

This drug is used clinically, as a racemic mixture of two enantiomeric forms. The l-form is a potent agonist at α_1 receptor while d-form is a potent α_1 receptor antagonist and also a powerful β_1 receptor agonist. Hence, the net cardiovascular effects of dobutamine (i.e., of the racemic form) are manifested as counterbalancing of α_1 receptor action by l- and d-forms with prominent β_1 receptor agonist actions of d-form. On heart, therefore, dobutamine has more selective inotropic than chronotropic effects without any significant change in peripheral vascular resistance and BP. As such it has been considered to be relatively selective β_1 agonist. Its actions do not appear to be a result of release of NE from sympathetic nerve endings, nor *via* DA-receptor action.

It is used in patients of heart failure (2–5 μg/kg/min, I.V. infusion) associated with myocardial infarction, cardiac surgery and for short-term management of acute congestive heart failure. Dobutamine increases cardiac output and stroke volume in such patients without affecting heart rate, peripheral resistance or blood pressure. Its half-life is about 2 min and therefore the steady state concentrations are achieved within 10 min of its I.V. infusion.

Adverse Effects. There may be a sharp rise in BP and heart rate, specially in patients with a history of hypertension. Being an inotropic agent, myocardial oxygen demand increases and hence angina may be precipitated or myocardial infarction may be aggravated. Tolerance may develop on prolonged use. Since the drug increases AV conduction, it should be used with caution in atrial fibrillation.

Dopexamine

It stimulates β_2 adrenoceptors and peripheral DA receptors and also inhibits neuronal uptake of NE. These actions result in an increased cardiac output, peripheral vasodilatation and an increase in renal and mesenteric blood flow. It is used to provide haemodynamic support in patients with congestive heart failure and shock. The most common side effect is tachycardia, transient hypotension and dyspnoea. It should not be used in patient with phaeochromocytoma.

Fenoldopam

It is a selective D_1 receptor agonist. It has no α or β receptor agonist activity. It is a peripheral arteriolar dilator and causes vasodilatation in coronary, renal and mesenteric arterioles. The drug is, therefore, useful in the short-term management of severe hypertension in patients with impaired renal functions where rapid reduction in BP is desired.

Adverse effects include reflex tachycardia, increase in intraocular pressure and headache.

Hypokalaemia has also been reported (because of diuretic action). Oral bioavailability is poor and hence it is usually given by intravenous route.

Non-catecholamines

α_1 Agonist Drugs

Phenylephrine and methoxamine (the prototype drugs) are directly acting vasoconstrictors and are selective activators of α_1 receptors.

Phenylephrine

It is an α_1 selective agonist. It lacks a hydroxyl group at 4-position on the benzene ring of epinephrine (hence a non-catecholamine; Fig.12.12). Being a non-catecholamine derivative, it is not metabolised by COMT and hence is longer acting than other catecholamine sympathomimetics.

An activation of α_1 receptor results in an increase in the peripheral vascular resistance and BP (which is associated with reflex bradycardia). It is mainly used as a nasal decongestant and as a mydriatic. However, it may be useful in some patients of hypotension or shock.

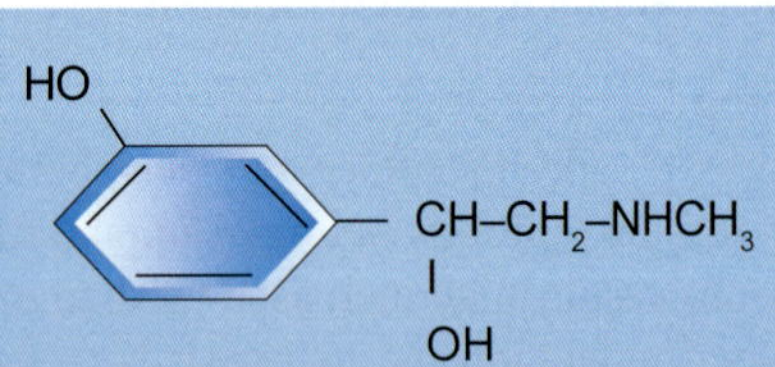

Fig 12.12 Chemical Structure of Phenylephrine.

Methoxamine: The pharmacological effects and uses of methoxamine are similar to those of phenylephrine.

Midodrine is a prodrug. Its active metabolite desglymidodrine has a selective α_1-receptor activity. It is used to treat postural hypotension. The main adverse effect is hypertension in supine position, hence dosing at the bed time should better be avoided.

Naphazoline, Oxymetazoline and Xylometazoline

These drugs are used as nasal decongestants in rhinorrhoea and to check epistaxis, in various nasal formulations. These are predominantly α_1 agonists. Oxymetazoline has some α_2 agonist action also (may cause hypotension).

Pseudoephedrine (a stereoisomer of ephedrine) and **phenylpropanolamine** are some other sympathomimetic non-catecholamines (though not specific α_1 receptor agonists) which are used most commonly in common cold oral formulations for the relief in nasal congestion. Because of the possibility that phenylpropanolamine increases the risk of haemorrhagic stroke (in young women and hypertensives), it has been withdrawn from many countries, including India. The mechanism of this potential adverse effect is not known.

α_2 Agonist Drugs

Alpha$_2$ receptors are located mainly presynaptically on the sympathetic postganglionic neuron and postsynaptically in blood vessels and brain. Stimulation of these receptors by NE or any α_2 agonist decreases further release of the neurotransmitter (NE). In the brain the α_2 receptors, whether present presynaptically or postsynaptically, decrease the central sympathetic outflow upon their activation by α_2 agonists (refer earlier text and Fig. 12.4). Hence α_2 agonists are primarily used for the treatment of hypertension. Surprisingly, many blood vessels possess postsynaptic α_2 receptors which promote vasoconstriction and hence rather produce hypertension. Therefore, some α_2 agonists (like clonidine), when given by I.V. infusion, may initially cause hypertension followed by a more prolonged hypotension which results from decreased central sympathetic outflow.

Clonidine

Clonidine belongs to an imidazoline group of antihypertensive drugs whose precise mode of action is still not clear. After I.V. injection (i.e., at higher concentration) clonidine produces a transient rise in BP (see above) but on oral administration (i.e., at low plasma concentration) it produces only the fall in BP. This is because, clonidine has lesser intrinsic activity on α_2 receptors present postsynaptically on vascular smooth muscle, at lower plasma concentrations. The antihypertensive effect of clonidine is a manifestation of the following concerted mechanisms:

a) It mainly stimulates α_2 receptors present at vasomotor center. Consequently, central sympathetic outflow is reduced, resulting in fall in BP and heart rate.
b) Recently two imidazoline receptors (I_1 and I_2) have been identified in brain and in periphery, respectively. It has been reported that I_1 receptor, to which clonidine binds and activates, is a G-protein coupled receptor which uses IP_3 and DAG as a second messenger system to modulate central α_2 receptor activity (to reduce central sympathetic outflow).
c) In addition, clonidine also activates the presynaptic α_2 receptors present on sympathetic postganglionic neurons and thus suppresses further release of NE from peripheral nerve endings.

The decreased central sympathetic discharge to the kidney also reduces renin release and decreases renal vascular resistance. Hence, clonidine is useful in hypertensive patients with poor renal functions.

Pharmacokinetics

Clonidine is well absorbed after oral administration (bioavailability nearly 100%). A transdermal delivery patch permits continuous administration of the drug as an alternative to oral therapy. The drug is released at an approximately constant rate for about a week. When the patch is removed, plasma concentrations remain stable for about 8 hrs and then decline gradually over a period of several days.

Therapeutic Uses

1. **Moderate Hypertension.** It is given orally (100 μg twice daily to a max. of 300 μg BD orally) usually along with a diuretic (to counteract sodium and water retention which leads to the development of tolerance). However, its side effects and the risk associated with rebound hypertension after its withdrawal limit its use as a first line antihypertensive (for details refer Chapter 19).
2. **To Control Diarrhoea in Diabetic Patients with Autonomic Neuropathy.** Stimulation of α_2 receptors in GIT decreases Na^+ and water retention and inhibits HCO_3^- secretion and reduces intestinal motility by inhibiting the release of ACh (Fig. 10.8). However, oral clonidine (not transdermal) causes orthostatic hypotension in such patients, which may limit its usefulness.
3. **In Prophylaxis of Migraine.** It reduces cerebral blood flow. Hence it was used for pro-phylaxis of migraine in smaller doses (25–75 μg) earlier. But better drugs are now available for this purpose.
4. **Management of Nicotine, Alcohol and Opiate Withdrawal.** Clonidine controls some of the adverse sympathetic effects associated with the withdrawal of opioids, alcohol and smoking and decreases craving for these drugs (for details refer Ch. 38).
5. **Preanaesthetic Medication.** It can be used preoperatively for its sedative, anxiolytic, and analgesic effects and to provide haemodynamic stability and to reduce anaesthetic requirements. **Dexmedetomidine** is a selective α_{2A} agonist which is used for preanaesthetic medication to provide preoperative sedation, analgesia, antianxiety effects and reduction in bronchial secretions. It is used to provide conscious sedation in ICU patients requiring mechanical ventilation for longer period. It also reduces the need for frequent opioid use, in cancer patients, for pain control.
6. **Menopausal Hot Flushes.** Transdermal patches of clonidine are useful for counteracting such symptoms.

Adverse Effects

Major adverse effects are: (1) Rebound hypertension after abrupt withdrawal of the drug (due to supersensitivity of the newly formed α_1 receptors). Therefore, the withdrawal of clonidine therapy should be gradual. (2) Dry mouth, (3) Sedation, (4) Nasal stuffiness, (5) Constipation, (6) Impotence and (7) Contact dermatitis, when using a transdermal patch of the drug.

Moxonidine and **rilmenidine**, the newer congeners of clonidine have a longer plasma half-life and are said to be selective for I_1 receptor rather than α_2 receptor. Rebound hypertension is much less frequent with these drugs, as omission of a single dose will not trigger the rebound.

Apraclonidine and Brimonidine

Apraclonidine and **brimonidine** are selective α_2 agonists which are used for the treatment of glaucoma. They reduce the formation of aqueous humor by their α_2 receptor agonist action (present on ciliary epithelium). These are potent ocular hypotensives which do not cross BBB and hence have least systemic effects (unlike clonidine which crosses BBB). These are primarily used to prevent an acute rise in intraocular pressure after laser trabeculoplasty.

Alpha Methyldopa

Methyldopa is a centrally acting antihypertensive (Chapter 19), which exerts its action *via* its active metabolite. Alpha methyldopa is metabolised by L-amino acid decarboxylase to α-methyldopamine in neuronal cytoplasm. It then enters into storage vesicle in place of DA and gets converted to *N*-methylnorepinephrine by dopamine-β-hydroxylase (Fig. 12.2 and 12.3; similar to NE). It is then stored in storage vesicles of adrenergic neuron. When the adrenergic neuron discharges its neurotransmitter, α-methyl NE is released, as a false neurotransmitter, in place of NE. However, the release of α–methyl NE, as false neurotransmitter, in the periphery is not responsible for its antihypertensive effect, because it is equipotent to NE as a vasopressor and as vasoconstrictor of peripheral arterioles and venules. It is now believed that α-methyl NE, rather acts in the brain to inhibit adrenergic neuronal outflow from the brain stem which is the principal mode of action for its antihypertensive effects. Since methyldopa reduces but does not abolish baroreceptor-mediated vasoconstriction, the frequency of postural hypotension is less.

Renin secretions are also reduced, but it is not a major determinant for its antihypertensive effects. Salt and water retention does occur, after prolonged use, which blunts its antihypertensive effect (pseudotolerance), but it can be overcome by concomitant use of a diuretic. Usual dose is 250 g TDS orally.

Some potential advantages of methyldopa include:

a) reduction in renal vascular resistance. Hence it is useful in hypertensive patients with renal insufficiency, and
b) reduction in ventricular hypertrophy. The drug is well tolerated by patients with diastolic dysfunctions in whom it reduces left ventricular mass.

However, potential side effects (mainly immunological and hepatotoxicity) are such that it is no longer a drug of choice in routine long-term management of hypertension except for hypertension during pregnancy as it is not only effective but safer too for both mother and the foetus.

Adverse Effects

Side effects, largely expected from its central mode of action, include: sedation (frequent but transient), dryness of mouth (inhibition of medullary centers that control saliva and partly due to nasal congestion which compels the patient to breathe through mouth), involuntary movements, gynaecomastia (in males) and galactorrhoea (in females) which occur due to interference with dopaminergic suppression of prolactin release. Reduction in libido is also secondary to sedation. Hepatotoxicity, at times associated with fever, though rare, is a serious toxic effect of methyldopa. Hepatic dysfunction, however, is reversible but it is advisable to avoid methyldopa in patients with hepatic disease. Methyldopa can cause haemolytic anaemia and development of positive Coombs test (due to auto-antibodies which are directed against the Rh locus on the patient's erythrocytes).

Guanfacine and Guanabenz: Their mode of action and adverse effects are similar to clonidine. These are rarely used because of no added advantage over clonidine.

Non-catecholamine β_1 Selective Agonists

There is hardly any drug in this group except for ***prenalterol*** which has been promoted for the reversal of β-blockade. The drug has more inotropic effect on heart with little chronotropic action. However, in synthetic catecholamine group, dobutamine which possesses selective β_1 agonist action, has already been discussed.

Non-catecholamine β_2 Selective Agonists

The drugs belonging to this group have preferential affinity for β_2 receptors compared to β_1 receptors. However, this selectivity is lost at higher concentration of these drugs. Structural modifications of these drugs have resulted either in lower rates of metabolism or enhanced oral bioavailability or both. Administration of these drugs by inhalation, in the form of aerosol, leads to an effective activation of β_2 receptors in bronchi. Consequently, there is less potential to activate cardiac β_1 receptors or to stimulate β_2 receptors in skeletal muscle which can cause palpitation and tremors when administered orally. The use of β_2 adrenergic agonists for the treatment of bronchial asthma is discussed, in detail, in Chapter 48.

Salbutamol (albuterol)

It is fairly selective β_2 agonist with relaxant effects on smooth muscles of bronchi and uterus. It has minimal cardiac stimulant effects and is safer than isoprenaline. Being a non-catecholamine it is not metabolised by COMT and thus exhibits longer duration of action than isoprenaline. For immediate relief of asthma it is given by oral inhalation from a metered dose inhaler (100 μg in single dose). It can also be given orally (2–4 mg TDS), intramuscularly or by slow I.V. injection. Sustained release tablets are also available. Inhalation causes fewer side effects than systemic administration. Salbutamol can also be used for the arrest of uncomplicated premature labour between 24 to 34 weeks of gestation by giving an intravenous infusion, but associated nausea and vomiting with risk of developing pulmonary oedema limits its use for this purpose. *Isoxsuprine* or *ritodrine* having more selective β_2 action on uterus is more preferred. Common side effects include tremors in hands, palpitations, headaches and hypokalaemia (after large dose).

Metaproterenol (orciprenaline)

It has lesser β_2 selective action than salbutamol and terbutaline but is resistant to methylation by COMT (like salbutamol). Uses and side effects are same as of salbutamol, but its use is declining (dose 10–20 mg TDS orally).

Terbutaline

Like salbutamol, it is also a β_2 selective bronchodilator. Being a resorcinol derivative, it is not metabolised by COMT and hence is longer acting. It is effective when administered orally, subcutaneously or by inhalation. It is used to relieve acute bronchospasm, as occurs in asthma, as a metered dose aerosol on an "as required, not regular, basis".

As with other β_2 agonists, tolerance may develop to terbutaline action if used regularly. With oral doses, onset of action is slow. It can also be used for the management of chronic obstructive pulmonary disease (COPD). Like salbutamol it may be used to arrest premature labour, but the side effects do not favour its use for this purpose. Other unlabelled use include treatment of unresponsive urticaria (to conventional antihistamines) where it is used along with ketotifen (e.g., in cold urticaria and idiopathic urticaria). Its inhaled powder formulations should be avoided as their pH is below 5.5, and thus may harm tooth enamel and cause tooth erosion. Its side effects are similar to salbutamol. Dose: 2.5–5 mg BD or TDS oral; 250 μg by inhalation as required.

Bambuterol

It is a prodrug of terbutaline which is slowly metabolised (longer acting, 24hr.). It has limited use only in chronic asthma. Dose 10-20 mg orally once a day in the evening.

Salmeterol and Formoterol

Salmeterol is a β_2-selective agonist with a prolonged duration of action (12 hrs) but with slower onset of action which makes it ineffective in acute attacks of asthma. It is rather preferred for the management of nocturnal asthma. Dose: 25 μg to 100 μg inhalation BD.

Formoterol is also a selective β_2-agonist with a longer duration of action (12 hrs) but has a quicker onset of action (within 5 min) and is therefore used to prevent the attacks of nocturnal asthma, prophylaxis of exercise-induced bronchospasm and COPD. Both these drugs have no anti-inflammatory action but can interact with inhaled glucocorticoids to improve asthma control. Dose 12–24 µg inhalation BD.

Pirbuterol

It has properties similar to salbutamol. Following inhalation, it exerts its effects within 10 min, which last for about 5 hrs.

Clenbuterol

It is selective β_2-agonist like salbutamol but is longer acting. It is known for its abuse by atheletes. β_2 agonists are known to increase the rate and the force of contraction of skeletal muscle to a varying extent. This is due to the long term changes produced by the continuous use of the drug in the expression of sarcoplasmic reticulum that control contraction-kinetics of skeletal muscle. Since, clenbuterol possesses robust sarcoplasmic anabolic properties, it is used illicitly by sportsmen to improve performance (doping agent).

Non-catecholamine β_3 Agonists

Mirabegron

It is an agonist at β_3 receptors located in the detrusor muscle of the urinary bladder. During the storage phase of the urinary bladder fill-void cycle, there is an enhanced sympathetic activity and the released NE by stimulating β_3 receptors in detrusor muscle increased the bladder capacity to accommodate more urine. Mirabegron, when administered orally in the doses of 50 and 100 mg mimics this effect of NE and is therefore approved for use in adults with overactive bladder suffering with urinary urge incontinence with or without urinary micturation frequency and nocturia.

In the high doses (≥200 mg dose), mirabegron may produce tachycardia and an increase in blood pressure due to activation of β_1 receptors. It should, therefore be used with caution in patients of uncontolled hypertention with or without angina. The drug is also not recommended in patients with end-stage renal disease or severe hapatic impairment.

The drug is transported and metabolised by multiple pathways, so there is a potential for drug interactions. It has been reported to increase the concentration of digoxin and to moderately inhibit the CYP 2D6 enzyme. The drug may increase the concentration of coadministered drugs metabolised by this enzymes (imipramine, metoprolol, tramadol).

Currently, there are limited comparative and long-term efficacy and safety data with this drug. It is only recommended when other uroselective antimuscarinic drugs are contraindicated, ineffective or not tolerated.

INDIRECTLY ACTING SYMPATHOMIMETICS

Their common characteristic features and the mode of action have already been described earlier. These agents do not have a direct stimulant action on postsynaptic adrenoceptors. These are taken up by neuronal membrane, and once inside the neuronal cytoplasm, these enter into the storages vesicle from where they displace NE from its store which in turn activates adrenoceptors (hence indirect action).

Repeated dosing of such drugs at short intervals leads to tachyphylaxis. These drugs cross BBB.

Tyramine

It is not used clinically. It is, rather, known for food-drug interactions which at times are alarming. Tyramine is found in cheese, beef, wine, beer, banana, yeast and yoghurt. Normally it gets metabolised by MAO present widespreadly in liver, GIT and other parts of body. But if the patient is taking MAO inhibitors (See Ch. 34) it can precipitate serious vasopressor episodes like hypertensive crisis, by releasing NE profusely from storage sites.

Amphetamine

It has a powerful CNS stimulant action in addition to peripheral α and β adrenoceptor effects (for details refer Ch. 35).

CNS Effects

d-isomer (dextroamphetamine) is 3 to 4 times more potent than l-isomer in exhibiting CNS stimulant effects which appear due to stimulation of cortical region and of reticular activating system. It stimulates the medullary respiratory cener, lessens the degree of CNS depression (by other drugs) and produces wakefulness, alertness and decreased sense of fatigue. The need for sleep may be postponed but cannot be avoided indefinitely. The performance of simple mental tasks is improved but is of no advantage because the number of errors increase due to overconfidence. Physical performance in athletes is improved and the drug is often abused for this purpose.

CVS Effects

The l-isomer is more potent than d-isomer in this regard. Amphetamine raises both systolic and diastolic BP and produces tachycardia followed by bradycardia. Arrhythmias may occur in large doses.

Effects on Smooth Muscles

Sphincter of urinary bladder constricts, hence difficulty in micturition occurs. It causes relaxation of gut and increases the tone of uterus, though effect varies.

Analgesia

Amphetamine has a mild analgesic effect which is not sufficiently pronounced to be therapeutically useful. However, amphetamine can enhance the analgesia produced by opiates.

Respiration

Higher dose of amphetamine may stimulate the respiratory centre, increasing the rate and depth of respiration.

Other Effects

Suppression of Appetite: Amphetamine suppresses appetite by depressing lateral hypothalamic feeding center. But tolerance to appetite suppression develops rapidly. Considering the side effects, the wisdom of its use as anorexiant is questionable.

Adverse Effets

1. Restlessness, tremors, hyperactive reflexes, irritability, insomnia, euphoria, hallucinations and sweating. Psychosis with high doses.
2. Palpitation, headache and cardiac arrhythmias.
3. Dry mouth, metallic taste, anorexia, abdominal cramps, and difficulty in micturition.
4. **Dependence and Tolerance**. Psychological dependence develops after prolonged use. Tolerance develops to its appetite suppressant effect but not for narcolepsy as patients of narcolepsy can be treated for years without any need to increase the dose. Withdrawal effects are opposite to its pharmacological effects and include fatigue, CNS depression, insomnia, and tremors.

Treatment of Toxicity. Amphetamine intoxication can be treated by acidification of urine with ammonium chloride or ascorbic acid. This increases its ionisation and prevents its reabsorption from renal tubule. Elimination is thus enhanced. Diazepam may be needed tocontrol CNS symptoms (see Ch. 38).

Therapetic Uses

1. **Narcolepsy**. Ampetamine in small dose improves narcolepsy and prevents attacks of daytime sleep. However, the drug should not be given after 4 p.m. as it will disturb the nocturnal sleep resulting in compulsions to have day time sleep.
2. **Attetion Deficit Hyperactivity Disorder (ADHD)**. This syndrome, in children, is characterised by impulsiveness, impaired interpersonal relationship, excitability and difficulty in sustaining attention resulting in loss in academic achievements. paradoxically, some children with this disorder respond well to low doses of amphetamine.
3. **Weight Reduction**. Available evidence does not support the use of amphetamine for this purpose.

Methamphetamine

It is closely related chemically to amphetamine. Low doses have predominantly central stimulant effects without significant peripheral actions. It has a high potential for abuse.

Methylphenidate

It is also an amphetamine analogue. Although a mild CNS stimulant, it has more prominent action on mental functions. Hence it is more effective than amphetamine in treating nacrcolepsy and attention deficit hyperactive disordes. Abuse potential is equal to amphetamine. In larger doses it produces convulsions. The use of methylphenidate is contraindicated in patients with glaucoma. Its dextro isomer dexmethylphenidate is better tolerated and more preferred to treat ADHD.

Pemoline

It is structurally similar to methylphenidate. It has prominent central stimulant effects with minimal effects on CVS. It has a longer plasma half-life. Hence it is used for the treatment of attention-deficit hyperactive disorder. Its polonged use is associated with dependence and hepatic damage.

Modafinil

Although not an amphetamine analogue, it blocks both NE and DA reuptake. It is used to treat narcolepsy. It does not produce insomnia, but improves wakefulness, and has no abuse potential.

SYMPATHOMIMETICS HAVING MIXED ACTION

Ephedrine

It is a noncatecholamine alkaloid obtained from *Ephedra vulgaris*. Its racemic form is used clinically. It has a direct agonist action on both α and β adrenoceptors. In addition, it enhances the relase of NE from sympathetic neuron. Epedrine is not destroyed by MAO and COMT and is therefore longer acting than E or NE. It crosses BBB and has a powerful stimulant action on CNS. The drug increases heart rate, cardiac output and blood pressure. Activation of β_2 receptors in the lungs promotes bronchodilation. Stimulation of α_1 receptor produces mydriasis with no cycloplegia. It nowadays has a very restricted use, e.g., to treat hypotension that may occur with spinal anaesthesia. It can be used orally for mild chronic asthma but the use has declined due to the availability of selective β_2 agonist. Untoward effects include hypertension (when administered parenterally), insomnia, and tachycardia. Repeated dosing, at short intervals, produces tachyphylaxis. ***Pseudoephedrine*** is a stereoisomer of ephedrine and is used as a nasal decongestant in several oral formulations. Since the drug has been illigally used to synthesize methamphetamine, the products containing pseudoephedrine have certain restrictions.

Mephentermine

Its pharmacological profile is similar to ephedrine but its use is restricted to maintain blood pressure in hypotensve states, for example, following spinal anaesthesia by giving slow I.V. injection. Adverse effects include CNS stimulation, hallucinations and convulsions (especially in overdosage). Dose: oral 10–20 mg/ BD; parenteral 15–60 mg I.V. infusion in 5% glucose.

ADRENOCEPTOR ANTAGONISTS

Adrenergic blocking drugs can be classified into two categories: ***adrenoceptor antagonists*** and ***adrenergic neuron blocking drugs***. ***Adrenergic receptor antagonists*** are devoid of intrinsic activity *per se* on adrenoceptors and instead exert effects by blocking the interaction of catecholamines or other sympathomimetics with adrenergic receptors. These are also called sympatholytics as they abolish (lyse) the respose to stimulation of sympathetic nerves but this term is lesser in use. As described earlier, adrenoceptors have been divided into three classes: Alpha (α), Beta (β) and Dopamine (D). Whereas drugs that block D-receptors peripherally are of lesser clinical significance (therefore not discussed here), those that block D-receptors centrally are important psychopharmacological agents and are discussed in Chapter 33. Similarly, ***adrenergic neuron blocking drugs***, that reduce the delivery of E and NE to the adrenergic receptors by disrupting catecholamine synthesis, storage or release are discussed in Chapter 13.

The α- and β-adrenoceptors have been classified into five subclasses: α_1, α_2, β_1, β_2, and β_3 . The pharmacology of these receptor agonists has already been described earlier. The pharmacology of non-selective and selective antagonists targeting these receptors is described below.

ALPHA-ADRENERGIC BLOCKERS

On the basis of their receptor selectivity and mode of their action, α-adrenoceptor antagonists may be classified as in Fig. 12.13.

Reversible Nonselective α–Adrenergic Blockers

Phentolamine and Tolazoline

These drugs are competitive antagonists at α-adrenergic receptors and have similar affinities for α_1 as well as α_2 receptors.

Cardiovascular Effects

Blockade of vasoconstrictor α_1 receptors in the periphery by phentolamine leads to vasodilatation, decrease in peripheral vascular resistance and in turn *hypotension*. The resultant fall in BP stimulates baroreceptor reflex causing sympathetic discharge. Since α_1 receptors are blocked, the sympathetic discharge stimulates β_1 receptors on the heart producing tachycardia. These drugs, being nonselective, also block presynaptic α_2 receptors which promote neuronal release of NE to produce more *tachycardia* and palpitation. The patients may also suffer from episodes of *postural hypotension*. In absence of efficient peripheral vasoconstriction in erect posture (due to a_1 blockade), there is a peripheral pooling of blood leading to *cerebral hypoxia*, vertigo and *fainting* which are characteristic features of *postural hypotension*. As discussed earlier, these drugs produce reversal of epinephrine vasopressor effect (Dale's vasomotor reversal phenomenon). Prior treatment with α_1-blocker prevents pressor response of epinephrine, hence the unopposed vasodilating β_2 effect is observed, i.e., the usual pressor response of epinephrine is reversed to vasodepressor response.

Other Effects

a) ***Nasal stuffiness*** results due to vasodilatation and congestion of nasal mucosa.
b) ***Miosis*** results due to loss of tone of radial muscles of iris and concomitant unopposed contraction of circular muscle.
c) ***Improved urine flow rates*** due to smooth muscle relaxation of bladder neck and prostate.
d) ***Failure of ejaculation and impotence*** due to inhibition of contractions of vas deferens and ejaculatory ducts.
e) ***Nausea, vomiting and diarrhoea*** due to partial inhibition of relaxant sympathetic influences on GIT, and increase in gastric secretions due to agonist action on H_2 receptors of histamine (mainly with tolazoline).

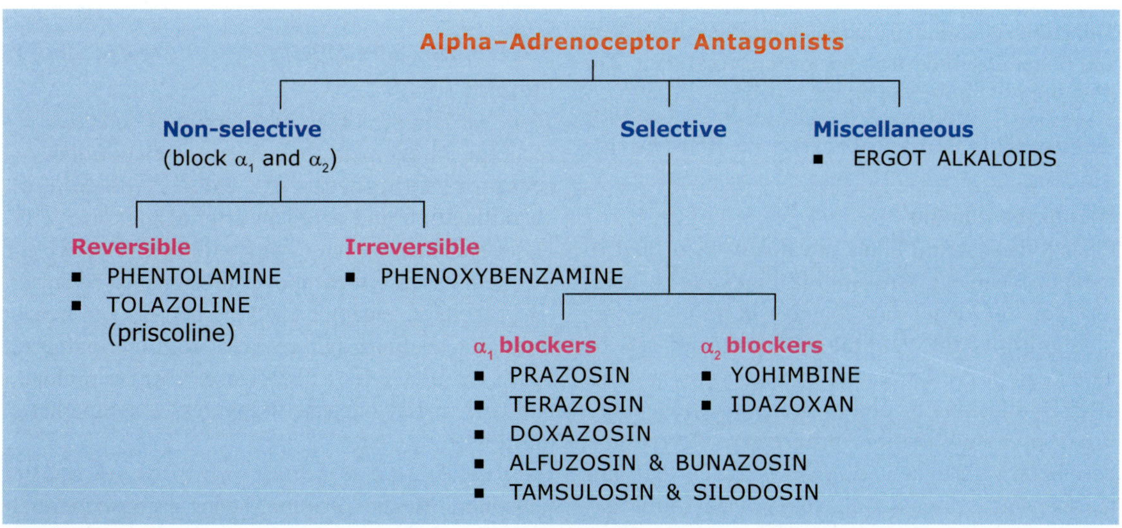

Fig 12.13 Classification of α-Adrenoceptor Antagonists

Therapeutic Uses

Phentolamine is poorly absorbed from GIT and is administered intravenously. It has an immediate onset but shorter duration of action.

a) **For the Diagnosis and Management of Phaeochromocytoma.** Phentolamine test can be performed to diagnose phaeochromocytoma-induced hypertension. However, its use is declining for such purpose. If after giving 5 mg of phentolamine (I.V.), the blood pressure falls by 25–35 mm of Hg, it is a potential case of phaeochromocytoma; and if less it is a case of essential hypertension. It is also used during operative manipulation of tumour to prevent hypertensive episodes.
b) **For Peripheral Vascular Disorders.** To counteract α-receptor mediated vasospastic component in the extremities as in Raynaud's syndrome and frostbite.
c) **To Prevent Dermal Necrosis.** Phentolamine can be used locally (S.C.) to prevent dermal necrosis after incidental extravasation of NE from I.V. infusion.
d) **To Treat Hypertensive Crisis** that follows abrupt withdrawal of clonidine or those resulting from interaction of ingested tyramine-containing food with MAO inhibitors.

Tolazoline is similar to phentolamine but is less potent and better absorbed from gastrointestinal tract. The drug is rarely used nowadays.

Irreversible Non-Selective α–Adrenergic Blockers

Phenoxybenzamine

Phenoxybenzamine binds covalently to α_1 and α_2 receptors causing irreversible blockade of these receptors for longer duration (20–48 hrs). The drug also inhibits the reuptake of released NE by adrenergic nerve terminals. The drug crosses BBB also. By blocking α_1 and α_2 receptors irreversibly, it causes vasodilatation, progressive decrease in peripheral resistance and *tachycardia* by the same mechanisms as discussed above. The tachycardia may be accentuated by blokdade of neuronal uptake of NE also. The drug exhibits Dale's vasomotor reversal phenomenon as discussed above. But the cardiovascular effects of an overdose of phenoxybenzamine cannot be reversed by catecholamines as the receptor binding is covalent and irrevesible and the effects cannot be surmounted by administering even increased amounts of agonist. This makes it a preferred drug for treating phaeochromocytoma. The drug causes *marked postural hypotension* with initial first few doses (first dose phenomenon) because of impairment of the compensatory vasoconstricting response in the periphery (as discussed above). Tolerance to this effect develops later. Other toxic effects include reversible inhibition of ejaculation, salt and water retention (can be corrected with diuretics), cardiac arrhythmias, sedation, fatigue and nausea.

Therapeutic Uses

a) **Treatment of Phaeochromocytoma.** The drug (1 mg/kg, slow I.V. infusion) controls episodes of severe hypertension during surgical manipulation of phaeochromocytoma. In cases of malignant phaeochromocytoma it can be given along with *metyrosine* (a competitive inhibitor of tyrosine hydroxylase – the rate limiting enzyme in the synthesis of NE & E).
b) To treat peripheral vascular disease like Raynaud's syndrome and frostbite (10 mg TDS orally).

Reversible, Selective α_1-AdrenergicBlockers

Prazosin

Prazosin is a prototype of a family of selective α_1 receptor antagonists (but does not distinguish α_1 receptor subtypes). It causes peripheral vasodilatation and a fall in arterial pressure with lesser tachycardia that occurs with non-selective α-blockers as described above, presumably because: (i) it lacks α_2 receptor blocking actions and hence does not promote NE release from sympathetic nerve terminals, (ii) it decreases cardiac preload, and (iii) partly because it suppresses sympathetic outflow from CNS.

It is also a potent inhibitor of cyclic phosphodiesterase enzyme, hence a consequential rise in cAMP in vascular smooth muscle could possibly contribute to its vasodilating effect.

Another favourable effect, of probable clinical significance, is an observed rise in the concentrations of high- density lipoproteins (HDL) and a decrease in low-density lipoproteins (LDL) and triglycerides. Being an α_1 selective antagonist it relaxes smooth muscle in the bladder neck, prostate capsule and prostatic urethra and hence improves urine flow in cases of benign prostatic hypertrophy.

Therapeutic Uses

The drug is well absorbed after oral administration. The plasma half-life is about 4 hrs.

1. **Treatment of Hypertension**. An interest has been focused for this use because α_1 adrenergic antagonists improve the lipid profile. However, the initial dose of prazosin should be 1 mg (orally) to be given at bed time to reduce the risk of postural hypotension that may follow after the first dose. The dose and the dose interval are then titrated upward depending on the blood pressure (see below).
2. **In the Treatment of Benign Prostatic Hyperplasia (BPH)**. Doses from 1 to 5 mg orally, twice daily can be used which is disadvantageous compared to newer α_1-receptor antagonists (see below).
3. **In the Patients of Raynaud's Disease**. Prazosin decreases the incidence of digital vasospasm but Ca^{2+} channel blockers are more preferred.

Adverse Effects

1. The major potential adverse effect of prazosin is marked *postural hypotension* (syncopal attack) at initial dose (first-dose phenomenon). For details, see above.
2. Impotence, nasal congestion, GIT upset and Na^+ and water retention are some common side effects of α_1 adrenergic blockers which are shared by prazosin also.

Terazosin and Doxazosin

Both of these drugs are α_1 adrenoceptor blockers like prazosin but with a longer duration of action. Both are well absorbed after oral administration. Plasma half-life of terazosin is 12 hrs, while that of doxazosin is 20 hrs which permit once daily dosage for the treatment of hypertension and benign prostatic hyperplasia (BPH). Terazosin (2–5 mg orally once daily) or doxazosin (1–4 mg orally, OD) has been found more effective than finasteride (a drug which inhibits conversion of testosterone to dihydrotestosterone) because of its faster action to improve urine flow. However, the combination works better in reducing the progress of disease because *finasteride* decreases prostate volume. Adverse effects are similar to prazosin.

Bunazosin and Alfuzosin

Both are orally effective α_1–adrenergic blockers and are similar to prazosin (subtype nonselective) in adverse effects and therapeutic uses. *Alfuzosin* (2.5 mg TDS orally or 10 mg slow release tab once daily) has a shorter plasma half-life (4 hrs) and hence needs twice or thrice daily dose requirement. It should be avoided in patients having hepatic impairment as it is primarily and extensively metabolised by liver. *Bunazosin* has slightly longer t½ but has no favourable profile than prazosin. Both are subtype nonselective. These drugs are primarily used in BPH.

Tamsulosin and Silodosin

These are selective α_{1A} receptor antagonists which are primarily located on bladder neck and urethra, rather than α_{1B} receptor subtype which are mainly located on blood vessels. ***Tamsulosin*** is more efficacious for the treatment of benign prostatic hypertrophy with little effect on blood pressure. Though plasma half-life is 8 hours, its sustained release capsules (0.2–0.4 mg) can be used for once daily dosing. This uroselective α_{1A} receptor blocker has a better oral bioavailability than prazosin. Abnormal ejaculation and intra-operative floppy iris syndrome (which creates problems during cataract operation) are the major side effects. It is usually given with *finasteride* or *dutasteride*. ***Silodosin*** is a weaker (4–8 mg/day, orally) but longer-acting analogue of tamsulosin.

Indoramin and Urapidil

Although indoramin has similar pharmacological actions as those of prazosin, it lacks any clinical usefulness due to its pharmacokinetic profile. It has lesser oral bioavailability (30%), undergoes extensive first-pass metabolism and has a shorter t½ (4 hrs). The role of urapidil in the treatment of hypertension is also not established because of its multiple effects. Besides being an α_1 antagonist (primary effect) it also has α_2-agonist, β_1-antagonist and 5HT-agonist action.

Alpha$_2$-Adrenergic Receptor Blockers

Yohimbine and Idazoxan

Yohimbine is a natural alkaloid from *Pausinystalia yohimbe.* Being lipid soluble, it crosses BBB. It also has 5HT antagonist action. It has no established clinical role. Theoretically it can be used to treat autonomic insufficiency by promoting NE release by blocking presynaptic α_2 receptor. Although efficacy is not clearly established yohimbine may be used to treat male sexual dysfunction and to treat diabetic neuropathy. It can also be used to treat postural hypotension. The drug can abruptly reverse the antihypertensive effects of an α_2 agonist like clonidine which seems to be an important drug interaction. Idazoxan is similar to yohimbine but also has a membrane stabilising action. However, its antidepressant activity is questionable though drug like mianserine, that has central α_2-receptor antagonist action, is used as an antidepressant.

Miscellaneous Non-Selective α-Adrenergic Blockers

Ergot Alkaloids

Ergot alkaloids (e.g., ergotamine and dihydroergotamine) exhibit a complex variety of pharmacological actions. Besides possessing competitive α-adrenoceptor blocking activity (both α_1 and α_2), these agents also act as partial agonist at α-receptors and at $5HT_2$ receptors. Some of these are oxytocics or dopamine receptor agonists. These have been discussed in detail in Chapters 24 and 41.

BETA-ADRENERGIC BLOCKERS

Beta-adrenergic receptor antagonists act on β_1 or β_2 receptor or on both of them and antagonise the effect of catecholamines which are mediated through these receptors. In addition, some of these drugs also possess membrane stabilising action (local anaesthetic action) and/or intrinsic sympathomimetic activity of their own on β_1 or β_2 receptors. Depending on their selectivity for β_1 or β_2 receptors, these can be classified as in Fig. 12.14.

Non-Selective (β_1+β_2) Blockers

Propranolol

It is a prototype non-selective β-antagonist, with all the actions, uses, adverse effects and contraindications characteristic of this class of drugs, except that it is not used to treat glaucoma (though it decreases intraocular pressure to some extent).

Though it is primarily used to treat hypertension and ischaemic heart disease, it has been reported to be of value in more than 8 non-cardiovascular disorders. It may also be noted that β-blockers have little effect on normal resting heart, but exhibit profound action when the sympathetic drive to the heart is high as during physical exercise or stress.

Cardiovascular Effects

The blockade of cardiac β_1 receptors results in decrease in heart rate, myocardial contractility, conduction velocity and cardiac output. Because of the decrease in the workload by heart, the myocardial O_2 demand is also reduced. The automaticity of the heart is also suppressed because of the inhibition of latent pacemakers (due to β_1-blockade). Consequent to this, the blood pressure falls. The total peripheral vascular resistance tends to rise initially because the vasoconstricting α_1 adrenoceptor response is no longer opposed by β_2-adrenoceptor (dilator) effects (since non-selective blockers also block β_2-receptors). Further, as reflex vasoconstriction is preserved (α_1 receptors are unhurt), postural hypotension is least troublesome as is seen with α-adrenoceptor blocking group of antihypertensive agents. Patients with hypertension (though not normotensive subjects) show a gradual fall in BP after chronic use of propranolol. Though cardiac β_1-receptor blockade is the main mechanism of its antihypertensive action, other mechanisms, of no lesser importance, that contribute to this effect are:

a) Decrease in renin release which reduces production of angiotensin II and aldosterone from adrenal cortex (β_1 mediated effect). However,

Beta-Adrenoceptor Antagonists

Non-selective ($\beta_1 + \beta_2$) blockers

- PROPRANOLOL*
- TIMOLOL
- SOTALOL
- NADOLOL
- PINDOLOL**
- OXPRENOLOL**

Selective β-blockers

Selective β_1-blockers

- METOPROLOL*
- ATENOLOL
- ESMOLOL
- ACEBUTOLOL**
- CELIPROLOL**
- BETAXOLOL
- BISOPROLOL
- NEBIVOLOL

Selective β_2-blockers

- BUTOXAMINE
- ICI 118551

Mixed (α and β) blockers

- LABETALOL*
- CARVEDILOL

* Drugs having membrane stabilising activity also.

** Drugs having membrane stabilising as well as intrinsic sympathomimetic action (β_1 agonist action).

Celiprolol has rather β_2 agonist action (besides β_1 antagonist action).

Both Celiprolol and Nebivolol induce endothelial release of nitric oxide and hence have direct vasodilating effect also.

Fig 12.14 Beta-Adrenoceptor Antagonists

pindolol which does not decrease renin release, is an effective antihypertensive.

b) Decrease in central sympathetic outflow. However, atenolol and sotalol have a poor brain penetrability, yet are effective antihypertensives.
c) Chronic decrease in cardiac output.
d) Blockade of the facilitatory effect of presynaptic β_2-receptors on NE release.

Cardiovascular effects of propranolol can be overcome by isoprenaline (β-agonist) which indicates that it is a competitive blocker at β_1-receptor. However, it cannot counteract cardiac stimulant action (myocardial contractility) of digoxin, Ca^{2+}, theophylline and glucagon which points to its selective action on β-receptors only.

Plasma lipid profile is worsened after long-term use of propranolol: total triglycerides and LDL-cholesterol tend to increase while HDL-cholesterol levels fall. Propranolol does possess the membrane stabilising (local anaesthetic type) and direct cardiac depressant (quinidine like) actions but this contributes little to its antiarrhythmic effects in usual doses.

Respiratory Effects

Airways resistance is least affected by β-blockers in normal subjects because their sympathetic bronchodilator tone is less. However, in asthmatic subjects, a non-selective β-blocker like propranolol, can cause severe bronchoconstriction. This danger is less with β_1-selective antagonists.

Metabolic Effects

In normal persons, propranolol has minimal effects on basal blood glucose levels. But it inhibits stress-induced or adrenaline-induced glycogenolysis, which acts as a safety device during episodes of hypoglycaemia (especially in insulin induced hypoglycaemia in diabetic patients). The drug also blocks adrenergically induced lipolysis and has an adverse effect on lipid profile (see above). It also masks the sympathetic manifestations (palpitation, tremors, sweating etc) of hypoglycaemia.

CNS Effects

Besides decreasing central sympathetic outflow (which contributes to its antihypertensive effects), it also produces sedation, lethargy and disturbances in sleep, after long-term use. Propranolol suppresses performance anxiety (e.g., anxiety prior to an interview) but this is due to peripheral rather than central action. In high doses it has antipsychotic effects but cardiac side effects limit its use.

Ocular Effects

Propranolol decreases formation of aqueous humour and thus reduces intraocular pressure especially in glaucomatous patients. Yet propranolol is seldom used for such purpose, firstly because it is less potent and secondly because its local anaesthetic action on cornea is highly undersirable (see under timolol).

Miscellaneous Effects

a) Propranolol increases synthesis and release of prostaglandins in selected vascular beds, as the hypotensive effect of the drug can be counteracted by aspirin group of analgesics.
b) It prevents platelet aggregation and promotes fibrinolysis to certain extent (see its use in myocardial infarction).
c) It reduces portal vein pressure in patients with cirrhosis (see its use under bleeding from esophageal varices).

Pharmacokinetics

It is completely absorbed orally but has low bioavailability as it is extensively metabolised by liver (undergoes first-pass metabolism). It is highly lipid soluble and crosses BBB. Its plasma half-life is short (t½ 4–6 hrs). It exists in two isomeric forms. l-Propranolol is 80–100 times more potent than d-propranolol in blocking β–adrenoceptor. Contrarily, d-form exhibits more quinidine like and membrane stabilising effects compared to l-form. Commercial preparations are racemic. Longer acting, sustained release preparations are available.

Therapeutic Uses

I. *Cardiovascular Uses*

(Remember : 2H-Hypertension, Heart failure; 2A-Angina, Arrhythmias; and MI-Myocardial Infarction, i.e., 2H-2A-MI).

1. **Essential Hypertension**: The drug is used alone or can be combined with either a diuretic or a α-adrenergic blocking drug. The fall in blood pressure, when used alone, is gradual and without postural hypotension. Dose 20–40 mg TDS orally or 80 mg sustained release tab. once a day.
2. **Congestive Heart Failure**: Although β-blockers can worsen the heart failure, nonetheless, it is now established that these may be beneficial in patients with mild to moderate heart failure (see Ch. 22). Introduced gradually with slow advancing doses over time and maintained for long term, these drugs retard the progression of CHF and prolong life. The benefit results from antagonism of damaging effects of cardiac β_1 receptor overactivity which promotes unfavourable remodeling of the myocardium (hence carvedilol or metoprolol are preferred).
3. **Angina Pectoris**: As it decreases workload on the heart, diminishes myocardial O_2 demand and increases exercise tolerance; hence β-blockers benefit patients having angina of effort. The drug should be given continuously and not merely when attack occurs. A judicious combination of propranolol with isosorbide dinitrate or mononitrate is able to prevent attacks of angina in nearly 85% of the patients. In Prinzmetal's angina where there is coronary spasm due to increased sympathetic activity without any fixed stenosis, β-blockers are contraindicated because blockade of β-receptors will unmask the α-receptor actions leading to more coronary spasm (see Ch.20). Dose: as above for hypertension.
4. **Cardiac Arrhythmias**: Propranolol is effective in all supraventricular tachycardias associated with high levels of circulating catecholamines as occurs with the use of certain general anaesthetics like halothane, in digitalis toxicity, phaeochromocytoma and thyrotoxicosis. The ventricular

ectopic beats associated with such conditions are also controlled. The beneficial effect is mainly due to an increase in refractory period of AV node and direct membrane stabilising action. β-blockade also reduces drive to cardiac pacemakers (see Ch. 21). Dose 40–80 mg BD orally.

5. **Myocardial Infarction**: β-blockers signi-ficantly decrease the incidence, recurrence and mortality in cases of MI after long-term use. Beneficial effects of propranolol, in addition to β-blockade, may also result due to prevention of platelet aggregation and promotion of fibrinolysis. β-blockers also prevent sudden ventricular fibrillation at the second attack of MI (dose 40-80 mg TDS orally). The choice of a drug is a pure β_1-antagonist without intrinsic sympathomimetic activity like atenolol or carvedilol.

II. ***Other Uses (Non-cardiovascular Use)***
(Remember : MAGH–Migraine, Anxiety, Glaucoma, Hyperthyroidism. PAw–Phaeochromocytoma, Alcohol withdrawal and EVB–Esophageal Variceal Bleeding, i.e., MAGH-PAw-EVB).

a) ***Migraine:*** Propranolol is effective for the prophylaxis of migraine (not for acute attack), the mechanism of which is uncertain. 20 mg TDS orally.

b) ***Anxiety Provoking Situations:*** Propranolol is used to reduce anxiety under conditions which provoke nervousness and panic, e.g., examination, interview etc. It blocks peripheral manifestations of anxiety (e.g., palpitation, tremors and sweating) which further aggravate anxiety. Propranolol is also used to treat essential tremors but provides no benefit in parkinsonian tremors. Dose 10–20 mg BD or TDS orally.

c) ***Glaucoma:*** β-blockers decrease intraocular pressure. Propranolol, however, is not used (see above). Other β-blockers like *timolol* and *betaxolol* are used topically for management of glaucoma (see Ch. 11, Table 11.2).

d) ***Hyperthyroidism:*** β-blockade reduces unpleasant symptoms of sympathetic overactivity (tachycardia, irregular cardiac rhythm, tremors, sweating and raised BMR). A nonselective agent (propranolol) is preferred to counteract both the cardiovascular (β_1 and β_2) effects and tremors (β_2). It may also inhibit the peripheral conversion of thyroxine to triiodothyronine (independent of β–receptor blockade). Dose 20 mg BD orally.

e) ***Phaechromocytoma:*** Propranolol may be given in combination with proper α-adrenoceptor blocker during removal of the tumour, to antagonise β_1 agonist effects of circulating catecholamines released from the tumour. Dose 20 mg TDS for 3 days before surgery.

f) ***Alcohol Withdrawal:*** It also produces beneficial effects in the treatment of patients undergoing alcohol withdrawal by reducing central sympathetic overactivity during the phase of withdrawal. Dose 20 mg BD or TDS orally.

g) ***Oesophageal Variceal Bleeding and Hepatic Portal Hypertension:*** Non-selective β-blockers like propranolol and nadolol reduce cardiac output (β_1 blockade) and induce splanchnic vasoconstriction (β_2-blockade allowing unopposed α-receptor mediated vasoconstriction). This reduces bleeding from esophageal varices. Portal pressure is also reduced by 40%. Dose 10–20 mg BD orally.

Adverse Effects and Contraindications

(Remember: 2B–Bronchoconstriction, Bradycardia; 2C–Cold extremities, CNS side effects; 2H–Heart failure, Hypoglycaemia; RH–Rebound Hypertension and ALP–Adverse Lipid Profile, i.e., 2B-2C-2H- RH & ALP).

1. **Bronchoconstriction**. This is of little significance in normal persons but in asthmatics, or in patients with bronchitis or emphysema this effect could be life-threatening *(contraindicated in bronchial asthma or in chronic obstructive lung disease)*.
2. **Bradycardia**. Lowering of HR to 55 beats/min, as it occurs with β-blockers at times, can lead to life-threatening bradyarrhythmias and heart block.
3. **Cold Extremities**. This results from a loss of β_2-receptor mediated cutaneous vasodilatation in the extremities (*contraindicated in Raynaud's disease*).

4. **CNS Side Effects**. Fatigue (due to reduced cardiac output and poor muscle perfusion), sleep disturbances, bad dreams and depression. Male patients may complain of sexual dysfunction.
5. **Heart Failure**. Cardiac patients always need a degree of sympathetic drive to support the heart to maintain proper cardiac output. β-blockers block this support and may aggravate heart failure (however, see above for their paradoxical use in CHF). AV nodal depression can lead to AV dissociation and may precipitate heart block (*contraindicated in heart failure*).
6. **Hypoglycaemia**. The sympathetic response to hypoglycaemia (release of glucose through glycogenolysis) is a safety device that warns the patients of diabetes to eat sugar, by producing symptoms like tachycardia, cold sweating and tremors. β-blockers mask these symptoms and delay recovery from hypoglycaemia. Hence, incipient hypoglycaemia may go unnoticed by the patient who may suffer from hypoglycaemic coma (*contraindicated in patients receiving insulin and oral hypoglycaemic drugs*).
7. **Rebound Hypertension and Anginal Attacks After Sudden Withdrawal**. After chronic therapy with β-blockers there is up-regulation in the number of β-receptors as a compensatory natural phenomenon. These newly formed β-receptors show hyper-responsiveness to even smaller release of catecholamines. Hence, there should be a gradual tapering of the doses instead of abrupt withdrawal.
8. **Adverse serum lipid profile**: (as discussed above).

Drug Interactions

1. ***Due to Pharmacokinetic Reasons***
   a) Al^{3+} salts, cholestyramine and colestipol decrease the absorption of β-blockers.
   b) Enzyme inducers (e.g., phenytoin, rifampin, smoking) decrease its plasma concentration.
   c) Cimetidine and hydralazine may increase its bioavailability.
   d) β-blockers impair the clearance of lignocaine and thus may increase its bioavailability.
2. ***Due to Pharmacodynamic Reasons***
   a) Digitalis and verapamil cause additive depression of SA node and AV conduction and can lead to cardiac arrest.
   b) Indomethacin and aspirin (other NSAIDs) can oppose the antihypertensive effects of β-blockers.
   c) Hypertensive patients treated with propranolol (a nonselective $\beta_1 + \beta_2$ blocker) are very sensitive to the pressor responses of adrenaline (present in local anaesthetic formulations), because simultaneous blockade of vasodilatory β_2 receptors (along with β_1) leads to unopposed vasoconstricting action of adrenaline on α_1 receptors.

Timolol (see Ch. 11, Table 11.3)

Orally absorbed, moderate first-pass metabolism, crosses BBB. Uses and side effects similar to propranolol.

Main Use: as eye drops to decrease raised intraocular pressure in cases of wide angle glaucoma, as it is devoid of membrane stabilising activity (see propranolol). It may be absorbed systemically from the ocular formulations to exhibit side effects.

Sotalol

It has low lipid solubility (lesser CNS effects), and negligible first-pass metabolism. Uses and side effects similar to propranolol. It has an additional K^+ channel blocking and class III antiarrhythmic property independent of β-blocking activity. Dose 80–320 mg BD orally.

Nadolol

Longer plasma half-life (20 hrs, administered 40 mg orally, once daily), does not cross BBB, least first-pass metabolism. Uses and side effects same as that of propranolol.

Non-selective β-Blockers With Intrinsic Sympathomimetic Activity

Pindolol and Oxprenolol

Although non-selective β-blockers, like propranolol, they possess inherent intrinsic sympathomimetic action also on β_1 and β_2 receptors. Daily doses for *pindolol* are 10 mg orally once daily and for *oxprenolol* are 20 mg orally twice or thrice a day (or 40 mg/day slow release preparation later as maintenance).

Though controversial, the benefits of this property are:

a) Lesser bradycardia and myocardial depression, hence may be useful in patients prone to bradycardia or those with low cardiac reserve as in CHF. These are less troublesome to asthmatics also, because of β_2-agonist action.
b) Rebound hypertension after withdrawal is less likely as β-agonist action of the drug itself prevents supersensitivity of up-regulated β-receptors.
c) Lipid profile is less worsened, compared to propranolol.

Disadvantages of intrinsic sympathomimetic activity are:

1. These drugs cannot be used in migraine prophylaxis as intrinsic β_2-agonist activity dilates cerebral blood vessels.
2. Less suitable for secondary proplylaxis of MI (see above for reasons).

Selective β_1 Blockers (cardioselective β-blockers)

Metoprolol, Atenolol, Bisoprolol, Nebivolol, Esmolol and Betaxolol

These drugs mainly block β_1 receptors in low and therapeutic doses but can block β_2 receptors also in high doses. Hence, though cardioselective, their selectivity is only relative to propranolol.

The advantages over non-selective blockers are:

a) These are safer in asthmatics, compared to propranolol, but they are not absolutely safe.
b) These are safer in diabetes as they cause less inhibition of glycogenolysis during hypoglycaemia (glucose release from liver is controlled by β_2 receptors). However, tachycardia in response to hypoglycaemia is blocked (β_1 blockade).
c) These are safer in patients with peripheral vascular disease (no β_2-blockade).
d) These have less deleterious effects on lipid profile.

Disadvantages of cardioselective blockers are:

a) Rebound hypertension after abrupt withdrawal of the drug, still remains a problem.
b) These are ineffective in controlling essential tremors (no β_2 blockade).

Metoprolol is completely absorbed after oral administration but bioavailability is less due to first-pass metabolism. Plasma half-life is 4 hrs. Extended release formulations are available for once daily administration. For treating hypertension the usual dose is 50-100 mg daily. Uses are similar to propranolol.

Atenolol does not cross BBB and has longer t½ compared to metoprolol and can be given once daily (25–50 mg once daily). Uses are similar to metoprolol.

Bisoprolol, like metoprolol, when used with ACE inhibitors, lowers overall mortality in chronic heart failure cases. It is commonly used for hypertension and angina (2.5–10 mg once daily orally). ***Nebivolol*** is a new highly selective β_1 blocker in the list. It also enhances NO production and release besides blocking β_1 adrenoceptors. It specifically lowers arterial blood pressure and reduces peripheral vascular resistance and is used for effective management of hypertension. Usual oral dose is 5–10 mg orally, once daily. ***Esmolol*** is an ultrashort-acting β_1 antagonist. It has plasma half-life of 8 to 10 min. Esmolol is given intravenously in urgent settings where β_1 blockade of short duration is desired, e.g., to terminate suprventricular tachycardia, episodes of atrial fibrillation, to control HR and BP during surgery or in critically ill patients in whom the drug can be withdrawn immediately if adverse effects like bradycardia, hypotension or heart failure appear. ***Betaxolol*** is available as eye drops for glaucoma (Ch.12, Table 12.3). Being selective β_1- blocker, it is less efficacious than timolol because 80% of β-receptors on ciliary body epithelium are β_2 subtype. However, it is better tolerated, has no membrane stabilising (local anaesthetic) effect, has cytoprotective action on retinal neurons, safer in asthmatic and diabetic patients and also facilitates drainage of aqueous humour by some unknown mechanism. Oral formulations are used for hypertension and angina.

Selective β_1-Blockers with Intrinsic Sympathomimetic Action

Acebutolol and Celiprolol

These offer combined advantages of pindolol group and atenolol group. They also have membrane stabilising action (of no clinical usefulness as this appears to be significant at high doses only). ***Acebutolol*** is well absorbed, but during first-pass metabolism in liver it gets converted into an active metabolite, *diacetolol,* which has a longer t½, (10–12 hrs). Hence it may be given as a single oral dose (400 mg/day). Also for treating ventricular arrhythmias. ***Celiprolol*** is well absorbed (bioavailability 75%). It has partial agonist action at β_2 receptors also. Besides, it also causes some direct vasodilatation by releasing nitric oxide. It is preferred for hypertensive patients having asthma. Dose 200–400 mg orally once daily.

Selective β_2-Antagonists

Butoxamine and ICI-118551

These drugs are used only as experimental tools in drug research and have no clinical utility.

Mixed (α+β) Antagonists

Labetalol and Carvedilol

Labetalol acts as a competitive antagonist at both α_1- and β-adrenergic receptors. It exhibits optical isomerism and has four diastereomers, each of which displays different relative pharmacological activity. The racemic mixture exhibits (a) selective blockade of α_1-adrenergic receptor, (b) blockade of β_1-receptor and (c) partial agonist activity (ISA) at β_2 receptor. The α_1 and β_1-blocking actions of labetalol contribute to the fall in BP. The intrinsic sympathomimetic activity (ISA) at β_2 receptors may contribute to peripheral vasodilatation and bronchodilatation (to a minor extent). Heart rate remains unaffected. It is orally effective, but undergoes first-pass metabolism, hence bioavailability is less (30%). Plasma half-life is also less (4–5 hrs). Main use is in hypertension in elderly patients where increased peripheral resistance is not desired.Usual dose is 100 mg orally a day; increased to 200 mg BD after 7–10 days. It is particularly useful in phaeochromocytoma and for controlling rebound hypertension after clonidine withdrawal. Postural hypotension and hepatotoxicity are the main side effects.

Carvedilol is also orally effective, undergoes significant first-pass metabolism (bioavailability 30%, t ½ 6–8 hrs). It is a β_1, β_2 and α_1 adrenoceptor blocker, but its β_1 and β_2 blocking effects are more prominent than α_1 blocking effects. Further, it also inhibits free radical induced lipid peroxidation and also inhibits vascular smooth muscle mitogenesis (independent of α or β adrenoceptor blockade). It also blocks L-type voltage-gated Ca^{2+} channels. These effects may prove to be cardioprotective in patients of CHF. The drug is used to treat essential hypertension also. Combined with conventional therapy, carvedilol reduces mortality in myocardial infarction. Adjustment in dosage is not necessary in renal patients as it is metabolised by liver. For hypertension/angina, usual dose is 6.25 mg orally twice a day and increased to 12.5 mg BD if needed (see Ch. 19 also).

Bucindolol and ***medroxalol*** are some $\beta_1 + \beta_2 + \alpha_1$ blockers but their superiority over carvedilol is doubtful.

CHAPTER 13 Ganglionic Stimulants, Blockers and Adrenergic Neuron Blocking Drugs

COMPETENCY PH1.13

Till now, we have discussed about the cholinomimetic drugs which activate muscarinic receptors, and anticholinergic drugs which antagonise the effects of ACh and cholinomimetic drugs at muscarinic receptors located on tissues innervated by cholinergic nerves. ACh is also released from preganglionic fibres to activate nicotinic receptors (N_N) present on sympathetic and parasympathetic ganglia and on adrenal medulla. There is no drug which can selectively activate or block the N_N receptors present on either the sympathetic or the parasympathetic ganglia.

The selective agonist at the nicotinic receptors (N_N) present at the autonomic ganglia are *dimethyl phenyl piperazinium* (DMPP) and *epibatidine* (obtained from the skin of South American frog); while the selective antagonists are *hexamethonium* and *trimethaphan*. *Nicotine* is, however, an agonist in small doses but antagonist in high doses.

Agonists act on the postsynaptic N_N receptors present on autonomic ganglia causing depolarisation and propagation of the EPSP down the postganglionic sympathetic or parasympathetic neuron to release NE or ACh respectively. Since they affect both the sympathetic as well as parasympathetic ganglia, their actions are nonselective. The net ultimate effect, therefore, would be a magnification of the dominant autonomic tone in that particular organ. For example, in GIT the predominant tone is parasympathetic, hence the agonist action would be the magnification of parasympathetic activity, like increase in GIT motility and tone etc.

Besides N_N receptors, there are also M_1 receptors at autonomic ganglia. These receptors play an important role in the modulation of EPSP generated by ganglionic stimulants (agonists). McNA-343 and *methacholine* are the agonists at M_1 receptors present at autonomic ganglia and their effects can be blocked by atropine-like drugs.

GANGLIONIC STIMULANTS

Nicotine (small doses), lobeline, dimethylphenyl piperazinium (DMPP) and tetramethyl ammonium (TMA).

Nicotine

It is water-soluble, colourless, volatile, highly toxic liquid obtained from the leaves of the tobacco plant *(Nicotina tobacum)*. Being an alkaloid, it is a highly basic substance. Although it has no therapeutic use, it will be discussed here in short, primarily because of its wide abuse in the society in the form of tobacco smoking and chewing. Although each cigarette contains about 20 mg of nicotine, the amount of nicotine absorbed from an average cigarette is about 1.5 mg. The rest of the amount simply gets burnt as side stream smoke and is also withheld in the filter of the cigarette. About 1.5 mg which is absorbed, provides the plasma nicotine levels to an extent of 130 to 200 nmol/lit. These values depend greatly on the type of the cigarette and on the extent of inhalation by the smoker. The fatal dose of nicotine is 40 mg.

The pharmacological actions of nicotine are dose dependent and in general are due to:

a) Initial stimulation of sympathetic or parasympathetic ganglia as well as of adrenal medulla (in low doses) followed by their paralysis due to persistent depolarisation (in high doses).
b) Stimulation of CNS (low doses) followed by its depression (high doses).
c) Depolarisation of neuromuscular junction (low doses) followed by its paralysis (high doses).

Other pharmacological effects of nicotine are:

a) Smoking causes enzymatic induction and thus increases the metabolism of many drugs like propranolol, benzodiazepines, tricyclic antidepressants, theophylline, nifedipine and heparin.
b) Smoking increases platelet aggregation, concentration of free fatty acids, LDL and VLDL in blood.
c) Except for increased bowel activity and tachycardia, tolerance develops to all effects of nicotine (particularly to CNS effects).

Adverse Effects

a) Besides nicotine, the cigarette smoke also contains irritant elements like pyridine, HCN, CO, CO_2, furfural and nitrosamine. Hence, cigarette smokers have increased incidence of oral, laryngeal, oesophageal and lung cancer.
b) Smokers have a higher incidence of hypertension, coronary artery disease and thromboangiitis obliterans.
c) Smokers suffer from chronic bronchitis and smoker's cough syndrome.
d) Smokers suffer from tobacco amblyopia, i.e., decrease in visual activity in central field.
e) Lady smokers suffer from a variety of reproductive disorders like pre-eclampsia, abortion, low birth weight of neonates, and fewer pregnancies.
f) Nicotine produces psychic dependence and withdrawal symptoms, which are characterised by headache, insomnia, anxiety, restlessness and constipation. ***Clonidine*** is a very effective drug for reducing withdrawal effects of nicotine and is considered superior to the buffered nicotine chewing gum, which is not suitable for nicotine dependent persons having cardiac ailments. Clonidine reduces craving for smoking and also antagonises insomnia (Ch.12 & 38). ***Nicotine transdermal patches*** are also available as an aid to smoking cessation, but with limited success, as they do not suppress carving for smoking. Moreover these are not suitable for cardiac cases. ***Bupropion*** (150–300 mg BD orally) is another atypical antidepressant drug that is used clinically for smoking cessation (Ch. 34 & 38). ***Varenicline*** is another very effective synthetic drug for cessation of smoking. It has a partial agonist-antagonist action on presynaptic N_N receptors located on dopaminergic neurons present in ventral tegmental area (VTA) covering nucleus accumbens, prefrontal cortex, amygdala and hippocampus. Activation of this mesolimbic-dopamine system (by nicotine) causes release of dopamine (DA) which promotes reinforcement and reward process leading to craving. The antagonist action of varenicline on these N_N receptors (present presynaptically on dopaminergic neurons) persists because of its longer half-life and therefore decreases the release of DA, with resultant lack in craving for smoking (N_N receptors are ion-channel coupled receptors. Activation of these receptors, whether present post-synaptic or presynaptic on cholinergic or any other neuron promotes, while blockade decreases the release of the concerned neurotransmitter from that neuron; see Ch. 10, heterotropic presynaptic innervation in relation to nicotinic receptors). Its usual dose is: Initially 0.5 mg once daily, then 1 mg BD from day 8 for 6 months. *Side effects* include nausea, headache, insomnia and depression (suicidal tendencies) which may limit its use in future.

Lobeline

It is also an alkaloid obtained from Indian tobacco, Lobelia. Its actions are similar to nicotine, but it is less potent. It has no therapeutic use.

Tetramethyl Ammonium (TMA)

It is a synthetic quaternary compound. Since it does not cross blood-brain barrier, it has least central effects. It is a specific ganglion stimulant (N_N receptors) and has negligible effect on myoneural junction (N_M receptors). It is used only as a pharmacological tool.

Dimethylphenyl Piperazinium (DMPP)

It is also a quaternary compound and is relatively specific ganglion stimulant like TMA but is more potent. Initial stimulant action of DMPP (and also of TMA) on ganglia is not followed by a blocking action (as observed with nicotine).

GANGLION BLOCKING DRUGS

Antagonists at N_N receptors, on the other hand, compete with ACh for the receptor site on the autonomic ganglia and thereby block the transmission of impulse from the preganglionic to the postganglionic neuron. Since they block both the sympathetic as well as the parasympathetic ganglia, release of NE as well as ACh is decreased at the effector organ from the postganglionic neuron. *Yet, the overall effect of ganglionic blockade would be like elimination of the dominant autonomic tone of the organ which is referred to. In short, the visible effects would now be characteristic of the less dominant tone (as the predominant tone has already been hurt).*

The drugs in this category include:

A) **Persistent Depolarising Blockers**
   Nicotine (high doses), anticholinesterases (high doses) and carbechol (high doses)
   These drugs are of no therapeutic utility. Their actions are non-specific as they depolarise (paralysis) the ganglia as well as the motor end plate.

B) **Non-Depolarising Blockers (Competitive Blockers)**
   i) *Quaternary ammonium compounds*:
      Tetraethyl ammonium (TEA), hexamethonium and pentolinium.
   ii) *Secondary or tertiary amines*:
      Mecamylamine, pempidine
   iii) *Monosulfonium derivatives*:
      Timethaphan

Among ganglion blocking drugs, only trimethaphan has some therapeutic usefulness. Rest all have no clinical relevance.

Trimethaphan

Trimethaphan is an ultrashort-acting ganglionic blocker. It is orally ineffective and hence given by slow I.V. infusion. It does not cross blood-brain barrier significantly. The relative autonomic tone and the effects of ganglionic blockade (by trimethaphan) on different organ systems are summarised in Table 13.1.

Therapeutic Uses

Since trimethaphan can stimulate the release of histamine, it should be used with CAUTION in patients having bronchial asthma and in those having history of allergy. Although therapeutic use of ganglionic blockers has declined, trimethaphan is still being used for the following purposes:

a) To control hypertension in patients with acute dissecting aortic aneurysm. Increased efficacy is obtained if the bed is tilted so that the legs are below the level of the heart.
b) Trimethaphan, as a slow I.V. infusion, may be used as an alternative to or in combination with sodium nitroprusside for the treatment of hypertensive emergencies and to produce controlled hypotension, to minimise blood loss during neurosurgery or in orthopaedic surgery or to facilitate surgery on blood vessels. Trimethaphan blunts the sympatho-adrenal stimulation caused by nitroprusside and reduces the required dosage.
c) Trimethaphan can be used in the management of autonomic hyper-reflexia. This results due to injuries in the upper spinal cord which leads to massive sympathetic discharge. The spinal reflexes get dominant because central inhibition of reflexes is lacking in such patients. Trimethaphan, being ganglionic blocker, successfully controls hyper-reflexia.
d) Trimethaphan can also be used for the emergency treatment of acute pulmonary oedema. For adverse effects of trimethaphan, refer Table 13.1 and its footnote. Trimethaphan preparation is not available in India.

ADRENERGIC NEURON BLOCKING DRUGS

These drugs markedly suppress the activity of adrenergic neuron by affecting the storage and release of NE but do not affect the normal functioning of α or β receptors. Hence, they do not affect (or may even potentiate) the response of exogenously administered directly acting sympathomimetics. On the contrary, the pharmacological effects of adrenergic neuron blocking drugs are antagonised by indirectly acting sympathomimetics (e.g., tyramine, ephedrine or amphetamine) and also by drugs like tricyclic antidepressants and cocaine which compete with them for their neuronal uptake (uptake-1).

Table 13.1 Usual Predominance of Sympathetic or Parasympathetic Tone at Various Effector Sites and Effects of Ganglionic Blockade

Effector Site	Predominant tone	Effect of ganglionic blockade (side effects)*
1. Arterioles**	Sympathetic	Vasodilation, increased peripheral blood flow, hypotension.
2. Veins**	Sympathetic	Dilation, peripheral pooling of blood, decreased venous return, decreased cardiac output (postural hypotension)
3. Heart (SA node)	Parasympathetic	Tachycardia (palpitation), decreased contractility
4. Eye		
a) Iris	Parasympathetic	Mydriasis (photophobia)
b) Ciliary muscle	Parasympathetic	Cycloplegia (blurred vision for near objects)
5. GIT		
a) Propulsive muscles	Parasympathetic	Reduced tone and motility (constipation)
b) Gastric and pancreatic glands	Parasympathetic	Decreased gastric and pancreatic secretions
6. Urinary bladder	Parasympathetic	Decreased tone, relaxation of detrusor muscle (urinary retention)
7. Male genital organs		
a) Vascular vessels of erectile tissue	Parasympathetic	Failure of erection (impotence)
b) Seminal vesicle and vas deferens	Sympathetic	Failure of ejaculation (impotence)
8. Lacrimal glands	Parasympathetic	Reduced lacrimation (dry sandy eyes)
9. Salivary glands	Parasympathetic	Reduced salivation (dryness of mouth)
10. Sweat glands	Sympathetic (in origin), cholinergic (in function)	Reduced sweating, but due to cutaneous flushing there is no hyperthermia (anhydrosis)

* The pharmacological effects of ganglion blockers represent the generally undesirable features (SIDE EFFECTS) which limit their therapeutic efficacy. Hence the common side effects are also summarised in this table and have been listed within parenthesis.

** Because of the blockade of ganglionic transmission, the peripheral sympathetic tone (being predominant) is decreased resulting in fall in blood pressure. The normal protective vasomotor reflexes, mediated through the baroreceptors and the sympathetic nervous system are also blocked. These are postural reflexes which normally prevent pooling of blood in the periphery. Hence, hypotension is more marked in standing posture than supine (postural hypotension). Moreover, because of venous dilation there is decrease in venous return and consequently decrease in cardiac output. This also aggravates peripheral pooling of blood (causing postural hypotension).

Peripherally Acting Adrenergic Neuron Blockers

Guanethidine and Guanadrel

Guanethidine is no longer used clinically because of its adverse effects. *Guanadrel* is a guanethidine derivative. It enters the neuron by uptake mechanism similar to NE. It then enters the storage vesicle from where it displaces NE (on weight by weight basis). When given orally, the NE release is slow which is metabolised by MAO present in the cytoplasm and by COMT present intracellularly. After sometime, the stores of NE get depleted and the vesicles get filled with guanadrel. The nerve impulse at this stage, releases rather guanadrel as "inactive substitute neurotransmitter". This is probably the principal mechanism for its antihypertensive effect. However, if guanadrel is given by fast I.V. injection, it produces a characteristic triphasic response. Initially, there is a fall in BP due to the membrane stabilising action on heart; thereafter there is hypertension due to faster release of NE by guanadrel (some of which can activate postsynaptic α_1 receptors), then there is a long-lasting fall in BP because NE stores have been depleted and it is now no more available on neuron stimulation. Hence, though guanadrel is used for the management of hypertension, it cannot be used for treating hypertensive crisis or for management of phaeochromocytoma because of its potential risk for massive NE release after fast I.V. injection. Due to prolonged adrenergic neuron blockade, the postsynaptic α_1 receptors usually show hypersensitivity (hence hyper-responsiveness to NE and directly acting sympathomimetics). The drug is orally absorbed, but does not cross BBB (hence no central action). It is administered in a regimen of twice daily doses.

Therapeutic Uses: Since better drugs (with no postural hypotension) are available, it is chiefly used as an additional drug in patients who have not achieved a satisfactory antihypertensive effect by two or more drugs.

Adverse Effects: Postural hypotension (lack of sympathetic compensation during standing). Sexual dysfunction is usually manifested as delayed ejaculation. Diarrhoea can also occur.

Drug Interactions: Drugs like tricyclic antidepressants, amphetamines, ephedrine and phenyl propranolamine can inhibit the effect of guanadrel (see above).

Bretylium

It is also a peripheral adrenergic neuron blocking drug. It was originally used to treat hypertension but because of poor gastric absorption and the development of tolerance during long-term therapy its use has been discarded.

However, it has been reintroduced for emergency settings, like ventricular fibrillation refractory to lidocaine or to electrical defibrillation. Besides interfering with the neuronal release of NE, it also has a direct antiarrhythmic action. It prolongs the ventricular action potential duration (APD) and effective refractory period (ERP), probably due to K^+ channel blockade. Thus, bretylium can reverse the shortened APD in ischaemic/infarcted ventricular tissue. The drug does not block Na^+ channels and hence does not depress automaticity, contractility and conductivity of the heart. It is a polar drug and thus does not cross BBB (no central effects). It is excreted unchanged in urine. For rapid termination of ventricular fibrillation a rapid bolus I.V. injection in a dose of 5 mg/kg is given over a period of 5–10 min. ***Adverse effects*** include postural hypotension, initial tachycardia (sudden NE release), otherwise bradycardia.

Peripherally as Well as Centrally Acting Adrenergic Neuron Blocking Drugs

Reserpine

Reserpine and other rauwolfia alkaloids are not used nowadays for treating hypertension because of their wide spectrum of side effects.

It inhibits vesicular dopamine uptake and decreases NE synthesis. It also inhibits vesicular NE uptake (after its neural uptake-1). Hence the NE available in neuronal cytoplasm gets metabolised by MAO. The net result is depletion of NE from storage vesicle with decreased noradrenergic neuron transmission. Chromaffin cells of adrenal medulla and central noradrenergic, dopaminergic and serotoninergic neuron functioning is also affected likewise and hence it depletes NE, DA and 5HT centrally also.

Adverse Effects

a) ***Central Side Effects***. Depression with suicidal tendencies, sedation, extrapyramidal manifestations (due to decreased DA levels in basal ganglia).
b) ***CVS Side Effects***. Na^+ and water retention, bradycardia, nasal congestion, postural hypotension.
c) ***GIT Side Effects***. Peptic ulcer (unopposed enterogastrin secretion due to decrease in 5HT levels). Dryness of mouth (nasal congestion compels breathing from mouth).
d) ***Endocrinal Side Effects***. Galactorrhoea in females (increased prolactin due to diminished DA levels) and gynaecomastia in males.
e) ***Other Side Effects***. Carcinoma breast in women, on long-term use.

CHAPTER 14

SECTION 3—DRUGS ACTING ON PERIPHERAL NERVOUS SYSTEM

Skeletal Muscle Relaxants

COMPETENCY PH1.15

The main clinical use of skeletal muscle relaxants ***(neuromuscular blocking drugs)*** is as an adjuvant in surgical anaesthesia to obtain relaxation of skeletal muscles, particularly of abdominal wall and lower limbs so that operative manipulations become easier. This situation minimises the risk of respiratory and cardiovascular depression besides shortening the post-anaesthetic recovery period because a much lighter level of anaesthesia is now sufficient. These drugs block the postsynaptic actions of ACh at motor end plate and are generally referred to as skeletal muscle relaxants or at times simply as muscle relaxants because smooth muscle relaxants are specifically designated as either antispasmodics or vasodilators or bronchodilators. Some muscle relaxants simply reduce spasticity in a variety of painful conditions (chronic back pain and myalgia). These are called ***spasmolytics.*** On the basis of their site and mechanism of action relaxants are classified as under.

I. PERIPHERALLY ACTING MUSCLE RELAXANTS

These act peripherally at neuromuscular junction (NMJ). They fall into two categories:

A) **Non-Depolarising Blockers (Competitive Blockers)**. These drugs prevent the access of ACh to N_M receptor of motor end plate and prevent its depolarisation. These include the following group of drugs:

Long Acting

a) **Isoquinoline Derivatives** : d-Tubocurarine (d-TC), Metocurine, Doxacurium
b) **Steroidal Derivatives**: Pancuronium, Pipecuronium

Intermediate Acting

a) **Isoquinoline Derivatives**: Atracurium, Cisatracurium
b) **Steroidal Derivatives**: Vecuronium, Rocuronium

Short Acting

a) **Isoquinoline Derivatives**: Mivacurium
b) **Steroidal Derivatives**: Rapacuronium

B) **Depolarising Blockers (Persistent Depolarisers)**. They produce an excessive depolarisation which persists for longer duration at NMJ primarily because they are resistant to hydrolysis by true AChE present in synaptic cleft. At present only a single depolarising agent is in clinical use:

- Succinylcholine (SCh)

II. CENTRALLY ACTING MUSCLE RELAXANTS (SPASMOLYTICS)

These drugs reduce skeletal muscle tone by a selective action in the cerebrospinal axis without altering consciousness. These belong to following categories:

Mephenesin Group: Carisoprodol, Chlorzoxazone, Chlormezanone, Methocarbamol
Benzodiazepine Group: Diazcpam, Clonazcpam
GABA Derivative: Baclofen
Central α_2-Agonist: Tizanidine
Miscellaneous Agents: Tolperisone HCl

III. DIRECTLY ACTING MUSCLE RELAXANTS (SPASMOLYTICS)

These directly interfere with the contractile mechanisms of voluntary muscle. At present only one clinically useful drug is available in this group:

- Dantrolene

IV. MISCELLANEOUS GROUP

Quinine, Botulinum toxins A and B, Gabapentin, Progabide, Riluzole, Idrocilamide

PERIPHERALLY ACTING MUSCLE RELAXANTS

Non-Depolarising Blockers

The first neuromuscular blocking drug that was found was curare, which the native hunters of South

America used to paralyse an animal while hunting. D-Tubocurarine (d-TC), the prototype non-depolarising agent, was ultimately introduced into clinical practice in early 1940s. It is now rarely used but a number of synthetic drugs, having distinct advantages, with same mode of action have been developed (see above).

Mechanism of Action

d-TC and other non-depolarising blockers are bulky quaternary compounds with two positively charged nitrogen (Fig. 14.1).

These drugs have an affinity for the N_M cholinergic receptors at the motor end plate but have no intrinsic activity over them. Being bulky molecules they shadow over (block) the N_M receptor and prevent its binding to ACh. As a result, necessary conformational change in the N_M receptor, which is needed for opening of sodium channel, is prevented. Therefore, in absence of end plate potential, the motor nerve impulses cannot elicit contractions and hence skeletal muscle relaxation ensues. They do not cause depolarisation by themselves but prevent end plate depolarisation by ACh (Fig. 14.2). The antagonism is surmountable (competitive) and hence the reversal of this type of block can be achieved with anticholinesterase drugs like neostigmine (Fig. 14.3).

At higher concentration these drugs block the Na^+ channels directly which augments the blockade. This leads to further weakening of neuromuscular transmission but at the same time reduces the ability of drug like neostigmine to reverse the actions of non-depolarising muscle relaxants.

Pharmacokinetics and Salient Features

- Non-depolarising skeletal muscle relaxants are quaternary compounds and hence they are polar and remain ionised at physiological pH. These are not absorbed when given orally. These are given intravenously but differ in their potency, rates of onset and duration of action (see Tables 14.2 and 14.3). In general, longer acting agents are more potent, requiring lower doses but the

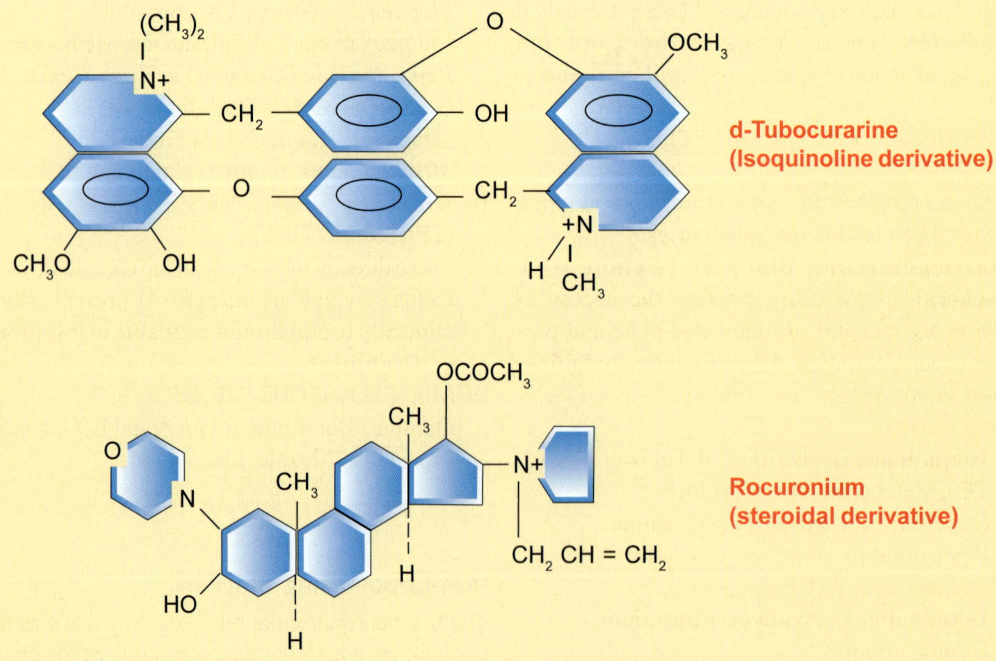

Fig 14.1 Structural Formulae of Representative Non-Depolarising Blockers.

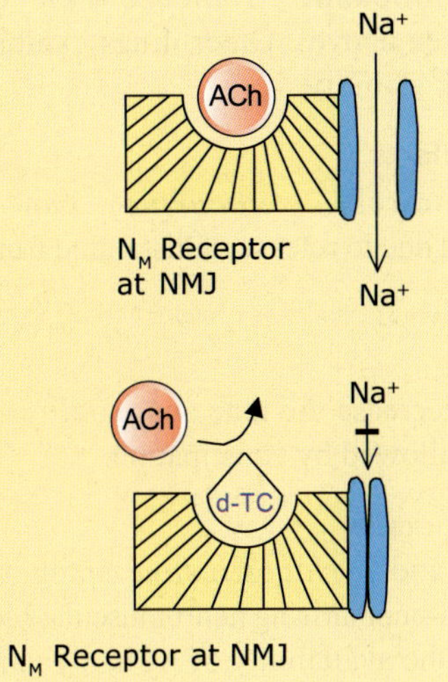

Fig 14.2 Mechanism of Action of Competitive Neuromuscular Blocking Drug.

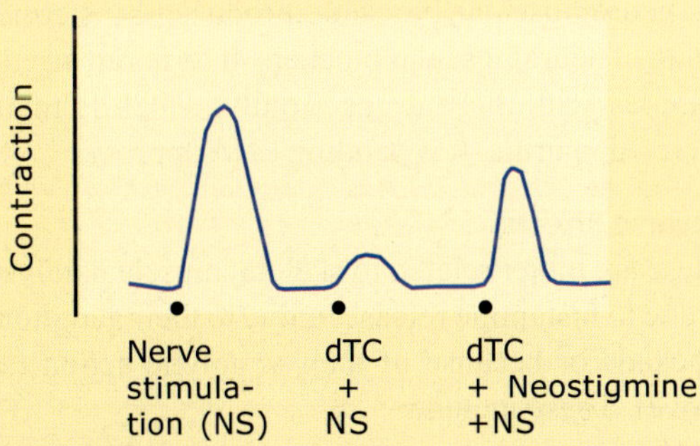

Fig 14.3 Reversal of Competitive Blockade Produced by d-TC with Neostigmine

necessity of administering them in low concentration delays their onset of action (except for pipecuronium).

- These have small apparent volume of distribution. The Vd is essentially confined to the extracellular fluid. Except for atracurium (see below), none of these drugs cross BBB. Hence they do not produce CNS toxicity. These drugs neither cross placental barrier and hence do not affect the newborn if used during caesarean section.
- The route of elimination bears an evident correlation with their duration of action (Tables 14.2 and 14.3).
  a) Drugs excreted by kidney have longer duration of action (35–100 min) (Table 14.2).
  b) Drugs eliminated by liver have an intermediate to shorter duration of action (Table 14.3).
  c) Drugs which are inactivated by plasma cholinesterase have a shorter duration of action, e.g., mivacurium (Table 14.3). However, because patients with renal failure have low levels of plasma cholinesterase, the duration of action of mivacurium may be prolonged in the patients with impaired renal functions.
  d) Some isoquinoline derivatives like atracurium and cis-atracurium are inactivated spontaneously in plasma by Hoffmann elimination (rupture of the ester containing bridge joining the two isoquinoline moieties). The drugs having this route of elimination are intermediate acting (Table 14.3). The main breakdown product of atracurium after Hoffmann elimination, is laudanosine. Though the latter is devoid of neuromuscular blocking properties, it crosses BBB and produces seizures (being CNS stimulant). Cis-atracurium is safer as it forms less laudanosine and releases less histamine.
- Steroidal neuromuscular blocking drugs, which are primarily metabolised by liver (e.g., vecuronium, rocuronium and rapacuronium), if given for several days as in ICUs, may show accumulation and cause prolonged paralysis. Their 3-OH metabolites are not only cleared slowly (longer t½), but are half as potent as the parent drug.
- Atracurium has an additional pharmacokinetic feature. It is chemically unstable at alkaline pH and hence its action becomes considerably briefer during respiratory alkalosis caused by hyperventilation.
- No pharmacogenetic variation in metabolism/response has been observed with non-depolarising blockers.

Pharmacodynamic Actions

The pharmacological characteristics of d-TC and their comparison with depolarising blocking drug succinylcholine (SCh) have been summarised in Table 14.1. The onest, duration, potency and important pharmacological features of non-depolarising blockers have been summarised in Tables 14.2 and 14.3 and compared with d-TC.

Skeletal Muscle Paralysis

After I.V. injection of these drugs motor weakness gives way to progressive flaccid paralysis. The fast moving smaller muscles like those of eyes, jaw, toes and larynx are affected first. Larger muscles like that of limbs and trunk are affected next. Finally, the intercostal muscles and then the diaphragm are paralysed. Recovery of muscles usually occurs in the reverse order. There is no muscle sore after the recovery (since it is a progressive flaccid paralysis).

Histamine Release

Benzylisoquinoline derivative like d-TC has a greater tendency to liberate histamine from mast cells. Others like *metocurine*, *mivacurium*, *doxacurium* and *atracurium* also release histamine but to a lesser extent (unless administered rapidly). Steroidal derivatives, e.g., *pancuronium*, *vecuronium*, *pipecuronium*, *rocuronium* and *rapacuronium* produce least histamine release (Tables 14.1, 14.2 and 14.3).

Ganglionic (N_N) and Cardiac Muscarinic (M_2) Receptor Blockade

At common clinical doses, d-TC and *metocurine* exhibit partial blockade of autonomic ganglia. Other benzylisoquinoline derivatives like *doxacurium*, *mivacurium*, *atracurium* and *cis-atracurium* exhibit least blockade (only at high doses). Steroidal derivatives do not block autonomic ganglia.

Only *pancuronium* has a vagolytic action (by blockade of M_2 receptors), which leads to tachycardia. Other drugs are devoid of vagolytic effects.

Cardiovascular Effects

d-TC (and to a much lesser extent *metocurine, mivacurium* and *atracurium*) produces hypotension mainly due to histamine release and partly due to ganglionic blockade. *Pancuronium* causes tachycardia (see above). Other drugs exhibit good cardiovascular stability.

Respiratory Effects

d-TC (and rarely *metocurine*) can cause bronchospasm due to release of histamine from mast cells.

Effects on GIT

These drugs decrease the tone and motility of GIT. Recovery is followed by constipation.

Reversal of Blockade

Neostigmine and *pyriodostigmine* antagonise or reverse the non-depolarising neuromuscular blockade by increasing the availability of ACh, by inhibiting true AChE present in the synaptic cleft, and also due to their direct nicotinic action at motor end plate. Reversal of neuromuscular blockade becomes necessary if longer acting or intermediate acting non-depolarising neuromuscular blocking agents are used. Short acting agents usually do not need reversal. *Sugammadex* is a newly introduced drug to reverse the neuromuscular blockade produced by steroidal group of neuromuscular blockers. It forms an inactive complex with these drugs rapidly, which is finally excreted in urine. It is pending FDA approval.

Adverse Effects

These are either related to skeletal muscle paralysis, or due to histamine release or due to their ganglionic blockade or because of their vagolytic action (see above). These include:

i) Hypoxia and respiratory paralysis: Which can be treated by artificial respiration and by giving neostigmine. However, neostigmine besides reversing the skeletal muscle blockade may also aggravate bronchospasm, hypotension and at times bradycardia. Hence, sympathomimetic amines like adrenaline may be given to support blood pressure and bronchodilation; atropine or glycopyrrolate may be administered to counteract muscarinic stimulation and antihistamines may be given to counteract the responses that follow histamine release.

Table 14.1 Comparative Features of Competitive and Depolarising Blockers

Parameters	d-Tubocurarine	Succinylcholine
1. Mechanism	Competitive blockade at N_M receptors	Persistent depolarisation of N_M receptors followed by their desensitisation
2. a) Potency b) Onset c) Duration	++ 4–5 min 30–50 min, no muscle sore	+ 1 min 5–6 min followed by muscle sore
3. Type of relaxation	Progressive flaccid paralysis	Initial fasciculations followed by flaccid paralysis
4. Effect of neostigmine	Reversal, i.e., antagonism	Potentiation of effect
5. Effect of neuromuscular blocking drugs	Potentiation of effect	No effect
6. Effect of hypothermia	Decreases effect	Increased effect
7. Histamine release	+ + (moderate)	Negligible
8. a) Blood pressure b) Cardiac muscarinic receptors	Hypotension No effect	+ Stimulates. Bradycardia in low doses; tachycardia in large doses
9. Respiratory effects	Bronchospasm	Nil
10. GIT effects	Constipation	Nausea, vomiting
11. Serum K^+ levels	No change	Hyperkalaemia
12. Intraocular pressure	No change	Raised
13. a) Pharmacogenetic variation in metabolism	Nil Mainly excreted through kidney	a) Metabolised by pseudocholinesterase. Hence persons having atypical pseudocholinesterase exhibit prolonged apnoea even with therapeutic doses of SCh
b) Other pharmacogenetic toxicity	Nil	b) Malignant hyperthermia

Table 14.2 Characteristic Features of Longer Acting Non-depolarising Neuromuscular Blocking Drugs*

Drug	Onset (min)	Relative potency to d-TC	Elimination	Pharmacological characteristics
d-Tubocurarine (d-TC)	4–5	1	Kidney 50% Bile 50%	Refer Table 14.1
Metocurine[2]	4–5	4	Kidney 80% Bile 20%	Isoquinoline derivative Dimethyl derivative of d-TC Lesser histamine release and ganglion blockade Greater safety ratio than d-TC
Doxacurium[1]	4–8	6	Mainly kidney 90%	Isoquinoline derivative Lesser histamine release and ganglionic blockade. Very good CVS stability, used for surgery of longer duration.
Pancuronium[2]	4–6	6	Kidney 80% Liver 20%	Steroidal derivative Low histamine release and ganglionic blockade. Good CVS stability. Inexpensive. Widely used in developing countries Produces tachycardia (vagal blockade).
Pipecuronium[2]	2–4	6	Kidney 80% Liver 20%	Steroidal derivative No histamine release or ganglionic blockade. Good CVS stability. Suitable for surgery of long duration.

* All these drugs have a duration of 35–100 min or more

1 Longest acting (90–120 min)

2 Longer acting (60–120 min)

Table 14.3 Characteristic Features of Intermediate and Short Acting Non-depolarising Neuromuscular Blockers

Drug	Onset (min)	Relative potency to d-TC	Elimination	Pharmacological characteristics
Atracurium*	2–4	1.5	Spontaneous nonenzymatic degradation, also by plasma ChE	Isoquinoline derivative. Inactivated in plasma by Hoffmann degradation and to some extent by plasma cholinesterase. Hence preferred in renal and hepatic insufficiency. Less histamine release Haemodynamically neutral.
Cisatracurium*	3–6	1.5 to 2.0	Spontaneous nonenzymatic degradation 100%	R-cis isomer of atracurium. No histamine release. Suitable for the cases of renal and hepatic insufficiency.
Mivacurium**	2–3	4	Plasma ChE	Isoquinoline derivative. Persons having atypical pseudo-cholinesterase show longer duration of activity and prolonged apnoea. Low histamine release and ganglionic blockade. Shortest acting, hence does not need reversal.
Vecuronium*	2–4	6	Liver 80% Kidney 20%	Steroid derivative. Cardiovascular stability better due to lack of histamine release and no ganglion blockade action.
Rocuronium*	1–2	0.8 to 1.0	Liver 80% Kidney 20%	Rapid onset, intermediate duration. Steroid derivative. Pharmacological profile similar to vecuronium.
Rapacuro-nium**	1–2	0.5	90%	Mainly liver Steroid derivative. Rapid onset, short duration, used for rapid sequence induction of anaesthesia and endotracheal intubation.

* Intermediate acting neuromuscular blocking drugs with duration of action between 25 and 50 min.
** Short acting neuromuscular blocking drugs with duration of action between 15 and 20 min.

ii) Hypotension, bronchospasm, and constipation (as discussed above). Pancuronium produces tachycardia.

Synergists and Antagonists

1. Anti-ChE agents like neostigmine and pyridostigmine are antagonistic to non-depolarising neuromuscular blockers (see above).
2. Hypothermia enhances the depolarising action of ACh. Hence, it antagonises the action of non-depolarising blockers.
3. Inhalational general anaesthetics (mainly isoflurane and halothane) decrease the sensitivity of the post-junctional membrane to depolarisation and therefore act synergistically with these agents. Hence their doses should be reduced if used with these anaesthetic agents.
4. Aminoglycoside group of antibiotics (like streptomycin, gentamicin, tobramycin) themselves produce neuromuscular blockade by decreasing ACh release from the preganglionic terminals by blocking P-type Ca^{2+} channels. Other antibiotics which by themselves have neuromuscular blocking properties include polymyxin-B, clindamycin and lincomycin. Tetracycline group of antibiotics also produce neuromuscular blockade by chelating Ca^{2+} ions. All these antibiotics act synergistically with competitive neuromuscular blockers.
5. In large doses, most local anaesthetics block neuromuscular transmission and can act synergistically with these drugs. Many other drugs like quinidine, propranolol, diltiazem, digitalis, diuretics and chloroquine can also be shown to act synergistically with these agents but not in therapeutic doses and hence these interactions are of no clinical significance.
6. Myasthenia gravis markedly augments the neuromuscular blockade by these drugs. Conversely, patients with burns and those with upper motor neuron disease require large doses of non-depolarising muscle relaxants, because proliferation of extrajunctional receptors, in such conditions, requires an additional amount of non-depolarising relaxant.

Depolarising Blockers (Persistent Depolarisers): Succinylcholine (SCh)

At present, only a single depolarising agent, succinylcholine, is in general clinical use. Pharmacological characteristics of SCh in comparison to d-TC have been summarised in Table 14.1. Its chemical structure is depicted in Fig. 14.4.

Mechanism of Action

Succinylcholine is an acetylcholine analogue which is hydrolysed by pseudocholinesterase but not by true AChE. Hence, only a small fraction of the original I.V. dose of SCh reaches the neuromuscular junction after being hydrolysed by pseudocholinesterase. At NMJ it acts like an excess of ACh and its actions persist for longer duration primarily because it is not degraded by true AChE. SCh reacts with N_M receptors of motor end plate, opens Na^+ channel and causes its depolarisation which then spreads and produces repetitive excitation of muscle motor units that results in transient muscle fasciculations. Both, SCh which is not metabolised by AChE and ACh released during action potential, now bind to the N_M receptors at motor end plate which is already depolarised. As a result the depolarised membrane remains depolarised and in absence of any repolarisation it becomes unresponsive to additional impulses. A flaccid paralysis therefore ensues (Fig. 14.5). This phase (phase I block) is rather augmented, not reversed, by AChE inhibitors like neostigmine.

However, with higher doses of SCh or following its prolonged infusion, the phase I block may get converted to a non-depolarising type phase II block. The transition from phase I block to phase II block is slow. After phase I block, even if the motor

$$(CH_3)_3.\overset{+}{N}.CH_2.CH_2.O.\overset{\overset{O}{\|}}{C}.CH_2.CH_2.\overset{\overset{O}{\|}}{C}.O.CH_2.CH_2\overset{+}{N}\,(CH_3)_3$$

Fig 14.4 Chemical Formula of Succinylcholine.

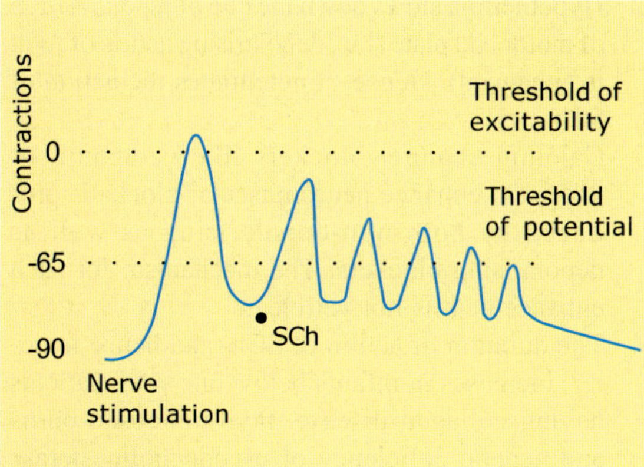

Fig 14.5 Phase I (depolarising block) by Succinylcholine

end plate gets repolarised it cannot be depolarised again because continuous exposure of N_M receptors to SCh have resulted in desensitisation due to persistent depolarisation. Whatever be the mechanism, the Na^+ channels behave as if they are in a prolonged closed state. The phase II block resembles that of non-depolarising block by d-TC and can be reversed by neostigmine.

Because of the uncertainty of this situation (transition of phase I to phase II block), a non-depolarising agent is preferred over SCh for anything other than short procedures. During short operative procedures, with usual clinical doses of SCh, the muscle relaxation results due to phase I block which is not transformed to phase II block (except in patients with atypical pseudocholinesterase, see below).

Pharmacokinetics

SCh also possesses two quaternary ammonium groups in its molecule (Fig. 14.4). Hence it is not absorbed if given orally and does not cross BBB or placental barrier. It is administered by I.V. route (0.75–1.5 mg/kg IV). The extremely brief duration of action of SCh (5–10 min) is mainly due to its rapid hydrolysis by plasma cholinesterase (pseudocholinesterase) present in liver and plasma. Its action is terminated by its diffusion away from the motor end plate into the extracellular fluid.

The activity of pseudocholinesterase actually influences the duration of action of SCh as it determines the amount of the drug that would reach the end plate. Neuromuscular blockade by SCh (also by mivacurium) may be prolonged in patients with genetic variant of plasma-cholinesterase (atypical pseudocholinesterase). An ability of this enzyme to metabolise SCh can be assessed by finding the "***dibucaine number***" of such patients. Dibucaine (a local anaesthetic) inhibits the normal enzyme by about 80% and atypical plasmacholinesterase only by 20% (i.e., the dibucaine number of a normal person is 80). Hence a dibucaine number of less than 80 shows the proportionate concentration of atypical enzyme.

Pharmacodynamic Aspects

- After a single I.V. dose of SCh, fasciculations, particularly over chest and abdomen, occur briefly but these are not troublesome in well anaesthetised patients. Complete relaxation occurs within 1–2 min and disappears within 5–10 min. Muscle soreness may follow the recovery and it occurs due to fasciculations induced damage to skeletal muscles. The sequence of paralysis, however, differs from d-TC. Twitches on cheek and abdomen appear first. Paralysis then spreads to neck, limbs, face, trunk and then to the respiratory musculature. Apnoea appears within 1 min, but is transient and lasts for 2–5 min. The onset and recovery being rapid, the sequence of paralysis is not that distinguishable.
- SCh stimulates ganglia due to its agonist action on N_N receptor. Histamine release is lesser than d-TC. Cardiovascular effects are manifested in the form of bradycardia (due to stimulation of vagal ganglia) and then tachycardia and hypertension (due to stimulation of sympathetic ganglia). Blood pressure, however, is not affected much, as the drug lowers BP also due to its muscarinic actions (vasodilatation).

Adverse Effects

1. **Hyperkalaemia**

   Efflux of intracellular K^+ occurs during depolarising blockade. This leads to slight rise in plasma K^+ levels (hyperkalaemia). In normal persons it has hardly any clinical relevance. However, the cases of burns, spinal injury and uraemia are very susceptible to hyperkalaemia which may precipitate arrhythmias or even cardiac arrest.

These cases have freshly denervated muscles and the N_M receptors show denervated supersensitivity (hyper-responsiveness).

2. **Malignant Hyperthermia**

   It is a genetically inherited condition, as an autosomal dominant trait, caused by a mutation of Ca^{2+} release channels of the sarcoplasmic reticulum. In such individuals, malignant hyperthermia may be triggered by SCh. As a result, there is persistent release of intracellular Ca^{2+} from the sarcoplasmic reticulum leading to persistent muscle contraction and increased heat production from the skeletal muscle (hyperthermia). These individuals have a higher susceptibility to malignant hyperthermia when a combination of general anaesthetic like halothane is used along with SCh (for treatment, see dantrolene).

3. **Masseter Muscle Rigidity**

   It is another genetically inherited condition caused by mutation of voltage-sensitive Na^+ channel. SCh in these susceptible individuals may complicate endotracheal tube insertion and airway management.

4. **Prolonged Apnoea**

   Persons having atypical pseudocholinesterase exhibit prolonged apnoea even with usual doses of SCh (see above).

5. **Increased Intragastric Pressure**

   Nausea and vomiting with SCh occur due to an increase in intragastric pressure as a consequence of fasciculations.

6. **Rise in Intraocular Pressure**

   The rise in IOP is short-lived (5–10 min) and occurs due to contractions of tonic myofibrils (extraocular muscle) and partly due to transient dilatation of choroidal blood vessels.

7. **Muscle Soreness**

   Muscle damage, due to fasciculations, has been verified by the occurrence of myoglobinuria following the use of SCh. Hence muscle soreness after the recovery is a common observation (see above).

Synergists and Antagonists

1. Neostigmine potentiates phase I block due to SCh (see above).
2. Hypothermia slows down the rate of repolarisation of motor end plate (i.e., depolarising action of ACh is enhanced). Hence, it potentiates the action of SCh.
3. Calcium channel blockers like verapamil or diltiazem enhance neuromuscular blockade produced by both non-depolarising as well as depolarising blockers. The mechanism for such enhancement is not yet clear.
4. The duration of action of SCh (and hence toxicity) increases in infants below one year, patients having collagen disease, thyrotoxicosis, burns and genetic deficiency of pseudocholinesterase (see above).

Therapeutic Uses of Neuromuscular Blocking Drugs

1. ***As an Adjuvant to General Anaesthesia***
   - To provide skeletal muscle relaxation during abdominal or throacic surgery and for endotracheal intubation.
   - To counteract laryngospasm during barbiturate anaesthesia.
   - To prevent reflex muscle contractions during surgery.

   Surgical procedures can be performed more safely and rapidly by employing peripherally acting neuromuscular blocking drugs. The selection of the drug depends on its onset of action, duration of blockade required, and on patient's hepatic, renal and haemodynamic status. For example, SCh or *mivacurium* are employed for brief procedures, e.g., endotracheal intubation, laryngoscopy, and bronchoscopy. *Mivacurium*, though a non-depolarising blocker, does not need reversal. For longer duration surgery, *pipecuronium* or *doxacurium* can be employed. For patients having renal or hepatic insufficiency, *atracurium* or *cis-atracurium* are preferred (inactivated in plasma by Hoffmann degradation). *Rocuronium* is preferred for renally compromised patients (metabolised by liver). In developing countries, evaluating the cost:benefit ratio, *pancuronium* is routinely employed.

2. ***To Prevent Trauma During Electroconvulsive Therapy***
   SCh with diazepam is used to prevent injuries or fractures due to excessive convulsions from ECT. This drug combination can also be used for reduction of fractures and other orthopaedic manipulations.
3. ***In Different Spastic Conditions***
   These can be used in spastic conditions like tetanus or status epilepticus which are not controlled by diazepam.
4. ***To Control Ventilation***
   These drugs eliminate chest wall resistance and ineffective spontaneous ventilation in patients having obstructive airway disease.

CENTRALLY ACTING MUSCLE RELAXANTS (SPASMOLYTICS)

These drugs reduce skeletal muscle tone by a selective action in the cerebrospinal axis without altering consciousness. In this section only those drugs which ameliorate some of the symptoms of skeletal muscle spasticity are being considered. Spasticity is characterised by an increase in tonic stretch reflexes and flexor muscle spasm along with muscle weakness. Such muscular rigidity is often associated with disease like cerebral palsy and multiple sclerosis, and involves abnormal function of bowel, bladder and skeletal muscle. Anti-skeletal muscle spastic drugs discussed here, control the symptoms of spasticity either by enhancing the activity of the inhibitory internuncial neurons of the reflex arc (e.g., *diazepam*, *baclofen*) or by interfering directly with skeletal muscle excitation-contraction coupling (e.g., *dantrolene*; see under directly acting muscle relaxants). Components involved in these processes and sites of drug action are shown in Fig. 14.6. A variety of other compounds belonging to mephenesin group (see classification) are also used to relieve acute local muscle spasm.

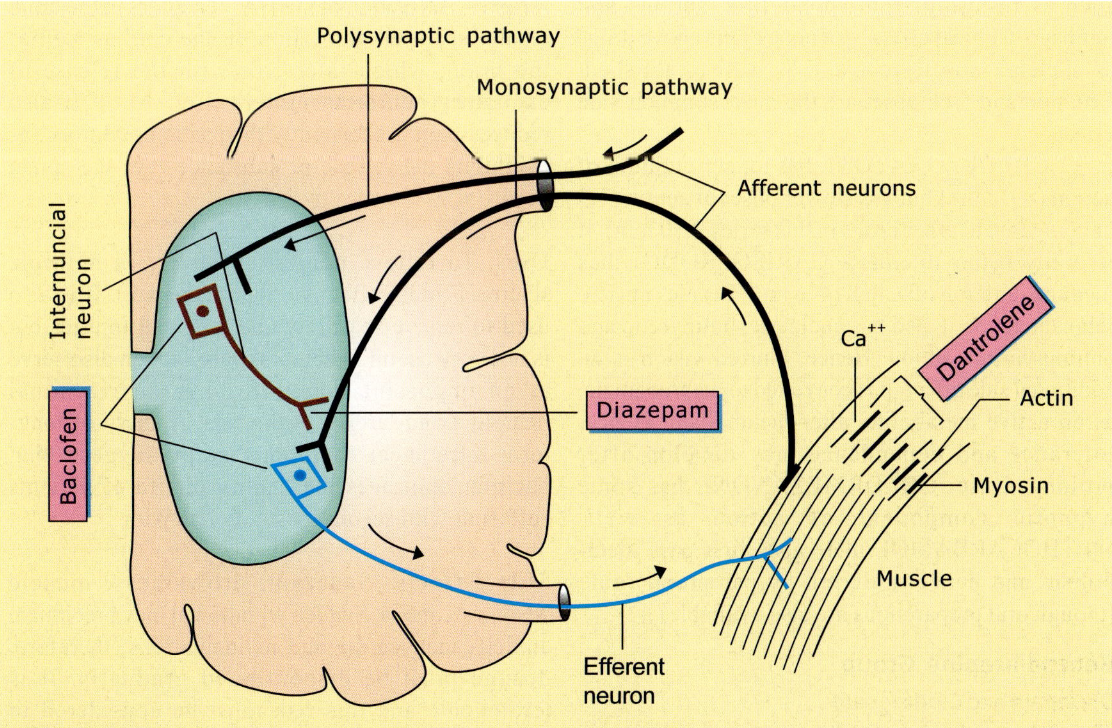

Fig 14.6 Cross Section of Spinal Cord Showing Components Involved in the Stretch Reflex Arc, with Postulated Sites of Action of Diazepam, Baclofen and Dantrolene.

Their mode of action is non-specific and is loosely described as depressants of polysynaptic reflexes at spinal level.

Both spinal and supraspinal polysynaptic reflexes are involved in the regulation of muscle tone. Monosynaptic pathways mediate stretch reflex. Drugs that inhibit spinal or supraspinal polysynaptic reflexes also inhibit polysynaptic pathways in the ascending reticular activating system, though to a lesser extent. Hence, all these drugs do have some sedative side effects.

Mephenesin Group

Carisoprodol, Chlorzoxazone, Chlormezanone and Methocarbamol

These drugs are believed to be spinal internuncial neuron blocking agents (at the level of brain stem). They preferentially inhibit polysynaptic reflexes without affecting monosynaptic (knee jerk) tendon reflexes. Exact mechanism of action is debatable. These are used to treat muscle spasm of local origin such as resulting from spondylitis, sprains and lumbago. Clinical efficacy of none of the above drugs as skeletal muscle relaxants is well established. Sedation and GIT upset are the most common side effects.

CHLORZOXAZONE has longer duration of action (8–12 hrs) but has slower onset of action (1.5 hr compared to other drugs in this series—30 min). It is orally better tolerated. CARISOPRODOL has medium duration of action (4–6 hrs). Besides muscle relaxant action it also has analgesic, antipyretic and antimuscarinic action. Hence, blurred vision is an additional side effect. It is converted to meprobamate, as an active metabolite, after metabolism. Hence, tolerance and dependence may develop after prolonged use. CHLORMEZANONE has some hypnotic component of action as well. METHOCARBAMOL undergoes first pass metabolism and hence preferred by parenteral route (though oral preparations are also available).

Benzodiazepine Group

Diazepam and Clonazepam

These drugs enhance GABA-ergic transmission in brain (see Chapter 32 also). They apparently act at all GABA synapses, but their site of action in reducing spasticity is supraspinal. These drugs inhibit both monosynpatic as well as polysynaptic reflexes and produce marked sedation. Diazepam/clonazepam probably facilitate $GABA_A$ mediated presynaptic inhibition of the release of excitatory neurotransmitters (Fig. 14.6). These drugs can reduce muscle spasm of almost any origin including local muscle trauma. These are particulary useful in spinal injuries, tetanus and rheumatic disorders associated with muscle spasm. Sedation is their major side effect.

GABA Derivative

Baclofen

It is an orally active GABA-mimetic drug which acts as a GABA agonist at $GABA_B$ receptors. The $GABA_B$ receptors are G-protein coupled receptors which hyperpolarise neurons by increasing K^+conductance and reducing Ca^{2+}conductance. Its muscle relaxant actions result from an action at the spinal level where it inhibits both monosynaptic and polysynaptic reflexes. Activation of $GABA_B$ receptors in the brain results in hyperpolarisation, in the cord as well as the brain, which interferes with the release of excitatory neurotransmitters (Fig. 14.6). It also reduces pain associated with spastic conditions, as it inhibits the release of substance-P in the spinal cord.

Uses: To relieve painful spasticity in multiple sclerosis (more effective than diazepam). It is also used to relieve spasticity due to spinal injuries but is not very useful in cerebral palsy. It can also serve as an important substitute to treat trigeminal neuralgia and tardive dyskinesia. A study of long-term intrathecal baclofen therapy suggests that baclofen improves the quality of life of patients suffering with severe spasticity and pain.

Side Effects: Sedation, drowsiness, muscle weakness, ataxia. Sudden withdrawal may precipitate anxiety, tachycardia and hallucinations; therefore, dosage must be discontinued gradually. It is teratogenic and this risk must be considered in pregnancy.

Central α_2 Agonist

Tizanidine

The ability of α_2 agonists to alter neuronal activity in the spinal cord resulted in the development of tizanidine for the treatment of spasticity. The drug antagonises spasticity at doses which hardly have any effect on blood pressure as compared to clonidine. It has significant α_2- adrenoceptor agonist effect in the spinal cord and inhibits the release of excitatory amino acids in spinal interneurons.

Tizanidine is widely used in the treatment of spasticity in multiple sclerosis. It is also effective in patients with amyotrophic lateral sclerosis. Spasticity due to neurological disorders and painful muscle spasm of spinal origin are also treated with tizanidine. Side effects include drowsiness, dry mouth, asthenia and sometimes hypotension. The drug is well tolerated orally, but undergoes first-pass metabolism.

Miscellaneous Agents

Tolperisone HCl

It is a centrally acting muscle relaxant with local anaesthetic properties. It inhibits reticulospinal reflex facilitation without affecting cortical functions. It improves peripheral blood flow. The circulatory effect is supposed to be based on peripheral mechanism and is independent from the cerebral centers of vasoregulation. This drug is used mainly for the treatment of elevated muscle tone and tension as well as for certain circulatory problems in the extremities. It reduces experimental hypertonia and decerebration rigidity.

Tolperisone is well absorbed from the small intestine. The peak plasma concentration occurs at 0.5 to 1 hrs after ingestion with t½ of 1.5–2.5 hrs. The average oral bioavailability is about 20% in human due to substantial first pass metabolism. High-fat meal increases the bioavailability.

It is indicated for the treatment of patients with acute muscle/musculoskeletal spasm in adults in the doses of 150 mg TDS alone or incombination with NSAIDs like Diclofenac sodium (50 mg). The drug is contraindicated in myasthenia gravis and for the treatment of perioperative pain in the setting of coronary artery bypass graft (CABG) surgery. It should not be used in patients of peptic ulcer and bronchial asthma.

DIRECTLY ACTING MUSCLE RELAXANTS (SPASMOLYTICS)

Dantrolene

Dantrolene is a phenytoin analogue but its site for antispastic action lies outside the CNS. It differs from the classical neuromuscular blocking drugs in that its action is distal to N_M receptors and the neuromuscular junction. Instead, it acts directly at the contractile mechanisms of voluntary muscle by reducing depolarisation-induced Ca^{2+} release from sarcoplasmic reticulum (Fig. 14.6). The muscle fibers still respond to nerve stimulus, hence the contractile responses are reduced but not absolutely abolished by dantrolene. The net result is muscle weakness rather than paralysis, which considerably neutralises the benefits from dantrolene. The drug also facilitates GABA which results in the depression of brain stem reticular functions and efferent motor neuron activity. Hence, it produces sedation but has no selective action on polysynaptic reflexes (like baclofen or diazepam). Cardiac muscle and smooth muscles are almost unaffected because the Ca^{2+} release from their sarcoplasmic reticulum occurs by a different mechanism.

It is used to treat spasticity resulting from upper motor neuron lesions such as those in spinal cord injury, multiple sclerosis and cerebral palsy but not in spasticity resulting from musculoskeletal injury, lumbago or rheumatoid disorders. It is a drug of choice for the treatment of *malignant hyperthermia* which is a genetically inherited condition, as an autosomal dominant trait. It is caused by a mutation of Ca^{2+} release channel of the sarcoplasmic reticulum. In such genetically predisposed individuals, malignant hyperthermia may be triggered by SCh and fluorinated anaesthetics. When it happens, there is a persistent release of Ca^{2+} with massive muscle contraction, lactic acid production (acidosis), and increased heat production from the skeletal muscle. Prompt treatment is essential to check Ca^{2+} release and to control acidosis and hyperpyrexia. This is accomplished by giving dantrolene I.V. starting with 1 mg/kg and repeating if necessary, to a maximum of 10 mg/kg.

The use of dantrolene in the treatment of neurolept-malignant syndrome has been found to be useful, although this syndrome does not appear to be due to abnormal Ca^{2+} release in skeletal muscle (see Chapter 33).

Orally it is poorly absorbed but absorption is consistent so that the plasma levels are proportional to the dose. Plasma half-life is 9–12 hrs. Major adverse effects are generalised muscle weakness, sedation, diarrhoea and occasionally hepatitis after prolonged use.

The pharmacological features of peripherally acting, centrally acting and directly acting skeletal muscle relaxants have been compared and summarised in Table 14.4.

Table 14.4 Comparative Features of Peripheral, Central and Directly Acting Muscle Relaxants

Parameters	Peripherally Acting (d-TC or SCh)	Centrally Acting (BZDs or Baclofen)	Directly Acting (Dantrolene)
Mechanism	Block neuromuscular transmission either by competitive blockade (d-TC) or by persistent depolarisation and desensitisation (SCh)	Selectively inhibit supraspinal (BZDs) or spinal (baclofen) polysynaptic reflexes which control and regulate the muscle tone	Reduces depolarisation-induced release of Ca^{++} from sarcoplasmic reticulum. Hence interferes with excitation–contraction coupling
Route	Usually given I.V.	Oral/Parenteral	Oral/Parenteral
Type of paralysis	Progressive, flaccid paralysis (d-TC) or fasciculation followed by flaccid paralysis (SCh). Loss of voluntary power	No paralysis, only decrease in muscle tone with no loss of voluntary power	No paralysis, only decrease in muscle tone with partial loss of voluntary power
CNS effects	Quaternary compounds Do not cross BBB	Cross BBB, produce sedation	Cross BBB, produce lesser sedation
Main use	During surgery, endo-tracheal intubation, laryngoscopy etc. BUT NOT IN MH or NMS	Spastic condts., tetanus, status epilepticus, neuro-logical spasms BUT NOT IN MH or NMS	Cerebral palsy, spinal cord injuries, ALSO FOR MH or NMS
Side effects	See text	Not serious, except sedation	Diarrhoea, hepatotoxicity

Key: d-TC–d-tubocurarine; SCh–Succinylcholine; BZDs–Benzodiazepines; MH–Malignant hyperthermia; NMS–Neuroleptic Malignant Syndrome.

MISCELLANEOUS GROUP

Quinine

It suppresses the neuromuscular transmission by decreasing the excitability of motor end plate. It occasionally benefits patients of myotonia congenita, torsion spasm and if taken at bed time, persons with nocturnal leg cramps.

Botulinum Toxin Type A and B

Botulinum toxins are neurotoxins produced by *Clostridium botulinum*, a spore-forming anaerobic bacillus. Botulinum toxin-A appears to affect only the presynaptic membrane of the cholinergic neuron at NMJ, where it prevents the Ca^{2+} -dependent release of ACh and produces a state of denervation leading to muscle relaxation.

Uses. For the treatment of strabismus and blepharospasm; for the temporary improvement in the wrinkles of the face in adult patients; the local injections of botulinum toxin-A are now finding increased use in the treatment of more generalised spastic disorders like cerebral palsy.

Botulinum toxin-B cleaves synaptic Vesicle Associated Membrane Protein (VAMP; synaptobrevin) which is responsible for the fusion of synaptic vesicle to the presynaptic membrane of the cholinergic neuron. Thus, by blocking ACh release it provides skeletal muscle relaxation. *Uses*. For treatment of cervical dystonia (spasmodic torticollis) in patients unresponsive to botulinum toxin-A.

Adverse Effects. Xerostomia, facial weakness, numbness, speech disorders, local injection site pain, dizziness, vertigo, dry eyes, and at times corneal ulceration due to reduction in blinking.

Other spasmolytic drugs include (i) **Gabapentin** (Ch. 39) which inhibits the high frequency voltage-activating Ca^{2+} channel currents by binding to L-type Ca^{2+} channel. It also increases the concentration of GABA in brain and is a $GABA_B$ receptor agonist. It is mainly an antiepileptic drug but is occasionally used to treat pain associated with multiple sclerosis (albeit in high doses); (ii) **Progabide** (Ch. 39) in another antiepileptic drug used as spasmolytic. It is both $GABA_A$ and $GABA_B$ receptor agonist but its use is restricted because of its hepatotoxicity and as it causes down-regulation of GABA receptors on prolonged use; (iii) **Riluzole** (Ch. 40) is a new drug, recommended for the treatment of amyotrophic lateral sclerosis (ALS). It decreases glutametergic trans mission in CNS, blocks postsynaptic NMDA type glutamate receptors and inhibits voltage dependent Na^+ channel. Usual dose is 50 mg BD orally, before meals. It is well tolerated but nausea or diarrhoea may occur; (iv) **Idrocilamide** is another new agent approved for the treatment for ALS. It acts intracellularly by inhibiting the release of calcium from the sarcoplasmic reticulum.

CHAPTER 15 Local Anaesthetics

COMPETENCY PH1.17

Local anaesthetics (LA) reversibly block the impulse conduction and produce a transient loss of sensation in a restricted region of the body. These drugs are preferred for performing minor surgery and unlike general anaesthetics, they neither cause a loss of consciousness nor need a proper maintenance of vital functions during the surgery.

SUSCEPTIBILITY OF NERVE FIBRES TO LOCAL ANAESTHETIC BLOCKADE

Although local anaesthetics are capable of blocking all types of nerves, different types of nerve fibres differ significantly in their susceptibility to LA blockade on the basis of their size and myelination. Thus, upon application of a LA to a nerve root, the smaller unmyelinated C fibres and B-fibres (which are lightly myelinated) are blocked first. Therefore, pain, temperature and touch sensation are blocked first while proprioception disappears in succession. The small type A-delta fibres, which are myelinated, are blocked next while larger and heavily myelinated A-alpha, -beta and -gamma fibres are blocked in the last. As a result, other modalities like skeletal muscle tone are lost in the end. The recovery takes place in reverse order.

The precise mechanism responsible for this apparent specificity of LA action on pain fibres is not known. However, the spacing of the nodes of Ranvier, which increases with the size of nerve fibres, seems to influence the conduction blockade by a LA. For myelinated nerves, at least 3 successive nodes must be blocked by the LA to block the impulse propagation. Hence, small fibres with closely spaced nodes may be blocked more rapidly compared to thick fibres where the nodes of Ranvier tend to be further apart.

CLASSIFICATION OF LOCAL ANAESTHETICS

The LAs can be classified as follows. Their pharmacological characteristics and therapeutic uses have been summarised in Table 15.1.

I. AMIDE TYPE

Ia. **Long Acting**
BUPIVACAINE, levo-BUPIVACAINE, ROPIVACAINE, DIBUCAINE

Ib. **Intermediate Acting**
LIDOCAINE (LIGNOCAINE), MEPIVACAINE, PRILOCAINE, ARTICAINE

II. ESTER TYPE

IIa. **Long Acting**
TETRACAINE (AMETHOCAINE)

IIb. **Intermediate Acting**
COCAINE

IIc. **Short Acting**
PROCAINE, CHLOROPROCAINE, BENZOCAINE*, PROPARACAINE (PROXYMETACAINE)*

III. **MISCELLANEOUS**
PRAMOXINE (PRAMOCAINE)*, DYCLONINE (DYCLOCAINE)*, OXETHAZAINE (MUCAINE)*.

*Used mainly for topical (surface) anaesthesia (Table 15.1).

Table 15.1 Pharmacological Characteristics and Uses of Different Local Anaesthetics[1]

Toxicity and Other Uses	Drug	Main LA Use and Pharmacological Properties
I. AMIDE GROUP		
Ia. Long Acting (Duration > 180 min)		
Toxicity: Prolongs QTc interval, induces ventricular tachycardia and ventricular arrhythmias because after blocking cardiac Na^+ channels during systole, it keeps them blocked even at the end of diastole (cumulative block due to slow dissociation). Its cardiac toxicity is enhanced further in presence of acidosis and hypoxaemia. Levobupivacaine is equally potent but less toxic than racemic bupivacaine. **Other Uses**: Nil	BUPIVACAINE and LEVO-BUPIVACAINE (Both 4 times more potent than lidocaine)	Used for infiltration, nerve block, epidural and spinal anaesthesia of long duration. Provides more sensory than motor block and has least placental transmission; hence gaining popularity for providing painless delivery. It has an intermediate onset of action. It should not be used for intravenous regional analgesia or for obstetrical paracervical block anaesthesia.
Toxicity: Less cardiotoxic than bupivacaine. It is available only as S-stereoisomer, which has inherently less affinity for cardiac Na^+ channels. R-isomer is toxic. **Other Uses**: Nil	ROPIVACAINE (Equipotent to bupivacaine)	Used for infiltration, epidural and regional anaesthesia. Continuous epidural ropivacaine is being used for relief of postoperative and labour pain. It is less cardiotoxic and more motor sparing than bupivacaine. It has an intermediate onset of action.
Toxicity: It is more toxic than bupivacaine **Other Uses**: It is a pseudocholinesterase inhibitor. It inhibits normal enzyme by 80% but atypical pseudocholinesterase (a genetic variant) by only 20%. Normal dibucaine number is 80. Values less than 80 indicate the proportionate concentration of atypical pseudo-cholinesterase (see Ch. 14).	DIBUCAINE (CINCHOCAINE)	It is very potent, longest acting LA having slow onset of action. It is mainly used as surface anaesthetic in anal canal and rectum and occasionally for spinal anaesthesia of longer duration. *Rarely used LA.*
Ib. Intermediate Acting (Duration 60–120 min)		
Toxicity: CNS side effects are frequently observed during therapy. These include dizziness, paraesthesia, and euphoria. Higher doses produce confusion, vertigo, tinnitus and nausea. Severe toxicity may	LIDOCAINE (LIGNOCAINE)	It is most widely used multi-purpose LA. It can be used topically on mucous membranes in the form of aqueous solutions, jelly, ointment or as viscous solution. It can be employed for

contd.

Toxicity and Other Uses	Drug	Main LA Use and Pharmacological Properties
precipitate seizures. Diazepam can be used to protect xylocaine induced seizures. Overdose toxicity includes cardiac arrhythmias, lowering of BP, coma and respiratory arrest. **Other Uses**: Administered intravenously for the management of ventricular arrhythmias occuring during myocardial infarction. Coadministration with propranolol impairs the clearance of lidocaine and enhances its toxicity.		infiltration, nerve block and for epidural anaesthesia. For spinal analgesia, a higher concentration (5%) made hyperbaric with 7.5% dextrose is used. It has a rapid onset of action which lasts for 1–2 hours. Intrathecal or epidural administration of lidocaine in combination with an opioid analgesic has a very synergistic effect. The mechanism is unknown, but this combination is gaining popularity in management of pain. Its transdermal patch is also available to relieve pain associated with post-herpetic neuralgia.
Toxicity: Similar to lidocaine **Other Uses**: Nil	MEPIVACAINE (Half as potent as lidocaine)	It is similar to lidocaine except that *it is not effective as a topical anaesthetic*. It can also be used for many purposes without epinephrine.
Toxicity: Similar to lidocaine except that one of its metabolites, orthotoluidine, is known to cause methaemoglobinaemia. Hence not used in obstetric practice because of its risk to produce neonatal methaemoglobinaemia. If it occurs it can be reversed by giving slow I.V. injection of methylene blue.	PRILOCAINE (Equipotent to lidocaine)	For the most part it is used for dental procedures & administered either by infiltration or nerve block. It is similar to lidocaine but does not cause vasodilatation; consequently it can be used without epinephrine (good choice for patients in whom epinephrine is contraindicated). With lignocaine it makes a EUTECTIC MIXTURE – a unique combination which can anaesthetise intact skin after surface application.[2]
Infection at the site of lumbar puncture. Mainly metabolised in liver but partly by plasma cholinesterase also (unique metabolism)	ARTICAINE (Almost equipotent to lidocaine)	Rapid onset of action (5 min). It is approved for dental and periodontal procedures but also used for epidural and spinal anaesthesia. Formulations for dental anaesthesia contain epinephrine.

contd.

Toxicity and Other Uses	Drug	Main LA Use and Pharmacological Properties
	II. ESTER GROUP	
	IIa. Long Acting (Duration > 180 min)	
Toxicity: It is more slowly metabolised compared to other ester group of LA, hence more toxic. Being a PABA ester it may antagonise the effects of sulfonamides. Intravenous doses may produce cardiac arrhythmias. **Other Uses**: Nil	TETRACAINE (AMETHOCAINE) (Four times more potent than lidocaine)	Used topically on the eye, nose, throat and tracheobronchial tree. When used in eye, it neither dilates pupil, nor paralyses accommodation, nor increases intraocular pressure (hence preferred). It is very suitable for spinal anaesthesia of long duration. It has a slow onset of action. Its highly lipophilic character and slower rate of hydrolysis, allows it to remain in the tissue surrounding the nerve for an extended period of time (hence longer acting than other ester type LAs).
	IIb. Intermediate Acting (Duration 60–120 min)	
Toxicity: It is a CNS stimulant drug, causes euphoria, delays fatigue and causes strong psychological dependence. It produces bradycardia, rise in BP, rise in body temperature, nausea and vomiting. **Other Uses**: Nil	COCAINE (Half as potent as lidocaine)	*It is no longer used now, as it is a protoplasmic poison and causes tissue necrosis*. It is never injected. Earlier it was used as ocular anaesthetic. *It is a vasoconstrictor, so mixing of adrenaline is not needed.*
	IIc. Short Acting (Duration 30–60 min)	
Toxicity: Bradycardia, vasodilatation, decrease in cardiac output, anxiety, restlessness and shivering. Hydrolysed to PABA and thus antagonises the action of sulfonamides. **Other Uses**: It forms poorly absorbable salt with benzylpenicillin called PROCAINE PENICILLIN, whose antibacterial actions last for more than 24 hours when given by I.M. route. Its amide derivative PROCAINAMIDE is used as class IA group of antiarrhythmics.	PROCAINE (One fourth as potent as lidocaine)	*No longer used*. It has slow onset of action. It is ineffective when applied topically. It is a vasodilator and hence addition of epinephrine is necessary to retard its absorption.

contd.

Toxicity and Other Uses	Drug	Main LA Use and Pharmacological Properties
Toxicity: Lesser toxicity compared to procaine because of faster metabolism. **Other Uses**: Nil	CHLOROPROCAINE (Slightly more potent than procaine)	It is a better and safer LA than procaine. It is used for infiltration, nerve block, caudal and epidural block. It has a rapid onset of action. It is not effective topically.
Toxicity: These have a poor penetration through mucous membrane or skin. Hence, least toxic. Both being PABA derivatives, can antagonise sulfonamide action locally. These are too toxic to be used as an injection anaesthetic.	BENZOCAINE and PROPARACAINE	THESE ARE USED AS TOPICAL (SURFACE) ANAESTHETICS. These are included in proprietary preparations of ointments, lozenges, and suppositories to relieve pain associated with ulcers, sore throat & inflammation in anorectal area. PROPARACAINE is preferred for short operative procedures in the eye, as it is non-irritating and least antigenic.
III. MISCELLANEOUS GROUP		
Toxicity: Safe, like benzocaine. Pramoxine is too irritating for eye, hence not used during ophthalmic surgery. These drugs should not be injected.	PRAMOXINE and DYCLONINE	These are unrelated to ester or amide type LA, hence useful in cases who are sensitive to LAs of these groups. These are SURFACE ANAESTHETICS like benzocaine.
Toxicity: Quite safe but overdoses may produce dizziness and drowsiness.	OXETHAZAINE (MUCAINE or OXETACAINE)	Used as surface anaesthetic. Although a basic drug, it remains mostly unionised in acidic medium. Hence, when swallowed along with antacids it affords symptomatic relief in gastritis, heart burn and in gastro-esophageal reflux by anaesthetising gastric mucosa despite acidity of the medium.

Key:

[1] Note that ester group of LAs have only one '*i*' (e.g., procaine, tetracaine, benzocaine), while amide group of LAs have two '*i*' in their spelling (e.g., lignocaine, bupivacaine, ropivacaine). *Etidocaine*, a longer acting LA of amide group, is rarely used nowadays.

[2] Eutectic mixture has a lower melting point than any of the two solids that are mixed. When lignocaine (2.5%) and prilocaine (2.5%) are mixed in equal proportions at 25°C the mixed melting point gets depressed which results in the formation of an oil. This oil is then emulsified in aqueous phase to form a cream. Usually, surface anaesthesia does not work well on intact skin, but this *eutectic mixture of local anaesthetics* (EMLA) has been used as an alternative to lignocaine infiltration. The cream can be applied under occlusive dressing for one hour before IV cannulation or skin grafting or for removal of unwanted facial hair by laser therapy. It produces complete anaesthesia, up to a depth of 5 mm, for a period of 1 hour after its removal.

MECHANISM OF ACTION

Local anaesthetic molecules consist of an aromatic part linked by an *ester* or *amide* bond to a basic amine side chain (Fig. 15.1). Benzocaine, however, has no basic amine side chain. The LAs are weak bases as they form salts with acids (e.g., lignocaine hydrochloride). These remain partly ionised at physiological pH. It is the unionsied form of the LA, which being lipophilic, is necessary for penetration through nerve membrane. Once inside the axon, it is the ionised form of the LA which is active at the receptor site. ***LAs block the voltage-gated Na^+ channels (see Ch.7) and consequently block the nerve conduction by reducing the permeability of Na^+ ions during depolarisation.***

The blocking action of LA is favoured by depolarisation. Thus, a resting membrane is much less sensitive to a LA than one that is repetitively stimulated. This phenomenon which is affected by the voltage gradient across the cell membrane is known as "voltage dependence". The voltage dependence of sodium channel opening, reflects conformational changes that result from the movement of voltage sensors due to difference in transmembrane potential. These voltage sensors are called as "gate charges" or simply as "gates". Hence, these channels are termed as "voltage-gated sodium channels."

The Na^+ channel has an Activation Gate (AG) on its extracellular site and an Inactivation Gate (IG) on its intracellular site. The voltage-gated Na^+

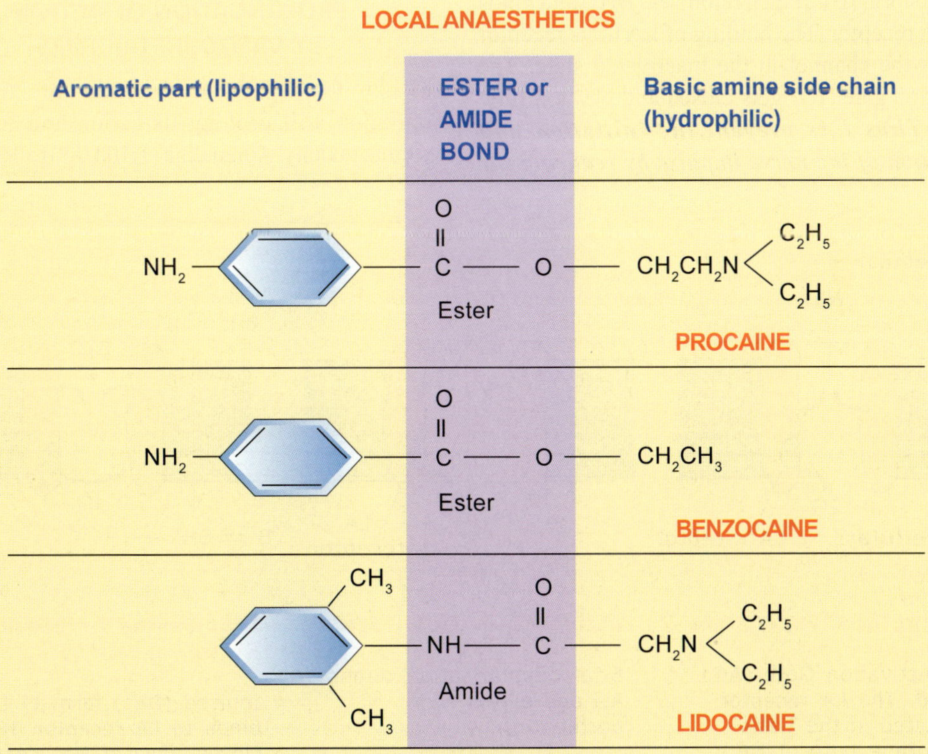

Key: Aromatic group (left), Ester or Amide group (shaded in between) and Amine side chain (right). Benzocaine is an exception, lacking an amine side chain.

Fig 15.1 Chemical Structures of Local Anaesthetics.

channels can exist in three functional states: **(1)** the *resting or the closed state* which prevails at the normal resting potential. In this state the activation gate is closed; **(2)** the *activated or the open state* which is favoured by brief depolarisation, that opens the activation gate to allow Na^+ ions to flow inside along concentration gradient; **(3)** the *inactivated or blocked state* resulting from a trap-door like occlusion of the channel by a floppy part of the intracellular region of the channel protein. The Na^+ ion flow ceases as soon as inactivation gate closes. After the action potential has passed, many Na^+ channels are in the inactivated state. These then revert to their resting state in a time dependent manner and become available for activation once more.

The LA-receptor is located in the trans-membrane pore of Na^+ channel in its intracellular half. The LA diffuses through the membrane in its unionised lipophilic form (B). It then reionises (BH^+) and binds to the LA receptor. The binding of LA to its receptor stabilises the channel in the inactivated state. The inactivation gate (IG) gets closed and Na^+ ion flow ceases. ***Thus LAs prevent the initiation and propagation of the nerve impulse by reducing the passage of Na^+ ions through voltage-gated Na^+ channels*** *(Fig. 15.2)*.

EFFECT OF pH ON LA ACTION

The LA action is strongly pH dependent, being more at alkaline pH and less at acidic pH. These drugs being weak bases remain partly ionised and partly unionised at physiological pH. The unionised form of LA is needed for its diffusion through axon membrane. Once inside the axon it is reionised and it is the cationic form (BH^+, Fig. 15.2) of LA which binds to LA receptor inside the channel. LA are less effective in infected tissue, because in infected area the extracellular pH is acidic. Hence in such an environment, LA remains predominantly ionised which results in their poor diffusion through the nerve.

PROLONGATION OF ACTION BY VASOCONSTRICTORS

Anything that delays the absorption of LA into the circulation will prolong its action and reduce its systemic toxicity. Adrenaline (1:100,000 to 1: 200,000;

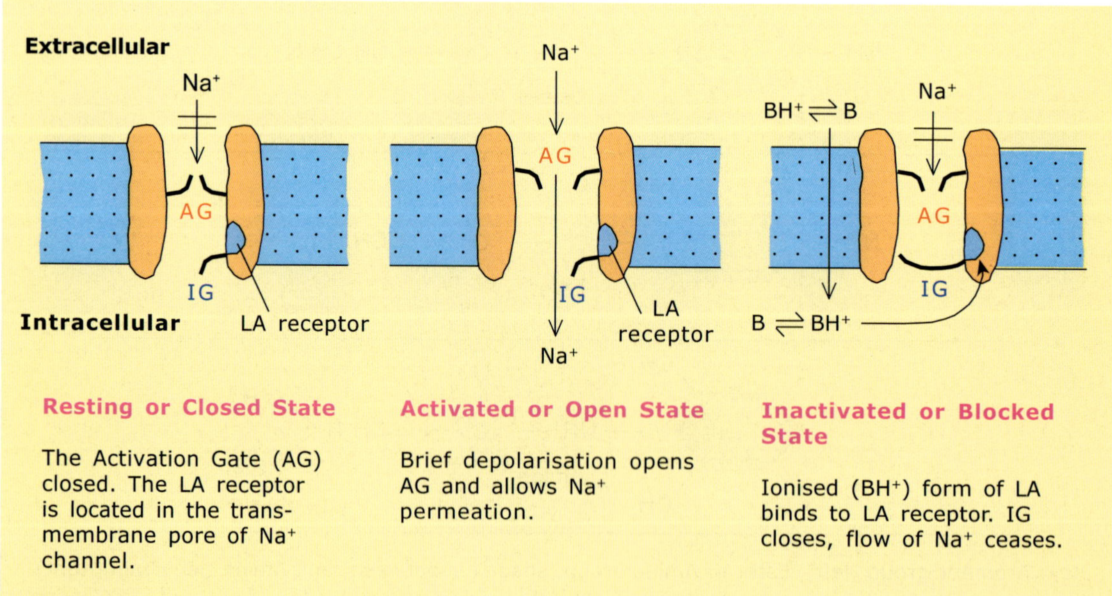

Fig 15.2 A Model of Voltage-Gated Na^+ Channel Depicting the Site and Mechanism of Local Anaesthetic Action.

in dentistry, 1:50,000 to 1:100,000), therefore, is most commonly used along with LAs as it doubles the duration of LA action.

Norepinephrine, being a powerful vasoconstrictor, is generally not preferred. A vasoconstrictor should not be used for nerve block of an extremity or end organ, e.g., on fingers, toes, nose and penis, because intense vasoconstriction will lead to total ischaemia and necrosis.

To avoid cardiac complications which may occur with the use of adrenaline, an alternative vasoconstrictor, ***felypressin*** (a synthetic vasopressin), can be used. It does not affect the heart rate, BP and may be preferable in patients with cardiovascular disease. Alternatively, prilocaine can also be used (see Table 15.1).

REVERSAL OF LA EFFECTS

Phentolamine mesylate (a non-selective α-adrenoceptor antoagonist) has been approved for the reversal of unpleasant effects (numbness, heavyness slurred speech, etc.) observed after administering LAs (with vasoconstrictors). The drug (0.4 mg/1.7 ml cartridge) is injected in the same manner (as of LAs) after the procedure, if the pain relief is no longer needed. Return of normal functions (e.g., speaking, smiling, eating, drinking and normal sensations) return within 50–80 min of the restorative procedure (compared to 130–160 min after the LA). Probably, phentolamine increases the local blood flow by blocking α_1-receptors at the site of injection which speeds up the removal of LA from its site to systemic circulation. This is because, by the time the procedure is over, and phentolamine reversal is performed, the epinephrine (added with LAs), no longer remains at the local tissues. The dose of phentolamine is so small (10 times less than antihypertensive dose) that it hardly has any effect on patient blood pressure.

PHARMACOKINETICS

The presence of the ester or the amide bond in a LA molecule governs its biotransformation and its liability to cause hypersensitivity reactions.

- The ester type LAs (e.g., tetracaine, chloroprocaine) are usually hydrolysed by plasma esterases (pseudocholinesterase) and also by liver esterases. As they are rapidly hydrolysed, they have a shorter duration of action. However, their action may be prolonged where there is genetic enzyme deficiency. The spinal fluid contains negligible esterases, hence intrathecal injection of ester type LA will exhibit prolonged duration of LA action.
- The amide type LAs (lidocaine, bupivacaine) are degraded by hepatic microsomes through N-dealkylation and subsequent hydrolysis. Consequently, the amide type LAs usually have a longer duration of action.
- Hypersensitivity reactions seem to occur most prominently in response to LAs of ester type (as they are metabolised to a potential allergen PABA or PABA derivatives). Allergic reactions to amide type of LAs are rare. Since ester group of LA are degraded to PABA, they antagonise the action of sulfonamides (Ch.53).
- After oral ingestion, both procaine and lidocaine undergo significant first-pass metabolism. Hence lidocaine is not used orally to combat cardiac arrhythmias.

USES OF LOCAL ANAESTHETICS AND TYPES OF LOCAL ANAESTHESIA

The local anaesthesia induced by a LA is designated according to the technique or anatomical site where it is injected or applied (Fig. 15.3).

Topical Anaesthesia

In topical (surface) anaesthesia, the sensory nerve endings are the chief nerve structures affected. It is restricted to mucous membranes, damaged skin surface, wounds or burns. Surface anaesthetics do not work well on intact skin (except eutectic mixture of lignocaine + prilocaine; see Table 15.1). The corneal surface, mucosa of mouth, nose, pharynx, trachea and urethra are easily anaesthetised. Surface anaesthetics can also be used to facilitate endoscopic procedures and to reduce pain of haemorrhoids or anal fissure. Solutions, ointments or cream of LAs can be applied to produce surface anaesthesia. LAs generally used for this purpose are tetracaine (2%), lidocaine (2–5%), eutectic mixture of lidocaine (2.5%) plus

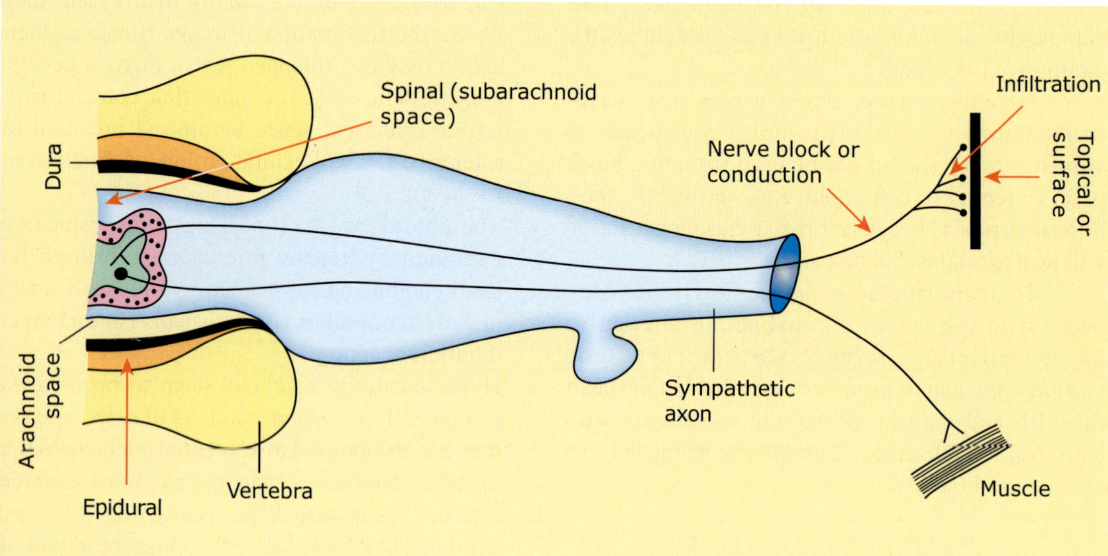

Fig 15.3 Sites of Application of Local Anaesthetics.

prilocaine (2.5%), benzocaine (5%), dyclonine (0.5–1%), and proparacaine (0.5-1%).

Infiltration Anaesthesia

Here the dilute solution of LA is injected under the skin to reach sensory nerve terminals. Infiltration is used for minor surgical procedures like incisions or excisions. Adrenaline or felypressin may be added to retard absorption (see following text). LAs most frequently used for infiltration anaesthesia are lidocaine (1-2%), bupivacaine (0.25%), ropivacaine (0.5–1%), mepivacaine (1–3%) and prilocaine (1–4%).

Conduction Block Anaesthesia

The LA is injected around the nerve trunk so that the area distal to the site of injection is anaesthetised. It is of two types:

a) Field Block

Here the LA is injected subcutaneously in the surrounding area of the nerve so that all other nerves coming to a particular field are blocked. Field blocks are applied to the scalp and anterior abdominal walls where the nerves travel superficially to supply the area.

b) Nerve Block

The LA is injected around anatomically localised nerve trunks, i.e., close to the mixed nerve. The block is usually described by adding the name of the anaesthetised nerve, e.g., radial nerve block, ulnar nerve block and trigeminal nerve block. Nerve block lasts longer than field block or infiltration anaesthesia.

The LA is never injected into the nerve as this would not only be painful but could lead to nerve damage. Instead, the LA is deposited as close to the nerve as possible. The LA then diffuses from the site of injection into the nerve where it acts.

For field block anaesthesia, the LAs used are the same as for infiltration anaesthesia. For nerve block anaesthesia, the choice of LA and its concentration depends on the type of the nerve to be blocked, the duration of anaesthesia required and the size and health of the patient. For block of 2 to 4 hrs, intermediate acting LAs like lidocaine (1.5%) or mepivacaine (1.5%) can be used. For longer duration of nerve block, bupivacaine (0.25–0.35%) can be used. Addition of epinephrine prolongs duration and lowers the plasma concentration of the intermediate acting LAs.

Central Nerve Block Anaesthesia

This includes EPIDURAL and SPINAL BLOCK anaesthesia.

a) Epidural Block Anaesthesia

Epidural block (also referred to as peridural block) is widely used to provide analgesia or anaesthesia in surgical and obstetric practice. It involves injecting a LA such as lidocaine, bupivacaine or ropivacaine alone or with a small dose of an opioid analgesic into the epidural space in the lumbar, thoracic or cervical regions to provide segmental analgesia. *Caudal block* is also an epidural block but in the caudal (sacral) region. Introduction of a cannula into the epidural space enables prolonged anaesthesia to be provided through the use of additional doses or continuous infusion of LA. A vasoconstrictor may also be added to reduce systemic exposure to the LA. A test dose at the intended site of injection is recommended before starting the procedure to ensure that the LA is not accidentally injected intravascularly or into the subarachnoid space.

b) Spinal Block Anaesthesia

It is also referred to as subarachnoid or intrathecal block anaesthesia or as spinal analgesia. It is produced by injecting a solution of a suitable LA like lidocaine (3 to 5%), tetracaine (0.3 to 0.5%) or bupivacaine (0.5 to 0.7%) in the spinal subarachnoid space between L2 and L3 or L3 and L4. The primary site of action is the nerve root in cauda equina rather than the spinal cord. It is used to anaesthetise lower abdomen and hindlimbs. Although vasoconstrictors are added to prolong the duration of the block, there is always a danger of restricting the blood supply to the spinal cord. Hence, this practice is not clinically useful. During late pregnancy, the inferior vena cava is already compressed leading to a decrease in the subarachnoid space. Hence, lesser amounts of LA are required to produce spinal anaesthesia.

The use of hyperbaric (in 7.5 to 10% glucose) or hypobaric (in distilled water) solution of a LA and proper positioning of the patient on the operating table permits manipulation of anaesthesia for various body areas. However, hypobaric solutions of LA are seldom used. With proper expertise, the complications of spinal anaesthesia are minimal except for headache, nausea and vomiting. However, respiratory paralysis, hypotension and *cauda equina syndrome* (loss of control over bladder and bowel sphincters) are a few rare complications that may occur.

Intravenous Regional Anaesthesia

It is also referred to as *Bier's block*, and is mainly used for the upper limb and for orthopaedic procedures. The limb is first elevated to ensure venous drainage and then tightly wrapped by an elastic bandage for maximal exsanguination. Tourniquet is then applied proximally and inflated just above the systolic BP. The elastic bandage is now removed and lidocaine (0.5%) is injected I.V., distal to the tourniquet. Normally the cuff is inflated for at least 20 min to minimise systemic toxicity. Prilocaine (0.5%) is also a preferred LA because of its higher safety index. Bupivacaine is avoided because of its higher cardiac toxicity.

ADVERSE EFFECTS

In general, the adverse effects are qualitatively similar for all LAs. If blood levels rise too high after their systemic absorption, adverse effects on different systems may be observed.

Central Nervous System

CNS effects at low doses include tongue numbness, sleepiness, mild headache, visual and auditory disturbances. At higher concentration, nystagmus and muscular twitching can occur. Profound CNS stimulation may lead to convulsions which may be treated by giving diazepam or thiopental intravenously. Cocaine, though rarely used, produces long lasting CNS stimulation and euphoria like amphetamine. It is widely abused drug causing dependence (see Ch 38). It is rarely used as LA.

Cardiovascular System

LAs block cardiac Na^+ channels and thus depress abnormal cardiac pacemaker activity, excitability and conduction. Excepting cocaine, most LAs produce hypotension.

Bupivacaine is cardiotoxic (Table 15.1) and can cause ventricular tachycardia and fibrillation. Cocaine blocks NE reuptake and hence produces vasoconstriction and hypertension. Lignocaine has a quinidine-like action on the heart and therefore is used in the treatment of cardiac arrhythmias (see Ch 21).

Blood

Administration of large doses of prilocaine may lead to an accumulation of the metabolite orthotoluidine, which oxidises haemoglobin to methaemoglobin. Higher levels of the latter leads to cyanosis. Reducing agents like methylene blue or ascorbic acid may be given intravenously to convert methaemoglobin to haemoglobin.

Allergic Reactions

The ester type LAs are metabolised to PABA derivatives which in turn are responsible for allergic reactions in a small percentage of population. Such allergic manifestations include contact dermatitis, rashes and asthma (rare). Amide group of LA do not metabolise to PABA derivatives and allergic reactions to these agents are rare.

DRUG INTERACTIONS

1. Hypertensive patients receiving therapy with *Propranolol* (a nonselective β_1+β_2 blocker) are very sensitive to the pressor (hypertensive) responses of adrenaline (present in lidocaine formulation); because simultaneous blockade of vasodilatory β_2 receptors (along with β_1) by propranolol, leads to an unopposed vasoconstricting action of adrenaline on α_1 receptors (Ch.12). On the contrary, drugs with prominent α_1-receptor blocking activity (e.g., *haloperidol*, an antipsychotic drug) may lead to rather hypotension if coadministered in high doses with lidocaine + adrenaline combination (due to unopposed β_2 effect after α-blockade).
2. Persons with acute alcohol intoxication need a bit higher dose of lidocaine + adrenaline combination for getting proper LA effects; because much of the vasoconstricting effects of adrenaline are rather neutralised by the cutaneous vasodilatory effects of alcohol. As a result, the availability of lidocaine at the desired site of action gets decreased (because of its increased systemic absorption).
3. Special care must be taken while giving an injection of lidocaine + adrenaline to a patient of cardiac failure who is taking *digoxin;* because in these patients, if the vasoconstrictor goes intravascularly, the chances of developing cardiac arrhythmias become high.
4. In coronary care units, where lidocaine is usually infused, in large doses, intravenously to treat ventricular arrhythmias, coadministration of *propranolol* can lead to lidocaine toxicity on two counts: (a) propranolol inhibits the metabolic oxidation of lidocaine and (b) propranolol also decreases the hepatic blood flow and thus diminishes its delivery to liver for metabolic degradation.

CHAPTER 16

SECTION 4—DRUGS AFFECTING RENAL AND CARDIOVASCULAR SYSTEM AND RELATED AUTACOIDS

Diuretics

COMPETENCY PH1.24, PH1.26

The main function of kidney is the excretion of waste products like urea, uric acid and creatinine. In the course of this activity, it also regulates the blood contents of NaCl and other electrolytes, as well as the volume of extracellular fluid to maintain homeostasis. It plays a crucial role in maintaining acid–base balance, and also serves other functions such as synthesis of local hormones like angiotensin, prostacyclin and erythropoietin. It is also involved in the hydroxylation of vitamin D.

In structure, each kidney consists of an outer cortex, an inner medulla and a hollow pelvis, which empties into the ureter. The functional unit of the kidney is nephron, of which there are about 1.3×10^6 in each kidney. The nephron consists of glomerulus, proximal convoluted tubule, loop of Henle, distal convoluted tubule and the collecting duct (Fig. 16.1).

Diuretic drugs increase the urinary output of electrolytes and water from the kidney by interfering with one or more reabsorptive processes occurring at different segments of the nephron. Hence, the initial discussion of this chapter begins with a description of those features of renal physiology which are prerequisite to the understanding of the pharmacology of diuretic drugs.

RENAL TUBULE TRANSPORT MECHANISMS

Approximately 16–20% of the blood plasma entering the kidneys is filtered from the glomerular capillaries into the Bowman's capsule. The filtrate is normally free of proteins and blood cells but contains other low-molecular-weight plasma components such as glucose, Na^+, K^+, Ca^{2+}, Cl^- and HCO_3^- plus amino acids and other organic solutes. Most of the filtrate is reabsorbed from the different segments of the renal tubule, as follows, with ultimate excretion of 1.5 litres of fluid as urine in 24 hrs (Fig. 16.1).

Proximal Convoluted Tubule (PT)

Approximately 85% of filtered $NaHCO_3$, 40% of NaCl and almost all of glucose, amino acids and other organic solutes are reabsorbed *via* specific transport systems in the *early part of the proximal tubule(PT).* About 60% of water is reabsorbed passively to maintain constant osmolality of PT fluid. If it were not for the extensive reabsorption of solutes and water in the PT, the body would have become rapidly dehydrated and lost its normal osmolarity. The bicarbonate reabsorption by the PT is dependant on carbonic anhydrase activity. The carbonic anhydrase (CA) enzyme is found in the brush border of the luminal membrane and also in the cytoplasm of PT cells. The function of CA is to catalyse the reaction of H_2O and CO_2 leading to the formation of H_2CO_3 which then spontaneously ionises to H^+ and HCO_3^-. The HCO_3^- are then transported into the interstitium together with Na^+ as $NaHCO_3$. As bicarbonate and other organic solutes have been largely removed from the tubular fluid, the NaCl present in the residual luminal fluid is predominantly removed from the *latter part of the proximal tubule.* The water is passively reabsorbed, in direct proportion to salt reabsorption in this segment.

Organic acid secretory systems are located in the middle third of the proximal tubule. These systems secrete a variety of organic acids such as uric acid, some antibiotics like penicillins and some diuretics like thiazide and loop diuretics.

Organic base secretory systems are localized in the early and middle segments of the proximal tubule, and secrete bases like creatinine and choline etc. These two secretory systems, therefore, account for several drug interactions, e.g., between diuretics and uric acid or diuretics and probenecid *(see following text)*.

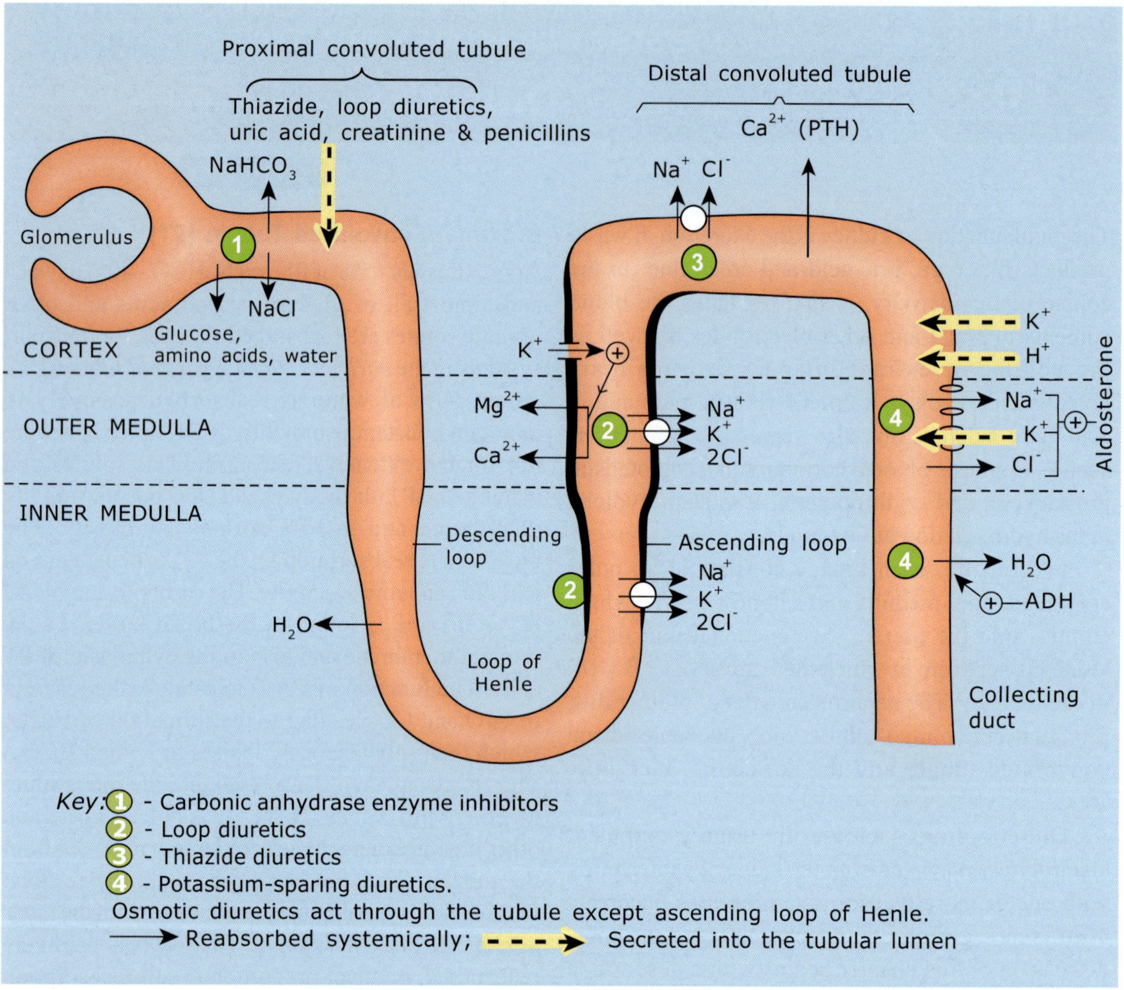

Fig 16.1 Normal Tubular Transport and Sites of Action of Diuretics.

Loop of Henle (LH)

The thin descending limb of LH does not participate in salt reabsorption, but being permeable to water it contributes to water reabsorption by osmotic forces created in the hypertonic medullary interstitium. This results in a tubular fluid with a three-fold increase in salt concentration.

The thick ascending limb of LH is referred to as diluting segment, firstly because this segment is impermeable to water and secondly because reabsorption of NaCl from this region further dilutes the filtrate. Active reabsorption of Na^+, K^+ and Cl^- is mediated by $Na^+/K^+/2Cl^-$ cotransporter system. In a cotransport system (or symport) the transport of one substance is coupled to that of another, both being transported across a membrane in the same direction (see Fig. 16.1 and Fig. 5.3).

The $Na^+/K^+/2Cl^-$ symport is electrically neutral because 2 cations are transported in lieu of 2 anions. However, from the basolateral side of the tubule, Na^+/K^+ ATPase is also pumping K^+ within the tubular cells. This leads to an accumulation of K^+ within the cell and subsequently promotes its back diffusion from the tubular cell into the lumen through potassium channels. Inside the lumen, the positive potential created by back diffusion of K^+ drives divalent cations – Mg^{2+} and Ca^{2+} – reabsorption *via* the paracellular pathway (between the space of tubular cells).

Thus loop diuretics which act at this site and inhibit NaCl reabsorption, by blocking the $Na^+/K^+/2Cl^-$ symport, also increase the urinary excretion of Mg^{2+} and Ca^{2+} in addition to Na^+.

Distal Convoluted Tubule

This segment of the tubule is also impermeable to water. About 10% of the filtered NaCl is reabsorbed from this site *via* a Na^+/Cl^- cotransport system which is electrically neutral and is sensitive to thiazide group of diuretics. Because there is no back diffusion of K^+, as happens in the ascending limb of LH, there is no lumen positive potential in this segment and, therefore, Ca^{2+} and Mg^{2+} are not driven out of the tubular lumen by electrical gradient. However, Ca^{2+} is actively reabsorbed from this segment. Both parathyroid hormone and calcitriol promote Ca^{2+} reabsorption. In contrast to the situation in the ascending limb of LH, where loop diuretics inhibit Ca^{2+} reabsorption (produce calciuria), thiazides rather enhance parathyroid hormone-regulated Ca^{2+} reabsorption from the distal convoluted tubule by some unknown mechanism *(see following text).*

Collecting Tubule

Several distal tubules empty into each collecting tubule and the collecting tubules then join to form the collecting ducts. The collecting tubule has two different types of cells: *the principal cells,* which reabsorb Na^+ and secrete K^+, and *the intercalated cells,* which secrete H^+. Unlike other segments of renal tubule, the principal cells of collecting tubule have Na^+ and K^+ channels, not cotransporters, in the luminal membrane. These cells are normally impermeable to water in the absence of antidiuretic hormone (ADH or vasopressin) and to Na^+ in the absence of aldosterone.

Aldosterone promotes Na^+ reabsorption to renal interstitium and K^+ secretion into the tubular lumen. Through its action on membrane aldosterone receptors it enhances the activity of both apical (luminal) membrane Na^+ channels (to allow transcellular passage of Na^+) and of the basolateral Na^+ pumps. There exists an important inter-relationship between Na^+ reabsorption and K^+ secretion at collecting tubule and both the processes are regulated by aldosterone. Na^+ that enters the principal cell from the tubular lumen is then transported to the interstitium blood *via* the basolateral Na^+/K^+ ATPase as in other nephron segments. This leaves the lumen with a negative electrical potential (due to loss of + ion). To compensate this, some Cl^- ions are driven from the tubular fluid toward the interstitium blood *via* the paracellular (in between the cells) pathway while K^+ ions are driven out of the principal cell towards the luminal fluid through the apical membrane K^+ channels.

The collecting tubule is responsible for only 2–5% of NaCl reabsorption by the kidney. Despite this, it plays a vital role in renal physiology and mechanism of action of diuretic drugs. Potassium-sparing diuretics such as *amiloride* inhibit apical (luminal) membrane Na^+ channels while *spironolactone* antagonises aldosterone actions.

The antidiuretic hormone (ADH) is secreted by the posterior pituitary gland. By stimulating V_2 receptors in the basolateral membrane of collecting tubule, ADH (or vasopressin) leads to an increase in the number of water channels in the luminal membrane with concomitant increase in the membrane permeability to water. In its absence, the low water permeability of collecting ducts would further enhance the hypo-osmolarity of the fluid coming from the distal tubule. As a result a large volume of hypo-osmolar urine would be excreted.

Role of Other Autacoids and Peptides in Regulating Renal Functions

Besides aldosterone, antidiuretic hormone (vasopressin), parathyroid hormone (PTH) and carbonic anhydrase enzyme which have a distinct role in regulating renal transport of various electrolytes, control of osmolality, volume of urine and maintenance of acid-base balance of body fluids (as discussed above), there are some other peptides and autacoids (discussed below) which also modulate the haemodynamics and excretory functions of kidney indirectly.

Natriuretic Peptides

The atrial natriuretic peptide (atriopeptin) is released endogenously from the atrium when the atrial pressure is high. It increases glomerular capillary pressure, by dilating afferent and constricting efferent arterioles, to promote Na^+ excretion and water diuresis. It also has direct tubular actions which include the inhibition of angiotensin II-stimulated Na^+ and water reabsorption in the proximal convoluted tubule and ADH-mediated water reabsorption in the collecting ducts.

Another peptide called *urodilatin*, similar to atriopeptin, is produced in distal tubule. It also promotes Na^+ excretion and water diuresis, but by acting on receptors on the luminal membrane of collecting ducts. The net result is to decrease blood volume and therefore to reduce atrial pressure (see also Ch. 17).

Prostaglandins

PGE_2 and PGI_2 (prostacyclin), the products of cyclo-oxygenase pathway, are also synthesised in the medulla and in the glomeruli respectively. They also modulate the haemodynamic and excretory functions of kidney. Factors that stimulate their synthesis include circulating angiotensin II, catecholamines, ADH and bradykinin, besides ischaemia and mechanical trauma (refer Ch. 25).

Under basal conditions, prostaglandins probably do not have much effect. But whenever vasoconstrictor agents like angiotensin II or noradrenaline are generated and released, the PGE_2 and PGI_2 try to neutralize the effects of these agents in kidney by increasing renal blood flow and causing excretion of Na^+. That is why the nonsteroidal anti-inflammatory agents, which inhibit prostaglandin synthesis, can cause a decline in renal perfusion and decreased excretion of both Na^+ and K^+. They can also exacerbate NaCl and water retention which is harmful to the patients of hypertension and heart failure (refer Ch. 26).

Angiotensin II

It is synthesised locally in vascular endothelial cells. It promotes Na^+ and water reabsorption from distal convoluted tubule. It also stimulates aldosterone release which further enhances tubular Na^+ reabsorption (refer Ch. 18).

DIURETIC DRUGS

Diuretics are the drugs that promote the excretion of Na^+ and water from the body by an action on the kidney. The increased water loss is actually secondary to the increased excretion of NaCl. This they achieve either by directly acting on different segments of the nephron or by indirectly modifying the contents of the urinary filtrate. Accordingly, they are classified as follows:

I. DIURETICS ACTING DIRECTLY ON DIFFERENT SEGMENTS OF THE NEPHRON

A) **Those Acting on the Thick Ascending Loop of Henle**: FUROSEMIDE, BUMETANIDE, TORSEMIDE, PIRETANIDE and ETHACRYNI-C ACID, INDACRINONE (uricosuric diuretic).

These are also called "Loop diuretics" or "High-ceiling diuretics".

B) **Those Acting on the Proximal (early) Part of the Distal Tubule**

(i) ***Thiazide Group***: HYDROCHLOROTHIAZIDE, CHLOROTHIAZIDE, BENZTHIAZIDE, POLYTHIAZIDE, BENDROFLUMETHIAZIDE and CLOPAMIDE.

(ii) ***Chemically Related Variants***: CHLORTHALIDONE, XIPAMIDE, INDAPAMIDE, METOLAZONE and QUINETHAZONE.

C. **Those Acting on Collecting Ducts and Tubules**: AMILORIDE and TRIAMTERENE

These are also called K^+-sparing diuretics.

D. **Aldosterone Receptor Antagonists at Distal (later) Part of the Distal Tubule and Collecting Tubule**: SPIRONOLACTONE, and EPLERENONE.

These too, are called K^+-sparing diuretics.

II. DIURETICS ACTING INDIRECTLY BY MODIFYING THE CONTENTS OF URINARY FILTRATE

MANNITOL and GLYCEROL

These are also called osmotic diuretics.

III. WEAK DIURETICS WHICH MAINLY HAVE NON-DIURETIC USE

Carbonic Anhydrase Inhibitors:
ACETAZOLAMIDE, DORZOLAMIDE, ETHOXZOLAMIDE, DICHLORPHENAMIDE, and METHA-ZOLAMIDE

A summary of the routes of their access into tubular lumen, their sites and mechanism of action has been provided in Figure 16.1 and Table 16.1. Their main pharmacological effects have been summarised in Table 16.2; while their diuretic and non-diuretic uses have been listed in Table 16.3.

DIURETICS ACTING DIRECTLY ON DIFFERENT SEGMENTS OF THE NEPHRON

Those Acting on the Thick Ascending Limb of Loop of Henle (LH)

Loop Diuretics/High-Ceiling Diuretics

The two prototype drugs of this group are ***furosemide*** and ***ethacrynic acid***. Organic mercurial diuretics also inhibit NaCl transport in the thick ascending LH; but they are of historical interest only and are no longer used because of their toxicity. Loop diuretics are the most powerful of all diuretics, capable of excreting 20–30% of Na^+ in the urinary filtrate. These are also called "high ceiling" diuretics because unlike other diuretics, their dose-response curve is steep and by increasing the dose, the maximal Na^+ excretion can even reach up to 30–40% in comparison to 10–12% caused by thiazides and 5–6% by potassium-sparing diuretics (Fig. 16.2).

When given by oral route these are readily absorbed from the GIT but may also be given by injection. Being highly protein bound these cannot pass through glomerulus. They are rather secreted through the proximal convoluted tubule by the organic acid transport mechanism. Subsequently, they reach their site of action—the luminal membrane of the thick ascending limb of LH. The fraction not secreted through proximal tubule is metabolised by liver. Given orally, they act within 1 hour; given I.V., they produce a peak effect within

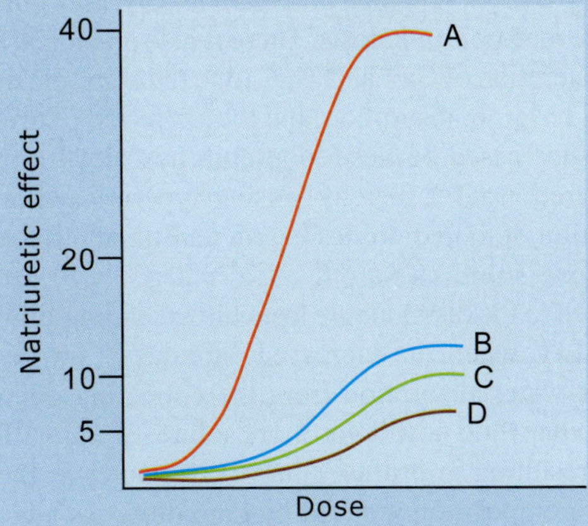

A—High-ceiling or loop diuretics
B—Thiazide diuretics
C—Osmotic diuretics
D—Potassium-sparing and Carbonic anhydrase inhibitors

Fig 16.2 Relative Natriuretic Efficacy of Diuretics

30 min. Their plasma half-life ranges from 30 min to 90 min and the duration of action 4–6 hours except torsemide (t½ 3.5 hours, duration of action 6 hours approx.). The relative potency order ranks as follows: *bumetanide > torsemide = piretanide > furosemide > ethacrynic acid.* Bumetanide is 40 times more potent than furosemide.

Mechanism of Action

These drugs act primarily on the thick segment of the ascending limb of LH inhibiting the reabsorption of NaCl out of the tubule into the interstitial tissue by inhibiting the $Na^+/K^+/2Cl^-$ cotransport carrier in the luminal membrane. Precisely speaking $Na^+/K^+/2Cl^-$ cotransport carrier protein exists in two isoforms. The secretory isoform is expressed on the basolateral membrane while the absorptive isoform is expressed at the luminal membrane of thick ascending limb of LH (also called as Cl^- binding site). The loop diuretics actually attach to the Cl^- binding site of this cotransport protein to inhibit the reabsorption of NaCl. Hence Na^+ and Cl^- are retained in the lumen and excreted. The increased Na^+ concentration now reaching the distal tubule promotes loss of H^+ and K^+. Loop diuretics, in high dose particularly, may thus produce metabolic alkalosis. There is also an increase in the excretion of Ca^{2+} and Mg^{2+} (due to inhibition of Ca^{2+} and Mg^{2+} reabsorption) but the excretion of uric acid is decreased because loop diuretics block uric acid secretion at PT, thereby causing hyperuricaemia. The action of loop diuretics has an additional effect, that more solutes (Na^+, K^+, Ca^{2+}, Mg^{2+}, Cl^-) are delivered to the distal tubule from the ascending limb of the LH, where its increased osmolarity further reduces water absorption from the collecting duct. The tubular fluid now holds more solutes along with water, resulting in profuse diuresis. Changes in the urinary composition induced by loop diuretics have been summarised in Table 16.2.

In addition to their prominent tubular transport inhibitory action they cause important changes in renal and systemic haemodynamics, probably because they induce renal prostaglandin synthesis. They transiently increase renal blood flow and also cause an increase in venous capacitance. As a result right ventricular filling pressure decreases even before the saluretic response becomes apparent. This ultimately provides quick relief in left ventricular failure and pulmonary oedema. Synthesis of PGE_2 and PGI_2 also contributes to Na^+ and K^+ excretion to some extent. Nonsteroidal anti-inflammatory agents, which inhibit prostaglandin synthesis, can interfere with the diuretic action of loop diuretics, particularly in patients of hepatic cirrhosis and nephrotic syndrome. Hyperglycaemic actions of loop diuretics are also observed, though less marked.

- BUMETANIDE is 40 times more potent than furosemide with lesser side effects. Its use is increasing because it may act in some cases not responding to furosemide. Dose 1–4 mg OD orally or 2–4 mg IM/slow IV.
- ETHCRYNIC ACID has practically gone out of use because of its ototoxicity and hepatotoxicity (which are greater than furosemide). Loss of K^+ is less marked but hypochloraemic alkalosis usually occurs.
- TORSEMIDE is 3 times more potent and longer acting than furosemide. Dose 2.5–5 mg OD orally or 5–10 mg OD orally in oedema.
- INDACRINONE (a uricosuric diuretic) is a ethacrynic acid analogue. It inhibits proximal tubular-uric acid absorption besides inhibiting Na^+ and Cl^- from the thick ascending LH. It is useful for the patients of gout requiring diuretic therapy where loop or thiazide diuretics are contraindicated.

Therapeutic Uses

1. The most important indications for the use of loop diuretics include oedematous conditions associated with congestive heart failure, cirrhosis of liver, and renal disease including nephrotic syndrome (as discussed above). Dose (furosemide) 40–80 mg slow I.V.
2. These can be used to treat hypertension (though thiazides are preferred) especially if it is complicated by renal impairment. Dose (furosemide) 20 mg OD orally or 40 mg every other day orally or 40 mg daily according to response.
3. Loop diuretics can increase the rate of urine flow and enhance K^+ excretion in acute renal failure. They may convert oliguric renal failure to non-oliguric failure which helps in management of renal failure.
4. These drugs can also be used to treat ingestion of toxic anions like Br^-, I^- or F^- because these are reabsorbed from the thick ascending LH. Normal saline may be administered during the therapy to replace urinary loss of Na^+ and Cl^- and to avoid extracellular fluid volume.
5. Mild hyperkalaemia can be successfully treated with loop diuretics as they enhance urinary excretion of K^+. This response is enhanced by simultaneous administration of NaCl and water.
6. **Non-diuretic Uses.** Loop diuretics can be used to treat mild to moderate hypercalcaemia because they increase Ca^{2+} excretion and urine flow; excess salt that is lost must, however, be replaced.

Adverse Effects

1. Loop diuretics can cause hyperuricaemia and precipitate the attacks of gout (as discussed above).

2. Hypercalciuria and hypomagnesaemia is a predictable consequence of the chronic use of loop diuretics as discussed above.
3. Loop diuretics cause hypokalaemia with hypokalaemic metabolic alkalosis (though more with thiazide diuretics; *see following text*) as they enhance the renal excretion of $K^+$and H^+. This can be reversed with K^+ replacement.
4. Ototoxicity (more with ethacrynic acid) can be caused by higher doses of loop diuretics, because they disturb the electrolyte composition of endolymph due to extrusion of Na^+ from endolymph to perilymph of the inner ear. These drugs also have a direct toxic action on the hair cells of internal ear. The risk is more in patients with impaired renal functions or in those receiving other ototoxic drugs like aminoglycoside antibiotics.
5. Hyperglycaemia (more with thiazides; *see following text*) can occur after chronic use of these drugs. Carbohydrate intolerance can be manifested due to inhibition of insulin release.
6. Hypersensitivity reactions in patients allergic to sulfonamides, can also occur. GIT disturbances, hepatotoxicity and at times pancreatitis can occur with ethacrynic acid. Myalgia may occur with bumetanide and piretanide.

Drug Interactions

1. Loop diuretics may enhance digitalis toxicity and can cause cardiac irregularities due to hypokalaemia.
2. Serum lithium levels may rise with loop diuretic therapy as they increase the reabsorption of Li^+ from the proximal tubule (PT).
3. Loop diuretics and aminoglycoside antibiotics exhibit additive ototoxicity and should not be used together.
4. Indomethacin and most NSAIDs, by inhibiting PGE_2 and PGI_2 synthesis, diminish the action of high-ceiling diuretics (see earlier discussion).
5. Probenecid competitively inhibits tubular secretion of furosemide at PT and therefore decreases its action.
6. Cotrimoxazole with loop diuretics increases the chances of thrombocytopenia.

Diuretics Acting on Proximal (Early) Part of the Distal Tubule

Thiazide Diuretics

The thiazides are most widely used of the diuretic drugs. They are sulfonamide derivatives but their chemical structure also resembles the carbonic anhydrase inhibitors like acetazolamide. *Hydrochlorothiazide* and *bendroflumethiazide* are prototype drugs. All thiazides affect the distal tubule and all have equal maximal diuretic effect, differing only in duration of action and potency (expressed in per milligram basis). Their potency rank order is as follows:

Polythiazide > Indapamide > Bendro-flumethiazide = Metolazone > Quinethazone = Hydrochlorothiazide = Chlorthalidone > Chlorothiazide.

Polythiazide is about 25 to 30 times more potent than hydrochlorothiazide; while chlorothiazide exhibits 1/10th of the potency of hydrochlorothiazide.

The rank order for their duration of action runs as follows:
Chlorthalidone > Polythiazide > Indapamide = Metolazone > Bendroflumethiazide > Hydrochlorothiazide > Chlorothiazide.

Chlorthalidone action lasts for more than 48 hours while that of chlorothiazide remains for 1.5–2 hours. When given by oral route, these are readily absorbed from the GIT. They are mainly secreted through the PT by the organic acid secretory mechanisms. Subsequently, they reach the site of action—early part of distal tubule. The longer acting agents have a high lipid solubility and consequently a higher aVd. They also undergo tubular reabsorption, which also prolongs their duration of action (Table 16.1).

Mechanism of Action

These drugs have a moderately powerful diuretic action causing excretion of 8–10% of Na^+ in the filtrate (Fig. 16.2). They decrease active reabsorption

Table 16.1 The Routes of Access, Sites and Mechanism of Action of Different Diuretics

Diuretic	Route of Access	Site of Action	Mechanism of Action
Loop diuretics	Organic acid secretory system at PT	Thick ascending LH	Inhibit $Na^+/K^+/2Cl^-$ Cotransport in luminal membrane.
Thiazide diuretics	Same as above	Early part of DT; also PT (clinically negligible)	Inhibit electro-neutral Na^+/Cl^- Cotransport.
Potassium-retaining diuretics			
▪ Amiloride group	Through organic base secretory system at PT	Latter part of DT and CT	Inhibit luminal mem. Na^+ channel and hence Na^+-K^+ exchange.
▪ Spironolactone	Through peritubular circulation	Same as above	Aldosterone receptor antagonist. Antagonises Na^+ retaining and K^+ excreting actions of aldosterone.
Osmotic diuretics	Glomerular filtration	PT, descending LH and CT	Passive H_2O reabsorption is reduced. H_2O is excreted with little Na^+
Carbonic anhydrase inhibitors	Secreted through PT	Mainly PT, also DT (subsidiary site of action)	Inhibit CA enzyme Increased excretion of HCO_3^-, Na^+ K^+ and H_2O

PT—Proximal tubule; LH—Loop of Henle; DT—Distal tubule; CT—Collecting tubule; CA—Carbonic anhydrase

of Na^+ and accompanying Cl^- by inhibiting electroneutral Na^+/Cl^- cotransport system (symport) operating in the early part of distal tubule (DT). When more sodium reaches the collecting duct from the DT, the high flow rate of the filtrate produced by these diuretics will also favour K^+ excretion by continually flushing it away, increasing the gradient from the principal cells to lumen. K^+ loss with these drugs is therefore significant.

In contrast to loop diuretics which increase the Ca^{2+} contents of the urine (hypercalciuria), thiazide diuretics decrease the Ca^{2+} concentration of urine by promoting its reabsorption. It has been postulated that the lowering of intracellular Na^+ (due to its excretion by thiazides) enhances Na^+/Ca^{2+} exchange in basolateral membrane which in turn promotes overall reabsorption of Ca^{2+}.

During diuresis with thiazides, the urine is rich in Na^+ and Cl^- but almost free of HCO_3^-. Thus there is increased concentration of HCO_3^- per unit volume of ECF because extracellular fluid volume is also reduced due to diuretic action. Furthermore, aldosterone stimulation in collecting tubule promotes hypokalaemia and H^+ secretion which stimulates HCO_3^- reabsorption from the PT. All these events lead to the development of hypochloraemic metabolic alkalosis due to thiazide diuretics.

Like loop diuretics, action of thiazides is also partly mediated by renal PGE_2 and PGI_2 synthesis. Hence the actions of thiazides can also be inhibited by NSAIDs as discussed above.

Thiazide diuretics also inhibit carbonic anhydrase (CA) enzyme in PT but it does not seem to contribute significantly to their diuretic action.

Therapeutic Uses

Diuretic Use (Oedematous Conditions): (1) As described under loop diuretics, these can also be used to relieve pulmonary oedema due to congestive heart failure, nephrotic syndrome and pregnancy. However, they should be avoided or used with caution in patients having oedema due to liver cirrhosis because hypokalaemia and hypochloraemic alkalosis may precipitate hepatic encephalopathy and even coma. Increased hypokalaemia aggravates alkalosis and generates more NH_3 which a cirrhotic liver cannot convert to urea. Hence coma may ensue. Further, thiazide diuretics increase protein catabolism. This increases amino acid levels in blood which a cirrhotic liver cannot metabolise. Hence tryptophan levels increase and can cross BBB to accumulate in brain leading to encephalopathy.

Usual doses: *Hydrochlorothiazide* (hypertension) 12.5–50 mg/day; for oedema 25–100 mg/day oral. *Clopamide* (hypertension) 10–20 mg/day; for oedema 20–40 mg/day oral. *Benzthiazide* (hypertension) 25 mg/day; for oedema 25–100 mg/day oral.

(2) In essential hypertension, thiazides are the first drugs to be used. The initial fall in blood pressure results from the decreased blood volume caused by diuresis, but the later phase seems to be caused by direct vasodilator effects (because diazoxide which is a thiazide chemically but a non-diuretic otherwise, also is a powerful vasodilating drug used in hypertensive emergencies). Many patients can be continued for years on smaller doses of thiazides alone with K^+ supplements. However, some patients also require additional medication such as β-adrenergic blockers. *Indapamide,* at low doses shows significant antihypertensive action with less metabolic disturbances.

Non-diuretic (non-oedematous) Use: (1) Thiazide diuretics have a paradoxical effect in diabetes insipidus, where they reduce the volume of urine. This they do by inhibiting cyclonucleotide phosphodiesterase enzyme and thus indirectly increase the 3,5-cyclic AMP levels even when ADH cannot generate 3,5-cyclic AMP directly. Hence membrane permeability of collecting tubule towards H_2O is increased and more water is reabsorbed from collecting ducts and distal end of distal tubule.

Another explanation is based on the decrease in extracellular fluid volume produced by thiazide diuretics, which leads to hyponatraemia. The latter condition stimulates Na^+ and water reabsorption from PT which in turn decreases delivery of the filtrate to the DT and also causes a decrease in urinary output. This hypothesis gathers support from the fact that a decrease in GFR by dehydration or by drug-induced hypotension also has beneficial effect. Dose (hydrochlorothiazide) up to 100 mg/day oral.

(2) The thiazides can be useful in treating idiopathic hypercalciuria because they inhibit urinary Ca^{2+} excretion. The effect is therefore beneficial for the patients suffering from renal calcium oxalate stones.

Adverse Effects

1. **Hypokalaemia**: Hyponatraemia produced by thiazides promotes the release of aldosterone which causes compensatory Na^+ retention and K^+ loss leading to hypokalaemia. In normal person it may lead to weakness, paraesthesia, fatigue and cramps but in patients receiving digitalis, it may aggravate digitalis toxicity. Also, in patients having severe liver disease, hypokalaemia may precipitate hepatic encephalopathy and coma (see above). Hence, thiazide diuretics are usually given along with potassium supplements or with a potassium-sparing diuretic.
2. **Hypochloraemic Alkalosis**: Thiazide diuretics cause hypochloraemic alkalosis with urine rich in chloride ions (for explanation, see above). This is not a major problem for normal person as it can be compensated by respiration.
3. **Hyperuricaemia**: Because they compete with uric acid secretion in the proximal tubule and may aggravate the attack of gout (see above).
4. **Hypercalcaemia**: They inhibit the secretion of Ca^{2+} and should be used with caution in cases of hyperparathyroidism (see above).
5. **Hyperglycaemia**: Thiazides stimulate glycogenolysis and also inhibit insulin secretion from the pancreas. This may exacerbate diabetes mellitus.
6. **Hyperlipidaemia**: They cause reversible increase in total cholesterol, LDL and triglycerides on chronic use.
7. **Erectile dysfunction** in males, which normalises after stopping the drug, is an idiosyncratic reaction observed with the use of thiazides.

8. **Hypersensitivity reactions** such as skin rashes, blood dyscrasias, and rarely pancreatitis, may also be observed with these drugs.

Drug Interactions

(1) Digitalis; (2) Lithium; (3) Probenecid and (4) Corticosteroids (as discussed under loop diuretics)

- CHLORTHALIDONE is as potent as hydrochlorothiazide but has a long duration of action (48 hrs). Therefore, it is often used to treat hypertension and is administered once daily. For mild hypertensives it can be given on alternate day. Dose 25–100 mg/day orally.
- INDAPAMIDE is a highly lipid-soluble, nonthiazide diuretic which is more potent and longer acting than hydrochlorothiazide. It is used to treat hypertension because it lowers the BP at a dose lower than that required for diuresis and produces lesser hypokalaemia, hyperglycaemia and hyperuricaemia. Dose 2.5–5 mg per day orally.
- METOLAZONE is also a non-thiazide diuretic which is more potent and longer acting than hydrochlorothiazide. It has a clinically useful response even in severe renal failure as it can produce Na^+ excretion in advanced renal failure. Dose (hypertension) 2.5–5 mg/day oral ; for oedema 5–20 mg/day orally.
- XIPAMIDE is a more potent and longer acting non-thiazide diuretic, but hypokalaemia is more prominent than with hydrochlorothiazide. Dose (hypertension) 20 mg/day; for oedema 40 mg/day orally.
- Typical thiazides like POLYTHIAZIDE and BENDROFLUMETHIAZIDE differ from hydrochlorothiazide only in potency and duration of action. Both are more potent and longer acting than hydrochlorothiazide. Dose (polythiazide): hypertension 2–4 mg/day; oedema 4 mg/day oral; (Bendroflumethiazide) 2.5–10 mg/day oral.

Potassium-Sparing Diuretics

a) Inhibitors of Na^+ Channels at Collecting Ducts

There are at present two drugs in this category—**amiloride** and **triamterene**. Both are secreted through organic base secretory system at the PT, and act by inhibiting the luminal Na^+ channels at distal part of DT and collecting tubules (CT). Blocking of these channels inhibits Na^+ reabsorption and K^+ excretion.

Mechanism of Action

By the time the filtrate reaches CT, most of the Na^+ has already been absorbed. When amiloride and triamterene block the epithelial Na^+ channels, reabsorption of Na^+ is prevented. As a result the lumen negative potential, which is the driving force for K^+ secretion reduces (*see previous text*). Therefore, while the net loss of Na^+ is minor, K^+ excretion is prevented indirectly to a significant level. The intercalated cells in CD possess an ATP-driven H^+ pump which secretes H^+ into the lumen. These drugs, by reducing the lumen negative potential, inhibit this pump and decrease secretion of H^+ concentration as well (leading to metabolic acidosis). Since their mode of action is independent of aldosterone, these have diuretic activity even in the patients of Addison's disease. Amiloride is not metabolised in liver and therefore is ten times more potent and longer acting compared to triamterene. Both are mildly uricosuric.

Therapeutic Uses

Diuretic Use: (1) To treat oedematous conditions including liver cirrhosis, as hyperkalaemia produced by them is advantageous in these situations. Combined with thiazides, they can be used to treat refractory oedema. (2) In combination with thiazides or loop diuretics they are used to treat hypertension, because they check hypokalaemia, a side effect of these diuretics. Dose (Amiloride) 5–10 mg/day; (Triamterene) 50–100 mg/day oral.

Non-diuretic Use: (1) Amiloride blocks Li^+ reabsorption through Na^+ channels in the CD principal cells and thus reduces lithium-induced polyuria. (2) When given as an aerosol, amiloride can be used to treat cystic fibrosis because it increases fluidity of respiratory secretion. (3) In situations of potassium loss.

Adverse Effects

1. Hyperkalaemia: These should not be given along with potassium supplements or with ACE inhibitors to avoid exacerbation of hyper-kalaemia.
2. Triamterene causes rise in blood urea, nausea, dizziness and muscle cramps. Being poorly soluble it can precipitate renal stones.
3. Amiloride causes diarrhoea and skin rashes (rarely).
4. Amiloride, if given by I.V. or I.M. route may decrease BP due to histamine release.

Drug Interactions

Potassium supplements and ACE inhibitors (as discussed above). NSAIDs can decrease the effects of these agents. Quinidine with amiloride may increase the risk of arrhythmias.

Aldosterone Receptor Antagonists

Spironolactone is an aldosterone receptor antagonist with a limited diuretic action, because it acts on the distal part of DT and collecting tubules (CT) from where only 3–5% of NaCl is absorbed. It is secreted through peritubular circulation. Its onset of action is slow but duration of action is longer (t½ 16–24 hrs), because its active metabolite *canrenone* also has similar effects. Spironolactone is mainly excreted through urine, but also through bile, and undergoes enterohepatic circulation which also contributes for its longer duration of action.

Mechanism of Action

Spironolactone competes for aldosterone receptors in the cells of distal tubule and collecting tubule. The drug-receptor complex is unable to attach to the requisite DNA. Therefore, the subsequent processes of transcription, translation and production of aldosterone's mediator proteins do not occur. The latter are responsible for opening of Na^+ channels. The result is inhibition of Na^+ reabsorption and concomitant decrease in K^+ secretion (as discussed above). Spironolactone has subsidiary actions in decreasing H^+ secretion and also uric acid excretion.

Therapeutic Uses

Diuretic Use: (1) In oedematous disorders due to primary hyperaldosteronism (Conn's syndrome) or in secondary hyperaldosteronism caused by hepatic cirrhosis complicated by ascites. (2) In hyper-tension, along with thiazide or loop diuretics to counteract hypokalaemia. Dose 25–100 mg BD oral.

Non-diuretic Use: (1) In congestive heart failure where it retards disease progression and reduces mortality. (2) In conditions of hypokalaemia.

Adverse Effects

(1) Hyperkalaemia (as discussed above); (2) Delays healing of peptic ulcers; (3) GIT disturbances, skin rashes, gynaecomastia, menstrual irregularities (but these incidences are rare; however, higher doses on chronic basis should be avoided).

Drug Interactions

Same as discussed under other K^+-sparing diuretics.

- EPLERENONE is a selective aldosterone antagonist but drug interactions are more. Besides those discussed under other K^+-sparing diuretics, it is a substrate for CYP3A4 and hence concurrent use of enzyme inhibitors like fluconazole, ketoconazole, erythromycin and verapamil lead to manifold increase in eplerenone concentration. Dose 50 mg once daily orally (dose to be reduced with concurrent use of CYP-3A4 inhibitors) (Table 16.2, 16.3).

OSMOTIC DIURETICS

These are the diuretics which act indirectly by modifying the contents of urinary filtrate by increasing the osmolarity. Water loss is, however, more than Na^+ loss. A common clinical example of osmotic diuresis is polyuria in diabetes mellitus. In such cases the filtered load of glucose from glomerulus exceeds the reabsorptive capacity of the tubule. The non-reabsorbed glucose now acts as osmotic diuretic causing polyuria.

Clinically used osmotic diuretics like *mannitol* (20–25% I.V.) or *glycerol* (1.5 g/kg orally)

Table 16.2 Electrolyte Changes in Urine and Plasma after Administering Diuretics

Diuretic Group	Urinary excretion of electrolytes and water						Effects on plasma contents
	Na^+	Cl^-	K^+	Ca^{2+}	$NaHCO_3$	Volume (H_2O)	
Loop diuretics	↑↑↑↑	↑↑↑	↑↑	↑↑↑ along with Mg^{2+}	±	↑↑↑	Hypokalaemia, Hypokalaemic metabolic alkalosis, Hyperuricaemia, Hypocalcaemia (Hypercalciuria), Hypomagnesaemia, Hyperglycaemia
Thiazide diuretics	↑↑↑	↑↑↑	↑↑	↓↓	±	↑↑	Hypokalaemia, Hypochloraemic alkalosis, Hyperuricaemia, Hypercalcaemia, Hyperglycaemia
Potassium-sparing diuretics	↑	↑	↓↓	↑	↓	↑	Hyperkalaemia, Metabolic acidosis (↑ in H^+ conc)
CA inhibitors	↑	±↓	↑↑	↑↑	↑↑	↑	Hypokalaemia, Acidosis Hypocalcaemia (Hypercalciuria)
Osmotic diuretics	↑	↑	±	±	±	↑↑↑ Mainly water	Transient ↑ in extracellular fluid volume and hyponatraemia

↑ Increase; ↓ Decrease; CA, Carbonic anhydrase

are pharmacologically inert substances that are filtered from glomerulus but incompletely reabsorbed or not reabsorbed at all by the nephron.

Mechanism of Action

Mannitol when given I.V., initially increases the osmolarity of extracellular fluid. To equalise this osmolarity, water shifts from intracellular space to extracellular space, which increases filtration load at glomerulus. Once within the nephron, their main effect is exerted on those parts of nephron that are freely permeable to water: the proximal tubule, the descending limb of LH and the collecting tubules. Due to the presence of non-reabsorbable inert mannitol, along with other electrolytes, the hypertonicity of the fluid inside the lumen increases. This inhibits water reabsorption from the tubule, and the volume of voidable urine increases. This has the secondary effect on reducing Na^+ reabsorption since its concentration within the tubule is lower (because of dilution) than it otherwise would be. High osmotic pressure of urine (due to non- reabsorbable mannitol) makes ADH less effective which further

Table 16.3 Therapeutic Uses of Diuretics

Diuretic	Therapeutic uses	
	Diuretic use	**Non-Diuretic use**
Loop diuretics	Oedematous disorders associated with CHF, liver cirrhosis and nephrotic syndrome. Hypertension with renal disease. Br, I^- overdose. Acute renal failure	Hypercalcaemia, also renal tubular acidosis
Thiazide diuretics	Oedematous disorders (except liver cirrhosis) Hypertension (essential)	Hypercalciuria Diabetes insipidus
Potassium-sparing diuretics a) Amiloride	Oedematous disorders inclusive of liver cirrhosis (secondary hyperaldosteronism). Hypertension (used with thiazide diuretics)	Lithium-induced polyuria Cystic fibrosis Hypokalaemia
b) Spironolactone	Same as above execpt that it can also be used in primary hyperaldosteronism (Conn's syndrome)	Congestive heart failure Hypokalaemia
CA inhibitors	Not used, self-limiting action. Sometimes with loop diuretics in cases of diuretic resistance	Glaucoma. Metabolic alkalosis. To treat urate calculi or cystinuria. High altitude sickness. Epilepsy
Osmotic diuretics	Acute renal failure	Cerebral oedema Raised intraocular pressure

helps diuresis. Therefore, the main effect of osmotic diuretics is to increase the amount of water, with a relatively small increase in Na^+ excretion.

Therapeutic Uses

To treat oliguria state in shock or crush injury and to prevent onset of renal failure in such cases. In the latter condition, the GFR is reduced and the absorption of NaCl and water from the PT is almost complete as a compensatory phenomenon. As a result all the distal parts of the nephron virtually get dried up, and urine flow ceases. Retention of fluid within the tubule by administering osmotic diuretics limits these effects and prevents onset of renal failure.

Non-diuretic Use: The intravenous administration of pharmacologically inert and non-reabsorbable mannitol increases plasma osmolarity, which results in a shift of intracellular fluid from the brain and eye. The osmotic diuretics are therefore used to treat acutely raised intracranial (cerebral oedema) and intraocular pressure (glaucoma). It has nothing to do with the kidney or resultant diuresis. In fact, the effect is lost as soon as mannitol appears in the urine.

Adverse Effects

There is transient expansion of extracellular fluid volume as a result of extraction of water from the intracellular compartment. Since diuretic effect will take its own time, this transient expansion of extracellular fluid volume and hyponatraemia may worsen the condition of cardiac failure, pulmonary oedema or both. If administered orally, mannitol causes osmotic diarrhoea. Hence it can be given orally in conjunction with activated charcoal to eliminate poisons or toxic substances from the GIT.

CARBONIC ANHYDRASE INHIBITORS

With the development of newer agents, the carbonic anhydrase (CA) inhibitors are now rarely used as diuretics. Yet, there are some specific applications of their use that will be discussed below. *Acetazolamide* is a typical prototype drug. Others include *dorzolamide, ethoxzolamide, methazolamide* and *dichlorphenamide*. These are secreted through S2 segment of PT which is also their site of action.

Mechanism of Action

CA inhibitors cause increased excretion of HCO_3^- with accompanying Na^+, K^+ and water (see earlier text under PT; Fig. 16.1). Due to CA inhibition at the distal part of distal tubule, the physiological mechanisms for the acidification of urine also fail. Hence the net result is excretion of alkaline urine containing $NaHCO_3$, $KHCO_3$ and water with mild metabolic acidosis. Because of metabolic acidosis and HCO_3^- depletion, the body tries to conserve Na^+ by enhancing its reabsorption from the remaining tubule segments in the nephron. As a result, with use over couple of days, the action of CA inhibitor becomes self-limiting.

Therapeutic Uses

Because of their self-limiting action, the major clinical applications of CA inhibitors involve sites other than kidney:

1. **Glaucoma**: The ciliary body of eyes normally secretes $NaHCO_3$ into the aqueous humour by a process similar to the reabsorption of $NaHCO_3$ from PT. Inhibition of CA, therefore, decreases aqueous humour formation by reducing $NaHCO_3$ concentration, and causes a decrease in intraocular pressure. *Acetazolamide* is given orally but *dorzolamide* and *brinzolamide* are instilled topically in eye (see Ch. 11). Thus systemic metabolic and diuretic effects are reduced. Dose (acetazolamide) 250 mg OD/BD, orally.
2. **Urinary Alkalinisation (to treat urate calculi and cystinuria)**: In the patients of leukaemia and lymphomas, chemotherapy causes hyperuricaemia due to rapid metabolism of nucleoproteins. Urate calculi, therefore, get precipitated in renal tubules and can lead to renal shutdown. CA inhibitors make urine alkaline in which urate calculi are soluble. Similarly, in certain genetic conditions, reabsorption of cystine gets drastically reduced and gets deposited in renal tubules. These are also soluble in alkaline urine produced by CA inhibitors.
3. **Metabolic Alkalosis**: CA inhibitors can be used to treat mild metabolic alkalosis as they produce hyperchloraemic acidosis.
4. **Epilepsy**: These can be used to treat petit mal epilepsy or can be tried as a last resort if patient is not responding to any kind of antiepileptic therapy. The mechanism is not clearly known. However, increased P_{CO_2} levels, as a result of metabolic acidosis, decrease the pH and thus may prevent convulsions (pH > 7.4 leads to convulsions). Alternatively, an increase in Cl^- ion concentration in plasma may provide a stabilizing effect on neuronal membrane by causing hyperpolarisation.
5. **Acute Mountain Sickness**: By decreasing cerebrospinal fluid formation and by decreasing its pH, CA inhibitors can enhance performance status of those mountain travelers who rapidly ascend high altitudes of more than 10,000 feet. Acetazolamide given once daily every night for 5 days before the ascent can prevent weakness, breathlessness, dizziness, nausea and at times cerebral and pulmonary oedema associated with high altitude sickness.
6. It has been found that the inhibition of CA by acetazolamide is also *useful in reducing respiratory work* in patients who are weaned from a respirator.

Adverse Effects

(1) Refractoriness after repeated use (as discussed above); (2) Hyperchloraemic acidosis (as discussed above); (3) Drowsiness and paraesthesia; (4) Hypokalaemia.

CHAPTER 17

Vasoactive Peptides and Nitric Oxide

COMPETENCY PH1.24

This chapter focuses on the vascular and other smooth muscle actions of the vasoactive peptides. These peptides include the *vasoconstrictor peptides* (angiotensin-II, vasopressin, endothelins, neuropeptide-Y and urotensin) and *vasodilator peptides* (bradykinin and related kinins, natriuretic peptides, vasoactive intestinal peptide, substance P, neurotensin, calcitonin gene–related peptide and adrenomedullin). Among these, angiotensin-II will be discussed in Chapter 18 and bradykinin and related kinins in Chapter 24. The pharmacology of remaining vasoconstrictor and vasodilator peptides as well as of nitric oxide (NO), which is a gaseous vasodilator, is discussed in this chapter.

VASOCONSTRICTOR PEPTIDES

Vasopressin (ADH, Antidiuretic Hormone)

Vasopressin, a nonapeptide hormone, is released by the posterior pituitary in response to rising plasma osmolarity or falling blood pressure. It promotes water reabsorption from the collecting duct (CD) of kidney and thus plays an important role in the long-term control of blood pressure (BP). Vasopressin also constricts blood vessels and can raise BP (hence the name vasopressin) but at higher doses than those required for maximal antidiuresis.

The terms *vasopressin, arginine vasopressin* (AVP) and *antidiuretic hormone* (ADH) are synonyms and used interchangeably. The mammalian ADH is 8-arginine-vasopressin (AVP). Its deficiency results in *diabetes insipidus*. Diabetes means "overflow" and insipidus means "tasteless". This disorder should not be confused with *diabetes mellitus* (meli = honey), a disorder of pancreas characterised by excretion of glucose in urine. Diabetes insipidus (DI) results from hyposecretion of ADH, and is usually associated with dysfunction of posterior pituitary or non-functional ADH receptors. Symptoms of DI include: excretion of large amounts of urine, dehydration and thirst. Bed wetting is common in afflicted children. Because so much water is lost through urine, a person with severe DI may die of dehydration if deprived of water. DI resulting from hyposecretion of ADH is called *central DI* (neurogenic or neurohypophyseal DI). It results due to head injury or tumour. It may also be idiopathic or familial. It is an ADH-responsive DI and can be treated by administering ADH through nasal spray. In contrast, *nephrogenic DI* is ADH resistant and results due to non-functional ADH receptors in collecting duct, although the hormone is present in normal amounts. About 25% of cases are idiopathic or familial. It may also occur due to drug or due to renal damage from heavy metal poisoning. In contrast to DI, there may be a state of increased ADH secretion also, which is characterised by syndrome of inappropriate secretion of ADH (SIADH). It may result from head injury, meningitis or encephalitis. It is characterised by low plasma osmolarity, water retention and dilutional hyponatraemia.

Regulation of Release of Vasopressin

ADH is released from the posterior pituitary in response to a decrease in plasma volume (hypovolaemia) or increase in plasma osmolality (which produces thirst). Pain, stress, anxiety, ACh, nicotine, morphine, indomethacin, chlorpropamide, carbamazepine and general anaesthetics also stimulate secretion of ADH (decrease in urine output). The osmoreceptors in hypothalamic nuclei, which are sensitive to the osmolarity of blood, regulate the release of ADH into blood. When osmolarity is increased (dehydration), ADH secretion is also increased (antidiuresis). Conversely, a reduction in osmolarity (overhydration) inhibits ADH release (increased urine output; Fig. 17.1). In certain chronic conditions where effective circulating blood volume is reduced as in CHF, cirrhosis of liver, and after prolonged use of diuretics, ADH release is stimulated through baroreceptors in left atrium, aorta and pulmonary vein. Angiotensin-II (in dehydration) also releases ADH.

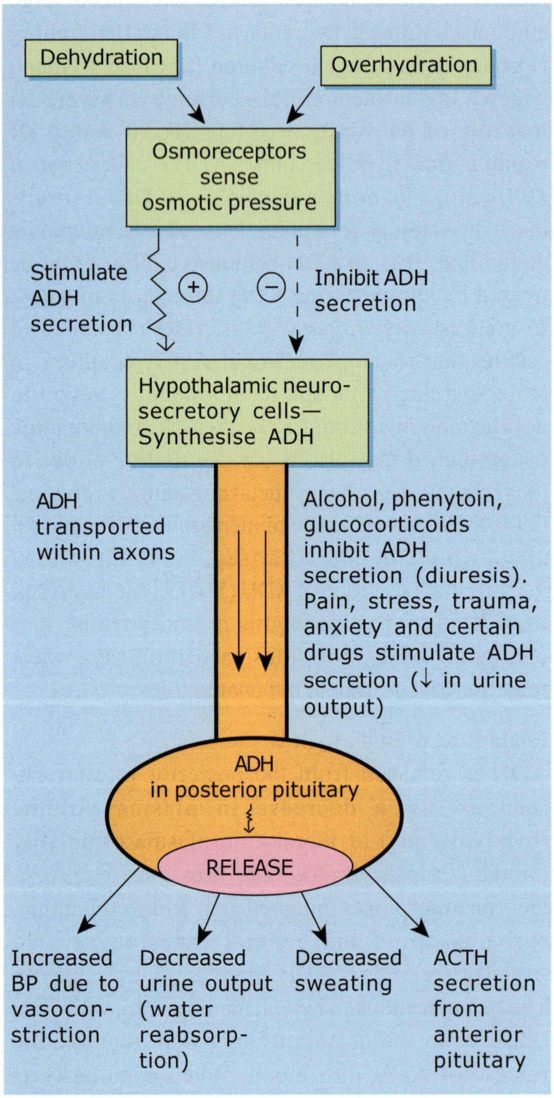

Fig 17.1 Regulation of Release and Effects of ADH.

On the other hand, ethanol, phenytoin and glucocorticoids inhibit ADH secretion. Lithium and demeclocycline partially antagonise ADH action by inhibiting cAMP formation. Their side effect (polyuria and polydipsia) has been utilised in patients suffering with syndrome of inappropriate (excess) ADH secretion (SIADH).

ADH Receptors

There are three classes of receptors for ADH: V_{1a}, V_{1b} and V_2 (some texts refer to as V_1, V_2 and V_3; (V_{1b} representing V_3). Antidiuretic action is mediated through V_2 receptors, occurs at low plasma concentrations of ADH and involves activation of adenylate cyclase in renal collecting ducts (CD). V_2 receptor activation also accelerates insertion of "preformed" aquaporin-2 channels into apical membrane of principal cells in CD, to increase renal conservation of water. V_{1a} and V_{1b} receptors are coupled to phospholipase-C/IP_3 system. Vasoconstriction is mediated through V_{1a} receptors and requires higher concentrations of ADH than that required for antidiuretic action. In the CNS, ADH acts as a neuromodulator and also as neurotransmitter. After getting released into the pituitary portal circulation, it promotes the release of ACTH from the anterior pituitary by acting through V_{1b} receptors. Vasopressin receptors are G-protein coupled receptors. The characteristic features of different vasopressin receptors have been summarised in Table 17.1.

ADH Receptor Agonists (Vasopressin Analogues)

Various analogues of ADH have been developed with an aim to increase the duration and specificity of receptor action.

VASOPRESSIN itself has a short duration of action (t½ 20 min). Its V_1/V_2 receptor actions are nonselective. It can be administered by any parenteral route or by intranasal application. If given orally, it is inactivated by trypsin.

DESMOPRESSIN has an increased duration of action (t½ 2 hrs, but action lasts for 10 hrs). It has V_2 receptor selective action and is usually given by any parenteral route or as nasal spray. It is now also

Table 17.1 Characteristic Features of Different Vasopressin Receptors

Characteristics	Vasopressin Receptors		
	V_{1a}	V_{1b}*	V_2
Location	Vascular and other smooth muscle, platelets[1] and hepatocytes[1], wider distribution	Anterior pituitary	Collecting duct cells of kidney, vascular endothelium
Function	Vasoconstriction. Visceral smooth muscle contraction. Platelet aggregation[1], Glycogenolysis[1]	ACTH release	Antidiuretic action
Mechanism	Release of Ca^{2+} through phospholipase C/IP_3-DAG pathway[2]	Same as for V_{1a}	Activation of adenylate cyclase in renal collecting duct (CD)

* In some texts it is designated as V_3 receptor

1 Physiological significance of such extrarenal receptors and the effects is not known

2 Also activates phospholipase A_2, release of arachidonic acid and hence synthesis of PGE_2. Since PGE_2 inhibits adenylate cyclase in CD, stimulation of PGE_2 synthesis by V_{1a} receptor reduces V_2 receptor mediated antidiuresis. Indomethacin, being a PGE_2 synthesis inhibitor enhances the antidiuretic response to vasopressin. V_{1a} receptor also activates proto-oncogene, through IP_3 DAG pathway and hence promotes the growth of vasuclar smooth muscle.

available as oral preparation but the doses are 10–15 times higher than intranasal dose. Desmopressin is 12–15 times more potent than vasopressin as antidiuretic. It has negligible V_1 receptor action.

TERLIPRESSIN is a prodrug of vasopressin and has an increased duration of action. It has low but prolonged vasopressor action (more selective V_1 receptor agonist) with minimal antidiuretic effects (V_2) and does not enhance fibrinolysis. Hence it is a preferred analogue of ADH for treating variceal bleeding.

FELYPRESSIN has a short duration of action. It has mainly vasoconstrictor action (V_1) and is used with local anaesthetics to prolong their action (see Ch. 15).

LYPRESSIN is 8-lysine vasopressin. Though less potent than vasopressin, it has a longer duration of action. *It is used in place of vasopressin for vasopressor (V_1) action.*

Therapeutic Uses

Based on V_1 Receptor Action

1) ***Bleeding Oesophageal Varices*** (Preferred drug: TERLIPRESSIN)

   V_1 receptor mediated constriction of mesenteric blood vessels and the resultant reduction of blood flow through the liver to the varices stops bleeding of oesophageal varices. Simultaneous addition of nitroglycerin with vasopressin (or terlipressin) reduces the cardiotoxic effects of vasopressin, while enhances the beneficial splanchnic effects of the drug. Terlipressin has lesser side effects than vasopressin. Dose: initially 2 mg followed by 1 mg every 6 hr I.V. until bleeding stops (max. 72 hr).

2) ***Miscellaneous Uses***
   a) V_1 receptor mediated contraction of intestinal smooth muscle is utilised to treat postoperative paralytic ileus and to drive out intestinal gases before abdominal radiography.
   b) Vasopressin (or terlipressin) can be used during abdominal surgery, in patients with portal hypertension to reduce the risk of haemorrhage.
   c) These drugs can also be used to prevent bleeding in acute haemorrhagic gastritis because of their V_1 receptor mediated vasoconstriction of the gastric vascular bed.

Based on V_2 Receptor Action (Preferred drug: DESMOPRESSIN)

1. ***Diabetes Insipidus (DI)***
   Only central DI (neurogenic or neurohypophyseal DI) responds to administration of desmopressin; nephrogenic DI does not, because ADH receptors on collecting ducts are non-functional. Treatment of central DI needs long-term therapy and therefore vasopressin is not suitable because of its short duration of action, besides V_1 receptor mediated side effects. However, desmopressin is also used to differentiate between neurogenic and nephrogenic DI. The urine volume is reduced and its osmolarity gets increased if DI is due to deficiency of ADH (central DI) but not when it is a case of nephrogenic DI (unresponsiveness of ADH receptors). The dose of desmopressin is then individually tailored on the basis of 24 hrs urine output. Dose: (oral) 100 μg TDS; (nasal) 10–40 μg/day; (I.V., I.M. or S.C) 1–4 μg/day.
2. ***Primary Nocturnal Enuresis***
   For this purpose desmopressin is used intranasally with restricted fluid intake and behavioural conditioning. Dose: (oral) 200–400 μg at bed time; (nasal) 20–40 μg at bedtime.
3. ***To Relieve Post–lumbar Puncture Headache***
   Due to its water retention property, it facilitates equilibration of fluid osmolarity in CNS.
4. ***Bleeding Disorders in Patients of Haemophilia A and von Willebrand's Disease***
   Desmopressin elevates factor VIII and von Willebrand factor and shortens bleeding time. However, tachyphylaxis to desmopressin develops after several days, due to depletion of factor VIII and von Willebrand factor storage sites, which limits its usefulness. Dose: 0.3–0.4 μg/kg slow I.V. (15–30 min) before surgery.

Adverse Effects

V_1 Receptor Mediated Adverse Effects

These effects are more with vasopressin, terlipressin and lypressin than with desmopressin. These include facial pallor (due to cutaneous vasoconstriction); nausea, abdominal cramps and an urge to defecate (due to increased intestinal motility); and precipitation of angina (due to constriction of coronary arteries). It is contraindicated in patients of hypertension and ischaemic heart disease.

V_2 Receptor Mediated Adverse Effects

Mainly, fluid retention and hyponatraemia may occur. Carbamazepine, indomethacin and chlorpropamide can potentiate the antidiuretic effects of desmopressin.

Common to Vasopressin and Desmopressin

Intranasal administration may cause irritation, ulceration and rhinitis. Urticaria, pruritus and other forms of allergy may occur, but rarely.

Vasopressin (ADH) Receptor Antagonists

There are two types of ADH receptor antagonists: (1) The peptide group of antagonists and (2) the non-peptide antagonists. Incidentally, the peptide antagonists antagonise all other actions of vasopression except for its antidiuretic effects. Hence, these are of hardly any clinical use.

Non-peptide ADH-receptor antagonists (the *vaptans*) have been introduced for the treatment of the conditions like SIADH. *Lithium* is effective but the toxicity outweighs its benefits. *Demeclocycline* can be used but it exhibits many side effects and several drug interactions. Moreover its antibacterial effects are not desired in this context. Hence, till date the restricted water intake is the only remedy for the treatment of SIADH.

Conivaptan (t½ 5–10 hrs) is the first non-peptide ADH receptor antagonist approved for the treatment of euvolaemic hyponatraemias (SIADH) and congestive heart failure where water retention, as a result of ADH excess, leads to dangerous hyponatraemia. But its disadvantages include: (1) Requirement of I.V. administration (not suitable for out patient settings); (2) Its non-selective action, i.e., it is an antagonist for both V_2 and V_{1a} receptors and (3) It cannot be administered concurrently with CYP3A4 inhibitors like ketoconazole, itraconazole, indinavir and ritonavir, etc. However, ***tolvaptan (t½ 12–24 hrs)*** a non-peptide orally active, selective V_2 receptor antagonists have been approved. Others like ***lixivaptan, satavaptan*** and ***mozavaptan*** are under submission for approval. By blocking V_2 receptors they prevent ADH-induced water reabsorption via aquaporin-2 channels in apical membrane of CD cells. These drugs are recommended to treat euvolaemic hyponatraemia and for water retention associated with SIADH, heart failure and cirrhotic ascites. Clinical trials reveal that ***tolvaptan*** also retards the vasopressin-driven growth of renal cysts in polycystic kidney disease. *Side effects* include, postural hypotension, hypokalaemia, polydipsia and polyuria.

Endothelins

These are very potent vasoconstrictor peptides derived from the endothelial cells of vasculature like nitric oxide (NO) and PGI_2. While endothelin (ET) is a potent endothelium-derived vasoconstrictor, NO and PGI_2 are two potent endothelium-derived vasodilators.

Biosynthesis, Release and Distribution (Fig. 17.2)

Three isoforms of ETs have been characterised. These are primarily ET-1 but two similar peptides ET-2 and ET-3 are also known. ET-1 is also present in brain and kidney. ET-1 is synthesised by a precursor prepro-ET which is processed to BIG-ET-1 and finally cleaved by an *endothelin-converting enzyme* to ET-1. This converting enzyme is a metalloprotease and is inhibited *phosphoramidon* and CGS 35066 (see following text). Stimuli to ET-1 synthesis in the endothelium include growth factors and cytokines (interleukin-1;TGF-β), angiotensin II, vasopressin and hypoxia. Inhibitors to ET-1 synthesis include NO, PGI_2 and atrial natriuretic peptide.

Endothelin Receptors and Responses

Two ET receptor subtypes ET_A and ET_B have been identified. ET_A receptors are primarily located on vascular smooth muscle (but not on the endothelium), brain, lungs, intestine, kidney and adrenal gland. ET_A receptor mediated responses mainly include vasoconstriction, broncho-constriction and aldosterone secretion. ET-1 preferentially activates ET_A receptors. ET_B receptors are primarily located on vascular endothelial cells (but not on the vascular smooth muscle) where they mediate vasodilatation through release of PGI_2 and NO. These receptors are also found in brain, intestine, kidney and adrenal gland. The physiological role of ET_B receptor is poorly understood.

When ET-1 is administered intravenously, there is a transient fall in arterial blood pressure initially (ET_B effect) followed by a prolonged rise (ET_A effect). As explained above, the depressor effect results from release of PGI_2 and NO from vascular endothelium, while the pressor response is a consequence of direct vasoconstriction of vascular smooth muscle. In heart ET-1 produces tachycardia, increase in force of contraction and coronary vasoconstriction. It also causes broncho-constriction, renal vasoconstriction and decrease in glomerular filtration. In endocrine system it releases renin, aldosterone and vasopressin (ET_A effect) and atrial natriuretic peptide (ET_B effect). Finally, ET-1 also stimulates mitogenesis in vascular smooth muscle cells and cardiac myocytes (long-term ET_A/ET_B mediated effect).

Both ET_A and ET_B receptor subtypes belong to the family of G-protein coupled receptors. As shown in Fig 17.2 and Table 17.2 the signal transduction mechanisms include an increase in

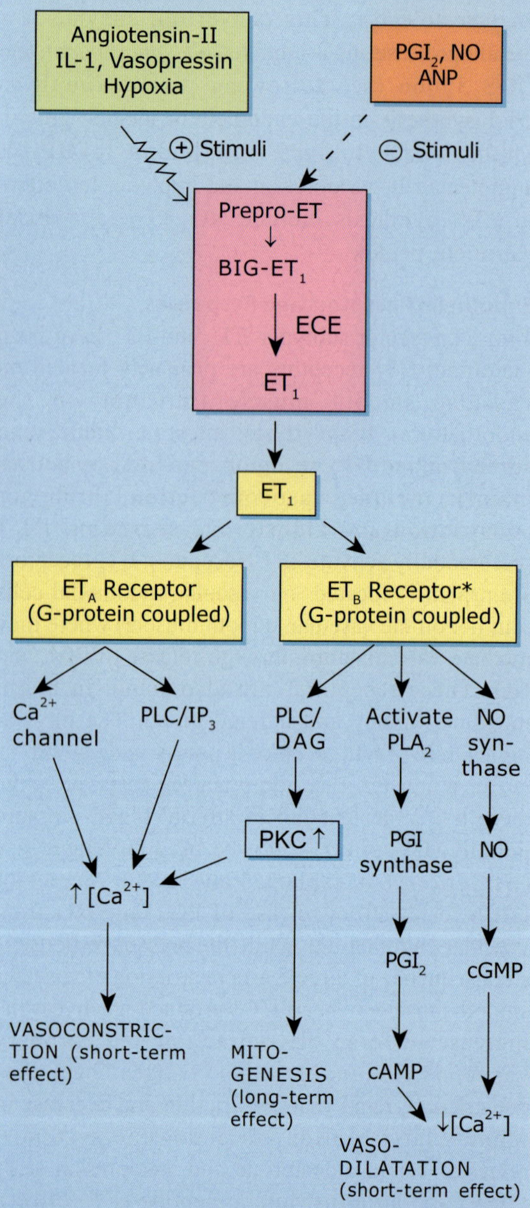

Key: IL-1—Interleukin-1; PGI_2—Prostaglandin I_2 (Prostacyclin); ECE—Endothelin-converting enzyme; PLC—Phospholipase C; PLA_2—Phospholipase A_2; NO—Nitric oxide; PKC—Protein Kinase C; ANP—Atrial natriuretic peptide. *Some reports suggest that $ET_{B\text{-}1}$ subtype causes vasodilatation by stimulating NO and PGI_2, while $ET_{B\text{-}2}$ mediates vasoconstriction

Fig 17.2 Biosynthesis, Release & Actions of ET_1 Through its Receptors.

intracellular Ca^{2+} concentration resulting from the increased influx of extracellular Ca^{2+} *via* opening of Ca^{2+} channels and through phospholipase-C/IP_3 pathway to produce vasoconstriction (ET_A response). In addition, there is an activation of phospholipase A_2 (which produces PGI_2) and of NO synthase (which generates NO) leading to transient vasodilatation (ET_B response). Lastly, activation of protein kinase-C through phospholipase-C/DAG pathway (combined ET_A/ET_B response) contributes to vasoconstriction and mitogenesis. The pharmacological characteristics of various endothelin receptors are summarised in Table 17.2.

ET Receptor Agonists and Antagonists

Many selective as well as nonselective antagonists have been developed and slowly finding place in clinical use. A non-selective antagonist ***Bosentan*** is active both intravenously and orally and blocks both the initial transient depressor (ET_B) and the prolonged pressor (ET_A) responses to I.V. ET. ***Bosentan*** and other non-selective agent, ***Macitentan*** have been found to lower pulmonary artery pressure and approved for the treatment of pulmonary hypertension in the doses of 62.5 mg BD and 10 mg OD, respectively. Out of the two selective ET_A antagonist, ***Ambrisentan** and **Sitaxsentan,*** the former has recently been approved for pulmonary hypertension (dose: 5 mg OD) and has shown efficacy and tolerability similar to the nonselective ET antagonists. All these drugs also have promise in heart failure and other indications for vasodilator drugs.

As discussed earlier, the formation of ET can be blocked specifically by ***CGS 35066*** and non-specifically by ***Phosphoramidon,*** the two endothelin-converting enzyme (ECE) inhibitors. Although the therapeutic potential of such drugs is similar to that of ET-receptor antagonists, their development as clinically useful agents is slow due to other off-target effects.

Adverse effects of ET-receptor antagonists include fall in BP, tachycardia, oedema, headache and gastric upset. The teratogenic effects of ET-receptor antagonists have also been reported. The

Table 17.2 Characteristic Features of Endothelin Receptors

Characteristics	Endothelin Receptors	
	ET_A	ET_B
Location	Vascular smooth muscle (++), Brain (+), Lungs (+), Kidney (+), Intestine (+), Adrenal gland (+)	Vascular endothelium (++), Brain (+++), Intestine (+++), Kidney (++), Adrenal gland (++)
	G-protein coupled	
Mechanism	Release Ca^{2+} from endoplasmic reticulum through PLC/IP_3 pathway; also through influx of extracellular Ca^{2+} via Ca^{2+} channels	Stimulate protein kinase-C through PLC/DAG pathway Also activate PLA_2 and NO synthase
Function	Vasoconstriction, Bronchoconstriction and Aldosterone secretion; also mitogenesis*	Vasodilatation Mitogenesis*
Agonist	$ET_1 > ET_2 > ET_3$	$ET_1 = ET_2 = ET_3$
Antagonist	Bosentan** and Macitentan**; Ambrisentan and Sitaxsentan	Bosentan**and Macitentan** IRL-1038

+++ High, ++ Moderate, + Low, * Both ET_A/ET_B mediated effect, ** Non-selective antagonist

major adverse effect of bosentan is elevation of serum transaminase levels (monthly monitoring of liver function test is necessary). Neither selective nor non-selective agonists are available yet for ET_A or ET_B receptor till date.

Neuropeptide Y

The neuropeptide Y (NPY) family of peptides consists of three members: NPY itself, pancreatic polypeptide and peptide YY. Among these, pancreatic polypeptide and peptide YY are both gut-endocrine peptides. NPY is widely distributed in the central and peripheral nervous system. In CNS it controls food and water intake, regulation of mood and central autonomic outflow. In the sympathetic nervous system, NPY is localised in noradrenergic neurons and functions both as vasoconstrictor and as cotransmitter with norepinephrine. NPY has a potent and prolonged vasoconstrictor action, including renal and cerebral vasoconstriction. Other CVS effects include positive chronotropic and inotropic actions on heart and hypertension. Multiple subtypes of NPY receptors, Y_1 through Y_6, have been identified. However, only Y_1, Y_2 and Y_5 receptors are of major concern in understanding the pharmacological effects of NPY. All these receptors (Y_1–Y_6) are G-protein coupled receptors, which involve mobilisation of Ca^{2+} and inhibition of adenylyl cyclase (decrease in cAMP).

Y_1 and Y_2 receptors are of major importance in cardiovascular and other peripheral effects of NPY. Selective agonist at Y_1 receptor are used only as research tools. The selective nonpeptide Y_1 receptor antagonists are: BIBP-3226 and SR-120107A. Out of these, BIBP-3226 has been extensively studied. It blocks the vasconstrictor and pressor responses to NPY, but has a short half-life.

SR-120107A is orally active and has a long duration of action.

Y_5 receptors are found mainly in CNS and are involved in the control of food intake. NPY is the potent orexigenic peptide in the brain. Activation of Y_5 receptors results in increased food intake and decreased energy expenditure. Y_5 receptor antagonists, therefore, have potential as anti-obesity agents.

Urotensin

Kidneys are the major source for circulating urotensin II but brain and spinal cord are also important sites of urotensin II expression. The prominent effects of urotensin II are regional vasoconstriction (primarily in arterial vessels) and cardiac depression. It has also been reported that urotensin II levels are increased in heart during end-stage heart failure but whether this increase was a cause or the consequence of heart failure is not clear.

Urotensin II receptors are widely distributed in brain, spinal cord, heart, vascular smooth muscle and kidneys. These are G-protein coupled receptors. The vasoconstricting effects of urotensin II are believed to be mediated by phospholipase-C/IP_3/DAG signal transduction pathway. A non- peptide urotensin receptor antagonist, ***palosuran***, has been developed for treatment of diabetic renal failure.

VASODILATOR PEPTIDES

Natriuretic Peptides (NPs)

NPs constitute a family of three cyclic polypeptides with natriuretic, diuretic, vasodilator and other properties: atrial (ANP), brain (BNP) and C-type (CNP). ANP (28-amino acid peptide) is synthesized in cardiac atrial tissue, BNP (32-amino acid peptide) is produced predominantly in ventricular myocardium, but to a lesser extent in atrial myocardium and brain, and CNP (22-amino acid peptide) is mainly expressed in the endothelium, CNS and bones. All three NPs exert their effects by combining with three NP receptors (NPRs): NPR-A (ANP_A), NPR-B (ANP_B) and NPR-C (ANP_C).

NPs Receptors

NPR-A (ANP_A) and NPR-B (ANP_B) are trans-membrane guanylyl cyclase (GC)-linked receptors. Binding of NPs (ANP, BNP or CNP) at extracellular domain of these receptors facilitates their dimerization and activation of GC, leading to production of cyclic GMP. The latter activates Protein Kinase-G that by lowering intracellular Ca^{2+} and dephosphorylation of MLCK produces vasodilation, natriuresis/diuresis, antihypertrophic and antifibrotic myocardial effects [renin-angiotensin-aldosterone system (RAAS) antagonistic actions]. ANP_A receptor has equal affinity for both ANP and BNP, which produce most of their effects through this receptor (Table 17.3).

NPR-C (ANP_C) Receptors have equal affinity for all NPs and is mainly located on vascular endothelium. This receptor has no known intrinsic enzymatic activity and is primarily involved in the bio-degradation of all three NPs. On binding with NPs, it dimerizes and gets internalized to metabolize the bound NPs in the cell (Table 17.3).

Biodegradation of NPs: Besides cell internalization by NPR-C (ANP_C) receptors, NPs are also biodegraded by a zinc-dependent enzyme called neutral endopeptidase (NEP 24.11), also known as neprilysin. Neprilysin is a metalloprotease and involved in the metabolism of a number of hetrogenous group of peptides like NPs, bradykinin, substance-P, adrenomedullin, VIP, CGRP, endothelin-1, angiotensin-II (Ang-II), etc.

Physiological Role of NPs: All NPs, especially ANP and BNP produce direct vasodilation, increase in glomerular filteration, natriuresis/dieresis, reduction in renin secretion in kidneys, and antihypertrophic and antifibrotic myocardial effects. CNP plays some autocrine and paracrine roles which are not clearly understood.

ANP and BNP synthesis and release is stimulated by an increase in cardiac wall stress during pressure or volume overload. Considerably higher levels of ANP and BNP have been noted in patients of heart failure (HF) that correlate closely with the severity of HF and other measures of left ventricular dysfunction like ejection fraction (EF), pulmonary wedge pressure and left ventricular end-dystolic volume.

Based on the physiological functions of NPs and the finding that NPs concentration is increased in HF patients, it was realized that NPs may have a potential role in the treatment of patients of systolic HF with reduced EF (HFrEF).

Sacubitril: An Inhibitor of Neprilysin

Since NPs (ANP and BNP) are potent vasodilator and natriuretic, and their release is activated by sympathetic stimulation, blood volume expansion, Ang-II, vasopressin and aldosterone; but vasodilatory and natriuretic/diuretic effects are antagonized by endothelins, Ang-II, aldosterone, it is an important proposition to block the biodegradation of NPs by inhibiting neprilysin or NEP. ***Sacubitril*** (AHU 377) is an orally active produrg medication that gets bioactivated by esterases to ***sacubitrilat*** (LBQ 657) which in turn inhibits neprilysin, an enzyme that degrades a number of endopeptides including NPs and Ang-II. As a consequence, use of neprilysin inhibitor, sacubitril would increase the levels of NPs as well as Ang-II, the latter being a vasoconstrictor may block the effect of the former as vasodilator thus cancelling the effects of its own consequences. As a result, efforts have been made to combine neprilysin with an AT-1 receptor antagonist (ARA).

Theoretically, neprilysin can be combined with an ACE-I to inhibit the formation of Ang-II. However, use of ACE-I may increase the concentration of bradykinin which may reduce the adverse effect of angioedema and dry cough. As a result combining neprilysin with ACE-I is not a good idea and when combined with an ARA, the adverse effects of ACE-I can be avoided.

Ang-II Receptor and Neprilysin Inhibitor (ARNI) is a new fixed dose combination (FDC) drug (LCZ 696) approved by the FDA which contains ***Sacubitril+Valsartan*** (an ARA) in 1:1 molar ratio in a sodium complex. The two components of this FDC assured that the effects of an increase in Ang-II (vasoconstriction and aldosterone release) as a consequence of neprilysin action are blocked by the valsartan. This dual-drug FDC represent a medication that act through inhibition of Ang-II receptors and neprilysin to modulate both the RAAS and vasoactive NPs simultaneously. Thus, ARNI is a therapeutic advancement that would benefit the patients of HFrEF addressing two of the pathophysiological mechanism of HF: activation of RAAS and decreased sensitivity to NPs.

After oral administration, the two components of ***FDC*** are separated to ***valsartan*** and ***sacubitril*** as individual drugs, the latter subsequently metabolized to its active form: ***sacubitrilat***. Peak concentration of both are reached at about the same time (1.5–4.5 hours) and steady-state levels of both are achieved after 2–3 days. **The sacubitril+valsartan FDC is available as tablets containing respectively 24+26 mg, 49+51 mg, 97+103 mg doses per tablet. Bioavailability of valsartan when administered as FDC is about 40% higher than when given alone**. Sacubitril is excreted in urine (50–68%), whereas valsartan is excreted mainly in faeces (86%).

As proof of concept, the results of PARADIGM-HF, a Phase III large outcome clinical trial conducted in 947 sites in 47 countries which compared the effect of sacubitril+valsartan FDC (200 mg BD) with enalapril (10 mg BD) in 8442 patients of HRrEF treated for 27 months has shown improved/superior cardiovascular endpoints (20% less risk of death or hospitalization for HF in patients given FDC when compared to the patients receiving enalapril). Based on the results of this large trial, US-FDA accorded its approval of FDC of sacubitril + valsartan for the treatment of patients of symptomatic HF.

Vasoactive Intestinal Peptide (VIP)

VIP is widely distributed in CNS and peripheral nervous system and is also present in GIT, heart, lung and kidneys. In CNS it functions as neurotransmitter or neuromodulator. In CVS it produces marked vasodilatation of coronary arteries and in most vascular beds, and exerts positive inotropic and chronotropic effects on heart.

Two subtypes of VIP receptors have been identified: $VPAC_1$ and $VPAC_2$ which are widely distributed in CNS and heart. Both are G-protein coupled receptors. Binding of VIP to these receptors

Table 17.3 Characteristics of Natriuretic Peptides Receptors

Characteristics	NPR-A (ANP_A)	NPR-B (ANP_B)	NPR-C (ANP_C)
Location	On the surface of target cells	Same as for ANP_A	Vascular endothelium
Ligand	ANP + BNP	CNP	ANP + BNP + CNP
Mechanism	Coupled to guanylyl cyclase, ↑ cGMP levels, ↓ in cytosolic free Ca^{2+} concentration	Same as ANP_A	Not clear
Function	As discussed for ANP and BNP	As discussed for CNP	Metabolic removal of ANP, BNP and CNP from circulation*

*Also called as "clearance receptor" for natriuretic peptides (NPs). Once the ANP_c receptor binds with NPs, the receptor and the bound peptides are internalised. The peptide is degraded enzymatically and the receptor is returned to the cell surface.

activates adenylyl cyclase and results in formation of cAMP which is responsible for its pharmacological actions described above. Specific agonists and antagonists are not yet available.

Substance P

This tachykinin group of peptides has three members: substance P, neurokinin A & neurokinin B. Substance P is present in CNS, GIT, blood vessels and skin. In CNS, it serves as neurotransmitter and plays a vital role in controlling anxiety, depression, emesis and nausea. In GIT it is an autacoid, and causes contraction of intestinal smooth muscles. In CVS, it is a potent vasodilator (by releasing NO from vascular endothelium) producing hypotension. Other effects include salivary secretions, natriuresis and diuresis.

Three G-protein coupled receptor subtypes have been identified: NK_1, NK_2 and NK_3. The predominant receptor for substance-P is NK_1. It is widely distributed in brain. Two orally-active NK_1 receptor antagonists—***aprepitant*** *and* ***netupitant*** (fosaprepitant & fosnetupitant, both lypholized salt for I.V. use)—have been found useful in preventing chemotherapy-induced nausea and vomiting *(Ch 28)*.

Neurotensin

Neurotensin is found to be present in brain, GIT and in the circulation. When administered in systemic circulation, it causes increased secretion of several anterior pituitary hormones, inhibits gastric acid and pepsin secretion, inhibits gastric motility, causes vasodilatation and increases vascular permeability.

Three subtypes of neurotensin receptors have been designated: NT_1, NT_2 and NT_3. Little is known about NT_3 receptors but NT_1 and NT_2 receptors belong to G-protein coupled receptor family.

Some neurotensin receptor agonists like PD 149163, which crosses BBB, is undergoing clinical trial as antischizophrenic and also as anti-Parkinsonism drug, because in CNS neurotensin has been found to govern dopamine neurotransmission. *Mechlinertant* has been developed as neurotensin receptor (NT_1) selective antagonist. Its therapeutic potential is not yet identified.

Calcitonin Gene-related Peptide (CGRP)

Like calcitonin (a calcium regulatory harmone of 32 amino acids) CGRP (a 37-amino acid peptide) is present in large quantities in the 'C' cells of the thyroid gland. CGRP was discovered accidentally while working on calcium regulation, researchers found that the same gene which encode calcitonin in thyroid gland can produce a different peptide in another organ like brain. It is now known that CGRP is a polypeptide from a tissue-specific alternative RNA splicing of the chromosome *11p15.2CALC1* gene, which also produces calcitonin and the calcium-lowering peptide katacalcin. However, CGRP which exist in both alpha and beta isoforms plays no role in Ca^{2+} homeostasis, rather it has both vasodilatory and nociceptive properties. CGRP is distributed in CNS (brain, spinal cord), pheripiral nerve fibres supplying to skin, GIT and urogenital system. When injected I.V., CGPR produces hypotension and tachycardia.

CGRP Receptor

CGRP acts through two colocalized protein molecules: **C**alcitonin receptor-**l**ike **R**eceptor (CLR) and a **R**eceptor **A**ctivity-**m**odifying **P**rotein (RAMP-1) which exist as heterodimer receptor. On binding with the CGRP ligand, these two proteins get dimerized and act in tandem to initiate receptor activity which produces various effects such as nociception & vasodilation. CGRP receptor functions are mediated by adenylate cyclase-cAMP mechanism.

Role of CGRP in Migraine

Based on the observations that (i) stimulating the trigeminal ganglion increased CGRP in cranial circulation; (ii) CGRP levels were elevated during migraine and that ***sumatriptan*** treatment returned CGRP to base line levels; and (iii) an infusion of CGRP in migraineurs produced migraine-like headache, CGRP has been implicated in the pathophysiology of migraine. An intensive research to develop CGRP blocking agents which can be used to treat or prevent migraine saw the birth of a number of CGRP receptor antagonists: ***Olcegepant*** (an I.V. formulation), ***Telcagepant*** (oral prepartation) [both not developed further due to issues of formulation in the former and off-site hepatotoxicity in the latter], ***Ubrogepant*** and ***Atogepant*** [both are being developed as oral dosage form, former for episodic and chronic migraine (EM, CM) and latter for EM prevention].

Anti-CGRP Monoclonal Antibodies (Anti-CGRP MAbs): *Erenumab*

Based on the polypeptide nature of CGRP and colocalized CLR-RAMP-1 protein structure of its receptor, a number of anti-CGRP MAbs have been developed as these may be more useful than the small molecule drugs. Migraine being a chronic recurrent headache, it was thought that MAb drugs administered S.C. will produce a long-lasting effect of weeks and months. Out of the four anti-CGRP MAbs, one, ***Erenumab***, a fully human MAb which block CGRP receptor has been approved by FDA (in 2018) for EM prophylaxis. Marketed by trade name AIMOVIG as prefilled autoinjector syringe, ***erenumab*** when injected in a dose of 70 mg S.C. in thigh, arm or abdomen skin: or 140 mg (administered as two consecutive 70 mg S.C. doses) is sufficient to relieve EM headache for one month. Except, injection site pain, constipation, muscle cramps and spasm in 1–3% cases, no other safety signals have been identified. The drug should not be used in children and in patients over 65 yrs of age and in pregnant women as safety and effectiveness has not been studied in such people.

The three other humanized anti-CGRP MAbs which are being developed against CGRP as ligand (not receptor) are: ***Eptinezumab*** (I.V. formulation for every 3-months administration), ***Fremenezumab*** and ***Galcanezumab*** (both for S.C. administration). All are in advanced stages of development in Phase II or III clinical trials in EM/CM patients. No major safety issues have been observed and all are potential candidates for FDA approval for different manifestations of migraine or cluster headache. A central 5-HT1F agonist, Lasmiditan (which inhibits the release of CGRP in brain) has been found to be effective in patients with moderate to severe migraine disability that remains unaffected by the prior use of triptan therapy (See Ch. 24, page 355).

Adrenomedullin

Like CGRP, adrenomedullin is member of calcitonin family of peptides. It is present in adrenal medulla, heart, vascular smooth muscle, kidney and lungs. It also circulates in blood as physiological antagonist to the vasoconstrictors like ET_1 and angiotensin II. Circulating adrenomedullin levels increase during vigorous exercise, in hypertensives, and in patients of renal failure and heart failure. Adrenomedullin is

Table 17.4 Physiological and Pathophysiological Role of Endogenous NO

System	Physiological effects	Pathophysiological effects	
		Overproduction	Inadequate production
Smooth Muscle (via eNOS)*	Vascular (vasodilation); Bronchial (bronchodilation); GIT (reduced GI motility)	Hypotension (septic shock) Ischaemia Reperfusion injury	Hypertension*, Atherosclerosis (e.g., in hyperlipidaemia, diabetes mellitus and ischaemic heart disease)
Cardiovascular (via eNOS)	Maintenance of vascular integrity; Inhibits monocyte adhesion and migration; Inhibits platelet aggregation; Inhibits smooth muscle and fibroblast proliferation; Anti-atherosclerotic action		
Central Nervous System (via nNOS and eNOS)	Neurotransmitter or Neuromodulator role; Increased cerebral blood flow; Nociception; Improved learning and memory	Neurotoxicity (e.g., ischaemic stroke, Huntington's disease, AIDS, dementia)	
Peripheral Nervous System (via nNOS** and eNOS)	Neurotransmitter in NANC neurons, Penile erection, ↑ in gastric emptying and pulmonary vasodilation	Portal cirrhosis	Erectile dysfunction; Hypertrophic pyloric stenosis** causing obstruction in gastric outflow; Bronchial asthma Renal failure
Immune system (via iNOS, large amounts of NO)	Antibacterial; Antiviral; Antifungal; Antiprotozoal and Antiparasitic effects; Tumorocidal; Apoptosis; Nonspecific immunity	Bacterial sepsis Transplant rejection Inflammation	—

* Mutant mice that lack the gene coding for eNOS are hypertensive, consistent with a role for NO biosynthesis in the physiological control of BP.

** Mutant mice that lack the gene coding for nNOS have grossly distended stomachs similar to human hypertrophic pyloric stenosis.

also a powerful vasodilator and causes long-lasting hypotension. It also causes reflex tachycardia and increase in cardiac output. It produces natriuresis and inhibits aldosterone and insulin secretion.

Adrenomedullin receptors are G-protein coupled receptors but incompletely defined and hence called *calcitonin receptor-like receptor*.

GASEOUS VASODILATORS

Nitric Oxide (NO)

Nitric oxide (NO; earlier called EDRF) is a simple, unique, gaseous, signaling molecule which readily diffuses across the cell membranes and regulates a wide variety of physiological processes.

Biosynthesis of Nitric Oxide (NO)

NO is synthesised from L-arginine and molecular O_2 by Nitric Oxide Synthase (NOS) enzymes. The NOS enzyme occurs in endothelial (eNOS), neuronal (n-NOS) and inducible (iNOS) isoforms. Two of them (eNOS and nNOS) are constitutively present in various tissues. The nNOS is found in peripheral and central neurons while eNOS is found in cardiac myocytes, platelets, osteoblasts, osteoclasts and renal mesangial cells besides endothelium. Both constitutive forms of NOS (nNOS and eNOS), require influx of extracellular Ca^{2+} into the cell and its binding to calmodulin (Cam) for their activation. Shear mechanical stress, acetylcholine, bradykinin and substance P which increase the cytoplasmic concentration of Ca^{2+} activate eNOS and nNOS. The subsequent generation of NO, in this case takes place in small amounts (picomoles). The duration of NO release is also short lasting. Inhibitors of eNOS and nNOS are L-nitroarginine methyl ester (L-NAME) and 7-nitroindazole, respectively.

On the contrary, iNOS is expressed on macrophages, Kupffer cells, fibroblasts, vascular smooth muscles and endothelial cells. It is induced in response to the pathological stimuli, e.g., invading microorganism and resulting cytokines (notably interferon-γ). Induction of iNOS is inhibited by glucocorticoids and by some cytokines, e.g., transforming growth factor-β. The iNOS activity, in contrast to nNOS and eNOS, is independent of intracellular Ca^{2+} concentration. However, the generation of NO, in this case, takes place in large amounts (nanomoles) and the duration of release is also long lasting. The eNOS is membrane bound enzyme, whereas nNOS and iNOS are cytosolic soluble enzymes. The expression of iNOS (on demand, during inflammation) is governed by transcription factors.

Nitric Oxide Donors

Some NO donors, e.g., oxygenated nitroprusside spontaneously generate NO, whereas organic nitrates and nitrites require the presence of a thiol compound such as cysteine to generate NO. Once generated, NO or its stable analogue R-SNO interacts with the haem moiety of soluble guanylate cyclase (GC), in the cytoplasm of cells, and promotes the conversion of GTP to cGMP (see Fig. 20.3).

The increase in cGMP causes vascular relaxation by reducing the $[Ca^{2+}]i$ and through dephosphorylation of myosin-light chain-PO_4 (MLC-PO_4) to MLC, which prevents interaction of myosin with actin, leading to smooth muscle relaxation. Some drugs, such as phosphodiesterase V inhibitors like ***sildenafil,*** prolong the duration of NO-induced cGMP elevation in erectile tissue and are used to treat erectile dysfunction.

Nitric Oxide Inactivators

Nitric oxide is inactivated by combination with the haem of haemoglobin or by oxidation to nitrite or nitrate which are excreted in urine or by the free radical, superoxide. The scavengers of superoxide anion such as superoxide dismutase, therefore, may protect degradation of NO, enhancing its potency and prolonging its duration of action. Interaction of NO with superoxide anion ($O_2^{\cdot}$) produces more toxic peroxynitrite ($ONOO^{\cdot}$) free radical which inactivates many -SH containing enzymes. Glutathione reduces such toxicity. In certain disease conditions like diabetes mellitus and atherosclerosis, vascular glutathione is decreased which may account for the increased incidence of cardiovascular complications in such disease. On the contrary, glutathione also interacts, under physiological conditions, with NO to generate a more stable S-nitrosoglutathione which serves as a longer-lasting adduct or carrier for NO. In presence of O_2, haem converts NO to nitrate and itself gets oxidised to methaemoglobin. Distinct from this inactivation reaction, NO bound to haem is relatively stable *in absence of oxygen.*

Cellular and Biochemical Effects of NO

Some beneficial physiological effects of NO are listed in Table 17.4. However, both deficiency (inadequate production) and excess (over production) of NO can lead to various patho-physiological complications. These are also summarised in Table 17.4.

Therapeutic Uses of Inhaled NO

1. Nitric oxide therapy is a preferred choice for new-born having persistent pulmonary hypertension.
2. Inhaled NO is used in adult and neonatal respiratory distress.

Adverse Effects: Methaemoglobinaemia (see above).

CHAPTER 18 Renin–Angiotensin System and Its Inhibitors

COMPETENCY PH1.26

Angiotensin and kinins belong to the family of autacoids (local hormones; autos = self, akos = remedy). Autacoids are produced in the tissues or endothelial cells and, after being released locally, they act at the site or near the site of their release. Endocrine hormones, on the other hand, are secreted from endocrine glands and released directly into the blood stream to act on cellular sites far away from the site of their release.

ANGIOTENSIN II (Ang-II)

Biosynthesis, Release and Metabolism

The pathway for the synthesis and metabolism of angiotensin II, the key autacoid of renin-angiotensin system, has been summarised in Fig. 18.1.

The main steps include (i) enzymatic cleavage of angiotensinogen by renin to form angiotensin I (Ang-I), (ii) conversion of Ang-I to angiotensin II (Ang-II) by angiotensin-converting enzyme (ACE or kininase II or peptidyl dipeptidase) and finally, (iii) angiotensin II is broken down by aminopeptidase giving rise to angiotensin III and angiotensin IV, respectively; both of which are further degraded into inactive fragments by a group of peptidases collectively called as angiotensinases.

Renin converts the circulating angiotensinogen to Ang-I. It is synthesised from prorenin in the kidney. Both prorenin and renin are stored in the juxtaglomerular cells of the kidney. Renin release is controlled by the following three mechanisms:

1. Decrease in renal perfusion which stimulates renin release. Reduction in the tension (stretch) within the wall of the glomerular afferent arteriole is believed to be the immediate stimulus.
2. A decrease of Na^+ concentration in the distal tubule leads to an increased renin secretion. The macula densa region monitors the osmolarity of tubular fluid and relays the stimulus to the juxtaglomerular apparatus to release renin.
3. Stimulation of β_1-adrenoceptors on the juxtaglomerular apparatus by norepinephrine (released due to sympathetic activity) and PGI_2 all increase renin release directly.

The plasma half-life of renin is very short (t½ 15 min). The rate at which the renin is secreted by the kidney is the primary determinant of activity of renin-angiotensin system. Drugs that inhibit renin release are discussed below under the section "drugs that inhibit renin secretion and release".

Angiotensinogen is a circulating α_2-globulin. It is synthesized and secreted by liver. The production of angiotensinogen is increased by glucocorticoids, oestrogens and thyroid hormones. It is also elevated during pregnancy. Mutations in the angiotensinogen gene have been reported to be linked to hypertension. Angiotensinogen has also been found in large quantities in amniotic fluid. Degradation of angiotensinogen by renin produces the decapeptide Ang-I.

Angiotensin I (Ang-I) has no appreciable biological activity *per se* but is converted to Ang-II by an angiotensin converting enzyme (ACE or kininase II or dipeptidyl carboxypeptidase/DPCP). Ang-II is a powerful vasoconstrictor *(see following text)*.

Angiotensin-Converting Enzyme (ACE) is a membrane bound enzyme present on the luminal surface of vascular endothelium and therefore remains in close contact with the circulation. It is particularly abundant in lung, which has a vast surface area of vascular endothelium. Therefore, the lung serves as the major organ for the production of circulating Ang-II. However, the ACE has also been identified on

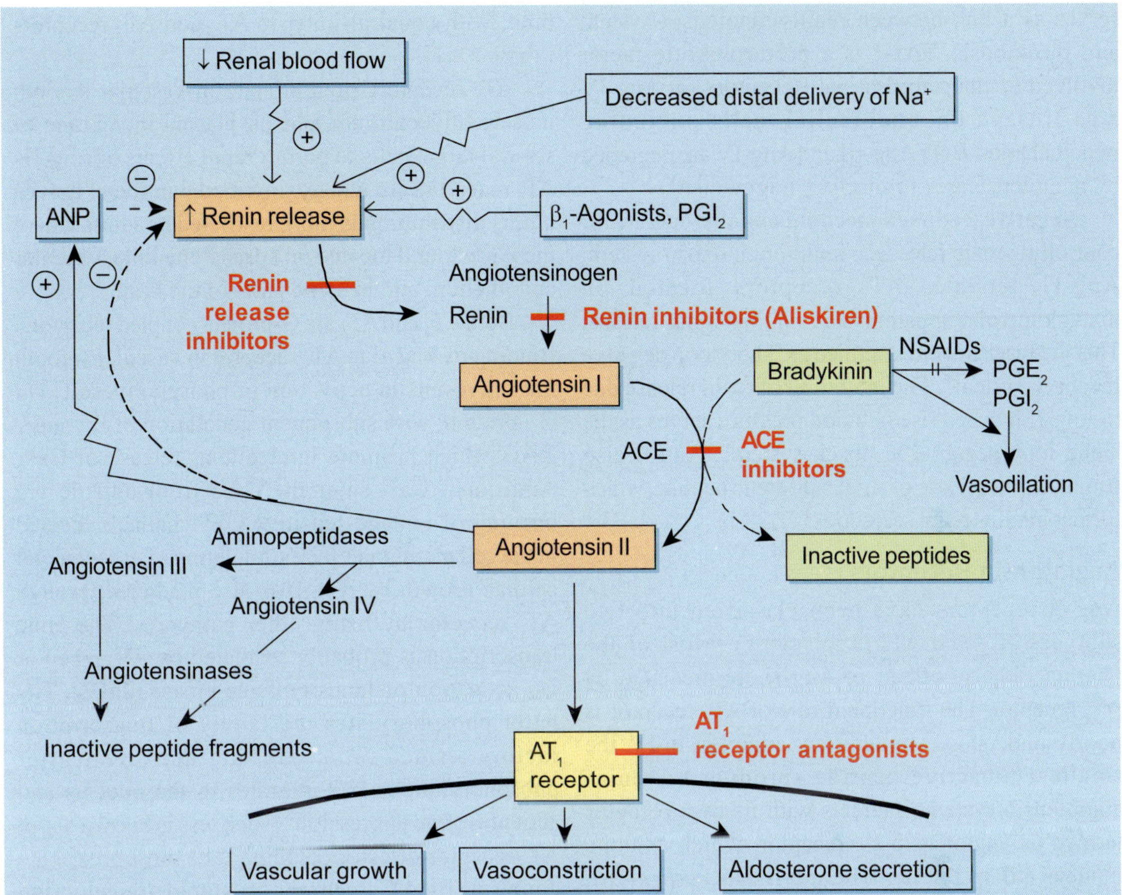

Key: ACE—Angiotensin-converting enzyme. ANP—Atrial natriuretic peptide. Inhibitors have been shown in red. Relationship with bradykinin has been shown in green.

Fig 18.1 Renin-Angiotensin System and Sites of Action of Drugs that Inhibit the Cascade.

epithelial cells of proximal tubule, small intestine and brain. Consequently, local formation of Ang-II can occur at different sites to provide local control independent of blood-borne Ang-II. ACE inactivates bradykinin into inactive peptides (Fig. 18.1 and Ch. 24). This further contributes to the antihypertensive actions of ACE inhibitors (by preventing degradation of bradykinin—a vasodilatory peptide; see below).

Angiotensin II (Ang-II) is the principal active local hormone of the *renin–angiotensin system*. Its prominent actions (discussed below) are vasoconstriction, vascular and myocardial growth and aldosterone secretion. It has a very brief plasma half-life (t½ 35–40 sec) and is metabolised by aminopeptidase A to angiotensin III (Ang-III) in plasma and numerous tissues. A small amount of Ang-II is also degraded to angiotensin IV (Ang-IV).

Angiotensin III (Ang-III) is about ¼th as potent as Ang-II in elevating blood pressure but it is now known that it is equipotent to Ang-II in aldosterone secretion. It also stimulates drinking (dipsogenic effect) and secretion of PAI-1 (see below).

Angiotensin IV (Ang-IV) has actions distinct from Ang-II. By activating its own receptors it secretes plasminogen activator inhibitor-1 (PAI-1) and thus serves as a link between renin-angiotensin system and thrombosis. PAI-1 is a prothrombotic factor involved in clot stabilisation. Receptors for Ang-IV are present on endothelial cells including hypothalamus. Both Ang-III and Ang-IV are degraded by angiotensinases to inactive fragments.

Negative feedback mechanisms also operate for controlling renin release in renin-angiotensin system. Ang-II activates AT_1 receptors located on juxtaglomerular apparatus and inhibits renin release. This feedback system is termed as "short loop negative feedback system". The inhibition of renin release due to Ang-II induced rise in blood pressure serves as the "long loop negative feedback system". Ang-II also stimulates the release of atrial natriuretic peptide, which further inhibits renin secretion (Fig.18.1).

Angiotensin Receptors

Ang-II receptors have been classified into two subtypes AT_1 and AT_2 (Table 18.1). Most of the pharmacological effects of Ang-II are mediated by AT_1 receptor. The functional role of AT_2 receptor is poorly understood. In addition, angiotensin IV, the smallest bioactive peptide product of renin-angiotensin system, interacts with its own receptor termed as angiotensin IV receptor, which exhibits minimal affinity for Ang-II or Ang-III *(see earlier text)*, but its significance is not yet known.

The nomenclature of angiotensin receptors as AT_1 and AT_2 appears to be misleading because these can be mistaken as the receptors for Ang-I and Ang-II, respectively. However, ang-II binds equally to both AT_1 and AT_2 receptors. Angiotensin IV interacts with its own AT_4 receptors. Ang-II also binds to recently identified AT_3 receptors but their role is not yet clear.

AT_1 and AT_2 receptors have been identified on the basis of their differential affinity for their antagonists. AT_1 receptors have a high affinity for ***losartan*** and a very low affinity for nonpeptide investigational antagonists PD123177; while AT_2 receptors have high affinity for PD123177, but a low affinity for losartan. Ang-II and *saralasin* (a partial agonist-antagonist) bind, with equal affinity, to AT_1 and AT_2 receptors (Table 18.1).

AT_1 receptors predominate in vascular smooth muscle, myocardium and on plasma membrane of several target cells to permit rapid effects of Ang-II. AT_2 receptors are widely distributed in foetal tissues but its distribution is more restricted in adults where these are found located on adrenal medulla, vascular endothelium and in some parts of the brain.

Both AT_1 and AT_2 are G-protein coupled receptors. Binding of Ang-II to AT_1 receptor in vascular smooth muscle results in activation of phospholipase-C *via* G_q protein, with subsequent generation of IP_3 and DAG which promote intracellular release of Ca^{2+}. Additional Ca^{2+} enter the cells from outside *via* opening of voltage-sensitive Ca^{2+} channels located in the cell membrane. The stimulation of vascular and cardiac growth by Ang-II is also mediated through AT_1 receptor by using other pathways. The gene transcription is probably regulated by AT_1 receptor *via* activation of Janus tyrosine kinase (**Jak2**). The latter phosphorylates the family of transcription factors termed *Stats*. Getting activated, after phosphorylation, *Stat* migrates to the nucleus and activates gene expression. Much less is known about AT_2 receptor-effector coupling. The most proximate coupling of AT_2 receptor to signal transduction system is mediated by G_i protein and includes activation of tyrosine phosphatases, K^+ channels, nitric oxide production and probably inhibition of Ca^{2+} channels.

Actions of Angiotensin II

AT_1 Receptor Mediated Responses

Renin-angiotensin system plays a major role in regulating arterial blood pressure as well as fluid and electrolyte balance. An overactivity of this system disturbs fluid and electrolyte balance and produces hypertension. The main actions of Ang-II include:

1. Generalised vasoconstriction, including efferent arterioles of kidney. The pressor response to Ang-II is accompanied with minimal reflex bradycardia as the peptide, through its central action, resets the baroreceptor reflex control mechanism of heart rate to a higher pressure. Pre-eclampsia is associ-

Table 18.1 Pharmacological Characteristics of Angiotensin Receptors***

Characteristic	AT_1 receptor*	AT_2 receptor**
Location	Vascular smooth muscle, myocardium; plasma membrane of target cells	***Foetus***: Widely distributed in all tissues ***Adults***: Adrenal medulla, vascular endothelium and in some parts of brain
Mechanism	Both are G-protein coupled receptors	
	Phospholipase C/IP_3/DAG–intracellular Ca^{2+} release, Activation of Ca^{2+} channels Activation of PKC and tyrosine protein kinase and transcription of specific genes (cell growth)	Coupled to Gi; Inhibition of Ca^{2+} channels. Activation of K^+ channels, tyrosine phosphatases and nitric oxide production
Function	Generalised vasoconstriction, cell growth in heart and arteries. Secretion of aldosterone. Reabsorption of Na^+ from proximal tubule and distal tubule. Enhances peripheral sympathetic activity.	- Vasodilatation - Antiproliferative - Apoptosis (program of cell death) - Foetal tissue development
Agonist	Angiotensin II*	Angiotensin II
Antagonist	Losartan, Valsartan Candesartan, Irbesartan Telmisartan, Olmesartan	PD123177

* Most of the pharmacological effects of angiotensin II are mediated by AT_1 receptor. The functional role of AT_2 receptor is poorly understood.
** AT_2 receptors get upregulated during heart failure and myocardial infarction.
*** There is unique receptor for AT-IV which has least affinity for AT-II or AT-III (see text).

ated with the development of agonistic antibodies against AT_1 receptors.

2. Increased release of E and NE from sympathetic nerve terminals and adrenal medulla by stimulating autonomic ganglia. This effect reinforces vasoconstriction and also increases the rate and force of contraction of the heart.
3. Secretion of aldosterone from the adrenal cortex. At higher concentrations, Ang-II also stimulates glucocorticoid biosynthesis.
4. Stimulation of Na^+ reabsorption from proximal tubule.
5. Stimulation of cell growth in the heart and arteries. Ang-II is mitogenic for vascular and cardiac muscle leading to cardiovascular hypertrophy. ACE inhibitors and Ang-II receptor (AT_1) antagonists prevent these morphological changes (remodeling) following myocardial infarction that would otherwise lead to congestive heart failure.

6. Stimulation of dipsogenic effects (drinking) and ACTH secretion, the physiological significance of which is not clear.

AT_2 Receptor Mediated Responses

Little is known about the AT_2 receptor mediated responses of Ang-II. However, foetal tissue development, anti-proliferative action, apoptosis (programmed cell death) and vasodilatation are some of the effects of Ang-II, which are believed to be AT_2 receptor mediated outcomes. AT_2 receptor–mediated vaso-dilatation appears to be nitric oxide (NO)-dependent and probably involves bradykinin-B_2 receptor-NO-cGMP pathway. Although AT_2 receptors are abundantly expressed in all tissues in foetal life of humans but they are meagerly present in adult life, and have been identified in vascular endothelium, adrenal medulla and some parts of the brain. AT_2 receptors are known to get upregulated in conditions of congestive heart failure and myocardial infarction.

INHIBITORS OF RENIN-ANGIOTENSIN SYSTEM

A summary of the agents that inhibit the renin-angiotensin system, with their sites of action, is provided in Figure 18.1. These drugs may block renin secretion, or renin action or the conversion of Ang-I to Ang-II by ACE. Another category of drugs belonging to this group is AT_1 receptor antagonists.

Blockers of Renin Secretion and Release

Beta-adrenoceptor blocking drugs inhibit the secretion of renin indirectly, by blocking the intrarenal and extrarenal β-receptors involved in neural control of renin secretion and release. Clonidine also inhibits renin secretion by reducing centrally mediated sympathetic activity.

Renin Inhibitors

Two orally active renin inhibitors—*enalkiren* and *remikiren*—which reduce plasma renin activity have been developed. However, their clinical efficacy in patients of hypertension has been disappointing because of their poor bioavailability (considerable first pass effect). Nevertheless, renin inhibition is becoming a new approach for the treatment of hypertension. ***Aliskiren*** is a new nonpeptide, orally active, direct renin inhibitor approved for the treatment of hypertension. It not only decreases plasma renin activity in hypertensive patients but also nullifies the renin rise as a result of ACE inhibition (feedback rise), or AT_1 receptor blockade or by diuretics. Its tolerability is akin to ACE inhibitors or AT_1 receptor antagonists but antihypertensive effects are remarkably greater because it blocks the catalytic activity of renin to cleave angiotensinogen to Ang-I, i.e., the very first step in the formation of Ang-II (Fig. 18.1). The drug can cause diarrhoea and hyperkalaemia as side effects. Despite these attractive claims (*single window service*), the downside is the recent reports that reactive renin secretion after its continued use limits its effectiveness.

Angiotensin-Converting Enzyme Inhibitors (ACEIs)

ACEIs not only block the conversion of Ang-I to Ang-II but also inhibit the degradation of vasodilatory peptide bradykinin (Fig. 18.1). Inhibition of bradykinin metabolism, by ACEIs, also contributes to their antihypertensive action. However, this property is also responsible for their characteristic side effects like cough and angioedema. They also inhibit aldosterone production and hence promote Na^+ and water excretion and K^+ retention.

Pharmacokinetics

Captopril was the first ACEI to be marketed. It was then followed by ***enalapril*** with effects similar to those of captopril. The latter is a prodrug, which on being hydrolysed by hepatic esterases, is transformed into an active ACEI, ***enalaprilat***. ***Lisinopril*** is a lysine derivative of enalaprilat and itself is a potent and an active ACEI. Rest all are prodrugs which are converted to their respective active metabolites due to hydrolysis by hepatic esterases enzyme.

In general, all ACEIs like ***ramipril, benazepril, perindopril, quinapril, trandolapril, fosinopril*** and ***moexipril***, differ with regard to their pharmacokinetic parameters as shown in Table 18.2. All ACEIs

Table 18.2 Comparative Features of ACE Inhibitors

ACEIs	Chemical group	Activity status	Duration of action	Dose schedule	Bioavailability reduced by
Captopril	SH	Active	8–12 hrs	25–50 mg BD	Food
Enalapril	Ester	Prodrug	< 24 hrs	2.5–40 mg OD	—
Lisinopril	Carboxy	Active	24 hrs	5–40 mg	—
Ramipril	Ester	Prodrug	> 24 hrs	1.25–20 mg	Food[1]
Benazepril	Ester	Prodrug	> 24 hrs	5–80 mg	Food[2]
Perindopril	Ester	Prodrug	> 24 hrs	2–16 mg	Food[3]
Quinapril	Ester	Prodrug	> 24 hrs	5–80 mg	Food[1]
Trandolapril	Ester	Prodrug	> 24 hrs	1–8 mg	Food
Fosinopril[5]	Phosphinate	Prodrug	> 24 hrs	10–80 mg	Food
Moexipril	Ester	Prodrug	> 24 hrs	7.5–30 mg	Food[4]
Imidapril	Ester	Prodrug	> 24 hrs	5–10 mg	Food[2]

Captopril and lisinopril are active by themselves. Others are inactive prodrugs until hydrolysed by hepatic esterases to their active form, e.g., enalapril to enalaprilat or ramipril to ramiprilat. [1] Only the rate but not the extent of its oral absorption is reduced by food. [2] Only slightly (30%) reduced by food. [3] The bioavilability of the active drug perindoprilat is reduced by food. [4] Markedly decreased by food; drug should be taken one hour before meals. [5] Except fosinopril which is eliminated by liver as well as kidney, all ACEIs are eliminated predominantly by kidney.

effectively block the conversion of Ang-I to Ang-II and, except for the difference in their pharmacokinetics, in clinical use these are interchangeable.

Therapeutic Uses

ACEIs decrease systemic vascular resistance without increasing heart rate. They also promote natriuresis. These are used to treat hypertension (see Ch. 19); to decrease morbidity and mortality in heart failure (Ch. 22) and left ventricular dysfunction after myocardial infarction. They are particularly useful in treating patients with diabetic nephropathy as they decrease proteinuria and stabilise renal functions. These are also useful in preventing the incidence of diabetic retinopathy in the patients of type I diabetes. ACEIs have been found to produce dramatic improvement in otherwise prognostically grim condition of scleroderma renal crisis.

Adverse Effects

1. Hypotension after the first dose, particularly in sodium-depleted patients (those using loop diuretics, or on salt restriction or suffering with GIT fluid loss). Preferably, the treatment should be initiated with small doses of ACEIs.
2. A dry cough, possibly the result of accumulation of bradykinin (Fig. 18.1) in the bronchial mucosa, is the commonest (5 to 20% of patients) persistent adverse effect. It is usually not dose related and occurs more frequently in women than in men. Once ACEIs are stopped, the cough disappears, usually within a week.

3. Patients with bilateral renal artery stenosis or with stenosis of the artery to a single remaining kidney, predictably develop renal failure if treated with ACEIs. Angiotensin II, by constricting the efferent arteriole, maintains the adequate glomerular filtration rate even when renal perfusion is low. Consequently, inhibition of ACE can induce acute renal insufficiency in such cases.
4. ACEIs may cause hyperkalaemia in patients with renal failure or in patients taking K^+-sparing diuretics, owing to reduced, Ang-II stimulated, aldosterone secretion.
5. Although ACEIs are not teratogenic during first trimester, continued administration of ACEIs during II and III trimesters of pregnancy carries the risk of foetal hypotension, anuria, renal failure, foetal malformations and even neonatal death (due in part to foetal hypotension). It is imperative, therefore, that once pregnancy is diagnosed, ACEIs should be withdrawn and an alternative antihypertensive therapy should be instituted.
6. Angioneurotic oedema, which may develop within 3-4 days of the initiation of the therapy, is not dose related. It may possibly involve accumulation of bradykinin and induction of tissue specific auto-antibodies. Once ACEIs are stopped the symptoms disappear within 24 hours.
7. Exceedingly rare but reversible minor adverse effects of ACEIs include, neutropenia, cholestatic type hepatotoxicity, glycosuria, proteinuria, altered sense of taste and allergic skin rashes. The latter two effects occur more frequently with captopril and are attributable to the presence of –SH group. Incidence of these adverse effects is negligible with long-acting ACEIs.

Drug Interactions

1. Non-systemic antacids reduce the bioavailability of ACEIs.
2. NSAIDs may impair the hypotensive effects of ACEIs by blocking bradykinin-mediated vasodilatation (see Ch. 24).
3. K^+-sparing diuretics or K^+ supplements may exacerbate ACEIs-induced hyperkalaemia.
4. Capsaicin may aggravate ACEIs-induced dry cough.
5. Plasma levels of lithium and digoxin may get elevated with concomitant use of ACEIs.

Angiotensin Receptor Antagonists (ARAs)

Saralasin, an earliest known peptide antagonist at AT_1 receptor inhibits the vasoconstrictor effects of Ang-II. However, it exhibits some partial agonist activity and, therefore, elicits some pressor responses also, particulary when circulating Ang-II levels are low. It must be administered intravenously, so it is not used clinically.

Attention was eventually focused onto the development of orally active non-peptide pure antagonists of AT_1 receptor. ***Losartan, Eprosartan, Valsartan, Candesartan, Irbesartan, Telmisartan,*** and ***Olmesartan*** are some orally active, potent and specific competitive antagonists of angiotensin AT_1 receptors. EXP 3174 is an active antihypertensive metabolite of losartan (another metabolite EXP 3179 has been shown to possess antiplatelet activity against collagen-induced platelet activation via blockade of GP VI receptor).

The rank order affinity of the AT_1 receptor for different ARAs is: candesartan > irbesartan > telmisartan = valsartan = EXP 3174 > losartan = eprosartan. The pharmacokinetic characteristics of these ARAs have been compared in Table 18.3.

All of the physiological effects of Ang-II, including release of aldosterone, are antagonised by ARAs. Although both ACEIs (described above) and ARAs block the renin-angiotensin system, ARAs differ from ACEIs in the following characteristics:

1. The ARAs have no effect on bradykinin metabolism (Fig. 18.1) and are therefore more selective blockers of Ang-II effects than ACEIs.
2. ACEIs may not suffice for the total elimination of Ang-II, because additional enzymes have been identified that are capable of forming Ang-II from Ang-I by alternative pathways. In contrast, ARAs are capable of blocking the effects of Ang-II regardless of any biochemical pathway for Ang-II formation.
3. Both group of drugs stimulate renin release. But ACE inhibition does not result in the increased levels of circulating Ang-II, while with ARAs this

Table 18.3 Pharmacokinetic Characteristics of Different Angiotensin Receptor Antagonists

Drug	Plasma half-life (hrs)	Plasma clearance	Dosage
Losartan	2.5–3	Renal/Hepatic[1]	50 mg OD
EXP 3174*	6–8	Renal/Hepatic[1]	—
Eprosartan°	5–8	Renal/Biliary[2]	400–800 mg OD/BD
Valsartan	9	Liver (70%)[1]	80–300 mg OD
Candesartan	9	Renal (30%) and Biliary (70%)[2]	8 mg OD
Irbesartan**	11–15	Biliary (80%)[1]	150–300 mg OD
Telmisartan	24	Biliary (90%)[1]	40–80 mg OD
Olmesartan	13	Biliary[1]	20–40 mg OD

* Active metabolite of losartan. ** Higher bioavailability (70–80%).
° Food decreases bioavailability. [1] Plasma clearance affected by hepatic insufficiency.
[2] Plasma clearance affected by both renal/hepatic insufficiency

increases circulating Ang-II levels. The resultant increased amount of Ang-II would now stimulate AT_2 receptors which are lying unblocked. This may be useful in view of the fact that activation of AT_2 receptor causes vasodilatation.

Despite these differences it is not yet clear if ARAs have any significant advantage over ACEIs.

Therapeutic Uses

Administration of ARAs decreases total peripheral resistance (afterload) and cardiac venous return (preload). Reduction of blood pressure occurs independently of the status of renin-angiotensin system, making them effective antihypertensives even in patients with normal to low activity of renin-angiotensin system. Longer-acting ARAs such as ***candesartan, irbesartan,*** and ***telmisartan*** seem to be more effective, than the shorter-acting antagonists, at providing 24-hour control of BP. ***Losartan*** is reported to be safe and very effective in the treatment of portal hypertension with cirrhosis of liver.

ARAs did not exhibit distinct advantage over ACEIs in reducing morbidity and mortality from congestive heart failure. However, like ACEIs, they also slow the progression of diabetic nephropathy. One ACEI, ***valsartan*** *has been shown to reduce the incidence of diabetes mellitus in subjects with impaired glucose tolerance test.*

The use of ARAs is generally restricted to patients who do not tolerate ACEIs. In clinical practice ARAs are reserved for patients of hypertension in whom ACEIs have to be withdrawn for the complaints of dry cough or angiooedema. These side effects are not caused by ARAs.

A combination of an ARA, ***valsartan+sacubitril,*** a ***neprilysin*** inhibitor (LCZ/696) has been approved for the treatment of symptomatic heart failure (See Ch. 17).

Adverse Effects

Unlike ACE Inhibitors

ARAs do not cause cough or angioneurotic oedema because they do not build up bradykinin levels as discussed with ACEIs. They do not produce dysgeusia (distortion of taste perception) either.

Like ACE Inhibitors

These can cause foetal toxicity and should be discontinued before second trimester of pregnancy. They may precipitate renal failure in patients with bilateral renal artery stenosis. ARAs can cause hyperkalaemia in patients with renal failure or in patients taking K^+ supplements or K^+-sparing diuretics. First-dose hypotension, in rare cases, may occur.

CHAPTER 19 Drug Therapy of Hypertension

COMPETENCY PH1.27

Hypertension (HT) has been, evidently, the most important contributing factor to cardiovascular disease, the leading cause of morbidity and untimely death. Sustained HT damages heart, kidney, blood vessels and brain which leads to ischaemic heart disease, congestive heart failure, renal failure and stroke. HT, therefore, is one of the most serious concerns of modern medical practice.

Primary Essential Hypertension: by convention, HT is categorized based on office measurements as **Stage 1** (140–159/90–99 mmHg) and **Stage 2** (greater than 160/100 mmHg). Cardiovascular morbidity and mortality increase as both systolic and diastolic blood pressures rise, but in individuals over age 50 years, the systolic pressure and pulse pressure are better predictors of complications than diastolic pressure. The prevalence of HT increases with age. Adequate blood pressure control reduces the incidence of acute coronary syndrome by 20–25%, stroke by 30–35%, and heart failure by 50%.

Prehypertension: data from the Framingham cohort study indicate that blood pressure bears a linerar relationship with cardiovascular risk down to a systolic blood pressure of 155 mmHg; based on these data, it has been suggested that indivuduals with blood pressures in the gray area of 120–139/80–89 mmHg be categorized as having "prehypertension". Because prehypertension often develops into HT (50% if affected individuals do so within 4 years), prehypertensive patients should be monitored annually.

Secondary Hypertension: When HT is secondary to a known organic disease such as phaeochromocytoma, renovascular disease, coarctation of aorta, Cushing's disease and primary aldosteronism, therapy is directed towards correction of the underlying disease. Incidentally, about 90% of the cases of HT are of unknown aetiology and are grouped as the cases having *essential hypertension* (so-called because it was originally thought that the raised BP was essential to maintain adequate tissue perfusion).

The risk factors for HT include smoking, hyperlipidaemia, diabetes and history of any cardiovascular disease. The risk of end organ damage due to HT is greater in black race. There is relatively less risk in premenopausal women as compared to men. Heredity contributes 30% in the cases of essential HT. Variations in the genes for angiotensinogen, angiotensin-converting enzyme (ACE) and the β_2 adrenoceptors on vascular smooth muscle appear to contribute in some cases of essential HT.

AUTOREGULATORY CONTROL OF BLOOD PRESSURE

Figure 19.1 summarises physiological mechanisms that control arterial blood pressure and shows sites at which antihypertensive drugs act. Arterial blood pressure is directly proportional to the product of cardiac output and the peripheral vascular resistance (PVR) and most antihypertensive drugs lower BP either by reducing cardiac output or by decreasing peripheral vascular resistance or both. Physiologically, the cardiac output as well as peripheral resistance are controlled mainly by three overlapping mechanisms:

a) The baroreflexes, mediated by the autonomic nervous system (upper half of Fig. 19.1)
b) The renin-angiotensin-aldosterone system (lower half of Fig. 19.1)
c) A local release of hormones from vascular endothelium, e.g., nitric oxide (NO) which dilates and endothelin 1 (ET-1) which constricts blood vessels (not shown in Fig. 19.1)

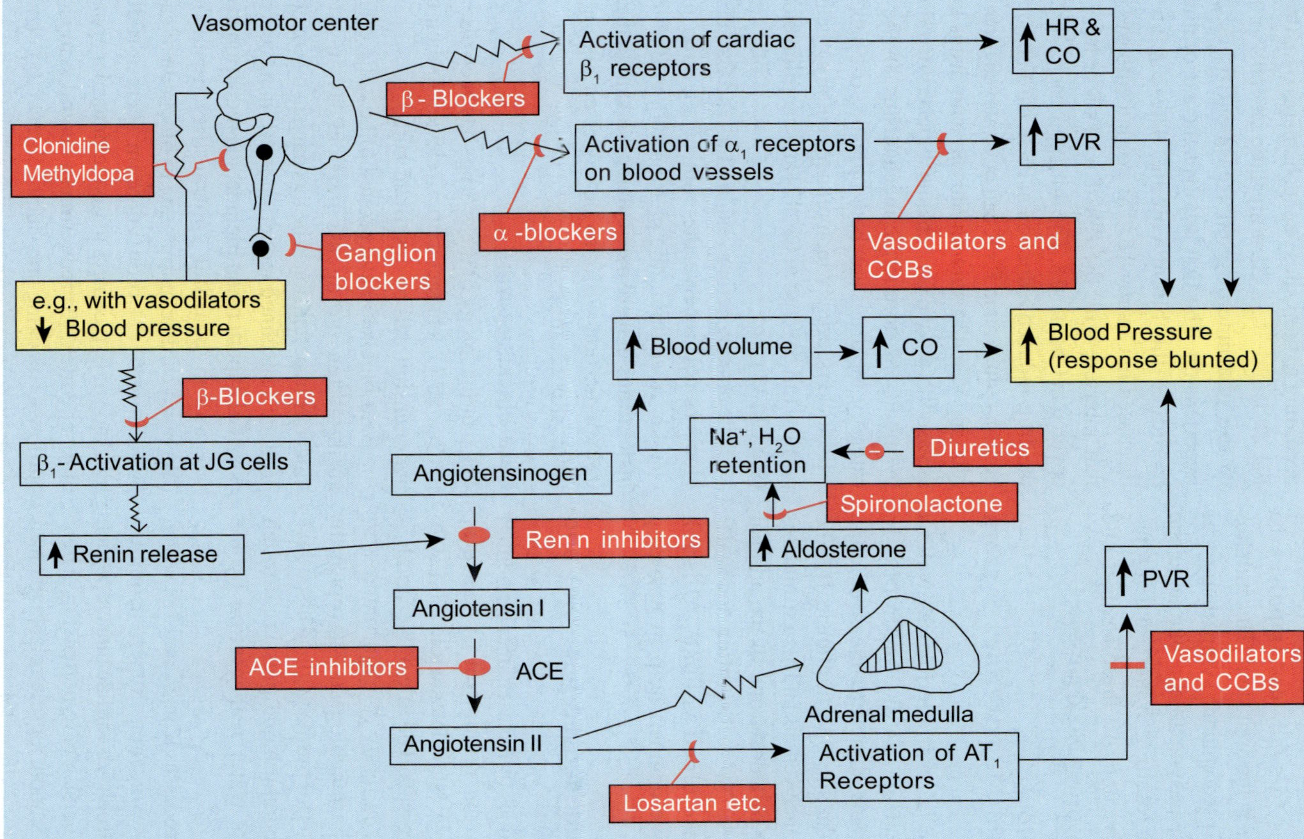

Key: HR—Heart rate; CO—Cardiac output; PVR—Peripheral vascular resistance; CCBs—Ca^{2+} channel blockers

Fig 19.1 Counter-Regulatory Responses to Fall in Blood Pressure and Sites of Action of Antihypertensive Drugs (in red bcx)

Autoregulatory Responses Through Sympathetic Nervous System

A fall in BP causes baroreceptors in the aortic arch and carotid sinuses to send less impulses to cardiovascular centres in the brainstem. This initiates a reflex response of predominant sympathetic and proportionately low parasympathetic output to the heart and vasculature resulting in increased cardiac output and vasoconstriction. All these changes end up in a compensatory rise in blood pressure.

Autoregulation Through Renin-Angiotensin-Aldosterone System (RAAS)

A decreased pressure in renal arterioles as well as sympathetic activation of β_1 receptors in juxtaglomerular apparatus, stimulates release of renin, which increases production of angiotensin II. The latter constricts resistance vessels and also stimulates synthesis and release of aldosterone in the adrenal cortex which stimulates Na^+ reabsorption and water retention, to increase blood volume. All such processes, in cohesive manner, help in restoring normal blood pressure (for details refer Ch. 18).

Role of Endothelium-derived Autacoids and Vasopeptides

Local release of hormones from vascular endothelium is also involved in the regulation of vascular resistance. For example, NO dilates while ET-1 (Ch. 17) constricts blood vessels. The role of NO and ET-1 in controling BP is currently of major interest to cardiologists and pharmacologists. Vasopressin released from the posterior pituitary gland also plays a major role in maintaining blood pressure through its ability to regulate water reabsorption by the kidney (Ch.17).

Some uncertain processes (Ch. 17 and 18) which lead to progressively worsening hypertension are remodeling and hypertrophy of cardiac muscle, which occurs in response to persistent hypertension. There is also proliferation of smooth muscle cells in the wall of resistance arteries that reduces the lumen diameter and increases the PVR.

ANTIHYPERTENSIVE DRUGS

The antihypertensive drugs can be classified according to their sites or mechanisms of action (see Fig. 19.1. and 19.2). There are three general approaches to the pharmacological treatment of essential hypertension. The first involves the use of diuretics to reduce the blood volume. These have been discussed in Chapter 16. The second employs drugs that interfere with the RAAS and these have been covered in Chapter 18. The third approach is aimed at the drug-induced reduction in PVR, cardiac output or both. A reduction in PVR can be achieved directly by relaxing vascular smooth muscle with drugs known as vasodilators and Ca^{2+} channel blockers or indirectly by modifying adrenergic mechanisms. In the latter category, the drugs are: beta-blockers, α-blockers, α + β-blockers, drugs which reduce central sympathetic outflow (all covered in Ch. 12) and ganglion blockers (see Ch. 13).

The directly acting vasodilators and Ca^{2+} channel blockers will receive the bulk of attention in this chapter. In addition, the pharmacology of all of the major drugs that are particularly relevant to their use in hypertension will also be reviewed highlighting their salient features (Fig. 19.2) only.

Beta-blocking Drugs

The pharmacology of these drugs has been discussed in Chapter 12; characteristics relevant to their use in hypertension will be described here.

Beta-blockers have proved to be quite effective antihypertensive agents particularly in mild to moderate hypertension. The mechanism by which they produce a sustained reduction in BP in patients with essential hypertension include: (1) reduction in heart rate and myocardial contractility, resulting in decreased cardiac output, due to blockade of cardiac β_1 receptors, (2) reduced renin secretion due to blockade of β_1 receptors in juxtaglomerular apparatus in renal cortex, (3) reduction in central sympathetic outflow by blocking presynaptic β-receptors centrally, (4) stimulation of prostacyclin synthesis in vascular beds, (5) blockade of peripheral facilitatory

ANTIHYPERTENSIVE DRUGS

- **β-Blockers**
  - Propranolol
  - Metoprolol
  - Atenolol
  - etc.
- **β + α Blockers**
  - Labetalol
  - Carvedilol
  - etc.
- **α-Blockers**
  - Prazosin
  - Terazosin
  - Doxazosin
  - Phenoxybenzamine
  - etc.
- **Central sympatholytics**
  - Clonidine
  - Methyldopa
- **Ganglion blockers**
  - Trimethaphan
- **Diuretics**
  - **Thiazides**
    - Hydrochlorothiazide
    - Chlorthalidone
    - Indapamide
    - etc.
  - **High-ceiling**
    - Furosemide
    - etc.
  - **K^+ sparing**
    - Spironolactone
    - Triamterene
    - Amiloride
- **ACE inhibitors**
  - Enalapril
  - Lisinopril
  - Ramipril
  - etc.
- **AT_1 antagonists**
  - Losartan
  - Candesartan
  - Irbesartan
  - etc.
- **Ca^{2+} channel blockers**
  - Verapamil
  - Diltiazem
  - Nifedipine
  - Amlodipine
  - Felodipine
  - etc.
- **Vasodilators**
  - **Arteriolar**
    - Hydralazine
    - Minoxidil
    - Diazoxide
    - Fenoldopam
  - **Arteriolar + Venous**
    - Sodium nitroprusside
- **Others**
  - Reserpine
  - Guanethidine
  - Not used nowadays

Fig 19.2 Summary of Antihypertensive Drugs in Use.

presynaptic β_2-receptors to reduce NE release and (6) increase in natriuretic peptide secretion caused by β-blockade.

Fall in BP produced by β-blockers seems to be somewhat paradoxical, because blockade of vascular smooth muscle vasodilatory β_2-receptors is expected to unmask or leave unopposed α-receptor mediated vasoconstrictor activity which is expected to increase rather than decrease blood pressure. With chronic use, the peripheral resistance, however, returns to the pretreatment levels or less because of overall reduction in cardiac output.

Beta-blockers are very popular antihypertensive drugs. They are well tolerated and serious side effects are seldom observed. Tolerance and orthostatic hypotension do not occur with these drugs. Earlier, these were employed as a first step in the management of essential hypertension. However, now these are often used in conjunction with a diuretic when monotherapy is not satisfactory. Although β-blockers do not usually cause salt and water retention, yet, clinical effectiveness improves when a diuretic is added with a β-blocker. Similarly, using a β-blocker in combination with a vasodilator is more advantageous from haemodynamic viewpoint. Reflexly mediated cardiac stimulation is a common feature of vasodilator treatment and may severely limit its antihypertensive effectiveness. A β-blocker prevents cardiac stimulation and thus preserves the effectiveness of the vasodilator. Further, vasodilator treatment initiates a reflex increase in plasma renin activity which is blunted by the use of a β-blocker. Contrarily, the vasodilator will prevent an increase in peripheral vascular resistance that results with the use of β-blockers. The combination of β-blockers, a diuretic and a vasodilator is very effective in patients who are resistant to other antihypertensive regimens. Besides HT, β-blockers are also used for the treatment of supraventricular tachyarrhythmias (Ch. 21), previous MI and angina pectoris (Ch. 20).

These drugs should not be used in those hypertensive patients who have concomitant insulin dependent diabetes, bronchial asthma or chronic obstructive pulmonary disease, Raynaud's phenomenon, variant angina and chronic congestive cardiac failure. *Adverse effects* include fatigue, lethargy, decreased libido and unfavourable lipid profile. There may be a rebound hypertension, tachycardia and anginal pain upon sudden withdrawal of β-blockers. Hence, they should not be discontinued abruptly. The withdrawal syndrome involves up-regulation and hyper-responsiveness of β-adrenoceptors (see Ch. 12).

The non-selective ($\beta_1 + \beta_2$) beta-blockers used in the management of essential hypertension include ***propranolol, sotalol, nadolol, pindolol*** and ***oxprenolol***. Their basic pharmacological profile is similar to prototype β-blocker propranolol. *Sotalol* has low lipid solubility (lesser CNS side effects) with negligible first-pass metabolism. It has an additional K^+ channel blocking and Class III antiarrhythmic property independent of β-blocking property (Ch. 21). *Nadolol* has longer half-life (t½ 20 hrs) and is administered once daily. It does not cross BBB and has least first-pass metabolism. *Pindolol* and *oxprenolol* possess some inherent intrinsic sympathomimetic actions (ISA) also. Hence they are useful in patients prone to bradycardia or those with low cardiac reserve. These are less troublesome to asthmatics because of their β_2 agonist action. Rebound HT after sudden withdrawal is less likely and lipid profile is less worsened compared to propranolol. ***Selective (cardio) β_1-blockers*** used for antihypertensive therapy include ***metoprolol, atenolol, esmolol, acebutolol, celiprolol*** and ***nebivolol***. Among these, *acebutolol* and *celiprolol* possess ISA (besides selective β_1 blockade). Hence, these offer all advantages of pindolol or oxprenolol group as cited above, besides being safe for the patients having concomitant diabetes or peripheral vascular disease (no β_2 blockade). Cardioselective β-blockers, as a rule, are safer than propranolol in hypertensive patients having concomitant asthma, diabetes, Raynaud's phenomenon and in those who have unfavourable lipid profile. However, rebound hypertension after abrupt withdrawal of the drug, still remains a problem (except acebutolol and celiprolol, because of ISA for β_2 receptors). *Atenolol* does not cross BBB and has longer duration of action than *metoprolol*. It can be given once daily. *Nebivolol* is a new hybrid drug possessing β_1 adrenoceptor blockade plus vasodilating properties (as it releases nitric oxide from vascular endothelium). *Esmolol* is an ultrashort acting β_1-adrenoceptor antagonist. It is given intravenously in urgent settings where β_1 blockade of short duration is desired, e.g., to terminate supraventricular tachycardia, episodes of atrial fibrillation or to control heart rate and BP during surgery. It can be withdrawn immediately if adverse effects like bradycardia, hypotension or heart failure appear. *Metoprolol* reduces mortality in patients of heart failure.

Mixed (α + β) Antagonists

The racemic mixture of ***labetalol*** exhibits (a) selective blockade of α_1 adrenoceptor, (b) inhibition of neuronal uptake of NE, (c) blockade of β_1 receptors, (d) partial agonist activity (ISA) at β_2 receptors and (e) some direct vasodilator properties. It is given orally to treat HT in elderly people where increased peripheral resistance is not desired. It is particularly useful in phaeochromocytoma and for controlling rebound HT after clonidine withdrawal. It is also employed for the treatment of black hypertensive patients because usually these patients are not adequately controlled by β-blockers. Postural hypotension and hepatotoxicity are main side effects. ***Carvedilol*** is a β_1, β_2 and α_1 adrenoceptor blocker but its β_1 and β_2 blocking effects are greater than its α_1 blocking effects. It is also used like labetalol. In addition, it inhibits free radical induced lipid peroxidation and also prevents vascular smooth muscle mitogenesis (independent of α or β adrenoceptor blockade). These effects may prove to be cardioprotective in patients of CHF (for details of dosage of β-blockers refer Ch. 12)

Alpha-Blockers

The classical α-blocker, ***phenoxybenzamine***, is non-selective. It binds covalently to both α_1 and α_2 receptors with the result that it produces correspondingly greater cardio-acceleration and tachycardia due to release of NE from sympathetic neuron by blocking α_2 receptors. The frequency of their use for treating primary hypertension has declined after the development of α_1-selective receptor antagonists like ***prazosin***, ***terazosin*** and ***doxazosin*** because these agents produce considerably less tachycardia than do non-selective α-antagonist.

These drugs reduce arterial pressure by dilating both the resistance and capacitance vessels. As expected, they share the risk of postural hypotension that may follow after the first dose. Retention of salt and water occurs when these drugs are administered without a diuretic. These drugs are more effective when used in combination with a β-blocker and a diuretic than when used alone. *Terazosin* and *doxazosin* have a longer duration of action than *prazosin* which permits once daily dosage for the treatment of primary HT.

Since these drugs do not significantly influence blood uric acid or glucose levels and are associated with favourable effects on lipid profile they may be useful in patients with concomitant complications such as gout, diabetes and hyperlipidaemia. These are also preferred in male hypertensive patients having benign prostatic hyperplasia (for details of dosage of α-blockers refer Ch. 12).

Centrally Acting Antihypertensive Agents

These agents reduce sympathetic outflow from vasopressor centre without affecting its sensitivity to baroreceptor control. Hence, their antihypertensive effects are unaffected by posture.

Methyldopa is an analogue of L-dopa and is converted to α-methyldopamine and α-methyl norepinephrine (similar to the biosynthesis of NE, Fig. 12.2 and 12.3). It is then stored in the storage vesicles of adrenergic neuron and then released as a false neurotransmitter in place of NE. It is now established that α-methyl NE stimulates central α_2 receptors to inhibit adrenergic neuronal outflow from the brainstem (primary mode of action). Renin secretions are also reduced but it is not a major determinant for its antihypertensive effects.

Because α-methyldopa lowers BP without compromising either renal blood flow or the glomerular filtration rate, it is particularly valuable in HT complicated by renal insufficiency. It is the drug of choice for treating HT during pregnancy as it is not only effective but safer too for both the mother and the foetus. Long-term therapy with α-methyldopa leads to fluid retention, oedema and plasma volume expansion. Hence, the drug should be used in conjunction with a diuretic. For other details and adverse effects refer Chapter 12.

Clonidine, after intravenous injection, produces a brief rise in BP followed by more prolonged hypotension; but on oral administration (i.e., at low plasma concentration) it produces only fall in BP. This is because, clonidine, at lower plasma concentration, has lesser intrinsic activity on postsynaptic α_1 receptors. The pressor response which appears at higher plasma concentration, is due to direct stimulation of α-adrenoceptors in arterioles. The antihypertensive effect of clonidine is exerted by activation of α_2 receptors at vasopressor centre. Consequently, central sympathetic outflow is diminished which results in fall in BP and HR. It has also been reported that clonidine binds to and activates imidazoline receptor (I_1) which may modulate the central α_2 receptor activity to mediate antihypertensive effects. Clonidine also activates the presynaptic α_2 receptors on sympathetic post-ganglionic neurons which suppresses further release of NE from peripheral nerve endings. The drug reduces renin release also and decreases renal vascular resistance. *The principal difference between clonidine and α-methyldopa is that clonidine acts directly on central α_2-adrenoceptors whereas α-methyldopa must be converted to α-methyl NE to exert its antihypertensive effects.*

Blood pressure lowering by clonidine results from reduction in central sympathetic outflow, which causes lowering of cardiac output due to decrease in HR and relaxation of capacitance vessels with a reduction in peripheral vascular resistance. It rarely causes postural hypotension. It is administered orally or applied as transdermal patch to treat mild to moderate HT. Since it causes salt and water retention, it is given usually in combination with a diuretic. A vasodilator can be added to the clonidine + diuretic combination to treat the cases of refractory HT. Such drug combination is not only effective but has distinct advantage because the reflex increase in HR and cardiac output that result from the use of vasodilator are negated by clonidine-induced decrease in HR and cardiac output. Like α-methyldopa, it is also useful for HT complicated by renal disease. However, clonidine is not used as a first-line antihypertensive drug because of its side effects and risk associated with rebound hypertension after its abrupt withdrawal (for side effects see Ch.12).

Moxonidine and ***rilmenidine***, the newer congeners of clonidine, have a longer plasma half-life and are said to be selective for imidazoline (I_1), receptor rather than α_2 receptor. Rebound hypertension is much less frequent with these drugs, as omission of a single dose will not trigger the rebound (dosage for α-methyldopa and clonidine have been provided in Ch. 12).

Diuretics

The sites of action within the kidney and the pharmacology of various diuretic drugs are discussed in Chapter 16. Na^+ contributes to vascular resistance by increasing vessel stiffness. These effects are reversed by diuretics or salt restriction. Initially, diuretics produce a mild degree of Na^+ depletion which leads to a reduction in blood volume and cardiac output. Later, the cardiac output returns towards normal while peripheral vascular resistance declines.

Thiazide Diuretics

When a diuretic therapy is indicated for the treatment of essential HT, the thiazide diuretics (hydrochlorothiazde, chlorothiazide, indapamide) are generally the drug of choice. These act on the early part of distal tubule and inhibit electroneutral Na^+/Cl^- cotransport. Many patients can be continued for years on smaller doses of thiazides alone with K^+ supplements. However, some patients may require additional medication such as β-blockers. ***Bendroflumethiazide***, ***polythiazide*** and ***chlorthalidone*** differ from ***hydrochlorothiazide*** only in potency and duration of action (see Ch. 16).

Indapamide is more potent and longer acting than hydrochlorothiazide and possesses some intrinsic vasodilator activity also. It reduces BP at a dose lower than that required for diuresis and produces lesser hypokalaemia, hyperglycaemia and hyperuricaemia. The main *adverse effects* of thiazide diuretics include hypokalaemia, hyperuricaemia, hypercalcaemia, hyperglycaemia, hyperlipidaemia and hypochloraemic alkalosis. These drugs can enhance digitalis toxicity due to hypokalaemia. Thiazides should be avoided in hypertensive cases with concomitant diabetes mellitus, gout, hyperlipidaemia, renal insufficiency (see below) and pregnancy. *Indapamide* can be used in diabetic hypertensives.

Loop Diuretics

These act primarily on the thick ascending limb of the loop of Henle by inhibiting the $Na^+/K^+/2Cl^-$ cotransport carrier in the luminal membrane. Examples include ***furosemide, bumetanide, torsemide*** and ***indacrinone***. Their relative potency order ranks as follows: bumetanide > torsemide > furosemide > indacrinone. These are not indicated in mild or moderate HT as rapid and greater diuresis causes severe reduction in blood volume and electrolyte imbalance. They are preferred in severe HT with cardiac and renal insufficiency. Loop diuretics promptly reduce pulmonary oedema in CHF due to rapid diuresis which results in the decrease in venous return and subsequently in the reduction in right ventricular output. These drugs can convert oliguric renal failure to non-oliguric failure which helps in management of renal failure. *Adverse effects* include hyperuricaemia, hypercalciuria, hypomagnesaemia and hypokalaemia (can potentiate digitalis toxicity). *Indacrinone* is useful for hypertensive patients having gout as it inhibits proximal tubular uric acid absorption also.

K^+-Sparing Diuretics

These are given usually in combination with thiazide diuretics to avoid excessive depletion of K^+. ***Amiloride*** and ***triamterene*** inhibit luminal membrane Na^+ channels (and hence Na^+-K^+ exchange) at collecting tubules. ***Spironolactone*** is an aldosterone receptor antagonist and hence antagonises Na^+ retaining and K^+ excreting actions of aldosterone. FK-453 is an investigational K^+-sparing diuretic. It causes brisk diuresis (like thiazides) with least K^+ loss. It is a selective adenosine (A_1) receptor antagonist. Concomitant use with ACE inhibitors should be avoided (Ch.18) (for dosage of these diuretics, refer Ch.16).

Angiotensin-Converting Enzyme Inhibitors

Angiotensin-converting enzyme inhibitors (ACEIs) not only block the conversion of angiotensin I to angiotensin II (Ang-II) but also inhibit the degradation of bradykinin (to promote vasodilation; see Fig 18.1 and Ch. 18). Ang-II is a vasoconstrictor and stimulates aldosterone release and thus promotes Na^+ retention. ACEIs therefore decrease peripheral resistance, lower blood pressure and produce mild natriuresis. These are the drugs of first choice for treating all grades of essential HT (with or without high plasma renin activity) as well as renovascular hypertension (except those with bilateral renal artery stensosis). They reduce BP without increasing the heart rate. Addition of a diuretic or a β-blocker improves their effectiveness. These are most useful antihypertensives in patients having diabetic nephropathy, left ventricular hypertrophy, CHF and in cases of post-myocardial infarction. A parallel system for conversion of Ang-I to Ang-II also exists in cardiac musculature which seems responsible for trophic changes such as cardiac hypertrophy. ACEIs reduce this post-MI myocardial remodeling. All ACEIs like ***enalapril, lisinopril, ramipril, benazepril, perindopril*** and ***quinapril*** effectively reduce BP and, except for their pharmacokinetic differences, in clinical use these are interchangeable. Except for enalapril and lisinopril which have duration of action of < 24 hrs and 24 hrs respectively, others have duration of action for > 24 hrs.

Adverse effects include: Hypotension after first dose, dry cough, angioneurotic oedema, hyperkalaemia, foetal hypotension with a risk of foetal malformations if administered during II and III trimester of pregnancy and altered sense of taste (for all details see Ch. 18).

Angiotensin Receptor Antagonists (ARAs)

Losartan, candesartan, irbesartan and ***valsartan*** are some orally active, potent and specific antagonists of angiotensin II receptors (AT_1 receptor). Except for losartan, others are longer-acting ARAs. Unlike ACEIs, ARAs have no effect on bradykinin metabolism (Fig. 18.1) and are therefore more selective blockers of Ang-II effects compared to ACEIs. Moreover, ARAs are capable of blocking the effects of Ang-II regardless of any biochemical pathway for Ang-II formation (see Ch. 18). Despite these differences it is not certain if ARAs have any distinct advantages over ACEIs. Therefore, their use is generally restricted to patients who do not tolerate ACEIs because of dry cough or angioneurotic oedema, both of which are bradykinin mediated. The *adverse effect* profile is similar to ACEIs, including the hazard to their use during pregnancy, with the exception of cough and angioedema. Losartan is also effective in portal hypertension due to cirrhosis of liver.

For dosage of these ACEIs and ARAs, refer Ch. 18.

Table 19.1 Properties of Voltage-Sensitive Ca^{2+} Channels

Voltage-Sensitive Calcium Channels				
Properties	**L (long lasting)**	**T (transient)***	**N (neuronal)**	**P/Q** & R****
Activation threshold	High	Low	High	High
Inactivation rate	Slow	Fast	Medium	Slow
Location	Cardiac and smooth muscle, SA node and AV node	SA node Thalamic and other neurons	Neurons in CNS and Secretory glands	Cerebellar and Purkinje neurons
Function	Regulate excitation–contraction coupling; Regulate pacemaker activity; Regulate conduction velocity	Regulate pacemaker activity; Regulate T current and repetitive spikes in thalamic nuclei	Modulate transmitter release	Modulate transmitter release
Blockers	Verapamil Dihydropyridine group of CCBs, Cd^{2+}	Flunarizine Ethosuximide Ni^{2+}	Cd^{2+} Gabapentin	Toxin from funnel web spider

* T channels are resistant to be blocked by most of CCBs except for the drugs shown

** Q channels have properties similar to P channels. Not much is known about R channels. The neuronal pharmacology of CNS is modulated by N, P/Q and R channels. This underlines the normally observed weak effects of L channel blockers on CNS functions — The terminology of these channels sounds quite melodious. **L** stands for *long lasting*; **T** for *transient*; **N** for *neither* long lasting *nor* transient but *neuronal*; **O** somehow has been *omitted* but **P** and **Q** follow as simple English alphabets; Next is obviously **R**.

Calcium Channel Blockers (CCBs)

Calcium channel blockers (CCBs) block voltage dependent L-type Ca^{2+} channels and thus reduce the frequency of the opening of these channels in response to depolarisation. The result is marked decrease in the transmembrane Ca^{2+} current in vascular smooth muscle, cardiac muscle, SA node and AV node (Table 19.1).

Types and Characteristics of Ca^{2+} Channels

Four types of Ca^{2+} channels have been described in the smooth and cardiac muscle.

1. **Voltage-Sensitive Ca^{2+} Channels**
   These are influenced by depolarising external stimuli, and are activated when membrane potential drops to - 40 mV or less. Five types of voltage-sensitive Ca^{2+} channels (L, T, N, P & Q) have been identified. Among these, the L-type Ca^{2+} channels (L for long-lasting) are dominant in cardiac and smooth muscles, and are blocked by CCBs. These channels get activated as well as inactivated at a slow rate. Properties of these channels have been summarised in Table 19.1. Each channel has a unique pharmacoresponsive profile.

CCBs exhibit voltage-dependent blocking action, i.e., they block more strongly when membrane is depolarised. Since they block more effectively in those cells in which Ca^{2+} channels are more active, these are also referred to as *use-dependent Ca^{2+} channels*.

The functioning of L-type Ca^{2+} channels and their blockade by CCBs resemble that of Na^+ channel and its blockade by local anaesthetics (for details refer Ch. 15, Figure 15.2). The voltage-gated Ca^{2+} channel has a voltage sensor or an activation gate (AG) on its extracellular site and an inactivation gate (IG) on its intracellular

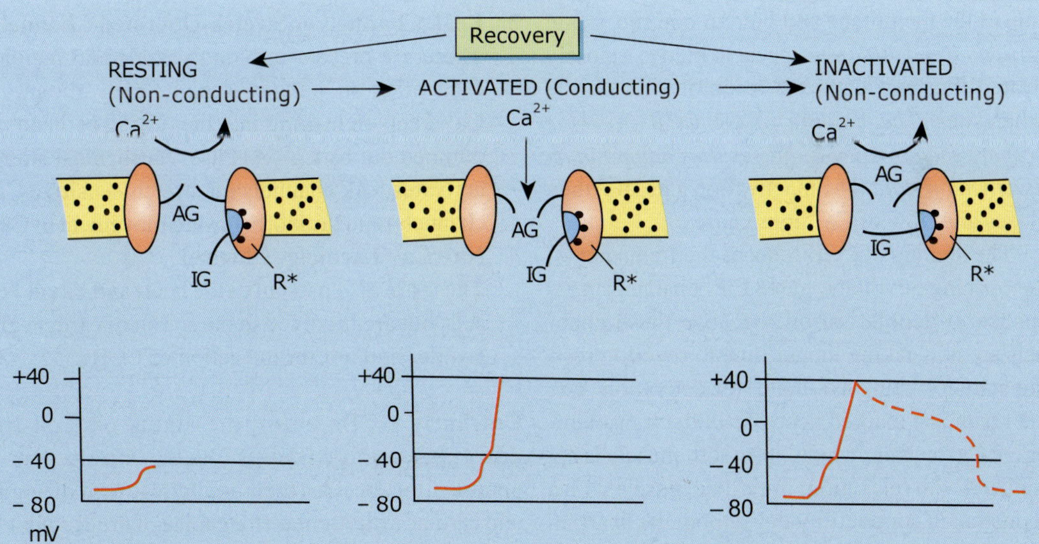

Key: AG—Activation gate; IG—Inactivation gate; R*—Receptor for CCBs with different binding sites. The part of AP during which most Ca^{2+} channels get completely or partly inactivated and not available for reactivation is shown by dashed line.

Fig 19.3 A Model of Voltage-Gated Ca^{2+} Channel Depicting the Site and Mechanism of CCBs Action

site (Fig. 19.3). These channels can exist in three functional states: (1) The *resting or closed state* prevails at the normal resting potential with activation gate (AG) closed; (2) *the activated or the open state* is favoured by the brief depolarisation which opens the activation gate and allows the Ca^{2+} to flow in along the concentration gradient and (3) the *inactivated or the blocked state* results from a trap-door like occlusion of the channel by a floppy part (IG) in the intracellular region. The Ca^{2+} ion flow ceases as soon as the inactivation gate (IG) closes.

After the action potential has passed, majority of Ca^{2+} channels pass to inactive state; these then revert to their resting state in a time dependent manner, and become available for activation again. The L-type Ca^{2+} channels are known to contain several stereoselective drug receptor sites for CCBs. These are located in the transmembrane pore of the L-channel in its intracellular half. ***Nifedipine*** and its analogues, act from the inner side of the membrane and bind to one site, while ***verapamil*** and ***diltiazem*** appear to bind to a closely related (but not identical) receptor sites on the other sites. *The binding of the CCBs to their proper receptor sites stabilises the channel in its inactivation state.* The inactivation gate (IG) then closes and flow of Ca^{2+} ions ceases.

The binding of CCB reduces the frequency of the opening of voltage-gated Ca^{2+} channels in response to depolarisation; because these channels are now taking longer time to revert to resting state for being available for activation. The net result is a marked decrease in the transmembrane Ca^{2+} current which in smooth muscle is associated with relaxation; in cardiac muscle with a reduction in contractility throughout the heart; in SA node with a decrease in pacemaker activity and in AV node with a decrease in conduction velocity.

Other type of voltage-gated Ca^{2+} channels (T, N, P/Q) are less sensitive to blockade by CCBs. Therefore, tissues in which these channel types are present (thalamic, cerebellar, Purkinje neurons and secretory glands) are much less affected by these drugs than are cardiac and vascular smooth muscles. In skeletal muscles, the Ca^{2+} is intracellular and hence CCBs are ineffective in skeletal muscles. Among these, T-channels (T for transient) open at a more negative potential (low threshold) and are present on SA and AV nodal tissue along with L-type Ca^{2+} channels.

2. **Receptor-Operated Ca^{2+} Channels**
   These channels increase the Ca^{2+} influx in response to NE, Ang-II, some hormones and tissue factors, independent of membrane depolarisation. NE contracts even depolarised aortic smooth muscle by promoting influx of Ca^{2+} through these channels and releasing Ca^{2+} from sarcoplasmic reticulum. CCBs also decrease Ca^{2+} entry through receptor-operated channel but to a much lesser extent. Their block can be reversed by the use of α_1 agonists that increase the transmembrane influx of Ca^{2+} through DAG-IP_3 pathway. The activity of these channels is also regulated directly by α_2 receptors.
3. **Leak Channels or Stretch-Operated Channels**
   These are present in blood vessels and increase Ca^{2+} influx on being stretched. Small amounts of Ca^{2+} keep on leaking into the resting cell and are pumped out by Ca^{2+} ATPase. Mechanical stretch activates leak channels (or stretch-sensitive Ca^{2+} channels) and promotes inward movement of Ca^{2+}.
4. **Na^+- Ca^{2+} Exchange Channel**
   These are also present in the heart and blood vessels, but are involved in the action of cardiac glycosides and not for the action of CCBs.

Currently CCBs enjoy the status of first-line antihypertensive drugs, used singly or in combination, besides their use in treatment of angina and cardiac arrhythmias (for choice of drugs refer Ch. 20 and 21). Their antihypertensive efficacy is comparable to that of β-blockers or ACEIs. The choice of CCBs in combination therapy is influenced by coexisting disease such as angina, asthma, diabetes and peripheral vascular disease (PVD). These drugs possess some distinct advantages relative to other vasodilators as follows:

1. Their relaxant effects on large arteries is more beneficial in elderly patients.
2. They improve arterial compliance and retard atherogenesis.
3. These can be used safely in patients with asthma (do not increase airway resistance), angina and PVD.
4. They do not have significant effects on release of renin and have no adverse effects on lipid profile, uric acid levels or glucose metabolism.
5. Postural hypotension, first dose effect or rebound phenomenon are not observed.
6. Tolerance associated with renal retention of fluids does not occur. Rather, an intrinsic natriuretic effect is often observed especially with nifedipine group of blockers.
7. They neither impair cerebral nor renal perfusion.
8. These neither impair male sexual activity nor the physical work capacity.
9. They have no adverse effects on foetus.

Classification of CCBs

I. **Dihydropyridines (DHPs)**
   a) **Ultra-short acting**: CLEVIDIPINE
   b) **Short acting**: NIFEDIPINE, NICARDIPINE and NIMODIPINE
   c) **Intermediate acting**: NISOLDIPINE, NITRENDIPINE, ISRADIPINE, LACIDIPINE, CILNIDIPINE and LERCANIDIPINE
   d) **Long acting**: FELODIPINE, BENIDIPINE and AMLODIPINE

II. **Non-dihydropyridines (Non-DHPs)**
   Short acting: VERAPAMIL, DILTIAZEM
   Long acting: BEPRIDIL

Pharmacological Characteristics

Among the three prototype drugs, ***verapamil*** is relatively cardioselective, ***nifedipine*** is relatively vascular smooth muscle selective while ***diltiazem*** exhibits intermediate selectivity. In brief, their pharmacological effects can be compared as follows:

- Cardiac depressant effects such as decrease in heart rate, contractility and conduction velocity: verapamil > diltiazem > nifedipine (Remember: **N**on-**D**HPs - have **N**odal **D**epressant effects)
- Coronary artery dilator effects, including dilatation of both epicardial and intramyocardial arteries, which prevent coronary spasm: nifedipine > verapamil > diltiazem
- Vasodilatory effects on peripheral and pulmonary blood vessels: nifedipine > verapamil > diltiazem (Remember: **DHPs - D**ecrease **P**eripheral vascular resistance).

All CCBs decrease heart rate (HR), contractility and conduction velocity to a varied extent. They also cause coronary vasodilation and reduction in peripheral arterial resistance (↓ in afterload). These have minimal effects on cardiac output or preload (no venodilation). Hence, these are commonly used to treat HT and angina. However, to treat different types of angina, the CCBs are not just interchangeable (see Ch. 20).

The non-DHPs, e.g., *verapamil* or *diltiazem* cause nodal depression more than peripheral vasodilation which makes these heart rate lowering (HRL) agents much closer to β-blockers, than DHPs. These properties reduce myocardial O_2 demand and make them suitable for treating angina, HT and supraventricular tachycardias. However, the non-DHPs differ from β-blockers pharmacologically in 3 aspects: 1) their mode of action; (2) their lack of effect on ventricular tachycardia (which is rather a contraindication for their use) and (3) no benefits in heart failure (rather contraindicated). The DHPs (*nifedipine group*) have more peripheral vasodilatory and coronary dilatory effects than nodal depression.

Restricting our discussion to HT, CCBs are excellent antihypertensive drugs in (1) low renin hypertensive patients, (2) elderly and South-African black patients and (3) in pregnancy as well. Their antihypertensive effect is independent of Na-intake or of concurrent use of NSAIDs (unlike ACEIs). In *hypertension with nephropathy,* both DHPs and non-DHPs reduce the BP remarkably but non-DHPs reduce proteinuria better than DHPs. In *diabetic hypertensives,* longer acting DHPs are reported to improve the clinical outcome. In fact, the 7th report of the Joint National Committee on Prevention, Detection, Evaluation & Treatment of High Blood Pressure has suggested that diabetes is a positive indication for the preferential use of CCBs. However, the current practice is to use a ACEI+ longer acting DHP+ a diuretic. The old controversy about the safety and efficacy associated with the use of short-acting CCBs has also been laid to rest after the findings that longer-acting DHPs are quite safe and efficacious antihypertensive and antianginal drugs.

DHP Group of CCBs

The short-acting capsular form of ***nifedipine*** was the first CCB of this group that was introduced to treat HT and angina. Soon, various clinical trials revealed that use of short-acting nifedipine is linked with poor outcomes in unstable angina that results due to abrupt vasodilation with reflex sympathetic activation leading to tachycardia and increased risk of ischaemia (↑ O_2 demand). Such baroreceptor- mediated sympathetic rebound can also aggravate the pre-existing left ventricular dysfunction. Earlier, short-acting nifedipine (10 mg, sublingually) was used in emergency management of severe hypertension. Later, it was associated with increased risk of myocardial infarction and mortality due to sudden fall in BP. The focus, therefore, changed to an introduction of extended-release formulation of nifedipine or truly long-acting DHPs (e.g., *amlodipine*) which are free of such dangers. Extended release formulation of nifedipine are now used for the treatment of HT and *exertional angina.* In addition, it has an intrinsic natriuretic effect and hence does not need an addition of a diuretic. Such preparations with a β-blocker (e.g., atenolol) are more suited to hypertensive-anginal patients. Antihypertensive dose for a sustained release preparation of nifedipine is 10–40 mg BD orally.

Adverse effects: The immediate release capsules of nifedipine cause headache, flushing and peripheral (ankle) oedema. The peripheral oedema in lower extremities results due to precapillary dilation and reflex postcapillary constriction which leads to an increased hydrostatic pressure. Headache results due to arteriolar vasodilation. Other side effects include tachycardia (see above) and reversible gingival hyperplasia (on prolonged use). Its negative inotropic effects are unsuited for patients with LV dysfunction.

Contraindications: Unstable angina (unless combined with β-blocker); LV failure; aortic stenosis and obstructive cardiomyopathy. ***Drug interactions***: Liver disease, enzyme inhibitors and grape fruit juice increase the plasma levels of nifedipine.

Amlodipine ($t_{1/2}$ 35–48 hr) because of its longer $t_{1/2}$, it can be given orally once a day. It has lesser first-pass metabolism, hence bioavailability is consistent. Day time fluctuations in blood levels are minimal and the antihypertensive effect lasts up to next morning. It has a slow but complete oral absorption, hence early side effects, related to vasodilatation, such as tachycardia, headache and flushing are largely avoided, but (like nifedipine) ankle oedema is quite troublesome. It is approved for effort angina as well as for hypertension. Dose 5–10 mg once daily orally. *Drug interactions*: virtually nil.

Contraindications: like nifedipine.

Felodipine $t_{1/2}$ (22–24 hr) like amlodipine it has longer $t_{1/2}$ but greater vascular selectivity than nifedipine. Once daily dose (5–10 mg oral) is sufficient. It is approved for long term treatment of hypertension.

Isradipine, nitrendipine, nisoldipine, cilnidipine, lercanidipine, lacidipine and ***benidipine*** are also vasoselective, intermediate acting, nifedipine derivatives. These have hardly any effect on AV node. Among these, ***isradipine*** ($t_{1/2}$ 8 hrs) is given in a dose of 2.5–5 mg BD orally, for HT. ***Nitrendipine*** ($t_{1/2}$ 8–12 hrs) can be given orally in dose of 20 mg once daily for HT and angina. ***Nisoldipine*** ($t_{1/2}$ 8–12 hrs) is indicated for HT in a dose of 20 mg OD orally. ***Lercanidipine*** ($t_{1/2}$ 8–10 hrs) is also a vasoselective CCB used to treat HT (10–20 mg OD orally). ***Benidipine*** is a CCB approved to treat HT and angina (2–4 mg OD or BD orally). It is claimed to inhibit cardiac remodeling. ***Lacidipine*** is a longer acting CCB used to treat HT (2–6 mg OD orally). It also slows down the progression of carotid atherosclerosis, limits the development of new metabolic syndrome and new diabetes, besides providing good vasoprotection. It causes least ankle oedema.

Cilnidipine is approved to treat HT and is claimed to be a renoprotective CCB.

Nicardipine ($t_{1/2}$ 4 hrs) is highly vasoselective drug. It has more pronounced coronary dilatation effect with lesser effect on cardiac contractility as compared to nifedipine. It is approved for both angina and HT. Dose (sustained release preparation) 30–60 mg BD orally.

Nimodipine ($t_{1/2}$ 2 hrs) is highly lipid soluble and crosses BBB. It shows higher affinity and selectivity for cerebral blood vessels and appears to reduce morbidity following a subarachnoid haemorrhage. Nimodipine is labeled for use in patients of migraine or those who have had a haemorrhagic stroke. (Dose: 60 mg, 6 hrly, for 21 days. Therapy to be started within 96 hrs of the stroke).

Clevidipine ($t_{1/2}$ 1 min) is an ultra short acting L-type CCB with a terminal $t_{1/2}$ of < 15 min when administered by I.V. infusion in a dose of 1–2 mg/hr. (2–4 mL/hr of 50 mg/100 mL solution).

The drug has been approved for urgent reduction of BP in patients of severe HT and in subjects with HT undergoing cardiac surgery to control perioperative and postoperative HT. When compared to other drugs to treat severe HT (180/115 mmHg) clevidipine infusion was found significantly more effective than sodium nitroprusside and glyceryl trinitrate infusion at keeping the BP within a target range in 30 min and was equally effective to nicardipine infusion. Most pataients can be switched to oral therapy within in 6 hrs of stopping clevidipine.

Non hypertensive patients undergoing cardiac surgery need monitoring, after prolonged infusion of clevidipine for atleast 8 hrs after the dosing is stopped. This is because of the risk of rebound HT. Common adverse effects of clevidipine in severe HT are headache, nausea and vomiting. Some of the adverse effects can be anticipated from its action, e.g., HT tachycardia and a negative inotropic effect which can exacerbate to heart failure.

Non-DHP Group of CCBs

Verapamil: The peripheral vasodilating effects of verapamil are accompanied by characteristic cardiac depressant effects like decrease in heart rate, conduction velocity and contractility. Verapamil has a more depressant effect on heart compared to diltiazem. The reflex tachycardia, a consequence of fall in BP, is blunted by direct negative chronotropic effect of the drug. It possesses a nonspecific α-adrenergic blocking action which may also contribute to peripheral vasodilatation. It is approved for use in angina (effort, vasospastic, unstable; Ch. 20), supraventricular tachyarrhythmias (Ch. 21), post-infarct protection and for mild to moderate hypertension. Dose: 120 mg BD or 80 mg TDS orally. *Side effects*: mainly constipation. Levels ↑ in liver or renal disease. *Contraindications*: sick sinus syndrome, AV conduction defects and heart failure. *Drug interactions*: Verapamil inhibits P-glycoprotein (digoxin transporter) and thus ↑ blood digoxin levels. It also inhibits CYP3A isoenzyme and thus ↑ blood levels of statins. With β-blokers, there is an additive sinus depression. Quinidine and disopyramide enhance negative inotropic potential.

Diltiazem: It is less potent coronary as well as peripheral vasodilator than nifedipine and verapamil. But, the suppression of automaticity at SA node and conductivity at AV node are of the same magnitude as of verapamil. However, the decrease in contractility is lesser than verapamil. Uses are same as of verapamil; side effect profile is low (no constipation). Contraindications and drug interactions are also same (but little or no effect on digoxin levels). Women are are more sensitive than men to its BP lowering effect. Dose : 60–120 mg BD oral; max 360 mg/day.

Bepridil: Like verapamil, it also blocks Ca^{2+} channels in cardiac cells. It reduces BP and heart rate in patients with exertional (stable) angina but also reported to improve left ventricular performance. Recent trials have revealed that it prolongs QTc interval and can produce serious arrhythmias (torsade de pointes in presence of hypokalaemia or bradycardia). Agranulocytosis has also been reported. Hence, it is not used commonly, except in patients who are refractory to all other therapy.

Vasodilators

The drugs discussed in this section are also referred to as ***direct vasodilators*** because the vasodilatation produced by them neither depends on innervation of the vasculature nor is mediated through receptors. The vasodilators decrease the total peripheral resistance (PR) and thus lower BP irrespective of the aetiology of HT. Majority of vasodilators (except sodium nitroprusside) relax arterial smooth muscle to a greater extent than venous smooth muscle and do not inhibit the reflex sympathetic activity; therefore, postural hypotension and impotence are not a problem. However, on chronic use their effectiveness is severely hampered by neuroendocrine and sympathetic reflexes that tend to counteract the fall in BP. Hence, the vasodilators are generally inadequate as the sole therapy for HT. All such inter-relationships have been discussed in earlier text and depicted in Figure 19.1.

Arteriolar Vasodilators

These include ***hydralazine***, ***minoxidil***, ***diazoxide*** and ***fenoldopam***. Two of these agents, hydralazine and minoxidil, are used orally for long-term outpatient therapy of HT. The other two, diazoxide and fenoldopam, are given parenterally to treat hypertensive emergencies.

COMMON FEATURES: These drugs produce vasodilatation by activating potassium channels present in arteriolar blood vessels. An increase in the K^+ conductance results in hyperpolarisation of cell membrane which causes relaxation of vascular smooth muscle. They have little or no effect on venous capacitance and do not inhibit reflex sympathetic activity. This limits the therapeutic usefulness of these drugs to such an extent that they are rarely used alone. These are usually administered in combination with a diuretic (to prevent Na^+ retention) and a β-blocker (to prevent the effects of reflex cardiac stimulation and hyper-reninemia). The triple combination provides a decrease in cardiac output (β-blocker), reduction in plasma volume (diuretic) and a decrease in TPR (vasodilator drug).

Hydralazine: The vasodilatation produced by hydralazine depends in part on the presence of an intact endothelium. This implies that, besides activating K^+ channels, vasodilatation due to hydralazine is partly endothelium dependent and may involve generation of nitric oxide and stimulation of cGMP. Increase in intracellular levels of cGMP are associated with vascular smooth muscle relaxation.

Hydralazine is well absorbed orally but undergoes first-pass metabolism. The maximum response comes within 30 min to 1 hour and its duration of effect lasts for about 6 hours. Interestingly, the duration of its effect is somewhat longer than its plasma half-life (t½ 1–2.5 hrs), because the drug is specifically accumulated in artery walls where it may continue to exert a vasodilator effect even when plasma concentration declines. Since N-acetylation of hydralazine is an important metabolic pathway, the genetically determined low activity of N-acetyl-transferase (slow acetylators) results in higher plasma levels of hydralazine. Conversely, in fast acetylators, the therapeutic effects may get decreased.

Hydralazine (25–50 mg BD, orally) is generally reserved for moderately hypertensive ambulatory patients in whom BP is not effectively controlled either by a diuretic or by a β-blocker. Hydralazine is generally not employed by I.V. route because the onset of action is hardly different than that of oral, and its therapeutic effects are also variable. ***Adverse effects*** are associated with vasodilatation and the reflex haemodynamic changes that occur in response to vasodilatation. These include headache, tachycardia, nausea, nasal congestion and anginal attack (due to tachycardia). These untoward effects of hydralazine are greatly reduced when it is administered in conjunction with a diuretic and a β-blocker. On prolonged use in high doses, it causes reversible disseminated lupus erythematosus like syndrome.

Minoxidil: It is an orally effective, more potent and longer acting vasodilator than hydralazine. Its vasodilator effects depend on its *in vivo* metabolism by hepatic enzymes to produce an active metabolite minoxidil sulfate which activates K^+ channel opening (see above). Maximum response comes within 1–2 hrs but the antihypertensive effects last for 12–24 hrs. This allows the drug to be administered only once or twice a day. Interestingly again, the therapeutic half-life of minoxidil is considerably longer than its plasma half-life (t½ 4 hrs). As has been suggested for hydralazine, this results either due to accumulation of drug itself or because of longer t½ of its active metabolite or both. It is primarily metabolised by liver and is not accumulated in patients with renal failure.

The major indications for the use of minoxidil are severe HT that may be life-threatening or HT associated with chronic renal failure or HT that is resistant to other forms of therapy (2.5–5 mg daily; gradually increased to 40–50 mg daily depending on response). ***Side effects*** are attributable to vasodilatation and reflex sympathetic activity and include headache, nasal congestion, tachycardia and precipitation of anginal attacks. These effects are of little clinical significance because the drug is almost always administered in combination with a β-blocker and a diuretic (see above). A more troublesome side effect, particularly in women, is the growth of body hair (hirsutism) because it activates a specific gene that regulates the hair shaft protein. This particular side effect has been capitalised upon and topical minoxidil is now marketed as a stimulant of hair growth for correcting male-type baldness. Minoxidil, therefore, illustrates how a side effect in women can be utilised for male's therapy.

Diazoxide: It is chemically related to thiazide diuretics but incidentally causes retention of Na^+ and water instead of diuresis. It opens K^+ channels to produce long lasting arteriolar dilatation with no effect on venules (see above). It lowers BP within 3–5 min after rapid I.V. injection. Slow I.V. injection or infusion is less effective as the drug exhibits rapid and extensive protein binding (90–95%). Long-term oral or parenteral use is not suitable because it causes hyperuricaemia, hyperglycaemia and fluid retention. It is metabolised both by liver and kidney. Plasma half-life (t½ 20–45 hrs) may therefore be further prolonged in patients with hepatic and renal insufficiency.

Diazoxide is used for the treatment of hypertensive emergencies such as malignant HT, hypertensive encephalopathy and eclampsia. It is frequently administered in conjunction with a diuretic and a β-blocker. Since diazoxide is not meant for long- term therapy, toxicities (Na^+ and water retention) associated with chronic use are rare, and are of little significance.

Fenoldopam: It acts primarily as an agonist of dopamine receptor (D_1) leading to dilatation of peripheral arteries and natriuresis. It has a poor oral bioavailability, a short elimination half-life (t½ 5 min) and a rapid onset of action. It is therefore, given by I.V. infusion for the short-term management of hypertensive emergencies. Additionally, in contrast to sodium nitroprusside, urine output, creatinine clearance, and Na^+ excretion are increased by fenoldopam. It may therefore, be useful in hypertensive emergency associated with impaired renal function. Concomitant use of a β-blocker and/ or a diuretic is not essential. However, caution is required for its use in patients in whom hypotension could be deleterious such as those with acute cerebral infarction or haemorrhage. The usual dose range is 0.1 to 1.5 μg/kg/minute.

As with other vasodilators, *the adverse effects* include reflex tachycardia, headache and flushing. However, it is not used for long-term therapy. Fenoldopam also increases intraocular pressure and should be avoided in patients of glaucoma. Hypokalaemia has also been reported and hence serum electrolytes should be monitored prior to and during therapy. BP and heart rate should be monitored for dose adjustments or dose increment.

Arteriolar + Venous Vasodilators

Sodium Nitroprusside: It is also called a nitrovaso-dilator as it releases nitric oxide *in vivo*. The pharmacological activity of the drug resides in its nitroso moiety. Sodium nitroprusside activates guanylyl cyclase either directly or through release of nitric oxide (NO). This results in an increase in the intracellular levels of cGMP which provides vascular smooth muscle relaxation.

It is a powerful, parenterally administered, vasodilator that dilates both arterial and venous blood vessels resulting in a decrease in peripheral vascular resistance and in venous return. The onset of its hypotensive effect is rapid (30 sec) after I.V. infusion (0.3 µg/kg/min, slowly raised to 0.5 µg/kg/min) and disappears within 10 min after discontinuation. It is administered by continuous I.V. infusion for the treatment of hypertensive emergencies. In hypertensive crisis which is not accompanied with heart failure, it decreases BP without affecting cardiac output (CO) significantly. But in patients with refractory heart failure, even in absence of HT, it improves ventricular performance by reducing preload (due to venodilatation) and also afterload (by arteriolar dilatation). Sodium nitroprusside has, therefore, special place in the treatment of severe HT with acute MI or LVF. The aqueous solutions of sodium nitroprusside are unstable and sensitive to light. Therefore, the solutions should be made up fresh before each administration and the bottle should be covered by a dark paper.

Other than headache, nausea and vomiting which quickly dissipate after the infusion is stopped, *serious toxicity* can occur due to accumulation of cyanide or thiocyanate. Sodium nitroprusside is converted in erythrocytes to cyanide which is then metabolised in liver to less toxic thiocyanate. The plasma half-life of thiocyanate is about 3 days. This may lead to metabolic acidosis and arrhythmias. Thiocyanate may accumulate particularly in patients with renal insufficiency, who cannot excrete thiocyanate at normal rate. Thiocyanate toxicity is manifested as psychosis, disorientation and convulsions. Delayed hypothyroidism may also occur owing to thiocyanate induced inhibition of iodide uptake by thyroid. Administration of sodium thiosulfate and hydroxycobalamine can be used to trap cyanide ions. Sodium thiosulfate acts as a sulfur donor and facilitates metabolism of cyanide to sodium thiocyanate which is excreted in urine. Hydroxycobalamine combines with cyanide ion to from nontoxic cyanocobalamine (see Ch.18).

Ganglion Blocking Agents

Owing to the frequency and severity of side effects and because of the availability of better antihypertensive agents, ganglion blockers are seldom used these days (Ch.13). However, a short acting drug **trimethaphan**, as a slow I.V. infusion, may be used as an alternative to or in combination with sodium nitroprusside for the treatment of hypertensive emergencies and to produce controlled hypotension to minimise blood loss during neurosurgery or to facilitate surgery on blood vessels. Trimethaphan blunts the symphatho-adrenal stimulation caused by sodium nitroprusside and reduces its required doses.

Miscellaneous Group

Reserpine

It is an alkaloid obtained from the roots of *Rauwolfia serpentina*. It was a popular antihypertensive of late 1950 and early 1960s, but nowadays it has historical importance only. It is now used as a pharmacological tool (see Ch.13).

Guanethidine

The availability of less toxic and more selective drugs has made guanethidine obsolete nowadays (For details see Ch.13). It is a polar compound and does not cross BBB. It is taken up into the sympathetic neuron by active amine uptake and later displaces NE from storage granules. It also blocks NE uptake by the axonal membrane. Chronic administration thus impairs NE release due to its depletion. Guanethidine is given orally in severe HT usually in combination with a diuretic and a vasodilator. Side effects include postural hypotension, diarrhoea (due to parasympathetic overactivity), inhibition of ejaculation, impotence, Na^+ and water retention leading to frank oedema.

TREATMENT OF HYPERTENSIVE URGENCIES & EMERGENCIES

Hypertensive urgencies and emergencies are situation in which BP must be rapidly reduced by

Table 19.2 The Drug of Choice and the Drugs to be Avoided in Hypertensive Patients With Concomitant Disease/Condition

Concomitant condition	Drugs of choice	Drugs to be avoided
Angina	β-Blockers; CCBs	Vasodilators
Asthma COPD	CCBs; Diuretics AT_1 receptor antagonists	β-Blockers; ACEIs
Benign prostatic hyperplasia	α-Blocker	CCBs
Congestive heart failure	Diuretics; ACEIs	Verapamil and other CCBs except Amlodipine; α-Blockers
Diabetes (insulin-dependent)	ACEIs; CCBs	β-Blockers; Diuretics
Hyperlipidaemia	ACEIs; CCBs; α-Blockers	β-Blockers (non-ISA); Diuretics
Isolated systolic HT in older patients	CCBs; Diuretics α-Blockers	—
Post-myocardial infarction	β-Blockers (non ISA); ACEIs	β-Blockers with ISA
Pregnancy	Methyldopa; Dihydropyridine group of CCBs; Cardioselective β-blockers (see text)	ACEIs; AT_1 receptor antagonists; Diuretics; Propranolol; Labetalol
Peripheral vascular disease	CCBs; α-Blockers	β-Blockers
Renal insufficiency	CCBs; Diuretics	K^+-sparing diuretics
Supraventricular tachycardia	Verapamil; Diltiazem	—
Thyrotoxicosis	β-Blockers (without ISA)	Drugs causing tachycardia

25 mmHg within 30 min to 1 hr to avoid the risk of severe morbidity and death. These include patients with asymptomatic severe HT (systolic BP > 220 mm Hg and/or diastolic BP > 125 mm Hg that persists after a period of observation) and those with optic disk edema, progressive target-organ complications, and serere perioperative HT. All these determine the seriousness of the emergency and the selection of the drug. Emergencies include *hypertensive encephalopathy* (headache, irritability, confusion and altered mental status due to cerebrovascular spasm), *hypertensive nephropathy* (haematuria, proteinuria, and progressive renal dysfunction due to renal arteriolar necrosis), *intracranial haemorrhage, dissecting aneurysm, pre-eclampsia-eclampsia, acute pulmonary oedema, unstable angina, myocardial infarction* or *malignant hypertension* (hypertension associated with vascular damage and papilloedema).

The initial goal in hypertensive emergency is to reduce the BP by no more than 25% (within few min to 1–2 hrs) and then toward a level of 160/100 mm Hg within next 2–6 hours. Subsequently, the BP can be reduced to normal levels using oral medication over several weeks. Rapid and complete normalisation of BP should be avoided because chronic HT is always associated with autoregulatory changes in cerebral blood flow. Thus a rapid normalisation of BP would lead to cerebral, coronary or renal ischaemia. A growing number of drugs used for the management of hypertensive crisis are discussed below.

Nicardipine: It is the most potent and longest acting parenteral CCB. It is the first line drug for hypertensive emergency. It is a vasodilator; dilates arterioles. It may cause reflex tachycardia; so esmolol or labetalol can be given along with it. It reduces BP within 1 hr in most of the patients. The beneficial effects are seen in haemorrhagic and ischaemic stroke. It can be given in hypertensive emergency due to aortic dissection and pre-eclampsia. It is the most commonly used drug with less side effects.

Sodium Nitroprusside is no longer the treatament of choice for emergency HT*. However, in combination with a beta-blocker, it is a reserved treatment of emergency HT in patients of aortic dissection.*

In most situations, appropriate control of BP is best achieved using combinations of clevidipine or nicardipine plus labetalol or esmolol.

Clevidipine: Intravenous clevidipine infusion produces a rapid and tight contol of severe HT by its effects on arterial vascular bed without any venodilator or myocardial depresent effects. Its use in HT emergency has already been discussed above.

Labetalol: This dual α- and β-blocking agent is useful in hypertensive emergencies associated with ischaemia, eclampsia, pre-eclampsia and at times phaeochromocytoma (I.V. infusion 2.5–25 μg/kg/min). It can be continued orally also after the crisis is over.

Esmolol: This short-acting β-blocker is useful for the treatment SVT but can be used for lowering acute rise of BP, especially when combined with nicardipine or clevidipine as used alone this β-blocker is weaker than labetalol. Such a combination would be useful in acute HT associated with aortic dissection and during myocardial ischaemia with episodes of tachycardia.

Fenoldopam: It is a peripheral dopamine (D_1) receptor agonist that elicits a dose-dependent reduction BP without evidence of tolerance, withdrawal /rebound HT or deterioration of renal function. This compound is useful in the treatment of hypertensive emergency associated with impaired renal function (see earlier text). Dose: I.V. infusion 0.2–0.5 μg/kg/min.

Nitroglycerin, intravenous: I.V. nitroglycerin should be reserved for patients of emergency HT with accompanying accut coronary syndrome .

Diazoxide: It is given in small I.V. bolus injection to treat hypertensive episodes of pre-eclampsia-eclampsia and is also preferred when myocardial reserve is low or in renal insufficiency. Its use is mostly obsolete.

Hydralazine: It can be used primarily in eclampsia and in children, but should be avoided in patients with coronary artery disease and aortic dissection (i.e., hypertension without cardiac complications). Generally obsolete these days.

Diuretics: Intravenous furosemide or bumetanide can be used as an adjunct, rather than a primary agent for hypertensive emergencies. These are useful in associated conditions like acute LVF, pulmonary oedema, CHF or cerebral oedema as in encephalopathy.

Phentolamine: This nonselective α-blocker is a drug of choice in hypertensive episodes associated with phaeochromocytoma, cheese reaction and clonidine withdrawal. Dose: 1–4 mg I.V. bolus injection.

When the BP has been brought under control, oral antihypertensives can be added as the parenteral drugs are tapered off over a period of 2–3 days. The subsequent therapy with oral antihypertensive drugs should invariably include a diuretic.The drugs of choice and the drugs to be avoided in hypertensive patients with comorbid conditions are given in Table 19.2.

MANAGEMENT OF HYPERTENSION

According to World Health Organization (WHO), 2021

WHO recommends initiation of pharmacological antihypertensive treatment of individuals with a confirmed diagnosis of hypertension and systolic blood pressure of ≥140 mm Hg or diastolic blood pressure of ≥90 mm Hg. Drug groups recommended: (1) thiazide and thiazide-like agents; (2) angiotensin-converting enzyme inhibitors (ACEIs)/angiotensin-receptor blockers (ARBs); (3) long-acting dihydropyridine calcium channel blockers (CCBs). WHO suggests combination therapy, preferably with a single-pill combination as an initial treatment. Antihypertensive medications used in combination therapy should be chosen from the above three drug classes: diuretics.

According to American College of Cardiology/ American Heart Association (AHA, European Heart Journal, 2022)

Criteria to start antihypertensive drugs: All adults with SBP ≥140 mm Hg or DBP ≥90 mm Hg. Adults with SBP 130–139 or DBP 80–89 mm Hg and CVD or a 10-year atherosclerotic CVD risk ≥10%, based on estimation using of the ACC/AHA Pooled Cohort Equations calculator. *Target reduction in BP*: A systolic/diastolic blood pressure <130/80 mm Hg target recommended for all adults with hypertension. *Drugs to be started*: For selection of a BP-lowering medication, treat with ≥1 drugs from the following classes: Diuretic, CCB, ACEI or ARB. Combination therapy is required in most patients with a starting SBP/DBP ≥20/10 mm Hg above the BP reduction target. Dual- and triple-drug therapy should include agents with different mechanisms of action.

According to Joint National Committee (JNC-8) Guidelines

Start with first line drug groups: ACEI or ARB or CCB or Thiazide diuretic (Not β blockers).

Stage I hypertension: Give thiazide or ACEI, ARB, CCB; review after 2–4 weeks, if BP not controlled; increase the dose or give combination therapy.

Stage II hypertension: Thiazide diuretic + ACEI/ARB/CCB. Alternatively, ACEI + CCB can be given.

Stepped Care Approach

If age of patient <55 years: start ACEI or ARB. If age of patient >55 years: start CCB or diuretic. If BP is not controlled; give ACEI/ARB + CCB or diuretic. Combination therapy: ACEI/ARB + CCB + Diuretic. In resistant hypertension: ACEI/ARB + CCB + Diuretic + β blocker/spironolactone/high dose thiazides can be given.

Rational Drug Combinations

1) Amlodipine + Lisinopril.
2) Amlodipine + Enalapril.
3) Lisinopril/Irbesartan + Hydrochlorothiazide.

Combinations to be avoided

a) β blocker + Diuretic: Risk of hyperglycaemia.
b) Verapamil + β blocker: Causes bradycardia.
c) ACEI+ ARB: Risk of hyperkalaemia.

CHAPTER 20 Drug Therapy of Angina Pectoris

COMPETENCY PH1.28

Slowly progressive insufficiency of coronary circulation is called ischaemic heart disease (IHD). It occurs as a result of atherosclerosis of large epicardial coronary arteries. Usually, atheromatous plaques are formed in the areas of flow disturbances such as bends in vessels or near branching. The plaques are often localized but coronary artherosclerosis can be diffused involving a long segment of the vessel. The parts of coronary artery affected by diffused atherosclerosis are particularly prone to vasospasm since endothelial function is impaired by atheroma as a result of reduced generation of nitric oxide. ***Angina pectoris*** (angere = to strangulate; pectus = chest) is a clinical manifestation of the reversible myocardial ischaemia and is most frequently experienced as suffocating substernal pain in the chest, over the heart, on exertion (precordial pain) which may radiate to left arm, neck or the jaw, and is relieved by rest.

The anginal pain occurs due to imbalance between the oxygen requirement and oxygen supply in the ischaemic area of myocardium. This imbalance results from an inability of the coronary blood flow to meet the metabolic demands of the myocardium (due to fixed narrowing of the coronary artery) and if vasospasm also occurs, angina may precipitate even at a lower work-load. If due to some co-existing conditions (e.g., anaemia, hypoxia, hypertension, hyperthyroidism and diabetes), the work-load of the heart increases and the oxygen supply from the blood becomes deficient to sustain the metabolic needs of the myocardium, the cellular viability of the heart is threatened and the above anginal symptoms appear.

In some people, ischaemic episodes may occur without producing angina pain. This is known as "silent myocardial ischaemia". It becomes dangerous because the person has no forewarning of an impending heart attack. More serious than myocardial ischaemia is myocardial infarction (MI), commonly called as "heart attack". Infarction means the death of an area of the tissue due to an interruption in blood supply. MI may result from a thrombus (stationary blood clot) or embolus (blood clot transported by blood) in the coronary arteries. The tissue distal to the obstruction dies and is replaced by a non-contractile scar tissue. The heart muscle, therefore, loses some of its strength. The after effects depend partly on the size and the location of the infarcted area. Besides damaging the normal heart tissue, the infarction may disrupt the conducting system of the heart and may cause sudden death by triggering ventricular fibrillation.

In ECG the IHD is manifested by an alteration in the direction of repolarisation. As a result, there is an elevation of ST segment in MI, or depression of ST segment when the heart muscle receives insufficient O_2. The T wave either gets flattened or inverted in IHD. The presence of Q waves of > 0.04 sec duration with a depth greater than 25% of the R wave amplitude is also a specific criteria for MI (Fig. 20.1).

Three forms of angina have been characterised:

1. ***Classical or Stable angina (Angina of effort or Exertional angina)***: This constitutes about 90% of angina cases. Attacks are provoked by exercise, emotion or meals. The ischaemia, caused by fixed atheromatous stenosis of larger coronary arteries, results in an accumulation of acidic metabolites, which stimulates myocardial pain-mediating nerve endings.
2. ***Crescendo or Unstable angina (Preinfarction angina)***: It is characterised by recurrent attacks of angina even with minimal exertion or even at rest due to progressive atheromatous narrowing of coronary vessel, or due to platelet aggregation at ruptured plaque, along with vasospasm. These patients need hospitalisation to prevent impending MI.

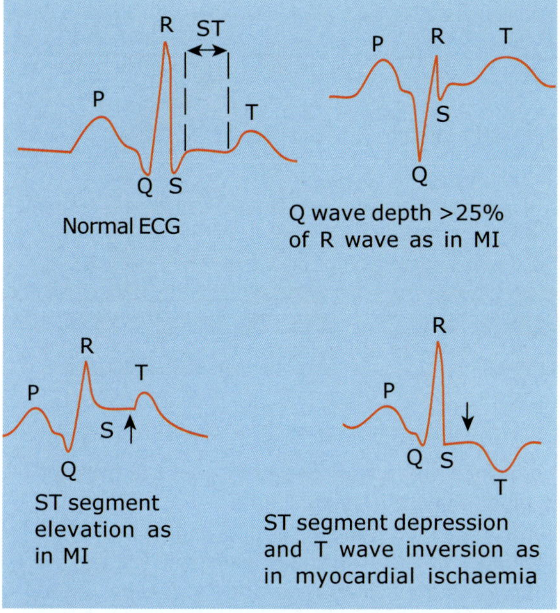

Fig 20.1 Effects of Mycoardial Ischaemia and Infarction on ECG.

3. ***Variant or Prinzmetal angina (Vasospastic angina)***: In this condition the pain appears even during rest or during sleep and is usually unrelated to exercise. It is due to recurrent localised coronary vasospasm that causes reduction in coronary blood flow. However, the coronary spasm may be superimposed with atheromatous stenosis. Vasospastic angina may deteriorate into unstable angina.

FACTORS AFFECTING CORONARY BLOOD FLOW, MYOCARDIAL OXYGEN SUPPLY AND DEMAND

The coronary blood flow is only 4% of the total cardiac output, but the oxygen extraction is 75% as compared to 25% in the systemic circulation. The coronary blood flow is facilitated by an increase in aortic diastolic pressure and by the decrease in coronary arteriolar resistance. The coronary flow occurs during the diastole only—the longer the diastole, better the coronary blood flow. On the contrary, an increase in ventricular pressure, myocardial fibre tension, heart rate, contractility and heart size will increase the oxygen demand of the myocardium.

The major determinants of coronary blood flow are the myocardial metabolic products which are generated locally due to ischaemia. A fall in arterial PO_2 causes hypoxia, which stimulates production of lactic acid, adenosine and PGI_2 all of which tend to produce vasodilatation around the ischaemic tissue as a compensatory phenomenon. If the other branch of the main coronary vessel is normal (unobstructed) and a powerful arteriolar dilator drug (e.g., dipyridamole, see following text) is administered, the arterioles of the normal vessel will be forced to dilate increasing the blood flow through a well-perfused area (where it is not required) at the cost of poorly perfused ischaemic area (where it is needed). Due to such decrease in coronary blood flow through obstructed branch, produced by arteriolar dilator drug, the anginal pain may even worsen. On the other hand, drugs that dilate veins and larger arteries more effectively than the resistance vessels (e.g., nitrates) reduce anginal pain. This apparent anomaly in the actions of dipyridamole and nitrates, has been explained on the basis of "coronary steal phenomenon" as described above (Fig. 20.2 A,B & C).

Coronary atherosclerosis or coronary spasm or thromboembolism decreases the coronary blood flow due to narrowing of the lumen of the coronary artery. However, this partial occlusion stimulates the opening of the collateral arteries between the epicardial and subendocardial region which try to meet the needed O_2 demand to some extent but not completely (Fig. 20.2 B).

ANTIANGINAL DRUGS

These can be classified as follows:

I. **ORGANIC NITRATES**

a) ***Rapid onset, short acting.*** Amyl nitrite; Nitroglycerine (glyceryl trinitrate)

b) ***Slow onset, long-acting.*** Isosorbide dinitrate (short acting by sublingual route); Isosorbide mononitrate, Erythrityl tetranitrate, Pentaerythritol tetranitrate.

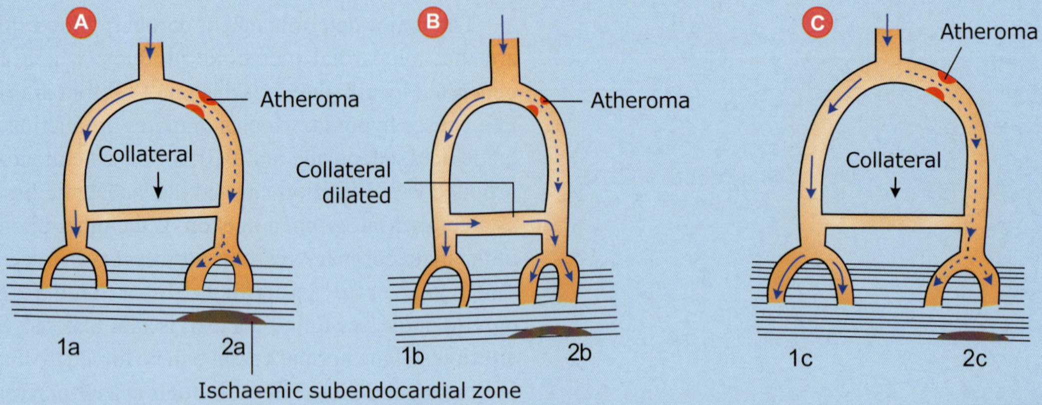

A—Untreated patient of angina. Arterioles of occluded branch are fully dilated in response to hypoxia (2a) in an attempt to compensate for the decreased blood flow to ischaemic area.
B—Drugs that dilate veins and larger arteries, dilate the collaterals, thus allowing more blood to the ischaemic region (2b) mostly by diverting blood from the normally perfused area (1b).
C—Powerful arteriolar dilating drug like dipyridamole, dilates arterioles and increases blood flow towards the normal area (1c) at the expense of ischaemic area (2c) where the arterioles are fully dilated anyway. This is termed as worsening of myocardial ischaemia due to ***"coronary steal phenomenon"***.

Fig 20.2 Phenomenon of 'Coronary Steal' and Opening of Collateral Arteries.

II. **CALCIUM CHANNEL BLOCKERS (CCBs)**
Verapamil, Diltiazem, Nifedipine, Amlodipine, Nicardipine, Nitrendipine, Isradipine and Benidipine

III. **BETA-BLOCKERS**
Propranolol, Atenolol, Metoprolol, Nadolol, Bisoprolol and Celiprolol

IV. **MISCELLANEOUS**
a) ***Potassium Channel Openers***: Nicorandil
b) ***Cytoprotective Drugs***: Trimetazidine, Ranolazine
c) ***Antiplatelet Drugs***: Aspirin, Ticlopidine, Clopidogrel, Dipyridamole, Cilostazol
d) ***Bradycardic Drugs***: Ivabradine
e) ***HMG-CoA Reductase Inhibitors***: Statins
f) ***Drugs for Peripheral Vascular Disease***: Naftidofuryl and Pentoxiphylline

ORGANIC NITRATES

Organic nitrates are polyalcohol esters of nitric acid whereas organic nitrites are esters of nitrous acid. Organic nitrate such as glyceryl trinitrate (or nitroglycerine) is a volatile oily liquid. It is kept in a tightly closed amber-coloured glass container as it loses potency due to light and adsorption to plastic surfaces. Isosorbide dinitrate, isosorbide mononitrate, erythrityl tetranitrate and pentaerythritol tetranitrate are solids. Organic nitrite such as amylnitrite is a highly volatile liquid that is administered by inhalation. Its use has been discontinued.

Mechanism of Action

The mechanism of action of nitrates is believed to involve nitrate receptors that are present in vascular smooth muscle. The nitrate receptors possess -SH groups which reduce nitrates to nitrite and nitric oxide (NO). The NO itself gets converted to an intermediate—reactive nitrosothiol (R.SNO)—which activates intracellular guanylate cyclase (GC) to convert GTP to cGMP (Fig. 20.3). The increase in intracellular cGMP results in vascular smooth muscle relaxation possibly through inhibition of Ca^{2+} entry *via* L-type Ca^{2+} channels or through decrease in Ca^{2+} release from sarcoplasmic reticulum. cGMP also facilitates the dephosphorylation of myosin-light chain-PO_4 (MLC- PO_4) to MLC, which prevents interaction of myosin with actin leading to vascular smooth muscle relaxation. Formation of PGE_2 or PGI_2 and membrane hyperpolarization may also contribute to its mode of action (Fig. 20.3).

Pharmacokinetics

The nitrates are inactivated in liver by glutathione-organic nitrate reductase. Therefore, their oral bioavailability is considerably less due to their first-pass metabolism. The sublingual route, which avoids first-pass effect, is therefore preferred. Despite the fact that therapeutic blood levels are reached within minutes after sublingual route, the total duration of action lasts for about 25–30 min. However, sustained release formulations or oral preparations in sufficient amount can be given to provide blood levels for a longer duration.

Amyl nitrite is now obsolete, because of its unpleasant odour and shorter duration of action. The dinitrate metabolites of nitroglycerine have much less vasodilator activity with a half-life of about 40 minutes. *Isosorbide dinitrate* is inactivated at one-sixth the rate of nitroglycerine. Their enzymatic denitration is followed by formation of glucuronide conjugation. The two metabolites—isosorbide-2-mononitrate and isosorbide-5-mononitrate—have longer half-lives (3 to 6 hours) and are, in part, responsible for therapeutic efficacy of the drug. *Isosorbide-5-mononitrate* has an excellent bioavailability (100%) as it does not undergo significant first-pass metabolism. It is available as plain tablet and as sustained release tablet both of which have a longer duration of action than isosorbide

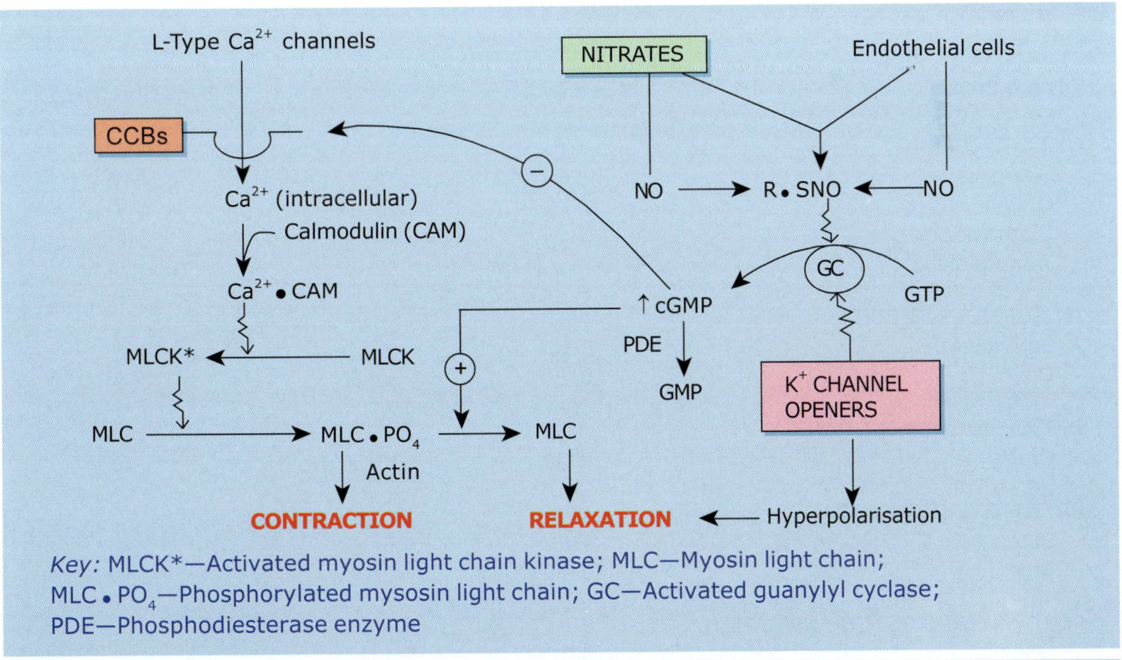

Fig 20.3 Mechanism of Action of Calcium Channel Blockers (CCBs), Organic Nitrates and Potassium Channel Openers.

dinitrate. Compared to *erythrityl tetranitrate*, *pentaerythritol tetranitrate* is inactivated at a slower rate by glutathione-organic nitrate reductase.

The dosage forms, onset of action and duration of effect of nitrates most commonly used in angina pectoris have been summarised in Table 20.1.

Pharmacological Actions

Although nitrates dilate both peripheral capacitance and resistance vessels, the effect on venous capacitance vessels predominates even in low doses. Dilatation of capacitance vessels leads to pooling of blood in veins and to a diminished venous return to the heart (*decreased preload*). Therefore, the diastolic pressure that distends the relaxed ventricular wall (i.e., ventricular end-diastolic pressure) is reduced. The benefit of decreasing preload is a reduction in O_2 demand, which makes these drugs useful in classical angina. However, because venous capacitance is decreased, postural hypotension or syncope may result.

A reduction in the ventricular pressure and heart size results in a *decrease in the myocardial wall tension*, which further decreases O_2 requirements. Since blood flow to subendocardium occurs primarily in the diastole, the reduction in the left ventricular end-diastolic pressure, induced by nitrates, reduces extravascular compression around subendocardial vessels and favours a *redistribution of coronary blood flow* to this area which is particularly vulnerable to ischaemia during anginal attacks. However, a fall in end-diastolic pressure causes reflex tachycardia to compensate reduced stroke volume. Although it is unlikely that nitrates have significant effects on the occluded coronary vessel, they cause selective vasodilatation of large epicardial vessels and help in redistribution of coronary blood flow to ischaemic subendocardial vessels *by opening up collaterals*, without increasing total blood flow.

At higher concentrations, nitrates also relax arteriolar smooth muscle, which leads to a decrease in total peripheral resistance and a decrease in aortic

Table 20.1 Dosage Forms, Onset of Action and Duration of Effect of Organic Nitrates used in Angina

Drug & Route	Dose (mg)	Onset (min)	Duration (hrs)
NITROGLYCERINE			
- Sublingual	0.5	2–5	0.25–0.5
- Oral*	5–15	20–30	4–8
- Ointment (2%)	–	15–30	3–8
- Transdermal	5–10 mg/24 hr	30–40	Max. 24 hr
ISOSORBIDE DINITRATE			
- Sublingual	5–10	5–15	1–2
- Oral*	10–20	30–60	2–4
ISOSORBIDE MONONITRATE			
- Oral*	20–40	15–30	6–10
ERYTHRITYL TETRANITRATE			
- Sublingual	5–10	5–15	2–4
- Oral	10–30	30	2–6
PENTAERYTHRITOL TETRANITRATE			
- Oral*	10–20	30	5–10

* Longer acting sustained release preparations are also available

resistance to left vertricular ejection (i.e., a *decrease in afterload*). The decreased resistance to ventricular ejection *may also reduce myocardial wall tension* and O_2 requirement. However, arteriolar dilatation by nitrates may also cause dilatation of cutaneous vessels leading to flushing of face. Analogously, dilatation of meningeal vessels causes throbbing headache, while dilatation of retinal vessels causes a rise in intraocular pressure.

In angina patients, nitrates increase the exercise tolerance because the same amount of exercise causes lesser increase in cardiac work. Nitrates may also increase the blood flow to ischaemic areas by inhibiting platelet aggregation. However, they do not provide clinical benefits, if used as platelet aggregation inhibiting drugs, in acute myocardial infarction.

Therapeutic Uses

Angina Pectoris: The dosage forms of organic nitrates available for therapeutic use, their usual dose, onset of action and duration of effect have been summarised in Table 20.1. The reduction in myocardial oxygen demand is the major mechanism of organic nitrates for the relief of pain in *angina of effort*. Nitrates benefit patients with *variant angina* (vasospastic angina) by relaxing the smooth muscle of the epicardial coronary arteries and relieving coronary artery spasm. Nitrates exert their beneficial effects in *unstable (preinfarct) angina*, both by dilating the epicardial coronary arteries and by simultaneously reducing myocardial O_2 demand. As noted above, nitrates (e.g., nitroglycerine) also decrease platelet aggregation and this effect may also contribute in the management of unstable angina.

Sublingual or oral nitroglycerine and other nitrates can be used either to terminate an acute attack of angina or for short-term prevention of angina. Nitroglycerine is the mainstay of therapy for relieving acute coronary vasospasm because of its rapid onset of action. Nitroglycerine ointment applied to the chest skin also acts within 15 min and may produce its effects which last for 3–8 hrs, although tolerance can be a problem with prolonged transdermal exposure to nitroglycerine. Therefore, a nitrate-free period of about 8 hrs between two applications should be kept to avoid development of tolerance. If anginal pain persists, the intravenous infusion (10 μg/min) of nitroglycerine (with BP monitoring) can be made which can be titrated upward as per need to a maximum of 200 μg/min until angina disappears. However, the set provided by the manufacturer should only be used because nitroglycerine is chemically incompatible with regular I.V. set-line material.

Heart Failure: Truly speaking, nitrates are being used more for CHF and acute LVF than for angina. Venous dilation by nitrates decreases preload while arteriolar dilation, with continued therapy, reduces afterload. This provide improvement in left ventricular function and regression of pulmonary congestion. Intravenous nitroglycerine is the preparation of choice in emergency but sublingual nitroglycerine or isosorbide dinitrate are most commonly used preparations.

Myocardial Infarction: It has been found that administration of appropriate doses of nitroglycerine intravenously (to avoid tachycardia) or transdermal application of nitroglycerine exerts a protective effect against myocardial infarction (MI) for a period of 72 hrs. Arrhythmias and early mortality can also be reduced. This beneficial new property of nitroglycerine is being exploited to prevent an impending MI. Nitrate therapy in the post-infarction period, however, provides relief from the anginal pain only.

Cyanide Poisoning: Cyanides ion (CN^-) chelate iron (Fe^{3+}) of cytochrome oxidase. This causes tissue anoxia, coma and death. *Amyl nitrite* or *sodium nitrite* (10 ml of 3% solution) convert haemoglobin into methaemoglobin (as a side effect). The latter traps CN^- (because of stronger affinity for CN^-) and gets converted to an unstable cyanomethaemoglobin. Cytochrome and other oxidative enzymes are thus protected from getting chelated by CN^-. Subsequent administration of sodium thiosulfate (50 ml of 25% solution I.V.) reacts with cyanomethaemoglobin and forms sodium thiocyanate which gets excreted through urine (see flow diagram).

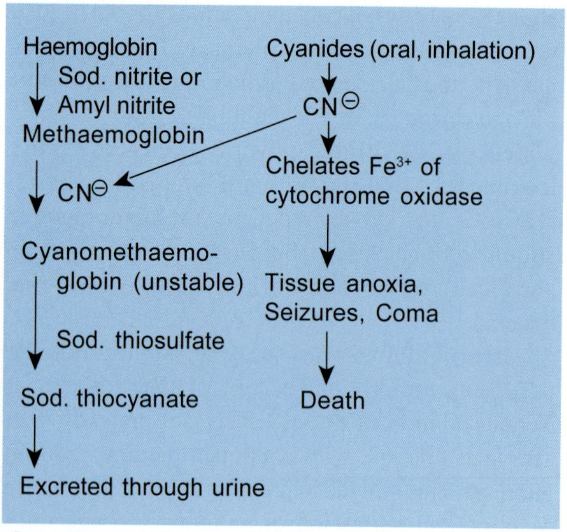

Oesophageal Spasm: Sublingual glyceryl trinitrate, taken before a meal promptly relieves pain due to oesophageal spasm.

Biliary Colic: As a spasmolytic, sublingual isosorbide dinitrate or glyceryl trinitrate can provide prompt relief from biliary colic.

Adverse Effects

1. These are direct extensions of therapeutic vasodilatation and include throbbing headache, flushing of face, palpitations and dizziness. The severity can be reduced by lying down posture. Nitrates are contraindicated if intracranial pressure is raised.
2. Clinically, no significant tolerance develops on intermittent use of nitrates for attacks of angina. However, if glyceryl trinitrate is used orally in sustained release form, or transdermally or by I.V. infusion without drug-free interval, *tolerance* develops more rapidly.

   In industries where glyceryl trinitrate is being manufactured, the factory workers suffer headache on Monday and Tuesday which gradually disappears by Friday due to development of tolerance. After enjoying their weekend on Saturday and Sunday when they return to their job on Monday, the headache reappears (hence the term Monday disease). A gradual decrease in the release of NO is partly responsible for development of tolerance to nitrates. Systemic compensation may also play a role in development of tolerance. These may include sympathetic stimulation and renin-angiotensin system activation. To prevent development of tolerance, the nitrate-free intervals should be provided every day.

   Though there is no evidence that physical dependence develops after the use of nitrates in therapeutic doses, yet sudden withdrawal after prolonged use has resulted in precipitation of coronary vasospasm and MI. Withdrawal of nitrates should be gradual.
3. While there is no direct proof that nitrates exhibit carcinogenicity in human beings, yet there is strong statistical correlation between the incidence of oesophageal and gastric carcinoma and the nitrate contents in food and water.

Drug Interactions

Sildenafil and other vasodilators potentiate the hypotensive action of nitrates (inhibit the metabolising enzyme PDE-IV and potentiate further release of cGMP; see Fig. 20.3 & Ch. 44). MI and sudden death have occurred.

CALCIUM CHANNEL BLOCKERS (CCBs)

All CCBs decrease heart rate, contractility and conduction velocity to a varied extent. They also provide coronary vasodilation and reduction in peripheral arterial resistance (↓ in afterload). Hence, besides HT, these are also used to treat angina. The non-DHPs (e.g., ***verapamil*** or ***diltiazem***) cause more nodal depression than peripheral vasodilation; while DHPs (***nifedipine*** group) have more peripheral vasodilatory and coronary dilatory effects than nodal depression (for detail refer Ch. 19). Hence, the heart rate lowering agents like non-DHPs are much closer to and as effective as β-blockers for the treatment of angina (as they ↓ myocardial O_2 demand). Among CCBs, of both groups, ***verapamil*** has the widest range of approved indications including all varieties of angina (effort, vasospastic and unstable), supraventricular tachycardias, post-infarct protection and hypertension. ***Diltiazem,*** with its low side effect profile, has advantages in the therapy of all sorts of angina, atrial tachycarida, flulter or fibrillation.

Among DHPs, only extended release preparation of ***nifedipine*** in combination with a β-blocker is approved for the treatment of effort angina (for reasons, see Ch. 19). Other DHPs that are used to treat effort angina or prinzmetal angina are all longer acting DHPs like ***amlodipine*** or ***benipidine*** or intermediate acting DHPs like ***nitrendipine*** and sustained release preparation of ***nicardipine.*** (For side effects, contraindications drug interactions, dosage refer Ch. 19).

BETA-BLOCKERS

The pharmacology of these drugs has been discussed in Chapter 12; the features relevant to their use in HT have been described in Chapter 19 and hence characteristics relevant to their use in angina will be discussed here.

Rationale for Their Use in Angina

The mechanism by which β-blockers provide relief in angina include, a reduction in heart rate and myocardial contractility due to blockade of cardiac β_1 receptors. This results in a decrease in cardiac output and a decrease in myocardial O_2 requirement, at rest and during exercise. They also prevent arrhythmias which may be precipitated by exercise or stress and decrease the magnitude of ST segment depression in ECG during exercise. These are considered as basal protective agents for most of the patients and are used with nitrates for chronic prophylaxis of effort angina (see below). They do not dilate coronaries.

The total coronary blood flow is rather reduced due to blockade of dilator β_2 receptors as well. However, the blood flow to ischaemic subendocardial area is not reduced due to favourable redistribution and decrease in ventricular wall tension. The mechanism responsible for an increase in the O_2 supply to subendocardium of ischaemic area is most likely related to the ability of β-blockers to increase the diastolic perfusion time, because the subendocardial blood flow and the flow distal to severe coronary artery stenosis occurs primarily during diastole. Finally, there is evidence that β-blockers inhibit platelet aggregation also.

Although all β-blockers are nearly equally effective in decreasing the frequency and severity of attack and increasing exercise tolerance in classical angina, cardioselective β_1-blockers like ***metoprolol*** or ***atenolol*** are more preferred. The non-selective β_1 + β_2 blockers like propranolol and nadolol can worsen prinzmetal angina, because an unopposed α-receptor mediated coronary vasoconstriction may aggravate coronary spasm (CCBs are preferred over β-blockers). Higher dose may even worsen classical angina by causing ventricular dilatation and prolonging systole, both of which tend to increase the O_2 demand. Other β-blockers used to treat effort angina are ***bisoprolol*** (a highly selective β_1-blocker which reduces mortality rate in heart failure) and ***celiprolol*** (a selective β-blocker with vasodilating property by releasing NO and because of its β_2 agonist actions also). The dosages of β-blockers for angina or HT are similar.

Abrupt withdrawal of β-blocker therapy in individuals with angina pectoris may precipitate an anginal attack and acute MI due to sudden increase in sympathetic tone of the heart. The mechanism underlying this adverse effect involves up-regulation of β-receptors that occurs following prolonged β-adrenoceptor blockade. If β-blockers have to be discontinued, such as before coronary bypass surgery, their doses should be tapered over 2–3 days.

The main undesirable effects of β-blockers in angina include an increase in end-diastolic volume with a consequent increase in ejection time. Increased end-diastolic volume indirectly increases myocardial O_2 requirements which blunts the beneficial effects of β-blockers if used as a single drug therapy for angina. Beta-blockers are contraindicated in patients with bronchial asthma, peripheral vascular disease, AV blockade, LVF and severe bradycardia. For other details refer Ch. 12.

BENEFICIAL ANTIANGINAL DRUG COMBINATIONS

The combined use of β-blockers and organic nitrates enhances the therapeutic effects of each and also minimises their side effects (Table 20.2).

The combination is very effective in the treatment of classical exertional angina. The Table 20.2 shows that their additive efficacy is basically a result of one drug blocking the adverse effects of the other on net myocardial O_2 consumption.

Table 20.2 Additive Efficacy of Nitrates and β-Blockers in the Treatment of Angina Pectoris

Parameters	Nitrates	β-Blockers	Combined Efficacy
1. Heart rate	↑	↓	± or ↓
2. Contractility	↑	↓	±
3. Arterial pressure	↓	↓	↓↓
4. End-diastolic volume	↓	↑	±
5. Ejection time	↓	↑	±
6. Coronary blood flow	↑	↓	± or ↑
7. Subendocardial ischaemic area blood flow	↑	± or ↑	↑
8. Collateral blood flow	↑	±	↑
9. Myocardial wall tension	↓	±	↓
10. Ventricular volume	↓	↑	±
11. Heart size	↓	↑	±

The above advantages may also be obtained by combining organic nitrates with calcium channel blockers (Table 20.3).

This combination may be valuable in variant angina, because nitrates decrease preload while

Table 20.3 Additive Efficacy of Nitrates and Ca^{2+} channel Blockers in the Treatment of Angina Pectoris

Parameters	Nitrates	Ca^{2+}-Blockers	Combined Efficacy
1. Heart rate	↑	↓*	± or ↓
2. Contractility	↑	↓*	±
3. Arterial pressure	↓	↓	↓↓
4. Preload	↓↓	±	↓↓
5. Afterload	↓	↓↓	↓↓
6. End-diastolic volume	↓	↑	± or ↓
7. Ejection time	↓	↑	±
8. Coronary blood flow	↑	↑	↑↑
9. Collateral blood flow	↑	↑	↑↑
10. Endocardial ischaemic area blood flow	↑	↑	↑↑
11. Myocardial wall tension	↓	↓	↓↓
12. Ventricular volume	↓	±	↓
13. Heart size	↓	±	↓

* Except for nifedipine which causes reflex increase in heart rate and contractility

CCBs decrease afterload. Therefore, their concurrent use may decrease cardiac work to an extent not possible by either drug alone. A combination of nitrates with nifedipine is generally advocated for patients of exertional angina with heart failure or sick sinus syndrome or AV nodal conduction defect but excessive tachycardia can be observed as side effect.

If a patient of angina is already being treated with optimal doses of verapamil or diltiazem, addition of a β-blocker such as atenolol would rather increase the risk of bradycardia, heart block or heart failure. However, if the patient is being treated with nifedipine, a reflex tachycardia limits its usefulness. A β-blocker may be a helpful addition in this situation which results in a lowering of heart rate and blood pressure with exercise. The commonly used efficacious combination is of amlodipine with atenolol.

In severe and resistant cases of classical angina all the three group of drugs, *viz,* organic nitrates + β-blocker + Ca^{2+} channel blocker (DHP group) can be used. Nitrates primarily decrease preload, CCBs decrease afterload while β-blockers decrease cardiac work.

MISCELLANEOUS ANTIANGINAL DRUGS

Potassium Channel Openers

K^+ ions control the resting membrane potential. Since intracellular concentration of K^+ is much higher (150 mM) compared to extracellular (4.5 mM), the K^+ channel openers cause an efflux of K^+ and hyperpolarisation. Such an effect indirectly opposes the opening of voltage-gated Ca^{2+} channels which require depolarisation above a certain threshold membrane potential for activation (Fig. 19.3). This results in a fall of cytosolic Ca^{2+} concentration with a reduction of cellular contractile activity at the myocardial and vascular level.

Types of Potassium Channels

The following types of K^+ channels have been identified. However, their exact role and sensitivity towards drugs have not been established yet.

Voltage-Gated K^+ Channels

These channels open when the cell is depolarised and therefore help in the process of repolarisation. These are present mainly in vascular and other smooth muscles. These channel openers produce relaxant effects on vascular smooth muscle and other smooth muscle such as tracheal, bronchial, intestinal, uterine, urinary bladder and of corpus cavernosum.

Calcium-Activated K^+ Channels

An increase in intracellular Ca^{2+} concentration causes opening of these channels. This facilitates an influx of K^+ and repolarisation of the cell. These are sensitive to a number of neurotransmitter actions such as 5HT, ACh and NE.

ATP-Sensitive K^+ Channels

These are present in cardiac muscle and β-cells of islets of Langerhans of pancreas. These K^+ channels close when intracellular concentration of ATP rises but open when it drops. Such K^+ channel openers act by antagonising the actions of intracellular ATP on these channels. Opening of these channels causes hyperpolarisation and relaxation of cardiac smooth muscle. These ATP-regulated K^+ channels are blocked by sulfonylureas such as glibenclamide (an oral hypoglycaemic drug). The blockade of these channels causes depolarisation of β-cells which stimulates insulin release.

Several other types of K^+ channels have also been identified, viz.,receptor-operated, Na^+ activated and cell volume sensitive K^+ channels which serve diverse functions and differ towards their sensitivities to different drugs.

K^+ Channel Openers (Therapeutic Uses)

K^+ channel openers or blockers are currently drawing considerable interest for their further therapeutic potential. Drugs like diazoxide, pinancidil, minoxidil and cromokalim are voltage-gated K^+ channel openers for blood vessels and cause membrane hyper-polarisation, leading to vasodilatation and a fall in BP. These are primarily used as antihypertensive drugs (Ch.19).

Nicorandil

It is an antianginal drug which activates ATP-sensitive K^+ channels and hyperpolarises vascular smooth muscle. It reduces pre- and afterload and produces coronary dilation. Since nicorandil carries a nitrate-like moiety, it also exerts a nitrate-like effect. Therefore, the drug combines an activation of K^+ channel with nitric oxide donor action. Its arterial vasodilator effects are attributed to K^+ channel opening whereas venodilator effects are due to nitrate-like activity. However, unlike nitrates, tolerance does not develop to its effects. Nicorandil increases coronary blood flow without causing coronary steal phenomenon and without producing significant cardiac effects on contractility, conduction, heart rate and blood pressure. It is used to treat vasospastic and chronic stable angina; dose 10–20 mg BD orally.

Side effects include flushing, palpitation, dizziness, headache, stomatitis, nausea and vomiting. Nicorandil is contraindicated in patients with cardiogenic shock, LVF with low filling pressure, and hypotension. It should not be used along with sildenafil as the hypotensive effects of nicorandil are potentiated by sildenafil.

Cytoprotective Drugs

Trimetazidine

It is a new Ca^{2+} channel blocker belonging to piperazine group. It is a type of cellular anti-ischaemic drug that has cytoprotective effects on myocardial energy metabolism. Trimetazidine prevents the degradation of membrane unsaturated fatty acids by lipid peroxidation and thus reduces myocardial O_2 demand. It also inhibits the superoxide cytotoxicity to protect the myocardium from the harmful effects of ischaemia. In the presence of ischaemia it maintains LV functions without affecting haemodynamics. It is indicated for stable (effort) angina, infarction sequelae and ischaemia of labyrinths as in Meniere's disease. Because it acts independent of BP reduction, trials are underway to use it in place of nitrates to allow free use of sildenafil in patients of angina with erectile dysfunction.

Ranolazine

Like trimetazidine, *ranolazine* was initially thought to act by inhibiting O_2-wasting fatty acid metabolism which takes place during myocardial ischaemia. Now it is clear that its main mode of action is through inhibition of inward sodium current during ischaemia. As a result the Ca^{2+} load in cardiac muscle is reduced indirectly via Na^+-Ca^{2+} exchanger. The drug prolongs excercise tolerance to angina but has no effect on heart rate or BP. Dose is 500 mg BD orally. It can safely be combined with CCBs, β-blockers or nitrates (but not with verapamil or diltiazem). The main side effect is prolongation of QTc interval, hence concurrent use of quinidine, dofetilide and sotalol should be avoided. It is metabolised by CYP3A4 and hence drugs like verapamil, diltiazem, ketoconazole, macrolide antibiotics, antiviral protease inhibitors can increase its plasma concentration (and hence QTc prolongation). It not only relieves angina but reduces the incidence of serious ventricular arrhythmias in patients with post-acute coronary syndrome.

Direct Bradycardic Agents

Ivabradine

Ivabradine (introduced in 2006) blocks hyper-polarisation-activated current (I_f) through Na^+-channels present in the SA node. These channels get activated during ischaemic episodes. Inhibition of I_f current by ivabradine decreases the myocardial O_2 demand by decreasing the heart rate. Its antianginal potency is equivalent to β-blocker or CCBs. There is no negative inotropic effect or reduction in BP nor any rebound on cessation of therapy (as with β-blockers). Chances for marked SA-node depression are also less because I_f current is only one of the several pacemaker currents at SA node (β-blockers and CCBs like verapamil affect all). *Side effects* are rare except unusual disturbance in nocturnal vision with flashing lights which may impair driving at night (I_f currents play important role in retina which also get blocked).

Antiplatelet Drugs

Aspirin therapy in low doses (75 to 325 mg daily) is effective in reducing the incidence of ischaemia in patients of coronary artery disease. However, concerns have been raised by recent reports that vasodilatory effects of ACE inhibitors are blunted by concomitant use of aspirin (Ch. 18).

Ticlopidine, clopidogrel and ***prasugrel*** are thienopyridine derivative antiplatelet drugs that do not appear to interfere with prostaglandin synthesis. All three agents act by inhibiting ADP pathway of thrombocytes (Ch. 51), i.e., these drugs inhibit binding of ADP to its receptors ($P2Y_1$and $P2Y_{12}$) irreversibly and reduce platelet aggregation. *Clopidogrel* has a safer toxicity profile compared to *ticlopidine* (lesser thrombocytopenia and leukopenia). It is equivalent to aspirin in the secondary prevention of stroke and extibits supra-additive synergism when used with the aspirin . All these drugs are used as prophylactic alone or as adjuvant drug for unstable angina pectoris and to prevent thrombosis in patients undergoing coronary artery bypass surgery. Ticlodipine is administered in the dose of 250 mg BD, clopidogrel is given initially in the loading dose of 300–600 mg followed by 75 mg OD and prassugrel is administered initially in the loading dose of 60 mg followed by 5–10 mg OD (for more discussion on these drugs refer Chapter 51).

Cilostazole is a phosphodiesterase-3 inhibitor which promotes vasodilation and inhibits platelet aggregation (↑ cAMP in vessel wall). It is used as an adjuvant in antianginal therapy but mainly reserved to treat intermittent claudication. It is metabolised by CYP3A4 and hence concurrent use of verapamil, diltiazem and ketoconazole etc should be avoided. Usual dose is 100 mg BD orally.

Dipyridamole inhibits adenosine deaminase and also phosphodiesterase which leads to an accumulation of adenosine and cAMP respectively. These mediators then inhibit platelet aggregation and may also stimulate release of PGI_2. It is a powerful coronary vasodilator. It has minimal effect on BP and cardiac work as venous return is not reduced. Though not useful as an antianginal drug it is being employed for prophylaxis of coronary and cerebral thrombosis in post-MI and post-stroke patients as well as to prevent thrombosis in patients with prosthetic heart valves (Ch. 51) where it is used along with warfarin. It is also given two days prior to open heart surgery to prevent platelet activation by extracorporeal bypass pump. ***Side effects*** include exacerbation of angina, headache, tachycardia and GIT distress. Theophylline may reduce the vasodilatory effects of dipyridamole.

Its therapeutic failure in angina has been explained on the basis of "coronary steal" phenomenon (Fig. 20.2). By dilating resistance vessels in the non-ischaemic zones, it diverts the already reduced blood flow away from ischaemic zone where it is most needed.

HMG-CoA Reductase Inhibitors

Statins

The supportive therapy for coronary artery disease has two key components, namely, the lipid-lowering agents (Ch.23) and antiplatelet agents (Ch. 26 & 51; see above also). The low density lipoprotein (LDL) target is 100 mg/dL or less which can be achieved by dietary modification plus statin therapy (e.g., with *atorvastatin* or *rosuvastatin*). These drugs also act in ways beyond regression of atheromatous plaque, e.g., by improving endothelial function, stabilising platelets or by inhibiting inflammatory response associated with atherogenesis (pleiotropic or non-lipid benefits).

DRUGS FOR PERIPHERAL VASCULAR DISEASE

Pentoxiphylline (oxypentifylline): It is a theo-bromine analogue and inhibits phospho-diesterase enzyme. It is a blood viscosity reducing agent and improves blood flow in ischaemic area through microcirculation.

Oral doses do not affect HR, total peripheral resistance and BP. It does not exhibit "coronary steal phenomenon". However, the overall benefits in anginal patients are only limited.

Its other uses are: To reduce peripheral claudication, non-haemorrhagic stroke; chronic cerebrovascular insufficiency; to improve symptoms like vertigo and memory defects; trophic leg ulcers; obstructive circulatory disturbances of retina; to improve sperm motility; diabetic neuropathy and in AIDS patients with increased TNF. Pentoxiphylline inhibits production of tumour necrosis factor-alpha

(TNF-α) in patients of AIDS. *Side effects* are mild and well tolerated. *Dose*: 400 mg BD orally. *Drug interactions:* It may increase anticoagulatory effects of warfarin and may increase serum levels of theophylline.

Other therapies include: **Cilostazole** (as discussed above), **Naftidofuryl** ($5HT_{2A}$ receptor antagonist) and **Levo-Carnitine** (which improves the metabolic status of skeletal muscle). These can be supplemented with statins for more beneficial results. All these drugs markedly improve the functional status of distance walking. ***Cyclandelate*** is sometimes used in cerebrovascular and peripheral vascular disorders (400 mg TDS orally).

DRUG THERAPY OF MYOCARDIAL INFARCTION

Myocardial infarction (MI) results from prolonged myocardial ischaemia, precipitated in most cases by an occlusive coronary thrombus at the site of pre-existing plaque. Less frequently, MI may also result from prolonged vasospasm or inadequate myocardial blood flow. Very rarely, MI may be caused by embolic occlusion, vasculitis or coronary artery dissection.

MI is the commonest cause of death as a result of mechanical failure of the ventricle or from arrhythmias which at times become unmanageable. About 25% of cases die even before hospitalisation. Myocardium cells survive on aerobic metabolism. If the supply of O_2 to cardiac myocytes drops below a critical value, their necrosis and apoptosis results. It appears that apoptosis (programmed cell death) is an adaptive process in hypoperfused region, sacrificing some endangered cardiac myocytes to avoid the arrhythmogenic disturbances inherent in necrosis. Nonetheless, prevention of irreversible ischaemic damage, following MI, by drugs and other supportive measures constitute some important aims of the therapy (Fig. 20.4).

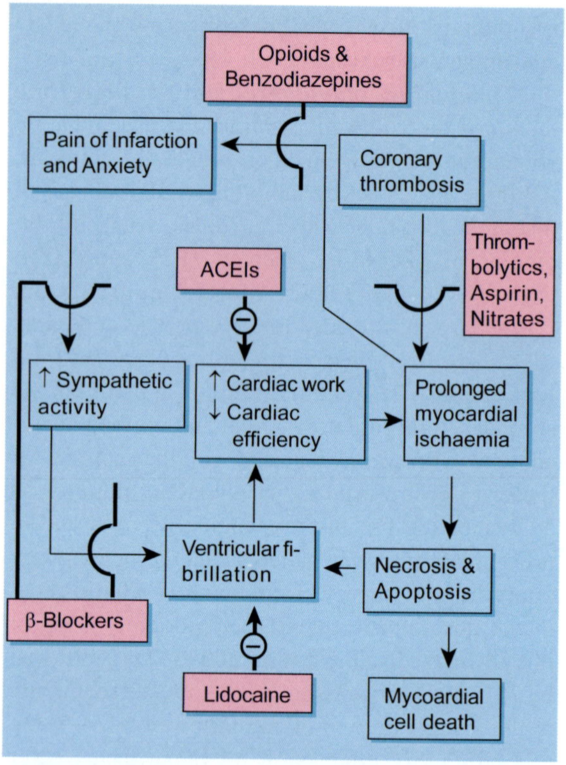

Fig 20.4 Effects of Mycoardial Infarction & Drugs Used for its Management.

The following is the generalised drug schedule for the treatment of MI.

Acute Myocardial Infarction

Aspirin

All patients with definite or suspected MI should receive aspirin at a dose of 160 mg or 325 mg at once regardless of whether thrombolytic therapy has been instituted or not. Patients having allergy with aspirin may be treated with ***clopidogrel*** 75 mg daily orally.

Thrombolytic Therapy

Thrombolytic therapy reduces mortality and limits infarct size in patients with acute MI. The greatest benefit occurs if treatment is initiated within the first 3 to 4 hours when a 50 to 60% reduction in the mortality can be achieved. The benefits decline rapidly thereafter; but a 10% reduction in the mortality can still be achieved up to 12–14 hours after the onset of chest pain. Six fibrinolytic (plasminogen activators) agents are available to achieve reperfusion of infarcted area (Ch. 51). Of these, ***streptokinase*** is less clot specific, produces rapid (but less effective) coronary artery opening with small differences in mortality rate compared to newer agents. Care should be observed if there is prior exposure, as it causes hypersensitivity reactions (including anaphylaxis) in 2% of cases. It is given by I.V. infusion. ***Anistreplase*** has most of the features akin to streptokinase including the potential to produce allergy and hypotension. ***Alteplase*** has been obtained through recombinant DNA technique. It is thrombus specific. It has a shorter $t_{1/2}$ and shows higher incidence of early reocclusion, thus necessitating concomitant use of I.V. heparin. ***Reteplase*** is also a recombinant tissue plasminogen activator related to alteplase but has a longer half-life and is administered as two bolus injection at 30 min apart. ***Tenecteplase*** is a genetically engineered mutant of alteplase. It has a longer half- life, increased fibrin sensitivity and increased resistance to plasminogen activator inhibitor-1. It is given as a single bolus injection. Except for streptokinase, all preparations are very costly. ***Urokinase*** is cheaper and is non-antigenic and does not produce hypotension. It is an enzyme prepared from cultured human kidney cells. It activates plasminogen directly. It is used in the patients of MI and for venous thrombosis and pulmonary embolism. It is given by slow I.V. injection. *Side effect:* fever during treatment.

Nitrates and Vasodilators

Nitroglycerine (GTN) is the agent of choice for recurrent ischaemia and is useful in lowering BP or relieving pulmonary congestion. Infused early, GTN may in addition limit infarct size and decrease mortality. Arteriolar, venous or a combined vasodilator such as nitroprusside can also be used.

β-Blockers

β-Blockers like ***metoprolol*** (5 mg I.V. every 5 min for 3 doses) in the early stages of MI, reduces infarct size, prevents reinfarction, reduces duration of ischaemia, incidence of ventricular fibrillation and chances of death. β-blockers should be continued if not otherwise contraindicated, to reduce risk for reinfarction, CHF and mortality. β-blockers should be avoided in patients whose HR is below 50 beats per minute, systolic BP is below 100 mm Hg, and in those suffering with asthma, CHF or AV block.

ACE Inhibitors

ACE inhibitors (Ch. 18), e.g., ***lisinopril*** or ***ramipril*** prevent remodeling of heart, reduce chances of subsequent CHF and afford long-term survival benefits.

Opioid Analgesics and Antianxiety Agents

A sublingual or I.V. nitrate also reduces pain besides benefitting in angina by relieving coronary artery spasm at the site of occlusion, with restoration of coronary blood flow. If pain is not relieved by giving two or three sublingual tablets of organic nitrates, ***morphine*** (4–8 mg) or ***pethidine*** (50–60 mg) can be given intravenously together with an antiemetic. Intramuscular injection should be avoided because a low cardiac output and poor tissue perfusion usually delay absorption. ***Diazepam*** or ***alprazolam*** can be given to reduce anxiety.

Anticoagulants

For prevention of thrombus extension, embolism and venous thrombosis, heparin (5000 units every 12 hrs S.C.) can be administered followed by oral anticoagulants on short-term basis. Low-molecular-weight heparins (e.g., ***dalteparin*** or ***enoxaparin*** are now more preferred than heparin) because these are less expensive, convenient to use (S.C.), do not require monitoring of activated partial thromboplastin time (aPTT) and carry lesser risk to cause thrombocytopenia.

General Measures

(1) Low flow O_2 therapy (2–4 L/min) should be given if oxygen saturation is reduced and dyspnoea occurs; (2) I.V. infusion of dopamine or dobutamine may be needed to increase pumping action of the heart; (3) Tachyarrhythmias can be treated with lignocaine or procainamide, but as it increases the risk of asystole and does not reduce mortality, this approach is no longer favoured; (4) Sinus bradycardia with low cardiac output can be treated with atropine 0.5–1 mg I.V.; (5). Among CCBs, only diltiazem (180–240 mg daily) can be used to prevent reinfarction and ischaemia in the subset of patients with non-Q wave MI. It is preferred as it causes less myocardial depression compared to verapamil and (6) Hypolipidaemic drugs can be added to control associated hyperlipidaemia.

CHAPTER 21 Drug Therapy of Cardiac Arrhythmias

COMPETENCY PH1.30

Cardiac arrhythmias are deviations from the normal pattern of cardiac rhythm. They include ***abnormalities in impulse formation*** (such as heart rate, its rhythm or site of impulse origin) and ***disturbances in impulse conduction*** (which disrupt the normal sequence of atrial and ventricular depolarisation). Cardiac rhythms that are too slow or too rapid or asynchronous can not only reduce cardiac output but at times may precipitate ventricular fibrillation. Though antiarrhythmic drugs are life saving in cardiac arrhythmias, many of them are hazardous. They can precipitate lethal arrhythmias by themselves if not judiciously used. As a rule, therefore, use of antiarrhythmic drugs for the treatment of asymptomatic arrhythmias should be avoided for this reason.

ELECTROPHYSIOLOGY OF CARDIAC RHYTHM

I) Impulse Generation and Transmission

There are two types of cardiac tissue:

a) ***Pacemaker or conducting tissue,*** which includes SA node, AV node, bundle of His and Purkinje fibres. All of these have pacemaker potential but SA node over-rides other pacemaker cells.
b) ***Myocardial contractile tissue,*** which includes atria and ventricles.

Two electrical sequences that make the heart chambers to fill with the blood and then contract to supply it to various organs are initiated by the conduction system of the heart. The first electrical sequence is the "impulse formation" and this takes place when an electrical impulse is generated spontaneously and automatically. The second sequence is "impulse transmission" which follows after the generation of impulse and signals the heart to contract.

The normal pathway of impulse conduction is as follows:

Internodal tracts → Atrial muscle → AV node

SA node → Internodal tracts → AV node → Bundle of His → Purkinje fibres → Ventricles

SA node in the wall of right atrium serves as the main pacemaker of the heart and initiates a spontaneous action potential (AP). Impulses generated by SA node trigger atrial contraction. Impulses then travel through internodal tracts to AV node, situated at the lower interatrial septum. At this site the impulses are delayed briefly to permit completion of atrial contraction. When the impulse reaches the bundle of His, it travels along the right and left branches located on either side of the intraventricular septum. From here the impulse then reaches Purkinje fibres which are a diffused network of bundle branches ending in the ventricular endocardial surfaces. Ventricular contraction occurs now.

II) Myocardial Action Potential

For cardiac contractions to occur, cardiac cells must depolarise and then repolarise through alterations in their ionic permeabilities (mainly of Na^+, K^+ and Ca^{2+}) across the cell membrane. The AP can be divided into five phases: *rapid depolarisation* (Phase 0), *early (or partial) repolarisation* (Phase 1), *plateau* (Phase 2), *rapid repolarisation* (Phase 3) and the resting phase called *slow diastolic depolarisation* (Phase 4).

The shape and characteristics of AP as well as the type of ionic permeability involved depend on the type of cardiac cell. For example, phase 0, 1, 2, and 3, are non-distinguishable in nodal tissue and phase-4 is the characteristic feature of these cells (discussed later).

Action Potential in Normal Atrial, Purkinje Fibres or Ventricular Cardiac Cells

The resting membrane potential in these non-autonomic cells lies near –90 mV. In these myocytes, the AP has 5 distinct phases (phase 0 to phase 4; Fig. 21.1).

PHASE 0 (*Rapid Depolarisation*): This results when Na^+ ions enter the cell through fast inward Na^+channels. The cell membrane's electrical charge changes from negative (-90 mV) to less negative (-80 mV) and finally to positive (+30 mV). The upstroke depolarisation ends as Na^+ inflow ceases. At this stage, the Na^+ channels become inactivated, i.e., they cannot be recruited to participate in generating a subsequent AP for a specified interval (for details see Ch. 15). This interval during which the myocyte cannot be stimulated is called the Absolute Refractory Period (ARP, discussed later).

PHASE 1 (*Early/Partial Repolarisation*): At this stage, as voltage-gated Na^+ channels close, potassium channels rapidly open. The cell therefore rapidly repolarises (membrane potential returns toward 0 mV). This produces a spike and dome configuration of AP.

PHASE 2 (*Plateau*): In this phase, voltage-sensitive L-type Ca^{2+} channels open (see Ch. 19), causing slow inward current. This is then balanced by the slow outward K^+ current, i.e., depolarisation = repolarisation (or $Ca^{2+} = 2K^+$). The cell membrane's electrical activity stabilises temporarily and the AP reaches a plateau. This is preceded by a notch at the beginning of the plateau phase (Fig 21.1).

PHASE 3 (*Rapid Repolarisation*): At this phase Ca^{2+} channels close, and K^+ channels open. K^+ are pumped out of the cell as the cell rapidly repolarises and resumes its initial negativity (–80 mV approximately). From phase 0 to phase 3 there has been a gain of Na^+ and loss of K^+. This imbalance is now corrected by Na^+-K^+ ATPase pump which restores the intra- as well as extracellular positive ion concentrations to their pre-excitation levels.

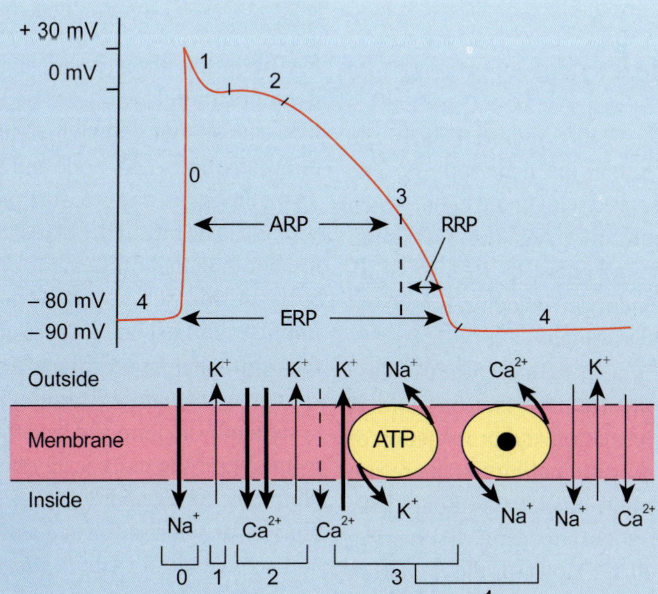

Fig 21.1 Ionic Movement Underlying Different Phases of Action Potential in Purkinje Fibres. Thick Arrows Represent Major Ionic Permeability

PHASE 4 (*Diastolic Depolarisation*): In phase 4, the ion balance is returned to normal by the, 1) Na^+ - K^+ ATPase pump (as discussed above), 2) Outward K^+ current and 3) Na^+ - Ca^{2+} ion exchanger which removes the remaing Ca^{2+} from the cell. The resting membrane potential of ventricular myocyte becomes stable and is held at –90 mV. It is during phase 4 that the Na^+ channels involved in atrial and ventricular myocyte depolarisation recover completely from inactivation and become available for activation again. Once depolarisation starts (phase 4 followed by phase 0), the myocardial cell remains refractory to other stimuli. This refractory period is subdivided into 3 phases: *Absolute, Relative* and *Effective Refractory Period.*

From phase 0 to mid phase 3, the cell does not respond to any stimulus. This period is called an ***Absolute Refractory Period* (ARP).** The cell's ability to repond to stimulus increases as repolarisation continues. Hence from midphase 3 to the end of phase 3, the cell can respond to strong stimulus. This is called ***Relative Refractory Period* (RRP).** The sum of these two refractory periods is called ***Effective Refractory Period* (ERP)** which depicts a minimum interval between two propagated responses (Fig. 21.1).

Action Potential in Nodal Tissues (SA Node and AV Node)

Unlike non-automatic cells, in nodal cells the maximum diastolic potential lies near –60 mV. The transmembrane AP observed with nodal cells, which are capable of automaticity, has the following characteristic features: (a) phase 0, 1, 2, & 3 are indistinguishable, (b) conduction velocity is slow, and (c) the refractory period is longer.

In nodal tissue, Ca^{2+} influx (not of Na^+) dominates the upstroke (depolarisation) and is largely responsible for initiation and propagation of AP (Fig. 21.2). Cardiac automaticity is therefore decreased by Ca^{2+} channel blockers. Automaticity means the ability of a cell to alter its resting membrane potential (–60 mV) towards the excitation threshold potential (TP, –40 mV) without the influence of any stimulus. When the membrane potential depolarises (less -ive) above the threshold (–40 mV) there is an inward Ca^{2+} current and an AP is generated. The steeper the diastolic depolarisation, closer to TP, the higher is the pacemaker rate.

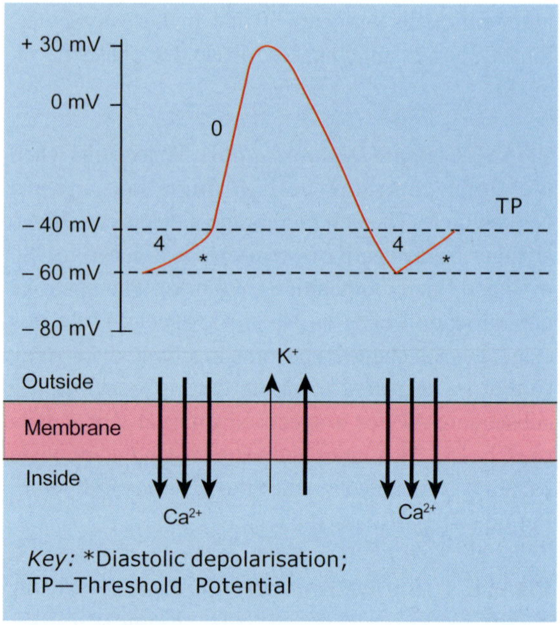

Fig 21.2 Ionic Movements Underlying the Action Potential in Nodal Cells.

SA node has the steepest and the fastest phase 4 depolarisation (Fig 21.2). Hence SA node normally over-rides other cells which also have the potential of automaticity (AV node and His-Purkinje system). The other cells can become pacemakers when their own intrinsic rate of depolarisation (phase 4) becomes greater than that of SA node or when the pacemaker cells within the SA node are depressed. When impulses fail to conduct across the AV node to excite the ventricular myocardium (e.g., during heart block), spontaneous depolarisation within the His-Purkinje system may acquire and lead the pacemaking activity to maintain the cardiac rhythm and cardiac output. Normally the AV node and His-Purkinje fibres undergo phase 4 depolarisation at a slower rate than SA node and work only as *latent pacemakers*. They do not undergo self-excitation but only receive the propagated impulses before reaching the TP. In all pacemaker cells the outward K^+ current during phase 4 is smaller, which keeps the cell with automaticity in a less negative potential (near depolarisation state, i.e., –60 mV). In other words, the depolarising inward Ca^{2+} currents are large enough to gradually depolarise the cell during diastole.

The rate of pacemaker discharge within these cells is influenced by sympathetic as well as parasympathetic activity. An increased sympathetic activity on the heart, through stimulation of β_1 receptors on pacemaker cells, makes the slope of diastolic depolarisation (phase 4) more steeper and hence increases the rate of pacemaker activity. Acetylcholine, on the other hand, stimulates M_2 receptors on SA node and decreases the slope of diastolic depolarisation. Hence parasympathetic activity at heart decreases the rate of pacemaker activity (Fig. 21.3). The release of ACh from cholinergic vagal fibres increases outward K^+ conductance in pacemaker cells. This results in a more negative potential or hyperpolarisation. Thus during vagal stimulation the threshold potential (TP) of the SA node is achieved more slowly and the heart rate is slowed.

III) Depolarisation and Repolarisation Waves as Shown in ECG

The conduction of impulse through different parts of the heart and the relationship of their APs with ECG has been shown in Figure 21.4.

P-WAVE: It is a small upward wave generated by atrial depolarisation (contraction after receiving impulse from SA node).

QRS-COMPLEX: Begins as a downward deflection (Q) and followed by an upright triangular wave (R) which then ends as a downward wave (S). It represents total ventricular depolarisation (contraction; phase O). QRS duration means the time required for all of the ventricular cells to be activated (i.e., the intraventricular conduction time).

T-WAVE: It is a dome-shaped upward deflection and represents ventricular repolarisation (phase 3). It occurs just before the ventricles start to relax. Repolarisation of atria is not evident in ECG as it is buried in the larger QRS complex generated by ventricular depolarisation.

PR (PQ) INTERVAL: It is a measure of conduction time from atrium to ventricle, i. e., from beginning of the P wave to the beginning of the QRS complex. In other words, it is the time required for an impulse to travel through atria → AV node → Purkinje fibre → ventricle.

ST-SEGMENT: Represents the time of the plateau phase of ventricular depolarisation (phase 2; it gets elevated in acute MI and depressed in angina).

QT-INTERVAL: It reflects the duration of the ventricular AP, and starts from phase 0 (depolarisation) and ends at phase 3 (i. e., end of repolarisation).

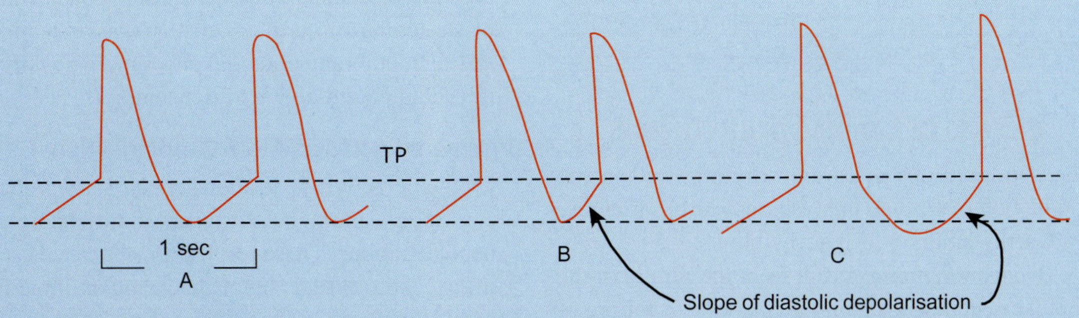

Key: A—Control, B—Norepinephrine, C—Acetylcholine

Fig 21.3 Effects of Norepinephrine and Acetylcholine on Spontaneous Diastolic Depolarisation (automaticity) at SA Node.

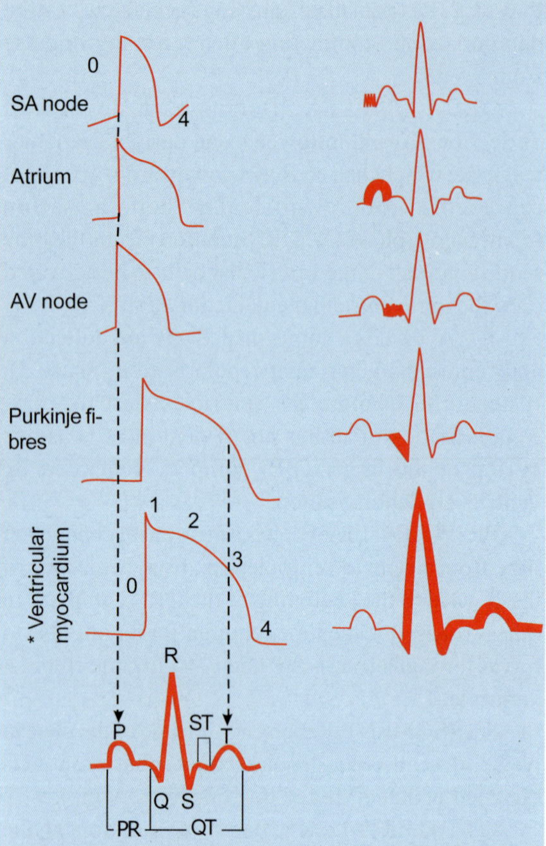

*Including endocardium and epicardium action potential. In the last right hand panel the thick portion of ECG is one contributed by respective tissue.

Fig 21.4 Action Potential–Electrocardiogram Relationship.

GENESIS OF CARDIAC ARRHYTHMIAS

The abnormalities in cardiac rhythm, and in the conduction of cardiac impulse, may result in either bradyarrhythmias or tachyarrhythmias.

Bradyarrhythmias result from the failure of the impulse generation within the SA node or failure of impulse conduction through AV node. Bradyarrhythmias include various kinds of heart block (e.g., AV block) and complete cessation of electrical activity, e.g., asystolic arrest. Normally, treatment of bradyarrhythmias requires permanent cardiac pacemaker as these are not amenable to drug therapy on long-term basis. Conversely, ***tachyarrhythmias*** can be satisfactorily managed by drugs. The commonest type of tachyarrhythmias are atrial fibrillation where the heart rate is completely irregular; and supraventricular tachycardia where the heart beat is rapid but regular. Sustained ventricular tachyarrhythmias are less common but more serious: they include ventricular tachycardia, extra systoles and ventricular fibrillation where the electrophysiological activity of ventricles is chaotic and cardiac output almost ceases.

Cardiac arrhythmias, due to any reason, lead to ***abnormal impulse generation, triggered activity and/or abnormal impulse conduction.***

1) Abnormal Impulse Generation

Abnormal impulse generation may stem from depressed automaticity of SA node which leads to escape beats and bradycardia. Conversely, there may be enhanced automaticity of SA node leading to sinus tachycardia. AV node, Purkinje fibres, atrial and ventricular cells also show spontaneous diastolic depolarisation and repetitive firing, if their membrane potential comes to about –60 mV. This leads to ectopic pacemakers in conducting system causing AV nodal rhythm, idioventricular rhythm or ectopic beats. Such ectopic pacemaker activity is encouraged by: (a) faster phase 4 depolarisation due to ischaemia, digitalis, catecholamines, acidosis, hypokalaemia or stretching of cardiac cells, (b) less negative resting membrane potential or (c) more negative threshold potential due to ischaemia.

2) Triggered Activity (After-Depolarisations)

Triggered activity (or after-depolarisations) occur when a normal AP triggers extra-abnormal depolarisations. These result from abnormal Ca^{2+} influxes into cardiac myocyte during or immediately after phase 3 of the ventricular AP and manifest as ventricular extra-systoles or tachycardia. The triggered activity, unlike abnormal automaticity, is not self-initiated or spontaneous, but it can be self-sustained and depends on the preceding AP. Two major forms of triggered rhythms are recognised: "delayed after-depolarisations" and "early after-depolarisation".

a) **Delayed After-depolarisations (DAD)**

Under the conditions of increased intracellular Ca^{2+} ions concentration, as seen in digitalis intoxication, a normal AP (after repolarisation) may be followed by a "delayed after-depolarisation" (DAD; Fig 21.5A). If this DAD reaches the threshold potential (TP), another triggered beat (or beats) may occur. DADs interrupt phase 4 of normal cardiac AP. These are exacerbated by fast heart rates and are responsible for arrhythmias resulting from digitalis toxicity, increased sensitivity of myocardium to catecholamines or myocardial ischaemia.

b) **Early After-depolarisations (EAD)**

In this type of triggered activity, phase 3 (repolarisation) of normal cardiac potential is interrupted (or plateau may be prolonged). Such after-depolarisations are categorised as "early after depolarisations" (EAD; Fig 21.5B). EADs markedly prolong cardiac repolarisation phase and therefore are associated with the development of polymorphic ventricular tachycardia with a long QT interval, known as *torsade de pointes* syndrome (French; meaning 'twisting of the points'. ECG is characterised by QRS complex of varying amplitudes as they twist along the baseline).

3) Abnormal Impulse Conduction

The third type of electrical disturbance of the heart involves defects in impulse conduction which can result from either one or combination of any of the three mechanisms: (a) conduction block, (b) re-entry phenomenon and (c) accessory tract pathways (Bundle of Kent or Wolff-Parkinson-White Syndrome).

a) **Conduction Block**

Incomplete or complete block of conduction can lead to partial heart block (dropped beats) or complete heart block (idioventricular rhythm). Severely depressed conduction may result in AV nodal block or His bundle branch block.

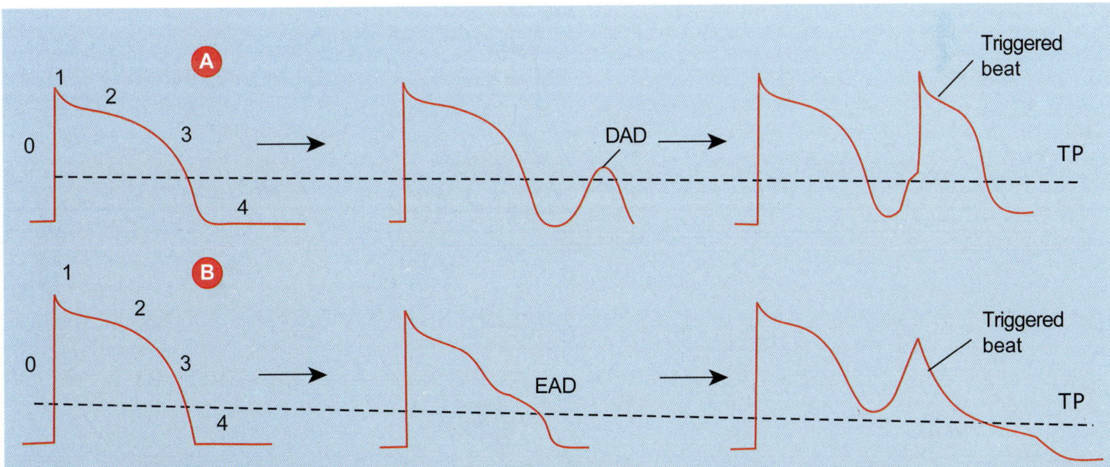

A) Delayed after-depolarisation (DAD) interrupting phase 4
B) Early after-depolarisation (EAD) interrupting phase 3
TP—Threshold potential

Fig 21.5 Two Forms of After-depolarisation.

b) **Reentry Phenomenon (circus movement of rhythm)**

It has been estimated that 80–90% of clinical arrhythmias occur due to reentry phenomenon. It is the underlying mechanism for various arrhythmias including premature beats, paroxysmal supraventricular tachycardia, atrial flutter and ventricular fibrillation.

Normally, the impulses from higher pacemaker centers are conducted unidirectionally through Purkinje system pathways that bifurcate to activate the entire ventricular surface. Physiologically, the conduction impulse splits, then passes through pathways 1 and 2 and excites the whole ventricle. The longer duration of ERP in the terminal Purkinje fibres prevents the impulses traversing within ventricular myocardium from reentering the Purkinje network in retrograde direction. Even if it does, it cannot reexcite the Purkinje fibres as they are still refractory due to longer ERP. Hence the impulses from pathway 1 and 2 collide and extinguish each other (Fig. 21.6A). The net result is the orderly activation of all ventricular myocardial fibres giving rise to normal APs in the respective regions and a normal ECG tracing.

In case of myocardial infarction or injury in one of the pathways, the impulses can pass through the unobstructed pathway but not through that pathway which has "unidirectional block" (an area of inexcitable cardiac tissue). The resting membrane potential of the blocked pathway is decreased due to the injury. Therefore, the impulse conducts slowly and decrementally and finally is blocked. That means, the antegrade impulse travelling toward the ventricular muscle is blocked (unidirectional block). The ventricular myocardium, however, has been depolarised from the impulse coming through unblocked Purkinje fibre pathway (Fig. 21.6 B).

This excitatory impulse traversing within the ventricular myocardium has not been terminated yet and therefore has all chances to reenter in a retrograde manner, though slowly, through the area of *unidirectional block* (in unidirectional block, the block is either in forward direction or in retrograde, i.e., backward

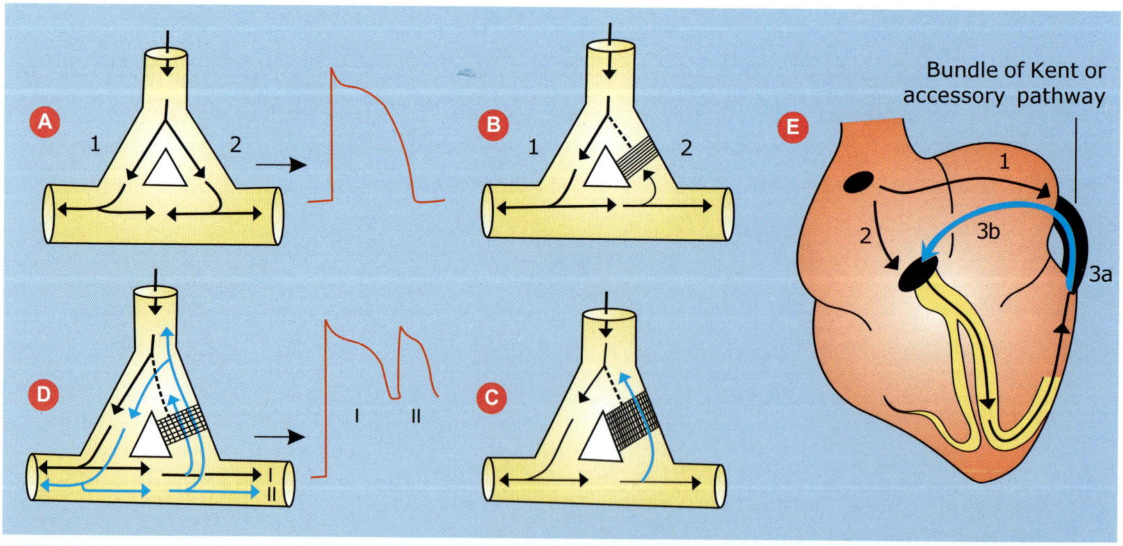

Fig 21.6 Normal Conduction (A) and Conduction Disorders As Might Occur in the Post-infarcted Myocardium Due to Reentry Phenomenon (B to D). Panel E Depicts Atrioventricular Reentrant Tachycardia in the Wolff-Parkinson-White Syndrome.

direction). Because retrograde conduction through "blockade" is slow, the cells of unblocked pathway "1" get time to recover and respond to the reentrant impulse, which depolarise the same tissue more than once producing an additional beat (ventricular premature contractions; Fig. 21.6 C). In case, this reentry mechanism becomes repetitive, a reentry circus phenomenon is established and a sustained reverberating arrhythmia such as ventricular tachycardia is generated which may end up in ventricular fibrillation (Fig. 21.6 D).

For reentry arrhythmias to develop, there must be a region of unidirectional block and a reentry impulse with slow conduction. In other words, the conduction time of the retrograde impulse, through the unidirectional block, should be more than the ERP of the cells which it is going to reexcite (See above).

c) **Accessory Tract pathways**
Patients with Wolff-Parkinson-White (WPW) syndrome exhibit an anatomically defined reentrant phenomenon. In these patients an accessory atrioventricular pathway (a sort of bypass tract called bundle of Kent) is present (Fig. 21.6 E). A premature atrial impulse faces unidirectional block in the accessory pathway (1) but propagates slowly through AV node and conducting system (2). After reaching the accessory pathway it reenters the atrium (3a) from where it can reenter the ventricle via the AV node (3b) and become self-sustaining to produce atrioventricular reentrant tachycardia in these patients (Fig. 21.6 E). Alternatively, the accessory pathway can also conduct impulses directly from the atria to the ventricles, bypassing the AV node. The impulse conduction through accessory pathway is far rapid than through AV node setting up the conditions of re-entrant tachyarrhythmias. The recurrences of such arrhythmias in WPW patients can be prevented by using drugs which prolong AV nodal refractoriness or by ablating the accessory pathway which obviates the need of long-term drug therapy.

POSSIBLE MECHANISMS OF ANTIARRHYTHMIC DRUG ACTION

The drugs which terminate cardiac arrhythmias may act by:

a) Suppressing the enhanced automaticity of pacemaker or non-pacemaker tissues by:
   i) *decreasing the rate of phase 0 depolarisation*
   ii) *decreasing the slope of phase 4 depolarisation*
   iii) *increasing the duration of Effective Refractory Period*
   iv) *making resting membrane potential more negative*
   v) *making threshold potential less negative.*
b) Abolishing reentry by further slowing the impulse conduction and thus converting the unidirectional block to bidirectional block. As implied, the antiarrhythmic drugs can also prevent reentry by increasing the ERP of cardiac fibres surrounding the region of reentrant circuit. Alternatively, the shorter the ERP in the depressed region, the less likely it is that unidirectional block will occur. Theoretically, accelerating the conduction, to make bidirectional conduction in place of unidirectional block, would also be effective in combating arrhythmias (see above). But no such drugs are available as yet.

DRUG THERAPY OF CARDIAC ARRHYTHMIAS

The Vaughan William's classification of antiarrhythmic drugs, is based on their mechanism of action. Accordingly these can be divided into the following categories: Class I to Class IV (Fig. 21.7).

A given drug may have multiple classes of action, e.g., amiodarone which has been classified as class III, shares the action of all the four classes. Certain antiarrhythmic drugs, e.g., adenosine and magnesium, do not fit readily into this classification and are described at the end of the chapter.

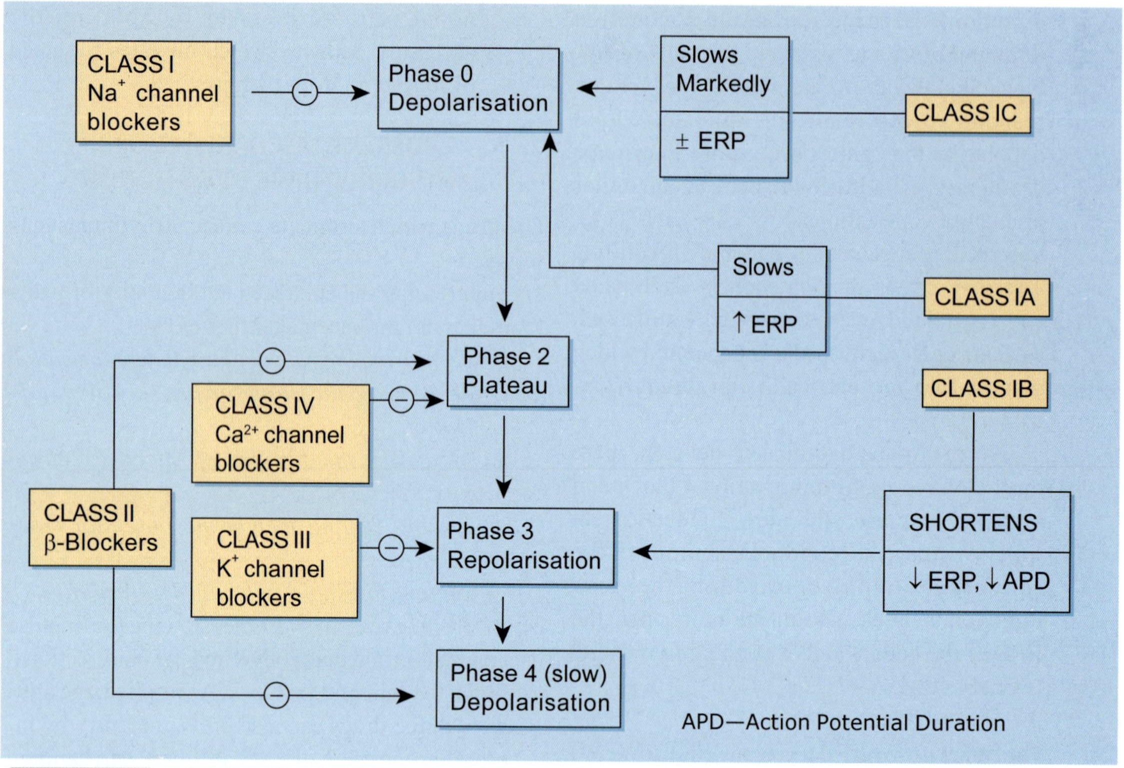

Fig 21.7 Classification and Actions of Antiarrhythmic Drugs.

Another descriptive classification is based on their clinical usefulness, e.g., (1) ***drugs used for supraventricular arrhythmias*** (adenosine, verapamil and diltiazem); (2) ***drugs used for ventricular arrhythmias*** (lignocaine, mexiletine and bretylium) and (3) ***drugs used for supraventricular as well as ventricular arrhythmias*** (amiodarone, β-blockers, disopyramide and procainamide etc).

Class I Antiarrhythmics

All drugs in this class block Na^+ channels just as local anaesthetics do. All of them reduce the maximum rate of depolarisation (MRD) during phase 0. These drugs suppress both normal Purkinje fibres and His bundle automaticity, resulting from myocardial damage, which permits the SA node to regain its role of the dominant pacemaker. Class I drugs bind to Na^+ channel more strongly when they are in the inctivated or open (i.e., activated) state, and less strongly when these are in resting state (see Fig. 15.2). Their inhibitory action therefore shows the property of "*use dependence*"; that means more frequently the Na^+ channels are activated the greater will be their block by these drugs. This characteristic property of Class I drugs enables them to block high frequency excitation of myocardium that occurs in tachyarrhythmias without preventing the heart from beating at normal frequency.

A rise in the threshold of action potential, by Na^+ channel blockers, means that in patients with implanted defibrillators a higher voltage would be needed to defibrillate the heart if these drugs are being used in such patients. Hence, the consequences of the use of Na^+ channel blocker should be taken into account before setting implanted defibrillators in these patients.

Based on the kinetics of their interactions with cardiac Na^+ channels and their effects on different phases of cardiac action potential, Class I drugs are subdivided as follows:

Class I A Drugs

QUINIDINE, PROCAINAMIDE and DISOPYRAMIDE (also AMIODARONE)

Mechanism

These drugs (a) ***slow the rate of rise of phase 0 of the AP***, (b) increase the ERP, (c) prolong the action potential duration (APD; prolong repolarization), and (d) increase the QRS and Q T interval. Furthermore, they also decrease the slope of phase 4 depolarisation in pacemaker cells other than SA node (Fig. 21.8). *These drugs block the open Na^+ channels > inactivated channels and have slow rate of dissociation (recovery) from them.* Slow recovery results in more suppression of cardiac conduction velocity.

Therapeutic Uses

They are used to prevent acute and chronic ventricular and supraventricular tachyarrhythmias, especially paroxysmal supraventricular tachycardia (PSVTs), premature ventricular contractions (PVCs), premature atrial contraction (PACs) and ventricular tachycardia (VT) (Fig. 21.8).

Individual Drugs

Quinidine: Because of the risk of ventricular proarrhythmias associated with its use, and the availability of several more efficacious drugs, quinidine is now seldom used. It shares all the pharmacological properties of quinine such as antimalarial, antipyretic and skeletal muscle relaxant actions. Quinidine has atropine-like (vagolytic) effects (i.e., increased AV conduction). Hence, its use in presence of rapid atrial rate (atrial flutter or fibrillation) can potentiate ventricular tachycardia. To prevent this, agents that slow AV node conduction (e.g., verapamil or digoxin) should be administered prior to the use of quinidine.

Hypokalaemic patients are usually unresponsive to the antiarrhythmic effects of quinidine (QT prolongation), whereas hyperkalaemia increases quinidine's efficacy.

The most common adverse effect of quinidine is diarrhoea (35%). In some patients its administration may cause reversible thrombocytopenia due to the formation of plasma protein-quinidine complex which evokes circulating antibodies against blood platelets. One serious side effect is "quinidine syncope" with loss of consciousness which results from ventricular proarrhythmias (possibly linked to *torsades de*

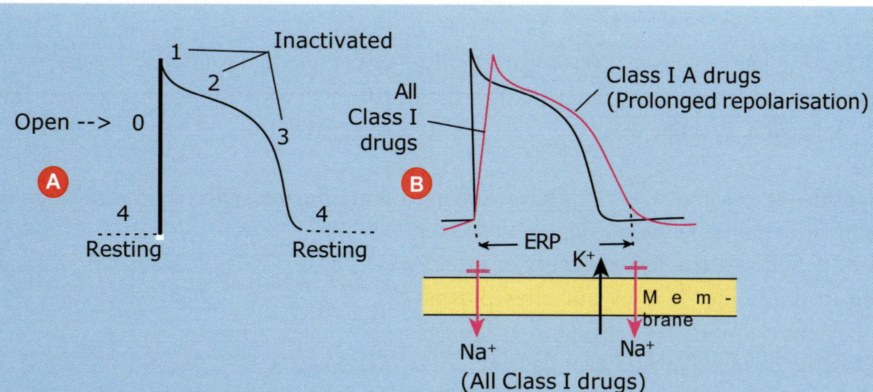

Fig 21.8 (A) Different states of Na^+ channels during the phases of action potential, (B) Electrophysiological Effects (magenta) of Gr. IA Drugs. ---- Resting, ▬ Open (activated), — Inactivated

pointes). Large doses of quinidine can produce a syndrome called "cinchonism" characterised by tinnitus, headache, nausea, blurred vision and vertigo.

Contraindications for quinidine use include: (1) AV block which may be further suppressed by quinidine leading to cardiac arrest; (2) Persons with QT prolongation, for the fear of developing *torsades de pointes* tachyarrhythmias; (3) CHF and hypotension, owing to its negative inotropic action on heart; (4) Digitalis intoxication and hypokalaemia which can potentiate the decrease in conduction velocity caused by quinidine; (5) Myasthenia gravis which might be aggravated due to its muscle relaxant action and (6) Embolism which may occur upon restoration of normal sinus rhythm after prolonged atrial fibrillation. To prevent this, anticoagulants may be administered prior to quinidine therapy.

Drug interactions with quinidine include: (1) Quinidine increases the plasma concentration of digoxin and precipitates digoxin toxicity (displaces digoxin from plasma protein binding sites; also decreases renal clearance of digoxin); (2) Enzyme inducers such as phenytoin and rifampicin can facilitate hepatic metabolism of quinidine and decrease its plasma concentration; while enzyme inhibitors like cimetidine can inhibit its hepatic metabolism and increase its plasma concentration and (3) Magnesium hydroxide and calcium carbonate elevate its plasma concentration by some unknown mechanism.

Quinidine is given in a dose of 200–400 mg orally, three times a day (I.V. no longer used; risk of cardiac failure, hypotension, syncope etc).

Procainamide: It is a procaine derivative, having actions similar to quinidine. It has relatively shorter duration of action and has lesser vagolytic effects compared to quinidine. It does not alter plasma levels of digoxin. With I.V. infusion it causes hypotension (blocks sympathetic ganglia; caution!). Hypersensitivity reactions are common and include drug fever, agranulocytosis, and lupus erythematosus syndrome (fatigue, arthralgia and myalgia). However, these are reversible and slowly disappear after discontinuation of drug. The incidence is more common in slow acetylators. Procainamide should be avoided in patients whose ECG shows prolonged QRS interval (i.e., severely depressed conduction) or prolonged QT interval (repolarisation). Like quinidine, it should also be avoided in AV-block, embolism and myasthenia gravis. For acute therapy, I.V. infusion of 1–1.5 g at a rate of 20–50 mg/min can be given. Once arrhythmias are terminated I.V. infusion can be followed at a dose-rate of 1.5–5 mg/min. Thereafter, long-term therapy can be instituted orally (150–300 mg TDS). Its major metabolite N-acetylprocainamide (NAPA) has class III antiarrhythmic property (prolongs ERP).

Disopyramide: It is used as an alternative to quinidine or procainamide. It is longer acting than other drugs of this class. It has both anticholinergic and direct depressant effects on SA node which antagonise each other so that at therapeutic plasma levels either there is no change or a slight increase in sinus heart rate.

Besides myocardial depression it can cause dry mouth, blurred vision, urinary retention and constipation (anticholinergic effects). It should be avoided in patients with benign prostatic hyperplasia and in those having glaucoma. However, incidence of side effects in long-term therapy are lower. It is contraindicated in patients with heart failure (due to its negative inotropic effects). It has no interaction with digoxin. Usual oral doses are 150 mg 6 hrly. In patients with renal impairment doses should be reduced.

Amiodarone: Discussed with Class III drugs.

Class I B Drugs

LIDOCAINE, PHENYTOIN, MEXILETINE and TOCAINIDE

Mechanism

These drugs have a nominal effect on the rate of rise of phase 0 of the action potential. ***They shorten phase 3 repolarisation, hence decrease the ERP as well as APD***. They have minimal effect on conductivity and contractility. Shortening of repolarisation results in a decrease or at times no effect on QT interval. The QRS interval is also unaffected. *These drugs block the inactivated Na^+ channels > open channels and have a rapid rate of association (block) and dissociation (unblock) with them.* Hence, Class I B drugs lack their effects on healthy myocardium and conducting tissue but can block Na^+ channels more in diseased myocardium where the cells are firing more frequently. They prolong the diastolic phase 4 depolarisation and thus allow time for the complete recovery of the myocardium (Fig.21.9). Like quinidine, they also abolish ventricular reentry tachycardias.

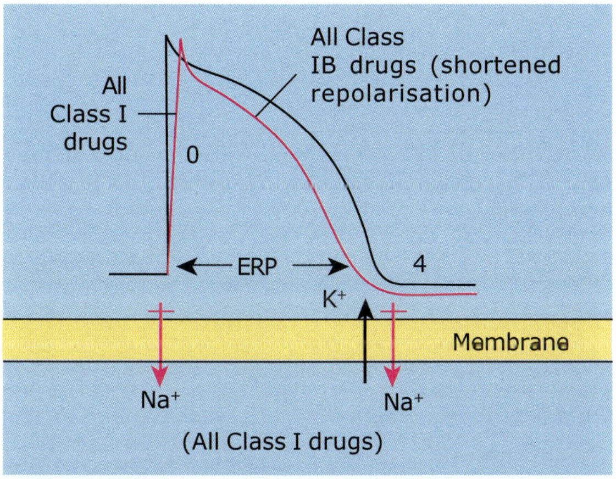

Fig 21.9 Electrophysiological Effects (magenta) of Class IB Drugs.

Therapeutic Uses

These drugs are commonly used for ventricular tachycardia (VT), PVCs and ventricular extrasystoles that result from acute MI or open heart surgery. Among these, phenytoin and lidocaine are best suited for treating arrhythmias associated with depolarisation (ventricular tachyarrhythmias or digitalis-induced arrhythmias), but not for the arrhythmias originating due to automaticity changes such as atrial flutter or fibrillation (see above).

Individual Drugs

Lidocaine: It is a most popular and commonly used local anaesthetic (Ch. 15). It is given by an I.V. infusion as a loading dose of 150–200 mg for 15 minutes followed by a maintenance infusion at the rate of 1–4 mg/min. Not more than 300 mg should be given in one hour. For emergency treatment of ventricular arrhythmias it can be given I.M. (300 mg to be repeated after 60–90 min if necessary). It is now felt that its current use "prophylactically for post-MI cases" is no longer justified. A recent analysis has shown an increase in the mortality in the group of patients receiving lidocaine prophylactically during MI as compared to placebo, possibly by increasing the incidence of asystole. It has an extensive first-pass metabolism in liver which precludes its oral administration. Since it is metabolised by liver, doses adjustment are needed in patients with liver dysfunction and CHF. It has no vagolytic effects (unlike quinidine). It is one of the least cardiotoxic drugs in Class I. Proarrhythmic side effets are uncommon with its use.

Extracardiac side effects include CNS effects like drowsiness, convulsions, slurred speech, confusion and paraesthesia. *Drug interactions* are less; the relevant being with phenytoin which increases cardiodepressant effects of lidocanie. β-Blockers like propranolol decrease the metabolism of lidocaine and increase its toxicity (decreases hepatic blood flow).

Phenytoin: It is reserved only to terminate digitalis-induced cardiac arrhythmias as it does not aggravate AV block, does not produce hypotension and can even be used when procainamide cannot be used because of widening of QRS complex. It has been reported that phenytoin is particularly useful in treating ventricular arrhythmias in children. Otherwise, its regular use as an antiarrhythmic agent has become obsolete (because I.V. injection damages the vein and causes hypotension. It is a potent enzyme inducer and hence more drug interactions). *For adverse effects and contraindications* refer Chapter 39. It is given by an intermittent I.V. administration. 100 mg is given I.V. every 5 min at a rate of 25–50 mg/min until arrhythmias disappear. The usual total effective dose is 700 mg.

Tocainide: It is structurally similar to lidocaine but can be administered orally. Although its uses are similar to lidocaine, some serious noncardiac side effects limit its usefulness as a preferred antiarrhythmic. These include nausea, dizziness, paraesthesias, numbness and tremors. Serious immune-based side effects such as pulmonary fibrosis, and blood dyscrasias such as agranulocytosis and thrombocytopenia may occur in about 3:1000 cases.

Mexiletine: It is an oral analogue of lidocaine, but there is no first-pass metabolism in liver. It is preferred for chronic treatment of ventricular arrhythmias associated with previous MI. Normally, a loading dose of 400 mg orally followed by a maintenance dose of 200 mg every 8 hours is given. Tremor is an early sign of mexiletine toxicity. Hypotension, bradycardia and widened QRS complex may develop during the therapy. Increasing plasma concentration may produce dizziness, ataxia and nystagmus. It is contraindicated in patients with AV block or with cardiogenic shock as it accelerates AV block. 450–750 mg of mexiletine orally per day provides significant relief in diabetic neuropathy (unlabeled use).

Class IC Drugs

FLECAINIDE, ENCAINIDE, PROPAFENONE and MORICIZINE

Mechanism

These drugs markedly decrease the rate of phase 0 depolarization in Purkinje and ventricular myocardial fibers. This produces marked slowing of conduction in all cardiac tissue with a minimal effect on ERP and action potential duration (Fig. 21.10). These drugs reduce automaticity, decrease AV conduction as well as contractility. Automaticity is decreased by a rise in threshold potential rather than a decrease in the slope of phase 4 depolarisation. They also retard reentry of retrograde as well as antegrade impulses. *These drugs block open Na^+ channels > inactivated ones but dissociate very slowly* (slower recovery compared to class IA drugs). Hence, these show prominent depressant effects on normal heart as well (hence proarrhythmogenic effects also).

Therapeutic Uses

They suppress PVCs and ventricular tachyarrhythmias which are refractory to other drugs. These (except moricizine) have also been shown to be effective in the treatment of supraventricular arrhythmias.

Since they markedly retard anterograde as well as retrograde conduction in the bypass tract of Wolff-Parkinson-White (WPW) syndrome, these are very useful for supraventricular arrhythmias especially in WPW syndrome.

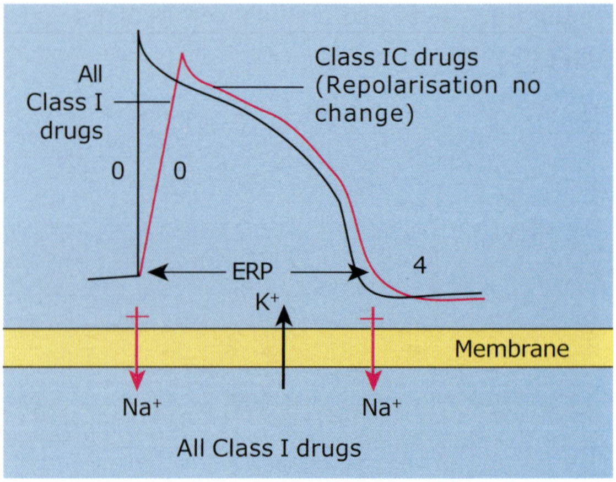

Fig 21.10 Electrophysiological Effects (magenta) of Class IC Drugs.

Individual Drugs

Flecainide and **Encainide**. The usual dose of flecainide is 100–200 mg twice a day orally. However, these drugs are proarrhythmogenic even when normal doses are administered to patients with sick sinus syndrome, preexisting ventricular tachyarrhythmias, or ventricular ectopy or with a previous MI. They have no antimuscarinic effects. These drugs are currently reserved for patients with life-threatening refractory ventricular arrhythmias, who do not have coronary artery disease. Likelihood of developing *torsades de pointes* is a serious drawback for these drugs. Other adverse effects include visual disturbances (spots before the eyes), dizziness, nausea and headache. These drugs may increase digoxin concentration on concurrent administration.

Propafenone: It has structural similarities with propranolol. The usual daily oral dose is 150–200 mg given at 8 hourly interval (to a max. of 900 mg/day). It has some β-blocking action and decreases AV conduction, hence contraindicated in CHF and bronchial asthma. Uses are same as described above. *Serious side effects* are proarrhythmogenic events. Other adverse effects are metallic taste, nausea and constipation. Concurrent administration of propafenone with digoxin or propranolol increases the serum concentration of these drugs.

Moricizine: It has properties of all the three subclasses but as it prolongs QRS interval, it has been placed with class IC drugs. It has a lower incidence of proarrhythmic effects. Usual dose is 200–400 mg orally at 8 hourly interval. Its use is reserved for documented refractory life-threatening ventricular arrhythmias. Side effects include GIT distress and dizziness. No clinically important drug interactions have been reported.

Class II Antiarrhythmics

PROPRANOLOL, ACEBUTOLOL, METOPROLOL and ESMOLOL

Mechanism

These drugs are β-adrenergic blockers that competitively block catecholamine-induced stimulation of cardiac β-receptors and ***depress phase 4 depolarisation of pacemaker cells*** (Fig 21.11). These drugs slow sinus as well as AV nodal conduction which results in a decrease in HR and prolongation in PR interval (atrial depolarisation). QT and QRS intervals are not altered significantly. *They increase the ERP and prolong the duration of AP* by decreasing conduction through AV node.

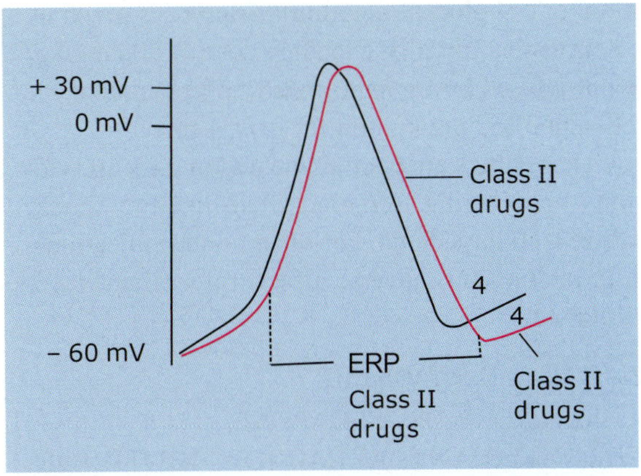

Fig 21.11 Electrophysiological Effects of Class II Drugs (magenta) on SA Node and AV node

Therapeutic Uses

Among the drugs in this class, propranolol, metoprolol, esmolol and acebutolol have been approved for antiarrhythmic use. For other uses of β-blockers refer Chapter 12, 19 and 20. *Propranolol*, *metoprolol* and *acebutolol* can be used to (a) control supraventricular arrhythmias (e.g., atrial flutter or fibrillation and PSVTs), (b) treat tachyarrhythmias caused by adrenergic stimulation (e.g., in hyperthyroidism and during anaesthesia), (c) suppress severe ventricular arrhythmias in prolonged QT syndrome, (d) treat digitalis-induced ventricular arrhythmias, (e) terminate PVCs in patients without structural heart disease, and (f) treat atrial fibrillation and WPW syndrome where digitalis is contra-indicated. *Esmolol* is used to treat supraventricular tachycardias. It has very short half-life (9 min) and has been used to control abnormal ventricular response to atrial fibrillation or flutter during or after surgery. *Metoprolol* and *acebutolol* being cardioselective are more efficacious. It has now been established that β-blockers can prevent recurrent infarction and sudden death in patients recovering from acute MI (Ch. 20).

For oral therapy, *propranolol* is given 10–80 mg TDS. For resistant ventricular arrhythmias, however, 1000 mg may be required. For emergency therapy it is given by slow I.V. infusion (1–3 mg in

50 ml of 5% glucose solution). *Esmolol* is given by I.V. infusion. Initially, a loading dose of 500 mg/kg/min is infused for 1 minute, followed by maintenance infusion of 50 mg/kg/min for over 4 min.

These drugs are contraindicated in patients with sinus bradycardia, AV block, cardiogenic shock, severe CHF or asthma. For other contraindications, drug interactions, adverse effects refer Chapter 12, 19 and 20.

Class III Antiarrhythmics

AMIODARONE, DRONEDARONE, VERNAKALANT, AZIMILIDE, IBUTILIDE, DOFETILIDE, BRETYLIUM and SOTALOL

Mechanism

Class III drugs block outward K^+ channels during phase 3 of AP. ***These drugs prolong the duration of AP without affecting phase 0 of depolarisation or the resting membrane potential. Instead, they prolong the ERP*** *(Fig. 21.12)*. QT and PR interval are prolonged but not the QRS interval.

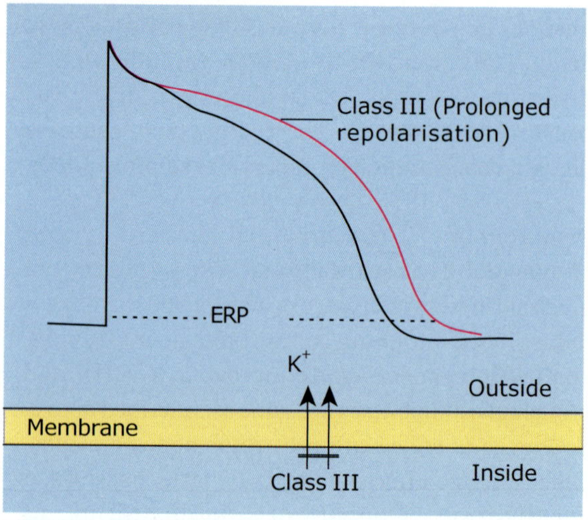

Fig 21.12 Electrophysiological Effects (magenta) of Class III Drugs

Therapeutic Uses

Amiodarone: It is an iodine-containing anti-arrhythmic agent. Besides possessing characteristics of class III drugs it also blocks Na^+ channels (like Class I A drugs), has mild β-blocking activity (like Class II drugs) and Ca^{2+} channel blocking actions (like Class IV drugs). Hence it decreases HR as well as AV nodal conductivity. Having broader spectrum of action, it has better efficacy with lower risk for developing *torsades de pointes* despite significant prolongation of QT interval. It has been recommended for the treatment of ventricular fibrillation, ventricular tachycardia and for the treatment of supraventricular arrhythmias such as atrial fibrillation (low doses 100–200 mg /day). Like β-blockers, it has been shown to reduce arrhythmic deaths in post-MI patients. Oral doses of usually 300–600 mg/day can be given as maintenance dose in ventricular tachycardia. For I.V. infusion a rapid loading dose of 150 mg is infused within 10 min. This is followed by slow infusion of 1 mg/min for 6 hrs (total 360 mg) and then a maintenance infusion of 0.5 mg/min for the remainder of the 24- hour period. *Cardiac adverse effects* include heart block with preexisting SA or AV node disease. *Extracardiac effects* involve dose-related pulmonary toxicity, hepatitis, photodermatitis and corneal microdeposits. It blocks peripheral conversion of T_4 to T_3, so may cause hypothyroidism; but being an iodinated compound may cause hyperthyroidism also. It also increases LDL levels.

Drug Interactions. It increases plasma levels of digitalis, diltiazem and quinidine. It increases pharmacological effects of β-blockers, Ca^{2+} channel blockers and warfarin.

Bretylium: It is an adrenergic neuron blocker introduced as antihypertensive (Ch. 19). It soon became obsolete because of poor bioavailability and development of tolerance. It has been reintroduced as antiarrhythmic for parenteral use. *Bretylium* should be given only in intensive care facilities for treating refractory life-threatening ventricular arrhythmias like ventricular tachycardia and ventricular fibrillation. I.M. therapy calls for administration of 5–10 mg/kg 6–8 hourly. For ventricular fibrillation, 5 mg/kg is given by rapid I.V. injection and repeated every 15–30 min. For ventricular arrhythmias 500 mg is diluted in 50 ml of 5% glucose solution and infused I.V. at a rate of 5–10 mg/kg over 8–10 minutes. *Main* *adverse effect* is postural hypotension. Nausea and vomiting can be minimized by slow infusion. Its use should be limited to a maximum of 5 days. Long-term use results in tenderness and swelling of parotid gland particularly at meal time. It is *contraindicated* in digitalis-induced arrhythmias and cardiogenic shock.

Sotalol: It is a non-cardioselective β-blocker and this effect is exhibited at doses below than that required for prolongation of APD. Thus, sotalol has both class II and class III actions. *Sotalol*, like amiodarone, is used to treat ventricular as well as supraventricular tachyarrhythmias. It decreases mortality associated with MI. Normally 80 mg are given orally twice daily (increased up to 640 mg/day slowly). It carries *side effects* and *contraindications* associated with β-blockade (Ch. 12, 19 and 20). It has proarrhythmic effects also, hence drugs that prolong the QT interval or cause hypokalaemia are contraindicated with its use.

Ibutilide: It is structural analogue of sotalol, having class III properties only. *The most important adverse effect* is excessive QT interval prolongation and *torsades de pointes*, hence continuous ECG monitoring for at least 4 hrs during its use is essential. It is contraindicated in hypokalaemia, hypomagnesaemia and pregnancy. It is rarely used.

Dofetilide: It is also a pure class III drug like ibutilide. *Adverse effects* and *contraindications* are same as for ibutilide. However, it shows lesser prolongation of APD at rapid rates and greater prolongation at slow rate which contributes to the risk of developing *torsades de pointes*. It is reserved for the treatment of atrial flutter and fibrillation. The usual dose is 0.5 mg orally twice daily. Doses have to be reduced for renally compromised patients.

Other Class III Agents

1. **Dronedarone** is an amiodarone-like drug without iodine atoms (no thyroid or pulmonary toxicity). It has a shorter t½ (1–2 days compared to months for amiodorone) and can be administered in dose of 400 mg, orally twice daily. The drug reduces mortality in the patients with atrial fibrillation (AF) and is used to prevent AF recurrences in patients with persistent AF.
2. **Vernakalant** is a mixed K^+ and Na^+ channels blocker used for the treatment of AF. It is contraindicated in advanced CHF and recent MI. It prolongs atrial ERP and slows conduction through AV node. Ventricular ERP is unaffected (less potent blocker of K^+ channel). Association and dissociation with Na^+ channels is faster, hence more effective in myocytes firing more rapidly. Given I.V. infusion 3 mg/kg over 10 min then 2 mg/kg over 15 min (if AF is not terminated).
3. **Azimilide** blocks both rapid and slow components of K^+ channels and is under trial to convert AF into normal sinus rhythm. It has low incidence of *torsades de pointes*.
4. **Tedisamil** is an upcoming class III antiarrhythmic K^+ channel blocker, for conversion of AF and atrial flutter to normal rhythm. It is given by I.V. infusion.

Class IV Antiarrhythmics

VERAPAMIL and DILTIAZEM

These Ca^{2+} channel blocking drugs have been described in detail earlier (Ch. 19 and 20). Dihydropyridines are not used as they may worsen arrhythmias.

Mechanism

They block both activated and inactivated L-type Ca^{2+} channels in myocardium resulting in a decrease in the rate of phase 4 depolarisation in SA node and AV node and slowed conduction through AV node. These drugs also prolong the ERP of AV node (Fig. 21.13). A decrease in inward Ca^{2+} current also occurs during upstroke, i.e., phase 0 of the AP. Ca^{2+} channel blockade in SA node and AV node results in an increase in PR interval. *Verapamil* has a stronger action on heart than vascular smooth muscle. *Diltiazem* exhibits mixed actions.

Therapeutic Uses

Both of these drugs are mainly used to treat supraventricular arrhythmias. These are first line agents for the suppression of PSVTs stemming from

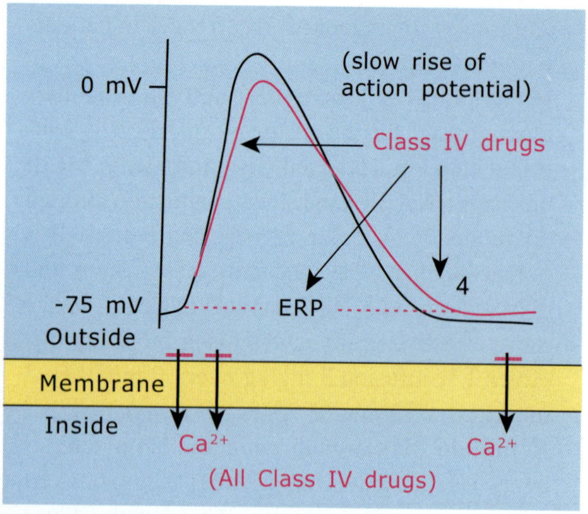

Fig 21.13 Electrophysiological Effects (magenta) of Class IV Drugs on AV Node.

AV nodal reentry and are preferred over older treatments (propranolol, digoxin and edrophonium). They can rapidly control the ventricular response to atrial flutter and fibrillation. To control PSVTs, ***verapamil*** is given orally in a dose of 80–120 mg three to four times a day. To control atrial arrhythmias it is given as 5–10 mg/hr continuous I.V. infusion till adequate response is obtained. For PSVTs usual dose of ***diltiazem*** is 30–90 mg every 6 hours orally. For atrial arrhythmias it is given as 5–15 mg/hr continuous I.V. infusion till adequate response is obtained.

Adverse Effects

Verapamil. A*dverse effects* include peripheral ankle oedema, constipation, and lassitude. It is contraindicated in patients with AV block, LVF, severe hypotension, sick sinus syndrome, CHF, WPW syndrome, hepatic or renal impairment. It is not to be given with β-blockers (aggravate bradycardia) or with digoxin (increases digoxin toxicity).

Diltiazem. It is similar to verapamil except that it decreases myocardial contractility to a lesser extent than verapamil. *Adverse effects, contraindications* and *drug interactions* are the same as described for verapamil (except constipation).

Miscellaneous Antiarrhythmics (which do not fit in the Class I–IV classification)

Adenosine

It is a naturally occurring nucleoside, normally present in all cells of the body. By stimulating adenosine receptors (A_1), it opens the G-protein coupled K^+ channels and inhibits SA nodal, atrial and AV nodal conduction. It terminates reentrant circuit through AV node and restores normal sinus rhythm in patients with PSVTs.

It is used for the conversion of acute supraventricular tachycardia to normal sinus rhythm especially when verapamil is ineffective. It is usually given as a rapid bolus I.V. injection in a 3 mg dose followed if necessary by a dose of 6 mg. Adenosine is highly efficacious for treating PSVTs and has an ultrashort half-life (10–20 sec). *The main adverse effects* are facial flushing, shortness of breath, bronchospasm, nausea and metallic taste but these side effects are normally short lived. *Drug interactions* include those with theophylline or caffeine which reduce its effectiveness, being adenosine receptor antagonist. On the other hand, its effects are potentiated by adenosine uptake inhibitors such as dipyridamole.

Magnesium

Magnesium sulfate is effective in terminating refractory ventricular tachyarrhythmias, particularly polymorphic ventricular tachycardia. Earlier, it was used for patients with digitalis-induced arrhythmias who were hypomagnesaemic. It is also useful in some patients with *torsades de pointes* even when serum Mg levels are normal. The proposed mechanisms for its antiarrhythmic effects are due to its influence on Na^+/K^+ ATPase, Na^+ channels , K^+ channels and Ca^{2+} channels. The usual dosage is 1 g (as sulfate) I.V. over 20 min and repeated once, if needed. *Overdose toxicity* includes loss of deep tendon reflexes.

Potassium

Both insufficient and excess potassium are potentially arrhythmogenic. Potassium therapy therefore is directed toward normalising K^+ gradient and K^+

Table 21.1 Choice of Antiarrhythmic Drugs for Some Commonly Encountered Arrhythmias

Arrhythmia type	Class I			Class II	Class III	Class IV	Miscellaneous
	IA	IB	IC				
Atrial flutter		–	–	PROPRANOLOL ESMOLOL	Amiodarone*	VERAPAMIL	Digoxin*
Atrial fibrillation		–	–	ESMOLOL PROPRANOLOL	AMIODARONE Dofetilide*	Verapamil	Digoxin* Anticoagulant therapy[1]
PSVTs	–	–	–	Propranolol* ESMOLOL	Amiodarone*	Verapamil* DILTIAZEM	ADENOSINE Digoxin*
Ventricular tachycardia	Quinidine* Procainamide*	LIDOCAINE	–	–	Sotalol* Amiodarone*	–	MAGNESIUM
Ventricular fibrillation		LIDOCAINE Mexiletine*	–	–	BRETYLIUM AMIODARONE	–	–
WPW syndrome			PROPAFENONE FLECAINIDE	Propranolol*	Amiodarone* Sotalol		
Torsade de pointes				Propranolol*			MAGNESIUM
Digitalis induced		LIDOCAINE PHENYTOIN		Propranolol			POTASSIUM

Drug names in capital letters denote drug of choice for acute therapy.
(*) indicates drug of choice for chronic therapy. Other drugs serve as alternatives.
[1]Reduces the risk of stroke that is associated with atrial fibrillation.

pools in the body. Normal K^+ levels help in reduction in conduction velocity, prolongation of refractory period and a decrease in automaticity, primarily in Purkinje fibres. Slight hyperkalaemia protects against arrhythmias arising after cardiac surgery. Correction of hypokalaemia can restore sinus rhythm without the use of antiarrhythmic drug. Hypokalaemia, if untreated, increases the risk of early and delayed after- depolarisation (DAD & EAD) and ectopic pacemaker activity, especially in presence of digitalis.

The choice of antiarrhythmic drugs in some commonly encountered arrhythmias is given in Table 21.1.

CHAPTER 22 Drug Therapy of Heart Failure

COMPETENCY PH1.29

The term heart failure literally means a condition in which the heart is unable to pump sufficient amount of blood to meet the metabolic demands of the body and also unable to receive it back because every time, after a systole, some residual blood remains in its ventricles. This condition, in the past, has been referred to as congestive heart failure due to oedematous state produced by the fluid retention leading to pulmonary as well as peripheral congestion. Nowadays, however, the term "heart failure" alone is used to reflect the clinical syndrome more precisely, because all patients do not necessarily present with fluid overload at the initial stage or on follow up evaluations (e.g., patients of high cardiac output type of heart failure associated with hyperthyroidism).

LOW OUTPUT *VERSUS* HIGH OUTPUT HEART FAILURE

Heart failure is a syndrome with multiple causes (MI, HT, angina, ventricular tachycardia, diabetes mellitus, hyperthyroidism and anaemia etc.), that may involve right ventricle, the left ventricle or both. Cardiac output (CO) in heart failure is usually low and the most common heart failure (HF) is a "low output cardiac failure" where the metabolic demands of the body are within normal limits, but the heart is unable to meet them.

"High output cardiac failure" occurs rarely. In some coexisting conditions (hyperthyroidism, anaemia and arteriovenous shunt), the metabolic demands of the body are excessive that even increased CO is insufficient to meet them. As compared to low output failure it should be treated by correcting the underlying cause.

LEFT SIDED *VERSUS* RIGHT SIDED HEART FAILURE (HF)

Signs and symptoms of HF usually result from the effects of blood backing up behind the failing ventricles (except in high output form of HF).

Left sided and right sided HF do not routinely exist as separate entities because, over time, right sided failure causes left sided failure and vice versa.

If the blood cannot be pumped adequately from the left ventricle to the peripheral circulation, a part of it will be retained in left ventricle during systole. Because of this accumulation, the left ventricle will be unable to accept blood from left atrium and the lungs. Hence, left sided HF is characterised by the presence of pulmonary congestion and oedema (presented as shortness of breath and dyspnoea).

On the other hand, when blood cannot be pumped from right ventricle into the lungs a part of it is retained in right ventricle. Because of this accumulation, the right ventricle will be unable to accept blood from the peripheral organs. Hence, right sided HF is characterized by peripheral oedema and/or juglar venous distension.

COMPENSATORY RESPONSES DURING HEART FAILURE

The failing heart evokes the following compensatory mechanisms to enhance the CO (CO = stroke volume x HR). If these mechanisms are able to restore the CO, the heart failure is said to be compensated. In long-term, however, these compensations rather increase the work load of the heart and cause worsening of cardiac performance (Fig. 22.1).

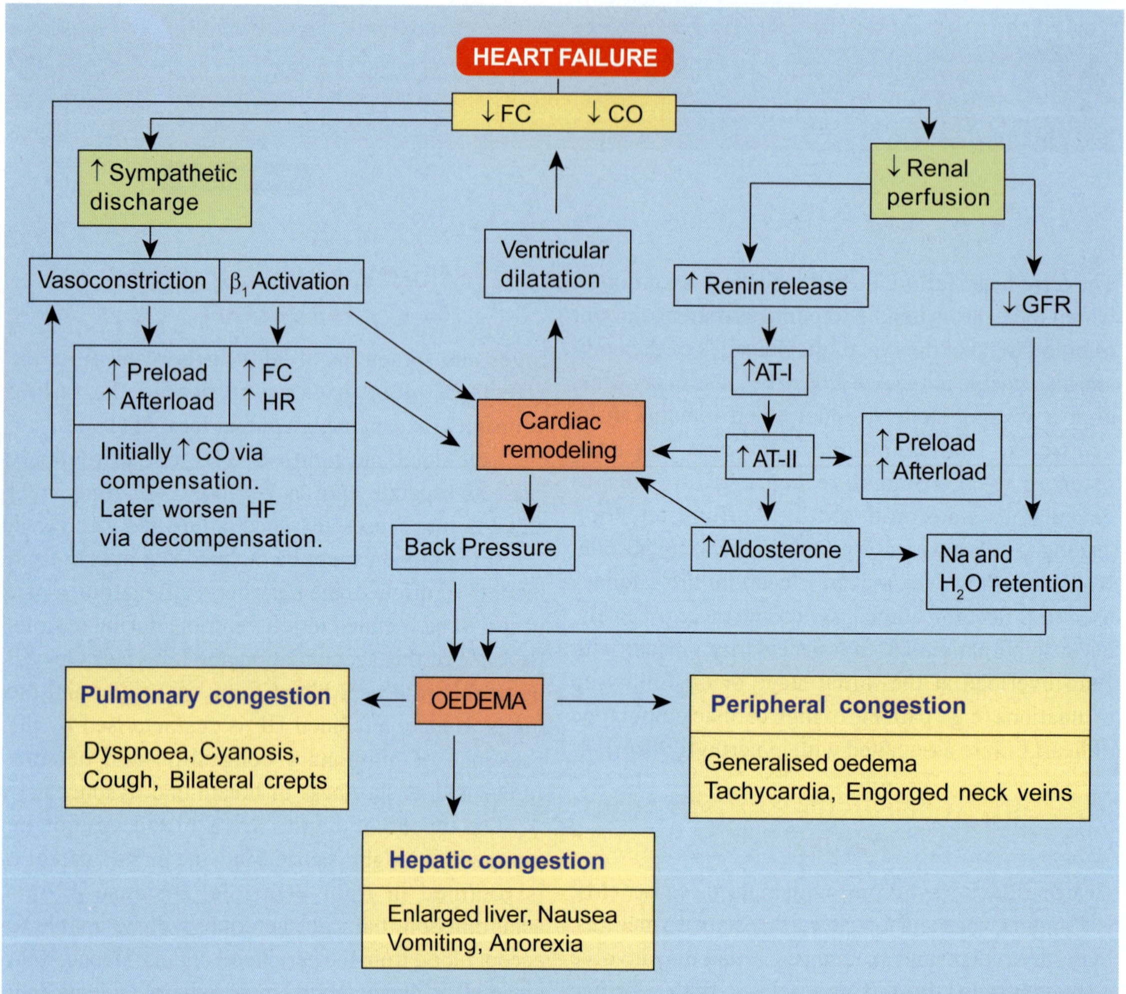

Fig 22.1 Sequence of Events and Compensatory Mechanisms in Heart Failure.

Increased Sympathetic Activity

Baroreceptors sense a decrease in BP and trigger activation of β_1-adrenoceptors in the heart resulting in an increase in heart rate (HR) and contractility. In addition, α_1 receptor mediated vasoconstriction enhances venous return which increases preload. The increase in HR, contractility and preload initially increases the CO. Vasoconstriction also increases arterial tone which results in an increase in afterload and a decrease in ejection fraction. CO finally decreases which reduces renal perfusion. After sometime, there is a down-regulation of β_1 receptors which negates the stimulatory effects of sympathetic discharge. Sustained increase in sympathetic activity, however, increases the work load on the failing heart and therefore contributes adversely to the cardiac performance ultimately.

Activation of Renin-Angiotensin-Aldosterone System (RAAS)

A fall in CO decreases blood flow to kidneys. This prompts renin release, synthesis of angiotensin II (Ang-II) and release of aldosterone (see Ch. 18). This results in an increase in peripheral vascular resistance (PVR) with Na^+ and water retention (Fig. 22.1). Thus blood volume increases and more blood reaches the heart (in preload). Since afterload also increases with increase in PVR, the heart is unable to pump this extra volume. The resulting fluid back-up between the left ventricle and the lungs, and up to right ventricle from peripheral circulation, causes pulmonary and peripheral oedema. HF is also associated with increased circulating levels of arginine, vasopressin and endothelin I which also promote vasoconstriction and fluid retention. Although atrial natriuretic peptide is also increased in HF, owing to increased arterial pressure, paradoxically it does not produce natriuretic or vasodilatory effects in patients of HF. Excessive compensatory neurohormonal activity, therefore, ultimately depresses cardiac functions.

Ventricular Remodeling

The most important intrinsic compensatory mechanism is myocardial hypertrophy with a resultant increase in a more spherical shape of the heart referred to as "cardiac remodeling" which means a type of dilatation other than that due to passive stretch of heart muscle. During remodeling there is proliferation of the connective tissue cells as well as of abnormal myocardial cells under the influence of Ang-II. Initially, the increase in muscle mass helps to maintain cardiac performance. But after the initial beneficial effects, hypertrophy can lead to ischaemic changes and alterations in ventricular geometry. The ventricular wall tension increases, mechanical performance of heart decreases and blood in both the ventricles is retained which ultimately worsens the remodeling process. Over time, the myocytes in the failing heart die through apoptosis leaving the remaining myocytes subject to even greater work load.

Hence, remodeling also, ultimately worsens the cardiac performance.

PHENOMENON OF DECOMPENSATED HEART FAILURE

After certain period, the compensatory mechanisms become exhausted and increasingly ineffective, entering a vicious circle of decompensation in which the compensatory mechanisms become self-defeating. As the strain continues, total peripheral resistance (TPR) and afterload increase, thereby decreasing the ejection fraction per heartbeat. Preload is also increased in HF because of increased blood volume and venous tone. Ultimately, a stage comes when the adaptive mechanisms fail to maintain the CO. The HF now is termed as "decompensated".

As the blood volume expands, the decompensated heart is unable to pump and produces signs and symptoms of HF like:

a) Pulmonary and peripheral oedema (as discussed above).
b) Dyspnoea with cyanosis, due to hypoxia as a result of inadequate oxygenation of blood.
c) Hepatomegaly due to hepatic congestion.
d) Cardiomegaly due to myocardial hypertrophy and cardiac remodeling.
e) Reflex tachycardia due to hypoxia and decreased CO induced sympathetic discharge.
f) Decreased urine formation due to renal congestion.
g) Decreased exercise tolerance and muscle fatigue due to diminished CO.

DRUGS USED IN HEART FAILURE (HF)

The therapeutic goal in the management of HF is to increase cardiac output (CO) anyhow. A better understanding of preload, afterload and myocardial contractility has encouraged the judicious use of the following drugs for the treatment of heart failure:

I. **Drugs with positive inotropic effects**
   a) ***Cardiac Glycosides***: DIGOXIN, DIGITOXIN and OUABAIN.
   b) ***Bipyridines or Phosphodiesterase Inhibitors***: INAMRINONE, MILRINONE, LEVOSIMENDAN and ENOXIMONE
   c) ***β-Adrenergic Agonists***: DOPAMINE, DOBUTAMINE and DOPEXAMINE

II. **Drugs without positive inotropic effects**

a) ***Diuretics***: BUMETANIDE, FUROSEMIDE, HYDROCHLOROTHIAZIDE, METOLAZONE and SPIRONOLACTONE

b) ***ACEIs***: ENALAPRIL, LISINOPRIL and RAMIPRIL (also AT receptor antagonist, e.g., LOSARTAN)

c) ***β_1-Adrenoceptor Antagonists***: BISOPROLOL, CARVEDILOL and METOPROLOL

d) ***Vasodilators***: HYDRALAZINE, SODIUM NITROPRUSSIDE, ISOSORBIDE DINITRATE and NESIRITIDE

e) ***Vasopressin Receptor Antagonists***: CONIVAPTAN and TOLVAPTAN

The basic pharmacology of β-adrenergic agonists (Ch. 12), β_1-adrenoceptor antagonists (Ch. 12, 19 & 20), diuretics (Ch 16 & 19), ACEIs (Ch. 18 & 19) and vasodilators (Ch. 19) has been discussed in detail in other chapters, hence these drugs will be discussed here only in context of the treatment of heart failure. Accordingly, the use of drugs, with positive inotropic effects, in the management of heart failure will be discussed in detail.

DRUGS WITH POSITIVE INOTROPIC EFFECTS

Cardiac Glycosides

Chemistry

If a sugar molecule is joined together with a non-sugar molecule by a ether linkage it is called a glycoside.

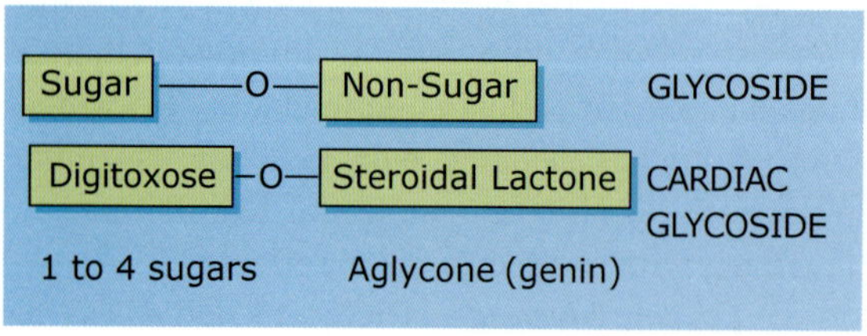

In cardiac glycosides the sugar part is 1 or 4 molecules of digitoxose while the non-sugar part (aglycone or genin) is a steroidal lactone. The pharmacological activity of cardiac glycosides resides in its non-sugar moiety called aglycone or genin. The sugar part, however, governs the pharmacokinetic characteristics such as lipid solubility and cell permeability.

Source

Leaves of *Digitalis lanata* provide two active principles—Digoxin and Digitoxin—while leaves of *Digitalis purpurea* (Fox glove) are the major source of digitoxin. Seeds of *Strophanthus gratus* provide two active glycosides—strophanthin-G and ouabain—while seeds of *Strophanthus kombe* yield primarily strophanthin-K.

Mechanism of Action

Normal Ionic Movements During the Contraction of Cardiac Muscle. The force of contraction of the cardiac muscle is directly related to the concentration of free cytosolic Ca^{2+}. Therefore, any drug that can increase the cytosolic Ca^{2+} levels can not only increase the force of contraction of heart muscle but can also increase the sensitivity of the contractile machinery to Ca^{2+}.

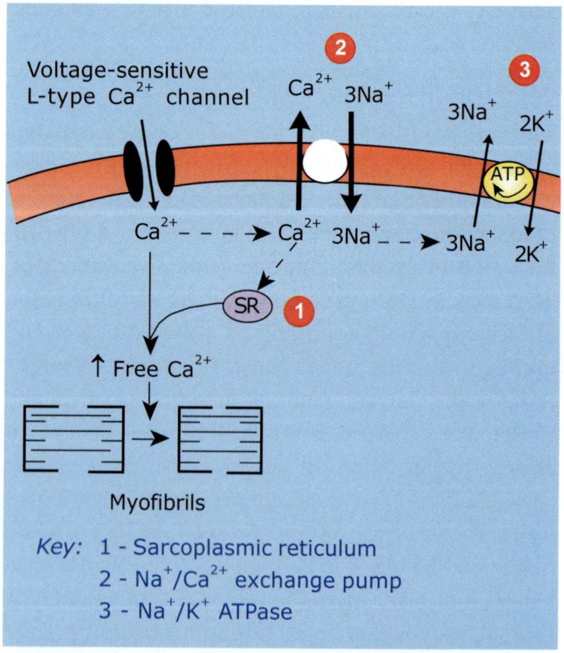

Fig 22.2 Normal Ionic Movement During Contraction of Cardiac Muscle.

Initially, the Ca^{2+} entry, through voltage-sensitive L-type Ca^{2+} channels, triggers the release of a much larger quantity of Ca^{2+} from the sarcoplasmic reticulum (and the mitochondria) by activating SR-Ca^{2+} release channel (ryanodine receptor). The increased Ca^{2+} concentration then initiates the contractile process. During restorative process of periodic contraction of cardiac muscle, Ca^{2+} ions are removed by reuptake into the sarcoplasmic reticulum by SR-Ca^{2+} ATPase (and mitochondria) as well as by its expulsion from the cell by a Ca^{2+}/Na^+ exchange pump. Intracellular Na^+ balance is then restored by Na^+/K^+ ATPase (Fig. 22.2).

Cellular Mechanism of Digitalis Action. Digitalis binds to and reversibly inhibits cardiac cell membrane associated Na^+/K^+ ATPase (Fig. 22.3). This leads to progressive accumulation of intracellular Na^+ and loss of intracellular K^+. Increase in the intracellular Na^+ concentration prompts the influx of Ca^{2+} from the outside and outflux of Na^+ from inside by Ca^{2+}/Na^+ exchange mechanisms. It should be noted that Na^+/Ca^{2+} exchanger normally extrudes Ca^{2+} in exchange for Na^+ (see above). However, in the presence of increased intracellular Na^+ concentration (as occurs under the effect of digitalis), it extrudes Na^+ in exchange of extracellular Ca^{2+}.

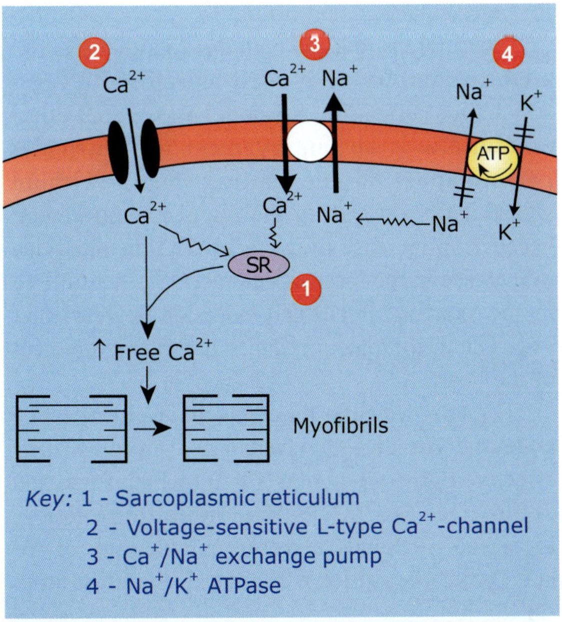

Fig 22.3 Cellular Mechanism of Digitalis Action.

There is also an increase in Ca^{2+} permeability through voltage-sensitive L-type Ca^{2+} channels, during plateau phase. Increased cytosolic free Ca^{2+} by these two mechanisms then triggers the release of more Ca^{2+} from sarcoplasmic reticulum and mitochondria. Digitalis also inhibits SR-Ca^{2+}-ATPase and thus reduces the reuptake of Ca^{2+} by sarcoplasmic reticulum.

Ultimately, the increased Ca^{2+} concentration in the cytosol triggers the contractile mechanisms of the failing heart. *In short, the inotropic action of digitalis results due to an increase in cytoplasmic Ca^{2+} concentration that enhances cardiac muscle contractility and ultimately the cardiac output (Fig.22.3).*

Higher serum K^+ concentration inhibits digitalis binding to Na^+/K^+ ATPase, therefore, hyperkalaemia can reduce digitalis toxicity while hypokalaemia will increase the risk of digitalis toxicity (tachyarrhythmias). Analogously, hypercalcaemia or hypomagnesaemia can increase the risk for digitalis-induced arrhythmias (magnesium actions are opposite of calcium).

Pharmacological Actions of Digitalis

Ventricular Function Curves in Normal Heart, in Heart Failure and After Digitalis Treatment

The three major determinants of cardiac function in the intact heart are preload (ventricular end-diastolic volume), afterload and myocardial contractility. When stroke volume, which is the measure of left ventricular performance, is plotted against left ventricular filling pressure (preload; Fig. 22.4) the resulting curve is termed as the left ventricular function curve (A). As per Frank Starling law, the stroke volume increases as the preload, or LV filling pressure, increases till 15 mm Hg. Beyond this point-A, there is plateau level of performance and preload greater than 25 mm Hg results in pulmonary oedema.

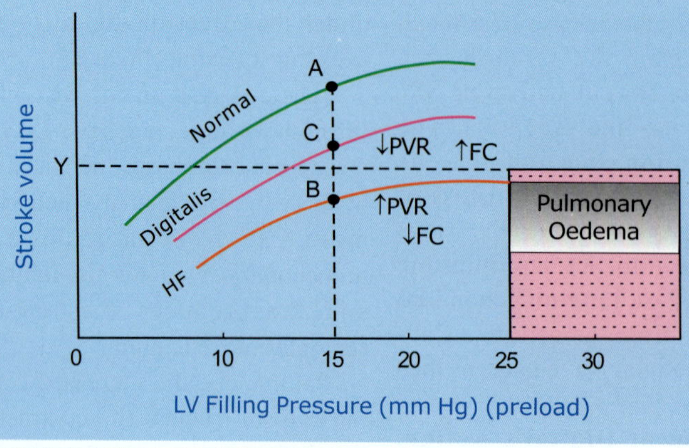

Fig 22.4 Ventricular Function Curves of Normal Heart, in Heart Failure and After Digitalis Treatment. PVR—Peripheral Vascular Resistance; FC—Force of Contraction

In heart failure, an increase in PVR and a decrease in contractility will provide a depressed LV function curve (B). Because this curve of the failing heart is lower, the plateau is reached at much lower values of stroke output. The downward shift of curve A to curve B shows that although the preload is same (15 mm Hg) but the stroke volume has dropped from 'Y' which is the minimal cardiac output (stroke volume) required to meet the normal metabolic needs of the body. In curve B even if preload increases to 25 mm Hg from 15 mm Hg, as a compensatory mechanism, there will only be a marginal improvement in the stroke volume. On the contrary, at this value of preload there would be exudation of fluid in the alveoli leading to pulmonary oedema (elevated pressure in the pulmonary capillaries pushes more fluid into the pulmonary interstitial space). As is clear with the curve 'B', the stroke volume is still not adequate to meet the metabolic needs of the patient having heart failure. Digitalis treatment shifts ventricular function curve 'B' to 'C' (more towards normal) by increasing contractility which in turn would lead to a decrease in PVR and preload.

Cardiac Effects of Digitalis. Effects of digitalis on normal heart are different than on the failing heart. In normal heart, digitalis increases force of contraction, and causes constriction of peripheral blood vessels. Heart rate and cardiac output (CO) are almost unchanged. In normal heart, digitalis has no effect on CO as the normal heart is emptying completely even otherwise. In heart failure, digitalis increases the contractility of the myocardium leading to an increase in cardiac output. Cardiac systole is shortened so that more time is provided for ventricular rest and filling.

Heart rate is reduced both due to direct (Na^+/K^+ ATPase inhibition) as well as indirect (vagal stimulation) effects on SA node. The overall effect of digitalis is an improvement in ventricular performance of the failing heart without significantly increasing the oxygen requirement; because an increase in myocardial O_2 demand due to increase in the force of contraction is neutralised by the reduction in HR and reduction in ventricular size, which ultimately reduces the O_2 requirement of the heart.

Digitalis decreases the conduction velocity of AV node and His-Purkinje system and prolongs their effective refractory period (ERP) by both vagal and extra-vagal (Na^+/K^+ ATPase inhibition) action. Increased ERP and decreased conductivity of AV node protects ventricles from atrial flutter or atrial fibrillation.

In relatively smaller doses, digitalis increases the conduction velocity and decreases the ERP of atrial muscle via vagal action while in high doses it increases automaticity and contractility but shortens the ERP of atrial muscle and ventricles causing extrasystoles, pulsus bigeminus and ventricular fibrillation.

Different parts of heart show different sensitivity towards digitalis as follows:

AV node>Atrial muscles>Purkinje fibres>Ventricles

Since cholinergic innervation is only up to AV node, the vagal effects of digitalis are more pronounced at AV node and atria than on Purkinje system or ventricles.

ECG shows prolongation of PR interval (delayed AV conduction), shortening of QT interval (shorter ventricular systole), depression of ST segment and inversion or disappearance of T wave. Later, extrasystoles, AV block and ventricular fibrillation appear as terminal events.

Extracardiac Effects of Digitalis

Blood Vessels. In normal persons, digitalis has direct vasoconstrictor effects. In heart failure, digitalis opposes compensatory sympathetic overactivity and causes a decrease in HR, decrease in PVR (↓ in afterload) and decrease in venous tone (↓ in preload). Since lesser blood reaches the heart, end-diastolic volume is reduced. There is no prominent effect on BP as it is secondary to the improvement in circulation.

Kidney. Diuresis occurs due to improvement in renal perfusion, which brings about a shift of oedematous fluid into circulation. Other contributing factors producing diuresis are: a decrease in compensatory sympathetic discharge, a decrease in activation of RAAS (↓ renin, ↓ Ang-II, ↓ aldosterone release and ↓ in salt and water retention).

GIT. The effects include anorexia, diarrhoea, nausea and vomiting (stimulation of chemoreceptor trigger zone).

CNS Effects. These include disorientation, hallucinations (in elderly), visual disturbance and aberrations of colour perception.

Pharmacokinetics

The pharmacokinetic characteristics of three typical cardiac glycosides—digoxin, digitoxin and ouabain—have been compared in Table 22.1.

Therapeutic Uses

Digoxin is the most commonly preferred drug amongst the three glycosides discussed above, even for the patients having hepatic insufficiency. Digitoxin is, however, preferred in the cases having renal impairment. Ouabain is reserved for acute heart failure. Slow digitalisation (Table 22.1) is always preferred to avoid cardiotoxicity. As digitalis has cumulative effect and exhibits smaller therapeutic window, it is always safer to prescribe a dose that provides digitalis plasma concentrations of 0.8 to 1.2 ng/ml. Such a dose reduces the incidence of side effects and optimises the benefits.

Congestive Heart Failure. Digitalis is a drug of choice for "low output heart failure" due to HT, IHD, or arrhythmias. It is not a suitable drug for "high output heart failure" due to thyrotoxicosis or arteriovenous shunt (see above). It provides relief from dyspnoea and cyanosis by subsiding pulmonary congestion. It increases urinary output and reduces oedematous fluid by increasing renal perfusion. Because it diminishes systemic venous pressure, engorged tender liver regresses and engorgement of neck veins disappears. With decreased end-diastolic fibre tension, heart size and O_2 demand of myocardium decreases. There is bradycardia and improved myocardial circulation with the development of a sense of well being.

Paroxysmal Supraventricular Tachycardia. It is a common arrhythmia due to reentry phenomenon taking place at SA or AV node. They frequently respond to digitalis favourably, because of reflex vagal activation which slows the conduction of impulses. However, adenosine or verapamil or β-blockers are more preferred these days as they take a shorter time for providing improvement. Digitalis is, now, reserved for preventing recurrences.

Atrial Flutter and Atrial Fibrillation. Atrial flutter (rate 200–300 beats/min) and atrial fibrillation (rate 500 beats/min) are effectively treated with

Table 22.1 Pharmacokinetic Profiles of Three Typical Cardiac Glycosides

Parameters	Digitoxin[1]	Digoxin[1]	Ouabain
1. Oral absorption	95%–100%	75%–90%[3]	0 (nil)
2. Administration	Oral	Oral	I.V.
3. aVd (L/kg)[4]	0.6	6–7	18
4. Protein binding	90	30	0 (nil)
5. Plasma half-life	6–7 days	38–40 hr	18–20 hr
6. Onset of action	2 hours	1/2 hour	Very rapid (given I.V.)
7. Duration of action	Very long	Intermediate	Short
8. Metabolised (%)	80 (liver)[2]	20 (liver)	0
9. Excretion	Mainly bile, also urine	Urine (unchanged)	Urine (unchanged)
10. Doses			
a) Digitalising dose	1.0 mg in 24 hr or 0.4 mg every 12 hr for total 3 doses orally	0.5–0.75 mg 8 hrly for total 3 doses orally	0.2–0.5 mg I.V. in cases of acute heart failure
b) Maintenance dose	0.1 mg single dose per day	0.25–0.5 mg per day	

[1] These digitalis preparations have cumulative effect
[2] Undergoes enterohepatic circulation which contributes to prolonged $t_{1/2}$
[3] About 10% of population harbour enteric bacteria which inactivates digoxin in the gut and reduces bioavailability
[4] Apparent volume of distribution

digitalis as it decreases conduction velocity and increases ERP of AV node. If the ventricular rate of 72–80 beats/minute (therapeutic end point) is not achieved by giving digitalis alone; a β-blocker or verapamil may be added.

Dilated Heart. Digitalis is still the most preferred drug for patients having dilated heart and low ejection fraction as it is helpful in restoring cardiac compensation. It is usually prescribed when the patient's condition is not controlled by diuretic or ACE inhibitor.

Digoxin therapy in HF, at present, remains controversial. Recent trials have failed to show any mortality benefits with digoxin use. A small mortality benefit may exist at blood levels below 1.0 ng/ml but recent reports reveal an increased mortality at higher blood levels that were earlier regarded as therapeutic. Besides, there are multiple factors governing its blood levels, efficacy and toxicity including numerous drug interactions.

Adverse Effects and Management of Toxicity

Cardiac Side Effects. These include bradycardia, partial or complete heart block, atrial or ventricular extrasystoles, coupled beats (bigeminy), ventricular fibrillation and fatal cardiac arrhythmias.

If cardiac arrhythmias develop, Ca^{2+}, Mg^{2+} and K^+ status should be corrected (see above). For brief runs of bigeminy, oral K^+ supplementation and withdrawal of digoxin may be sufficient. If arrhythmias are more serious, parenteral K^+ and lidocaine may be administered (see Ch. 21). Propranolol can be used for ventricular or supraventricular tachycardia, provided AV block is absent. Atropine can be used to control sinus bradycardia and different degrees of AV block. If there is a severe digitalis intoxication, measurement of serum K^+ levels are misleading as these are found elevated because of K^+ loss from intracellular compartments of various tissues and skeletal muscles.

Since automaticity also gets depressed at toxic doses, use of any antiarrhythmic drug could be fatal. Such patients can be saved by administering digitalis antibodies, e.g., Digibind Fab fragments (digitalis immune Fab). Although these antibodies are raised against digoxin, these also recognise digitoxin and ouabain. A 40 mg vial of these antibodies neutralises 0.6 mg of digoxin stored in the body. These are extremely useful in reversing severe intoxication with most glycosides.

Extracardiac Side Effects. ***GIT***: Anorexia, nausea, vomiting, diarrhoea and abdominal cramps.

CNS: Headache, fatigue, neuralgia, blurred vision, loss of colour perception (as discussed above)

Endocrinal: Gyanecomastia in males (but very rare).

Management of extracardiac side effects requires no more than reducing the dose of digoxin.

Contraindications

- Hypokalaemia enhances digitalis toxicity as it potentiates its binding to Na^+/K^+ ATPase.
- In children below 10 years and in elderly patients with hepatic or renal impairment, because such patients are more sensitive to digitalis action.
- Myocardial infarction; except when heart failure is accompanied with atrial flutter or fibrillation.
- Hypothyroidism, because of slower elimination (or more cumulation) of digoxin.
- Myocarditis or grossly damaged myocardium, because of the risk of developing arrhythmias.
- Wolff-Parkinson-White syndrome, because in such cases digitalis may enhance transmission through accessory pathway and may increase the probability of conduction of arrhythmic atrial impulses to ventricle leading to ventricular fibrillation.

Drug Interactions

These are summarised in Fig. 22.5

Phosphodiesterase Inhibitors (Bipyridines)

To this category belong ***inamrinone*** (also called as *amrinone*), ***milrinone*** and ***levosimendan***. These bipyridine derivatives are also referred to as non-glycoside, non-sympathomimetic inotropic agents. By inhibiting phosphodiesterase isozyme-3, which is specially located in cardiac myocytes and vascular smooth muscle, these drugs increase the amount of cAMP by preventing its degradation to AMP (Fig. 22.6). As a result, there is an increase in myocardial contractility along with vasodilatation (hence also called *inodilators*). These are administered initially in loading dose by I.V. infusion followed by slow maintenance infusions in normal saline. These drugs are unstable in dextrose solution. Because of the fluid balance concerns, this becomes a potential problem and a drawback in patients of heart failure.

The toxicity of ***inamrinone*** includes nausea, vomiting, dose-dependent thrombocytopenia and arrhythmias as ventricular rates may get increased in patients with atrial flutter or fibrillation. ***Milrinone*** is safer than inamrinone but it can also potentiate arrhythmias occurring in CHF. Renal impairment can prolong the plasma half-life of milrinone. Minor side effects include headache and tremors.

Levosimendan, like milrinone, inhibits phospho-diesterase isozyme-3 (causing vasodilation), but also sensitizes the contractile mechanisms of cardiac smooth muscles to Ca^{2+}.

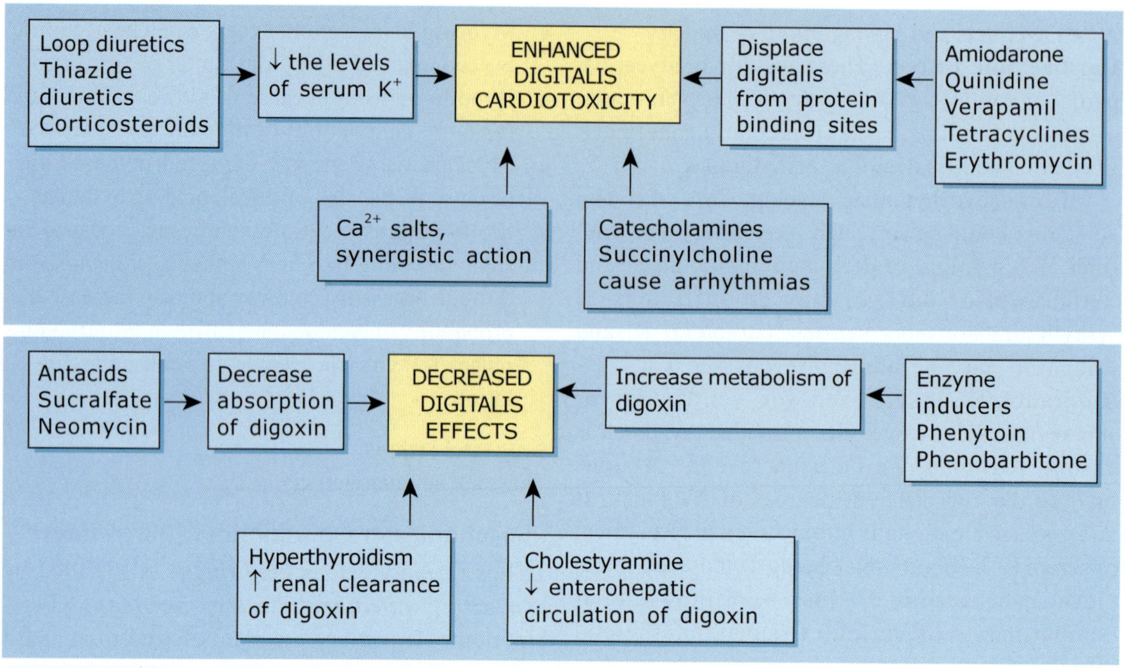

Fig 22.5 Digoxin Drug Interactions

Enoximone is another congener of inamrinone given I.V. in case of acute heart failure. As with inamrinone there is risk for developing arrhythmia but it is better tolerated and improves the physical mobility and quality of life in these patients (central stimulatory effects of increased cAMP).

The usefulness of these inotropic drugs in CHF is quite limited. Milrinone, however, is used intravenously only for acute HF, or for an exacerbated HF on short-term basis. Thus the role of such inotropic drugs appears to be limited to patients with symptoms and signs of low cardiac output (primarily with hypoperfusion and deteriorating renal functions) and those who fail to respond to I.V. diuretics. In some selected cases, milrinone may help in maintaining patients awaiting cardiac transplantation.

β-Adrenergic Agonists

β-Adrenergic stimulation improves cardiac performance through positive inotropic effects. β_1 agonists lead to an increase in intracellular cAMP which results in the activation of protein kinase. Slow Ca^{2+} channels are then phosphorylated by protein kinase which increases Ca^{2+} flow into the myocardial cell causing increased force of contraction of heart muscle (Fig. 22.6).

Dobutamine (Ch.12) is the most commonly used inotropic agent, other than digitalis. On heart, dobutamine has more selective inotropic than chronotropic effect without any significant change in peripheral resistance and BP. As such it has been considered to be relatively selective β_1 agonist. Its actions do not appear to be a result of the release of NE from sympathetic nerve endings, nor via dopamine receptor action. Its half-life is about 2 min and therefore must be given by I.V. infusion (5–10 μg/kg/min). The steady state concentrations are achieved within 10 min of its I.V. infusion. It is used for short-term management of acute HF and for patients of HF associated with MI or cardiac surgery. It increases cardiac output (CO), and therefore urinary output, and stroke volume without affecting HR, TPR or BP. Being an inotropic agent it increases myocardial O_2 demand, and hence angina may be precipitated or MI may be aggravated. Tolerance may develop on repeated use. Since the drug increases AV conduction,

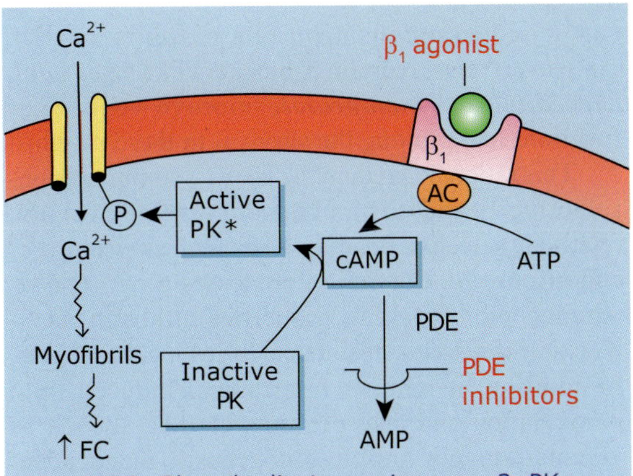

Fig 22.6 Mode of Action of β-Agonists and Phosphodiesterase Isozyme-3 Inhibitors in Heart Failure.

it should be used with caution in atrial fibrillation. As it increases BP it should be avoided in patients with a history of HT.

Dopamine (Ch.12), when given by I.V. infusion in low doses (2–5 μg/kg/min), acts on D_1 receptors in kidney and causes dilatation of renal blood vessels resulting in an increase in GFR, renal blood flow and urinary output. In therapeutic doses (5–10 μg/kg/min), it also stimulates β_1 receptors resulting in an increase in CO but the TPR is unchanged, due to simultaneous renal and splanchnic vasodilatation through stimulation of D_1 receptors. However, in high doses (above 10 μg/kg/min) it then activates α_1 receptors also, which causes vasoconstriction with an increase in TPR and pulmonary pressure. This may nullify the beneficial effects of dopamine in HF. Dopamine is used in the treatment of low cardiac output HF with compromised renal functions (advantages of increased CO with renal vasodilatation). However, the BP, HR and urinary output should be continuously monitored not only to adjust the dose but to achieve the desired beneficial effects.

DRUGS WITHOUT POSITIVE INOTROPIC EFFECTS

Diuretics

Diuretics and their mechanism of action has already been discussed in detail in Chapter 16 and 19. Loop diuretics like ***bumetanide*** and ***furosemide*** promptly reduce pulmonary oedema due to rapid diuresis which results in the decrease in extracellular fluid, decrease in venous return, and subsequently in the decrease in the right ventricular output (ventricular preload). These reductions have two useful effects: reduction in oedema (and its adverse effects) and reduction in cardiac size which leads to an improvement in pump efficiency. Though widely used, loop diuretics do not influence the primary disease process in CHF.

The addition of ***spironolactone*** to digitalis and an ACE inhibitor significantly improves survival among patients with chronic/severe HF. Spironolactone, being aldosterone antagonist, enhances diuresis by promoting Na^+ and water excretion (while retaining K^+) and prevents myocardial as well as vascular fibrosis which is responsible for pathological remodeling of the heart. There is now an evidence for the existence of aldosterone receptors on cardiac myocytes which explains the usefulness of spironolactone in cardiac remodeling. Hyperkalaemia is a major risk during the therapy with spironolactone and requires serum K^+ monitoring. Gynaecomastia may occur in male patients, after long-term use of spironolactone.

Thiazide diuretics (***hydrochlorothiazide*** and ***metolazone***) are used less frequently in HF. However, in advanced CHF, after chronic use, resistance develops to loop diuretics. If such a situation arises, hydrochlorothiazide or metolazone or spironolactone may be added with loop diuretics to overcome this problem. For mild HF, hydrochlorothiazide + spironolactone are sufficient. For refractory HF, ***chlorthalidone*** can be especially useful thiazide type diuretic. It may also be given along with spironolactone for deriving additional benefits (as discussed above) and to prevent hypokalaemia.

Angiotensin-Converting Enzyme Inhibitors (ACEIs) and Angiotensin Receptor Antagonists (ARAs)

ACEIs are now considered as the agents of first choice in the pharmacological management of HF. ACEIs have already been discussed in detail in Chapter 18 and 19. These drugs not only block the conversion of angiotensin I (Ang-I) to angiotensin II

(Ang-II) but also prevent the breakdown of bradykinin to promote vasodilatation (reduce afterload). They also decrease aldosterone secretion and hence reduce salt and water retention. This decreases venous return and preload. The decrease in preload and afterload improves cardiac output. Most important of them all, they prolong the survival by preventing pathological remodeling of the heart and blood vessels, an adverse consequence of HF. ACEIs also reduce the death rate due to arrhythmias, MI and stroke. These are very useful in decreasing the damaging effects of left ventricular dysfunction in the patients of CHF whose ejection fraction (EF) is less than 35% (HFrEF). Nonetheless, ***enalapril*** (2.5 mg twice daily and worked up to 10 mg twice daily), ***lisinopril*** (2.5 mg to 5 mg once daily, worked up to 20 mg once daily) and ***ramipril*** (2.5 mg once daily, worked up to 10 mg once daily) are most commonly used.

Combination of ***spironolactone*** with ACEIs provides more beneficial effects and further reduces mortality. Ang-II is not the only stimulus to aldosterone secretion and after prolonged treatment with ACEIs, circulating aldosterone levels return toward normal, a phenomenon called "***aldosterone escape***". Hence, the combination maintains beneficial effects which otherwise may decline after chronic use of ACEIs alone.

AT_1 receptor antagonists (ARAs) like ***losartan*** (Ch. 18 and 19) also appear to have similar but limited beneficial effects. However, the consensus opinion for their use is to try an ACEI as the first line therapy before using ARAs like ***losartan*** or ***valsartan***. A fixed-dose combination of ***valsartan*** + ***sacubitril*** ARNI (**A**ngiotensin **R**eceptor+**N**eprilysin **I**nhibitor) has been approved by the US-FDA for the treatment of HFrEF (See Ch. 17 for details).

β_1-Adrenoceptor Antagonists

The detailed pharmacology of β-blockers has been described in Chapter 12, 19, 20 and 23. As a general rule, β-blockers are contraindicated in CHF. Heart failure patients have a decreased cardiac output (CO). Since CO is equal to stroke volume (SV) multiplied by heart rate (HR), an increased HR would be necessary to maintain an adequate CO in the presence of decreased SV as observed in HF. As a result, a decrease in HR and cardiac contractility produced by β-blockers would be expected to produce acute cardiac decompensation, in patients of HF.

Nevertheless, certain β-blockers like ***bisoprolol, carvedilol*** and ***metoprolol,*** improve ventricular functions and prolong the survival in these patients.

This rationale favours the use of a combined non-selective β and α-blocker, *carvedilol* over the relatively selective β_1 antagonists such as *metoprolol* and *bisoprolol*. Carvedilol possesses β_1, β_2, and α_1 adrenoceptor blocking properties although its β-blocking effects are greater than its α-blocking effects. In addition, it inhibits free radical induced lipid peroxidation and also prevents cardiac as well as vascular smooth muscle mitogenesis, independent of its α or β-adrenoceptor blocking effects. The suggested mechanism for the favourable effects of carvedilol, bisoprolol and metoprolol in the patients of HF include reduction in cardiac remodeling and blunting of the adverse effects of higher circulating levels of catecholamines including apoptosis β_1 effect and vasoconstriction α_1 effect.

Vasodilators

These agents reduce pulmonary congestion and increase cardiac output by reducing preload and/or afterload. Vasodilators can be divided into arteriolar dilators (e.g., ***hydralazine***), venous dilators (e.g., ***nitroglycerine*** and long-acting nitrates) and arteriolar as well as venous dilators (e.g. ***sodium nitroprusside***). These are discussed in Chapter 19. The vasodilators are useful in acute HF as they provide a reduction in preload (due to venodilatation) or a decrease in afterload (due to arteriolar dilatation) or both. They also prevent remodeling of the heart. The choice of the vasodilator depends on patient's signs and symptoms. In patients of HF with dyspnoea, venodilators like ***nitroglycerine*** or long-acting nitrates are preferred because these may reduce the filling pressure and ultimately the pulmonary congestion. Conversely, in patients having low left ventricular output, an arteriolar dilator such as ***hydralazine*** may be useful in increasing cardiac output.

However, patients having severe chronic failure are benefited by a combination of ***hydralazine*** (to reduce afterload) and a ***long-acting nitrate*** (to reduce preload). The combination is useful in patients in whom ACEIs are contraindicated or are not tolerated.

Nesiritide, which is a recombinant form of human

B-type natriuretic peptide, has been introduced for use in acute HF. This recombinant form of naturally occurring hormone secreted by the ventricles, increases cGMP in vascular smooth muscle (similar to nitric oxide) and therefore reduces venous as well as arteriolar tone. It is used in patients with acutely decompensated HF associated with dyspnoea at rest. Hypotension is its most common adverse effect.

Vasopressin Receptor Antagonists

Vasopressin (ADH) is released in response to increased plasma osmolality, decreased arterial pressure and reduced cardiac filling (Ch.17). Among the vasopressin receptors, V_1 receptors mediate vasoconstrictor actions of vasopressin, while V_2 receptors mediate its antidiuretic action. ***Conivaptan*** is a mixed V_1+V_2 receptor antagonist which has been approved for a small subset of the patients having acute heart failure with hyponatraemia. ***Tolvaptan*** is an oral V_2- antagonist.

Vericiguat

cGMP plays a major role in the regulation of vascular tone, cardiac contractility and cardiac remodelling. Heart failure is associated with impaired NO synthesis and decreased sGC activity, which may contribute to myocardial and vascular dysfunction. Vericiguat stimulates soluble guanylate-cyclase (sGC), the intracellular receptor for endogenous nitric oxide (NO), which catalyzes cyclic guanosine monophosphate (cGMP) production. Vericiguat is highly bound to plasma proteins. Vericiguat is used for adults with symptomatic, chronic heart failure. Adverse effects: Nausea, vomiting, hypotension, anaemia and allergic reactions.

AHA/ACC/HFSA Guideline for the Management of Heart Failure, 2022 (Table 22.2)

A guideline offers updated recommendations for the assessment and management of heart failure (HF). The guideline is issued by the *American College of Cardiology (ACC)*, the *American Heart Association (AHA)* and the *Heart Failure Society of America (HFSA)*. It is updated latest in 2022.

Other salient features of guideline: In chronic heart failure, sodium-glucose cotransporter-2 inhibitor like dapagliflozin reduces hospitalization and cardiovascular mortality irrespective of the presence of type-2 diabetes mellitus. For hyperkalemia due to ACEI, potassium binders like patiromer, sodium zirconium and cyclosilicate can be used to improve outcome. For patients with symptomatic (NYHA class II & III) stable chronic HF, *Ivabradine* can be beneficial to reduce HF hospitalization and cardiovascular death. It is a sinoatrial node modulator that selectively inhibits the I_f current in the heart. In selected high-risk patients with HF, oral soluble guanylate cyclase inhibitor *vericiguat* may be considered to reduce HF hospitalization and mortality.

Table 22.2 Classification and treatment of heart failure

AHA*/ACC stage	NYHA**	Description	Treatment
Stage A	**Pre-failure**	No symptoms but risk factors are present	Treat obesity, hypertension, diabetes, hyperlipidemia
Stage B	**I**	No limitation of ordinary activities, Symptoms with severe exercise	ACEI/ARB, β blocker, Diuretic
Stage C	**II**	Slight limitation of activity, symptoms with marked activities	Add spironolactone/eplerenone digoxin, nitrates, hydralazine, Ivabradine
	III	Symptoms with mild physical activities	
Stage D	**IV**	Severe symptoms even at rest/ refractory HF	Heart Transplant, left ventricular assist device

*American College of Cardiology/American Heart Association classification. **NYHA: New York Heart association classification 2022. Risk factors include hypertension, myocardial infarct, diabetes

CHAPTER 23

Drug Therapy of Dyslipidaemia

COMPETENCY PH1.31

Ischaemic cardiovascular and cerebrovascular diseases are leading cause of morbidity and mortality the world over, specially in developed and developing countries. As the major cause for the development of ischaemic diseases is related to dyslipidaemia and resulting atherosclerosis, these are also called **a**thero**s**clerotic **c**ardio**v**ascular **d**iseases (ASCVDs). Disorders of the metabolism of lipoproteins, including lipoprotein over-production and deficiency are classified as dyslipidaemias. These may manifest in one or more of the following ways:

a) Elevated total cholesterol (CH) levels
b) Elevated low density lipoprotein (LDL) cholesterol levels
c) Elevated triglyceride (TG) levels
d) Decreased high density lipoprotein (HDL) cholesterol levels

The term *dyslipidaemia* is, nowadays, preferred over *hyperlipidaemia* or *hyperlipoproteinaemia* because a low plasma concentration of high density lipoprotein cholesterol (HDL-C) is rather harmful and *vice versa*. If the metabolic disorders of lipoproteins (↑ LDL or ↓ HDL) are due to genetic reasons, these are termed as *primary dyslipidaemias* and if the disorders are secondary to some disease (diabetes mellitus, hypothyroidism or hypopituitarism) these are called *secondary dyslipidaemias*. *Hyper-lipaemia* denotes increased levels of triglycerides (TGs), a leading cause of acute pancreatitis. *Dyslipidaemia* ultimately contributes to the pathogenesis of ASCVDs.

Before discussing the metabolism of lipoproteins and the treatment of lipoprotein disorders, it would be pertinent to mention briefly about lipids, lipoproteins, apolipoproteins, lipoprotein receptors and various lipolytic and other enzymes involved in the metabolism of lipoproteins.

LIPIDS

Lipids are heterogeneous group of compounds related to fatty acids, which are insoluble in water and are stored in the body as a source of energy. These are of three types:

Simple Lipids

These are esters of *fatty acids* and *alcohol*. The dietary fatty acids may be (i) *saturated fatty acids* (SFAs) such as lauric and palmitic acids, which have sizeable effect of raising blood CH. Most animal fats and hydrogenated vegetable oils like 'Dalda' have SFAs; (ii) *monounsaturated fatty acids* (MUFAs) which have one double bond in their structure, e.g., oleic acid and palmitoleic acid. These occur largely in olives and nuts and are useful compared to SFAs, as they help in lowering of LDL and VLDL; (iii) *polyunsaturated fatty acids* (PUFAs) which have 2 or more double bonds in their structure, e.g., linolenic acid and arachidonic acid. All PUFAs have a hypolipidaemic effect. PUFAs are abundant in corn oil, safflower oil, fish oil; (iv) *trans-fatty acids* (TFAs) such as elaidic acid or trans-oleic acid are also unsaturated fatty acids in trans-geometry. These are generated during hydrogenation of PUFAs and MUFAs. These are present in some commercial vegetable oils and are harmful as they raise LDL cholesterol and lower HDL cholesterol.

Compound Lipids

These are also esters of fatty acids and alcohol as described above but possess certain other groups in their structure and thus named accordingly, e.g., sulfolipids and phospholipids.

Neutral Lipids

These are non-polar lipids such as triglycerides (TGs), cholesterol (CH) and cholesterol esters (CE). Triglyceride is a glycerol with all the three OH groups linked to fatty acids. Cholesterol is a lipid which chemically is a sterol but not a fat. Neutral lipids are transported into circulation, in solubilised form, with the help of lipoproteins.

LIPOPROTEINS

Lipoproteins are spherical particles of water-soluble proteins, that transport neutral lipids (TG, CH and CE) through body fluids.

TG and CE constitute the non-polar hydrophobic core of the lipoprotein (Fig. 23.1). Since the core of lipoprotein (LP) is hydrophobic in character, it is surrounded by a hydrophilic surface coat of phospholipids, unesterified CH and specific proteins called apoproteins. The hydrophilic surface coat makes the LP molecule soluble in plasma and acts as an interface between the plasma and the core components. Apoproteins (Apo) also play a crucial role in the regulation of lipid transport/exchange and in lipoprotein metabolism.

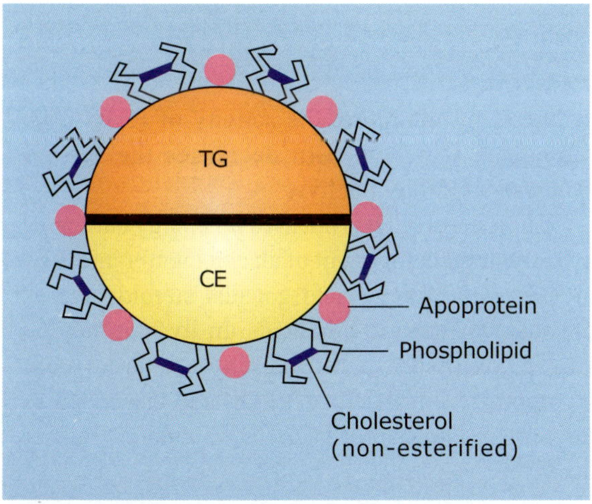

Fig 23.1 Structure of a Lipoprotein

Types of Lipoproteins (LPs)

LPs have been classified on the basis of their densities, diameter, TG and CE contents into 5 major classes: Chylomicrons (CM), Very Low Density Lipoprotein (VLDL), Intermediate Density Lipoprotein (IDL), Low Density Lipoprotein (LDL) and High Density Lipoprotein (HDL).

There is yet another LP particle, similar in composition to LDL, but with an additional Apo-A besides Apo-B100. This LP, called *Lipoprotein*-(a) [LP(a)] is now firmly linked with increased risk of atherosclerosis. LP(a) is a homologue of plasminogen but lacks plasminogen's enzymatic activity. It is a competitive inhibitor of plasminogen at its receptors at endothelial cells. Hence, the fibrinolytic enzyme *plasmin* is not generated. Instead, thrombosis is promoted. LP(a) also stimulates smooth muscle cell proliferation and inhibits 'transforming growth factor-B', thereby increases the plaque mass in arteries. Hence, compared to LDL, LP(a) has greater atherogenic potential. The rank order of different LPs for their density, diameter, TG and CE content and atherogenicity is as follows:

DENSITY : HDL>LP(a)>LDL>IDL>VLDL>CM
DIAMETER : CM>VLDL>IDL>LDL>LP(a)>HDL
CE CONTENT : LP(a)=LDL>IDL>HDL>VLDL>CM
TG CONTENT : CM>VLDL>IDL>LDL>LP(a)=HDL
ATHERO-GENICITY : LP(a)>LDL>VLDL=IDL=CM>HDL*

*HDL is rather antiatherosclerotic lipoprotein

APOPROTEINS (Apos)

Apoproteins (Apos) are the surface proteins present on various lipoproteins. Their function is to provide structural stability to the lipoprotein and to determine its metabolic fate by transporting its lipid contents to verious tissues and finally to liver. In doing this, some of the apoproteins are exchanged between different types of lipoproteins. The composition of various lipoproteins and the apoproteins which they carry are listed in Table 23.1. Apoprotein-B48, synthesised in GIT and found in CM and CM remnants (CMR), is responsible for their assembly and secretion. Apo-B100, synthesised in liver and found in VLDL, IDL and LDL, is responsible to deliver lipids to artery wall. HDL carries many apoproteins, but manily A,C and E, which play a crucial role in *reverse cholesterol transport* from peripheral cells and artery wall, ultimately to liver (see following text).

Table 23.1 Composition of Various Lipoproteins and the Apoproteins which They Carry

Lipoproteins	Core Lipids	Apoproteins*
From Diet		
CM	TG > CE	B48, C, E, A
CMR	TG < CE	- do -
From Hepatocyte		
VLDL	TG > CE	C, B100, E
IDL	TG = CE	- do -
LDL	CE	B100
HDL	CE (+PL)	A, C, E

* Listed according to their importance.
CM—Chylomicron; CMR—Chylomicron remnant; VLDL—Very low density lipoprotein; IDL—Intermediate density lipoprotein; LDL—Low density lipoprotein; HDL—High density lipoprotein; TG—Triglycerides; CE—Cholesteryl esters; PL—Phospholipids

NORMAL LIPOPROTEIN METABOLISM

An understanding of the normal lipoprotein metabolism (Fig. 23.2) and the pathophysiology of various hyperlipidaemic states is essential prior to making a rational choice for drug treatment of dyslipidaemia.

The liver is the central place for lipoprotein metabolism. It derives CH from 3 sources: (1) delivery of dietary CH from CMRs (as discussed below), (2) endocytosis of low density lipoprotein (LDL) cholesterol through LDL receptors (as discussed below), and (3) biosynthesis from acetyl-CoA involving HMG-CoA reductase enzyme (3-Hydroxy-3-methyl glutaryl-coenzyme A-reductase). In this process acetyl-CoA is reduced to mevalonic acid (a precursor to CH synthesis; see following text). A small amount of CH is also absorbed from the gut either after dietary intake or by enterohepatic circulation of bile salts. This CH is also taken up by hepatocytes. A high intracellular CH in the hepatocytes provides a negative feedback for CH synthesis by inhibiting the activity of HMG-CoA reductase, which in turn decreases the further synthesis of CH by the liver.

Cholesterol (CH) is not used for energy but serves as a structural component of all cell membranes, as a precursor for adrenal and gonadal steroids and as precursor of hepatic bile acids. In liver, it may be stored, oxidised to bile acids or alternatively incorporated into HDL or VLDL and resecreted as lipoprotein-cholesterol back into circulation, as per need (Fig. 23.2).

Transport of Exogenous (Dietary) Lipids

In the intestinal mucosa, dietary TG and CH are incorporated into the core of chylomicrons (CM). The surface coat of CM is composed of phospholipids, Apo-B48, Apo-C, E and A. The CM is then transported to the circulation via the thoracic duct. In the plasma, Apo-C is also transferred to CM from HDL (Fig. 23.2). Apo-C mediates hydrolysis of TG (in CM) by activating lipoprotein lipase (LPL) enzyme present on the capillary endothelial cells. The free fatty acids

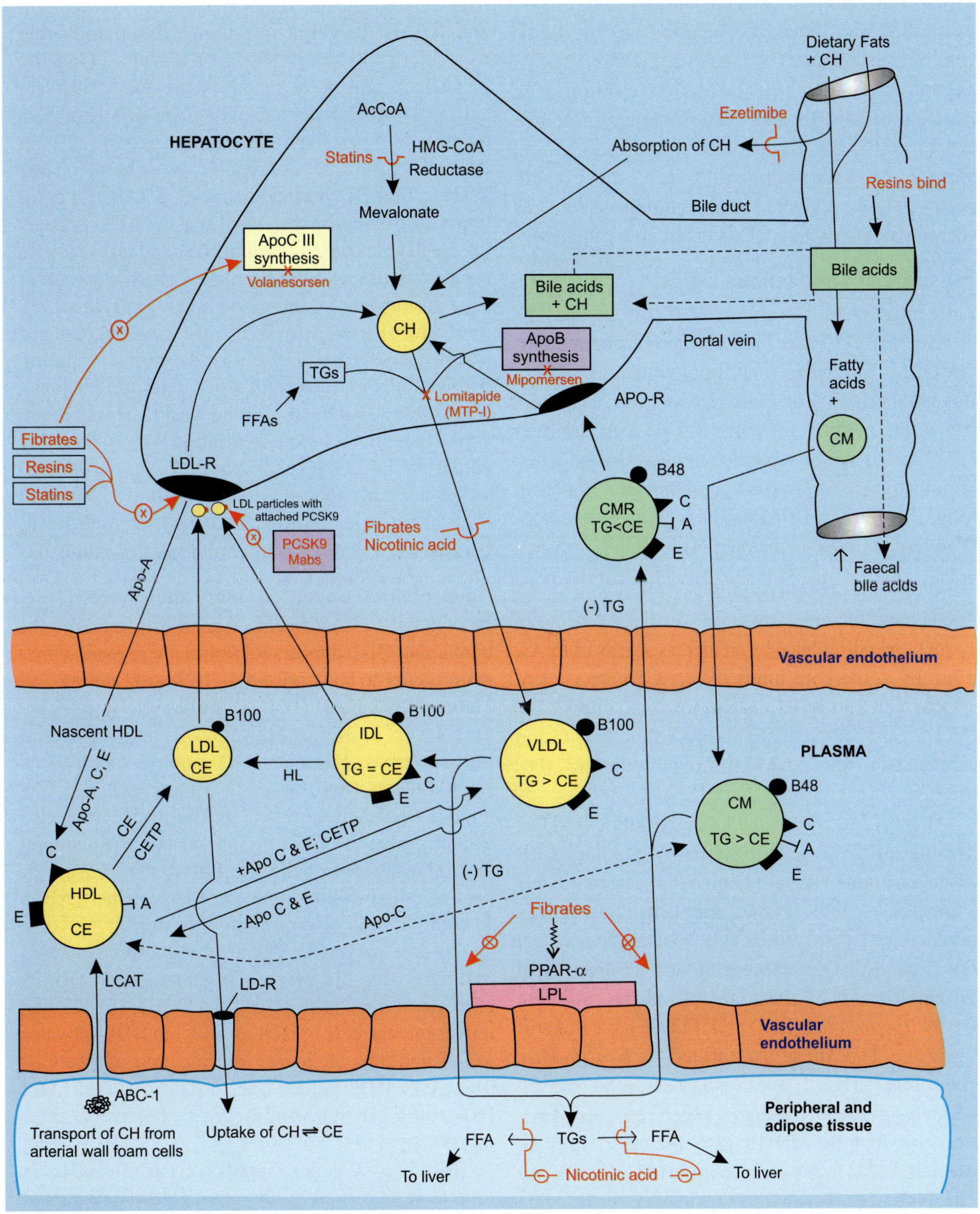

Fig 23.2 Normal Lipoprotein Metabolism and Sites of Action of Drugs Affecting the Metabolism. For Abbreviations, See Text.

(FFAs) thus formed provide energy for muscle contraction and metabolic functions of the body. After delivering the TGs to adipose tissues, the CM are converted to cholesterol-rich chylomicron remnants (CMRs) which bind to apolipoprotein-E receptor (APO-R) present on liver and endocytosed to serve as a dietary source of CH. As a net result, dietary TGs are delivered to fat and muscle cells (as fatty acids) and dietary CH is taken up by the liver.

Transport of Endogenous Lipids

While intestinal mucosa secretes TG-rich CMs, the liver secretes TG-rich VLDL through endogenous transport. The endogenous lipid transport system conveys lipids (TG and cholesteryl ester, CE) from liver to the peripheral tissues and back to the liver (Fig. 23.2). It can be separated into two subsystems: The atherogenic Apo-B100 lipoprotein guided system (for VLDL, IDL and LDL) and the antiatherogenic Apo-AI governed lipoprotein system (for HDL).

Apo-B100 Lipoprotein Guided System

VLDL particles are synthesised in liver when TG production is stimulated by an increased flux of FFAs. In the liver, the core lipids (TG > CE) are packed together with Apo-B100 and phospholipids into VLDL which is then secreted into plasma where Apo-C and E are added to nascent VLDL from circulating HDL particles.

After VLDL is released into circulation its TGs, (like that of CM) are hydrolysed by capillary LPL present on luminal surface of blood vessels of various tissues. FFAs, thus formed, are utilised as energy source. After hydrolysis of TGs, VLDL particles get converted to VLDL remnants. If these remnants still contain some TGs, these are called *intermediate density lipoproteins* (IDL) and if these have none or negligible TGs these are termed as *low density lipoprotein* (LDL). IDL can either enter the liver by endocytosis *via* LDL receptor (which recognise Apo-E on the surface of IDL as a receptor ligand). Alternatively, it may get converted to LDL by hydrolysis of its TG contents by hepatic triglyceride lipase (HTGL or hepatic lipase, HL). Apo-B100 is the only apoprotein and CE is the main core lipid in LDL, as other apoproteins (Apo Cs and E) are transferred back to HDL after the major amount of TGs of VLDL and IDL is delivered to adipose tissue and other tissues after hydrolysis by LPL enzyme. Half-life of LDL in plasma depends on the availability (or activity) of LDL receptors, which are largely present on liver and peripheral tissues that require CH for their metabolic needs. Apo-B100 present on the surface of LDL particles acts as a LDL receptor ligand for this purpose. Most plasma LDL is taken up by liver and the remainder is delivered to peripheral tissues which utilise CH as a precursor for steroidogenesis. Increased levels of plasma LDL cholesterol and Apo-B100 are risk factors for atherosclerosis (as LDL can be deposited in arterial wall as foam cells to form atherosclerotic plaques). The role of VLDL in atherogenesis is less certain while the atherogenic potential of IDL is probably equal to LDL. One species of LDL, *lipoprotein(a)* which contains apoprotein-a has also been found in atherosclerotic plaques and may contribute to coronary artery disease by inhibiting thrombolysis.

Apoprotein-AI Governed Lipoprotein System

In contrast to atherogenic Apo-B100, the Apo-AI containing HDL appears to be antiatherogenic. Other apoproteins on HDL are Apo-AII, Apo-C and Apo-E. Nascent (precursor) HDL is synthesised by intestine and liver and contains mainly Apo-AI and phospholipids. Nascent HDL acquires much of its lipid contents from the surface monolayers of CM and VLDL when they undergo lipolysis. HDL also acquires free CH from peripheral tissues including arterial wall foam cells. A cholesterol transporter protein called ATP-binding cassette protein-1 (ABC-1) facilitates this important first step in "reverse cholesterol transport". The acquired free CH is then esterified by the circulating enzyme lecithin-cholesterol acyltransferase (LCAT) and the CE then moves into the core of HDL. Apo-CI in HDL activates LCAT and thus facilitates esterification of free CH. The CE of HDL is then transferred to VLDL, LDL, IDL and CMR with the help of cholesteryl ester transfer protein (CETP).

Much of CE, so transferred from HDL, is ultimately delivered by the recipient lipoproteins to liver by endocytosis via LDL receptor or Apo-R. HDL mediated "reverse cholesterol transport" from arterial wall foam cells to liver is thought to be primary mechanism by which HDL protects from atheroselerosis. In addition, HDL also protects LDL from oxidative processes (by enhancing antioxidant enzyme activity). Low levels of HDL cholesterol and Apo-AI are associated with consequential elevations of Apo-B100 containing LPs [including LP(a)] which deliver CE to the vessel wall, and increase the risk for atherosclerosis.

LIPOPROTEIN DISORDERS

As discussed earlier, the excess LPs in plasma are phagocytosed by macrophages for disposal. When too much of LPs have to be degraded in this manner, CH gets deposited in arterial walls as atheromas and in skin and tendons as xanthomas. Elevated TG levels are associated with pancreatitis. Since TGs are mainly carried in VLDL, an increase in TGs is manifested as increased VLDL levels. Similarly, CH is mainly carried by VLDL and LDL, therefore increased CH levels are exhibited by an increased VLDL and LDL levels.

Hyperlipoproteinaemias can be classified as:

A) ***Primary Hyperlipoproteinaemias***: (i) these can be familial or genetic due to single gene defect, OR (ii) can be multifactorial or polygenic which have multiple genetic, envirnonmental, dietary and physical activity related causes.

B) ***Secondary Hyperlipoproteinaemias***: These hyperlipoproteinaemias are associated with some disease, e.g., diabetes, myxoedema, nephrotic syndrome, chronic alcoholism or drugs like oral contraceptives & β-blockers, etc.

Important features of the major types of hyperlipoproteinaemias and drugs used for their treatment are summarised in Table 23.2. The desirable plasma lipid levels for treatment guidelines as per National Cholesterol Education Program (2004) are provided in Table 23.3.

PHARMACOTHERAPY OF HYPERLIPIDAEMIAS/DYSLIPIDAEMIAS

Lifestyle changes are the first step for decreasing the risk for atherosclerosis and consist of healthy diet (low fat + high roughage), weight control, increased physical activity and smoking cessation. Successful lifestyle changes including dietary therapy can reduce total CH by 25% depending on the compliance and the metabolic basis of dyslipidaemia. When these measures fail to meet the desired goals, drugs therapy should be initiated. Clinical guidelines recommend the drug therapy to be started along with lifestyle changes in patients with ASCVD or in patients having LDL greater than 130 mg/dL (currently > 100 mg/dL).

The Pharmacotherapy of dyslipidaemias can be divided into following two categories which utilize different classes of drugs.

I. ***Therapies that Target Atherogenic Lipoproteins***

II. ***Therapies that Target High Density Lipoprotein (HDL)***

I. *Therapies that Target Atherogenic Lipoproteins*

(A) **Well-established Anti-dyslipidaemic Therapies**

1) **HMG-CoA Reductase Inhibitors (Statins)**: Atorvastatin, Simvastatin, Lovastatin, Pravastatin, Fluvastatin, Rosuvastatin, Pitavastatin
2) **Bile Acid-Binding Resins**: Cholestyramine, Colestipol, Colesevelam
3) **Inhibitors of Intestinal Absorption of Cholesterol**: Ezetimibe, Stanol Esters
4) **Lipoprotein Lipase (LPL) Activators (Fibrates)**: Gemfibrozil, Bezafibrate, Fenofibrate, Ciprofibrate
5) **Inhibitor of Lipolysis and VLDL Secretion from Adipose Tissue**: Niacin (Nicotinic acid)

(B) **Newly Developed Anti-dyslipidaemic Therapies**

6) **Proprotein Convertase Subtilisin/Kexin Type 9 (PCSK9) Inhibitors**: Alirocumab, Evolocumab
7) **Inhibitor of Apolipoprotein B Synthesis**: Mipomersen

8) **Microsomal Triglyceride Transfer Protein (MTP) Inhibitor**: Lomitapide
9) **Apolipoprotein C-III Synthesis Inhibitor**: Volanesorsen
10) **Miscellaneous Agents**: Gugulipid and fish oil derivatives.

II. ***Therapies that Target High Density Lipoprotein (HDL)***

1. **Cholesteryl Ester Transfer Protein (CETP) Inhibitors**: Dalcetrapib, Torcetrapib, Evacetrapib, Anacetrapib.

Pharmacotherapy of Dyslipidaemias: An Overview

Atherogenic lipoproteins include CH-rich LDLs and the catabolic remnants of TG-rich lipoproteins such as VLDL and IDL. Isolated or combined increase of any of these when accompanies with a decrease in HDL particles leads to different manifestion of primary or secondary dyslipidaemias or hypercholestrolaemias (Table 23.2) and constitute the leading cause of ASCVDs.

Various classes of lipid lowering agents (as classified above) are usually recommended for the treatment of dyslipidaemic ASCVDs. Each one of them act by targetting different intracellular or cells surface proteins or molecules that predominantly lower LDL-C and to a varied extent increase HDL-C or both. These are described in following discusstion.

It is important to note that *first five classes of these agents in the Category I (A) of drugs belong to **well-established antidyslipidiaemic therapies***, which have comparatively well-defined actions and effects and have proven their clinical potential. But still in some patients could not fulfil the desired lipid-lowering goals, especially in those having homo- and heterozygous FH which are difficult to treat, particularly the former. Intensive research in the area has identified and developed some new drugs which have provided hopes for the treatment of such difficult-to-treat cases of dislipidaemia and has been described as ***newly developed anti-dyslipidaemic therapies*** *(Category I [B] drugs)*.

I. ***Therapies that Target Atherogenic Lipoproteins***

(A) **Well-established Anti-dyslipidaemic Therapies**

1. HMG-COA REDUCTASE INHIBITORS (STATINS)

These antihyperlipidaemic agents competitively inhibit the HMG-CoA reductase enzyme (which converts HMG-CoA to mevalonic acid) and therefore deplete the intracellular supply of CH by inhibiting its biosynthesis (Fig. 23.2). To compensate for decreased CH biosynthesis, the liver now responds by increasing the uptake of plasma LDL by increasing the number of LDL receptors (upregulation). Thus, the desired and the beneficial reduction in the plasma LDL levels is achieved. Low intracelluar levels of CH also decreases secretion of VLDL, and because IDL, the CH rich VLDL remnants are also taken up by LDL receptors, statins also produce a moderate lowering of TGs level (30%). However, HDL-C is only slightly increased (5–10%). Basically, statins are the most powerful drugs which cause dose-related reduction in LDL levels ranging from 20–60%. *Lipoprotein(a) levels are not altered by the available statins.*

Unfortunately, treatment with statins has some limitations. After prolonged use even increased doses of statins give diminishing results. For example, after prolonged use, there is only 6% additional decrease in LDL levels even after doubling their dose. Thus, despite treatment, a significant proportion of patients do not achieve their target lipid goals. The observed ceiling-dose effect after continued use of statins occurs due to "feedback compensatory induction" of HMG-CoA reductase enzyme which now tends to increase CH biosynthesis. This autoregulatory increase in CH biosynthesis due to feedback induction of HMG-CoA reductase favours rather down-regulation of LDL receptors after sometime.

Different statins differ in their potency. On a mg-for-mg basis the potency order for reduction in LDL-C is: *Pitavastatin* > *Rosuvastatin* > *Atorvastatin* > *Simvastatin* = *Lovastatin* >

Table 23.2 Types of Hyperlipoproteinaemias and their Drug Treatment

Type*	Elevation in lipoprotein	Elevation in lipids		Risk of atherosclerosis	Drug treatment
		TG	CH		
I	CM	+++	+/N	No	None
IIa	LDL	N	++	High	Statins ± Anti PCSK9 Mab/± Lomitapide/ ± Mipomersen; Resins ±; Ezetimibe
IIb	VLDL and LDL	++	++	High	Statins ± Anti PCSK9 Mab/± Lomitapide/ ± Mipomersen; Fibrates; Niacin; Ezetimibe
III	Remnants of VLDL and CM	++	++	Moderate	Fibrates; Niacin
IV	VLDL	+++	+/N	Moderate	Fibrates; Niacin
V	VLDL and CM	++	+/N	No	None; Niacin if needed

Key: CM—Chylomicron; CH—Cholesterol; TG—Triglycerides

* ***Type I*: Familial Hyperchylomicronaemia**. Absence of Lipoprotein lipase (LPL). TG in CM, therefore, cannot be utilised.

***Type IIa*: Familial Hypercholesterolaemia**. Deficiency of LDL receptors. LDL and IDL are taken up very slowly by liver and extrahepatic tissues.

***Type IIb*: Familial Combined (Polygenic) Hyperlipidaemia**. Similar to IIa except VLDL is also increased. Hence increased CH as well as TG. Caused by deficiency of LDL receptors as well as overproduction of VLDL by liver.

***Type III*: Familial Dysbetalipoproteinaemia**. Overproduction or under-utilisation of IDL due to mutant Apo-E (same with CM remnants); hence a rise in TG as well as CH levels.

***Type IV*: Familial Hypertriglyceridaemia**. Over production and/or decreased removal of VLDL resulting into raised TG levels and mildly raised normal CH levels. Patients with this disorder are more common and are frequently obese, diabetic, hyperuricaemic and/or with ischaemic heart disease. Most of them are alcoholic. LDL levels are normal.

***Type V*: Familial Combined Hypertriglyceridaemia**. Increased production or decreased clearance of VLDL and CM; usually a rare genetic defect; resulting into raised TG with mildly raised or normal CH level. LDL is normal.

Pravastatin > *Fluvastatin*. Serum triglyceride reduction by statins occurs in a rank order of: *Atorvastatin* > *Pravastatin* > *Rosuvastatin* = *Simvastatin* > *Lovastatin* > *Fluvastatin*. Serum HDL-C increase by statins takes place in a rank order of: *Pravastatin* >*Simvastatin* > *Rosuvastatin* = *Lovastatin* = *Fluvastatin* > *Atorvastatin*. Plasma half lives of these drugs range from 1 hr to 3 hrs, except for *atorvastatin* and *rosuvastatin* which have long half- lives of 14 hrs and 19 hrs, respectively. Because CH biosynthesis takes place predominantly at night, HMG-CoA reductase inhibitors—atorvastatin and rosuvastatin having long half life can be taken anytime of the day if a single daily dose is

Table 23.3 Optimal Plasma Lipid Levels for Treatment Guidelines as per US National Cholesterol Education Program (NCEP, 2001) 2004: Revision of Adult Treatment Panel (ATP)-III

Plasma lipids	Desirable	Border-line	High
Total CH	< 200 mg/dL	200–239 mg/dL	>240 mg/dL
LDL-C	<130 mg/dL*	130–159 mg/dL	>160 mg/dL
HDL-C	> 40 mg/dL for men >50 mg/dL for women		>60 mg/dL for both
TGs	<150 mg/dL	150–199 mg/dL	>200 mg/dL

Key: CH—Cholesterol; LDL-C—LDL-Cholesterol; HDL-C—HDL-Cholesterol; TG—Triglycerides.
*Current trend is to keep its levels below 100 mg/dL in high risk and below 70 mg/dL in very high risk patients

taken; all the rest drugs should be taken in the evening: lovastatin with the evening meal to facilitate its absorption, whereas other drugs can be taken without any regard to meal. The usual starting dose (mg/day) for various statins is: ***pitavastatin*** (2 mg, never use more than 4 mg/day), ***atorvastatin*** (10 mg), ***rosuvastatin*** (in Asians 5 mg; others 10 mg), ***lovastatin*** (20 mg), ***simvastatin*** (20–40 mg), ***pravastatin*** (20–40 mg) and ***fluvastatin*** (40 mg).

With the possible exception of pravastatin, pitavastatin, rosuvastatin and atorvastatin—which also lower TGs levels significantly—the statins are generally used to lower LDL-C in familial or multifactorial hypercholesterolaemia (type IIa) or combined FH (type IIb). Recent studies also suggest that use of statins may lower the risk of stroke, dementia and Alzheimer's disease, may improve bone density in postmenopausal women and even prevent prostate cancer. These broad actions may be related to their pleiotropic effects which are unrelated to their lipid lowering actions. Some of these actions include: (1) improved endothelial function, (2) reduced vascular inflammation, (3) antithrombotic action, (4) enhanced fibrinolysis, (5) immune suppression, (6) reduced platelet aggregation, and (7) stabilisation of atherosclerotic plaque. ***Adverse Effects***. The statins are usually well tolerated. Muscle pain and liver dysfunction can be seen in 1 to 2% of patients. Another relatively common side effect (1–2% of cases) is myositis, i.e., inflammation of skeletal muscle accompanied by pain, weakness with elevated serum creatine kinase levels. If the drug is not discontinued, rhabdomyolysis, i.e., disintegration of muscle with myoglobinuria and resultant renal shutdown may be a rare but extreme toxic outcome. Why statins should cause myopathy in not clear. By inhibiting CH synthesis, statins probably alter muscle cell composition and their electrial properties. Lovastatin and simvastatin cross blood-brain barrier and can cause sleep disturbances. Other drugs do not.

Drug Interactions. The risk of muscle damage is said to increase when statins are simultaneously used along with fibrate (gemfibrozil), niacin or cyclosporine. Fluvastatin is safest in this regard. Drugs like itraconazole, cyclosporine and erythromycin which inhibit CYP3A4 can vastly increase plasma levels of many statins (except fluvastatin and rosuvastatin) and thus increase the risk of their toxicity. Drugs that induce CYP3A4 system, such as phenytoin, on the other hand, can accelerate their metabolism and suppress their blood levels. Fluvastatin and rosuvastatin are metabolised by CYP2C9 system and therefore drugs such as ketoconazole, metronidazole and amiodarone which inhibit this enzyme system can increase their toxicity. Warfarin utilises this enzyme system for its own metabolism and hence warfarin toxicity may be increased if these drugs are used simultaneously. Unexpectedly, grape fruit juice inhibits intestinal degradation of statins and can result in 8–10-fold increase in the levels of lovastatin, simvastatin and atorvastatin. Pravastatin is neither metabolised by CYP3A4 nor by CYP2C9 but is metabolised by sulfate conjugation and therefore shows least drug interactions.

Contraindication: (1) Liver disease with persistently elevated serum transaminases;

(2) Pregnancy and during lactation because CH is essential for foetal development.

2. BILE ACID BINDING RESINS

The bile acids are synthesised in the liver, from CH and then secreted into the duodenum to aid absorption of dietary fat. These are then reabsorbed and returned to the liver through portal circulation (Fig. 23.2). Bile acid binding resins are nonabsorbable anion exchange resins that complex with negatively charged bile acids in the small intestine. The resin + bile acid complex is non-absorbable and gets excreted through the faeces, thus preventing the bile acids from returning to the liver by enterohepatic circulation. To make up for this loss (of bile acids), the biosynthesis of bile acids from CH increases, leading to partial depletion of hepatic CH pool. The intracellular CH depletion in the liver results in an up-regulation of LDL receptors and consequently LDL-C from the blood is cleared more rapidly with a fall in circulating levels of LDL. There is a small rise in the levels of HDL-C and TGs (because bile salts physiologically suppress hepatic TG production). However, on long- term use they not only ↑ TGs but also tend to induce HMG-CoA reductase in liver (due to ↓ in intrahepatic CH levels). This negates their desirable effects and makes them unsuitable as monotherapy.

Available bile acid binding resins are ***cholestyramine***, ***colestipol*** and ***colesevelam***. These are the drugs of choice for type IIa, i.e., familial hypercholesterolaemia. If used to treat type IIb, i.e., familial combined hyperlipidaemia (where VLDL is already raised, Table 23.2), they may be used along with niacin. Other uses include relieving of pruritius in patients surffering with cholestastis and bile salt accumulation. Because they bind to digitalis glycosides, these resins can also be used for digitalis toxicity. Cholestyramine and colestipol are available in granular form to be taken orally (16 g daily). The granular resin is mixed with water or juice and allowed to hydrate for 2 min and is taken with meals. Hence palatability of these drugs is a big problem. ***Colesevelam*** is a recent addition to this class of drugs. It is available as 625 mg tablet and is administered as 6 tablets per day. It has a better patient's compliance than other two drugs.

Adverse Effects: These include, constipation (which can be usually offset by increasing the fiber intake in diet), exacerbation of pre-existing haemorrhoids and GIT distress.

Drug Interactions: Absorption of fat-soluble vitamins and of folic acid can be impaired. Cholestyramine and colestipol bind to digoxin, tetracyline, statins and thiazide diuretics and hence an interval of 3–4 hrs is necessary between these drugs and resins. Colesevelam is devoid of such drug interactions.

3. INHIBITORS OF INTESTINAL ABSORPTION OF CHOLESTEROL

Cholesterol in the intestine reaches both from the diet and secretion through bile. ***Ezetimibe*** not only inhibits the intestinal absorption of CH but also inhibits enterohepatic reabsorption of CH excreted in the bile. The net loss of CH, in turn, accelerates the uptake of LDL from the plasma *via* LDL receptors.

Ezetimibe acts by inhibiting Niemann-Pick C1 like 1 (NPC1L1) protein, an intestinal brush border transporter involved in the absorption of CH. *Ezetimibe* reduces total CH, LDL-C, (20%), TGs (8%) and Apo-B while increases HDL-C (3%). It can be given orally (10 mg/day OD; t½ 22 hrs) as a monotherapy or in combination with statins to treat type IIa (FH) and type IIb (combined FH) (Table 23.2).

The combined therapy of ezetimibe with a statin is more effective. It is because when the intestinal CH absorption is reduced by ezetimibe, a derease in the hepatic CH content occurs to which liver respond by a compensatory increase in the synthesis of CH that partially offsets the lipid-lowering benefit of ezetimibe. By combining a statin with ezetimibe, this compensatory increase in hepatic CH synthesis is thus prevented. By this logic a *vice-versa* situation will also be true where a decreased synthesis by a statin in the liver may offset its lipid-lowering effect by a compensatory increase in the intestinal CH absorption. Combining ezetimibe with statin then would prevent this compensatory enhancement in CH absorption from the intestine.

Adverse drug effects are rare, except GIT discomfort. However, it should be avoided in patients with liver dysfunction. Ezetimibe can increase the plasma concentration of cyclosporine which should be monitored when the two drugs are given together.

Plant Stanol Esters (present in food products) are also used for inhibiting the absorption of lipids from the intestine. Plant Stanol Esters (present in margarine spread) are least absorbable, more safe and effective than ordinary plant sterols in decreasing CH absorption and serum LDL concentrations. The esterification of plant stanols with fatty acids, from vegetable oils, provides stanol esters and being soluble in dietary fats, these are incorporated into food products like margarine.

Plant Stanol and Esters are structurally similar to CH but are more hydrophobic. As a result these molecules displace CH from micelles and their by increase the excretion of CH in the faeces. The plant sterols and stanol are themselves poorly absorbed. Based on their mechanism gram quantities of these agents are required to reduced plasma LDL-C concentrations by 15%.

4. LIPOPROTEIN LIPASE (LPL) ACTIVATORS: PEROXISOME PROLIFERATOR-ACTIVATED RECEPTOR-ALPHA (PPAR-α) AGONISTS (FIBRATES)

Several structurally related fibrates are at present available for clinical use. These are ***gemfibrozil, ciprofibrate, fenofibrate*** and ***bezafibrate***. The fibrates activate a *nuclear receptor (transcription factor)* termed as *peroxisome proliferator activated receptor-α* (PPAR-α). This receptor belongs to steroid hormone receptor superfamily. Activation of PPAR-α leads to: (1) an increased expression of lipoprotein lipase (LPL) located in the vascular endothelium to catalyse enhanced hydrolysis and removal of TGs from VLDL (↓ TG levels), (2) a decreased expression of APO-CIII (a LPL inhibitor) to enhance LPL activity, and (3) an increased expression of APO-AI which facilitates the *reverse cholesterol transport* to HDL.

Fibrate drugs typically lower VLDL-TGs by >40% and increase plasma HDL-C by >10%. Additionally these agents have been demonstrated to lower plasma fibrinogen levels and to shift LDL to a larger, less dense phenotype which has considerably weak atherogenic potential.

Fibrates are well absorbed from GIT. Their absorption is enhanced when taken with food. Plasma half-life of gemfibrozil and bezafibrate is short, while that of fenofibrate is long (20 hrs).

The fibrates are the drugs of choice for treating hypertriglyceridaemias, particularly those associated with low levels of HDL-C. These are mainly used to treat two hyperlipidaemias—familial hypertriglyceridaemia (type IV) in order to prevent pancreatitis and dysbetalipoproteinaemia (type III). Type IIb hyperlipoproteinaemia, however, requires the use of niacin with fibrates to lower both LDL and VLDL. These drugs are also used for reducing the risk of ASCVD in patients who have a triad of increased LDL-C, low HDL-C and elevated TGs and whose lipidaemia has not responded to lifestyle changes or other pharmacological agents. However, the ability of fibrates to prevent ASCVD is uncertain. Most clinical trial have demonstrated that fibrates do not significantly lower the risk of fatal MI or total mortality. For this reason some experts suggest the use of niacin, rather than a fibrate, to control dyslipidaemia in patients who have not responded to other drugs.

Fenofibrate is uricosuric and is used where hyperuricaemia coexists with hyperlipidaemia. Usual doses are: ***Bezafibrate***: 200 mg BD or TDS orally or 400 mg once daily (extended- release formulation); ***fenofibrate***: 200 mg OD or 160 mg OD (improved bioavailability formulation); ***Gemfibrozil*** : 600 mg BD before meals.

Adverse effects. Include GIT distress, reversible myopathy and increase in blood levels of aminotransferases or alkaline phosphatase. The risk of myopathy increases when these are used with statins. Fibrates increase the risk for cholesterol gallstones.

Drug Interactions. Their use with statins require caution as the co-medication therapy may increase the risk of myositis and rhabdomyolysis. Fibrate drugs potentiate the action of coumarin anti-coagulants.

5. INHIBITORS OF LIPOLYSIS AND VLDL SECRETION FROM ADIPOSE TISSUE

Nicotinic acid (*Niacin*, but not niacinamide) has three special features as a hypolipidaemic drug: (a) it has several beneficial effects on serum lipoproteins: decreases VLDL, LDL and LP (a) and increases HDL-C, (b) it is inexpensive, and (c) it has numerous acute and chronic side effects.

When administered in pharmacological doses (1.5–3 g/day), niacin reduces the level of plasma TGs by 40%, VLDL by 35%, reduces LDL-C by 10–15%, and increases the HDL-C by upto 25%. Therefore, niacin is particularly useful in treating Type IIb and Type IV hyperlipoproteinemias in which both VLDL and LDL are elevated. Since it can both lower TGs and elevate HDL, it is useful in patients at increased risk for ASCVD, i.e., those having high plasma TGs with low HDL (in fact the only drug which can raise HDL-C that effectively).

The precise mechanism of these effects allthough remains uncertain. Recent studies have identified a G protein-coupled receptor on adipose cells that appears to be the target for niacin action Stimulation of this receptor by niacin decreases hormone-sensitive lipase activity in adipocyte, leading to reduced peripheral tissue TG catabolism which results in decreased flux of FFAs to the liver (Fig. 23.2). The liver normally utilises FFAs as a major sources for TGs synthesis, which are then utilised for VLDL production. LDL is derived from VLDL in the plasma. Therefore, a decrease in synthesis of TGs in liver leads to a reduction in plasma VLDL along with LDL concentration. Niacin is known to decrease the catabolism of APO-I and thus prolongs its t½ and thereby increases the concentration of plasma HDL. Niacin also boosts secretion of tissue plasminogen activator and lowers plasma fibrinogen and hence can reverse some of the endothelial dysfunction that contributes to thrombosis associated with hypercholesterolaemia. In addition, the drug shifts LDL particles to larger sizes which have lesser atherogenic potential. *It is also the only drug that significantly reduces LP(a) levels*. Used alone, niacin can decrease TG levels by 40%, LDL levels by 25% but increases HDL-C by 25–30%.

Adverse Effects. The major adverse effects of niacin are cutaneous "hot flushing" and pruritus (itching). The flushing is mediated by the G protein-coupled niacin receptor and involves the release of PGD_2 and PGE_2 within the skin. It can be reduced significantly by premedication with aspirin (81–325 mg/day) or laropiprant (20 mg), a potent, highly selective PGD_2 receptor (DP) blocker. A fixed-dose combined pill containing ***nicotinic acid*** (1.0 g) plus ***laropiprant*** (20 mg), is also available to mitigate hot flushing effect of niacin. These adverse effects usually disappear after several weeks of niacin. Extended-release formulations of niacin are associated with less hot flushing than the immediate-release dosage forms.

Other adverse effects observed with niacin include: hyperuricaemia impaired insulin sensitivity, hypatotoxicity, and the potentiation of statin-induced myopathy. Hyperuricaemia may precipitate gout. Impaired insulin sensitivity may prcipitate diabetes in susceptible patients and due to this reason niacin should be used with caution in diabetic patients.

(B) Newly Developed Anti-dyslipidaemic Therapies

6. PROPROTEIN CONVERTASE SUBTILISIN/ KEXIN TYPE 9 (PCSK9) INHIBITORS

PCSK9 is a physiological enzyme ligand of LDL-receptor (LDL-R) which when binds along with LDL-C to it, facilitates its lysosomal degradation inside the hepatocyte. This enzyme thus decreases the number of LDL-R on the surface of liver cells and consequently increases the plasma concentration of LDL-C and apoB. Some studies in humans revealed that when LDL-R degradation is reduced by genetic loss-of-function of PCSK9, the incidence of ASCVD is reduced by 88%.

The physiological mechanism that removes LDL particles from the plasma is via LDL-R located on the surface of hepatocytes. The circulating plasma LDLs bind to LDL-R to form complexes that are endocytosed into the liver cell. The lower intracellular pH dissociates LDLs from the LDL-R, leaving the receptor to recycle back to the cell surface. The dissociated LDL particles enter the lysosome where they are degraded. The CH that is released during LDL degradation is metabolized by the hepatic cell. It has been estimated that each LDL-R recycles between intracellular compartments and the cell surface about 150 times.

When an LDL particle interact with an LDL receptor to which PCSK9 is already bound, a complex consisting of PCSK9+ LDL-R + LDL particle is formed. This complex enters the cell, where PCSK9 prevents LDL from dissociating from the LDL-R and the entire complex (including the LDL-R) is directed towards lysosomes for degradation. This prevents the LDL-R from recycling back to the cell surface, thus reducing the number of cell surface LDL-R, decreasing the removal of LDLs from plasma, and consequently increasing the plasma concentration of LDL-C in long term.

This observation leads to a hypothesis that if PCSK9 is prevented from binding to LDL-R, it may result in an increased number of LDL-R on the liver cells and thereby more catabolism of LDL-C and its subsequent reduction in the plasma.

Two fully human **m**onoclonal **a**nti**b**odies (Mabs) that target the LDL-R interacting domain of PCSK9 for the treatment of patients with heterozygous FH or clinical ASCVD who require additional therapy beyond life-style control and maximal statin therapy. These include ***evolocumab*** and ***alirocumab***, which are administered by S.C. route and can lower LDL-C and apoB by 50-72% with a reduction in plasma PCSK9 activity upto 80%. These drugs have been well tolerated in short-term clinical trials and in post-marketing surveillance no major adverse effects were reported. Both drugs have been approved for clinical use in patients with hetero-(HeFH) and homozygous FH (HoFH) with or without ASCVD which as such are difficult to treat, especially the latter.

It is pertinent to mention that PCSK9 is also involved in the degradation of many receptor targets (e.g., LDL-R, apoE-R2, VLDL-R, and LRP1) that are also receptors for viruses, such as human rhinovirus and hepatitis C virus. This suggests that the incidence of viral infections needs to be monitored closely in patients who are being treated with PCSK9 inhibitors. ***Inclisiran*** is approved by the US-FDA for hyperlipidaemia. It inhibits the synthesis of PCSK9 within hepatocytes. It is given subcutaneously. It is used to treat heterozygous familial hypercholesterolaemia or clinical atherosclerotic cardiovascular disease as an add-on therapy. Adverse effects: Nausea, diarrhoea, allergy, injection site reaction and arthralgia.

7. INHIBITOR OF APOLIPOPROTEIN B SYNTHESIS: *MIPOMERSEN*

ApoB is the main protein component of all atherogenic lipoproteins. In its absence, VLDLs and their catabolic products, LDLs cannot be formed. Inhibition of apoB synthesis has the potential to reduce the concentration of apoB-containing lipoproteins in people with hetero- and homozygous FH who lack functional LDL-R and thus do not respond to agents such as statins and PCSK9 inhibitors that lower the level of apoB-containing lipoproteins by increasing the number of LDL receptors on the cell surface.

Mipomersen is an **a**nti**s**ense **o**ligonucleotide (ASO) that inhibits apoB-100 synthesis in the liver. In a small 28-week clinical trail a 200 mg once weekly dose of mipomersen administered S.C. has been observed to reduce apoB levels by 33–54%, LDL-C levels by 34%–52%, and Lp(a) levels by 24%. The noted adverse effects with the agent included severe injection site reactions (72–97%), flu-like reactions (25–29%), headache in 15–31%, and liver enzyme elevation in 3–17% of subjects.

Mipomersen has been approved for the treatment of homozygous FH with restrictions (as applicable to lomitapide also, see below) as the drug will only be available through the restricted Kynamro (brand name of the drug) **R**isk **E**valuation and **M**itigation **S**trategy (REMS) program because of the risk of hepatotoxicity. Under the program, only certified health care providers can prescribe the drug, and only certified pharmacies may dispense the medicine.

8. MICROSOMAL TRIGLYCERIDE TRANSFER PROTEIN INHIBITOR: *LOMITAPIDE*

Microsomal **T**riglyceride Transfer **P**rotein (MTP) is the protein responsible for transferring TG to apoB in the liver and intestine to form apoB-containing lipoproteins (VLDL, LDL). MTP inhibition has the potential to reduce the concentration of apoB-containing lipoproteins in people with HoFH who lack functional LDL receptors and thus do not respond to agents such as statins and PCSK9 inhibitors.

Lomitapide is a small molecule that on binding to MTP, inhibits it from transfering the lipids to apoB. As a consequence apo B is destroyed and lipoproteins secretion is inhibited. The drug has been approved for oral treatment of people with homozygous HoFH. In a small 78-week study treatment with lomitapide in such patients was observed to reduce the concentration LDL-C by 42–50% at week 26. The common ADRs observed with the drug were GIT symptoms (which included diarrhea, nausea, vomiting, dyspepsia, and abdominal pain), elevation of liver transaminases, and an increase in liver fat.

The drug has been advised to start with a low dose of 5 mg daily initially and gradually escalating to doses of 10,20,40, upto 60 mg, based on tolerability and acceptable liver enzyme levels.

Lomitapide has been approved with restrictions (as applicable to mipomersen also, see above) as the drug will only be available through the restricted Juxtapid (brand name of the drug) **R**isk **E**valuation and **M**itigation **S**trategy (REMS) program because of the risk of hepatotoxicity. Under the program, only certified health care providers can prescribe the drug, and only certified pharmacies may dispense the medicine.

9. APOLIPOPROTEIN C-III SYNTHESIS INHIBITORS: *VOLANESORSEN*

Apolipoprotein C-III (ApoC-III) is a pro-inflammatory protein which is synthesized mainly in the liver and circulates in plasma as a component of all lipoprotein particles. It inhibits LPL which reduces the lipolysis of TG-rich lipoproteins and increases the concentration of plasma TG. It also inhibits hepatic lipase and thus reduces the catabolism and hapatic uptake of atherogenic TG-rich lipoprotein remnants.

Fibrates are also known to reduce the concentration of apoC-III, an effect that may contribute to the ability of these agents to reduce ASCVD events in people with hypertriglyceridaemia.

A more targeted approach to reduced plasma levels of apoC-III has been provided by the development of **Volanesorsen**, an **a**ntisense **o**ligonucleatide (ASO) of apoC-III synthesis. When people with severe hypertriglyceridaemia, including those with a deficiency of LPL, are treated with this inhibitor, the resulting decrease in plasma level of apoC-III is accompanied by a major reduction in plasma TG levels and a substantial increase in concentration of HDL-C.

The long term effects of inhibiting apoC-III synthesis on patients with ASCVD risk remain to be established.

10. MISCELLANEOUS AGENTS: GUGULIPID AND FISH OIL DERIVATIVES

1. **Gugulipid**: It is a drug devloped at Central Drug Research Institute, Lucknow (India). It consists of Z and E guggul sterones isolated from "guggul gum". The oral administration of guggul gum exerts hypolipidaemic effects by inhibition of CH biosynthesis and also by enhancing the rate of excretion of CH. Dosage recommended is 25 mg tablet three times a day. There is reduction of total CH, LDL-C with an elevation of HDL-C. Modest lowering of TGs also occurs after continued use. It is well tolerated. Loose stools are the only side effect. It has no teratogenic or carcinogenic effects.

2. **Fish Oil Derivatives (Omega-3 Fatty Acids)**: Fish oil contains **p**oly**u**nsaturated **f**atty **a**cids (PUFAs) namely **e**icosa **p**enta-enoic **a**cid (EPA) and **d**ocosa **h**exa-enoic **a**cid (DHA). These are used as prophylaxis in high-risk patients of coronary artery disease with hyperlipidaemia because of their membrane stabilising and antioxidant action. These are usually formulated with vitamin E. EPA is also available as ethyl easter of the acid or ***Icosapent ethyl*** as oral dosage form of 1 g capsule.

COMBINATION DRUG THERAPY

The combination of two lipid-lowering drugs is very useful in the treatment of severe hyperlipoproteinaemia, particularly with homo- and heterozygous FH (type IIa) in whom single drug therapy often fails to achieve satisfactory plasma levels of LDL-C. The commonly used drug combinations are as follows:

1. BILE ACID BINDING RESIN plus a FIBRATE: Recommended for familial combined hyperlipidaemia (type IIb). There is, however, increased risk of cholelethiasis.
2. BILE ACID BINDING RESIN plus NIACIN: Effective in familial hypercholesterolaemia (type IIa) and also in familial combined hyperlipidaemia (type IIb). The resin has acid neutralising action also, which reduces gastric irritation caused by niacin.
3. STATIN plus BILE ACID BINDING RESIN: Highly effective in reducing LDL-C in patients of FH (type IIa). Statins should be given either one hour before or four hours after the resin to ensure proper absorption.
4. BILE ACID BINDING RESIN plus NIACIN plus STATIN: Specially useful in patients with severe disorders due to elevated LDL (type IIa and IIb).
5. NIACIN plus STATIN: An efficacious combination for familial combined hyperlipidaemia (type IIb) and familial hypercholesterolaemia (type IIa) and for those having ↑ LDL and ↓ HDL.
6. STATINS plus EZETIMIBE: Synergistic combination for treating primary hypercholesterolaemia and can also be used for the treatment of individuals with homozygous FH (type IIa), who are high absorbers and low synthesisers of CH.
7. STATIN plus a FIBRATE: for high-risk patients on statin therapy who have elevated TG level as their primary lipid abnormality. However, patients treated with this combination, must be carefully watched for myopathy (up to 2% incidence). Nevertheless, the judicious and careful use of this combination has conferred more benefits than harm.
8. STATIN plus a ANTI-PCSK9 Mab (alirocumab or evolocumab): Synergistic combination for treating primary hypercholesterolaemia and can also be used for the treatment of individuals with homozygous FH (type IIa), who are high absorbers and low synthesisers of CH.

II. *Therapies that Target High Density Lipoprotein (HDL)*

The concentration of HDL-C is a powerful inverse predictor of the risk of having an ASCVD event. Increasing the concentration of HDL in plasma with HDL infusions, or by overexpressing apoA-I, reduces atherosclerosis in mice and rabbits. In a proof-of-concept study in humans, infusion of a preparation of **r**econstituted **h**igh-**d**ensity **l**ipoproteins (rHDLs) reduced coronary atheroma burden as assessed by intravascular ultrasonography. HDLs also have several potentially cardioprotective properties that include:

1. facilitation of efflux of cholesterol from macrophages and inhibition of vascular inflammation,
2. antioxidant and antithrombotic effects,
3. Increase in the synthesis in, and secretion of insulin from the pancreatic β cells, and an improvement in insulin sensitivity,
4. enhancement of endothelial function, and
5. promotion angiogenesis.

It is important to understand that the cholesterol transported in HDLs does not protect against ASCVD. Rather, if HDLs do protect, it is probably a consequence of one or more of the functions of

HDLs. It is possible that in some disease states, and after treatement with some HDL-raising agents, HDLs may be dysfunctional, in which case the concentration of HDL-C may no longer be a marker of HDL function. Only long term studies with already developed and yet to be developed HDL raising drugs will provide the proof of this concept.

Some of the drugs which belongs to this category are described in the following discussion.

1. CHOLESTERYL ESTER TRANSFER PROTEIN (CETP) INHIBITORS: DALCETRAPIB, TORCETRAPIB, EVACETRAPIB, ANACETRAPIB

Cholesteryl **E**ster **T**ransfer **P**rotein (CETP) is a glycoprotein that is synthesized in the liver and on secretion in the plasma promotes bidirectional transfers of both CE and TG between all plasma lipoprotein particles in processes that result in the equilibration of these lipids between different lipoprotein fractions (Fig 23.2). Since most of the CEs in plasma are formed by **l**ecithin–**c**holesterol **a**cyl**t**ransferase (LCAT) in a reaction that takes place primarily in HDLs, and most TG enters plasma as a component of VLDLs or chylomicrons, the effect of the equilibration facilitated by CETP is a net mass transfer of CE from the HDL fraction to the potentially proatherogenic non-HDL lipoproteins and a net mass transfer of TG from TG-rich VLDLs and chylomicrons into the HDL and LDL fractions. This equilibration process of lipids ultimately would result in a net increase in the plasma concentration of HDL-C.

The idea that CETP could be a target for antihyperlipidaemic therapy came from the observations that rodents lack CETP and are naturally resistant to the development of atherosclerosis. In contrast to rodents, rabbits like humans have a high level of CETP activity and both species are extremely susceptible to the development of diet-induced atherosclerosis. Inhibiting CETP in rabbits with a CETP ASO or by administration of the small molecule CETP inhibitors (dalcetrapib, torcetrapib) was observed to reduce the development atherosclerosis.

Encouraged by these observations, since the year 2000, several CETP inhibitors **dalcetrapib**, **torcetrapib**, **evacetrapib**, **anacetrapib** were synthesized and put to clinical trial in 2007. Among them, ***anacetrapib*** provided encouraging results by increasing HDL-C by 129% with a statin-like decrease in LDL-C, suggesting that CETP inhibition can be a potential target for raising HDL-C and decreasing the incidence of ASCVD risk. After niacin, CETP inhibitors were the agents which exclusively produced such a large increment in the HDL-C.

However, clinical trials with other three CETP inhibitors although did produce a desired increase in HDL-C, did not reduce ASCVD events, rather trocetrapib was observed to cause harm by increasing the BP and other vascular damaging effects. It was suggested that the latter are not the class effect of CETP inhibitor trocetrapib but the drug specific off-target effects develped due to endothelial dysfunction and increased synthesis of aldosterone initiated by the agent. The above clinical trial results have clouded the hope of developing CETP inhibitors to successful antihyperlipidaemic agents.

A currently undergoing clinical trial involving 30,000 people with another CETP inhibitor ***anacetrapib*** [**R**andomized **Ev**aluation of the **E**ffects of **A**nacetrapib through **L**ipid Modification (REVEAL; clinical Trial. Gov. NCT01252953)] has upto now shown very encouraging results.

TRIPHOSPHATE-CITRATE LYASE (ACL) INHIBITOR

Bempedoic acid

Bempedoic acid is approved drug by the US-FDA for hyperlipidaemia. It inhibits adenosine triphosphate-citrate lyase (ACL) and cholesterol biosynthesis. ACL is an enzyme upstream of HMG-CoA reductase in the cholesterol biosynthesis pathway. Hence, ACL inhibitor lowers LDL-C by inhibiting cholesterol synthesis in the liver. It is used to treat adults with heterozygous familial hypercholesterolaemia or established atherosclerotic cardiovascular disease who require additional lowering of LDL-C level. Adverse effects: Abdominal pain, muscle spasm, hyperuricaemia, elevated liver enzymes and upper respiratory tract infection.

CHAPTER 24

SECTION 5—DRUG THERAPY OF INFLAMMATION & RELATED AUTACOIDS

Histamine, Serotonin, Ergot Alkaloids & Bradykinin

COMPETENCY PH1.16

Like other endogenous peptides (Ch. 17 and 18) and eicosanoids (Ch. 25), histamine, serotonin and bradykinin are also categorised as autacoids or local hormones (autos = self; akos = remedy). Autacoids are produced by the tissues or endothelial cells which, after being released locally, act at the site or near the site of their release. Histamine, serotonin or bradykinin, hardly have any therapeutic application but their agonists and antagonists do have some clinical utility and, hence, their basic and clinical pharmacology has been discussed in this chapter.

HISTAMINE

Histamine is a naturally occurring imidazole derivative. It is widely distributed in skin, GIT mucosa, lungs, brain, cerebrospinal fluid and bone marrow. It is also a component of some venoms and sting secretion.

Biosynthesis, Storage, Release and Metabolism

Histamine is formed by decarboxylation of the amino acid L-histidine. This reaction is catalysed by the enzyme histidine decarboxylase (Fig. 24.1). Histidine decarboxylase enzyme has a very wide distribution, e.g., in most of the tissues, mast cells, GIT mucosa and in certain actively growing tumours. Activators of histidine decarboxylase enzyme are gastrin, nicotine, stress or even infection. Its selective inhibitor is *α-fluoromethyl histidine* which is used only as a research tool.

Mast cells are the predominant site of storage for histamine in most of the tissues. In these mast cells histamine is held in intracellular granules complexed with an acidic protein and heparin of high molecular weight (macroheparin). In blood, histamine is stored in basophils which resemble mast cells only morphologically, but are of haemopoietic origin. The non-mast cell histamine is stored in histaminocytes in the stomach and in histaminergic neurons in the brain. Replenishment of histamine contents of mast cells or basophils, after its secretion, is a slow process which may take even weeks; whereas turnover of histamine in gastric histaminocytes (non-mast cells) is very rapid because many substances (see above) can activate histidine decarboxylase enzyme in the non-mast cell tissues to form more histamine. The newly formed histamine, therefore, is continuously released rather than stored.

The stores of histamine from the mast cells can be released by any of the following mechanisms:

a) **Immunologic Release**: Initial exposure to allergen (A in Fig. 24.2) leads to the production of IgE antibodies which then bind to their respective IgE specific receptors present on tissue mast cells or blood basophils. Re-exposure to allergen leads to cross-linking of mast cell membrane bound IgE (i.e., one antigen attatches to two IgE antibodies on the surface of the mast cell). This union causes degranulation of cytoplasmic granules and release of histamine with other allergic mediators (Fig. 24.2). This type of release requires energy and Ca^{2+}. Histamine released by this mechanism is a mediator in immediate (type I) allergy.
b) **Chemical and Mechanical Release**: Chemical or mechanical mast cell injury causes degranulation of mast cell and histamine release. Certain drugs like morphine, succinylcholine, d-tubocurarine and radiocontrast media directly replace histamine from heparin-protein complex, within the mast cells, by a non-receptor action. After exocytosis, the histamine-heparin-protein complex is exposed to extracellular cations (Na^+ or Ca^{2+}) where histamine is displaced

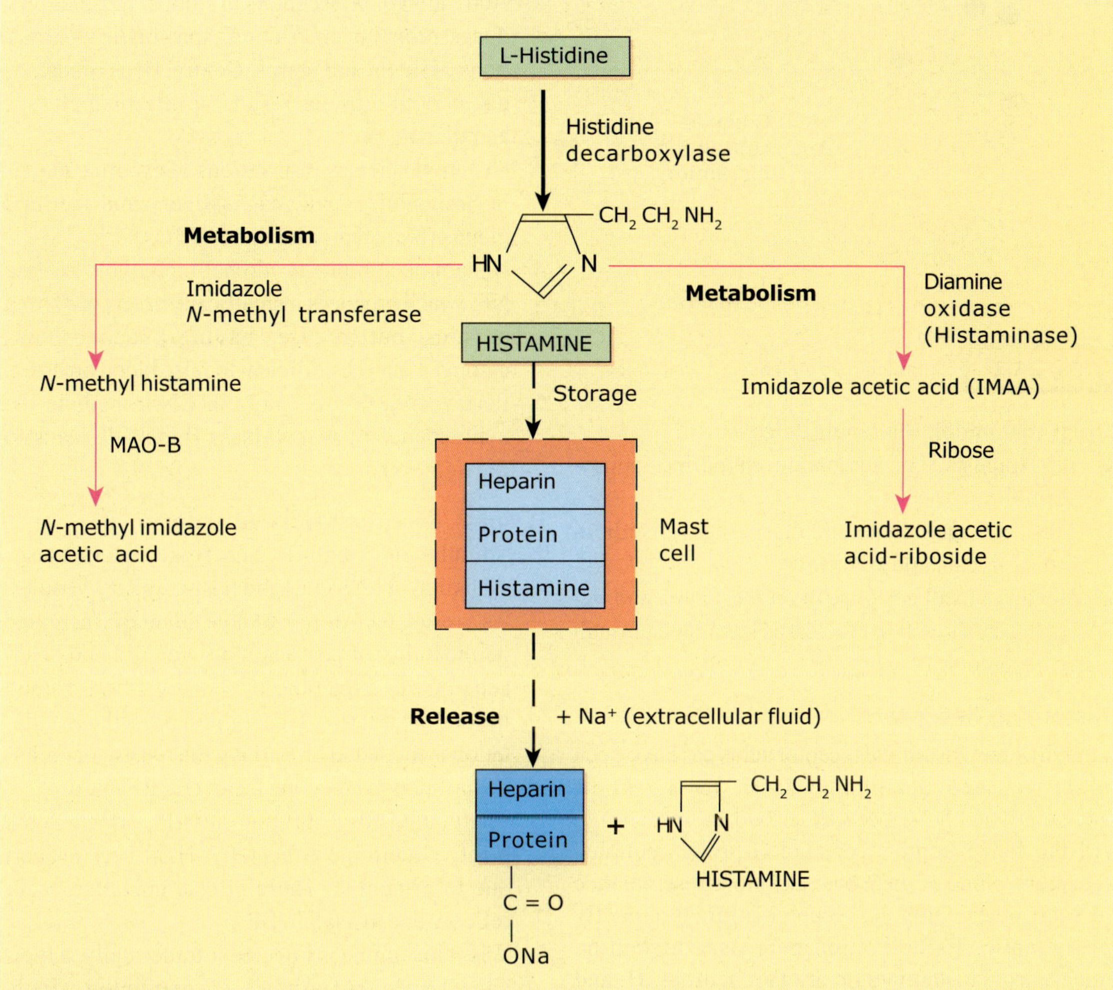

Fig 24.1 Biosynthesis (black arrows), Storage, Release (broken arrows) and Metabolism (magenta arrows) of Histamine.

and released after cationic exchange with Na^+ or Ca^{2+} (Fig. 24.1). Histamine is only one of the several potent physiological mediators that are released from the mast cells; other substances such as serotonin and leukotrienes also contribute to the overall hypersensitivity reaction and anaphylactic shock.

Histamine is metabolised by *histaminase* to imidazole acetic acid (IMAA) and by *N*-methylating enzyme *imidazole-N- methyltransferase* (followed by MAO-B) to *N*-methylimidazole acetic acid (Fig. 24.1). IMAA is then excreted in urine as an amino acid conjugate.

Drugs or Chemicals that Liberate Histamine

- Morphine, d-tubocurarine, trimethaphan, polymyxin-B, succinyl choline, hydralazine, dextran, polyvinyl pyrolidone (PVP), detergents, substance P, bradykinin, radiocontrast media and compound 48/80.
- Heat, cold, exposure to sunlight and X-rays.
- Proteolytic enzymes—trypsin and chymotrypsin
- Venoms

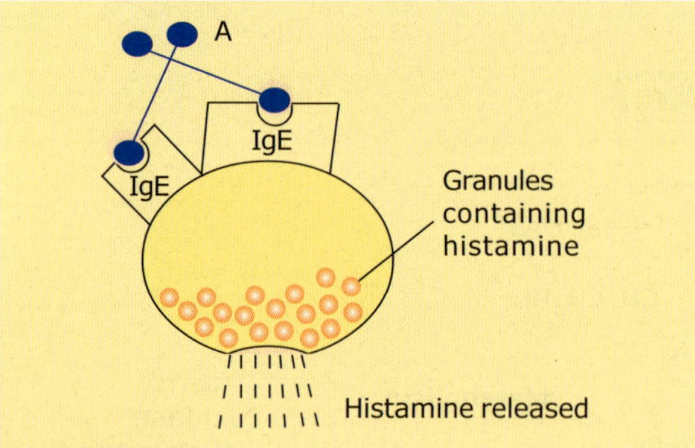

Fig 24.2 Immunologic Release of Histamine

Drugs that Inhibit Histamine Release

- β_2 - Agonists, e.g., adrenaline, ephedrine, isoproterenol
- Mast cell membrane stabilisers, e.g., disodium cromoglycate and ketotifen.
- Negative feedback control on mast cells and basophils by the action of released histamine through H_2 receptors.

Histamine Receptors

Four different histamine receptor subtypes have been identified and designated as H_1 to H_4. Their characteristics have been described in Table 24.1. All the four receptor types are G-protein coupled receptors. None of them bear any close resemblance to each other. Only H_3 receptor is predominantly presynaptic. Its activation decreases histamine release from histaminergic or other neurons. H_1 and H_2 receptors are postsynaptic and are located on cell membrane of neuro-effector junction (NEJ). H_4 receptors are located on blood cells such as eosinophils, neutrophils and CD4 -T cells. They may modulate production of these cell types or may play a role in chemotaxis of white blood cell. Till date only the H_1 and H_2 receptor agonists or antagonists have been the targets of drug research.

Pharmacological Actions of Histamine

H_1 Receptor Mediated Actions

1. Histamine is a powerful stimulant of sensory nerve endings mediating pain and itching. This H_1 mediated effect is an important component of urticarial response to insect bites and stings.
2. Activation of H_1 receptors in smooth muscles produces bronchoconstriction, spasmodic contractions of ileum and uterus. Contractions of intestinal smooth muscles results in intestinal cramps and diarrhoea.
3. Histamine increases secretions of exocrine glands in bronchioles, pancreas, salivary and lacrimal glands (H_1 receptor mediated effect).
4. Histamine stimulates adrenal medulla to release NE, which produces insignificant effects in normal persons; but in cases having phaeochromocytoma it may be sufficient to raise blood pressure.
5. Postsynaptic H_1 receptors in CNS, mediate the maintenance of wakefulness (blockade leads to drowsiness).

H_1 and H_2 Receptor Mediated Actions

1. Stimulation of both H_1 and H_2 receptors causes dilatation of arterioles and post-capillary venules. As a result, there is remarkable fall in BP, increased permeability of post-capillary venules and headache due to stretching of sensory fibers around the cranial arteries. Histamine-induced vasodilatation is mediated, in part, by the release of endothelium-derived relaxing factor (EDRF; NO).
2. There is positive chronotropic (H_2 effect) and a positive inotropic effect ($H_1 + H_2$ effect) on heart due to histamine. These effects may also occur reflexly due to a fall in BP.
3. When histamine is injected intradermally, a typical "triple response" is produced. It is characterised by an immediate reddening of the skin (FLUSH), formation of oedematous patch (WHEAL) and a red irregular halo surrounding the wheal (FLARE). *Flush* results due to dilatation of small vessels and capillaries, *wheal* due to increased permeability of the post-capillary venules while *flare* is a consequence of axon reflex causing vasodilatation through the release of vasodilatory neuromediator (local concentration of histamine can depolarise efferent axonal nerve ending). Earlier, triple response was considered to be a H_1 receptor mediated response; recent evidence, however, suggests that H_2 receptors are also involved.

Table 24.1 Characteristic Features of Histamine Receptors

Receptor type	Distribution and function	Post-receptor mechanisms	Agonists	Antagonists or inverse agonist
H_1	Smooth muscle (intestine, bronchi and uterus) - CONTRACTION Blood vessels - VASODILATION - ↑ CAPILLARY PERMEABILITY CNS - NEUROTRANSMITTER Sensory nerve endings - PAIN, ITCHING	G_q protein coupled, PIP_2 hydrolysis ↑ IP_3, ↑ DAG Release of Ca^{2+}	Histaprodifen	Mepyramine* Triprolidine Chlorpheniramine Cetirizine
H_2	Gastric glands - ACID SECRETION Blood vessels - VASODILATION - ↑ CAPILLARY PERMEABILITY Heart- ↑ HR, ↑ FC Brain - NEUROTRANSMITTER	G_s protein coupled ↑ cAMP	Dimaprit Amthamine	Cimetidine* Ranitidine Nizatidine Famotidine
H_3	Brain-presynaptic ↓ HISTAMINE, ↓ NE ↓ ACh RELEASE Lung, spleen, gastric mucosa ↓ HISTAMINE RELEASE, ↓ SECRETIONS Blood vessels VASODILATION	G_i protein coupled ↓ cAMP ↓ Ca^{2+} influx Opening of K^+ channels	R-α-methyl histamine Imetit	Iodophenpropit Clobenpropit* Thioperamide* Tiprolisant (Pitolisant)*
H_4	Eosinophils Neutrophils CD4 T cells Chemotaxis of WBC Production of blood cell types	G_i protein coupled ↓ cAMP ↓ Ca^{2+} influx	Imetit Clozapine	Thioperamide*

*Inverse agonist

In addition to flush, wheal and flare, transient pain and itching also result from the effects of histamine as described above. Severe hypersensitivity reaction may also occur suddenly following injection of histamine. This is called *anaphylactic shock* which is characterised by bronchospasm, angioneurotic oedema and hypotension. It is life threatening and requires prompt medical intervention.Cardiovascular responses to high doses of histamine are thought to be mediated by both H_1 and H_2 receptor action, as the combination of both H_1 and H_2 receptor blocking agents is more effective in blocking cardiovascular responses of histamine.

H_2 Receptor Mediated Actions

Histamine is a powerful stimulant of gastric acid secretion, an effect produced by activation of H_2 receptors on gastric parietal cells. Histamine also stimulates secretions in small and large intestine but gastric pepsin secretion and intrinsic factor production are affected to a lesser extent.

H_3 Receptor Mediated Actions

1. In the CNS as well as ANS, the presynaptic H_3 receptors serve as feedback inhibitors for the release of histamine, NE and ACh. Activation of H_3 receptors present on sympathetic nerve terminals in the heart decreases NE release (heterotropic presynaptic receptor interaction). Hence it helps to prevent arrhythmias and cardiac damage that may result from NE discharge during stress or ischaemia.
2. H_3 receptor activation by histamine rather inhibits gastric acid release and blocks certain inflammatory processes (counterbalancing of H_2 activation in needful situations).

Clinical Uses, Toxicity and Contraindications of Histamine

Today, the main clinical use of histamine is as a positive control injection for skin allergy testing. All other uses are outdated or hazardous. *Adverse effects* include, flushing, hypotension, headache, wheal formation, bronchoconstriction, gastric acidity and intestinal cramps. It is contraindicated in patients of asthma and peptic ulcer.

H_1-Receptor Agonists

Betahistine is a H_1 receptor agonist. In a dose of 8–16 mg BD orally, it is used to treat episodes of vertigo as it causes vasodilatation and improves the blood flow to labyrinth and brain stem. Being H_1 receptor agonist, it may aggravate peptic ulcer and bronchial asthma.

H_1-Receptor Antagonists

These drugs are competitive antagonists at H_1 receptor and are classified as either first or second generation antihistamines. Their clinical classification and pharmacological characteristics have been provided in Table 24.2. The *first generation drugs* are short to intermediate acting, more sedating and are likely to have more antimuscarinic side effects. The *second generation drugs* have longer duration of action, have poor permeability to BBB and are, therefore, least sedating, besides being devoid of autonomic side effects.

Pharmacokinetics

Though most of H_1 antagonists, irrespective of their groups, are metabolised in liver by microsomal system, some of the second generation agents (terfenadine and astemizole) are metabolised by specific CYP3A4 subtype of P- 450 enzymes. Hence, drugs like ketoconazole and erthromycin which inhibit CYP3A4 microsomal enzyme can provide elevated plasma levels of both the antihistamines leading to the development of life-threatening arrhythmias (*torsade de pointes*). Hence, both astemizole and terfenadine are no longer used in most of the countries.

In second generation H_1 antagonists, ***cetirizine*** is an active metabolite of ***hydroxyzine*** (I generation drug). The l-isomer, ***levocetirizine,*** is more potent and less sedating than cetirizine. ***Fexofenadine*** and ***desloratadine*** are active metabolites of terfenadine and loratadine, respectively, and are claimed to be less toxic and more potent. The reduction in therapeutic

Table 24.2 Clinical Classification & Pharmacological Characteristics of H_1-Receptor Antagonists

Name	Adult dose (oral)	Duration of action (hrs)	Anticholinergic activity	Remarks
FIRST GENERATION ANTIHISTAMINES				
HIGHLY SEDATIVE				
Dimenhydrinate	25–50 mg	4–6	+++	Anti–motion sickness activity
Diphenhydramine	25–50 mg	4–6	+++	- do -
Doxylamine	1.5–25 mg		++	Used as "Sleep Aid"
Hydroxyzine	25–50 mg	4–6	+++	Antiemetic
Promethazine	10–25 mg	4–6	+++	Antiemetic
MODERATELY SEDATIVE				
Pyrilamine	25–50 mg	4–6	+	Also as "Sleep Aid"
Cyproheptadine	4 mg	4–6	++	Antiserotonin effects
Pheniramine	25–50 mg	4–6	+++	—
Clemastine	2–6 mg	12	+++	—
MILD SEDATIVE				
Meclizine	25–50 mg	12–20	++	—
Chlorpheniramine	4–8 mg	4–6	+	
Cinnarizine	25–75 mg	6–8	++	Used for vertigo. Also a Ca^{2+} channel blocker
Triprolidine	2.5–5 mg	4–6	+	—
SECOND GENERATION ANTIHISTAMINES*				
Astemizole	10 mg OD	24	-	
Fexofenadine	120-180 mg OD	12	-	
Cetirizine	10 mg OD	12-24	-	
Loratadine	10 mg OD	24	-	
Desloratadine	5 mg OD	24	-	Anti-inflammatory action also
Levocetirizine	5 mg OD	24	-	
Ebastine	10 mg OD	24	-	
Olopatadine	0.2% Eye drops	24	-	Used for ocular itching with allergic conjuctivitis

* All are non-sedating. Terfenadine is no longer used.

effectiveness that is observed when antihistamines are given for longer periods is probably related to an induction of microsomal P-450 enzymes. Individuals with hepatic impairment may eliminate these antihistamines slowly. Children tend to eliminate antihistamines faster than adults.

Pharmacological Characteristics and Therapeutic Uses

1. Both the groups of H_1 antagonists are used to prevent or treat the symptoms of allergic rhinitis and urticaria. For atopic dermatitis, however, first generation H_1 antagonists are preferred because of their additional sedative effects and for their better control of itching. For hay fever and chronic urticaria, non-sedating second generation drugs are preferred. The newer drugs in this series, though expensive, exhibit sedation in only 5–7% of the subjects. In all these conditions, histamine is the primary mediator and hence their use is quite efficacious. However, in bronchial asthma, several mediators are involved besides histamine. Therefore, these drugs, irrespective of their group, remain almost ineffective.
2. Although angioedema during anaphylaxis is precipitated by histamine, there are other peptide kinins which keep it maintained later. Hence H_1 antagonists alone are not effective under such situation; rather, adjuvant drugs like glucocorticoids (I.M.) and adrenaline (S.C.) are also needed along with supportive measures such as O_2 inhalation.
3. Many of the I generation H_1 antagonists have some additional pharmacological effects which are not mediated through H_1 receptor (Table 24.2). For example, antimuscarinic activity in most of them (though a side effect) may account for their effectiveness in combating motion sickness (***dimenhydrinate, diphenhydramine, cyclizine*** and ***meclizine***). Some of them are used as antiemetics (***hydroxyzine*** and ***promethazine***) while ***doxylamine*** in some formulations (e.g., ***doxinate***) is used to prevent nausea and vomiting due to pregnancy (being least teratogenic among all drugs). All first generation H_1 blockers have some degree of sedation as a rule. Never-the-less, this side effect is sufficiently prominent in some drugs (***doxylamine*** and ***pyrilamine***) to make them useful as over-the-counter sleeping aids. Favourably, no compulsive use has been reported with these agents. Second generation drugs are, however, least sedative.
4. Recent II generation antihistamine, ***desloratadine***, has been found to inhibit non-histamine mediated release of various inflammatory substances also and this may account for its better effectiveness in combating allergic conditions.
5. Besides pharmacological effects and related therapeutic uses discussed above, I generation H_1 blockers exhibit only limited effectiveness in suppressing parkinsonian symptoms (***diphenhydramine*** and ***promethazine***). Some of them (***pyrilamine, promethazine*** and ***diphenhydramine***) possess local anaesthetic actions also. However, none of these is clinically used as antiparkin-sonism agent or as local anaesthetic. Only ***cyproheptadine***, a first generation H_1 antagonist, has notable antiserotonin effects (discussed later).

Adverse Effects and Drug Interactions

Despite the fact that the most common side effects like *sedation* and *antimuscarinic actions* have been utilised for therapeutic purposes, these two effects constitute the most common undersirable actions when H_1 antagonists are used to treat allergic conditions. An additive effect on alertness and motor skills results if alcohol or another CNS depressant drug is taken along with these drugs. Antimuscarinic effects caused by them include *dry mouth, urinary retention* and *constipation*, which may aggravate with concomitant use of other antimuscarinic drug or tricyclic antidepressants. Drug allergy especially with topical agents may also occur. *Tolerance* to their actions may also develop after prolonged use. *Teratogenic effects* of ***hydroxyzine, cyclizine*** and ***meclizine*** have been reported in some animal species but not in humans. Toxic doses of H_1 antagonists may lead to even excitement, hallucinations, convulsions and coma.

As discussed above, enzyme inhibitors like ketoconazole, chloramphenicol or erythromycin elevate the plasma levels of some II generation drugs such as ***astemizole*** and ***terfenadine***. This may induce *torsade de pointes* type of fatal cardiac arrhythmias.

Fexofenadine, an active metabolite of terfenadine does not produce *torsade de pointes* type of cardiac arrhythmia.

H_2-Receptor Antagonists

These are discussed in Chapter 27. Currently available H_2 antagonists are ***cimetidine, ranitidine, famotidine*** and ***nizatidine***. Among these, cimetidine has become obsolete and has been replaced by newer H_2 blockers named above. These drugs compete with histamine for H_2 receptors and block gastric acid secretion and some cardiovascular effects of histamine (Table 24.1). They have minimal effects on H_1 receptors while have no effect on H_3 or H_4 receptors. They not only inhibit gastric acid secretion, induced by histamine, gastrin, cholinergic stimulation and food, but also promote healing of duodenal ulcers. However, relapses are likely to occur when treatment with H_2-receptor antagonists is stopped. Their rank order of potency is nizatidine > famotidine > ranitidine > cimetidine.

- These are used to treat hyperacidity, duodenal and gastric ulcers, reflux oesophagitis and Zollinger-Ellison syndrome.

The major drawbacks of the earlier drug ***cimetidine*** were antiandrogenic effects and hepatic enzyme inhibition, thereby causing gynaecomastia in males, galactorrhoea in females and various drug interactions. Cimetidine enhances the activity of most of the drugs when used concomitantly. These side effects are minimal with ***ranitidine*** and absent in ***famotidine*** and ***nizatidine***. Side effects with the latter two drugs are rare and mild.

H_3- and H_4-Receptor Antagonists

After the availability of H_2 or H_4 ligands a great interest has been evoked to findout their therapeutic potential. An inverse H_3-receptor agonist, ***tiprolisant***, has been observed to reduce sleep cycles and weight gain, and to cause behavioural and convulsive changes. As a result it and yet to be discovered H_3 -receptor antagonists or inverse agonist may find a place in the treatment of narcolepsy, obesity, psychosis and seizure disorders. It is worth mentioning that some the available antipsychotic drugs have binding affinity for H_3- receptor.

H_4 receptors have been shown to play a role inflammatory conditions by virtue of their presence on the membrane of eosinophils and mast cells. Although no selective H_4 ligand is available, some H_1 antagonists (e.g., cetirizine, loratidine, diphenhydramine) have been found to block H_4 receptors as well and such agents may find a place in the treatment of chronic inflammatory conditions like bronchial asthma, pruritis, allergic rhinitis and certain pain conditions

Histamine Release Inhibitors

Cromolyn sodium (disodium cromoglycate) and ***nedocromil sodium*** prevent the degranulation of mast cells, that results from immunological triggering by antigen-IgE interaction, and thereby prevent the release of histamine and other inflammatory mediators from these mast cells. These drugs have a wide variety of inhibitory effects on many other cell types also, including eosinophils, neutrophils and monocytes.

- *Cromolyn sodium* and *nedocromil sodium* are used as pulmonary inhalants in the treatment of bronchial asthma (Ch. 48). Nasal and ophthalmic formulations of cromolyn sodium are used to reduce the symptoms of allergic rhinitis and conjunctivitis. *Side effects* include throat irritation, coughing and wheezing which can be prevented by pretreatment with β_2 adrenoceptor agonists. Serious side effects are rare.

Pemirolast is also a mast cell stabiliser but with anti-inflammatory properties. ***Ketotifen fumarate*** is a H_1 receptor antagonist with mast cell stabilising properties. All are available for systemic as well as ophthalmic use.

5-HYDROXYTRYPTAMINE (5-HT; SEROTONIN)

5-Hydroxytryptamine (5-HT) has diverse pharmacological and physiological roles in the body which include as a neurotransmitter in CNS, as a regulator of smooth muscle function in CVS and GIT and as regulator of platelet function, besides other subsidiary roles in several functions. As a matter of fact it is an autacoid mediator without portfolio, which is discharging its responsibilities with full freedom and yet enjoying freedom from all responsibilities. This chapter deals with the biosynthesis, distribution, metabolism and possible physiological roles of 5-HT in the periphery. Its role in the CNS and its relationship to psychiatric disorders has been discussed in Chapters 30, 33 and 34.

Distribution, Biosynthesis, Release and Metabolic Degradation of 5-HT

Structures rich in 5-HT are (a) GIT enterochromaffin cells (90%) and myenteric plexus where it serves as a prokinetic agent and neurotransmitter, (b) platelets where it diffuses inside from plasma by active transport, and is released at the site of damage after platelet aggregation, and (c) in lungs, bone marrow, pineal gland (as a precursor of melatonin) and CNS (as neurotransmitter).

5-HT is formed by dietary tryptophan which is converted to 5-hydroxytryptophan by tryptophan hydroxylase and then to 5-hydroxytryptamine (5-HT) by a nonspecific aromatic L-amino acid decarboxylase (also called dopa decarboxylase). 5-HT is then stored in 5-HT containing cells such as enterochromaffin cells and neurons as cotransmitter together with various peptide hormones such as somatostatin, vasoactive intestinal peptide and substance P.

Degradation occurs through oxidative deamination by MAO, to 5-hydroxyindole acetaldehyde followed by its oxidation to 5-hydroxyindole acetic acid (5-HIAA) (Fig. 24.3). 5-HIAA is excreted in urine.

5-HT Receptors

At present, there are seven main types (5-HT_1 to 5-HT_7) of serotonin receptors. Of these, 5-HT_1 and 5-HT_2 are subdivided further. With a total of 14 (types plus subtypes) receptors identified so far, 5-HT receptors have beaten the record of all receptors for their diverse characteristics (Table 24.3).

5-HT_1 receptors are located mainly in CNS. They function as inhibitory presynaptic receptors (autoreceptor) and belong to the family of G-protein coupled receptors linked to adenylate cyclase. Their

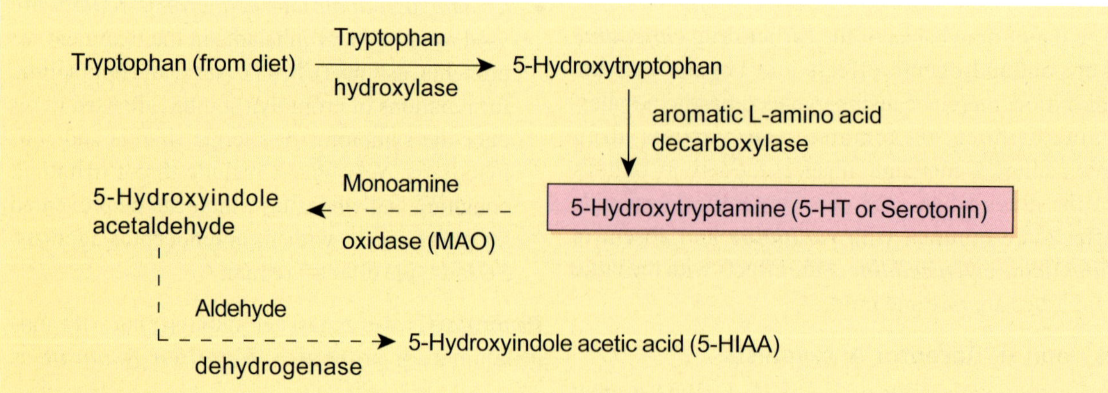

Fig 24.3 Biosynthesis and Metabolism of Serotonin. Biosynthesis: solid arrows; Metabolism: broken arrows.

Table 24.3 5-HT Receptor Types, Subtypes and Their Characteristic Features

Receptor types	Distribution	Function	Receptor mechanism	Agonist (subtypes)	Antagonist (subtypes)
5-HT_1 and subtypes	Mainly CNS and cerebral blood vessels	Presynaptic (auto-receptor); affects mood and behaviour; cerebral vasoconstriction	GPCRs (G_i) ↓ cAMP	Buspirone (5-HT_{1A}; PA); Sumatriptan (5-HT_{1D})	Spipirone (5-HT_{1A}); Ergotamine (5-HT_{1A-1D}; PA)
5-HT_2 and subtypes	CNS, Smooth muscles, Platelets	Smooth muscle contraction, Platelet aggregation; Excitation	GPCRs (G_q) ↑IP_3↑DAG	LSD (non-selective)	Ketanserin (5-HT_{2A}) Methysergide (5-HT_{2A-2C}) Clozapine, risperidone (5-HT_{2A-2C}) Cyproheptadine (5-HT_{2A})
5-HT_3	CNS (area postrema); PNS; ENS	Excitation of nociceptive neurons; anxiety; Emesis	5-HT gated ion channel	2-methyl-5-HT	Ondansetron Granisetron
5-HT_4	CNS (Hippocampus) ENS	Excitation ↑GI motility	GPCR (G_s) ↑ cAMP	Metoclopramide Cisapride Mosapride Tegaserod	GR-113808

Key: GPCRs—G-protein coupled receptors; ENS—Enteric nervous system; PNS—Peripheral nervous system; PA—Partial agonist

activation decreases cAMP. These are of 6 subtypes. Among these, 5-HT_{1A} and 5-HT_{1B} are involved in the regulation of mood and behaviour (Ch. 30, 33 and 34). Activation of 5-HT_{1D} receptor mediates cerebral vasoconstriction. ***Sumatriptan***, a 5-HT_{1D} receptor agonist, is therefore used for the treatment of migraine. The precise physiological role of other receptors is not known. Only in cerebral blood vessels, the vasoconstriction is mediated by 5-HT_1 receptors; in other vessels vasoconstriction is caused by activation of 5-HT_2 receptors (see below).

5-HT_2 receptors are located in the periphery (smooth muscles and platelets) and to a certain extent in CNS. These are also G-protein coupled receptors but are linked to IP_3 and DAG production (instead of cAMP). These are of 3 subtypes. Smooth muscle contraction and vasoconstriction of most vessels is mediated through 5-HT_{2A} receptors. Hence, their physiological role becomes important during asthma and vascular thrombosis (as these are distributed in platelets also). Other receptor subtypes have limited role.

5-HT_3 receptors occur in peripheral nervous system, especially on nociceptive afferent neurons and neurons of ENS. 5-HT_3 receptors are exceptional in being directly linked to membrane ion-channels, and have no involvement of any second messenger. 5-HT effects on these receptors are excitatory, e.g., it evokes pain when injected locally. 5-HT_3 receptors are also located in the area postrema and on activation cause emesis. 5-HT_3 receptor antagonists like ***ondansetron, granisetron*** and ***tropisetron*** possess good antiemetic effects (Ch. 28).

5-HT_4 receptors occur in ENS as well as in CNS. Effects are stimulation of peristalsis and gastric emptying. These are G_s protein coupled receptor which stimulate adenylate cyclase and increase cAMP formation. 5-HT_4 receptor agonists, ***metoclopramide*** and ***cisapride***, are used as antiemetic and to stimulate gastric emptying (Ch. 28).

Little is known about the precise physiological role of the remaining 5-HT_5, 5-HT_6 and 5-HT_7 receptors.

Pharmacological Actions of 5-HT

The actions of serotonin are mediated through a large number of receptors which possess diverse characteristics. Hence, generalisations of serotonin actions on receptor basis, as we did for histamine, becomes difficult. Instead, it is easier to discuss its actions on specific tissue and organ system.

Central Nervous System

5-HT is an important neurotransmitter in CNS (Ch. 30). 5-HT is involved in the regulation of mood, behaviour, sleep, depression, pain perception, sexual activity, thermoregulation and in the hypothalamic control of the release of pituitary hormones. 5-HT is also synthesised in pineal gland where it is precursor for the synthesis of melatonin, a melanocyte stimulating hormone, which influences sleep. Injected 5-HT (I.V.) does not cross BBB.

Cardiovascular System

5-HT directly causes contraction of vascular smooth muscle (including intracranial vessels), except in skeletal muscles and heart where it causes vasodilatation and bradycardia. When injected I.V, it produces a typical triphasic response. There is an early sharp fall in HR and BP. The bradycardia is mediated by vagal outflow to the heart and can be blocked by atropine. The hypotension is a consequence of the decrease in cardiac output that results due to bradycardia. Thereafter, there is a rise in BP due to peripheral vasoconstriction and increase in cardiac output. Finally, there is a sustained phase of hypotension due to dilatation of blood vessels of skeletal muscles. 5-HT, however, is not involved in physiological regulation of BP.

Serotonin causes blood platelets to aggregate by activating 5-HT_{2A} receptors and this aggregation is followed by further release of 5-HT. If the endothelium is damaged, this release from the adherent platelets causes vasoconstriction which impairs blood flow. Platelet derived 5-HT, therefore, plays important role in vascular diseases.

Gastrointestinal Tract

5-HT stimulates peristalsis and gastric secretions (*via* 5-HT_4 receptors). Activation of 5-HT_4 receptors in ENS causes increased ACh release which mediates a prokinetic (motility enhancing) effect of 5-HT and also of some selected 5-HT_4 receptor agonists like

cisapride and ***mosapride*** (Ch. 28). Overproduction of 5-HT, as in carcinoid tumour (a tumour of enterochromaffin cells) is associated with severe diarrhoea.

Miscellaneous Effects

1. Serotonin, like histamine, stimulates perception of pain and itch by activating 5-HT$_3$ receptors on afferent nerve endings.
2. 5-HT constricts bronchial smooth muscles by facilitating ACh release from bronchial vagal nerve endings. Hyperventilation may result due to stimulation of bronchial sensory nerve endings by 5-HT.
3. 5-HT reduces food intake and also has an anorexigenic effect.

5-HT Receptor Agonists

Serotonin has no clinical application as a drug. However, its receptor subtype selective agonists are of some therapeutic value. Notable among these are :

1. ***Buspirone*** group of antianxiety agents belonging to non-benzodiazepine group (Ch. 32). These are partial agonists of 5-HT$_{1A}$ receptors in CNS.
2. ***Sumatriptan*** and its congeners are selective agonists at 5-HT$_{1D}$ receptors, which being cerebral vasoconstrictors, have emerged as most effective drugs for the treatment of acute migraine attacks.

   The mechanism of their action, side effects and pharmacokinetics have been summarised in Table 24.4.

   Usual dosage are: ***Sumatriptan***: 25–100 mg single oral dose to a maximum of 200 mg per day. Orally it is less effective. For better results 8 mg S.C. Inj. can be given, which can be repeated only once in 24 hr, or 5–20 mg as nasal spray to a maximum of 40 mg in 24 hr. ***Almotriptan***: 6.25–12.5 mg single oral dose to maximum of 25 mg per day. ***Eletriptan***: 20–40 mg single oral dose to a maximum of 80 mg per day. ***Naratriptan***: 1–2.5 mg single oral dose to a maximum of 5 mg per day. ***Zolmitriptan***: 1.25–2.5 mg single oral dose to a maximum of 10 mg per day. ***Rizatriptan***: 5–10 mg single oral dose to a maximum of 30 mg per day.

   Lasmiditan, a 5-HT$_{1F}$ receptor agonist (which inhibits the release of CGRP in CNS) has been found to be effective in patients with moderate to severe migraine which remains unaffected by the prior use of triptan therapy.
3. ***Cisapride*** and ***renzapride*** are selective 5-HT$_4$ receptor agonists which increase GIT motility and are used to treat gastroesophageal reflux (Ch. 27, 28). ***Tegaserod*** is a new 5-HT$_4$ agonist which is used to treat irritable bowel syndrome with constipation (Ch. 28).
4. ***Dexfenfluramine*** is a nonselective 5-HT receptor agonist. It also blocks 5-HT transporter and inhibits 5-HT uptake. It was earlier used as an appetite suppressant (see above). It has now been withdrawn because of its cardio- as well as neurotoxicity (Ch. 12). Similarly, ***sibutramine*** also inhibits 5-HT transporter and prevents 5-HT reuptake. It is used to suppress appetite in the management of obesity (see Ch. 72).
5. ***d-Lysergic acid diethylamide*** (LSD; Ch. 35) is another non-selective 5-HT receptor agonist. It is a potent hallucinogen and a drug of abuse.

5-HT Receptor Antagonists

The salient features of drugs, used clinically as 5-HT antagonists, are described below:

Ketanserin is mainly a 5-HT$_{2A}$ receptor antagonist. It is an effective antihypertensive drug with only mild side effects such as dizziness, tiredness, nausea and dry mouth. Its α_1 adrenoceptor blocking action appears to be responsible for its antihypertensive effects rather than 5-HT$_{2A}$ receptor blockade. This drug also blocks 5-HT$_{2A}$ receptor on platelets and antagonises platelet aggregation caused by 5-HT.

Sarpogrelate, a selective 5-HT$_{2A}$ antagonist was develop as an inhibitor of platelet aggregation and vasoconstriction induced by the 5-HT.

The pharmacological affects of these two drugs may be utilized in symptomatic relief in vasospastic condition like Raynaud's disease.

Ritanserin, a congener of ketanserin, is a more selective 5-HT_{2A} antagonist. It has insignificant α_1 blocking action. It reduces thromboxane formation and increases bleeding time presumably by inhibiting platelet aggregation. However, their preparations are not available.

Ondansetron, dolasetron and ***granisetron*** are 5-HT_3 receptor antagonists and are very efficacious for treating chemotherapy-induced emesis (Ch. 28).

Clozapine, olanzapine, quetiapine and ***risperidone*** (Ch. 33) are atypical antipsychotic agents which have varying 5-HT_{2A} and 5-HT_{2c} receptor blocking action in addition to being dopamine receptor antagonist (though to a lesser extent compared to typical neuroleptics).

Methysergide belongs to ergot group of alkaloids. It is a potent 5-$HT_{2A\text{-}2C}$ antagonist with some non-selective action on 5-HT_1 receptors also. It is neither emetic nor oxytocic like other ergot alkaloids. Though its use is declining, it was used for migraine prophylaxis earlier.

Cyproheptadine has 5-HT_{2A} receptor antagonist action on smooth muscles in addition to H_1 receptor blocking effect (see earlier text). It also has mild anticholinergic activity and CNS depressant property. The antiserotonin activity of cyprohep-tadine is utilised in controlling GIT manifestations of carcinoid and postgastrectomy dumping syndrome, migraine prophylaxis and to increase appetite in children to promote weight gain. However, cyproheptadine is not a preferred treatment for such conditions these days.

Partial Agonist/Antagonist at 5-HT Receptors

Ergot Alkaloids

Ergot alkaloids, on the basis of their pharmacological characteristics and receptor actions, are hard to classify anywhere. Because majority of them possess partial agonist-antagonist actions at 5-HT receptors, these are discussed here, in this chapter, even though their advocated use in the treatment of migraine is on decline.

These alkaloids are produced by fungus *(Claviceps purpurea)* which infects cereal crops and is responsible for sporadic poisoning incidence. The most important alkaloids in this group are ***ergotamine*** and ***dihydroergotamine*** (both partial agonist/antagonist at 5-HT_1 receptor) and are used in acute attack of migraine; ***methysergide*** (partial agonist/antagonist at 5-HT_2 receptor) which, earlier was used for migraine prophylaxis and for the treatment of carcinoid syndrome; ***bromocriptine*** which is used in parkinsonism and other endocrine disorders (being dopamine receptor agonist); and ***ergometrine*** (a uterine stimulant and 5-HT_2 receptor agonist) which is used in obstetric practice to prevent postpartum haemorrhage (Ch. 41). The common side effects are nausea, vomiting and vaso-constriction. Ergot alkaloids are therefore contraindicated in pregnancy, peripheral vascular disease, coronary artery disease and hypertension.

Drug Treatment of Migraine

Migraine is a common debilitating headache, affecting 10–15% of population, the pathophysiology of which is still debatable. Migraine can usually be distinguished from two other related types of headaches—the *cluster headache (or migrainous neuralgia)* and *tension headache*—by its clinical and other characteristics. In short, *migraine* is a pulsatile, throbbing pain; *cluster headache* is a distressing, sharp but steady pain while *tension-type headache* is a dull headache with a persistent tightening feeling in the head. There are two types of migraine headache:

1. ***Classic migraine (migraine with aura)***: In this type, the pulsatile throbbing headache is preceded by neurologic symptoms called aura which can be visual, sensory with or without speech or motor disturbances. Most common pro-dromal symptoms are visual which appear 20–30 min prior to the onset of headache. About 15–20% of the migraine patients suffer from classic mi-graine.
2. ***Common migraine (migraine without aura)***: It is a severe, unilateral, pulsating headache that typi-cally lasts from 2 hrs to 3 days. These headaches are often aggravated by physical work and are accompanied by nausea, vomiting, intolerance to light and sound. In both the types of migraine, women are three times likely to suffer than men.

At times, a unilateral focal tenderness or local oedema is also observed in both the types of migraine.

Pathophysiology of Migraine

The postulated pathogenesis of migraine and sites of action of antimigraine drugs are shown in Fig. 24.4.

Irrespective of the aetiology of migraine, there is a strong evidence to implicate 5-HT in its pathogenesis for the following reasons:

- There is a sharp increase in the urinary excretion of 5-HIAA (a major 5-HT metabolite) during the migraine attack.
- Majority of antimigraine drugs are either 5-HT receptor agonists or antagonists.

Antimigraine Drugs

The drugs used to treat migraine are summarised in Table 24.4, while their possible sites of action are shown in Fig. 24.4. Prophylactic drugs are used during the asymptomatic phase of the migraine, i.e., between attacks when no symptoms are evident. These are a mixed bag of drugs and the mode of action for majority of them is poorly understood. Drugs for treating acute attack are appropriate when attacks are infrequent. Among them ***ergotamine*** is used in prodromal phase; ***analgesics*** with ***metoclopramide*** in headache phase; while ***sumatriptan*** (or any triptan) can be used for both the phases.

Atogepant

Atogepant is approved drug for migraine. During attack of migraine, calcitonin gene-related peptide (CGRP) level is acutely elevated. Atogepant is an antagonist of the calcitonin gene-related peptide receptors and prevents actions of CGRP. It is effective orally, used to prevent episodic migraine attacks. Adverse effects: Nausea, constipation, decreased appetite, fatigue and sleepiness.

Erenumab

It is a human monoclonal antibody that binds to the calcitonin gene-related peptide receptors. It is given subcutaneously for the prevention of migraine. Adverse effects: Muscle spasm, rash, angioedema, injection site pain and hypertension.

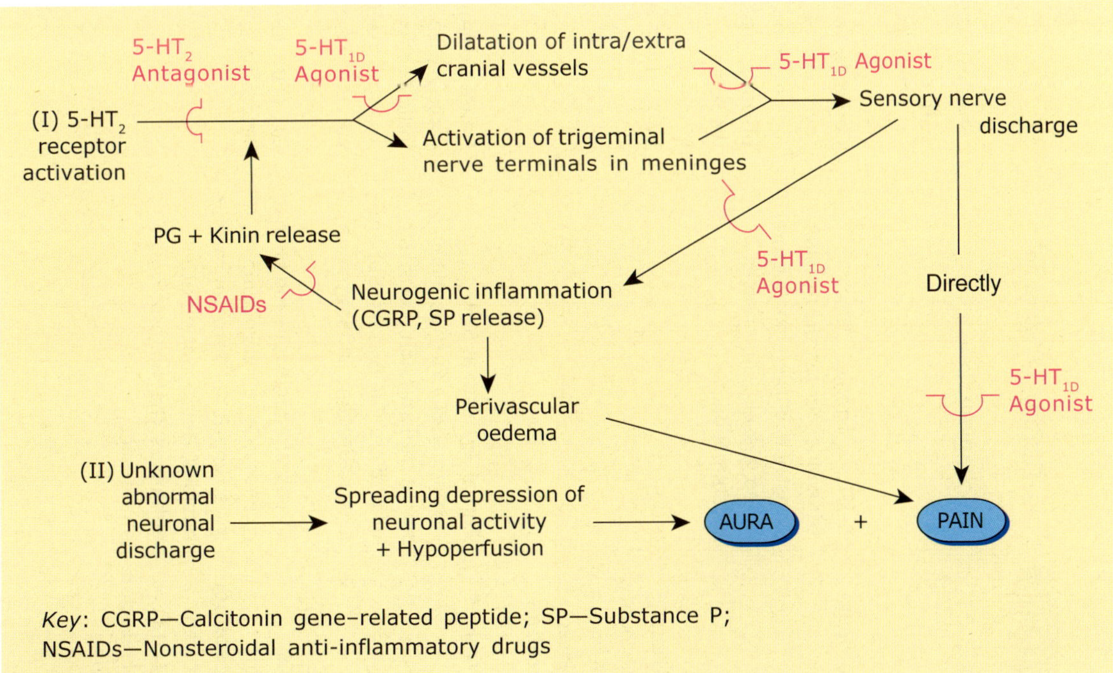

Fig 24.4 Postulated Pathogenesis of Migraine.

Table 24.4 Drug Therapy of Migraine

Drug	Mechanism	Side effects	Remarks
		For Acute Attack	
Sumatriptan	$5\text{-}HT_{1D\text{-}1B}$ agonist. Block trigeminal nerve transmission. Constricts dilated extracranial blood vessels. Suppresses inflammation.	Coronary vasospasm; risk of myocardial infarction, contra-indicated in coronary artery disease. Paraesthesia, muscle weakness.	Poor oral bioavailabililty; given S.C. or as nasal spray. Oral doses are high. Shorter half-life, does not cross BBB. Effective in 70% cases.
Naratriptan Zolmitriptan Almotriptan Eletriptan Rizatriptan	- do -	Lesser than sumatriptan	Improved oral bioavailability. Lesser oral dose. Cross BBB. Not much difference in $t_{1/2}$
Ergotamine*	Partial agonism at $5\text{-}HT_{1D\text{-}1B}$ receptors. Blocks trigeminal nerve transmission. Constricts dilated cranial vessels. Suppresses neurogenic inflammation.	Nausea, vomiting, uterine contraction, coronary vasoconstriction, contra-indicated in pregnancy, coronary artery disease and peripheral vascular disease.	Poor oral bioavailability. Caffeine 100 mg enhances its absorption. Effective but avoided because of side effects.
NSAIDs Aspirin Paracetamol Naproxen Diclofenac with Metoclop-ramide	Inhibit prostaglandin and kinin release due to neurogenic inflammation. Metoclopramide, besides being antiemetic, enhances the absorption of analgesics.	GIT disturbances and bleeding. For details refer Ch. 26	For migraine without aura; usually taken till the attack passes off.

contd.

Drug	Mechanism	Side effects	Remarks
For Prophylaxis of Migraine			
Propranolol Nadolol Timolol	β-adrenoceptor blockers; Mechanism uncertain	Bronchoconstriction; Fatigue. Contraindicated in asthmatics.	Used orally. Very effective, frequently used.
Cyproheptadine	5-HT_{2A} receptor antagonist. Also blocks H_1 receptors and muscarinic receptors.	Sedation, weight gain.	Given orally, low efficacy, rarely used.
Flunarizine*	Weak but cerebroselective Ca^{2+} channel blocker. Inhibits Na^+ channels also. Reduces intracellular Ca^{2+} overload due to cerebral hypoxia.	Sedation, constipation, flushing, dry mouth.	Given orally (5–10 mg once daily). As effective as propranolol. Reduces severity of attacks and prevents recurrences.
Clonidine	α_2-adrenoceptor agonist. Reduces cerebral blood flow. Mechanism unknown.	Dry mouth, sedation, constipation.	Given orally, efficacy doubtful.
Tricyclic anti-depressant Amitriptyline	5-HT uptake blocking property is causally related to the prophylactic effect.	Dry mouth, blurred vision, constipation, urinary retention, postural hypotension, weight gain.	To be taken orally at bedtime. Quite effective but avoided due to side effects. Effective even in persons who are not depressed.
Divalproate sodium	GABA-ergic mechanism	Weight gain, hair loss, tremors, hepato-toxicity, pancreatitis, Pregnancy Category D drug	Given orally
Topiramate	Uncertain mechanism	Metabolic acidosis, acute myopia, angle-closure glaucoma	Given orally
Erenumab	Anti-CGRP Receptor monoclonal Antibody (Fully human)	Injection site pain, muscle cramps, and spasm, constipation	Administered by S.C. injection (70 mg) once monthy for Episodic Migraine

Eptinezumab

Eptinezumab, a humanized immunoglobulin G1 (IgG1) monoclonal antibody, which binds to the CGRP ligand and blocks CGRP binding to its receptors. It is approved for the prevention of migraine in adults.

Ubrogepant

Ubrogepant binds to calcitonin gene-related peptide receptors and acts as an antagonist. It is a US-FDA approved drug for acute migraine with or without aura. *Adverse effects*: Nausea, somnolence, dry mouth and allergic reaction.

Rimegepant

Rimegepant is approved for the treatment of acute attack of migraine in adults. It is a calcitonin gene-related peptide receptor antagonist. *Adverse effects*: Nausea, rash, urticaria and dyspnoea.

Lasmiditan

Lasmiditan binds with high affinity to 5-HT1F receptors. It is used for acute attack of migraine. It acts as an agonist on 5-HT1F receptors. *Adverse effects*: Paraesthesia, dizziness, fatigue, nausea, vomiting and muscle weakness.

Galcanezumab

(A humanized monoclonal antibody), binds to calcitonin gene-related peptide (CGRP) ligand and blocks its binding to the receptor.

Fremanezumab

Fremanezumab is a humanized monoclonal antibody (IgG) that selectively targets both the α and β isoforms of CGRP. It is used subcutaneously for the prevention of migraine in adults. Adverse effects: Injection site reaction, pain, induration and erythema.

KININS (BRADYKININ)

Kinins are a group of potent vasodilator peptides. Three kinins have been identified in mammals: *bradykinin, lysyl-bradykinin (kallidin)* and *methionyl-lysyl-bradykinin (Met-Lys-bradykinin).* **Bradykinin** is a nonapeptide, kallidin is a decapeptide while Met-Lys-bradykinin is an undecapeptide (its role is not clear). *Substance P* is also a kinin, but belongs to tachykinin family of peptides. It is an undecapeptide, discussed in Chapter 17.

Biosynthesis and Degradation of Bradykinin

The pathway for the formation and metabolism of bradykinin is shown in Fig. 24.5.

Bradykinin is formed enzymatically by the action of plasma kallikrein (kininogenase) on high-molecular-weight kininogen (HMW kininogen). HMW kininogen is a plasma α_2- globulin. Kallikrein is a glycoprotein which is produced in liver as pre-kallikrein, and transferred to plasma. Plasma pre-kallikrein is activated to kallikrein by Hageman factor. Tissue kallikrein does not need activation.

Bradykinin is rapidly degraded (t½ < 1 min) in lungs and other tissues. The main enzymes that inactivate bradykinin and kallidin are called kininases. One of these, *kininase II,* is the same as *angiotensin-converting enzyme* (ACE, Ch 18) and is found mostly in lungs. Another enzyme *kininase I* is a carboxypeptidase, which is synthesised in liver and is present in serum. It converts bradykinin to des-Arg-bradykinin, which is a bradykinin receptor (B_1R) agonist (see below). It is further degraded to inactive peptides by other peptidases.

Bradykinin Receptor: Agonists and Antagonists

There are two main subtypes of bradykinin receptors: ***B_2 receptors*** which are constitutively present on

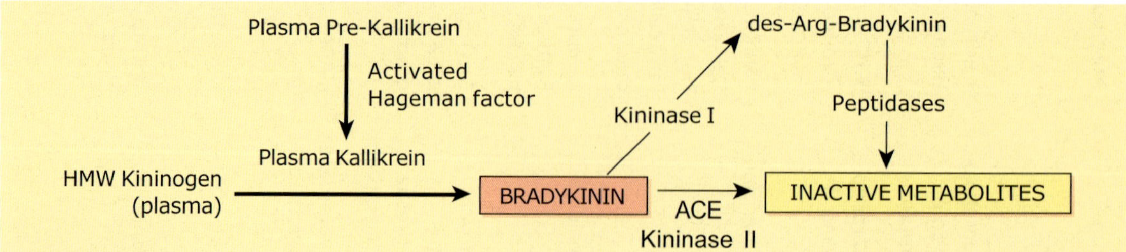

Fig 24.5 Biosynthesis (Thick Arrows) and Metabolism (Thin Arrows) of Bradykinin

visceral smooth muscle, vascular endothelium and sensory nerve endings (i.e., wider distribution). B_2R mediate the majority of bradykinin actions. ***B_1receptors*** (B_1R) which are induced within few hours at the site of inflammation and tissue damage. In the terminology, 'B' stands for bradykinin and not for beta-adrenoceptor.

B_2 receptor is a G_q-protein coupled receptor which activates phospholipase C (IP_3/DAG cascade). Selective agonist is bradykinin (but not des-Arg-bradykinin). ***Icatibant*** is a selective antagonist of ***B_2R***. ***B_1R*** is also a G-protein coupled receptor. However, its signaling mechanisms are not yet clear. These receptors are upregulated by inflammation, tissue damage and also by release of cytokinins and endotoxins. Selective agonists is des-Arg-bradykinin (but not bradykinin). ***des-Arg-Icatibant*** is a selective antagonist of ***B_1R***.

Pharmacological Actions of Bradykinin

Cardiovascular System

Bradykinin is a potent vasodilator, ten times more potent than histamine. Vasodilatation (B_2 action) results due to release of EDRF (NO), PGE_2 and PGI_2 and partly due to arteriolar vasodilatation. When injected I.V., it causes flushing, throbbing headache and a fall in BP for a short duration.

Smooth Muscles

Bradykinin causes, as compared to histamine, slow and sustained contractions of various smooth muscles (B_2 effect) of intestine, uterus and bronchi (brady = slow; kinin = movement).

Endocrine and Exocrine Glands

The bradykinin may diffuse from several glands, including pancreas, kidney, gall bladder, intestine, sweat and salivary glands, to act as local modulators of blood flow to these organs. Kinins stimulate epithelial ion transport and fluid secretions in bronchi, GIT, gall bladder and salivary glands (B_2 effect).

Sensory Nerves

Bradykinin stimulates pain nerve endings, when injected intradermally. It elicits pain by stimulating nociceptive afferents in skin and viscera. It produces redness, local warmth, swelling and pain and plays an important role in inflammation (B_2 effect).

Physiological Role of Bradykinin

It is involved in (a) maintenance of BP, (b) mediation of inflammation and pain, (c) production of hyperaemia in various glands, (d) maintenance of tissue growth and repair, (e) maintenance of sperm motility and (f) closure of ductus arteriosus.

Therapeutic Uses

Aprotinin

Bradykinin *per se* has hardly any clinical use. However, ***aprotinin***, a nonspecific kallikrein antagonist is administered to patients undergoing coronary bypass surgery in order to minimise bleeding (aprotinin also inhibits plasmin and hence inhibits fibrinolysis to reduce operative blood loss).

Icatibant

It is structurally similar decapeptide analogue of bradykinin. Due to substitution of five non-proteogenic amino acids, it resists degradation by metallo-protease: **N**eutral **E**ndo**P**eptidase (NEP), amino-peptidases and carboxypeptidases. It is selective kinin B_2 receptor (B_2R) antagonist as it possesses higher affinity for B_2R than bradykinin itself. ***Icatibant*** is effective in cutaneous, abdominal and laryngeal attacks in **H**ereditary **A**ngio**E**dema (HAE). HAE is characterized by oedematous attacks of subcutaneous and submucosal tissues which can cause swelling, itching and urticaria-like skin lesions and life-threatening laryngeal oedema.

Icatibant is approved for the treatment of acute attacks of bradykinin-mediated HAE which occurs due to hereditary **C1** (esterase) **INH**ibitor (C1INH) deficiency. Adverse effects include injection-site reactions like itching, oedema, burning and hypersensitivity manifestations. Due to its vasodilatory effect, since bradykinin is responsible for cardio-protective effects in myocardial ischemia, ***Icatibant*** must be used with caution in patients of ischemic heart disease, angina pectoris or after stroke.

Icatibant can also be used in the treatment of acquired angioedema and ACE-I-induced angio-edema. It was argued that during ACE-I administration, there is a continued bradykinin accumulation on the B_2R leading to its desensitization, resulting into inefficacy of ***Icatibant*** as B_2R antagonist. It is useful in ACE-I-induced angioedema.

CHAPTER 25 Prostaglandins, Leukotrienes and Platelet Activating Factor

COMPETENCY PH1.16

Prostaglandins (PG) is the generic name for a group of closely related, cyclic, oxygenated, 20 C-atom containing unsaturated fatty acids. These are considered to be derived from a hypothetical parent acid called *prostanoic acid* which is a 20 C-atom containing fatty acid with a five membered cyclopentane ring. Prostanoic acid does not occur in the nature.

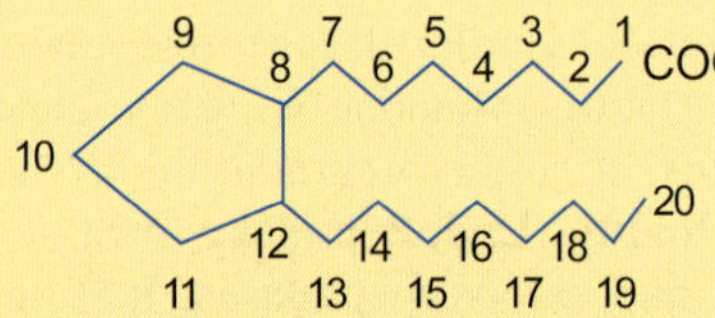

Hypothetical prostanoic acid

PG is not just one substance, but a whole family of compounds (PGA, B, C, D, E and F) and are formed in most of the tissues. Earlier it was obtained from the prostate and was saddled with the misnomer "prostaglandin". The inflammatory mediators derived from the membrane phospholipids are called *"eicosanoids",* which include PGs, thromboxanes, leukotrienes and platelet activating factor (PAF). The eicosanoids are derived from *arachidonic acid* which is also called *eicosa tetraenoic acid.* It is a 20 C-atom containing unsaturated fatty acid having four double bonds (eicosa = 20 C-atom; tetraenoic = 4 double bonds).The term *prostanoids* includes only PGs and thromboxanes.

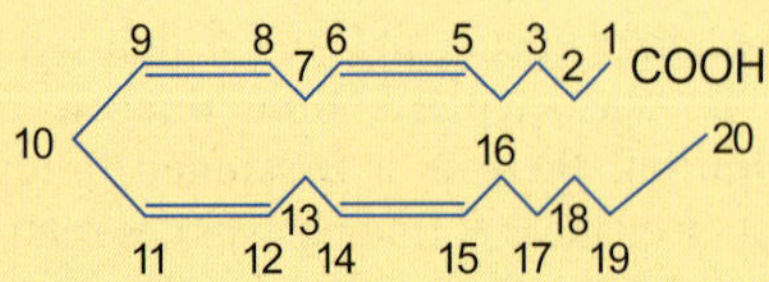

Arachidonic acid (eicosa tetraenoic acid)

The nomenclature of eicosanoids (particularly of PGs) is a bit confusing. These are the derivatives of arachidonic acid. All prostaglandins have a cyclopentane ring with a double bond between C-13 and C-14 and a OH group at C-15. The subscript "2" denotes that the PG has a total number of two double bonds in the side chain (inclusive of that between C13-C14). The subscript "α" denotes that the orientation of the OH group at 9-position of cyclopentane ring is above the plane of that ring.

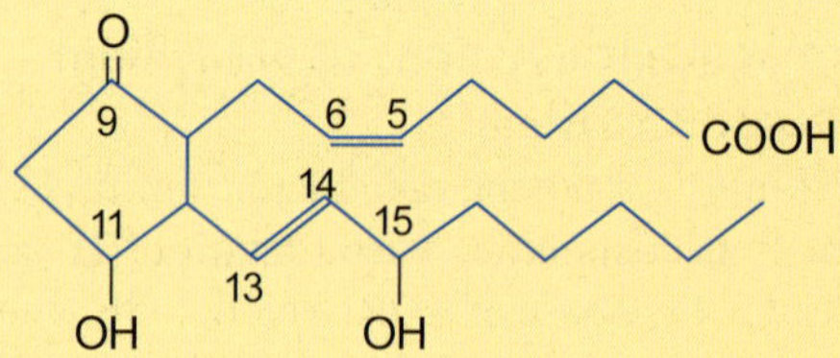

PGE_2

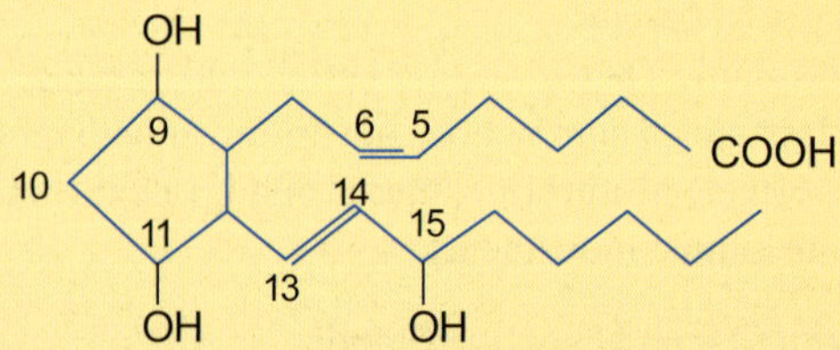

$PGF_{2\alpha}$

The names of the first two PGs were assigned on their method of separation: PGE from **E**ther and PGF from phosphate buffer (**F**osfat in Swedish language). PGA and PGB were so named because the former was stable in **A**cid while the latter in **B**ase. The alphabets like D,H,I were later suffixed to PGs in a random manner. PGE_2 has a C=O group at position-9 and a OH group at position-11 of cyclopentane ring while $PGF_{2\alpha}$ has OH groups at both of these positions.

BIOSYNTHESIS OF EICOSANOIDS
(COMMON FEATURES)

The flow chart (Fig. 25.1) outlines the biosynthetic pathways of various eicosanoids as well as the exact steps where the clinically useful drugs block these pathways. With suitable stimuli (physical, chemical, neurological or humoral, e.g., bradykinin), the enzyme phospholipase A_2 (PLA_2) is activated which liberates arachidonic acid from the membrane phospholipids. At least three PLA_2 (cardiac PLA_2, cytosolic PLA_2 and secretory PLA_2) mediate arachidonic acid release from membrane lipids.

Following its release, the arachidonic acid is oxygenated and cyclised by four separate routes: the *cyclo-oxygenase pathway*, the *lipoxygenase pathway*, the *cytochrome P-450 epoxygenase pathway* and the *isoprostane pathway.* Out of these four pathways, the last two pathways are of little significance and hence have been omitted from Fig. 25.1.

Biosynthesis of PGs and Thromboxane A_2 (Cyclo-oxygenase Pathway)

Two unique cyclo-oxygenase (COX) enzymes (COX-1 and COX-2; also known as PGH synthase -1 and -2, respectively), then convert arachidonic acid into different prostanoids (i.e., PGs and thromboxanes). COX-1 is constitutively expressed (i.e., it is always present in most of the cells); while COX-2 is inducible in inflammatory cells by an inflammatory stimulus (e.g., endotoxins, cytokines and tumour promoters). The two isozymes also differ in their functions. COX-1 has "house-keeping" functions, e.g., gastric cytoprotection and regulation of vascular responses. COX-2 is involved in normal renal development and vascular prostacyclin (PGI_2) production. COX-2 is the predominant cyclo-oxygenase at the sites of inflammation but not at sites such as GIT and platelets.

A new COX isozyme (COX-3) has also been identified recently. In humans, COX-3 mRNA is expressed most abundantly in cerebral cortex and the heart. It is selectively inhibited by paracetamol. It is involved in pain perception and fever but not in inflammation (not shown in Fig. 25.1).

A majority of ***Non Steroidal Anti-Inflammatory Drugs*** (NSAIDs) exert their analgesic-anti-inflammatory effects by inhibiting the activity of COX-1, while drugs like *celecoxib* or *rofecoxib* preferentially inhibit COX-2. The steroidal anti-inflammatory drugs like *prednisolone* or *dexamethasone* rather inhibit phospho-lipase A_2, by producing PLA_2 inhibitor—lipocortin. They also inhibit COX-2 gene expression.

Both the COXs promote oxygenation and cyclisation of arachidonic acid to yield PGG_2 which is then rapidly modified by peroxidase moiety of COX to PGH_2. PGH_2 being highly unstable, gets quickly converted to prostaglandins (PGE_2, $PGF_{2\alpha}$ and PGD_2), prostacyclin (PGI_2) and thromboxane A_2 by separate pathways as shown in Fig. 25.1. In platelets, the pathway leads to thromboxane A_2 (TXA_2); in vascular endothelium it leads to prostacyclin (PGI_2) and in mast cells to PGD_2, while in vasculature, GIT, lungs and other tissues to PGE_2 ($PGF_{2\alpha}$ is formed mainly in smooth muscles of GIT, bronchi, uterus and blood vessels).

All prostanoids, then rapidly undergo oxidative metabolism to their corresponding inactive metabolites. The half-life of most PGs in circulation is less than one minute.

Biosynthesis of Leukotrienes (Lipoxygenase Pathway)

Leukotrienes are the products of lipoxygenase pathway. Lipoxygenases are soluble enzymes located in cytosol and are found in lungs, platelets, mast cells and white blood cells. In the term leukotrienes, "leuko" signifies that they were first found in leukocytes; while "trienes" depicts that they contain a conjugated triene system of double bonds. 5-Lipoxygenase is the main enzyme which is involved in the synthesis of leukotrienes. As a first step (Fig. 25.1), 5-lipoxygenase adds a hydroperoxy group at C-5 in arachidonic acid to give 5-hydroperoxy-eicosatetraenoic acid (5-HPETE). It is then converted to LTA_4. The latter, in turn, can be converted either to LTB_4 or to a series of cysteinyl

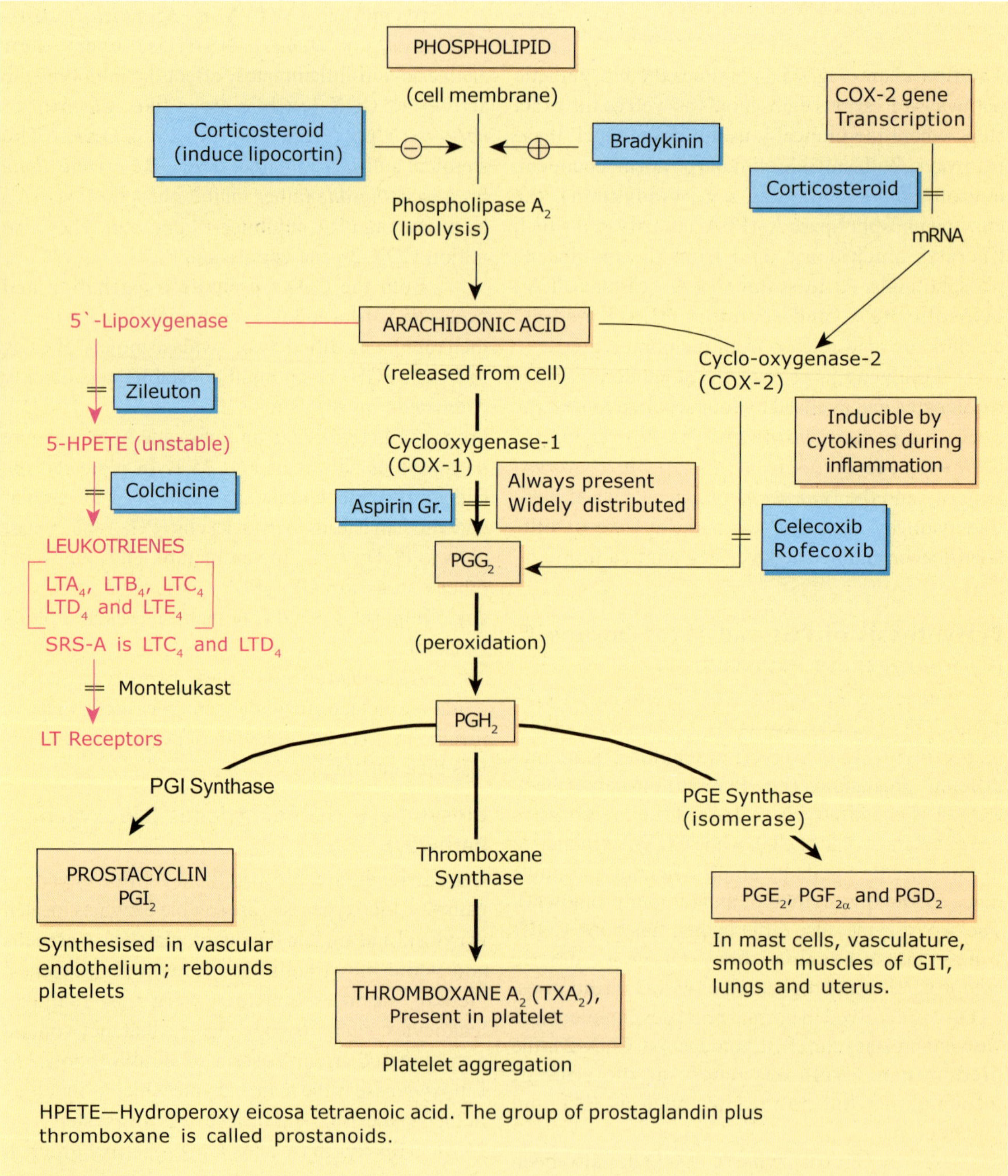

Fig 25.1 Prostaglandin, Thromboxane and Leukotriene Biosynthesis.

leukotrienes LTC_4, LTD_4 and LTE_4 which are also called as peptido-leukotrienes. LTC_4 and LTD_4 are potent bronchoconstrictors and are primary component of the ***S****low* ***R****eacting* ***S****ubstance of* ***A****naphylaxis* (SRS-A), that is secreted in asthma and anaphylaxis.

LTB_4 is produced mainly by neutrophils, while LTC_4, LTD_4 and LTE_4 are formed mainly in eosinophils, mast cells, basophils and macrophages. LTB_4 is metabolised to 20-hydroxy LTB_4 while LTC_4 and LTD_4 are metabolised and excreted as LTE_4 in the urine.

BIOSYNTHESIS OF PLATELET ACTIVATING FACTOR (PAF) AND ITS PHARMACOLOGICAL ACTIONS

PLA_2 can not only give rise to arachidonic acid but also to lysoglyceryl-phosphoryl choline (lyso-PAF), which is the precursor of another lipid mediator of inflammation called ***platelet activating factor (PAF;*** not shown in Fig. 25.1). Since PAF exhibits actions on a variety of different cells at exceedingly low concentration and is an important mediator in inflammation and allergies, the term PAF seems to be misleading. Nevertheless, it is generated and released from most inflammatory cells, when these are stimulated, *and also from platelets on stimulation, with thrombin* (hence may be the name).

PAF is derived from membrane bound acyl-PAF by PLA_2 activity, resulting in the formation of precursor lyso-PAF (besides formation of eicosanoids through arachidonic acid). Lyso-PAF, on acetylation by AcCoA, provides PAF (Fig. 25.2). PAF is degraded through deacetylation by acetyl hydrolase to lyso-PAF which is then acetylated again to provide acyl-PAF. The latter gets incorporated in the membrane to be recycled.

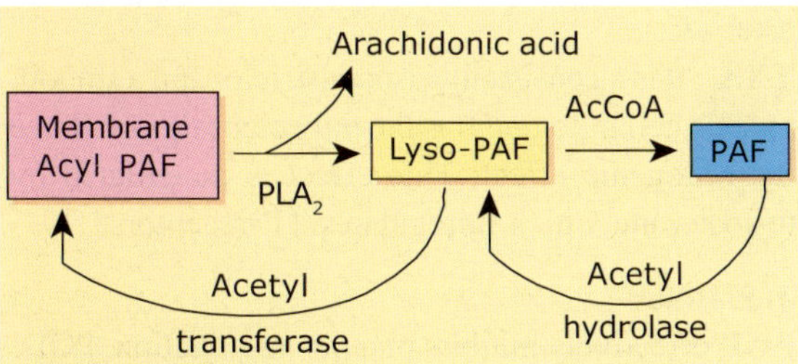

Fig 25.2 Biosynthesis and Breakdown of PAF

Pharmacological actions include vasodilatation, increased vascular permeability, chemotactic to eosinophils and neutrophils (i.e., stimulates neutrophils to aggregate and to stick to vascular endothelium and induces degranulation of eosinophils), activation of leucocytes, activation and aggregation of platelets (through release of TXA_2) and bronchoconstriction. It is implicated in inflammation and in bronchial hyper-responsiveness (and also in delayed phase of asthma). PAF produced by foetus at final term may be involved in progression of labour. PAF is most potent peptic ulcerogen.

The PAF receptor is a G-protein coupled receptor which exerts pharmacological actions through intracellular messengers IP_3 /DAG leading to Ca^{2+} release. Some actions are mediated through release of PGs, TXA_2 and LTs, which may be considered as its extracellular messengers. Glucocorticoids inhibit PAF synthesis.

BASIC PHARMACOLOGY OF PROSTANOIDS (PGs & TXA_2)

Prostanoid Receptors

Based on the five classes of natural prostanoids (PGD_2, PGE_2, $PGF_{2\alpha}$, PGI_2 and TXA_2), there are five main classes of prostanoid receptors which are termed as DP, EP, FP, IP and TP receptors, respectively. The EP receptors are further subdivided into four subgroups as EP_1, EP_2, EP_3 and EP_4. All of these receptors are G-protein coupled receptors, which utilise IP_3 /DAG or cAMP transducer mechanisms. Their characteristics are summarised in Table 25.1.

Pharmacological Effects of Prostanoids

The PGs, PGI_2 and TXA_2 have a vast variety of effects on vascular, gastrointestinal, reproductive and bronchial smooth muscles. Other targets include

Table 25.1 Pharmacological Characteristics of Prostanoid Receptors

Receptor type	Endogenous ligand	G-protein II messenger	Function
DP	PGD_2	G_s; ↑ cAMP	Inhibits platelet aggregation; Vasodilatation; Relaxation of GIT, bronchial and uterine muscle
EP_1	PGE_2 (also $PGF_{2\alpha}$)	G_q; ↑ IP_3 ↑ DAG	Bronchoconstriction; GIT smooth muscle contraction
EP_2	PGE_2	G_s; ↑ cAMP	Bronchodilatation; Vasodilatation; GIT smooth muscle relaxation; Stimulation of intestinal fluid secretion
EP_3	PGE_2	G_i; G_s; G_q ↑ or ↓ cAMP ↑ IP_3, ↑ DAG	Inhibition of gastric acid secretion; Increased gastric mucus secretion (cytoprotective action); Contraction of pregnant uterus and GIT smooth muscle; Inhibition of lipolysis and of Autonomic neurotransmitter release
EP_4	PGE_2	G_s; ↑ cAMP	Not much known; Vasodilatation, Maintenance of patent ductus
FP	$PGF_{2\alpha}$	G_q; ↑ IP_3 ↑ DAG	Contraction of uterus and GIT smooth muscle; ↓ intraocular pressure
IP	PGI_2	G_s; ↑ cAMP	Inhibits platelet aggregation; Vasodilatation; Renin release; Natriuresis
TP	TXA_2	G_q; ↑ IP_3 ↑ DAG	Causes platelet aggregation, Vasoconstriction; Bronchoconstriction, smooth muscle cell mitogenic

platelets, kidneys, endocrine organs, adipose tissue and CNS.

1) Cardiovascular System

PGE_2: Causes vasodilatation in most vascular beds. When injected I.V. it produces a fall in BP. It has weak positive inotropic effect on heart and increases cardiac output slightly. It also increases capillary permeability. It is continually produced in ductus arteriosus during foetal life and keeps it patent.

$PGF_{2\alpha}$: Potent vasoconstrictor for large arteries and veins. It has little effect on BP, heart rate, cardiac contractility or capillary permeability. It is not a smooth muscle cell mitogen (see TXA_2).

PGI_2: It is uniformly vasodilator and is more potent hypotensive than PGE_2. It keeps the patency of ductus arteriosus.

TXA_2: It is a consistent vasoconstrictor and a smooth muscle cell mitogen. It is the only eicosanoid to have the mitogenic effect. This effect is potentiated by testosterone which upregulates TP-receptors.

2) Platelets

PGI_2 effectively inhibits platelet aggregation. PGD_2 and PGE_1 also have antiaggregatory actions but **PGE_2** has inconsistent effects. **TXA_2** is a potent platelet aggregator. Working together with PGI_2, it maintains the integrity of the vascular endothelium, preventing platelets to aggregate and stick to the arteriolar walls. Because platelets lack nuclei (and hence DNA), they cannot continually synthesise COX-1 and therefore a limited amount of COX-1 and TXA_2 persists only up to the lifetime of platelet (approx. 7 days). This contrasts with the vascular endothelial cells, which have nuclei and therefore can produce new COX-1 (and therefore PGI_2) on regular basis. This property of platelets has been exploited by using low doses of aspirin for the prevention of coronary thrombosis (see Ch. 26).

3) Uterus

Both **PGE_2** and **$PGF_{2\alpha}$** uniformly contract pregnant as well as nonpregnant uterus *in vivo,* but **$PGF_{2\alpha}$** is more potent than **PGE_2**. *In vitro,* however, PGE_2 relaxes nonpregnant but contracts pregnant uterus while $PGF_{2\alpha}$ consistently contracts both. At term, PGs, in low doses, soften cervix and make it more yielding. PGs produced by foetus, at term, may be involved in initiation and progression of labour. Primary dysmenorrhoea is attributable to increased endometrial synthesis of PGE_2 and $PGF_{2\alpha}$ during menstruation, with uterine contractions which lead to ischaemic pain. Aspirin group of drugs, therefore, are highly effective in relieving dysmenorrhoea in most women (see Ch. 26).

4) Bronchial Muscle

PGE_2 and **PGI_2** cause relaxation of bronchial smooth muscle. **$PGF_{2\alpha}$** and **TXA_2** (also PGD_2 though TP receptor) induce contractions of respiratory muscles. Asthma may also be attributed to an imbalance between bronchoconstrictor PGs ($PGF_{2\alpha}$, TXA_2 and LTs) on one hand and bronchodilator PGs (PGE_2, PGI_2 and PGE_1) on the other. The dilator PGs also inhibit histamine release. In some individuals, aspirin induces asthma because of the shift in arachidonic acid metabolism from COX-pathway (blocked by aspirin) to leukotriene pathway. Leukotrienes are very powerful bronchoconstrictors.

5) Gastrointestinal Tract

PGE_2 markedly reduces acid secretion in the stomach. **PGI_2** also inhibits acid secretion but to a lesser extent. Both PGE_2 and PGI_2 also increase mucus production and mucosal blood flow, i.e., PGE_2 and PGI_2 are antiulcerogenic. The ulcerogenic action of aspirin group of drugs is probably due to the loss of this cytoprotective influence.

The longitudinal muscle of the gut is contracted by **PGE_2** (via EP_3 effect) and by $PGF_{2\alpha}$ (via FP effect). **PGE_2** also increases water and electrolyte secretions in intestines. Hence colic with watery diarrhoea are important side effects of PGE_2. **PGI_2** opposes propulsive activity of PGE_2 and does not produce diarrhoea. PGs seem to play some important role in colonic cancer and regular intake of aspirin, therefore, reduces the risk of colonic cancer.

6) Kidney

Renal medulla produces substantially more PGs compared to renal cortex. Both **PGE_2** and **PGI_2** cause natriuresis, renal vasodilatation and inhibit ADH action to promote water clearance. In addition, PGE_2 decreases Cl reabsorption. Both facilitate β_1 adrenoceptor stimulated renin release. **TXA_2**, however, causes renal vasoconstriction, and perhaps an ADH-like effect (but kidneys synthesise very little TXA_2). Loop diuretics, e.g., furosemide, produce a part of their effect through stimulation of COX activity to produce vasodilator PGE_2 and PGI_2. That is why, patient's response to a loop diuretic diminishes if a COX-inhibitor like indomethacin is administered concurrently (see Ch. 16 and 26).

7) Male Reproductive System

There is about 20 times more PGE (**PGE_1** and **PGE_2**) than **$PGF_{2\alpha}$** in a fertile semen. TXA_2 and LTs are not found in semen. Testosterone promotes prostaglandin production while large doses of aspirin decrease PG contents of seminal fluid. PGE_1, due to its smooth muscle relaxing effect, enhances penile erection (see Ch. 44). It increases sperm motility from vagina to uterus.

8) Central Nervous System

No clear cut physiological role of PGs in CNS has yet been established. Nonetheless, PGE_1 and **PGE_2**

are pyrogenic (via EP_3 receptor action). Their synthesis is blocked by aspirin. In some animal species PGD_2 induces sleep. **$PGF_{2\alpha}$** is not pyrogenic (unless given exogenously). PGD_2 and TXA_2 are also not pyrogenic. PGs probably function as neuromodulators in the brain as they inhibit the release of NE from postganglionic sympathetic nerve endings.

9) Peripheral Nerve Endings

Both **PGE_2** and **PGI_2** sensitise pain receptors at afferent nerve endings to mediators of pain (histamine, 5-HT and bradykinins) at the inflammatory site and amplify algesia.

10) Endocrine System

PGE_2 facilitates the release of growth hormone, TSH, ACTH, FSH, LH and prolactin. However, PGE_2 analogues, *per se* have no significant effect on the release of these hormones. It also has insulin-like effects on carbohydrate metabolism.

11) Bone Metabolism

PGE_2 plays some role in osteoporosis that occurs at menopause as it stimulates bone resorption.

12) Eye

$PGF_{2\alpha}$ (via FP receptor action) and also **PGE_2** lower the intraocular pressure by increasing the outflow of aqueous humour from the anterior chamber *via* the uveoscleral pathway.

13) Cancer

PGE_2 is considered to be the principal pro-oncogenic prostanoid, which promotes polyp formation (colon carcinogenic). TXA_2 is another likely pro-carcinogenic mediator (see use of aspirin Ch. 26).

Therapeutic Uses of Prostanoids and Their Analogues

PGs are not popular drugs in clinical practice because of their limited availability, unstability, shorter half- life, cost, adverse effects and parenteral route of administration. Yet, some analogues are gaining popularity for following indications:

1) Abortion

PGE_2 and **$PGF_{2\alpha}$** and their analogues are used to terminate pregnancy and to induce cervical ripening in pregnancy. These prostaglandins are used for first and second trimester abortion and appear to soften the cervix, before abortion, by increasing proteoglycan content and changing the collagen characteristics. PGs or its derivatives in current practice are:

Dinoprostone: It is a synthetic **derivative of PGE_2** which is administered vaginally for inducing abortion in second trimester of pregnancy and for ripening of the cervix for induction of labour at full term. Its plasma half-life is 2.5–5 min. Its use for menstrual regulation or for early abortions (1–2 weeks after last menstrual period) is usually avoided because of the chances of prolonged vaginal bleeding and severe menstrual cramps.

Misoprostol: It is a **PGE_1 derivative** which is given orally for abortifacient purpose. It is used with ***mifepristone*** (an antiprogestin, Ch 43) to induce abortion in the first few weeks of pregnancy. Vaginal, route of administration is associated with increased incidence of sepsis.

Carboprost: It is a **$PGF_{2\alpha}$ derivative** which is usually administered by intra-amniotic injection for inducing second trimester abortions. The drug is now least preferred because of its serious toxicity such as cardiovascular collapse, chances of anaphylactic shock and pulmonary hypertension.

2) Facilitation of Labour, Cervical Priming and Post-partum Haemorrhage

Oral **PGE_2** is superior to oral oxytocin analogues and is as effective as I.V. oxytocin in augmenting labour and to check postpartum haemorrhage.

Dinoprostone **(PGE_2 derivative)**, however, is less effective than oxytocin as it is for vaginal administration. Vaginal PGE_2 or dinoprostone can also be used to soften the cervix before inducing labour. Oral $PGF_{2\alpha}$ causes more GIT toxicity than PGE_2. Though clinical benefits have not been documented, PGs can be preferred over oxytocin for inducing labour in women with pre-eclampsia, eclampsia or with cardiac or renal disease as they have diuretic and natriuretic effects. In intrauterine foetal death, **PGE_2** alone or with oxytocin seems to cause evacuation effectively.

Carboprost **($PGF_{2\alpha}$ derivative)** has been successfully used to control postpartum haemorrhage when oxytocin or methyl ergonovine are of no avail.

3) Healing of Peptic Ulcer

PGE_1 and **PGE_2** have remarkable cytoprotective effects against peptic ulcers. ***Misoprostol*** (a stable PGE_1 analogue) is orally administered in a dose of 200 μg four times daily for this purpose. This and other **PGE_2 analogue** ***(enprostil)*** are used for healing peptic ulcer in patients of NSAIDs-induced ulcers or in persons who are chronic heavy smokers.

4) To Prevent Platelet Aggregation

As discussed above, TXA_2 promotes platelet aggregation and PGI_2 inhibits it. **PGI_2** derivative ***(epoprostenol)*** can be used to prevent platelet aggregation in extra-corporeal circulation such as renal dialysis and cardiopulmonary bypass. **PGE_1** and **PGI_2**, in smaller amounts, can also be used for storage of platelets for transfusion.

5) To Treat Pulmonary Hypertension

A **PGI_2 preparation** ***(epoprostenol),*** lowers peripheral, pulmonary and coronary resistance. By providing I.V. infusion, the drug has been used to treat pulmonary hypertension. A longer-acting **PGI_2 analogue**, ***treprostinil*** has been approved for use in pulmonary hypertension by I.V, S.C and inhalation route.

6) For Patency of Ductus Arteriosus

Both **PGE_2** and **PGI_2** are responsible for maintaining the patency of foetal ductus arteriosus. **PGE_1** being vasodilator and inhibitor of platelet aggregation also plays the same role. In certain types of congenital heart disease, like pulmonary artery stenosis, it becomes essential to maintain the patency of neonate's ductus arteriosus prior to or during surgery. This is done by giving I.V. infusion of ***alprostadil*** (**PGE_1**) or ***epoprostenol*** (**PGI_2** preparation).

7) Peripheral Vascular Disease

PGE_1 or PGI_2 infused I.V. can promote ulcer healing in acute intermittent claudication. ***Beraprost*** is a stable oral **PGI_2 derivative** which is given thrice a day for treating peripheral vascular disease.

8) For Treating Glaucoma

Ocular drops of ***latanoprost*** (a stable, long-acting **$PGF_{2\alpha}$ derivative**) has shown efficacy similar to timolol in reducing intraocular pressure (*via* FP receptor action). Other drugs in this series include ***bimatoprost, travoprost*** & ***unoprostone (see ch. 11).***

9) Miscellaneous Uses

a) ***Male impotence:*** Intracavernosal injection or uretheral suppository of ***alprostadil*** (**PGE_1**) is used to treat erectile dysfunction. Side effects include pain but priapism is less common.

b) ***To reduce infarct size:*** Intravenous infusion of **PGI_2** ***(iloprost),*** in the immediate post-MI period, can help reducing the infarct size but efficacy is doubtful.

c) ***Bronchial asthma:*** Areosolised PGE_2 effectively aborts the acute attack of asthma but clinical utility is limited because of coughing as side effect.

Side Effects of Prostanoids

Abortifacient PGs exhibit dose-related adverse effects such as vomiting, diarrhoea, fever and broncho-constriction. Hypotension, syncope, dizziness and flushing can also occur which may be related to the vasomotor and vasovagal effects of **PGE_2**. The intra-amniotic injection of ***carboprost*** (**$PGF_{2\alpha}$ derivative**), to induce second-trimester abortions can cause anaphylactic shock and cardiovascular collapse. $PGF_{2\alpha}$ has a greater gastrointestinal toxicity than PGE_2. $PGF_{2\alpha}$ should be used with caution in persons having asthma.

Prolonged treatment with ***alprostadil*** **(PGE_1)**, for maintaining the patency of ductus arteriosus, should be avoided as it may lead to ductus fragility and rupture.

Misoprostol **(PGE_1)** and ***enprostil*** **(PGE_2 analogue)**, used for the treatment of peptic ulcer, usually cause GIT discomfort and diarrhoea. However, these side effects are dose related. Recently, dose-dependent hyperostosis and bone pain has been reported in patients having liver disease, if these drugs are used on a long-term basis. This results due to PGE induced, EP_4-receptor mediated increase in osteoclast and osteoblast activity. Recurrent renal Ca^{2+} oxalate stones may be another problem due to PGE-induced hypercalciuria.

$PGF_{2\alpha}$ analogues (latanoprost and bimatoprost) used for treating glaucoma, produce blurred vision, brown pigmentation of iris and dryness in eyes.

BASIC PHARMACOLOGY OF LEUKOTRIENES

Leukotrienes play a role in numerous physiological functions. Specific receptors and actions of leukotrienes include the following:

Leukotriene Receptors

Receptors for leukotrienes are termed as LT-receptors: ***BLT receptors*** for LTB_4 and ***cys-LT receptors*** for LTC_4, LTD_4 and LTE_4. All LT receptors are GPCRs and function through IP_3 /DAG transducer mechanism.

Pharmacological Actions of Leukotrienes

1) Blood

LTB_4 is a potent chemoattractant for neutrophils (BLT_1 receptor action) while cysteinyl-leukotrienes (LTC_4 and LTD_4) are potent chemoattractants for eosinophils. LTC_4 and LTD_4 also promote eosinophil adherence, degranulation and oxygen radical formation.

2) Heart and Blood Vessels

LTC_4 and LTD_4 reduce myocardial contractility and coronary blood flow (cardiac depression). These are potent chemoattractants for vascular smooth muscle cells and may play a role in myointimal proliferation that occurs after vascular injury such as that caused by angioplasty.

3) GIT Smooth Muscle

LTB_4 causes neutrophil chemotaxis that has been associated with inflammatory bowel disease. The colonic mucosa of patients with inflammatory bowel disease contains increased amounts of LTB_4.

4) Bronchial Smooth Muscle

The actions of LTs within the pulmonary system include: bronchoconstriction, increased permeability and increased mucus secretion (cys-LT_1 and cys-LT_2 receptor action). The cysteinyl-LTs (LTC_4, LTD_4 and LTE_4) are mainly involved in causation of asthma. LTE_4 is less potent compared to LTC_4 and LTD_4 but it is longer acting.

5) Inflammation

LTB_4 is an important mediator in all types of inflammation. LTB_4 can be found in inflammatory conditions, including rheumatoid arthritis, psoriasis and ulcerative colitis.

Leukotrienes Synthesis Inhibitors and Receptor Antagonists

Zileuton: It is 5-lipoxygenase enzyme inhibitor and thus blocks formation of all leukotrienes and prevents all LT-induced responses. It is used as antiasthmatic-anti-inflammatory agent. It has a shorter duration of action and exhibits hepatotoxicity. These limitations have restricted its use.

Zafirlukast, ***Montelukast***, ***Pranlukast*** and ***Iralukast***: These are cys-LT_1 receptor (or LTD_4 receptor) antagonists. These agents reduce bronchospasm and associated symptoms that are mediated through LTs. These can be given orally and are indicated for prophylactic therapy of asthma mainly as an alternative to inhaled glucocorticoids (especially children who comply poorly with inhaled therapies). Side effects are mild GIT upset and headache. Sudden withdrawal of glucocorticoids in patients taking zafirlukast has precipitated a Churg-Strauss syndrome (eosinophilia and vasculitis). Montelukast is safer in this regard.

CHAPTER 26 Nonsteroidal Anti-inflammatory Agents, Drugs for Gout and Antirheumatoid Drugs

COMPETENCY PH1.16

Pain is whatever a person says it is and exists wherever a person says that it exists. There are two components in pathophysiology of pain: (i) the peripheral component in which nociceptive afferent neurons are activated by noxious stimulus and (ii) the central component through which afferent inputs generate a pain sensation. There are two main classes of pain: (i) integumental pain (i.e., superficial, related to skin, muscle and joints) and (ii) visceral pain (i.e., deep seated, related to heart, stomach, kidney and gall bladder). The physiological peripheral pain receptors are the free nerve endings which get sensitised by different proinflammatory autacoids like bradykinin, prostaglandins, histamine, 5-HT and interleukins (as discussed in Ch. 24 & 25). The **N**on-**S**teroidal **A**nti-**I**nflammatory **D**rugs (**NSAIDs** or non-narcotic or non-opioid analgesics), are more effective against pain associated with inflammation (i.e., for integumentary pain). Narcotic analgesics (or opioid analgesics related to morphine) are mainly used to treat deep seated visceral pain (Ch. 37).

This chapter deals with the drugs used to treat pain, fever and inflammation. Other anti-inflammatory drugs considered in this chapter are antirheumatoid agents and drugs used to treat gout. Although glucocorticoids are the main steroidal anti-inflammatory agents (Ch. 42), the nonsteroidal anti-inflammatory drugs (NSAIDs), of which aspirin is the prototype, are among the most widely used therapeutic agents some of which are often taken without prescription for minor aches and musculoskeletal pains. The common characteristics of all the NSAIDs are as follows: (i) none of them is a steroid; (ii) all of them are analgesic-antipyretic and, barring paracetamol, all are anti-inflammatory; (iii) they do not produce CNS depression, respiratory depression (in therapeutic doses) and do not cause drug dependence (like opioid analgesics); (iv) they have dose-dependent uricosuric action, and (v) they act by inhibiting prostaglandin synthesis, except nimesulide which has some other modes of action as well; and nefopam which does not act through PG synthesis inhibition (see following text).

CLASSIFICATION OF NSAIDs

I) **Nonselective Irreversible Inhibitors of COX** (COX-1 > COX-2): Aspirin (acetylsalicylic acid), Sodium salicylate, Sulfasalazine, Olsalazine, Methylsalicylate

II) **Nonselective Reversible Inhibitors of COX** (COX-1 = COX-2): Oxyphenbutazone, Indomethacin, Sulindac, Ibuprofen, Ketoprofen, Flurbiprofen, Naproxen[2], Mefenamic acid, Tenoxicam[1], Piroxicam[1], Ketorolac, Tolmetin, Oxaprozin[1], Diflunisal[2], Diclofenac, Aceclofenac, Nepafenac.

III) **Weak Inhibitor of COX-1 < COX-2 Plus Other Modes of Anti-inflammatory Action**: Nimesulide (5 to 10 fold COX-2 selective)

IV) **Preferential COX-2 Inhibitors** (10 to 20 fold COX-2 selective): Meloxicam[2], Etodolac, Nabumetone[2]

V) **Selective COX-2 Inhibitors** (>50 fold COX-2 selective): Rofecoxib[2], Celecoxib[2], Valdecoxib[2], Etoricoxib[2], Parecoxib[2]

VI) **COX-3 Inhibitor (?) or Reversible Inhibitors of Hypothalamic COX-1**: Paracetamol, Metamizol (Analgin)

VII) **NSAIDs Which do not Inhibit Prostaglandin Synthesis**: Nefopam, Diacerein

[1] Plasma half-life of more than 50 hrs.

[2] Plasma half-life of 10 to 30 hrs.

MECHANISM OF ACTION

When a tissue is injured, from any cause, prostaglandin (PG) synthesis in that tissue increases.

PGs have two major actions: **(1)** they are mediators of inflammation which also sensitise pain receptors at the nerve endings, lowering their threshold of response to stimuli and **(2)** they allow other mediators of inflammation, e.g., histamine, 5-HT and bradykinin etc., to intensify the activation of the sensory nerve endings. Naturally, a drug that prevents the synthesis of PGs is likely to be effective in relieving pain due to inflammation of any kind. NSAIDs, although structurally heterogeneous, possess a common mode of action which is to inhibit the cyclo-oxygenase (COX) enzyme in the arachidonic acid cascade to prevent the synthesis of prostanoids (PGs, PGI_2 and TXA_2; see Fig. 25.1).

Mainly there are two types of cyclo-oxygenase enzymes, namely COX-1 and COX-2. A third form, COX-3, has also recently been identified. COX-1 is constitutively expressed, i.e., it is always present in most of the cells. Majority of traditional NSAIDs in current practice are nonselective inhibitors of both COX-1 and COX-2, though they vary in the degree of COX inhibition (see classification). ***Aspirin*** and its derivatives cause an irreversible inactivation of COX, acting on both COX-1 (including that present in GIT and platelets) and COX-2. With others, COX inhibition, though nonselective, is reversible. It now appears that their analgesic-antipyretic and antiplatelet aggregation effects are mediated through inhibition of COX-1; while the anti-inflammatory action is mainly related to their inhibition of COX-2. Their unwanted effects in GIT are largely a result of their inhibition of COX-1. In the group of nonselective reversible inhibitors of COX, most have selectivity for COX-1. However, some drugs such as ***piroxicam, tenoxicam, mefenamic acid derivatives, diclofenac sodium, sulindac*** and ***diflunisal*** exhibit less than five fold selectivity for COX-2 also.

COX-2 is not constitutively expressed; rather it is inducible in inflammatory cells by an inflammatory stimulus (e.g., endotoxins, cytokines and tumour necrosis factor-α). It is a predominant COX at the site of inflammation but not at the sites such as GIT and platelets. Drugs with a selective inhibition of COX-2 are ***celecoxib, parecoxib, valdecoxib*** and ***etoricoxib*** These have more than 50-fold selectivity for COX-2. These are potent and safe anti-inflammatory drugs as they have lesser GIT side effects. However, they lack antiplatelet aggregatory effects (COX-2 is absent in platelets). There are other NSAIDs like ***meloxicam, etodolac*** and ***nabumetone*** which exhibit 10–20 fold COX-2 selectivity and therefore are classified as preferential COX-2 inhibitors. ***Nimesulide*** is a unique NSAID in the sense that beside having about 10 fold selectivity for COX-2 it has some other modes of anti-inflammatory action also. Reactive oxygen radicals (superoxides) produced by neutrophils and macrophages play a prominent role in tissue damage. ***Nimesulide*** (also ***sulindac***) has a strong oxygen free radical scavenging effect, along with COX-1 and COX-2 inhibitory activity, which may further help in its anti-inflammatory activity by preventing tissue damage. Nimesulide also inhibits PAF synthesis, TNF_α release and metalloproteinase activity in cartilage.

A new COX isozyme (COX-3) has also been identified recently. In humans, COX-3 mRNA is expressed most abundantly in cerebral cortex and the heart. COX-3 is involved in pain perception and fever but not in inflammation. It is a splice variant of COX-1 isoform. ***Paracetamol*** is reported to be a selective COX-3 inhibitor. Paracetamol (acetaminophen) is one of the most commonly used non-narcotic analgesic-antipyretic agents. It has negligible anti-inflammatory action. Another explanation offered for the lack of anti-inflammatory action is its poor ability to inhibit COX-1 in the presence of peroxides which are generated peripherally at inflammatory sites (by the leukocytes) but are not produced in hypothalamus. It does not inhibit COX-2.

NONSELECTIVE IRREVERSIBLE INHIBITORS OF COX

Aspirin

Pharmacologically Useful Actions and Therapeutic Uses

Analgesia

By inhibiting the PG synthesis, aspirin blocks the pain-sensitising mechanisms induced by bradykinin,

TNF_{α} and interleukins. It relieves integumental pain associated with inflammation and tissue injury, but is relatively ineffective in severe visceral (e.g., renal colic, biliary colic or intestinal colic) and ischaemic pain (e.g., in MI). Some evidence supports its central action at subcortical level which raises the threshold to pain perception. However, there is no sedation, no tolerance or drug dependence on its use.

THERAPEUTIC USES: It is used for headache, backache, toothache, myalgia, neuralgia, dysmenorrhoea, rheumatoid arthritis and pain of cancer metastases in bone. Relief in headache probably results also due to a marked reduction in PG-induced cerebral vasodilatation. Effective analgesic-antipyretic dose is 300–600 mg, 6 to 8 hourly.

Antipyretic Action

Aspirin reduces body temperature in fever but does not affect normal body temperature. By inhibiting both COX-1 and COX-2, it reduces PG synthesis in the hypothalamus and resets the "hypothalamic thermostat". During fever, due to infection or inflammation, bacterial endotoxins release IL-1 from the macrophages. This stimulates the generation of PGEs which cause elevation of the set point of temperature in the hypothalamus. Once there has been a return to the normal set point, the temperature regulating mechanisms such as sweating and cutaneous vasodilatation then operate to reduce fever.

THERAPEUTIC USES: In the analgesic doses described above it is effective in reducing fever of any origin. In higher doses, 75–100 mg/kg/day (in divided doses), it is effective in reducing rheumatic fever.

Anti-inflammatory Effects

Anti-inflammatory actions of aspirin also result due to inhibition of PG synthesis. A decrease in vasodilator PGs (PGE_2 and PGI_2) means lesser vasodilatation and indirectly less oedema. Besides inhibiting PGE_2 and PGI_2, aspirin also stabilises leukocyte lysosomal membrane and increases the resistance of connective tissue mucopolysaccharides to prevent the spread of inflammation.

THERAPEUTIC USES: In higher doses (3–6 g/day or 75–100 mg/kg/day) it can be used to treat osteoarthritis, rheumatoid arthritis and rheumatic fever. However, the progression of underlying disease in such cases is not affected. Further, such large doses of aspirin are poorly tolerated for longer period. The newer NSAIDs are therefore preferred by most clinicians.

Inhibition of Platelet Aggregation

Thromboxane A_2 enhances, while PGI_2 decreases platelet aggregation. Aspirin irreversibly inactivates COX-1. Theoretically, it should reduce both TXA_2 synthesis in platelets as well as PGI_2 synthesis in vascular endothelium. However, if low doses of aspirin (75–100 mg) are used, it irreversibly inhibits TXA_2 production by inhibiting COX-1 of platelets for their total life span (7 days). This is because, the platelets lack nuclei and cannot synthesise COX. Such small doses do not affect PGI_2 synthesis in the widely distributed vascular endothelium which can regenerate COX if at all inhibited to some extent. Consequently, low doses of aspirin given intermittently are sufficient to decrease the synthesis of TXA_2 without drastically reducing PGI_2 synthesis.

Controversy exists about the use of low doses of aspirin (75–100 mg/day) to inhibit platelet aggregation. In fact, urinary metabolites of TXA_2 keep on increasing in patients who had MI, even when they were receiving low-dose aspirin. At this dose, though, TXA_2 synthesis in platelets remains inhibited, its synthesis and availablity through other cells like monocytes and eosinophils continues. Hence, some clinicians prefer a moderate dose of aspirin (325 mg/day) to prevent thrombotic events in cases of MI.

THERAPEUTIC USES: Aspirin is used to lower the risk of reinfarction in post-MI and post-stroke patients. Aspirin reduces "transient ischaemic attacks", risk for deep vein thrombosis and pulmonary embolism.

Relief in Dysmenorrhoea

Levels of PGEs in menstrual flow and that of $PGF_{2\alpha}$ in circulation are raised in dysmenorrhoea.

Menstrual cramps result due to intermittent ischaemia of the myometrium while ischaemia results due to PG-induced uterine contractions. Aspirin decreases uterine PG levels to provide relief in myometrium ischaemia.

THERAPEUTIC USE: Aspirin provides excellent relief in dysmenorrhoea. Excess flow is also normalised.

Closure of Ductus Arteriosus

During foetal circulation, ductus arteriosus is kept patent by PGE_2 and PGI_2. This synthesis is switched off at birth for time being and the ductus closes. Low doses of aspirin can bring about this closure by inhibiting PGs synthesis, if this fails to occur at birth.

Miscellaneous Effects and Therapeutic Uses

Aspirin provides benefits in not only pain and inflammation but in increasing number of other conditions as well:

a) **Colonic and Rectal Cancer**. Regular and sustained use of aspirin is reported to reduce the risk of colonic and rectal cancer. However, COX-2 inhibitors may be more effective as colonic tumours express large quantities of COX-2.
b) **Pre-eclampsia**. Aspirin (100 mg/day) benefits in pre-eclampsia by selectively suppressing TXA_2 production.
c) **Alzheimer's Disease**. There is some evidence now that regular intake of small doses of aspirin lowers the risk and retards the onset of Alzheimer's disease.
d) **Familial Colonic Polyposis**. Aspirin in low doses suppresses polyp formation in colon and provides symptomatic relief in this rare disorder.
e) **Niacin Induced Cutaneous Flush and Pruritus**. This probably is mediated through PGs and can be reduced significantly by premedication with low doses of aspirin (See Ch. 23).
f) **To Slow down Catract Progression**. Aspirin (also paracetamol and ibuprofen) have been reported to slow down cataract formation by protecting the proteins of the lens against non-enzymatic glycosylation and carbamylation. However, the doses used were higher (50 mg/kg to 100 mg/kg of body weight).

Pharmacologically Unwanted (Adverse) Effects

Gastric Mucosal Damage

PGE_2 and PGI_2 inhibit gastric acid secretion, stimulate mucus and bicarbonate formation and dilate mucosal blood vessels. Aspirin inhibits COX-1 and therefore nullifies these gastro-protective effects of PGs. Hence, common GIT side effects include dyspepsia, diarrhoea, nausea, vomiting, gastric bleeding and even necrosis and ulceration. Besides inhibiting PG synthesis, local "ion-trapping" of aspirin also plays a significant role in gastric mucosal damage. Aspirin, being a weakly acidic drug, remains unionised in gastric acid juice and can enter the gastric mucosal cells by passive diffusion. Once inside, it ionises (cellular pH 7.2) and becomes trapped, being indiffusible. This "ion-trapping" in gastric mucosal cells also enhances its gastric toxicity. COX-2 inhibitors and paracetamol cause significantly less damage (see following text and Ch. 25).

Effect on Respiration and Acid-Base Balance

These effects are dose dependent. Aspirin in therapeutic doses causes only a mild uncoupling of oxidative phosphorylation which leads to a mild increase in O_2 consumption and CO_2 production. The concomitant stimulation of respiration washes out CO_2 and hence shortly, P_{CO_2} levels become normal. The acid-base balance, therefore, is not disturbed in therapeutic doses.

As plasma levels of aspirin increase (400–500 μg/ml) there is hyperponea due to direct stimulation of respiratory centre. P_{CO_2} levels get decreased and ***"respiratory-alkalosis"*** results. This leads to ***"salicylism"*** which is a mild complication characterised by headache, vertigo, tinnitus, hyperventilation, nausea and vomiting. Renal mechanisms compensate for the respiratory alkalosis by increasing the excretion of HCO_3^- from the kidney so that the normal acid-base balance is again restored. However, if treatment of *salicylism* is necessary, systemic acidifying agents like ascorbic acid or ammonium chloride may be given along with I.V. fluids.

At plasma levels of 500 μg–1 mg/ml, aspirin causes medullary depression and hence respiratory depression. Pco_2 levels, therefore, become elevated. Since plasma HCO_3^- reserves are already depleted, in compensating respiratory alkalosis earlier, moderate toxicity called ***"respiratory acidosis"*** results.

Plasma levels above 1 mg/ml of aspirin cause severe and lethal toxicity in the form of ***"metabolic acidosis"***. Three mechanisms simultaneously operate and culminate in metabolic acidosis: (1) plasma pH being already acidic, aspirin is hydrolysed to free salicylic acid, (2) due to depression of vasomotor centre and failure of renal functions, there is accumulation of metabolic acids like H_3PO_4 and H_2SO_4, and (3) due to an absolute uncoupling of oxidative phosphorylation, there is decrease in ATP formation and derangement of carbohydrate and fat metabolism. This leads to an accumulation of lactic acid, pyruvic acid and acetoacetic acid. Symptoms of metabolic acidosis include, loss of vision, hyperpyrexia, vasomotor collapse, renal and respiratory failure, dehydration, convulsions, coma and ultimately death. *Hyperpyrexia due to aspirin, which itself is an antipyretic, sounds paradoxical.* However, during metabolic acidosis, there is an absolute uncoupling of oxidative phosphorylation which leads to increased oxygen consumption and consequently an increased liberation of energy. Because of absolute uncoupling, this energy cannot be utilised to couple inorganic phosphates to energy rich organic phosphates (ATP). This unutilised energy gets manifested as *hyperpyrexia* during metabolic acidosis.

Infants show greater incidence of metabolic acidosis compared to adults because: (1) children have low protein binding capacity, hence plasma concentration of free drug increases swiftly, (2) children in fever are more acidotic and underhydrated. This further increases plasma concentration of free salicylic acid and (3) two features of salicylism—tinnitus and headache—are usually missed in infants because of their inability to describe these features. As a result the stage of respiratory alkalosis is usually missed which then swiftly passes on to metabolic acidosis.

Increase in Bleeding Tendency

Long-term use of aspirin decreases prothrombin levels by decreasing proconvertin (factor V). Hence, it prolongs prothombin time and increases bleeding tendency. Aspirin should be stopped one week before surgery and is contraindicated in haemophilia.

Hypersensitivity

With inhibition of COX by aspirin, there is consequent diversion of arachidonic acid to 5'-lipoxygenase pathway leading to an increase in the formation of leukotrienes. Leukotrienes are potent broncho-constrictors and some of them are primary component of the slow reacting substance of anaphylaxis. Anaphylactoid reaction to aspirin includes bronchial asthma, skin rashes, rhinitis and angioneurotic oedema. Drugs like ***zileuton***, which blocks 5-lipoxygenase enzyme prevents intolerance to aspirin (Ch. 25).

Effect on Uric Acid Excretion

Low doses of aspirin (< 2 g/day) decrease uric acid excretion and antagonise uricosuric effect of probenecid. High doses (> 5 g/day) increase uric acid excretion (uricosuric effect). However, aspirin is not a suitable drug for gout mainly because such high doses are not tolerated and also because better drugs are now available for treatment of gout.

Renal Effects

Therapeutic doses of aspirin, in normal person, pose little threat to kidney functions; but in susceptible patients (with CHF, hepatic cirrhosis and renal disease) it causes acute, but reversible renal insufficiency. This results through the inhibition of PGE_2 mediated compensatory vasodilatation that occurs in response to angiotensin II (Fig. 18.1). Chronic aspirin consumption in such cases can cause "analgesic nephropathy", characterised by chronic nephritis and renal papillary necrosis.

Reye's Syndrome

There is an association between aspirin intake and *Reye's syndrome*, which is a rare and at times fatal disorder in children. It is characterised by liver damage and encephalopathy which occurs when they are recovering from febrile viral infection. Hence, paracetamol and not aspirin, should be preferred in fever of unknown origin in children below 12 years.

Drug Interactions

If given concomitantly with warfarin, aspirin can cause a hazardous increase in the risk of bleeding by displacing warfarin from plasma protein binding sites. Aspirin interferes with the effect of uricosuric drugs like *probenecid* and *sulfinpyrazone,* and since low doses of aspirin by themselves reduce uric acid excretion such combination should not be used in gout.

Salient Features of Other Nonselective Irreversible Inhibitors of COX

- METHYL SALICYLATE: For external use only as a counter-irritant. Used in balms. Also known as "oil of wintergreen".
- SALICYLIC ACID: It is keratolytic agent used for local treatment of corn and warts.
- SODIUM SALICYLATE: It is a non-acetylated derivative of aspirin. Seldom used, being much less potent than aspirin.
- SULFASALAZINE: It is poorly absorbed after oral administration but is cleaved into 5-aminosalicylic acid (5-ASA) and sulfapyridine by the bacteria in the colon. It is used to treat ulcerative colitis (an inflammatory bowel disease). Enteric coated tablets are used to treat rheumatoid arthritis (see following text). OLSALAZINE is an analogue of sulfasalzine.

NONSELECTIVE REVERSIBLE INHIBITORS OF COX

The salient features of some commonly used NSAIDs of this group are summarised below:

- DIFLUNISAL: m-Difluorophenyl derivative of aspirin. More potent anti-inflammatory-analgesic than aspirin, but has no antipyretic action (does not cross BBB). It is not metabolised to salicylic acid and hence no salicylism. Seldom used except, at times, for cancer pain with bone metastases.
- INDOMETHACIN: Indole derivative. Inhibits phospholipase A_2 also, and has some immunosuppressive actions as well. More potent than aspirin. Effective in gout but preferred in ankylosing spondylitis. Produces more GIT upset and is less tolerated. Contraindicated in psychiatric cases and in epilepsy (causes hallucinations, convulsions, vertigo and confusion in higher doses). Also contraindicated in pregnancy. Dose 25 mg BD or TDS.
- OXYPHENBUTAZONE: Now obsolete. More toxic, GIT upset, peptic ulcer and bone marrow suppression. Oxyphenbutazone is an active metabolite of phenylbutazone.
- IBUPROFEN: Adverse effects less than aspirin. Better tolerance but hypersensitivity can occur. Dose 400 mg TDS.
- KETOPROFEN: Same as ibuprofen with additional lysosomal stabilising action. Inhibits both COX-1 and 5 lipoxygenase but is not superior than other NSAIDs. Dose 50 mg BD or TDS.
- FLURBIPROFEN: Not superior to aspirin or ibuprofen. Dose 50–100 mg TDS. Also available as eye drops for postoperative anti-inflammatory effects and as gel for topical application.
- DICLOFENAC SODIUM/POTASSIUM: Moderate potency with moderate risk of GIT side effects. 99.5% protein bound, *hence not suitable for I.V. use*. Dose 50–100 mg orally TDS. It also reduces superoxide generation at inflammatory sites. Topical use as gel and ophthalmic use as drops. It has been implicated in the increased risk of myocardial ischaemia and infarction.
- ACECLOFENAC: Same as diclofenac, but longer acting. Dose 100 mg BD orally. 99% protein bound, *hence not suitable for I.V. use.*
- NAPROXEN: Longer acting. Moderate potency with moderate risk of GIT side effects. Also inhibits leukocyte migration. Also useful in gout. Dose 250 mg BD. Available as gel for topical use.
- OXAPROZIN: Longer acting. Preferred for osteoarthritis and rheumatoid arthritis. Less side effects. Dose 1200 mg once daily.

- MEFENAMIC ACID: Besides COX-1 inhibition, it has PG receptor antagonist action also. Inhibits leukotriene levels as well, by inhibiting phospholipase A_2. Very effective in dysmenorrhoea, besides osteoarthritis. Diarrhoea and skin reactions are likely. Dose 250–500 mg TDS.
- SULINDAC: Less toxic but less potent than indomethacin. Prodrug, converted into an active sulfide metabolite which has longer duration of action. Dose 150–200 mg BD.
- TOLMETIN: Moderately toxic. Efficacy equal to ibuprofen. Dose 400 mg TDS.
- KETOROLAC: Mainly used as eye drops for seasonal allergic conjunctivitis. Orally it can be used in a dose of 10–20 mg QID for short-term management of pain except for obstetric analgesia. Continuous use for >5 days is not recommended.
- PIROXICAM and TENOXICAM: Both are longer acting. Given orally 20 mg once daily. Inhibit activation of neutrophils and decrease IgM rheumatoid factor. Thus, these drugs can inhibit inflammation by different ways. However, GIT side effects and rashes are common. Also available as gel for local application.
- NEPAFENAC ophthalmic is a NSAID, prodrug, converted to amfenac which inhibits COX-1, COX-2 and prostaglandin synthesis. It is used for pain & inflammation associated with cataract surgery. One drop is administered before surgery and continued for 14 days after surgery. Adverse effects are decreased visual acuity, redness, conjunctival oedema, increased IOP and ocular discomfort.

WEAK INHIBITOR OF COX-1 & COX-2 WITH OTHER MODES OF ANTI-INFLAMMATORY ACTION

NIMESULIDE: Relatively weak PG synthesis inhibitor with COX-2 selective inhibition more (5–10 fold) than COX-1. Other mechanisms implicated are: reduced superoxide generation, free radical scavenging action, inhibition of PAF synthesis and of metalloproteinase activity in cartilage (thus preventing its breakdown). Causes no bronchospasm (suitable for asthmatics) and shows no cross tolerance to aspirin. It is contraindicated in cases of hepatic impairment specially in children <5 years. Dose 100 mg BD. Also available as gel for local application.

PREFERENTIAL COX-2 INHIBITORS (10–20 FOLD COX-2 SELECTIVE ACTION)

- ETODOLAC: Lesser GIT toxicity, otherwise no superiority over other established NSAIDs. However, more potent than aspirin. Dose 200–400 mg TDS or QID.
- MELOXICAM: Longer acting. Less toxic than piroxicam and other NSAIDs. Dose 7.5–15 mg once daily.
- NABUMETONE: Longer acting. A prodrug, converted to an active acetic acid derivative in liver. Antipyretic action more marked than aspirin but adverse effects are less. Dose 500–1000 mg once daily.

SELECTIVE COX-2 INHIBITORS (>50 FOLD COX-2 SELECTIVE)

These drugs selectively inhibit COX 2 isoenzyme which is induced at the site of inflammation without affecting the action of COX-1 present in GIT and platelets (see above). Selective COX-2 inhibitors, called **coxibs**, have analgesic, antipyretic and anti-inflammatory actions similar to that of non-selective NSAIDs but with lesser GIT side effects. Likewise COX-2 inhibitors do not have any impact on platelet aggregation and therefore are devoid of the useful cardioprotective effects of traditional NSAIDs like aspirin. On the other hand, on long-term use, COX-2 inhibitors can reduce whole body PGI_2 production without affecting TXA_2 contents of platelets, and thus disturb the cardioprotective PGI_2:TXA_2 ratio. An increase in TXA_2 concentration may exert prothrombotic influence and enhance the risk of myocardial ischaemia and infarction during long-term use of coxibs. For this reason FDA and DCGI have withdrawn ***rofecoxib*** from being marketed as NSAID.

But in patients who do not require platelet inhibition, COX-2 inhibitors seem to be an attractive alternative to classical NSAIDs because of their gastroprotective action. Hence, prior to their use, a risk to benefit ratio between gastroprotection and cardioprotection should always be considered. For their long-term use prophylactic simultaneous use of low doses of aspirin can be considered. Indeed, in a "Celecoxib Long-term Arthritis Safety Study (CLASS)" no increase in cardiovascular risk (compared to classical NSAIDs) was found when aspirin was allowed with celecoxib. However, since COX-2 is constitutively present in the kidney, recommended doses of COX-2 selective inhibitors may cause renal toxicity similar to traditional NSAIDs. COX-2 inhibitors are mainly used to treat osteoarthritis, rheumatoid arthritis, as well as dysmenorrhoea and familial colonic polyposis (see above). These may also be used in gouty arthritis and acute musculoskeletal pain.

CELECOXIB, VALDECOXIB and ETORICOXIB: Plasma half-lives for celecoxib, valdecoxib and etoricoxib are 11, 11 and 22 hrs respectively. The recommended dosage in arthritis are: celecoxib 100–200 mg BD; valdecoxib 10–20 mg once daily and etoricoxib 60–90 mg once daily. Celecoxib and valdecoxib, being sulfonamide derivatives, may cause skin rash. Etoricoxib is structurally related to diclofenac, hence hepatic functions should be watched carefully. Occasional oedema and mild hypertension are common side effects to all coxibs. The toxicity profile of all coxibs is almost similar and they are clinically interchangeable except for their pharmacokinetic characteristics.

PARECOXIB is a COX-2 inhibitor to be used for short-term management of post-operative pain (as an alternative to opioids). It is a prodrug of valdecoxib, but given by parenteral (40 mg deep IM or I.V) route. Adverse effect: mild hepatotoxicity.

COX-3 INHBITORS (?) OR REVERSIBLE INHIBITORS OF HYPOTHALAMIC COX-1 VARIANT

Paracetamol (acetaminophen)

Paracetamol is an active metabolite of phenacetin (now withdrawn because of toxicity). It is one of the most commonly used non-narcotic analgesic-antipyretic agents with negligible anti-inflammatory action.

Recent evidence suggests that paracetamol may act by inhibiting COX-3 in CNS (a splice variant of COX-I isoform). COX-3 is involved in pain perception and fever but not in inflammation. COX-3 mRNA is expressed abundantly in cerebral cortex. Another explanation offered for its lack of anti-inflammatory action is that paracetamol poorly inhibits COX-1 in the presence of superoxides which are generated in periphery at inflammatory sites by leukocytes, but not in hypothalamus where the thermostat set point of body temperature lies. Paracetamol does not stimulate respiration or affect acid-base balance. It does not produce gastric mucosal damage nor affects platelet aggregation. It is not uricosuric either and does not inhibit COX-2.

Indications

Paracetamol is indicated for mild to moderate pain such as headache, myalgia and postpartum pain. For analgesic purposes, it is a preferred drug in patients allergic to aspirin, in patients with haemophilia or with a history of peptic ulcer or bronchial asthma. It is preferred to aspirin in children with viral infection (to avoid danger of Reye's syndrome). Usual dose is 500 mg TDS.

Adverse Effects

In therapeutic doses, it is quite safe and well tolerated. However, nausea or skin rashes may occur occasionally. A reversible but mild increase in hepatic enzymes may occur in absence of jaundice.

Acute Paracetamol Poisoning

Acute toxicity due to paracetamol can occur in children who at this age have lower glucuronide conjugation ability than adults; or in adults, in whom hepatic functions are compromised or in chronic alcoholics in whom there is cytochrome P-450 enzyme induction. The mechanism of toxicity and its treatment is summarised in Fig. 26.1.

Toxic doses of paracetamol cause a serious hepatotoxicity and renal toxicity. Normally, paracetamol is metabolised by glucuronide and sulfate conjugation (major pathway). However, *N*-acetyl-p-benzoquinone imine is a highly toxic minor metabolite formed by cytochrome P-450 enzymatic system (minor pathway). The little amount of the metabolite so formed from the therapeutic doses of paracetamol gets detoxified by glutathione conjugation. With toxic doses of paracetamol (4–5 g/day) larger amounts of this toxic metabolite are formed which cannot be handled and detoxified through glutathione conjugation. Instead, this metabolite forms covalent bonding with hepatic and renal cellular proteins causing necrosis and cell death. Treatment should be started early within 16 hours of paracetamol ingestion. Vomiting should be induced or gastric lavage done. Activated charcoal should be given orally to prevent further absorption. Drug treatment includes administration of *N*-acetycysteine (I.V.) or methionine (orally). Both have SH groups like glutathione. They replenish the stores of glutathione in liver and also themselves conjugate with this toxic metabolite and thus prevent its covalent bonding to hepatic and renal cellular proteins.

Metamizol (Analgin)

This pyrazolone derivative is good analgesic-antipyretic with lesser anti-inflammatory action. It is relatively safer except for producing GIT irritation and at times agranulocytosis. Dose 500 mg BD or TDS orally.

NSAIDs WHICH DO NOT INHIBIT PG SYNTHESIS

Nefopam

It is an atypical NSAID which does not act by PG inhibition (mechanism of action is uncertain). It is used for short-lasting musculoskeletal pain not responding to other NSAIDs. It can also be used for postoperative, dental and cancer pain. It produces

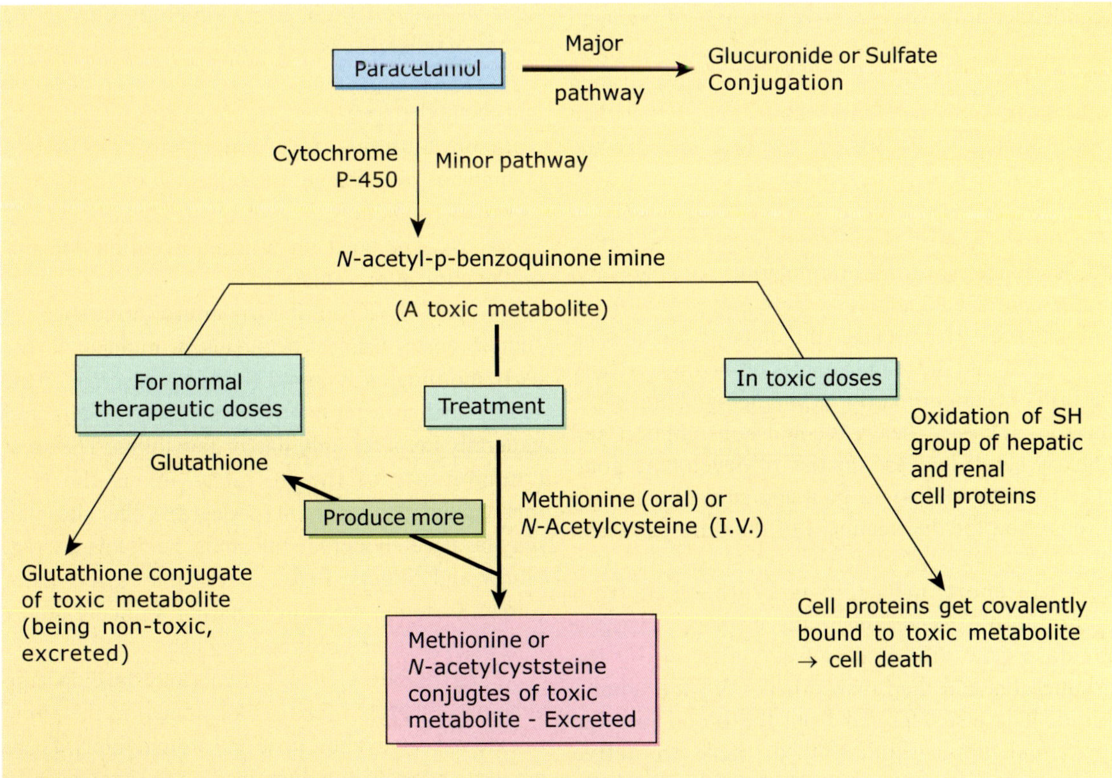

Fig 26.1 Mechanism of Paracetamol Poisoning and its Treatment.

atropine like (dry mouth, urinary retention and blurred vision) and sympathomimetic side effects (tachycardia, tremors and nervousness). Nausea and vomiting are dose dependent. It is contraindicated in patients of MI and epilepsy. Dose is 30 mg TDS.

Diacerein

It is also an atypical NSAID, which inhibits interleukin-1 (IL-1), an important cytokine implicated in osteoarthritis (instead of inhibiting PG synthesis). Dose: 50 mg once a day. Adverse effects: diarrhoea and discolouration of urine. Drug interactions: antacids, prokinetic drugs like metoclopramide and laxatives.

DRUG TREATMENT FOR GOUT

Gout is a metabolic disorder which is always preceded by hyperuricaemia. Uric acid is a waste product produced during metabolism of purines (RNA and DNA subunits). A person who suffers from gout either produces excessive amounts of uric acid or is unable to excrete normally. The result is a build up of uric acid in blood. This excess uric acid then reacts with sodium to form sodium urate, which then accumulates in soft tissues. Typical sites are the kidneys, cartilage of joints and ears. In gouty arthritis, the sodium urate crystals are deposited in the soft tissues of the joints. The crystals irritate the cartilage, causing inflammation, swelling and acute pain. Eventually, the crystals destroy all the joint tissues. If untreated, the ends of articulating bones fuse and the joint becomes immovable. Gouty arthritis occurs primarily in middle aged and older persons. Obesity, heavy alcohol consumption and dietary habits increase the risk of developing gout. The pathophysiology of gout and sites of action of drugs used for the treatment of gout are shown in Fig. 26.2.

In short, uric acid is synthesised from xanthine by the action of the enzyme xanthine oxidase. The uric acid is freely filtered by the glomerulus and then reabsorbed from the tubular fluid. It is also secreted from the blood into the proximal tubule fluid. Both of these are active energy-requiring processes. Both the synthesis as well as reabsorption of uric acid (from the tubule fluid) can be affected by drugs (see below).

With hyperuricaemia, there is precipitation of urate crystals in the synovial fluid. This triggers the inflammatory process involving the infiltration of granulocytes that phagocytise the urate crystals. This process generates free radical metabolites, which damage tissue, resulting in the release of a proteolytic enzyme—a glycoprotein—which further aggravates the inflammatory changes by the release of lactic acid in the synovial tissue. The resultant increase in an "acidic pH" fosters further deposition of urate crystals. Another precipitating factor is the release of lysosomal enzymes that causes more joint destruction and precipitation of urate crystals in synovial fluid. Therefore, the chronic hyperuricaemia is the basic cause of gout. The hyperuricaemia may be primary or secondary. Principally, for therapeutic purposes, patients with *primary hyperuricaemia* (and gout) can be classified as "overproducers" or "underexcretors" of uric-acid. *Secondary hyperuricaemia* (and gout) develops during the course of other disease (leukaemias, lymphomas and polycythaemia, specially when treated with radiation and chemotherapy) or as a result of some drug therapy (thiazide diuretics, furosemide, ethacrynic acid, ethambutol, pyrazinamide and ethanol), or due to some disorders (diabetic ketoacidosis, lead poisoning and psoriasis). The need for drug intervention depends on the clinical presentation.

ACUTE GOUT: It is a painful arthritic attack of sudden onset, usually occurring at night or in the early morning as synovial fluid is readsorbed. This severe arthritic pain progressively worsens and generally involves only one or few joints. The most common site of the initial attack is the first metatarsophalangeal joint (podagra). Other sites that may be affected include the ankle, heel, knee, wrist, elbow and fingers. Later attacks may affect more joints. Systemic symptoms during an acute attack may include fever, chills and malaise.

CHRONIC GOUT: Patients may develop large subcutaneous tophi (chalk like stones) in the pinna of external ear, eyelids, nose and around joints. There are urate crystals in kidney leading to renal disease. Chronic hyperuricaemia leads to the development

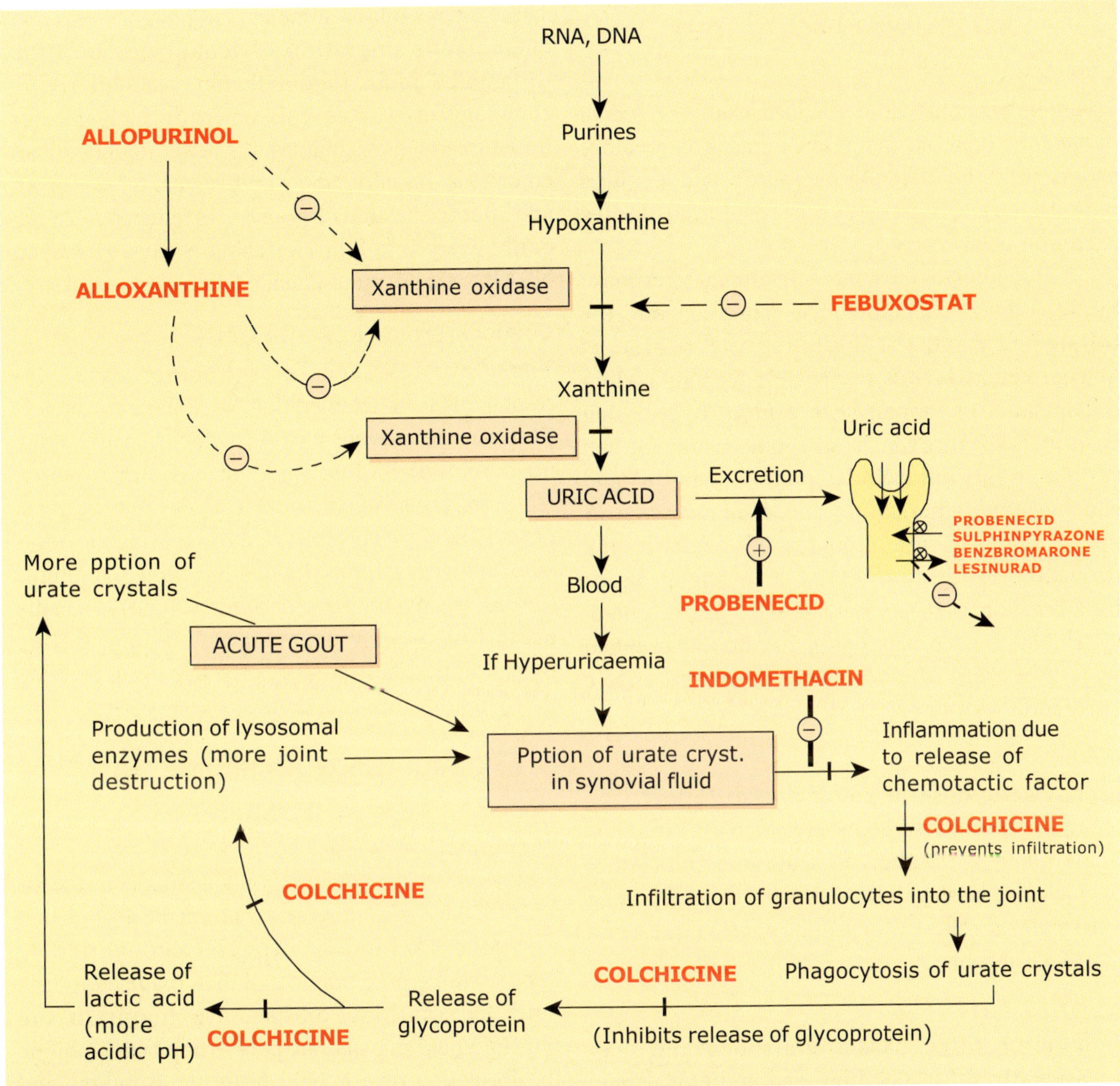

Fig 26.2 Pathophysiology of Gout, and Sites of Action of Drugs Used in Gout

of tophi in the synovia and various periarticular locations. Eventually, articular cartilage may be destroyed resulting in joint deformities. The clinical manifestation is pain and stiffness in the joints which persists in between the attacks.

CLASSIFICATION OF DRUGS USED IN GOUT

I) **DRUGS USED IN ACUTE GOUT** : **(a)** ***Which Inhibit Neutrophil Migration into the Joints:*** COLCHICINE, **(b)** ***Which Inhibit Inflammation and Pain:*** NSAIDs, PREDNISOLONE

II) **DRUGS USED IN CHRONIC GOUT** : **(a)** ***Uric Acid Synthesis Inhibitors:*** ALLOPURINOL, FEBUXOSTAT, **(b)** ***Uricosuric Drugs:*** PROBENECID, SULPHINPYRAZONE, BENZBROMARONE, LESINURAD **(c)** ***Uricase-mimetic Agents:*** PEGLOTICASE

DRUGS USED IN ACUTE GOUT

Colchicine

Colchicine is an alkaloid obtained from *Colchicum autumnale.* It has no analgesic or anti-inflammatory action. It has no effect on blood uric acid levels as it neither inhibits the synthesis nor promotes excretion of uric acid.

It suppresses the gouty inflammatory response by: (a) preventing granulocyte migration into the inflammed joint, (b) inhibiting the release of glycoprotein, which is responsible for aggravating inflammation by forming lactic acid and by releasing lysosomal enzymes which cause joint destruction and (c) binding to intracellular protein 'tubulin' and causing depolymerisation and disappearance of microtubules in granulocytes. As a result, the migration of granulocytes into the area of inflammation is not only distorted but prevented. Colchicine treated neutrophils develop a "drunken walk". Colchicine undergoes enterohepatic circulation.

Indications and Dosage

Prophylactic dose of colchicine for alleviating recurring episodes of gouty arthritis is 0.5 mg/day. For terminating the attack of acute gout, initial dose of colchicine is 1 mg, followed by 0.5 mg every 3 hrs, until pain is relieved or troublesome nausea and diarrhoea appear.

Adverse Effects

Colchicine often causes diarrhoea and may occasionally cause vomiting and abdominal pain (neurogenic stimulation of gut motility). Acute intoxication leads to bloody diarrhoea, throat pain, respiratory depression, haematuria and oliguria. Chronic toxicity may produce agranulocytosis, peripheral neuritis and myopathy.

NSAIDs in Acute Gout

Strong anti-inflammatory drugs like ***indomethacin, naproxen, piroxicam*** and ***diclofenac potassium*** (except aspirin, salicylates and tolmetin) have been successfully used to treat acute gouty episodes. These agents inhibit urate crystal phagocytosis and chemotactic migration of leukocytes into the inflammed joint. Indomethacin, particularly, is commonly used as the replacement of colchicine, for initial treatment of gout, as it is better tolerated than colchicine. Initially, 50 mg orally every 6 hrs is given and after the desired response, it is reduced to 25 mg orally every 6 to 8 hrs for about 5 days. However, NSAIDs are not recommended for long-term use.

Corticosteroids in Acute Gout

These are reserved for refractory cases not responding to or not tolerating NSAIDs or colchicine. Systemic steroids are usually avoided because of the need for larger dose and the ensuing toxicity. However, prednisolone (40–60 mg/day) can be given initially for 3–5 days followed by tapering the doses over 2–3 weeks. Intra-articular injection of a soluble steroid (hydrcocotisone or prednisolone) is usually preferred over suspensions or crystalline preparations. These are very effective in suppressing the symptoms of acute gout.

DRUGS USED FOR CHRONIC GOUT

Uric Acid Synthesis Inhibitors

Allopurinol

Purines which are not incorporated into nucleic acids and also those which are derived from the degradation of nucleic acids are ultimately converted to hypoxanthine or xanthine and then oxidised to uric acid by xanthine oxidase, to maintain the physiological size of urate pool. Allopurinol inhibits the formation of uric acid from hypoxanthine and xanthine by inhibiting the enzyme xanthine oxidase. Allopurinol itself is short acting competitive inhibitor of xanthine oxidase but its major metabolite alloxanthine is a long acting ($t\frac{1}{2}$ 24 hrs) non-competitive inhibitor of xanthine oxidase which mainly contributes for the inhibition of uric acid synthesis (Fig. 26.2).

Allopurinol, therefore, reduces the concentration of the relatively insoluble urates and uric acid in tissues, plasma and urine and decreases the size of urate pool. The deposition of urate crystals in tissues (tophi) is reversed and formation of renal stones is inhibited. Allopurinol is neither analgesic nor anti-inflammatory, nor an anticancer drug, despite being a purine antimetabolite.

Therapeutic Uses

Allopurinol has a longer duration of action (see above) and needs to be given only once daily (start with 100 mg/day, gradually increase at weekly intervals to 300 mg/day). Allopurinol is indicated for the following:

a) Chronic gout, in patients with gouty tophi or nephropathy. It is ineffective in the treatment of acute gout and indeed makes it worse,
b) In patients whose 24 hrs urinary uric acid excretion exceeds 1.1 g,
c) When uricosuric drugs cannot be used because of allergic or other reasons,
d) For recurrent renal urate stones,
e) In secondary hyperuricaemia due to cancer chemotherapy, radiation or thiazide diuretics,
f) During the treatment of blood dyscrasias and other myeloproliferative disorders where cell destruction creates a high urate load leading to formation of renal calculi and
g) Apart from gout, allopurinol is also used as an adjuvant with sodium stibogluconate in the treatment of kala-azar as it inhibits *Leishmania* by altering its purine metabolism.

Adverse Effects

a) Acute attacks of gouty arthritis may get precipitated in the beginning because rapid lowering of plasma urate by any means may precipitate acute gout, probably by causing the dissolution of tophi. To prevent such acute attacks, colchicine or indomethacin should be given during the initial period of therapy with allopurinol;
b) Hypersensitivity reaction, at times, may be severe, e.g., exfoliative skin rash, arthralgia, fever, lymphadenopathy and hepatitis; and
c) GIT distress, nausea, peripheral neuritis and cataract formation (deposition of allopurinol in lens).

Drug Interactions

a) It interferes with the mobilisation of hepatic iron stores; hence haematinics should be avoided during allopurinol therapy,
b) Allopurinol reduces the metabolism of 6-mercaptopurine (an antimetabolite used in cancer chemotherapy) and also that of azathioprine (an immunosuppressant drug used to prevent organ transplant rejection). Xanthine oxidase, which is inhibited by allopurinol, is also needed for the metabolism of these drugs. Hence their doses should be reduced to one-fourth. Allopurinol also enhances the effects of cyclophosphamide, another anticancer drug,
c) It can potentiate the actions of oral anticoagulants and of theophylline by inhibiting their metabolism,
d) Higher incidence of hypersensitivity reactions has been reported if ampicillin is used concomitantly with allopurinol and
e) It should be used with caution during pregnancy, in elderly and in children.

Febuxostat

It is a recently introduced potent and selective inhibitor of xanthine oxidase (compared to allopurinol) and thereby reduces the formation of uric acid (Fig. 26.2). Dose 40–120 mg once daily. It is used for the treatment of chronic gout or secondary hyperuricaemia and is very useful during the intercritical period of gout. *Adverse effects:* Liver dysfunction, diarrhoea, headache. It is very suitable drug for the patients intolerant to allopurinol as it does not produce hypersensitivity reaction seen with allopurinol.

Uricosuric Drugs

Patients of hyperuricaemia can be divided into two categories—*overproducers* or *underexcretors of uric acid.* As discussed above it is logical to use allopurinol in former cases. For underexcretors of uric acid, uricosuric drugs are used.

Probenecid

Probenecid is neither analgesic nor an anti-inflammatory drug. It acts by promoting the excretion of uric acid by inhibiting its active reabsorption from the renal tubule (Fig. 26.2). As the urinary excretion of uric acid increases, the size of urate pool decreases and tophaceous deposits of urate are reabsorbed with relief of arthritis.

Therapeutic Uses

As with allopurinol, it is used for chronic gout and is given with plenty of water and with urinary alkaliniser to prevent formation of renal urate calculi. It should not be given during acute attack of gout unless a cover of NSAIDs (e.g., indomethacin) has been provided. It can also be used to treat secondary hyperuricaemia due to drugs and disease but allopurinol is preferred. Aside from gout, it is also used to prolong penicillin or cephalosporin levels to treat various infections. Dose: 250 mg BD orally then 500 mg BD after one week.

Adverse Effects

Less common except GIT distress and allergic dermatitis. Dyspepsia is the frequent side effect. Toxic doses can lead to nephrotic syndrome and convulsions.

Drug Interactions

a) Low doses of aspirin block uricosuric action of probenecid,
b) Inhibits biliary excretion of rifampicin and
c) It inhibits urinary excretion of penicillins, cephalosporins, methotrexate and indomethacin.

Sulfinpyrazone

It is structurally related to phenylbutazone but has neither analgesic nor anti-inflammatory action. Like probenecid, sulfinpyrazone in subtherapeutic doses prevents secretion of uric acid into tubular fluid; but in therapeutic doses, it powerfully prevents reabsorption of uric acid, increasing its excretion in the urine. Initial dose is 100–200 mg/day orally, increasing over 2 weeks to 600 mg/day to be continued till serum uric acid levels become normal. Thereafter, the maintenance dose may be kept as little as 200 mg/day. During initial therapy, adequate fluid intake is necessary to prevent urate crystalluria. If urate load is high, a urinary alkaliniser may be added.

In chronic gout, its results are comparable to probenecid. Its uricosuric action is additive with probenecid but blocked by salicylates. It inhibits metabolism of warfarin and sulfonylureas.

Adverse effects are mainly gastrointestinal and its use is contraindicated in peptic ulcer. Hypersensitivity reactions are rare.

Benzbromarone

It is a more potent uricosuric drug that can be used in patients who are either allergic or refractory to probenecid or sulfinpyrazone or in patients with renal insufficiency where GFR is as low as 25% of the normal. It is a reversible inhibitor of the tubular reabsorption of uric acid like other uricosuric drugs. It is effective in a single dose which is as little as 60–80 mg/day. Preparations that combine benzbromarone with allopurinol are more effective than either drug alone. However, its uricosuric action is antagonised by sulfinpyrazone or aspirin. Side effects are rare except for GIT distress.

Lesinurad

It is a URAD-1 (Urad transporter-1 present in proximal tubule and is involved in uric acid absorption inhibitor. It is used in the treatement of gout in combination with xanthine oxidase inhibitor, allopurinol in the doses: lesinurad 200 mg+allopurinol 200 mg per day or lesinurad 200 mg+allopurinol 300 mg per day.

Uricase-mimetic Agents

Pegloticase

Uricase or urate oxidase enzyme, normally absent in humans and some higher primates, is involved in converting uric acid to allantoin. Allantoin is highly soluble and can be easily eliminated by the kidney (Fig.26.2 does not depict this step as humans are devoid of this enzyme). **Pegloticase** is a recombinant uricase that has been covalently linked to methoxypolyethylene glycol to increase its circulating half-life (t½ 6–14 days) and reduce immunogenicity. It is a rapidly acting drug, eliciting a peak decline in uric acid level whithin 24–72 hrs. When administered in a dose of 4–12 mg by I.V. infusion, pegloticase decreases the levels of uric acid for up to 21 days, enabling it to be dosed every 2 weeks.

Gout flare can occur during treatment with this drug, especially during the first 3-months. An NSAID or colchicine prophylaxis can prevent such a flare of acute gout. Common ADRs reported with the dosing of pegloticase are nausea, headache, anaemia, arthralgia, msucle regidity and nephrolithiasis. Incidence of haemolytic anaemia has been reported in patients with glucose-6-phosphate dehydrogenase (G-6-PD) deficiency because of the formation of H_2O_2 as a result of uricase activity of the drug; thus this drug should be avoided in G-6-PD deficient patients.

ANTIRHEUMATOID DRUGS: DISEASE MODIFYING ANTIRHEUMATOID DRUGS (DMARDs)

Rheumatoid arthritis (RA) is an immunologic disease that not only affects mobility but the quality of life as well. NSAIDs offer only symptomatic relief in inflammation and pain but have little effect on the progression of bone and cartilage destruction, where cytokines IL-1, IL-6 and TNF_α play a major role in pathogenesis. Interest has therefore emerged to find out drugs which antagonise the effects of these proinflammatory cytokines, so as to arrest or slow down the progress of joint destruction by modifying the pathogenesis of disease itself. The drugs most frequently used for such therapy are called "**D**isease **M**odifying Anti**R**heumatoid **D**rugs (DMARDs)". The DMARDs cover a wide variety of drugs with different chemical groups and with different modes of action, but none of them is able to halt the long-term progression of the disease. Hence the term "disease modifying" seems to cause more confusion than understanding.

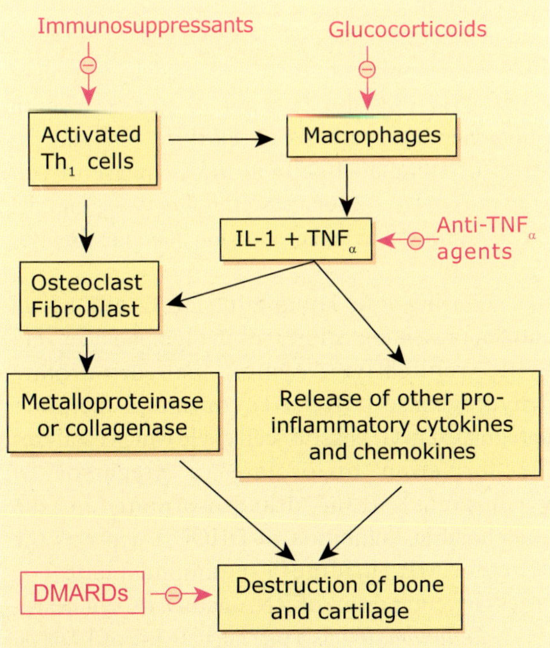

Fig 26.3 Pathogenesis of Rheumatoid Joint Damage and Sites of Action of Antirheumatoid Drugs.

Some cytokines (IL-1, IL-6 and TNF_α) are found in high levels in synovial fluids of patients of RA and activate synovial cells to proliferate and synthesise metalloproteinases and collagenases resulting in degradation of cartilage and stimulation of bone resorption. TNF_α and IL-1 also induce the expression of adhesion molecules resulting in further recruitment of inflammatory cells and release of additional cytokines. Majority of DMARDs neutralise the effects of proinflammatory cytokines. The sites of action of various DMARDs are shown in Fig. 26.3.

TNF_α Blocking Drugs

Although a wide range of cytokines are expressed in the joints of RA patients, TNF_α plays a major role in joint destruction. Its actions are manifold. For example, TNF_α activates the release of nitric oxide which causes vasodilatation and increased vascular permeability. Platelet activation and adhesions are also increased by TNF_α, causing local blood vessel occlusion. These TNF_α effects result after binding to two different "membrane bound TNF receptors ($TNFR_1$ and $TNFR_2$)". These receptors are bound to fibroblasts, neutrophils and vascular endothelial cells. Besides these, there are "soluble form of TNF_α receptors" which are present in serum and synovial fluid. The following three drugs which interfere with TNF_α, by different mechanisms, are used for the treatment of RA.

Etanercept

It is a genetically engineered fusion protein (not a monoclonal antibody) composed of two soluble TNF p75 receptor moieties linked to Fc portion of human IgG_1. This soluble fusion protein serves as an exogenously administered soluble TNF_α receptor which prevents TNF_α from binding to membrane bound TNF receptors (TNFR$_1$ and TNFR$_2$). The drug does not discriminate between TNF$_\alpha$ and TNF$_\beta$ (lymphotoxin). Because TNF$_\beta$ is important in modulating cellular immune response to infection and tumour, there is some concern about the long-term use of etanercept (see adverse effects).

The drug is given S.C. in a dosage of 25 mg twice a week. It is longer acting (serum half-life 115 hours). It is used to treat RA, juvenile arthritis and psoriatic arthritis. It is also used in treating sarcoidosis, Wegener's granulomatosis and scleroderma, though efficacy is controversial. Recent clinical trials showed that the combination of ***etanercept*** with ***methotrexate*** provide greater clinical benefits than either drug alone. Upon discontinuation of *etanercept*, the symptoms of arthritis generally reappear within a month.

Etanercept is well tolerated. Although anti-etanercept antibodies may appear in some patients, it does not appear to interfere with its efficacy. Other less common side effects include drug-induced lupus and activation of latent tuberculosis or opportunistic infections in some patients. At the site of S.C. injection, local pain, swelling or itching may appear.

Infliximab

It is a chimeric (25% mouse and 75% human) monoclonal antibody that cross-links with soluble as well as membrane bound TNF$_\alpha$ receptors and inhibits activated T-cells and macrophage function. Consequently, macrophage and T-cell functions are down-regulated which prevents the release of other proinflammatory cytokines (IL-1, 6 and 8, collagenase and metalloproteinases).

In treating RA it is given by I.V. infusion in a dose of 3–5 mg/kg at 0, 2 and 6 week interval. I.V. infusion should be given over a period of not less than 2 hrs. It can be administered at an interval of 8 weeks thereafter. It is used to treat RA, and has been approved for treating Crohn's disease (increased levels of TNF$_\alpha$ are found in faecal samples of the patients of Crohn's disease). It is being used for treating other diseases also including juvenile chronic arthritis, psoriatic arthritis, Wegener's granulomatosis and sarcoidosis. In RA, a regimen of ***infliximab*** plus ***methotrexate*** is clinically more beneficial than either drug alone.

Adverse effects include upper respiratory tract infections, nausea and headache. Infliximab may also be associated with activation of latent turberculosis and opportunistic infections. Infusion site reaction may occur. Long-term use of infliximab may be associated with the development of anti-infliximab antibodies but not when the drug is used with methotrexate.

Adalimumab

Adalimumab is a recombinant human anti-TNF monoclonal antibody. Its mechanism of action, clinical use and adverse effects profile is similar to infliximab. It has lesser immunogenicity than infliximab. It is given 40 mg S.C. every other week and has a plasma half-life of 9–14 days. Combination with methotrexate is clinically more beneficial.

Immunomodulators

Leflunomide

Leflunomide acts through its active metabolite A77-1726 which inhibits dihydro-orotate dehydrogenase (DHODH) enzyme leading to a decrease in ribonucleotide synthesis (↓ UMP levels) and the arrest of stimulated cells in the G$_1$ phase of cell growth (Fig. 26.4). As a result, *leflunomide* inhibits T-cell proliferation and production of autoantibodies by B-cells.

During RA, stimulation of T-cells by an antigen presenting cell drives the lymphocytes into their replicative cycle. Dihydro-orotate dehydrogenase (DHODH) enzyme is therefore upregulated in G$_1$ phase of cell cycle which catalyses the formation of orotate (a precursor of pyrimidines) from dihydro-orotate in the mitochondria. Inhibition of DHODH deprives the cell of UMP (uridine-5'-monophosphate)—a necessary component of RNA and DNA synthesis.

Leflunomide has a plasma half-life of 19 days. It also undergoes enterohepatic circulation. *Leflunomide*, therefore, is given in a loading dose of 100 mg daily (orally) for three days initially,

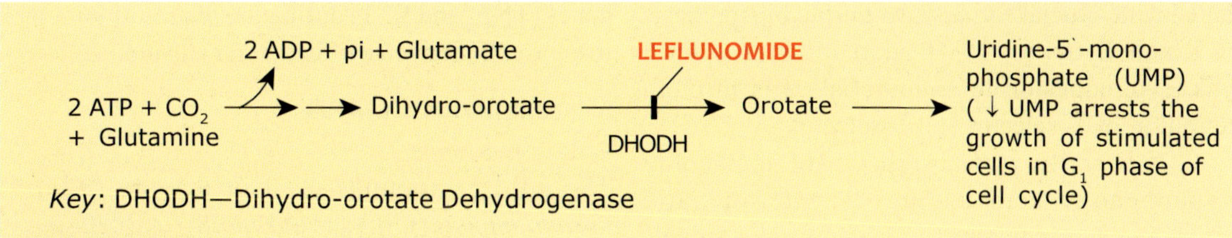

Fig 26.4 Site of Action of Leflunomide.

followed by 10–20 mg OD. It is used for the treatment of RA. Its clinical efficacy has been rated equal to methotrexate but with faster benefits.

Adverse effects include diarrhoea, headache, nausea, rashes, mild alopecia and elevation in hepatic transaminases. It is contraindicated during pregnancy and lactation. Cholestyramine can be used to increase the clearance (or to decrease toxicity) of leflunomide.

Methotrexate

Methotrexate is a folic acid antagonist with cytotoxic and immunosuppressant activity and with potent antirheumatoid action. It is commonly a first-choice DMARD. It has a rapid onset of action, acts at much lower doses than those needed in cancer chemotherapy and has fewer side effects compared to other DMARDs. It acts by inhibiting aminoimidazole-carboxamide ribonucleotide transformylase (AICAR) and thymidylate synthetase. This inhibits replication and function of T-cells (and possibly of B-cells) because of selective inhibition of DNA synthesis.

For RA, methotrexate is used in a dose of 15–25 mg weekly (orally). It can also be used for juvenile chronic arthritis, psoriasis, psoriatic arthritis, Wegener's granulomatosis and subacute lupus erythematosus.

Adverse effects include nausea, mucosal ulcers and progressive dose-related hepatotoxicity (enzyme elevation) but cirrhosis is very rare. Other side effects are breathlessness and pseudo-lymphomatous reaction. The toxicity can be prevented by giving leucovorin 24 hrs after weekly dose of methotrexate.

Cyclosporine

Cyclosporine inhibits IL-1 and IL-2 receptor production. It also inhibits macrophage-T cell interaction and T-cell responsiveness. It is used in doses of 3–5 mg/kg/day (in 2 divided doses). Its major *adverse effect* is nephrotoxicity which is accentuated with NSAIDs, diltiazem, potassium-sparing diuretics and by enzyme inhibitors. Other toxicities involve hypertension, hyperkalaemia, hepatotoxicity, hirsutism and gingival hyperplasia. *Its routine use has been discarded.*

Azathioprine (AZA)

AZA is prodrug for 6-mercaptopurine (6-MP). The slow conversion of AZA to 6-MP and its final conversion to 6-thio GTP provides a counterfeit product which gets falsely incorporated into DNA of lymphocyte, making it nonfunctional. Hence, T-cell activation and proliferation is prevented. AZA is used in organ transplant rejection, rheumatoid arthritis and inflammatory bowel disease. *Its use in RA is on decline because of toxicity.* ***Major side effects*** include bone marrow depression, leukopenia, thrombocytopenia, alopecia, increased risk of herpes simplex and varicella infection, neoplasia, hepatotoxicity and GIT toxicity. Given along with corticosteroids, it has a steroid sparing effect, for which it is primarily used these days.

Mycophenolate Mofetil (MMF)

It is a semisynthetic fungal antibiotic. Its active metabolite, mycophenolic acid, inhibits proliferation of both T and B lymphocytes and reduces the production of cytotoxic T cells by inhibiting cytosine monophosphate dehydrogenase (an enzyme crucial for *de novo* purine biosynthesis in T and B-cells). MMF also interferes with leukocyte adhesion to endothelial cells through inhibition of E-selectin and P-selectin.

It is orally well absorbed. The metabolite mycophenolic acid undergoes enterohepatic circulation and is finally eliminated by the kidney. In a dose of 2 g/day, it is reserved for patients with severe RA that is not adequately controlled by other DMARDs, *but the efficacy is doubtful.* MMF exhibits GIT, haematopoietic and hepatic toxicity profile similar to azathioprine.

Glucocorticoids

Although symptomatic relief is dramatic, there is reluctance to use systemic glucocorticoids for RA because of adverse effects (for details, refer Ch. 42). However, their use is justified in the following circumstances:

- To provide immediate relief in inflammation during the spell required for DMARDs to act, or to buy time to change the DMARD or dose.
- To effectively suppress severe inflammation, e.g., in patients with vasculitis or rheumatoid lung while the patient awaits response from a remission inducing drug.
- To add prednisolone (7.5 mg/day) to the standard DMARD treatment to reduce the rate of joint destruction in moderate RA of less than 2 year duration.
- Intra-articular injection of triamcinolone, hydrocortisone, prednisolone or dexamethasone is advocated when there is involvement of one or two major joints with marked pain, swelling and immobility. Clinical benefit of a single injection lasts for weeks. Injections in one joint should not exceed 2–3 per year.

Immunosuppression by glucocorticoids involves both their effects on the immune response and their anti-inflammatory actions. They inhibit the clonal proliferation of Th_1 cells through decreasing the transcription of the gene for IL-2. However, they also decrease the transcription of many other cytokine genes (TNF_α and IL-1) during the phases of immune response. For adverse effects refer Chapter 42.

Miscellaneous DMARDs

Gold Compounds

The gold compounds used in RA are ***sodium aurothiomalate*** (I.M.) and ***auranofin*** (oral). *Because of their toxicity, the use of gold salts is on decline.* Gold alters the morphology and functional capabilities of human macrophages. Cell-mediated immune reactions are suppressed leading to a reduction in circulating rheumatoid factors and ESR. It prevents joint destruction and induces healing of bony erosions. ***Aurothiomalate*** also reduces lysosomal enzyme activity, reduces histamine release from the mast cells and suppresses the phagocytic activity of polymorphonuclear leukocytes. ***Auranofin*** also inhibits the release of PGE_2, LTB_4, IL-1 and TNF_α.

Gold salts tend to accumulate in synovial fluid, liver, kidney, spleen, lymph nodes and bone marrow. The half-life is 7 days initially but increases with treatment. So the I.M. gold is given in 50 mg dose first at weekly and then at monthly intervals. Oral gold is given in 6 mg doses every day. The oral form of the gold is less effective in RA compared to I.M. gold.

The unwanted effects are dermatitis, stomatitis, exfoliative dermatitis, hepatitis, albuminuria, peripheral neuropathy, pulmonary fibrosis, thrombocytopenia and neutropenia. Adverse effects with auranofin are less frequent and less severe.

Penicillamine

Its D-isomer is effective in treating RA *but seldom used* because of toxicity (Ch. 68). Moreover the effect takes weeks to start and the desired response is not seen for several months. It is a metal chelator also.

Hydroxychloroquine Sulphate (HCQS)

Hydroxychloroquine is primarily an antimalarial drug but because it traps free radicals, suppresses T-lymphocyte responses to mitogens, stabilises lysosomal enzymes and decreases leukocyte chemotaxis, it is useful in patients of RA.

It is less efficacious than gold and is preferred in milder non-erosive RA. It does not retard the progression of bone damage. The response in RA does not appear until a month or two after the drug is started. Like chloroquine it may precipitate corneal deposits and opacity but with HCQS it is less common.

Other effects include rashes, greying of hair, myopathy and neuropathy. Aside RA, it is also used both for systemic and discoid lupus erythematosus. Usual dose: 200 mg BD orally.

Sulfasalazine

Sulfasalazine is a drug which is primarily used in ulcerative colitis because of its anti-inflammatory actions. It is metabolised to sulfapyridine and 5-aminosalicylic acid (5-ASA) in the colon by bacterial action. Sulfapyridine is absorbed systemically and appears to be the active component in treating RA (unlike ulcerative colitis in which 5-ASA acting locally in colon is the active component).

Sulfasalazine decreases rheumatoid factor levels and suppresses the generation of superoxide free radicals and cytokine release by inflammatory cells.

Sulfasalazine half-life is 6–15 hours. The usual oral dose is 500 mg daily for 7 days, increased by 500 mg every week to a maximum of 3 g/day in 2–3 divided doses. It is effective in RA, juvenile chronic arthritis and ankylosing spondylitis. Its efficacy is similar to hydroxychloroquine but is better tolerated than gold and is a better alternative to even methotrexate for early or milder cases of RA.

The common side effects are GIT disturbances, malaise, headache and rashes. About 30% of patients discontinue the drug because of GI intolerance and headache. A reversible decrease in sperm count has also been reported. Reversible leucopenia and methaemoglobinaemia may occur but is rare.

Upadacitinib

Upadacitinib is a disease-modifying antirheumatic drug (DMARD) and approved by US-FDA for the treatment of rheumatoid arthritis to slow down disease progression. It is a Janus kinase (JAK)1-selective inhibitor, which is an essential downstream cell signalling mediator of pro-inflammatory cytokines like IL-6, IL-2 and IL-15. It is given orally. It can be used in psoriatic arthritis, atopic dermatitis and ankylosing spondylitis. *Adverse effects*: Nausea, vomiting, neutropenia, cough, elevated creatine phosphokinase and allergic reactions.

Baricitinib

Baricitinibis a Janus kinases (JAK) pathway inhibitor (blocks JAK1 and JAK2) and blocks further signalling. It has anti-inflammatory effects. It is used for adults with moderately to severely active rheumatoid arthritis who have inadequate response to other drugs. *Adverse effects*: Anaemia, neutropenia, liver dysfunction and increased lipid level.

CHAPTER 27

Treatment of Gastric Acidity, Peptic Ulcer and Gastroesophageal Reflux Disease

COMPETENCY PH1.34

A localised loss of gastric as well as duodenal mucosa leads to the formation of peptic ulcer, a term that includes both gastric as well as duodenal ulcer. Peptic ulcer arises when the normal mucosal defense mechanisms (mucus, mucosal blood flow, formation of HCO_3^- and PGE_2) are impaired or overpowered by the damaging factors (acid, pepsin, NSAIDs and *Helicobacter pylori*). Ulcers occur 5 times more commonly in the duodenum, and 95% of them are found in duodenal bulb or in pyloric channel. Benign gastric ulcers are located most commonly (60%) in the antrum. However, some are located (25%) at the junction of antrum and the fundus of lesser curvature. A gnawing, dull, "hunger like" pain in epigastric region is reported by 80–90% of the patients of peptic ulcer. About half of these patients report a relief of pain after taking food or antacids. There may be a presence of occult blood in faeces (or may be melaena). Barium meal X-ray shows the presence of ulcer crater. The old dictum "No acid-No ulcer" does not seem tenable now, because majority of peptic ulcers are also caused by infection with the bacterium *Helicobacter pylori*.

PHYSIOLOGY OF ACID SECRETION (FIG. 27.1)

Gastric acid is secreted by the parietal cells in gastric mucosa. The basolateral membranes of these cells contain receptors for the three main stimulants of acid secretion, namely gastrin (from antral G-cells), histamine from enterochromaffin-like cell (ECL cells) and acetylcholine (from vagal efferents). Histamine binds to the H_2 receptor, resulting in an increase in intracellular cAMP; while ACh and gastrin exert their effects by causing an increase in cytosolic Ca^{2+}. Both cAMP and cytosolic Ca^{2+} activate protein kinases which in turn stimulate acid secretion through H^+/K^+ ATPase (the proton pump) located on the canalicular surface of parietal cells. To start with, Cl^- is actively transported through the canaliculi into the lumen of the stomach. This Cl^- secretion is accompanied with K^+ which is then exchanged for H^+ within the cell by proton pump (P). H^+ then combines with Cl^- to form HCl, which is secreted into the gastric lumen. The carbonic anhydrase (CA) enzyme catalyses the reaction of water and carbon dioxide to form carbonic acid (H_2CO_3) which then dissociates into HCO_3^- and H^+. These H^+ ions are used for the production of HCl by the proton pump. Bicarbonate ions exchange across the parietal cell for Cl^- ions which are then utilised for the formation of HCl. The bicarbonate ions are ultimately trapped in the mucus, creating a gel like protective layer over the mucosal surface. ACh release from the postganglionic vagal fibres can stimulate gastric acid secretion directly by activating muscarinic M_3 receptor located on parietal cells or through activation of M_1 receptors present on ECL cells which are major sources for histamine release also. Gastrin released from G-cells of the antrum can also stimulate histamine release from ECL cells. Thus, ECL cells are the major source of gastric histamine release needed for acid secretion and that histamine has an obligatory role to play, as a final chemostimulator, in all modes of acid secretion. The chief or peptic cells, found primarily in the gastric fundus, synthesise and secrete pepsinogen, the inactive precursor of the proteolytic enzyme pepsin. The acidic pH < 2.0 within the stomach cleaves pepsinogen to an active pepsin. Too much of pepsin activity erodes gastric mucosa, to form peptic ulcer.

The gastric defense mechanisms, against peptic ulcers, include the presence of prostaglandins (PGE_2 and PGI_2) in the gastric mucosa, the presence of mucin layer over the gastric epithelial cells and the secretion of HCO_3^- into the mucin layer. PGE_2 produced by gastric mucosa, inhibits acid secretion by inhibiting cAMP formation (in parietal cells). In

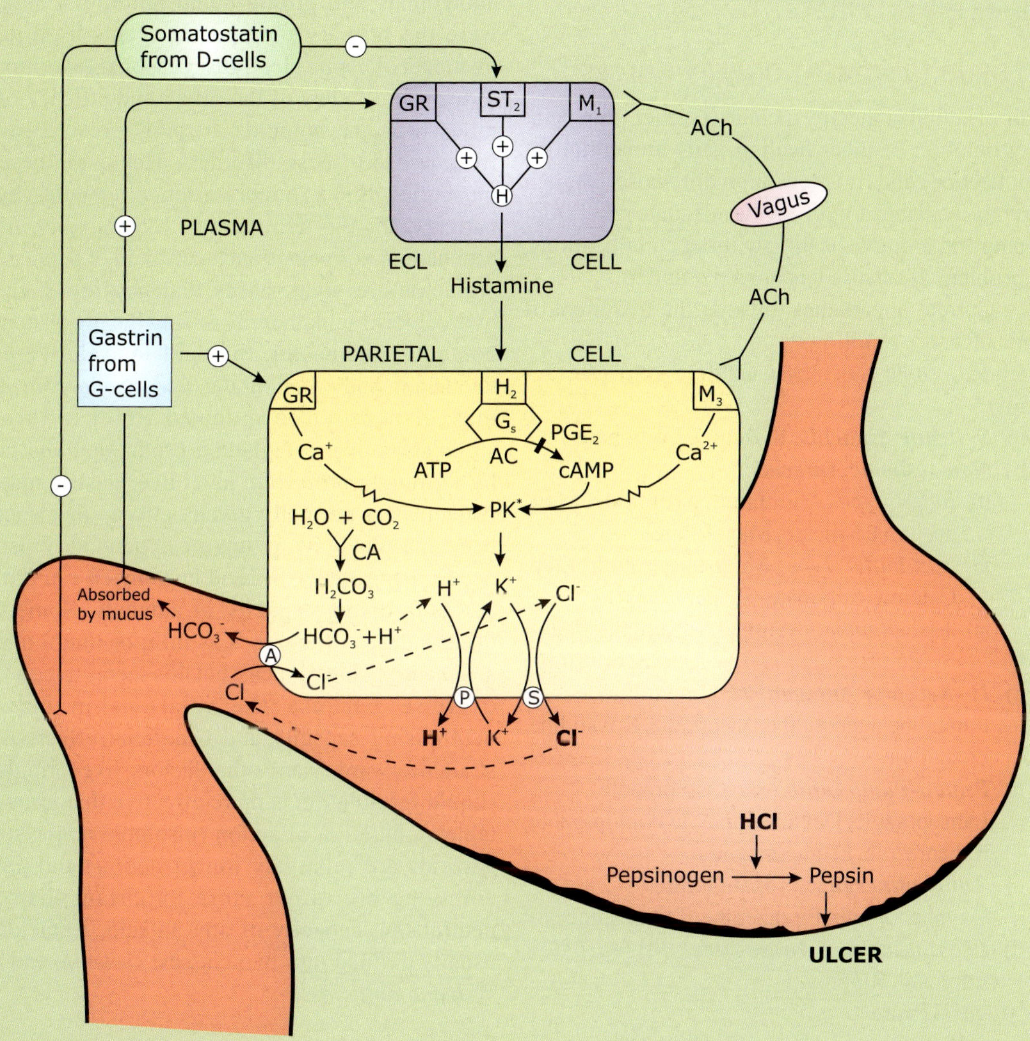

Key: GR—Gastrin receptor; ST_2—Somatostatin receptor; P—Proton pump (H^+/K^+-ATPase); S—Symport carrier for K^+ and Cl^-; A—Antiport carrier for HCO_3^- and Cl^-; CA—Carbonic anhydrase; PK*—Protein kinase activated; AC—Adenylate cyclase; H—Histamine (its receptor H_2); ECL—Enterochromaffin like cells

Fig 27.1 Physiological Aspects of Gastric Acid Secretion and Peptic Ulcer Formation

addition, PGE_2 enhances mucosal blood flow and stimulates secretion of mucus and bicarbonate. The physiological regulation of gastric acid secretion is shown in Fig. 27.1.

DRUG TREATMENT OF PEPTIC ULCER

Goals of antiulcer therapy include (i) relief from pain, (ii) promotion of ulcer healing, (iii) prevention of complications and (iv) prevention of relapse. Though currently available drugs provide adequate relief from the pain and promote healing without complications, the problem of relapse has eluded solution.

Current approaches towards the treatment of peptic ulcer are as follows:

I. **Drugs Which Neutralise Gastric Acid (Antacids)**
   a) ***Systemic Antacids***: Sodium bicarbonate
   b) ***Non-systemic Antacids***:
      i) *Buffer Type:* Aluminium hydroxide, Magnesium trisilicate, Magaldrate
      ii) *Non-buffer Type:* Magnesium hydroxide, Calcium carbonate
      iii) *Miscellaneous:* Alginates, Simethicone

II. **Drugs Which Reduce Gastric Acid Secretion**
   a) ***H_2-Receptor Antagonists***: Cimetidine, Ranitidine, Famotidine, Nizatidine, Roxatidine, Loxatidine
   b) ***Proton-Pump Inhibitors***: Omeprazole, Lansoprazole, Dexlansoprazole Pantoprazole, Rabeprazole, Esomeprazole
   c) ***Anticholinergics***: Propantheline, Oxyphenonium, Pirenzepine, Telenzepine
   d) ***Prostaglandin Analogues***: Misoprostol, Enprostil, Rioprostil

III. **Mucosal Protective Drugs**
   Sucralfate, Colloidal bismuth subcitrate, Ranitidine bismuth citrate

IV. **Ulcer Healing Drugs**
   Carbenoxolone

V. **Anti-*Helicobacter pylori* Drugs**
   Amoxicillin, Clarithromycin, Tetracycline, Metronidazole, Ranitidine bismuth citrate, Bismuth subsalicylate and Proton-Pump Inhibitors (combinations).

ANTACIDS

Prior to the introduction of histamine H_2-receptor antagonists and proton-pump inhibitors, antacids were the primary therapeutic agents used in the treatment of peptic ulcer, gastroesophageal reflux and dyspepsia. In view of the safety and efficacy of the modern drugs, antacids are now prescribed less frequently for these disorders. However, these are most often used as nonprescription remedies, by the patients, for the treatment of hyperacidity, reflux esophagitis, dyspepsia and acute pain of peptic ulcer. Antacids are weak bases that neutralise gastric hydrochloric acid, thereby raising the pH of stomach contents, decreasing the acid load delivered to duodenum and *reducing the activity of pepsin*. They may also promote mucosal defense through stimulation of prostaglandin production and partly by forming a protective layer over gastric mucosa. Antacids are normally given between meals and at bed time when symptoms of hyperacidity usually occur; the presence of food in stomach can prolong the neutralising capacity of antacids. Some texts discuss doses of antacids as mEq or mmol of their acid neutralising capacity but this seems to be a futile exercise because the relationship between neutralising capacity and beneficial effects is not straightforward. Many other factors, like formulation (liquid formulation is more effective than chewable tablets), duration of action (insoluble non-systemic antacids are relatively longer acting) and gastric emptying are rather more important than acid neutralising capacity of any antacid. Antacids are usually divided into two classes: *systemic* and *non-systemic antacids*.

Systemic Antacids

Sodium bicarbonate is an example of systemic antacid. It acts rapidly, has a brief duration of action and raises the pH of gastric secretions to about 7.4. On neutralising gastric HCl, it forms CO_2 and NaCl. Formation of CO_2 results in gastric distension and belching that can be dangerous if ulcer is near perforation. Unreacted alkali is readily absorbed from the GI lumen and can raise the pH of blood (systemic alkalosis) and also of urine. Absorption of NaCl may increase sodium load and may exacerbate fluid retention in patients of hypertension, CHF and renal insufficiency. A sudden rise in gastric pH (up to 7.4) and the release of CO_2 promotes gastrin release which causes "***rebound acidity***". Given in sufficient quantity for longer time they can produce healing of duodenal ulcers but are less effective in gastric ulcers. However, in view of its side effects, described above, it should not be prescribed for long-term use, nor it should be given to patients of hypertension, CHF and renal failure.

Non-systemic Antacids

These are poorly absorbed from GI tract and do not disturb systemic acid-base balance nor do they elevate urinary pH. These are further classified as *buffer type* and *non-buffer type antacids*.

Buffer Type Antacids

Aluminium hydroxide, ***Magnesium trisilicate*** and ***Magaldrate*** constitute some examples of this group. These have slow onset but longer duration of action and raise the gastric pH to 3.5 to 4 (the pepsin activity is inhibited at around pH 4). Hence "rebound acidity" is not a problem with these antacids.

Both ***aluminium hydroxide*** and ***magnesium trisilicate*** neutralise gastric HCl to form aluminium chloride and magnesium chloride, respectively which further react with intestinal bicarbonates to form aluminium carbonate and magnesium carbonate. Hence HCO_3^- are not available for systemic absorption as these have already been utilised for this reaction. Secondly, NaCl formed in this process gets reabsorbed to compensate the loss of Cl^- during gastric acid neutralisation. Consequently, buffer type non-systemic antacids do not disturb the acid-base balance of the body.

$Al(OH)_3$ causes constipation because of (i) formation of aluminium phosphate, (ii) smooth muscle relaxant action of Al^{3+} and (iii) mucosal astringent action of aluminium salts in general. Further, as it binds to PO_4^{3-} in intestine and prevents its absorption, hypophosphataemia may occur. Thus, $Al(OH)_3$ can also be used to treat hyperphosphataemia and phosphate stones.

$$Al(OH)_3 \xrightarrow[\text{Stomach}]{\text{HCl}} AlCl_3 \xrightarrow[\text{Intestine}]{HCO_3^-,\ PO_4^{3-}} Al_2(CO_3)_3 + AlPO_4 + NaCl$$

$$2MgO.3SiO_2.nH_2O \xrightarrow[\text{Stomach}]{\text{HCl}} MgCl_2 + SiO_2$$

$$MgCl_2 \xrightarrow[\text{Intestine}]{HCO_3^-} MgCO_3 + NaCl$$

Magnesium trisilicate, as discussed above, does not disturb acid-base balance also. SiO_2, formed during neutralisation reaction, forms a gelatinous coating over gastric mucosa and prolongs the antacid effect. However, both $MgCl_2$ and $MgCO_3$ produced during the reaction cause diarrhoea, as a side effect. *Since magnesium salts cause osmotic diarrhoea and aluminium salts cause constipation, these two agents are, therefore, commonly administered together in most branded formulations to minimise the impact on bowel movements.*

Magaldrate is a hydrated complex of aluminium-magnesium hydroxide sulfate: $Al_5Mg_{10}(OH)_{31}(SO_4)_2.nH_2O$. When it reacts with HCl it rapidly releases aluminium hydroxide and magnesium hydroxide. The freshly released $Al(OH)_3$ is in the more reactive unpolymerised form. It is an effective buffer-type non-systemic antacid with prompt and sustained neutralising action.

Non-Buffer Type Antacids

Calcium carbonate and ***magnesium hydroxide*** constitute the examples of non-buffer type, non-systemic antacids. These are powerful antacids with fast onset of action, and raise gastric pH > 7.

$$CaCO_3 \xrightarrow[\text{Stomach}]{\text{HCl}} CaCl_2 \xrightarrow[\text{Intestine}]{HCO_3^-,\ \text{Stearates}} CaCO_3 + \text{Cal. Stearate} + NaCl$$

(constipation)

Like $NaHCO_3$, ***calcium carbonate*** may cause belching due to liberation of CO_2 (albeit at a slower rate than $NaHCO_3$). Like $NaHCO_3$, excessive doses of $CaCO_3$ if given along with milk can lead to hypercalcaemia, renal insufficiency and metabolic alkalosis (called ***milk-alkali syndrome***). Acid rebound with $CaCO_3$ is marked because of sudden rise in gastric pH and partly because $CaCl_2$ itself is a stimulant for gastrin release. $CaCO_3$ causes constipation due to formation of calcium stearate in intestine.

Magnesium hydroxide neutralises HCl promptly and is an efficacious antacid. It also brings gastric pH up to 7.

$$Mg(OH)_2 \xrightarrow[\text{Stomach}]{\text{HCl}} MgCl_2 \xrightarrow[\text{Intestine}]{HCO_3^-} MgCO_3 + NaCl$$

Acid rebound with $Mg(OH)_2$ is mild and brief compared to $CaCO_3$. Liberation of $MgCO_3$ causes diarrhoea (see above). Because no CO_2 is generated, belching does not occur. It is usually given along with aluminium hydroxide (see above for reasons).

Drug Interactions

1. By forming inert complexes, Al^{3+}, Ca^{2+} and Mg^{2+} group of antacids decrease the absorption and therefore bioavailability of tetracyclines.
2. Antacids, usually should not be given within 2 hrs of administration of tetracyclines, fluoroquinolones, itraconazole, digoxin or iron salts.
3. Al^{3+} group of antacids decrease the bioavailability of phosphates, iron salts and digoxin. Magnesium salts also decrease the absorption of digoxin.
4) By raising gastric pH and ionisation, antacids decrease the absorption of acidic drugs like barbiturates, phenytoin and NSAIDs.

Miscellaneous Adjuvant to Antacid Preparations

Simethicone (dimethyl polysiloxane)

It is a silicon polymer and therefore has water repellant properties. It acts as an antifoaming agent and reduces gastric flatulence. It aids proper dispersion of antacid in gastric contents, coats ulcer surface, prevents hiccups and reduces flatulence. It is pharmacologically inert and is not absorbed from GIT. It is also used in topical skin preparations to prevent bed sores. It is also called activated dimethicone.

Sodium Alginate (Alginic acid)

Alginates are hydrophilic colloidal carbohydrate derivatives extracted from brown sea weeds. These are used along with antacids or a H_2-receptor antagonist, such as ranitidine, for the management of heart burn and gastroesophageal reflux disease (GERD). Sodium alginate is a prototype. It reacts with gastric acid to form a viscous gel (termed as raft) which floats at the top of gastric contents. This foam/raft, then acts as mechanical barrier to reduce heart burn and the effects of gastric reflux. Recent preparations of antacids usually contain buffer type antacids (Al^{3+}+Mg^{2+}) along with sodium alginate.

H_2-RECEPTOR ANTAGONISTS

H_2-receptor antagonists continue to be prescribed commonly for acid-peptic disease. Their safety record eventually led to their availability as "over-the-counter" drugs. However, with recognition of the role of *H. pylori* in peptic ulcer and the advent of more efficacious (albeit costlier) proton-pump inhibitors (PPIs), the use of H_2 blockers has declined markedly.

Mechanism of Action

The H_2 blockers competitively inhibit H_2 receptors on the parietal cells and suppress basal and food-stimulated acid secretion. They have relatively specific action and do not inhibit H_1 or H_3 receptor. By blocking the H_2 receptors of gastric parietal cells, they block the actions of histamine released from ECL cells through gastrin or vagal stimulation. These also inhibit direct stimulation of parietal cells by gastrin or ACh. They markedly reduce gastric acid secretion for a longer duration and also decrease pepsin production but for a shorter period.

H_2 antagonists block more than 90% nocturnal acid but only 60–70% of day-time food-stimulated acid secretion. Recommended doses maintain at least 50% inhibition up to 10 hr; hence, these drugs are usually given on twice daily basis. The clinical comparison of H_2-receptor blockers has been provided in Table 27.1. ***Cimetidine*** is a prototype; other H_2 antagonists in use are ***ranitidine***, ***famotidine***, ***nizatidine***, ***roxatidine*** and ***loxatidine***. Use of *cimetidine* is, however, obsolete.

Clinical Uses

Clinical uses of H_2-receptor antagonists include: **(a)** gastroesophageal reflux disease (GERD), **(b)** duodenal and gastric ulcer disease, **(c)** NSAIDs-induced ulcers; though PPIs are preferred if NSAIDs have to be continued, **(d)** prevention of stress related gastric bleeding, **(e)** prevention of ulcer recurrence, **(f)** Zollinger-Ellison syndrome; though PPIs are more preferred and its definitive treatment is surgical, and **(g)** H_2 blockers can also be used to treat chronic urticaria as they increase the efficacy of H_1 antagonists.

The dosage schedule of different H_2 blockers, in use, have been detailed in Table 27.1. Loxatidine (not included in this table) is a new powerful non-competitive H_2 blocker which almost totally blocks gastric secretion. Its clinical superiority over other H_2 blockers is yet to be ascertained.

Adverse Effects

(1) These are extremely safe drugs—headache, fatigue, myalgia and constipation may occur, but rarely, **(2)** Mental status changes may occur with I.V. cimetidine but not with other blockers, **(3)** Endocrinal effects are often seen with cimetidine as it inhibits binding of dihydrotestosterone to androgen receptors (impotence in males); inhibits metabolism of estradiol and increases serum prolactin levels (gynaecomastia in males and galactorrhoea in females) on long-term use. These endocrinal effects do not occur with other H_2 blockers, **(4)** H_2 blockers reduce the secretion of intrinsic factor but no vitamin B_{12} deficiency occurs even after prolonged use, and **(5)** They cross placental barrier but have no harmful effects on foetus. These are also secreted into breast milk. However, these should be avoided during pregnancy and lactation.

Drug Interactions

(1) Antacids reduce the absorption of all H_2-blockers; hence, a gap of at least 2 hours should be kept in between the administration of these two drugs and **(2)** Drug interactions are more common with *cimetidine* as it is a potent inhibitor of CYP1A2, CYP2C9, CYP2D6 and CYP3A4. Hence, plasma half-lives of warfarin, theophylline, phenytoin, quinidine, β-blockers, tricyclic antidepressants, benzodiazepines, Ca^{2+} channel blockers, oral hypoglycaemic agents, metronidazole and alcohol may be prolonged. Negligible interactions occur with other H_2-blockers.

PROTON-PUMP INHIBITORS (PPIs)

Proton-pump inhibitors (PPIs) are now the most widely used drugs for peptic ulcer and related disorders, because of their outstanding efficacy and safety. ***Omeprazole*** is a prototype while ***esomeprazole***, ***lansoprazole***, ***Dexlansoprazole***, ***pantoprazole*** and ***rabeprazole*** were introduced later. All are substituted benzimidazoles. Though given orally, most of the PPIs are now available for parenteral use. Since these are acid labile and can be destroyed by gastric acid, they are available in enteric coated (EC) formulations.

Mechanism of Action

All PPIs are prodrugs as their active entity is a "sulfenamide cation" that is formed within the gastric parietal cells. During their passage through alkaline intestinal lumen, the enteric coating dissolves and the prodrug is absorbed from intestine. Being weak bases, these are lipid soluble in alkaline milieu, and therefore get absorbed by passive diffusion across lipid membrane of the small intestine.

Due to its high concentration in the blood it gets secreted into the parietal cells' canaliculi. Once these agents reach the parietal cell canaliculus, are exposed to acidic environment and get rapidly ionised, and concentrated (because being ionised they are get trapped and cannot diffuse back). In parietal cells they undergo a molecular rearrangement to an activeachiral moiety, i.e. "sulfenamide cation". PPIs-

Table 27.1 Clinical Comparison of H_2 Receptor Blockers

Features	Cimetidine	Ranitidine	Famotidine	Roxatidine	Nizatidine
▪ Relative potency	1	5	30	8	5
▪ Bioavailability (%)	80	50	50	> 90	> 90
▪ Cytochrome P-450 inhibition	++++	+	0	0	0
▪ Endocrinal effects	++++	0	0	0	0
Doses for					
▪ 50% acid inhibition	400–800 mg	150 mg	20 mg	75 mg	150 mg
▪ Duodenal or gastric ulcer	800 mg HS 400 mg BD	300 mg HS 150 mg BD	40 mg HS 20 mg BD	150 mg HS 75 mg BD	300 mg HS 150 mg BD
▪ GERD	800 mg BD	150 mg BD	20 mg BD	75 mg BD	150 mg BD
▪ NSAIDs-ulcers	400 mg BD	150 mg BD	20 mg BD	75 mg BD	150 mg BD
▪ Stress related GIT bleeding or in ZE syndrome	50 mg/hr infusion	6.25 mg/hr infusion or 50 mg I.V. every 6-8 hr	1.7 mg/hr infusion or 20 mg I.V. every 12 hr	75 mg slow I.V. every 12 hr	Not available
▪ Prevention of recurrence	400 mg HS	150 mg HS	20 mg HS	75 mg HS	150 mg HS

Key: GERD—Gastroesophageal reflux disease. ZE—Zollinger-Ellison syndrome.
Use of cimetidine has declined these days due to availability of better H_2 blockers.

Sulfenamide (active form) makes a covalent disulfide bond with the SH group of the proton pump, thereby inactivating it irreversibly and shutting off the acid secretion. PPIs also inhibit gastric mucosal carbonic anhydrase and reduce HCO_3^- secretion in mucus. A new PPI (***tenatoprazole***) has been developed, which is not a benzimidazole, but a imidazopyridine derivative. It has a longer t½ than other PPIs and therefore inhibits nocturnal acid secretion effectively. It is pending approval for the treatment of GERD. An absolutely new class of PPIs is also under development. These will be called potassium competitive acid pump blockers (P-CABs). These agents block gastric acid secretion by competitive binding to potassium site of H^+/K^+- ATPase (see Fig. 27.1).

Pharmacokinetics

Their comparative bioavailability is shown in Table 27.2. The presence of food decreases their bioavailability significantly. Theoretically therefore, they should be administered on an empty stomach. However, in the fasting state only 10% of proton pumps are in an active state, rest are in dormant state and optimal binding to PPIs occurs when pumps are secreting actively. Hence, the best way to administer these drugs is to give in the morning just before taking breakfast so that their peak serum concentration coincides with the maximal activity of proton pumps. These drugs have short serum half-lives (1–2 hr) but the duration of acid inhibition lasts up to 24 hr (as PPIs are irreversible inactivators of proton pump and at least 18 hr are needed for the synthesis of new H^+/K^+- ATPase pumps). There is a biological lag of 3–4 days before a full acid inhibiting activity of PPIs is achieved. Similarly, it takes 3–4 days again for the return of normal acid secretion once PPIs are withdrawn. PPIs undergo rapid first pass and are metabolised by liver. However, dose reduction is needed only when there is severe liver impairment. The I.V. formulation of pantoprazole has similar characteristics to its oral formulation, but is given over 24 hr as a continuous infusion.

Clinical Uses

In contrast to H_2-antagonists, PPIs inhibit both fasting and food-stimulated acid secretions, because they block the final pathway of acid secretion—the proton pump itself. The clinical comparison of PPIs with their dosage schedules has been provided in Table 27.2.

The clinical uses of PPIs include: **(1)** Duodenal and gastric ulcer disease, **(2)** Gastro-esophageal reflux disease (GERD), **(3)** NSAIDs-induced ulceration, **(4)** Prevention of ulcer recurrence, **(5)** Zollinger-Ellison (ZE) syndrome, though definitive treatment is surgical, and **(6)** *H. pylori* associated ulcers: PPIs promote eradication of *H. pylori* by raising the intragastric pH which helps in lowering the minimal inhibitory concentration (MIC) of antibiotics used against *H. pylori*. The most effective regimen of *H. pylori* eradication is a combination of two antibiotics and a PPI given twice daily (see following text and Table 27.3). After completion of the therapy, the PPI is usually continued once daily for 4–6 weeks to promote and ensure ulcer healing.

Adverse Effects

(1) PPIs are quite safe, yet diarrhoea, headache and abdominal pain may occur, although rarely, **(2)** They cross placental barrier but are not teratogenic. However, their safety during pregnancy and lactation has not been established, **(3)** They inhibit absorption of vit. B_{12} on prolonged use. However, vit B_{12} deficiency does not occur in 6–8 weeks treatment. Nonetheless, they decrease Ca^{2+} absorption and may aggravate osteoporosis, **(4)** Gastric acid serves as an important barrier to bacterial colonisation of the stomach and small intestine. Hypochlorhydria produced by PPIs, theoretically, should increase the risk of enteric infections due to Shigella, Salmonella and by bacterial strains that have the potential to convert ingested nitrates into carcinogenic nitrites and nitrosamines. Phase IV clinical trials till date have not provided any evidence that this is a real clinical hazard, and it is absolutely unlikely with their short-term use, i.e., up to 8 weeks, **(5)** A concern has arisen that long-term use of PPIs may increase the risk of gastric neoplasia. When the secretion of gastric HCl is suppressed, the feedback inhibitory role of somatostatin over gastrin release is endangered. Hence, gastrin levels rise 2- to 4-fold in patients taking PPIs. Gastrin is a trophic hormone that causes hyperplasia of ECL cells which may transform into carcinoid tumours. This may be true in rats, but there is no real evidence, as yet, for these being clinically hazardous drugs, and **(6)** In patients of *H. pylori*–associated peptic ulcers, long-term use of PPIs may increase the risk of chronic inflammation of gastric body. This may culminate into atrophic gastritis and intestinal metaplasia—the known risk factors for gastric adenocarcinoma. However, surveillance studies till date have not provided any evidence that this is a real risk in their use.

Table 27.2 A Clinical Comparison of Proton-Pump Inhibitors

Features	Omeprazole	Esomeprazole[a]	Lansoprazole[a]	Pantoprazole[a]	Rabeprazole[a]
▪ Bioavailability (%)	55	70	85	77	52
Doses for					
▪ Duodenal* and gastric ulcers*	20 mg OD 40 mg OD	20 mg OD 20 mg OD	15 mg OD 30 mg OD	40 mg OD 40 mg OD	20 mg OD 20 mg OD
▪ GERD*	20 mg OD	20 mg OD	30 mg OD	40 mg OD	20 mg OD
▪ NSAID* ulcers	20 mg OD	20 mg OD	30 mg OD	40 mg OD	20 mg OD
▪ ZE syndrome	60–120 mg daily**	60–120 mg daily**	60–120 mg daily**	40–240 mg daily**	60–120 mg daily**
▪ *H. pylori* eradication	20 mg OD or BD	40 mg OD or BD	30 mg OD or BD	40 mg BD	20 mg BD
▪ Prevention of recurrences*	20 mg OD	20 mg OD	15 mg OD	40 mg OD	20 mg OD

* Therapy continues for 6–8 weeks, ** In two equally divided doses, [a]These PPIs are also available in I.V. dosage forms

Drug Interactions

Clinically significant drug interactions with PPIs are rare. However, these may include: **(1)** A decrease in gastric acidity due to PPIs may decrease the absorption of ketoconazole and digoxin, **(2)** Omeprazole, esomeprazole and lansoprazole inhibit CYP2C19 and CYP3A4 and therefore may enhance the effects of warfarin, phenytoin, carbamazepine and benzodiazepines by decreasing their metabolism (but inhibition is much less than cimetidine). Lansoprazole, though a weak enzyme inducer, may also enhance the elimination of theophylline and **(3)** Rabeprazole and pantoprazole exhibit no significant drug interaction.

ANTICHOLINERGICS

Until the advent of H_2-receptor antagonists and PPIs, antimuscarinic drugs were mainly used to treat peptic ulcer. Among them, classical quaternary antimuscarinic drugs like ***propantheline*** and ***oxyphenonium*** were more preferred because they do not cross BBB and therefore offer lesser side effects; but being non-selective antimuscarinic drugs, they still retained other side effects like blurred vision, dry mouth, constipation and urinary retention. These drugs block basal secretions (fasting phase) more effectively than that stimulated by food. Besides this, by increasing the gastric emptying time, they rather prolong the exposure of ulcer bed to gastric acid which makes them unsuitable for treatment of peptic ulcer. Since they delay gastric emptying and relax lower oesophageal sphincter, they can rather exacerbate the condition of GERD by allowing the reflux of acid-mixed food into the oesophagus.

However, some selective M_1 receptor blockers such as ***pirenzepine*** and ***telenzepine*** are being used in Canada and Europe for the treatment of peptic ulcer. These drugs probably act by blocking M_1 receptor at paracrine cells in gastric mucosa (see Ch.11). These drugs effectively heal as well as prevent the recurrence of duodenal ulcers. At therapeutic doses, the usual side effects like dry mouth, blurred vision, constipation and urinary retention were relatively low, while CNS side effects were absent (as these drugs do not cross BBB). Telenzepine is 25 times more potent than pirenzepine. Both drugs are not available in India and USA.

PROSTAGLANDIN ANALOGUES

Prostaglandins play an important role in gastric defense mechanisms against peptic ulcer. PGE_2 produced by gastric mucosa, inhibits acid secretion by inhibiting cAMP (in parietal cells) and gastrin release from antral cells. In addition, PGE_2 enhances mucosal blood flow and stimulates the secretion of mucus and bicarbonates. ***Misoprostol*** (a stable methyl analogue of PGE_1) in a dose of 200 µg orally, four times a day, is used and approved for healing of peptic ulcer in patients using NSAIDs and in persons who are chronic heavy smokers. However, even for this indication it has not received any wide-spread acceptance mainly because of its adverse effects and a need for multiple daily dosing (plasma half-life 25–30 min). Moreover, PPIs are equally effective and better tolerated than misoprostol for this indication. ***Enprostil*** and ***rioprostil***, which are stable PGE_2 analogues, also offer no additional advantage.

The commonest side effect occurring with misoprostol is diarrhoea and colicky pain because it increases water and electrolyte secretions in intestine. Other GIT effects include nausea, vomiting and flatulence. Headache and dizziness can occur. It should not be given to patients who are pregnant or who may become pregnant because it can cause uterine contractions. No significant drug inter-actions are, however, reported.

MUCOSAL PROTECTIVE DRUGS

Sucralfate

It is an aluminium salt of sulfated sucrose. In acidic environment (pH < 4), it polymerises by cross-linking of molecules and forms a sticky-like gel over ulcer crater which acts as acid-resistant physical barrier. Dietary as well as mucosal proteins also get adsorbed over this coat forming another layer to provide further resistance. There is some evidence to suggest that it also stimulates mucosal PGE_2 synthesis and HCO_3^- secretion. It is also believed to bind epithelial as well as fibroblast growth factors which promotes mucosal repair. It promotes ulcer healing, though it has no acid neutralising action and delays gastric emptying. Incidentally, it is not effective in preventing or healing NSAIDs-induced ulcers. Its superiority over H_2-blockers and PPIs is questionable. Sucralfate is administered in a dosage of 1 g four times daily, as it keeps adhering to ulcer crater for 6 hr. It is virtually devoid of side effects, as it remains unabsorbed. However, it binds phosphate ions in intestine. Hence hypo-phosphataemia may occur. Antacids should not be given with sucralfate because its polymerisation occurs in acidic media only (efficacy would be reduced). Sucralfate adsorbs tetracylines, fluoroquinolones, H_2 blockers, phenytoin and digoxin and decreases their absorption.

OTHER USES: In glycerine paste it is used for stomatitis. Its gel is used for burn dressing and bed sores. In slightly higher doses it may be used to prevent phosphate stones in kidney. Its preparations with surface local anaesthetic are also available.

Colloidal Bismuth Subcitrate and Bismuth Subsalicylate

In gastric acidic media, colloidal bismuth subcitrate forms an acid-resistant protective coating over ulcer base. It is reported to stimulate PGE_2, mucus and bicarbonate secretion. It also dislodges *H. pylori* from the surface of gastric mucosa and has direct antimicrobial activity against this ulcer-causative organism. It is administered in a dosage of 120 mg orally four times a day. It heals peptic ulcer within

4–8 weeks of treatment. Many duodenal ulcers which did not heal after H_2 blocker treatment, get healed by subsequent 4 weeks treatment with colloidal bismuth. Colloidal bismuth has an excellent safety profile, except that it causes blackening of stool and darkening of tongue. Prolonged use may lead to bismuth toxicity (osteodystrophy and encephalopathy), albeit rarely. Antacids should not be taken concomitantly with colloidal bismuth as they decrease its efficacy. Another bismuth salt in clinical use is ***ranitidine bismuth citrate*** which upon hydrolysis by gastric acid releases bismuth as well as ranitidine. Currently bismuth salts are used as one of the agents in an anti-*H. pylori* treatment regimen (see Table 27.3).

ULCER HEALING DRUGS

Carbenoxolone Sodium

Its use as an antiulcer drug has become outdated because of the adverse effects (mineralocorticoid like side effects such as hypertension, Na^+ and water retention and hypokalaemia) and availability of better drugs.

ANTI-*HELICOBACTER PYLORI* DRUGS

Peptic ulcer, although a multifactorial disease, also occurs due to colonisation of duodenal mucosa by *H. pylori*. About 90% cases with duodenal ulcers, 60–70% cases of gastric ulcers and probably 50% cases of non-ulcer dyspepsia are *H. pylori*–positive individuals. It has become widely accepted as a cause of chronic atrophic gastritis. *H. pylori* is also a risk factor for gastric adenocarcinoma and to some extent for non-Hodgkin's lymphoma affecting stomach. This bacterium, unlike others, is able to survive in the acidic gastric environment by its ability to produce urease, which hydrolyses urea into ammonia. Ammonia neutralises gastric HCl to create a neutral protective cloud over the bacteria. Secretion of ammonia by *H. pylori*, on the other hand, disturbs the normal negative feedback mechanisms which cause more secretion of gastric acid through release of more gastrin in response to food. *H. pylori* also produces various other proteolytic enzymes such as proteases and lipases which further decrease the important mucosal defence by degrading mucus layer and damaging lipid containing epithelial cell membrane leading to chronic inflammation of gastric and antral mucosa and ultimately ulcers.

H. pylori infection can be detected by "urea breath test" but this test may provide false-negative results if used after the treatment with PPIs. Since *H. pylori* becomes less virulent in absence of acid, a combination of antibiotics with PPIs is more efficacious in eradicating *H. pylori*. PPIs also exhibit antimicrobial properties (against *H. pylori*) *in vitro* and lower the minimal inhibitory concentrations (MIC) of antibiotics against *H. pylori*. All PPIs, except pantoprazole, have been approved, by FDA, in various combinations of antibiotics for eradication of *H. pylori*.

Although several 2-drug, 3-drug and 4-drug combination regimens, with their duration of treatment, have been prescribed, none of them can be proclaimed as an optimal regimen for eradication of *H. pylori*. Some of these are outlined in Table 27.3, but the best eradication mechanism has not been established yet and the number of regimens being tried is large. Eradication rate is lower in cigarette smokers.

The combination therapy for 14 days provides the greatest efficacy compared to 7–10-day short-term regimen. An efficacious combination should provide an eradication rate of > 90%. The **dual therapy** is outdated and is not recommended these days as eradication rate with these drugs is around < 80%. The **triple therapy** has comparable success rates that are desired. For better compliance the dose regimens have been kept as twice a day. Failure of *H. pylori* eradication with triple therapy is usually due to infection with a resistant organism. **Quadruple therapy** should then be considered as next step. A new **sequential therapy** has also been introduced which has demonstrated 90% eradication rate with good patient tolerance (Table 27.3). In summary, *H. pylori* eradication therapy is indicated for duodenal and gastric ulcer (not associated with NSAIDs use), mucosa-associated lymphoid tissue (MALT) type lymphoma and for non-ulcer dyspepsia but not for GERD. Comparison between H_1 and H_2 antagonists are given in Table 27.4.

Table 27.3 Preferred Therapies for Eradication of *H. pylori* Infection*

Drug Combinations	Dose and Frequency
TRIPLE THERAPY (14 days)	
Omeprazole (or Lansoprazole)	20 mg (30 mg) BD
plus Clarithromycin	500 mg BD
plus Amoxicillin	1 g BD
Or	
Metronidazole**	500 mg BD
Ranitidine Bismuth Citrate	400 mg BD
plus Tetracycline	500 mg BD
plus Metronidazole**	500 mg BD
Or	
Clarithromycin	500 mg BD
QUADRUPLE THERAPY (14 days)	
Omeprazole (or Lansoprazole)	20 mg (30 mg) OD
plus Bismuth Subsalicylate	2 Tabs (525 mg) QID
plus Metronidazole**	250 mg QID
plus Tetracycline	500 mg QID
SEQUENTIAL THERAPY (10 days)	
For 1–5 days	
Omeprazole (or Lansoprazole)	20 mg (30 mg) BD
plus Amoxicillin	1 g BD
Followed by days 6–10	
Omeprazole (or Lansoprazole)	20 mg (30 mg) BD
plus Clarithromycin	500 mg BD
plus Tinidazole	500 mg BD

* After completion of any therapy, treatment with PPIs (once daily) is continued for another 4–6 weeks to promote ulcer healing.

** Kits available in India contain tinidazole in place of metronidazole

Table 27.4 Compare and contrast H_1 and H_2 Antagonist

Feature	H_1 antagonist (Promethazine)	H_2 antagonist (Ranitidine)
Histamine receptor blocked	H_1	H_2
Antagonist to other receptors	Muscarinic (M_1)	None
Anticholinergic side effects	Present	Absent
Sedation	Yes	No
Anti-emetic effect	Present	Absent
Effect of CNS depressant	Excessive sedation	No effect
Effect on gastric acid	No effect	Reduced
Use	Allergy	Peptic ulcer

CHAPTER 28 Antiemetics, Prokinetic Agents and Drugs for Irritable Bowel Syndrome

COMPETENCY PH1.34

Vomiting means expulsion of gastric contents through mouth due to mass antiperistalsis. It is often preceded by *nausea* which means an uneasy feeling in anticipation of vomiting. In between these two stages there is a series of weaker and unproductive vomiting movements called *retching*. Vomiting can be a valuable, life saving, physiological response to the ingested toxic substances. However, it is also an unwanted side effect of radiation and cancer chemotherapeutic agents. It also occurs in early pregnancy, during migraine attack and due to motion sickness. Vomiting results due to stimulation of vomiting center (VC) which is located in the lateral medullary reticular formation. Efferent fibres from this center, when stimulated, cause stimulation of phrenic nerve supplying to diaphragm and of somatic nerve supplying the abdominal muscles to promote emesis.

EXCITING INPUTS AND NEUROTRANSMITTER ROLE IN EMESIS

Proper pharmacological managment of vomiting requires understanding of neurotransmitter involvement in emesis (Fig.28.1).

1. The major afferent inputs to vomiting centre are routed through chemoreceptor trigger zone (CTZ; or area prostema) which is located at the end of IV ventricle. Since CTZ lies outside of the BBB, it can freely monitor for toxic and emetogenic stimuli circulating in blood or CSF and can relay this information to VC to trigger nausea and vomiting. The CTZ is rich in dopamine (D_2), serotonin (5-HT_3), muscarinic (M_1), histamine (H_1), opioid (μ) and NK_1, receptors which could be the targets for existing and newer antiemetic drugs.
2. The vestibular apparatus generates impulses during motion sickness which reach VC mainly *via* cerebellum. Vestibular apparatus is rich in muscarinic (M_1) and histaminic (H_1) receptors.
3. Vagal and splanchnic afferents in the GIT mucosa are rich in 5-HT_3 receptors. Irritation of GIT mucosa by irritants, chemotherapeutic agents, radiation therapy, endogenous toxins and poisons lead to a release of mucosal serotonin from enterochromaffin-like cells (ECL cells) which activate these 5-HT_3 receptors. This propagates vagal afferent inputs to nucleus tractus solitarius (NTS) for onward transmission to VC. NTS is rich in histamine (H_1), cholinergic (M_1) and serotonin (5-HT_3) receptors.
4. Transmitter mediators in the cerebral cortex (higher centers) are poorly understood. However, cortical cannabinoid (CB_1) receptors have been implicated. Muscarinic (M_1), histaminic (H_1), serotonin (5-HT_3) and Neurokinin-1 (NK_1) receptors have been identified at the vomiting center. Histamine through activation of H_1 receptors has a permissive role to play, as an excitatory neurotransmitter, in all sorts of emesis.

TYPES OF EMESIS AND ANTIEMETIC DRUGS

Motion Sickness

Motion sickness can result during space flights, taking off and landing of an aeroplane, viewing of a moving horizon or waves of the sea from the dock of a rolling ship. Since it is a labyrinthine vomiting *via* stimulation of vestibular nuclei, one can use a H_1- receptor antagonist or a centrally acting anticholinergic drug (see Fig. 28.1).

Hyoscine (or scopolamine) transdermal patch or 0.6 mg orally 30–60 min before journey, can be used prophylactically or 0.2 mg I.M. can be used if motion sickness has started. Side effects are least at this dose but higher doses may cause common anticholinergic effects like blurred vision, dryness of mouth, cycloplegia, sedation and sleepiness (For preparations, see Ch.11).

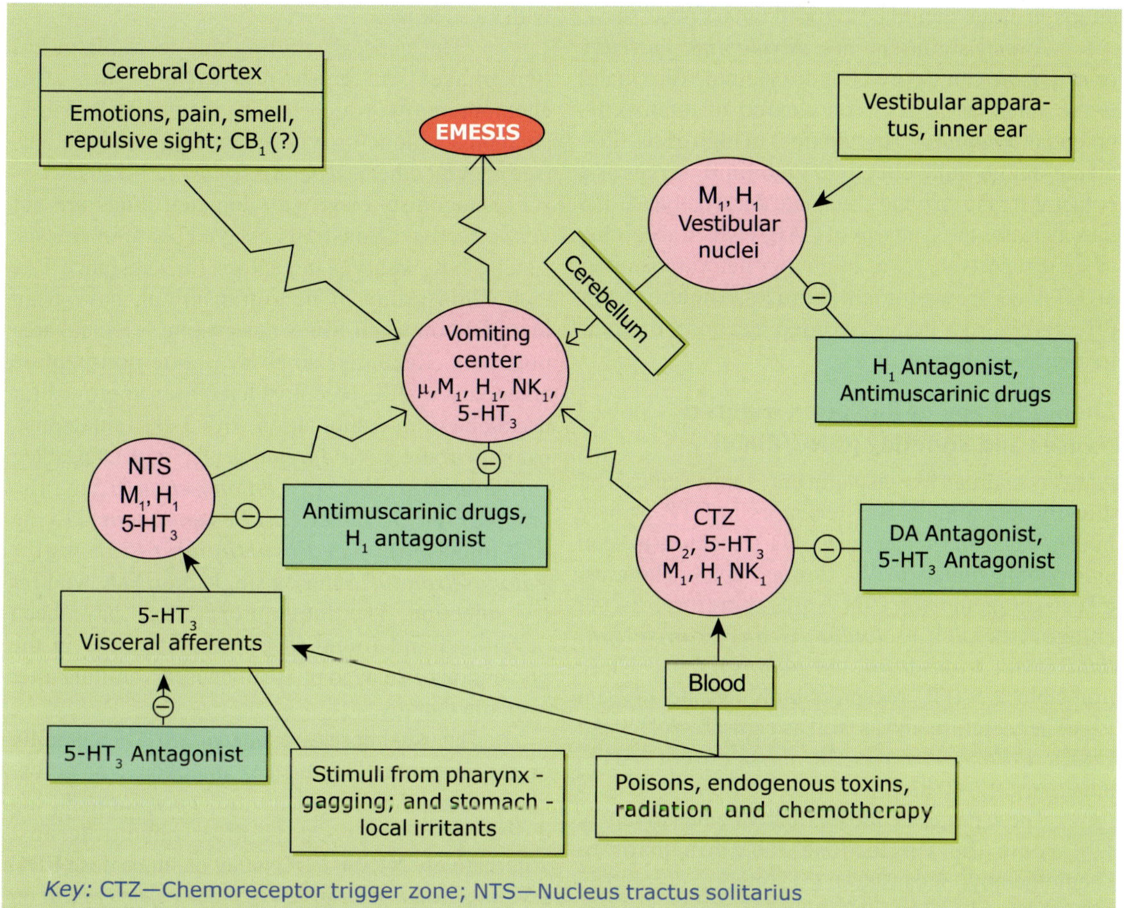

Fig 28.1 Neurotransmitters Involved in the Process of Vomiting, and Probable Sites of Action of Antiemetic Drugs.

H_1 antagonists (Ch. 24), with anticholinergic properties are particularly useful for prevention or treatment of motion sickness. ***Diphenhydramine*** (or ***dimenhydrinate***), ***cyclizine*** or ***meclizine*** are commonly used drugs for the prevention of motion sickness and for treatment of vertigo due to labyrinth dysfunction. A non-neuroleptic phenothiazine, ***promethazine***, because of its antihistaminic-anticholinergic properties also possesses potent antimotion sickness activity. As discussed earlier, these drugs are associated with common anticholinergic side effects besides sedation. ***Cinnarizine*** is another antivertigo drug which can also be used for the prevention of motion sickness. It is an antihistamine having additional anticholinergic, antiserotonin and Ca^{2+} channel blocking properties. By inhibiting the influx of Ca^{2+} from endolymph into the vestibular apparatus it blocks further mediation of labyrinthine reflexes.

Morning Sickness (vomiting during pregnancy)

It results in the first trimester of pregnancy due to the effect of increased oestrogen levels on CTZ. It persists for few weeks and then subsides. However, in some cases there may be hyperemesis gravidarum leading to dehydration which needs proper drug treatment, although drugs should be avoided unless necessary.

Among antihistamines, ***doxylamine, cyclizine*** or ***meclizine*** can be used but doxylamine (doxinate) is the safest as it has been cleared of teratogenic potential. ***Vitamin B_6*** (pyridoxine) in high doses (20–60 mg/day) is quite effective. Vitamin B_6 serves as a cofactor for the enzyme glutamate decarboxylase and thus increases the synthesis of GABA which according to some reports serves as inhibitory neurotransmitter at CTZ. D_2 receptor antagonists, though work effectively, are better avoided because of their teratogenic potential.

Chemotherapy or Radiation Induced Nausea and Vomiting (CINV/RINV)

Anticancer drugs like cisplatin may induce emesis by directly activating 5-HT_3 receptors in CTZ or may bind to vagal and splanchnic 5-HT_3 receptors to send emetogenic signals to VC through NTS. The most effective agents for CINV are, therefore, 5-HT_3 antagonists such as ***ondansetron, granisetron, dolasetron, tropisetron*** and ***palonosetron.*** These drugs block 5-HT_3 receptors both peripherally (on vagal nerve terminals) as well as centrally (NTS and CTZ). *Palonosetron* is the most potent 5-HT_3 antagonist (t½ 40 hrs).

These drugs are most effective when given by I.V. route (as single dose), 30 min prior to chemotherapy: ondansetron 0.15 mg/kg; dolasetron 1.8 mg/kg; granisetron 10 μg/kg; and palonosetron 0.25 mg. These doses may be repeated every 24 hrs. For less emetogenic chemotherapeutic agents and for radiotherapy, the oral doses may be effective: ondansetron 8 mg BD, granisetron 2 mg/day and dolasetron 100 mg/day. The efficacy of 5-HT_3 antagonists is enhanced by the concurrent administration of ***dexamethasone*** (basis unknown) or ***prochlorperazine/metoclopramide /domperidone*** (for additional D_2 blocking effects) and/or ***diazepam*** (for enhancing the inhibitory effects of GABA on CTZ—see above).

5-HT_3 antagonists have an excellent safety profile. However, headache, constipation, abdominal discomfort and rashes (especially after I.V. injection) may occur. Dolasteron may prolong QT interval and should be avoided in patients having prolonged QT. No significant drug interactions have been reported with these drugs.

The nausea-vomiting due to cisplatin has two phases: *an acute phase* (0–24 hrs after chemotherapy), which can be treated with 5-HT_3 antagonists alone or with other drug combinations (see above); other is *a delayed phase* (25–120 hrs). 5-HT_3 antagonists even with adjuvant drugs are not very effective against this delayed phase of emesis. Lately, NK_1 subtype receptors for substance-P, a tachykinin group of neurotransmitter, have been identified on vagal fibres innervating NTS and area postrema. Recently, some synthetic non-peptide antagonist of NK_1 receptors have been approved for use alone or in combination with 5-HT_3 antagonist, palonosetron, e.g.: (i) ***Aprepitant*** (125 mg): Oral tablet; (ii) ***NEtupitant*** (300 mg) + ***PAlonosetron*** (0.5 mg): an oral **NEPA**-FDC tablet; (iii) ***Fosaprepitant*** (115 mg I.V. injection); (iv) ***Fosnetupitant*** (235 mg) + ***Palonosetron*** (0.25 mg): a single dose FDC vial for I.V. injection. The above preparations have been developed and found to be very effective in the prevention of delayed phase of nausea-vomiting after cisplatin therapy.

The usual doses are: ***aprepitant*** 125 mg orally or ***fosaprepitant*** 115 mg I.V. injection 1 hr before chemotherapy followed by oral ***aprepitant*** 80 mg daily for next two days after chemotherapy. Alternatively **NEPA-FDC** tablet or single dose **FDC I.V.** injection can be given in place of ***aprepitant*** on day one followed by oral **NEPA** tablet for next two days. These drugs are given along with ***dexamethasone*** in the dose of 4–8 mg BD for 4 days starting from day one of chemotherapy and continued for next 3 days.

For many years, ***metoclopramide*** (5–10 mg TDS oral or I.M. every 6 hrs), a dopamine (D_2) receptor blocker acting on CTZ, enjoyed the status of most widely used antiemetic drug to treat chemotherapy induced or radiation induced nausea-vomiting. Later it was found that its prokinetic effects (see below for details), also contribute to its effectiveness in chemotherapeutic induced nausea-vomiting. Metoclopramide efficacy is improved while incidence of side effects is reduced when it is combined with other agents, like ***diphenhydramine*** (a H_1 receptor antagonist) + ***dexamethasone*** (a corticosteroid) + ***lorazepam/diazepam*** (an antianxiety agent).

Domperidone (10–40 mg TDS oral), is another D_2 receptor antagonist with antiemetic and prokinetic effects like that of metoclopramide. Though its antiemetic efficacy is lesser than metoclopramide, its principal advantage over metoclopramide is the lack of extrapyramidal CNS side effects: restlessness, dystonias, and parkinsonian symptoms because of its poor penetration to CNS. The efficacy of domperidone in chemotherapy/radiation-induced emesis is improved when it is combined with other agents like ***prochlorperazine*** (a phenothiazine group of neuroleptic-antiemetic) + ***diphenhydramine*** (a H_1 blocker) + ***dexamethasone*** (a corticosteroid).

Postoperative Nausea and Vomiting

Postoperative nausea-vomiting (PONV) are complications in 30–40% of patients receiving general anaesthesia. Women undergoing gynaecological surgery are particularly at a greater risk (60–80%) in experiencing such type of vomiting. 5-HT_3 receptor antagonists because of their better reliable index, are generally preferred to prevent or treat postoperative nausea and vomiting. Antihistamines (promethazine and diphenhydramine) and the prokinetic drugs with D_2 receptor blocking action (metoclopramide and domperidone) are also used but with a limited success.

Phenothiazines, which are primarily used as antipsychotic agents, can also be used for their antiemetic properties in postoperative nausea and vomiting. The most commonly used agents are ***prochlorperazine*** (5–25 mg oral, TDS or 12.5 mg, I.V.) and ***promethazine*** (12.5–25 mg BD or TDS oral or I.V.). Prochlorperazine has D_2 receptor and muscarinic receptor blocking action. Promethazine is a potent antihistaminic and anticholinergic drug.

Butyrophenone group of antipsychotics (e.g., ***droperidol***) can also be used to treat postoperative nausea and vomiting by giving I.V. or I.M. injection. In antiemetic doses it is extremely sedating and both prochlorperazine as well as droperidol, can precipitate extrapyramidal side effects and postural hypotension. Droperidol should not be used in patients who show prolongation of QT interval in their ECG because further prolongation of QT interval may lead to tachyarrhythmias, though rarely.

Vomiting of Varied Origin and Adjuvant Antiemetics

Drug-induced vomiting, and raised intracranial pressure induced emesis are some examples of vomiting of varied origin whose pharmaco-therapy is still unresolved.

Vomiting in patients due to brain injury, cerebral tumour or hydrocephalus increases CSF pressure which is possibly responsible for neurotransmitter-related activation of receptors present on CTZ. However, which neurotransmitter is responsible to cause this type of emesis is not known, except for 5-HT because 5-HIAA levels in CSF are raised in patients with raised intracranial pressure. Recently, role of CB_1 receptors has also been implicated.

Nabilone and ***dronabinol*** (delta-9-THC) are analogues of 9-tetrahydrocannabinol (9-THC). The latter is the active principle of *Cannabis sativa*, and has antiemetic properties but disorienting and hallucinogenic effects limit its clinical usefulness. Nabilone and dronabinol are however less hallucinogenic with better antiemetic efficacy against moderately emetogenic chemotherapeutic agents. They probably act by stimulating CB_1 subtype of cannabinoid receptors present on neurons around vomiting center. Since their antiemetic effect is antagonised by naloxone, it is believed that they might be inhibiting endorphins (or μ receptors) in vomiting centre. Dronabinol is administered at an initial dose of 5 mg/m² given 2 hrs before chemotherapy and then at every 4 hrs afterwards, for a total of 4 to 6 doses. It can also be used for vomiting refractory to other antiemetics but it is not helpful in emesis due to raised intracracranial pressure where correction of cause is more beneficial. Because of its appetite stimulant action it is also used in AIDS-related anorexia. A combination therapy with phenothiazines (***prochlorperazine***), provides the synergistic antiemetic action with reduced side effects of both the drugs. *Adverse effects* of nabilone and dronabinol include euphoria, dysphoria, sedation, hallucination, dry mouth, increased appetite, tachycardia and orthostatic hypotension.

EMETICS

Emetics are used for deliberate production of emesis for treatment. They may act centrally by stimulating CTZ or may work as reflex emetics. Commonly used emetics are *apomorphine* and *ipecacuanha*. ***Apomorphine*** is a semisynthetic morphine derivative which stimulates dopamine receptors at CTZ. It is administered parenterally (S.C. or I.M.). If vomiting does not occur, the second dose should be avoided. Larger doses produce convulsions and respiratory depression. ***Ipecacuanha*** (syrup ipecac) is procured from the roots of *Cephalis cuanha*. It stimulates CTZ and also works as a reflex emetic (active principle: emetine). It is administered orally and is safer than apomorphine. Ingestion of ***sodium chloride solution*** and ***mustard powder*** also serves as domestic substances to produce emesis.

Emetics are contraindicated in hypertension, peptic ulcer, pulmonary tuberculosis, uraemia and pregnancy. Emetics should be avoided in case of corrosive poisons because an increase in intragastric pressure may lead to perforation. These should also be avoided in cases of poisoning due to petroleum products because of the danger of producing lipoid aspiration pneumonia.

PROKINETIC DRUGS

Prokinetic agents **(1)** stimulate GIT motility; **(2)** increase lower oesophageal sphincter pressure (hence useful for GERD); **(3)** speed-up gastric emptying (hence useful for gastroparesis); **(4)** stimulate small intestine (hence beneficial for postoperative paralytic ileus and colonic pseudo-obstruction); and **(5)** enhance colonic transit (hence useful for treating constipation). In current practice, prokinetic agents mean the drugs that enhance the coordinated activity among the various segments of the gut to propel the luminal contents.

Physiology of Gut Motility

The Enteric Nervous System (ENS) is organised into two types of network of neurons called plexus (Fig. 10.11). One is myenteric (Auerbach's) plexus which is found between the circular and longitudinal muscle layers and is responsible for motor control (peristaltic reflex). Another is submucosal (Meissner's) plexus which is located below mucosal epithelium and regulates secretions. The primary neurotransmitter of the myenteric motor neuron is ACh (Fig. 28.2).

These neurons receive inputs from both ascending and descending interneurons (relay system) which are of two types: excitatory (ACh) and inhibitory (NO). Mucosal stimulation leads to release of serotonin from enterochromaffin cells (EC) and by neurons of myenteric plexus. It acts as an autacoid and affects both motor activity as well as secretion. Serotonin action appears to be mediated

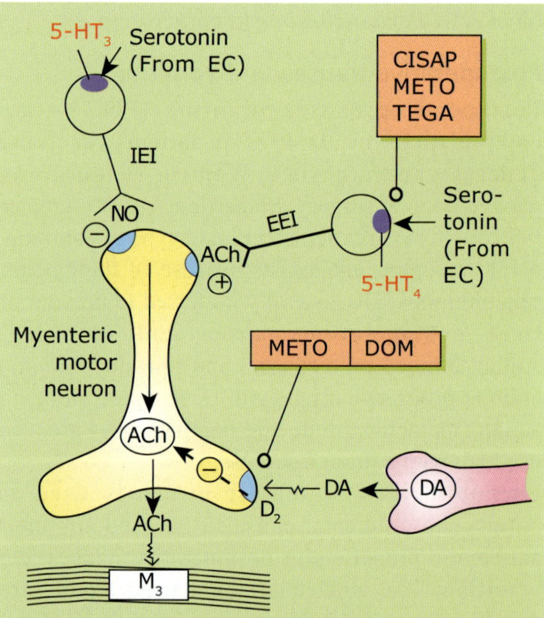

Key: EC—Enterochromaffin cells; ACh—acetylcholine; DA—dopamine; METO—metoclopramide; DOM—domperidone; CISAP—cisapride; TEGA—tegaserod; NO—nitric oxide; M_3, D_2, 5-HT_3 and 5-HT_4 are respective receptors; IEI—Inhibitory ENS interneuron; EEI—Excitatory ENS interneuron.

Fig 28.2 Modulation of Gastrointestinal Motility by Prokinetic Agents.

principally *via* 5-HT_3 and 5-HT_4 receptors which are present on the inhibitory and the excitatory interneurons, respectively, that synapse with cholinergic myenteric motor neuron. The latter neuron (i.e., excitatory) when excited induces smooth muscle contraction *via* release of ACh and when the inhibitory neuron is activated there is relaxation *via* dampening the release of ACh from primary cholinergic motor neuron. Dopaminergic neurons also make a synapse with the primary cholinergic neuron (Fig. 28.2). Dopamine (DA) acting through D_2 receptors present on the cholinergic neurons inhibits the release of ACh *via* heterotropic presynaptic receptor interaction (see Ch. 10).

Motilin is another polypeptide hormone secreted by ECL cells of duodenum and jejunum. Motilin receptors have been identified on intestinal smooth muscle cells, activation of which induces potent contractile movements in the upper gastrointestinal tract, increases lower esophageal sphincter (LES) tone and stimulates pepsin secretion.

Metoclopramide

Metoclopramide is a D_2 receptor antagonist, 5-HT_3 receptor antagonist and 5-HT_4 receptor agonist. Due to blockade of D_2 receptors, dopamine loses its inhibitory control over ACh release from the primary cholinergic neuron in myenteric plexus (Fig.28.2). It has now been ascertained that central D_2 action of metoclopramide is clearly responsible for its antiemetic effects and that its prokinetic activity contributes only partly. The major mechanism responsible for its prokinetic effects is *via* activation of 5-HT_4 receptors present on excitatory interneurons (see earlier text and Fig. 28.2), which enhances ACh release from primary cholinergic neurons in myenteric plexus. Thus it increases LES tone, facilitates gastric peristalsis and speeds-up gastric emptying. However, colonic motility remains unaffected (not enhanced). 5-HT_3 receptors on inhibitory interneurons are also blocked by metoclopramide but in high doses only. Thus the release of NO is also suppressed, which indirectly facilitates ACh release from the primary motor neuron. However, this mechanism seems to contribute little towards its prokinetic effects.

Metoclopramide is used as antiemetic (see earlier text) and as gastrokinetic agent to accelerate gastric emptying prior to giving emergency general anaesthesia in case the patient has taken food less than 4 hrs before, to facilitate duodenal intubation and to relieve diabetes associated gastric stasis. Metoclopramide also affords relief in mild gastroesophageal reflux disease (GERD) but PPIs/H_2 blockers are more preferred (Ch. 27) because it is not effective in erosive oesophagitis. The drug may also succeed in stopping presistent hiccups.

Metoclopramide, being a central/peripheral D_2 receptor blocker, produces sedation, muscle dystonias and in higher doses may induce extrapyramidal side effects, galactorrhoea (in females) and gynaecomastia (in males).

Domperidone

Its mechanism of action is similar to meto-clopramide. It is a peripheral D_2 receptor blocker which is structurally related to haloperidol (but has got no antipsychotic activity). It is pharmacologically related to metoclopramide, but its antiemetic efficacy is lower than that of metoclopramide. It is also used to prevent the emetic side effects of levodopa or bromocriptine without affecting their therapeutic efficacy as anti-parkinsonism drugs. Other indications are also similar to metoclopramide (see above).

Cisapride, Mosapride, Zacopride and Renzapride

This group of prokinetic drugs is devoid of D_2 receptor blocking properties; nor do they act on CTZ and hence they facilitate GIT motility with no antiemetic effects. These drugs act mainly through 5-HT_4 agonist action which promotes ACh release from myenteric plexus aided by 5-HT_3 antagonism which depresses inhibitory transmission and thus also facilitates ACh release indirectly from myenteric plexus (Fig. 28.2).

Cisapride (10–20 mg oral TDS) facilitates gastric motility, throughout the GIT including the colon, hastens gastric emptying, improves LES tone and oesophageal peristalsis. Primary indication for cisapride is GERD (but PPIs/H_2 blockers are preferred). Other indications include non-ulcer dyspepsia, impaired gastric emptying and constipation, though usefulness is debatable.

Adverse effects include abdominal cramps and diarrhoea. Though side effects are mild, the safety of cisapride has been questioned as it prolongs the QT interval and predisposes to ventricular fibrillation in high doses. It is also a cytochrome CYP3A4 enzyme inhibitor. Hence when coadministered with the drugs which also inhibit the same enzyme, significant rise in cisapride plasma levels results that may lead to prolongation of QT interval and ventricular arrhythmias. Such drugs include fluconazole, ketoconazole, erythromycin, clarithromycin and some antidepressants like nefazodone. For this reason it has been withdrawn in USA but is still available in several countries, including India.

The other congeners like ***mosapride*** (5 mg oral TDS), ***renzapride*** and ***zacopride*** do not cause QT prolongation or arrhythmias. Their pharmacological characteristics, mode of action, indications and side effects are similar to cisapride (except QT prolongation).

Macrolides (motilin agonists)

Macrolide antibiotics, like ***erythromycin, azithromycin*** and ***clarithromycin,*** directly stimulate motilin receptors on GIT smooth muscle (see above), and promote upper gastrointestinal motility, increase the LES tone and stimulate small intestinal contractility. In contrast to cisapride they have no effect on colonic motility. A standard dose of erythromycin used for gastric stimulation is 40 mg I.V. or 200–250 mg orally TDS. It can be used to improve gastric emptying in patients with diabetic gastroparesis and in small bowel dysmotility such as seen in pseudo-obstruction. However, tolerance develops rapidly to its prokinetic effects, and its antibiotic effects are absolutely undesirable in gastrokinetic context.

Miscellaneous Agents

- ***Prucalopride*** is a safest analogue of cisapride and is a highly selective 5-HT_4 receptor agonist. It is used to treat severe constipation but its long-term effficacy and safety has not been established.
- ***Loxiglumide*** is a CCK_1 receptor antagonist that has been developed to improve and speed up gastric emptying and GIT motility. Cholecystokinin (CCK) is a gastrointestinal hormone that is released from the intestine in response to meal, and slows down gastric emptying (Ch.27).
- ***Amisulpride***: Dopamine (D_2) receptors are located in the chemoreceptor trigger zone (CTZ) which is involved in emesis. Amisulpride is a selective dopamine-2 (D_2) and dopamine-3 (D_3) receptor antagonist. It is a US-FDA approved drug for the prevention of postoperative nausea and vomiting (PONV), either alone or in combination with an antiemetic of a different class. Given 5 mg as a single IV dose at the time of induction of anesthesia. *Adverse effects* arc increased prolactin level, chills, hypotension, hypokalaemia and infusion site pain.

DRUGS FOR IRRITABLE BOWEL SYNDROME (IBS)

Irritable bowel syndrome (IBS) is manifested by a variety of gastrointestinal symptoms including disordered bowel habits (constipation, diarrhoea or both) in association with abdominal pain and bloating. Hence the patients generally fall into two categories: ***Constipation-dominant-IBS*** or ***diarrhoea-dominant-IBS.***

The mainstay of the treatment for IBS is directed towards relieving abdominal pain and discomfort plus improving the bowel disorder. For patients of diarrhoea-dominant IBS, antidiarrhoeal agents (see below) are used while for patients of constipation-dominant IBS, fibre supplements are administered orally with enough water-intake. This reduces strain during defaecation by softening of the stool. However, if bloating or abdominal discomfort is exacerbated, osmotic laxative, e.g., milk of magnesia (Ch. 29) may be substituted in place of fibre diet. Several other agents, that are generally used to treat IBS, are discussed below.

Antidiarrhoeal-Antispasmodic Drugs

In patients of diarrhoea-dominant IBS, ***loperamide*** or ***diphenoxylate*** are preferred over other opioid antidiarrhoeals like codeine, to avoid CNS side effects

(Ch. 37). ***Fedotozine*** is a recently developed opioid which is peripherally κ-receptor selective antagonist. Being devoid of CNS effects, it can be given to chronic patients in whom prolonged medication is anticipated. To provide relief from abdominal pain or discomfort "antispasmodics" such as ***dicyclomine*** and ***hyoscyamine*** are commonly used. These agents work primarily by inhibiting M_3 cholinergic receptors in the enteric plexus and on smooth muscles. At low doses these have minimal side effects but at higher doses they exhibit significant anticholinergic side effects such as dryness of mouth, blurred vision, urinary retention and constipation. However, their efficacy in IBS is doubtful and hence these are not used that frequently. ***Mebeverine*** is a reserpine analogue which directly suppresses colonic hypermotility. It is devoid of usual anticholinergic side effects observed with commonly used antispasmodics.

Antidepressants

In recent years, an increasing emphasis has been laid on the pharmacological treatment of visceral sensitivity towards pain in patients of IBS. Low doses of tricyclic antidepressants (e.g., ***amitriptyline*** or ***desipramine*** 10–25 mg OD) do not affect mood but hamper central processing of visceral afferent information. Their anticholinergic properties also help in reducing gastrointestinal motility and secretion which in turn reduces the frequency and liquidity of stools.

5-HT$_3$ Receptor Antagonists

Although the biological basis of visceral hyperalgesia in IBS patients is not clear, a possible role of 5-HT$_3$ receptor has been suggested. Of all the currently identified 5-HT receptors, only 5-HT$_3$ receptor is an ionotropic receptor belonging to the nicotinic-acetylcholine super-family of receptors. 5-HT$_3$ receptors in GIT activate visceral afferent pain sensation from the gut to CNS. Blockade of 5-HT$_3$R inhibits colonic motility by decreasing the ion-permeability besides inhibiting unpleasant pain sensation.

Alosetron is a potent and selective 5-HT$_3$ antagonist that has been used to treat women with diarrhoea-dominant abdominal pain-associated IBS, who have failed to respond to conventional therapy. Somehow, the efficacy in man has not been established. In dosage of 1 mg OD or BD, it reduces all symptoms of IBS, including pain and diarrhoea. Like ondansetron, it prolongs total colonic transit time by inhibiting colonic hypermotility. However, like ondansetron it is not used as antiemetic. On the other hand, ondansetron is not used for treating IBS. This relative difference between these two 5-HT$_3$ antagonists seems paradoxical and needs elucidation.

Usual side effects of alosetron are constipation, sleep disorders and abdominal discomfort. However, constipation induced by alosetron may result into fatal ischaemic colitis. The drug has to be discontinued immediately if constipation or symptoms of ischaemic colitis occur. Reinitiation of the drug after treating ischaemic colitis is also not advisable. From the year 2000, the FDA has restricted its use in women with diarrhoea-dominant IBS not responding to other therapies.

5-HT$_4$ Receptor Agonists

Tegaserod is the peripheral 5-HT$_4$ receptor agonist that binds to mucosal 5-HT$_4$ receptors and promotes gastric emptying and facilitates small and large bowel transit. *Tegaserod* (6 mg BD) is being used for the treatment of patients with constipation-predominant IBS. It also reduces sensitivity as well as severity of pain and bloating in such patients. However, its bioavailability is only 10% and food further reduces its bioavailability. Hence, it should be taken before meals. It should be avoided in patients having severe hepatic and renal impairment.

Because of the increased incidences of heart attack and stroke (observed in post-marketing studies), tegaserod has been withdrawn from many countries including India.

Chloride Channel Activator

Lubiprostone, a prostanoic acid derivative, has been approved for treating women with constipation-dominant IBS. In men its usefulness has not yet been proved. It activates Cl^- channels in the small intestine to promote intestinal secretions and motility. It can be used on long-term basis but on stoppage the constipation reappears to pretreatment stage. Usual dose is 8 μg BD orally. Side effects include nausea; contraindicated in pregnancy.

Miscellaneous Agents

- ***Clonidine***, an α_2-adrenergic receptor agonist, can also decrease visceral hyperalgesia and reduce distension-induced pain. It also enhances salt and water absorption from the intestine and hence prevents diarrhoea. It, therefore, can be used in diarrhoea-dominant IBS but its blood pressure lowering effects limit its use.
- ***Buspirone***, an anxiolytic drug with a partial agonist action on brain 5-HT_{1A} receptors, can also reduce gastric and colonic sensitivity to distension and can be used as an adjuvant drug in the treatment of IBS.
- Other agents being used are CCK_1 receptor antagonists ***loxiglumide*** and ***dex-loxiglumide*** (see above) and ***sumatriptan*** a 5-HT_1 receptor agonist, but with little clinical success.
- ***Methylnaltrexone*** and ***alvimopan*** are two selective inhibitors of peripheral μ-receptors which may be used to antagonise opioid-induced constipation or to correct postoperative ileus in hospitalised patients; but their cardiovascular toxicity limits their use.

Tenapanor

Tenapanor is approved by the US-FDA for irritable bowel syndrome with constipation. It is a locally-acting small molecule inhibitor of the sodium/hydrogen exchanger isoform 3 (NHE3), an antiporter expressed on the apical surface of enterocytes in the small intestine and colon which is involved in sodium-fluid homeostasis. By inhibiting this antiporter, tenapanor causes retention of sodium within the lumen of the intestine results in an osmotic gradient that draws water into the lumen and softens stool consistency. It is given orally. Highly plasma protein bound drug (99%). Adverse effects: Abdominal pain, nausea or vomiting, difficulty in breathing, weakness, numbness and tingling in hands and feet.

CHAPTER 29 Drugs for Constipation, Diarrhoea, Inflammatory Bowel, Biliary & Pancreatic Disease

COMPETENCY PH1.34

Constipation means delayed passage of faeces through the intestine with defaecation process remaining normal. Evacuation is often associated with straining and is usually incomplete.

Dyschezia means derangement of defaecation process which may result due to (1) pain arising from haemorrhoids or fissure, (2) presence of hard dehydrated faecal matter in the rectum or (3) sudden cessation of a habitual use of a purgative.

Normal defaecation clears only the descending colon, whereas purgatives empty the entire colon. Thus after the successful use of purgative, a few days are needed before the normal defaecation process restarts. During this phase, the patient feels psychologically constipated and takes the purgative again. A vicious cycle now builds up which is difficult to break. This leads to the development of "cathartic or purgative-habit". It is again a misbelief that the retention of faeces results in auto-intoxication due to absorption of toxins from the colon. It is not so; because it has been observed that the headache and the feeling of being sick, due to constipation, also result by artificial distention of sigmoid colon and rectum by plugging with cotton or by an inflated balloon. Hence, these symptoms are simply due to the physical presence of the faecal matter and not by its chemical toxicity.

Majority of cases suffer with only functional constipation which can be corrected by: **(1)** An increase in the roughage (fibrous content) in the daily diet; **(2)** An increase in daily fluid intake; **(3)** An increase in physical activity; **(4)** Not neglecting the nature's call; **(5)** Adjusting the daily routine; **(6)** Selecting alternative drugs which cause lesser constipation as side effect. Certain drugs like morphine, anticholinergics and aluminium or calcium group of antacids are known to cause constipation as side effect, and **(7)** Correcting the underlying pathology; as vitamin B_1 deficiency, hypothyroidism, diabetes mellitus and Parkinson's disease etc., are some factors leading to constipation.

If all these non-therapeutic measures fail, laxative or purgatives can be used. Earlier many terms were being used as synonyms for the drugs used to relieve constipation. Their meaning and rank order of effectiveness is provided below:

Aperient (to get rid off) < *Laxative* (to loosen) < *Emollient* (to smooth and soften) < *Evacuant* (to empty) < *Purgative* (to clean) < *Cathartic* (to utterly clean).

Intensity of their action, however, depends on dose. A purgative in smaller doses can work as laxative and *vice versa*; while a purgative in higher doses can act as cathartic and *vice versa*. Hence such a classification has been dropped. Only two terms are now being used:

LAXATIVES, which result in elimination of soft semisolid stool and PURGATIVES, which provide more watery evacuation. However, these terms are used interchangeably and pharmcodynamic outcome effects are many times in distinguishable. In this text only the term purgative has been used.

PURGATIVES

Purgatives are used for complete colonic cleansing prior to

Purgatives are used: (1) to treat constipation, (2) to avoid undue straining at defaecation in cases having hernia, haemorrhoids or cardiovascular disease, (3) before or after any anorectal surgery or gastrointestinal endoscopic procedures, (4) for postoperative or post-MI bed-ridden patients, (5) to flush out worms after the use of an anthelminthic drug, and (6) to prepare the bowel before surgery or abdominal X-ray and may be needed for neurologically impaired patients.

1. Bulk-Forming Purgative

Examples: Wheat bran, Psyllium husk, Ispaghula husk, Semisynthetic cellulose such as carboxy-methyl cellulose and polycarbophils (synthetic fibers).

Site and Mode of Action: These are luminally active, hydrophilic, indigestible vegetable fibres. They stimulate peristalsis and defaecation reflexes by increasing faecal bulk due to their water absorbing and retaining capacity.

Dosage and Latency Period: Adequate amount of water must be taken with all bulk-forming laxatives. Choice of the agent is a matter of personal preference. Effect appears within 1 to 3 days. Bran powder or husk can also be sprinkled over stewed food.

Side Effects and Comments: These are not absorbed, and are quite safe. However, bacterial digestion of vegetable fibres within the colon may lead to bloating and flatus causing abdominal discomfort.

2. Osmotic Purgatives

Examples: **(A) Saline purgatives***:* Magnesium sulfate, Magnesium hydroxide (milk of magnesia), Sodium sulfate and Sodium phosphate; **(B) Polyethylene glycol (PEG)**—Electrolyte osmotic purgative. *Osmotic purgatives lead to watery evacuation;* **(C) Lactulose (10 g/15 ml), Sorbitol**.

Site and Mode of Action: All of them act on small as well as large intestine.

A) ***Saline purgatives*** are soluble inorganic salts which increase the faecal bulk by retaining water by osmotic effect, thus increasing peristalsis indirectly. Magnesium salts also release cholecystokinin which further helps in increasing intestinal secretions and peristalsis.

B) ***Polyethylene glycol (PEG)***—Electrolyte osmotic purgative contains a nonabsorbable polyethylene glycol (PEG) which is a sugar that retains water by virtue of its high osmotic nature. It is used in a form of a balanced isotonic solution prepared by adding sodium chloride, sodium sulfate, sodium bicarbonate and potassium chloride. The isotonic solution of PEG is so designed that no electrolyte shift occurs across the intestinal wall. Therefore, the preparation is safe for all patients.

Dosage and Latency Period: Milk of magnesia, being tasteless, is the most commonly used saline purgative. Other salts have an unpleasant taste. 30 ml of its 8% w/w suspension is given in the morning because it is quite effective. Its effects come within 2–3 hrs. PEG—Electrolyte osmotic purgative is ingested orally. 4 liters of this solution should be ingested over 2–3 hours for complete colonic cleansing prior to GIT endoscopic procedures. For treatment of chronic constipation smaller doses of this solution can be used (300–500 ml daily in the morning or 17 g of the powder in 8 ounces of water per day). The latency period is 2–3 hrs.

Side Effects and Comments: The saline purgatives should be ingested with enough water, because being irritants these may induce vomiting. The hyper-osmolar agents may lead to intravascular fluid depletion and electrolyte disturbances. These should never be used on long-term basis and should be avoided in hypertensives and in cases of CHF. Magnesium salts should not be used for prolonged period in patients with renal insufficiency due to the risk of hypermagnesaemia, as about 20% of ingested magnesium is normally absorbed.

C) Lactulose (10 g/15 ml), Sorbitol.

Site and Mode of Action: It is also luminally active, nonabsorable-indigestible disaccharide (sugar). It increases faecal bulk by hydrophilic action and also due to osmotic action.

Dosage and Latency Period: It is given in a dose of 10 g BD or TDS with plenty of water to produce 2 or 3 soft stools per day. Latency period is 1–3 days.

Side Effects and Comments: It is non-toxic and is also suitable for long-term use. Flatulence is common, cramps may occur in few. Some patients may feel nauseated due to its peculiar sweet taste.

Lactulose is also used for the treatment of hepatic encephalopathy. For this purpose a dose of 20 g TDS orally is needed. In hepato-encephalopathy there is a severe hepatocellular damage because of which the portal blood is directly shunted to systemic circulation.

Hence, several toxic metabolites from the colon (e.g., NH_3) get accumulated in the blood leading to CNS toxicity. Lactulose is degraded to lactic acid and converts NH_3 to ionised NH_4^+ salt which is then excreted.

3. Lubricant Purgative

Example: Liquid paraffin.

Site and Mode of Action: It is also a luminally active agent. It is pharmacologically inert viseous liquid which contains mineral oil. It is a faecal lubricant and stool softener as it retards water absorption from the stool.

Dosage and Latency Period: It is given as 15–30 ml per day at bed time. Latency period is 1–3 days.

Side Effects and Comments: It is not palatable but can be given in emulsified form or with juices. Frequent use leads to the deficiency of fat-soluble vitamins (A, D, E & K) as they are carried away with stool in emulsified form. Forcible administration can lead to aspiration lipid pneumonia. It also delays the healing of enteric fistula. Though *used only occasionally* it is useful where straining at defaecation is to be avoided.

4. Surfactant Purgative

Example: Dioctyl sodium sulfosuccinate (Docusate sodium).

Site and Mode of Action: It is again a luminally active agent and is an anionic surfactant which softens the stool by decreasing the surface tension of fluids in the bowel. It also acts as a wetting agent for the bowel, because by emulsifying the colonic contents it facilitates the mixing of water into fatty substances of the faeces.

Dosage and Latency Period: 100–400 mg orally per day (in divided doses). It is a mild laxative, specially indicated when straining at defaecation is to be avoided. Latency period is 1–3 days.

Side Effects and Comments: It is not absorbed and hence non-toxic. Being bitter in taste, it can cause nausea. Cramps and abdominal pain may occur. Hepatotoxicity may occur after prolonged use. It increases the absorption of liquid paraffin, hence should not be given together.

5. Irritant Purgatives

Examples: **(A) Anthraquinone group**: Senna, Cascara and Aloe; **(B) Organic irritants**: Phenolphthalein, Bisacodyl (and its suppository); Sodium picosulfate; and **(C) Oils**: Castor oil. *Irritant purgatives provide soft semifluid stools.*

Site and Mode of Action: All of them stimulate peristalsis by irritant action on intestinal mucosa. They also stimulate colonic electrolyte and fluid secretion by altering the absorptive and secretory activity of the mucosal cells. *Aloe, senna* and *cascara* occur naturally in plants. ***Senna*** is most commonly used. These plant purgatives contain anthraquinone glycosides. On reaching the colon, the bacteria degrade them to the active principle—"anthrol"—which either acts locally or is absorbed into circulation. After being excreted through bile it then stimulates small intestine.

The primary site of action of *organic irritants* is in the colon. ***Bisacodyl*** is metabolised in the intestine into an active deacetylated metabolite. In the colon ***sodium picosulfate*** is also converted to an active metabolite which stimulates peristalsis and promotes water and electrolyte accumulation. ***Castor oil*** itself is non-irritant. It is hydrolysed in intestine by pancreatic lipase to ricinolic acid which increases the intestinal motility.

Dosage and Latency Period: Calculated on the basis of ***Senna glycosides:*** Sennoside A and B; these are given in a dose of 12–25 mg (approx) at bed time. Effect comes within 6–8 hours. ***Phenolphthalein*** (though seldom used now) is given in a dose of 60–130 mg at bed time. The effect appears within 6–8 hrs. ***Bisacodyl*** is given in a dose of 5–10 mg at bedtime. The effect appears within 8–10 hrs. Suppositories (10 mg) are also available. ***Sodium picosulfate*** is administered in a dose of 5–10 mg at bed time. It is usually effective within 6–8 hrs. ***Castor oil*** (because of unpalatability and side effects) is seldom used these days. Usual dose is 15–25 ml in the morning as the effect appears within 3 hrs.

Side Effects and Comments: Senna glycosides are secreted through milk, hence should be avoided in lactating mothers. These glysosides turn urine colour to yellowish-brown (acidic urine) or to red (alkaline urine). Chronic use leads to a characteristic brown pigmentation of the colon known as "melanosis coli". It is contraindicated in pregnancy to avoid pelvic congestion. All anthraquinones can produce abdominal cramps and nausea. About 15–20% of ***phenolphthalein*** undergoes enterohepatic circulation and hence exhibits prolonged action. It turns urine reddish-pink, if alkaline. Skin rash may occur (but rarely). Its use has drastically declined because of the reports about its cardiac toxicity and carcinogenicity.

Bisacodyl, is however, quite safe, except for occasional abdominal cramps and skin rashes. Prolonged use or overdosage of ***sodium picosulfate*** can cause colonic atony and hypokalaemia. ***Castor oil*** is no longer a favoured purgative because of its unpalatability, frequent cramping, after-constipation, and risk for damaging intestinal mucosa. It is contraindicated in pregnancy (to avoid pelvic congestion). However, its purgative action is self limiting because irritant action of ricinolic acid increases peristalsis, which sweeps away the remaining castor oil.

For other drugs, to treat constipation, refer irritable bowel syndrome (Ch. 28).

ANTIDIARRHOEAL AGENTS

Diarrhoea is an abnormal increase in the frequency and the liquidity of stools. Increased motility of GIT and the decreased ability of intestine to absorb water from the stool are the major factors in the causation of diarrhoea. Treatment of specific-infective diarrhoeas needs proper diagnosis and appropriate drug treatment by selecting proper antibiotic or an antiprotozoal drug or a combination of both. Similarly, diarrhoea due to underlying pathology or endocrinal disorders can be treated by correcting the underlying cause. *However, for the symptomatic relief of non-specific diarrhoeas, the following category of drugs can be used:*

Antimotility and Antisecretory Agents

1. Opioid Agonists

The drugs which fall in this category are ***loperamide, diphenoxylate, difenoxin*** (an active metabolite of diphenoxylate) and ***racecadotril***. These drugs act by stimulating peripheral μ (mu) as well as δ (delta) receptors present on small and large intestine. Activation of μ receptor decreases motility; while activation of δ receptors decreases intestinal secretions. Although all opioids such as morphine or codeine have antidiarrhoeal effects, their CNS effects and dependence liability limit their usefulness. ***Loperamide*** is an OTC drug among opioid agonists that does not cross BBB and has neither analgesic effects nor any addiction liability. As an antidiarrhoeal agent it is 40 times more potent than morphine. The usual adult dose is 4 mg followed by 2 mg after each loose motion to a maximum of 16 mg/day (onset of action: 1–2 hrs; duration of effect: 6–12 hrs). However, for chronic diarrhoeas it is commonly given as 2–4 mg TDS. ***Diphenoxylate*** or its active metabolite ***difenoxin*** are other opioid agonists that have no analgesic properties. However, higher doses have CNS depressant effects and exhibit dependence liability after prolonged use. As an antidiarrhoeal agent it is more potent than morphine but less potent than loperamide. The most popular formulation (LOMOTIL) contains ***diphenoxylate*** (2.5 mg) with small doses of ***atropine*** (0.025 mg) to discourage abuse potential. Atropine, besides providing antispasmodic effects, prevents the possible abuse of diphenoxylate because undesirable effects of atropine would appear prior to the pleasurable effects of the opioid, if the dose is increased for abuse. Usual dose is 2 tabs TDS or QID.

These drugs have been shown to be effective against traveler's diarrhoea or to prevent non-specific diarrhoea; but replacement of fluids through ORS (see below) is still the mainstay for such therapy.

In the recommended doses, these drugs are well tolerated, except for some milder side effects like abdominal discomfort and dry mouth. These drugs should not be used in patients with colitis in order to avoid development of megacolon. These medications should be avoided in patients suffering from acute bacterial diarrhoeas associated with high fever or blood in stool because of the potential of these drugs to decrease the clearance of the pathogens and to enhance the subsequent systemic invasion of these organisms. These should not be used in children below 2 years of age (danger of paralytic ileus).

Racecadotril is a new antidiarrhoeal drug that belongs to this group. It is the enkephalinase inhibitor that increases local concentration of enkephalins in intestinal mucosa which then stimulate μ and δ opioid receptors (like loperamide) to produce antidiarrhoeal effects. Side effects are mild and include nausea, constipation and headache. It is secreted through breast milk and hence should be avoided in lactating mothers. No significant drug interactions have been reported.

2. Anticholinergics

Anticholinergic drugs like ***hyoscyamine*** and ***dicyclomine*** decrease bowel motility which results in an increase of fluid absorption, back from the intestinal tract, and a decrease in abdominal cramps. However, these drugs are not used as a sole antidiarrhoeal drug but are used in combination with adsorbents or opiates. Adverse effects include the usual anticholinergic effects.

3. α_2-Adrenergic Receptor Agonists

Clonidine (0.1 mg BD, oral) facilitates absorption, inhibits secretion of fluids and electrolytes as well as increases the intestinal transit time. Clonidine and substitutes may have a special role in the treatment of diabetic diarrhoea and in diarrhoea caused by opiate withdrawal. However, its blood pressure lowering effects are the major limiting factors for its use as a routine antidiarrhoeal agent.

4. Octreotide

It is a synthetic octapeptide analogue of somatostatin (Ch. 41). It has a longer half life (1.5–2 hr) compared to somatostatin (3 min). It is much more potent (more than 40 times) than somatostatin in inhibiting the secretion of growth hormone, glucagon, insulin and VIP. However, its antidiarrhoeal effects involve the inhibition of the release of 5-HT, gastrin, secretin, CCK, motilin and pancreatic polypeptide. It reduces GIT motility, intestinal fluid and electrolyte secretion, pancreatic secretion and gall bladder contractions. It is, therefore, mainly used to treat secretory diarrhoeas associated with carcinoid tumours and VIP secreting tumours as well as to treat acromegaly and to prevent variceal bleeding (as it decreases hepatic blood flow). It may be given subcutaneously in a dose of 100 mcg BD or TDS. In low doses (50 mcg S.C.) it rather stimulates GIT motility. Side effects depend on duration of treatment. A short-term therapy leads to slight nausea, abdominal discomfort and pain at the site of injection. Long-term therapy can lead to gall stone formation and hypothyroidism. Impaired pancreatic secretion may cause steatorrhoea which can lead to fat-soluble vitamin deficiency.

The new analogs of octreotide are ***lanreotide***, ***seglitide*** and ***vapreotide***. Out of these lanreotide has longer duration of action of about 4 weeks.

Telotristat Ethyl

Telotristat ethyl is used orally for carcinoid syndrome diarrhoea. It is a rare condition with neuroendocrine tumours, which can produce excessive serotonin leading to diarrhoea, flushing and broncho-constriction. Telotristat ethyl is an inhibitor of enzyme tryptophan hydroxylase required for the synthesis of serotonin. It is used in combination with somatostatin analogue therapy.

Adsorbent Drugs

Kaolin is a hydrated magenisum-aluminium silicate while ***pectin*** is a sort of indigestible purified carbohydrate obtained from apple. Both the agents adsorb bacteria, enterotoxins and fluid to increase the consistency of faecal matter. Pectin being demulscent, coats the inflammed GIT mucosa also. ***Kaolin-pectin combination*** had been a popular formulation before, but seldom used now.

Bismuth subsalicylate reduces stool frequency and liquidity in acute diarrhoea due to inhibition of PG synthesis and Cl^- secretion by its salicylate counterpart. Bismuth has some antimicrobial effects, binds to enterotoxins and also provides protective coating over inflammed gastric mucosa. It is now rarely used because the doses required for relief are large and need to be administered frequently. Being not absorbed, adsorbents have minimal side effects except constipation. Bismuth subsalicylate causes blackening of stool (mistaken for melaena) and darkening of tongue because of a reaction between bismuth and the sulfide (produced by bacteria) to form a black bismuth sulfide.

No adsorbent drug (discussed above) should be taken within 2 hrs of other medication, because it may decrease the absorption of other orally administered drugs.

Miscellaneous Agents

Lactobacillus sporogens are intended to replace the normal bacterial flora that is lost during acute diarrhoea or due to the use of antibiotics. These are also used as an adjuvant therapy for aphthous stomatitis and diarrhoea.

Lactase is indicated for individuals who have insufficient amount of lactase in the small intestine. Lactase is an enzyme responsible for digesting lactose, a common disaccharide present in the dairy products. In absence of lactase, lactose draws water into the GI tract and causes diarrhoea. The dose is 1–2 capsules of lactase taken with milk.

Non-Pharmacological Measures Fluid and Electrolyte Replacement (Oral Rehydration Therapy; ORT)

During diarrhoea, a glucose-coupled sodium transport continues in the intestine which causes water and electrolyte losses through stools. Hence, glucose-electrolyte solutions are simple, effective and cheaper oral therapy to treat a vast majority of watery diarrhoea. However, if fluid loss is severe and/or severe vomiting persists, there may be a need for I.V. fluids before oral maintenance rehydration therapy can be pursued. Oral rehydration solution (ORS) replaces the fluid or electrolytes what the body has lost due to diarrhoea. The ***glucose-based*** ORS can easily be made at home as per WHO standard formula:

Sodium Chloride	3.5 g
Potassium Chloride	1.5 g
Sodium Citrate	2.9 g
Glucose	20.0 g
Water	1 L

Total osmolarity 311 mmol/L

The higher sodium content of WHO formulation is based on approximate sodium loss in adult diarrhoea. However, low-sodium glucose-based formulations may be preferred in infants and children whose faecal losses of sodium are less. The WHO has recommended the replacement of standard 311 mmol/L formula by the new 245 mmol/L formula.

Sodium Chloride	2.6 g
Potassium Chloride	1.5 g
Sodium Citrate	2.9 g
Glucose	13.5 g
Water	1 L

Total osmolarity 245 mmol/L

For mild to moderate diarrhoea in adults, approximately 2–3 liters of any one of the ORS cited above should be consumed within first 4 hrs. Thereafter, simply the ongoing losses are to be replaced.

Carbonated soft drinks, tea, coffee, powdered drinks and hypertonic juices should be avoided in diarrhoea because these make diarrhoea worse and do not contain the electrolytes needed.

The ***cereal-based*** ORS has the advantage of controlling diarrhoea much more effectively than the *glucose-based* ORS. This may be because undigested starch is fermented in the colon to short chain fatty acids which stimulate sodium and water absorption back from the colon. Further, rice powder has 7% protein which on hydrolysis yields amino acids that too stimulate colonic salt and water absorption. The commonly used ***rice-based ORS*** formula is as under:

Precooked rice flour	10.15 g (extruded)
Sodium Chloride	0.94 g
Sodium Citrate	0.20 g
Potassium Citrate	0.44 g
Water	200 ml

TREATMENT OF INFLAMMATORY BOWEL DISEASE

Ulcerative colitis and Crohn's disease are the two important diseases among the inflammatory bowel diseases. The pathogenesis of these diseases involves immune mechanism and an imbalance between proinflammatory and anti-inflammatory cytokines. The main drugs used in the treatment of ulcerative colitis and Crohn's disease are the aminosalicylates and corticosteroids, though recent introduction of certain immunosuppressants and anti-TNF$_\alpha$ drugs constitute some novel therapies for the treatment of inflammatory disease. Antidiarrhoeals should be avoided in active and severe ulcerative colitis as they can lead to dilatation of colon and its perforation.

Ulcerative Colitis

Aminosalicylates

Sulfasalazine, olsalazine and ***balsalazine*** contain a 5-aminosalicyclic acid (5-ASA) moiety bound by an azo (N=N) bond to an inert moiety or by another 5-ASA molecule. In ***sulfasalazine***, 5-ASA is bound to sulfapyridine; in ***balsalazine*** 5-ASA is bound to an inert carrier 4-aminobenzoyl-β-alanine, while in ***olsalazine*** two 5-ASA molecules are joined to each other. Azo compounds, in general, are least absorbed in stomach and small intestine. When they reach terminal ileum and colon, the colonic bacteria split the azo compound by an azoreductase enzyme that releases 5-ASA in higher concentration at the desired site of action. Sulfapyridine released from sulfasalazine (along with 5-ASA) is absorbed, acetylated in liver and excreted in urine. By contrast, the breakdown product of balsalazine, after azoreduction is not absorbed but excreted as such in faeces. These components of the drug molecule merely serve as an inert carrier for 5-ASA and have no therapeutic action in colitis. 5-ASA (the active moiety) has only topical anti-inflammatory action (not systemic). The generic name of 5-ASA is ***"mesalamine"***.

Patients intolerant to sulfasalazine or balsalazine usually tolerate olsalazine which contains two 5-ASA molecules joined together by an azo bond. Most of the adverse effects of sulfasalazine are attributable to its associated sulfapyridine moiety. ***Mesalamine*** with pH-sensitive coating has been introduced which releases 5-ASA directly in the terminal ileum and the colon. It is claimed to be a more efficacious formulation with lesser side effects.

5-ASA inhibit the synthesis of prostaglandins by inhibiting cyclo-oxygenase, like salicylates, as well as inhibit the production of cytokinins. 5-ASA also inhibits the activity of nuclear factor-kB which is an important transcription factor for pro-inflammatory cytokines. It also suppresses the generation of superoxide free radicals.

Sulfasalazine group of drugs induce as well as maintain the remissions in patients of ulcerative colitis. 5-ASA suppository or enema is useful in patients with ulcerative colitis confined to rectum or distal colon but if ulcerative colitis extends up to proximal colon, systemic use of these drugs is more beneficial. Oral dose of sulfasalazine is 1 g 6 hrly until remission occurs; thereafter 1 g BD for maintenance. Sulfasalazine group of drugs are also useful as disease modifying antirheumatoid drugs (DMARD, see Ch. 26). Balsalazine is given as 2.25 g TDS orally followed by 1.5 g BD for maintenance. pH-sensitive mesalamine is given as 800 mg orally TDS and then 400 mg TDS for maintenance.

Their *adverse effects* are due largely to the presence of carrier molecule and include headache, anorexia, nausea-vomiting, allergic reactions like skin rash, fever and lymphadenitis. Sulfasalazine in high doses or on prolonged use can lead to reversible oligospermia and male infertility. Sulfasalazine impairs folate absorption. Dietary supplements of folic acid are usually required to compensate the needs. Other formulations of ASA are better tolerated than sulfasalazine. However, olsalazine may stimulate secretory diarrhoea which can create diagnostic confusion in patients with inflammatory bowel disease.

Immunosuppressants

1. Glucocorticoids

Prednisone and ***prednisolone*** have been the mainstay of the treatment for acute/severe exacerbations of inflammatory bowel disease. These have an intermediate duration of action allowing once daily dosing. When ulcerative colitis is restricted to the left hemicolon, exacerbations that do not respond to 5-ASA alone can normally be controlled by steroid retention enema. The foam-based formulations appear to coat the colonic mucosa more effectively than the aqueous formulations. Moderately severe attacks of ulcerative colitis should be treated with systemic glucocorticoid, administered orally. Oral prednisone in a starting dose of 40 mg once a day or prednisolone 60 mg once a day are considered as standard dose regimen. Higher doses have not been more beneficial. The anti-inflammatory response appears within 2 weeks. Once remission has been attained, the doses can be tapered down over a period of 6–8 weeks. If there is no improvement, immunosuppressants and/ or infliximab may be used to induce remission (see below). 5-ASA may then be used for the maintenance therapy, as corticosteroids are not useful for maintenance. The mechanism of action and the side effects of glucocorticoids are detailed in Chapter 42.

2. Cyclosporine

Cyclosporine may induce remissions in case of severe ulcerative colitis unresponsive to corticosteroids. It causes pronounced suppression of proinflammatory transcription factors. It is given in a dose of 2–4 mg/kg/day I.V., until remission is attained. Later for maintenance therapy, *azathioprine* is often substituted as cyclosporine is not effective for maintenance therapy. Renal functions should be closely monitored while using cyclosporine as it is nephrotoxic (Ch. 69).

3. Azathioprine and 6-Mercaptopurine

These are purine antimetabolites that have immunosuppressive properties (Ch. 69). Azathioprine is a prodrug yeilding 6-mercaptopurine (which is azathioprine without a side chain). Both these drugs can be used interchangeably. Azathioprine is given in a dose of 2.5 mg/kg/day while 6-mercaptopurine is given in a dose of 1.5 mg/kg/day. Both get converted to active metabolites having longer half-life. As a result the therapeutic effects of azathioprine are delayed by about 6–8 weeks. Hence, it is not effective for inducing remission in patients of ulcerative colitis. These drugs are primarily used for maintenance of remission for ulcerative colitis. Azathioprine or 6-mecraptopurine may allow dose reductions or elimination of steroids in patients of ulcerative colitis.

The toxicities of these drugs are dose related and include nausea, vomiting, bone marrow depression and hepatotoxicity. Hence, liver function tests and blood counts should be monitored intermittently. Pancreatitis, which probably is a hypersensitivity reaction, can occur in about 5% of the cases. Risk of teratogenicity appears to be negligible. 6-Mercaptopurine is better tolerated than azathioprine.

Allopurinol markedly inhibits the metabolism of these purine analogues. Hence the dose of 6-mercaptopurine or azathioprine should be reduced appropriately in patients receiving allopurinol.

Crohn's Disease

Ulcerative colitis and Crohn's disease have several overlapping features and so do the drugs used for their treatment which also share many properties that are beneficial in both the disease conditions. Ulcerative colitis is confined to the colon and the inflammatory processes, which are usually superficial and involve the distal portions, can extend for a variable length proximally. Crohn's disease on the contrary can affect both the small as well as large instestine and, although less commonly, any other segment of GIT which can be complicated further by intestinal strictures, fistula and intra-abdominal abscess.

Treatment depends on the site of disease. Management of colonic Crohn's disease is very similar to that of ulcerative colitis treated with 5-ASA and corticosteroids. Sulfasalazine group of drugs are ineffective in small bowel Crohn's disease because these drugs liberate 5-ASA in the colon. In more severe disease, corticosteroids are needed to induce remission but are of little value in maintaining remission. ***Budesonide***, a potent topically active corticosteroid, can also be administered either orally or as enema but with a little success as even a delayed release formulation has a very poor bioavailability. However, enteric-coated budesonide has been recently introduced to treat ileocaecal Crohn's disease. Dose: 9 mg/day for 12 weeks. There is no supportive evidence to prove that cyclosporine is effective in Crohn's disease. Other drugs which are beneficial in the management of Crohn's disease are as under:

1. Anti-TNF_α Drugs

Infliximab, Adalimumab and Certolizumab

Increased levels of TNF_α are found in faecal samples of the patients of Crohn's disease. ***Infliximab*** is a chimeric (25% mouse + 75% human) monoclonal antibody that cross-links with soluble as well as membrane bound TNF_α receptors and inhibits T-cells and macrophage functions. Consequently, the release of other proinflammatory cytokines (IL-1, 6 and 8; collagenase and metalloproteinases) is prevented. It is administered in a dose of 5–10 mg/kg by I.V. infusion at 0, 2 and 6 week interval. A single dose of infliximab induces remission in approximately 40% of patients with Crohn's disease resistant to conventional therapies. An additional dose after 8 weeks appears to produce long-lasting remission. ***Adalimumab*** is a recombinant 100% human anti-TNF_α monoclonal antibody. Its mode of action is similar to infliximab. It is given subcutaneously (160 mg, 80 mg and 40 mg at 0, 2 and 4 weeks, respectively) and has a longer plasma half-life. It has lesser immunogenicity and side effects compared to these drugs. For adverse effects profile of these drugs refer Chapter 26. There is no substantial proof about the efficacy of infliximab in ulcerative colitis. Like adalimumab, ***certolizumab*** also is a recombinant monoclonal (95% human) antibody with similar mode of action. It is given as 400 mg (S.C.) at 0, 2 and 4 weeks interval. Certolizumab, as it lacks Fc protion in its structure, does not produce antibody-mediated apoptosis and complement-mediated cytotoxicity of cells expressing membrane-bound TNF_α.

2. Methotrexate

Methotrexate is useful in controlling relapse of Crohn's disease unresponsive to corticosteroid or azathioprine. It is a cytotoxic agent (Ch. 67) with pronounced immunosuppresive (Ch. 69) and anti-inflammatory properties (Ch. 26). 15–25 mg I.M. or S.C. injection of methotrexate every week appears to be effective in steroid-dependent Crohn's disease but not in ulcerative colitis. However, its adverse effects on long-term use, including bone marrow suppression, pulmonary and hepatic fibrosis limit its use in Crohn's disease.

3. Antibiotics

In contrast to ulcerative colitis about 50% of patients with colonic Crohn's disease respond to ***metronidazole*** and/or ***ciprofloxacin***. However, adverse effects as a consequence of long-term therapy (Ch. 65) limit their usefulness. Certain bacterial strains (e.g., *Bacteroides*) are pro-, while some (e.g., *Lactobacillus*) are anti-inflammatory. Hence, probiotics have also been used as adjuvants in the management of Crohn's disease.

4. Anti-Integrin Monoclonal Antibody

Integrin and selectins are two different classes of adhesion molecules found on the surface of leukocytes and on vascular endothelium, respectively. During inflammatory process circulatory leukocytes get adhered to vascular endothelium and subsequently penetrate through the vessel wall into other tissues. The α-4 subunit of integrins is involved in binding of leukocytes to the vascular adhesion molecules. ***Natalizumab*** is a humanised monoclonal antibody against α-4 subunit of integrin and their subsequent migration into surrounding tissue. Though withdrawn in 2005, due to controversial reports about its association with progressive multifocal leukoencephalopathy (PML), it was reintroduced later for restricted use in patients of Crohn's disease who did not respond to other therapies. Dose: 300 mg every 4 weeks by I.V. infusion. Concomitant use of other immuno-suppressant drugs is contraindicated (reactivation of latent human polyomavirus leading to PML).

DRUGS USED IN PANCREATIC INSUFFICIENCY

Pancreatic enzymes supplements, which normally contain a mixture of amylase, lipase and proteases, are the mainstay of the treatment of the pancreatic enzyme insufficiency which is most commonly caused by cystic fibrosis, chronic pancreatitis or pancreatic resection. Exocrine pancreatic enzyme deficiency leads to fat and protein indigestion which in turn causes steatorrhoea, azotorrhoea, vitamin deficiency and weight loss.

Most commonly used preparation is ***pancrelipase*** which has a more powerful lipolytic and proteolytic activity compared to pancreatin. Since pancrelipase is acid-labile, its enteric coated formulation is used. The non-enteric formulation should be used along with H_2-blockers or PPIs (to reduce chances of its gastric acid destruction). It is given in a dose that provides 30,000 Units of lipase activity post-meal; addition of H_2 blocker or PPI may improve response. The enteric-coated tablet should be swallowed and not chewed, not only to prevent gastric acid destruction of pancrelipase, but to avoid the risk of producing oropharyngeal mucositis caused by the enzyme itself. Higher doses should not be used in patients with cystic fibrosis as they may cause ileocaecal and large bowel strictures.

Pancreatin is another preparation commonly used in developing countries. It is obtained from pig pancreas and contains amylase, trypsin and lipase. It is much less potent than pancrelipase. Its properties and side effects are similar to pancrelipase.

Miscellaneous Enzymes

Papain is obtained from raw papaya while ***pepsin*** powder is prepared from gastric mucosa of pigs, cattle or sheep. Both have proteolytic activity which helps in degradation of proteins into peptides of low molecular weight. Pepsin maintains its activity in acidic medium (pH 1–5). It is used along with HCl or glutamic acid as an adjunct in the treatment of gastric hypochlorhydria or to treat digestive enzyme deficiency. ***Diastase*** and ***takadiastase*** are amylolytic enzymes (amylase) obtained from fungus *Aspergillus oryzae*. It hydrolyses polysaccharides to sugars.

These enzymes are sometimes also used in pancreatic insufficiency but efficacy is doubtful.

DRUGS FOR CHOLESTEROL GALLSTONES

Cholesterol (CH) remains dissolved in bile with the help of bile salts. A high CH:bile salt ratio favours crystallisation of CH in bile leading to gallstone formation. ***Ursodeoxycholic acid*** (***ursodiol***) is the only available agent for dissolution of gallstone. It is a minor constituent of human bile (but major bile acid in the bear, hence the prefix *urso*). It is effective only in a functional gall bladder. If the bile is not entering the gall bladder, it would not be able to solubilise the stones.

Ursodiol (ursodeoxycholic acid) promotes dissolution of gallstones because: **(1)** It inhibits absorption of cholesterol from intestines, **(2)** It reduces CH secretion in the bile, shortly after the initiation of the drug therapy, **(3)** It lowers saturation index of bile so that it is no longer lithogenic and **(4)** It promotes solubilisation of gallstone by liquid crystal formation.

Ursodiol in a dose of 7–10 mg/kg/day usually dissolves small non-calcified CH stones (<10 mm dia) in gall bladder in 50% of patients but its use beyond 2 years is not justified. It is also effective for the prevention of gallstones in obese patients undergoing rapid weight loss therapy. Ursodiol 13–15 mg/kg/day (in 4 divided doses after some food) is useful in patients with early primary biliary cirrhosis (reduces liver function abnormalities and improves liver histology). **Ursodiol** may produce diarrhoea. About 30% of cases may have stone recurrence.

CHAPTER 30

SECTION 7—DRUGS ACTING ON CENTRAL NERVOUS SYSTEM

Neurotransmission in Central Nervous System & Types of Mental Disorders

COMPETENCY PH1.19

This chapter introduces fundamental principles regarding actions of various neurotransmitters and modulators onto their respective receptors along with an organisation of CNS which will be viewed from anatomical, functional or chemical perspectives. Specific therapeutic approaches to neurologic and psychiatric disorders are discussed in subsequent chapters of this section.

ORGANISATION OF CNS

The brain is basically a super computer, operating through chemical neurotransmission. It is concerned with every happening in the body right from specialised functions like circulation, digestion and respiration to modulation of psychic processes such as emotional feelings, our attitude, thoughts and memory including a balanced co-ordination between them.The brain is protected by a specialised system of capillary endothelial cells known as blood-brain-barrier (BBB). The role of BBB is to **(1)** preserve the internal environment of the brain and to maintain the desired concentration of nutrients and to regulate the levels of circulating neurotransmitters such as E, NE, ACh, 5-HT and dopamine (DA) as well as to **(2)** protect the brain tissue, both from toxic substances that may circulate in the blood and also from neurotransitters like E, NE, ACh and DA which were released peripherally to provide systemic peripheral effects but could bind to CNS receptors to cause adverse effects if their access was permitted. The BBB does not cover all parts of the brain. The circumventricular organs not covered by BBB include: area postrema (beneath the floor of fourth ventricle, i.e., area of chemoreceptor trigger zone and vomiting centre), pineal gland, pituitary gland, median eminence and the choroid plexus capillaries (for detail refer Ch. 6).

The major anatomical divisions of the brain include *cerebrum* (cerebral cortex or cerebral hemispheres), subcortical region which includes *thalamus* and *hypothalamus* (collectively called diencephalon); the *mid brain* (the upper segment of brainstem); the *hind brain* composed of *pons*, *medulla* and *cerebellum* (the brainstem) and the *spinal cord* (Fig. 30.1).

The *cerebrum* (cerebral cortex) is the largest part of the human brain and is divided into left and right hemispheres. Left hemisphere is associated with logic and reasoning while the right hemisphere with creativity. The cerebral cortex consists of four regions: (a) the *frontal cortex,* which is associated with higher cognitive functions and long-term memory storage. The posterior part of this frontal cortex, called *primary motor cortex*, controls fine movements; (b) the *parietal lobe,* which integrates and processes sensory information from touch, muscle stretch receptors and joint receptors. Hence it is also called *somatosensory cortex;* (c) the *temporal lobe,* which is involved in auditory functions and language and also processes sensory information originating from ears and vestibular organs; and (d) the *occipital lobe,* which is involved in visual processing and receives information from visual pathways and hence also referred to as "visual cortex". Major cholinergic and dopaminergic pathways pass through cerebral cortex region.

The *thalamus* has both sensory and motor functions. It is a relay center for sensory pathways to the cortex. It is concerned with appreciation of pain, temperature and crude touch sensation. The *hypothalamus* is involved in homeostasis, emotion, thirst, hunger, circadian rhythm and control of autonomic functions. It also controls pituitary gland. *Limbic system* (also called emotional brain) consists of *hippocampus* (involved in learning and memory), the *amygdala* (associated with emotions, fear and memory) and the *ventral tegmental area* or *nucleus accumbens* (involved in addiction). In short, the limbic system consists of structures beneath the cerebral cortex that control emotions and instincts

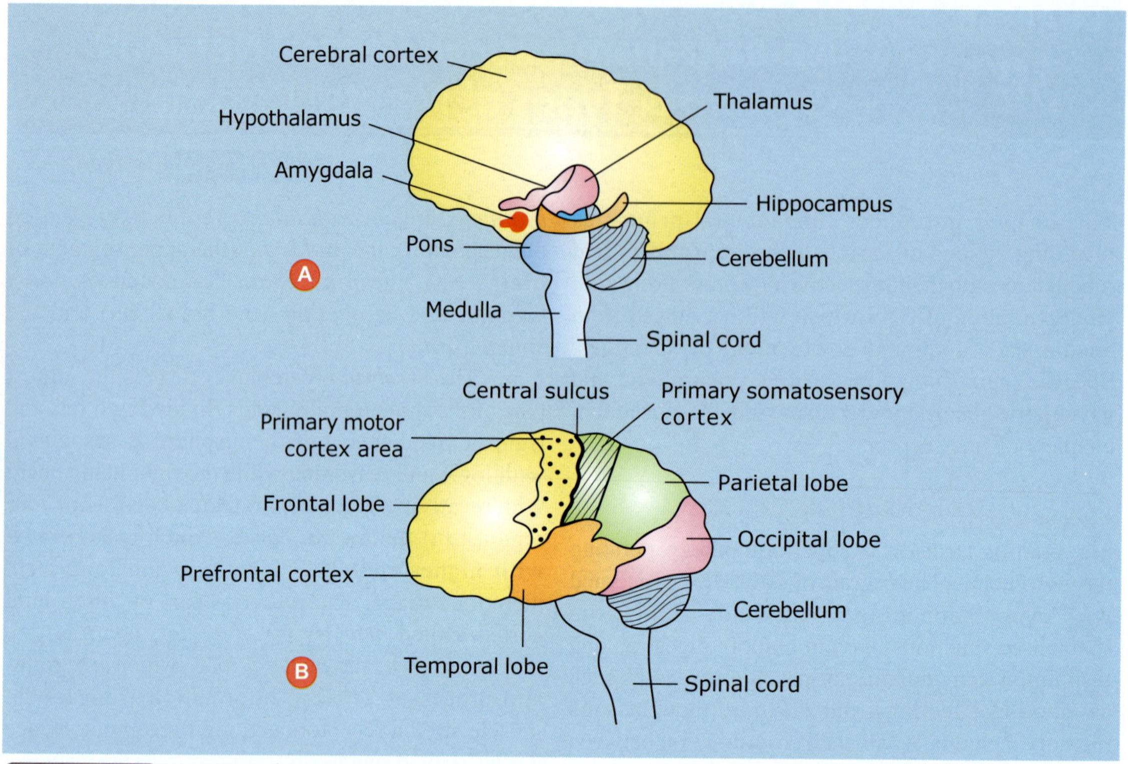

Fig 30.1 (A) Anatomical Structures in the Brain. (B) Regions of Cerebral Cortex.

along with motor and visceral activities. The *basal ganglia* which is the part of extrapyramidal system consists of *corpus striatum* (caudate nucleus + putamen + globus pallidus) and *substantia nigra*. It provides extrapyramidal control of skeletal muscle tone and its coordination with posture. Its degeneration produces tremors and rigidity. It contains the major dopaminergic pathways of the CNS.

The *reticular formation* is a heterogenous mass of cell bodies embedded in a network of dendrites and axons located in the central core of medulla, pons and midbrain. It is a diffused multisynaptic system. A complex inter-related group of pathways coursing through the reticular formation is called *reticular activating system* (RAS). It is intimately concerned with sleep-wakefulness cycle and for coordination of gaze and eye movements. All sensory information courses through the RAS. It also controls the muscle tone, posture and such vital functions as respiration and circulation. It has the major monoamine containing neurons of the brain.

The *medulla* and *pons* (including midbrain) are referred to as *brainstem* and are involved in vision, hearing and in body movements. The *medulla* regulates vital functions such as breathing and heart rate while the *pons* is concerned with motor and sensory control and plays a vital role in consciousness and sleep. The *cerebellum* is associated with the control of vestibular functions, body posture and balance. Cerebellum and brainstem relay information from the cerebral cortex and the limbic system to the spinal cord. The *spinal cord* integrates the sensory and motor reflexes and also controls the muscle tone.

NEUROCHEMICAL TRANSMISSION IN CNS

The basic process of synaptic transmission in CNS is essentially the same as that operating in the periphery (Ch. 10,11 and 12). Four processes may occur in relation to nerve transmission within the CNS: the *neurotransmission*, the *neuromodulation*, the *neuromediation* and *mediation through neurotropic factors*. Analogously such chemical secretions are termed as *neurotransmitters, neuromodulators, neuromediators* and *neurotropic factors*, respectively.

The ***neurotransmitters*** are released into the synaptic cleft to *rapidly stimulate* or *inhibit* the postsynaptic neurons (or receptors). Neurotransmission is the process by which an impulse is transmitted across the synapse between the two neurons. Several criteria must generally be fulfilled for a substance to be accepted as a neurotransmitter. For instance, the transmitter must be synthesised in the presynaptic nerve terminal, stored in synaptic vesicles, released from presynaptic terminal on nerve stimulation and should be rapidly inactivated after its action is over. In addition, an exogenous application of this substance should produce the same effects as does its endogenous release. These are discussed below, in detail.

Neuromodulators are released by neurons and also by astrocytes and act either to slow or enhance the *pre- or postsynaptic responses*. These have a latent action of longer duration and arise from the neurons as well as from non-neuronal cells. They are neither stored nor released like neurotransmitters but may increase or decrease their efficacy without participating directly as neurotransmitter. In general, neuromodulation relates to *synaptic plasticity* which means long-term changes in synaptic transmission, connectivity and efficacy following pathological damage (as in epilepsy or drug dependence) or following physiological alterations in neuronal activity (as in learning and memory). Examples of neuromodulators include CO_2, locally released adenosine, some purines, peptides, prostaglandins, arachidonic acid metabolites and nitric oxide (NO). Neuromodulation also involves short-term events like neuronal gene transcription and even alteration in synaptic activity of one neurotransmitter by another.

Neuromediators are actually second messengers like cAMP, cGMP and inositol triphosphate (IP_3), which play a crucial role in the elicitation of postsynaptic responses produced by neurotransmitters.

The ***neurotropic factors*** are mainly released by CNS neurons, astrocytes and microglia. These act over a longer time scale than neuromodulators to regulate the growth and morphology of neurons. They also control long-term changes in brain (e.g., synaptic plasticity, remodeling and phenotype characteristics) mainly by affecting gene transcription by acting through tyrosine kinase–linked receptors. Examples include cytokines, chemokines and growth factors (nerve growth factor, insulin–like growth factors, transforming growth factor α and β and platelet-derived growth factor etc.).

In addition, there are some neurosecretions that are released into the blood circulation and then act on distant target organs. These are called ***neurohormones***; for example, hypothalamic hormones that are released into hypothalamo-pituitary portal circulation (Section 8).

CNS NEUROTRANSMITTERS AND THEIR RECEPTOR INTERACTIONS

Within the CNS, acetylcholine, biogenic amines, amino acids, peptides and purines represent the main class of neurotransmitters. Here we discuss interactions of various neurotransmitters with postsynaptic receptors. Presynaptic receptors (autoreceptors) also play an important role in the modulation of neurotransmitter release from the presynaptic terminals. The presynaptic release of the neurotransmitter in CNS is regulated either by homotropic or by heterotropic receptor interaction in a manner similar to that in periphery (Ch. 10,11 and 12). Activation of the presynaptic receptors in the CNS can result either in inhibition (muscarinic, α_2 adrenoceptors and DA receptors) or in enhancement of the respective neurotransmitter release (nicotinic and β_2-adrenoceptors).

Acetylcholine (ACh)

ACh is primarily a peripheral neurotransmitter but cholinergic neurons are widely distributed in CNS particularly in cerebral cortex, ascending reticular system, cerebellum and spinal cord. They also appear as local circuit neurons in basal ganglia and limbic system (Ch. 40). Both muscarinic and N_N receptor subtypes have been identified in CNS. ACh is thought to modulate arousal, respiration, motor activity, vertigo and memory. Centrally acting antimuscarinic drugs are useful in the management of Parkinson's disease (Ch. 40) or in prevention of motion sickness (Ch. 11). Contrarily, anticholinesterases such as *tacrine, donepezil* and *rivastigmine* are used to improve cognitive deficits related to Alzheimer's disease (Ch. 40).

Biogenic Amines

Dopamine, norepinephrine, epinephrine, 5-HT and histamine are the primary members of this class.

Dopamine (DA)

DA is the most important of the biogenic neurotransmitters in the CNS (Ch. 10 & 12). The most important central dopaminergic pathway is in the tuberobasal ventral hypothalamus (that innervates the median eminence) and the intermediate lobe of pituitary (that plays an important role in prolactin release and regulation of several hypothalamic-hypophyseal functions; see Ch.41). Another very important dopaminergic neurons projection in the brain covers substantia nigra, ventral tegmental areas to limbic cortex and other limbic structures, amygdala, caudate and putamen (Ch. 33 and 40). Parkinson's disease is characterised by a marked reduction in the concentration of DA in basal ganglia (Ch. 40), while in schizophrenia there is dopaminergic overactivity in mesolimbic-mesocortical-mesofrontal pathway, which controls behaviour (Ch. 33). DA is primarily an inhibitory neurotransmitter. Its deficiency causes extrapyramidal disturbances (Ch. 33 and 40).

Five DA receptors (D_1 to D_5) have been identified. Among them D_1 and D_5 belong to one group while D_2, D_3 and D_4 belong to other. D_1 and D_5 stimulate the release of cAMP by activation of adenylyl cyclase and also stimulate phosphatidyl inositol (PIP_2) hydrolysis. These receptors are coupled to G_S protein (metabotropic receptors). *D_1 receptor* is located in the region of putamen, nucleus accumbens and in olfactory tubercle, i.e., in the nigrostriatal pathway. Its inhibition causes extrapyramidal disorders. *D_5 receptor* is found in hypothalamus and hippocampus.

Its exact role is not clear. *D_2, D_3 and D_4 receptors* inhibit cAMP release, block Ca^{2+} channels and open K^+ channels. These are coupled to G_i proteins. *D_2 receptor* is distributed in striatum, substantia nigra and pituitary. It is involved in the control of behaviour, voluntary movements, prolactin release and in other endocrine consequences. *D_3 receptor* is distributed in midbrain, nucleus accumbens and hypothalamus while *D_4 receptor* is distributed in the frontal cortex, medulla, and midbrain, i.e., in mesocortical pathway. Some of the atypical neuroleptics possess D_3 and D_4 antagonist properties (Ch. 33) but their exact role in schizophrenia cannot be fully established unless specific or predominantly D_3 or D_4 receptor antagonists are made available for evaluation as neuroleptics. A byproduct of illicit opioid manufacture, known as MPTP (Ch. 40), has been shown to cause selective destruction of nigrostriatal dopaminergic neurons and produce Parkinson-like syndrome in opioid addicts.

Norepinephrine (NE) and Epinephrine (E)

These neurotransmitters and their receptors have already been discussed earlier (Ch. 10 & 12). All noradrenergic receptors (α and β subtypes) are metabotropic receptors (G-protein coupled). NE constitutes about 30% of total CNS catecholamines and is a neurotransmitter of brainstem neurons within locus ceruleus (pons and the neurons of reticular formation) with projections to cortex, cerebellum and spinal cord. Primarily NE is the neurotransmitter of postganglionic neurons of the sympathetic nervous system. In CNS, NE is thought to modulate affective disorders (depression), learning, memory, arousal and pain perception. In contrast to DA and NE, concentration of epinephrine in CNS is quite low (5–12% of NE content). It is localised primarily in cell bodies of reticular formation but the precise role of epinephrine in CNS is still debatable.

5-Hydroxytryptamine (5-HT)

5-HT and its receptors have been detailed in Chapter 24. Serotoninergic neurons are found primarily near the midline raphe nuclei of the brainstem and project to the cortex, cerebellum and the spinal cord. Surprisingly, in humans, about 90% of the total serotonin in the body is found in enterochromaffin cells in the GIT and the remaining 10% is shared by platelets and the brain; yet, brain serotonin has been implicated as a potential neurotransmitter in the mediation of a wide variety of brain functions. 5-HT is thought to modulate sensory pathways (nociception) and homeostasis. Serotoninergic systems play an important role in schizophrenia (Ch. 33), depression (Ch. 34), temperature regulation and eating disorders (Ch. 24) and are the targets of many drugs for treating these disorders. In addition to its presumed role as a neurotransmitter in CNS, 5-HT is synthesised also in the pineal gland where it serves as a precursor for the synthesis of melatonin presumably by an action within hypothalamus.

5-HT acts on more than a dozen receptor subtypes (Ch. 24). Except for 5-HT_3 receptor which is an ionotropic receptor, all of these receptors are metabotropic (G-protein coupled) receptors. 5-HT_{1A} receptor agonists (e.g., buspirone) are used to treat anxiety disorders (Ch. 32); 5-HT_{1D} receptor agonists (e.g., sumatriptan) are used to treat migraine and cluster headaches (Ch. 24); $5\text{-HT}_{2A/2C}$ receptor antagonists (e.g., clozapine) are used to treat schizophrenia (Ch. 33); while 5-HT reuptake inhibitors (SSRIs, e.g., fluoxetine) are used to treat depression and obsessive-compulsive disorders (Ch. 34).

Histamine

Histaminergic neurons originate from posterior hypothalamus. These neurons project upward to cerebral cortex, the limbic system, caudate, putamen and globus pallidus. Downward projections of these neurons include brainstem structures, substantia nigra, dorsal raphe, cerebellum and spinal cord. Neurochemical evidence also reveals histamine binding sites (H_1 receptors) in various regions of the brain. Histaminergic neurons and postsynaptic central H_1 receptors play a major role in arousal. Blockade of these receptors is thought to account for sedation experienced after taking antihistamines like chlorpheniramine and diphenhydramine. Other possible roles for histamine include regulation of food and water intake, body temperature, hormone release and sleep. Detailed information on histamine is available in Chapter 24.

Amino Acids Neurotransmitters

***Glutamate** and **aspartate** are the main excitatory amino acids (EAAs) in the CNS.* They are capable of depolarising the neurons. ***GABA** is the main inhibitory transmitter in the brain.* ***Glycine** is also an inhibitory transmitter* but in the spinal cord and the brainstem only. Both GABA and glycine are capable of hyperpolarising the neurons. Normally a balance between excitatory inputs (mostly glutamatergic) and inhibitory inputs (mainly GABAergic) determines the prevailing level of neuronal activity in limbic system and RAS in the brain. If the balance swings in favour of GABA, anxiety and nervousness are decreased while sedation, amnesia, muscle relaxation and ataxia appear. In contrast, a reduction in GABAergic activity elicits arousal, precipitates anxiety, insomnia and restlessness.

Gamma-Aminobutyric Acid (GABA) as Neurotransmitter

GABA is the major inhibitory neurotransmitter in mammalian CNS. It is present fairly uniformly in brain. There is only a little amount in periphery. GABA is primarily synthesised from glutamate by the enzyme L-glutamic acid-l-decarboxylase (GAD). It is subsequently metabolised by GABA

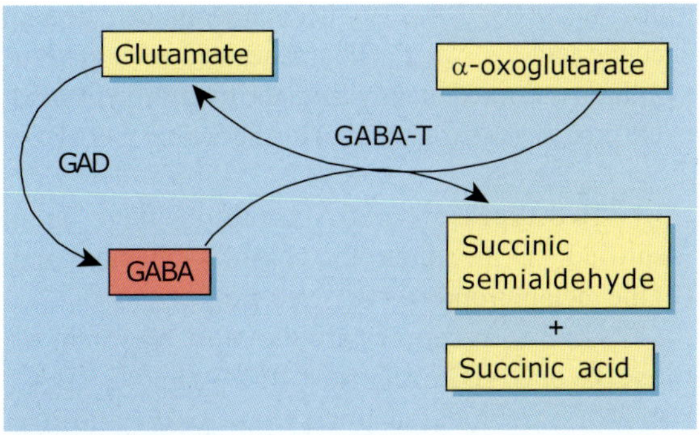

Fig 30.2 Synthesis & Metabolism of GABA

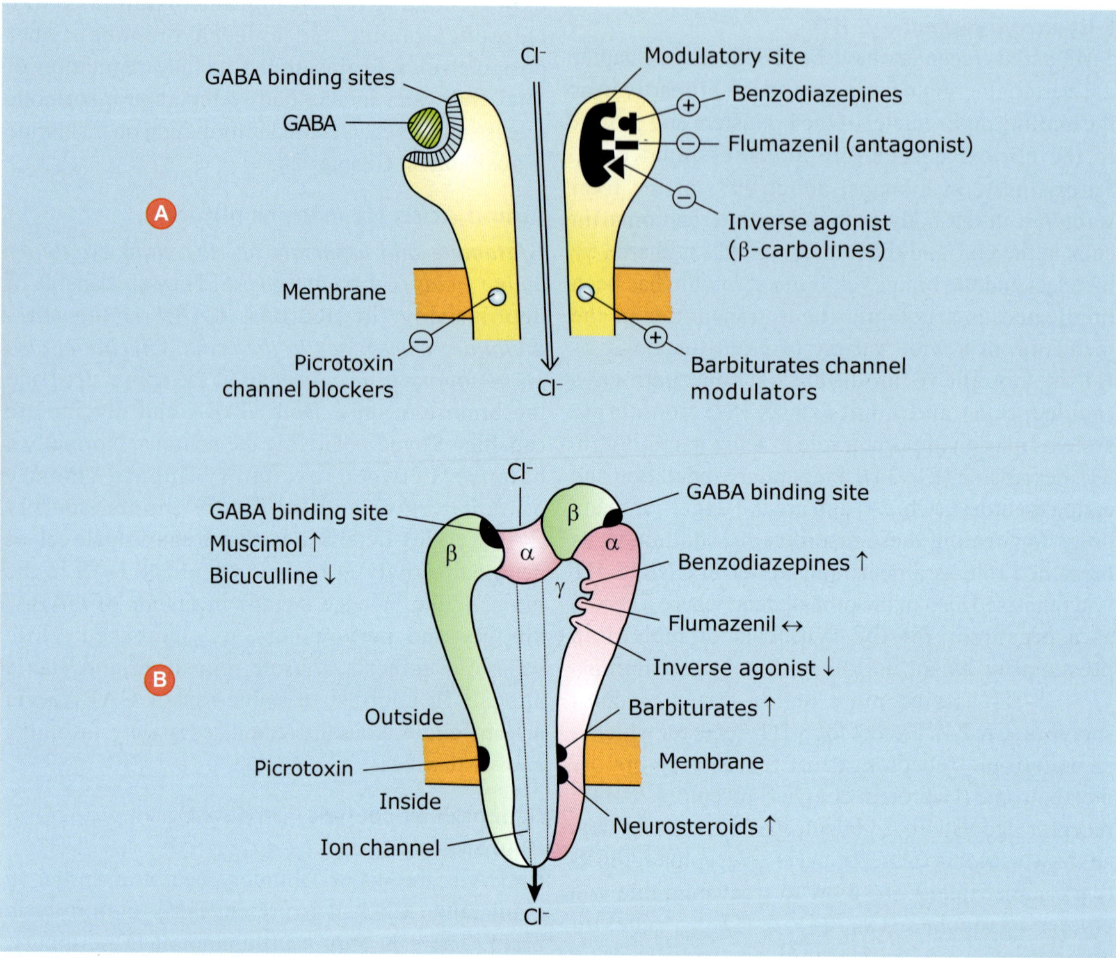

Fig 30.3 A Hypothetical Model of $GABA_A$ Receptor–Chloride Ion Channel Complex and Sites of Various Drugs Action

transaminase (GABA-T) to succinic semialdehyde and succinic acid (Fig. 30.2). Glutamate needed for GABA synthesis is formed mainly from the tricarboxylic acid cycle product (α-oxoglutarate) by the action of GABA-T.

Two types of GABA receptors have been identified: (1) the ionotropic $GABA_A$ receptors and (2) the metabotropic $GABA_B$ receptors.

$GABA_A$ receptors are the most prevalent of these two GABA receptor subtypes. $GABA_A$ receptors are located postsynaptically and are directly linked with Cl^- ion channel opening which causes hyperpolarisation and reduction in the membrane excitability. *Muscimol* is an agonist at $GABA_A$ receptor, while the convulsant *bicuculline* is an antagonist and interferes with GABA binding to $GABA_A$ receptor (Ch. 35). $GABA_A$ receptor has several different accessory binding sites (Fig. 30.3A & B) that include:

- The neurotransmitter GABA-binding site.
- The modulatory sites to bind *benzodiazepines* (BZDs), their antagonist such as *flumazenil* and inverse agonist such as *carbolins*.
- The modulatory as well as blocking site at Cl^- ion channel as for *barbiturates* and *picrotoxin*.

$GABA_A$ receptor has a pentameric structure assembled from five sub-units selected from seven polypeptide classes (α, β, γ, δ, ε, θ, ρ). The major isoform of the $GABA_A$ receptor in the brain consists of 5 subunits (two α_1; two β_2 and one γ_2 subunit). It has been found that binding of GABA with its site, located between α_1 and β_2 subunits, triggers Cl^- channel opening with resultant membrane hyperpolarisation; while the binding site for BZDs lies between α_1 and γ_2 subunits. This facilitates GABA binding to its receptor sites and increases the frequency of chloride channel opening. The benzodiazepine binding site is also labeled as *benzodiazepine receptor*. In addition, coexpression of individual γ-subunit variants (γ_1, γ_2, γ_3) with α and β subunits results in varying modulatory sites for antagonists and inverse agonists at BZD receptor. Studies involving genetic manipulations of $GABA_A$ receptors in rodent models reveal that α_1 subunits in $GABA_A$ receptors mediate sedation, amnesia and possibly antiseizure effects of BZDs, while α_2 subunits are involved in their antianxiety and muscle relaxant properties. Further studies on transgenic mice have led to the findings that a recently identified α_5 subunit is involved in at least some of the memory impairment caused by BZDs.

The adjacent site between α and β subunits of $GABA_A$ receptors, are the functional receptors that respond to barbiturates but not to BZDs. In therapeutic doses barbiturates act on these channel modulatory sites of $GABA_A$ receptor and potentiate the GABA-mediated inhibitory effects by *increasing the duration* (not the frequency) of Cl^- channel opening. However, at higher concentration, barbiturates directly increase Cl^- ion conductance, i.e., GABA mimetic action in absence of GABA. Convulsants like *picrotoxin* block the Cl^- ion channel directly. Some neurosteroid anticonvulsants like *ganaxolone* act on a selective and a separate modulatory site on the $GABA_A$ receptor complex and increase Cl^- ion conductance. A model of $GABA_A$ receptor complex and the sites of action of different agents on the receptor are shown in Figure 30.3 A & B. Additional information is available in chapters 32 and 39.

$GABA_B$ receptor, unlike $GABA_A$ receptor, is not modulated by BZDs or barbiturates. It is present at the lower levels in the CNS than the $GABA_A$ receptor and is not linked to Cl^- channel. It is a G-protein coupled receptor. Its activation decreases cAMP formation. These receptors cause pre - and postsynaptic inhibition (hyperpolarisation) by inhibiting Ca^{2+} channel opening and increasing K^+ conductance. The peripherally acting skeletal muscle relaxant, *baclofen*, is a $GABA_B$ receptor agonist and is used to treat spastic disorders. The competitive antagonist for $GABA_B$ receptor is *saclofen* but it is not yet in clinical use.

Glycine

Glycine is an inhibitory neurotransmitter, enriched in medulla, spinal cord, the lower brainstem and perhaps in retina. Glycine receptor is structurally and functionally similar to $GABA_A$ receptor and is directly linked to Cl^- ion channel. The native *glycine receptor (strychnine-sensitive glycine receptor)* is a pentameric structure and both the glycine and strychnine-binding sites appear to be located on the same α subunit. The convulsant drug strychnine is a competitive antagonist at glycine receptor (Ch. 35), while tetanus toxin acts mainly by preventing the glycine release causing excessive reflex hyper-excitability and violent muscle spasm (lock jaw).

Interestingly, the activation of NMDA receptors requires low concentration of glycine along with glutamate (see below). The binding sites of both (glutamate and glycine) are different but both have to be occupied for the receptor channel to open. This is surprising, because glycine is primarily recognised as an inhibitory neurotransmitter (while at NMDA receptor, as coagonist to glutamate, it facilitates excitation; see below). This effect of glycine is "strychnine-insensitive" suggesting a mechanism involving allosteric regulation of the NMDA receptor complex through a separate glycine binding site on this receptor (Fig. 30.5). It has been suggested that the main effect of glycine is to prevent desensitisation of the NMDA receptor during prolonged exposure to agonist. Glycine probably accelerates the recovery of the receptor from its desensitised state rather than blocking the onset of desensitisation.

Glutamate Receptors

Synthesis, Storage and Release of Glutamate (GLU)

In brain GLU is synthesised in the nerve terminals from two sources: from glucose *via* the Krebs cycle and transamination of oxoglutarate (Fig. 30.2) and from glutamine that is synthesised in the glial cells (Fig. 30.4). GLU is then stored in the synaptic vesicles and released by Ca^{2+} dependent exocytosis. After its release and action GLU is recaptured from the synaptic cleft by neuronal type GLU-transporters (GTn) into the neuron and by glial type transporters (GTg) into the glial cells. Glial glutamate is then converted to glutamine by the enzyme glutamine synthetase. Glutamine subsequently enters the nearby neuron to replenish the glutamate after hydrolysis by mitochondrial glutaminase (Fig. 30.4). Therefore, glutamine serves as a pool of inactive transmitter within glial cells and act like a ball-boy in the tennis court, who returns the ball back to the player for fresh service.

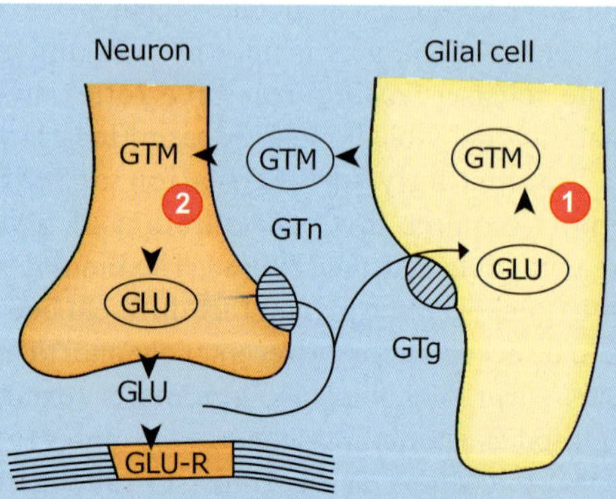

Key: GLU-R—glutamate receptor; GTM—glutamine; GTn—glutamate transporter neuronal type; GTg—glutamate transporter glial type; (1) glutamine synthetase; (2) glutaminase.

Fig 30.4 Synthesis, Storage, Release and Metabolism of Glutamate

Glutamate (GLU) and **aspartate** (ASP) are the two excitatory neurotransmitters widely concentrated in cortex, basal ganglia and sensory pathways. Besides acting as neurotransmitters they also play an important role in the intermediary metabolism in neural tissue, e.g., in detoxification of ammonia in brain, as building blocks in the synthesis of peptides and proteins and as a precursor for the inhibitory neurotransmitter GABA (Fig. 30.2). With the development of more selective agonists and antagonists, five different types of excitatory glutamate receptors have been identified in the CNS. These are: NMDA (**N**-**m**ethyl-**D**-**a**spartate); AMPA (α-**a**mino-3-hydroxy-5-**m**ethylisoxazole-4-**p**ropionic **a**cid); Kainate (isolated from sea weeds); AP-4 (1,2-diamino-4-phosphobutyrate) and ACPD (1-**a**mino**c**yclo**p**entane-1,3-**d**icarboxylic acid) receptors. The first three of these (NMDA, AMPA and Kainate) are ionotropic receptors (linked to Ca^{2+} channels in case of NMDA and to Na^+ in case of AMPA and kainate receptors). The fourth, i.e., AP-4 receptor, appears to be an inhibitory autoreceptor about which more details are awaited. The fifth receptor, activated by ACPD, is a metabotropic (G-protein coupled) receptor which modulates inositol-phosphate metabolism and thus Ca^{2+} release. Their names have been assigned because these experimental agents are the specific agonists which activate them. *Glutamate is an agonist to all of them*. Most excitatory synapses contain both NMDA and rest non-NMDA receptors on the post-synaptic membrane.

NMDA Receptors

Out of all the glutamate receptors, the NMDA receptors have become a major focus of attention because these are involved in a wide range of both neurophysiological and pathological processes—as important and diverse as memory acquisition, development of synaptic plasticity, epilepsy and the neuronal excitotoxicity due to cerebral ischaemia.

NMDA receptor is a pentamer, composed of two different subunits NR-1 and NR-2. It is a ligand-gated ion channel receptor having high permeability to Ca^{2+} (also to Na^+). It has a wider distribution in brain (spinal cord, hippocampus, cerebral cortex and glial cells). There appear to be at least six pharmacologically distinct binding or modulatory sites through which different agents can alter the functioning of NMDA receptor:

1. *GLU (or NMDA) binding site* promoting the opening of Ca^{2+} and Na^+ channels;

2. *The modulatory site that binds glycine.* This site should not be confused with glycine-binding site of glycine inhibitory receptor, which is strychnine sensitive. GLU is virtually ineffective unless the modulatory site that binds glycine is also occupied. This modulatory site is not blocked by strychnine (see above). *Kynurenic acid*, that occurs exclusively in glial cells, is an endogenous antagonist to this site. Thus glial cells may play an active role in supporting synaptic transmission during activation of NMDA receptors;
3. *A polyamines (spermine and spermidine) regulatory site* which also facilitates NMDA receptor channel opening. An investigational drug *eliprodil* blocks their action;
4. *A site within the channel that binds phencyclidine (PCP site)* and related noncompetitive antagonist (e.g., *ketamine*) which act most effectively when the receptor channel is activated (open channel block). *Dizocilpine* and *memantine* are also the channel blockers but have better permeability through BBB;
5. *A voltage-dependent Mg^{2+} binding site.* At resting membrane potentials, the NMDA channel is blocked by Mg^{2+}, but this block is overcome if the cell is depolarised; and

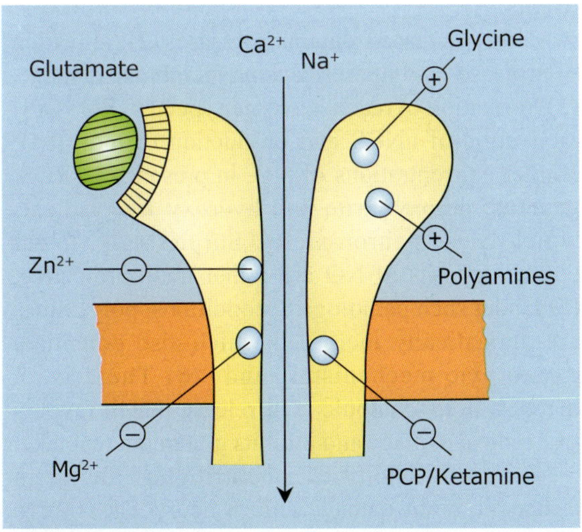

Fig 30.5 Hypothetical Model of NMDA Receptor. (For abbreviations see text.)

6. *A voltage-independent Zn^{2+} ion binding site near the mouth of the channel.* Zn^{2+} produces voltage- independent inhibitory action on NMDA receptor ion channel.

A hypothetical model of NMDA receptor with sites of action of different agents are shown in Figure 30.5

AMPA and Kainate Receptors

Both AMPA and kainate receptors mediate fast excitatory synaptic transmission primarily associated with influx of Na^+ ions through Na-channels. Both are different than NMDA receptor but are hard to be distinguished from each other. Hence, some texts collectively call them as *non-NMDA receptors* (to simplify).

AMPA receptors are pentamers consisting of $GLUR_{1-4}$ subunits (representing variations associated with alternative splicing and RNA editing). AMPA receptors lacking $GLUR_2$ subunit have much higher permeability to Ca^{2+} than others. AMPA and *quisqualate* are the preferred agonists for AMPA receptor, while CNQX (6-cyano-7-nitroquinoxaline-2,3-dione) is a selective AMPA receptor antagonist. Kainate receptors are also pentamers but consist of $GLUR_{5-7}$ subunits plus KA_{1-2} subunits. *Domoate* and *kainate* are the preferred agonist to kainate receptor. While NBQX (2,3-dihydro-6-nitro-7-sulfamoyl-benzoquinoxaline) is a selective antagonist of kainate receptor. Trials with these agonists and antagonists have so far proved disappointing.

Metabotropic Glutamate (ACPD) Receptors

These receptors act indirectly on ion channels *via* G-proteins. Till date eight subtypes of ($GLUR_{1-8}$) metabotropic glutamate receptors have been identified but no agonist or antagonist has yet been reported to be specific for any of these receptor subtypes. The recent researches suggest an important role of these receptors in both synaptic transmission and synaptic plasticity. The most exciting new development is the finding that activation of metabotropic $GLUR_5$ is probably responsible for cocaine self-administration and craving, and that the reinforcing properties of cocaine are absent in mice lacking metabotropic $GLUR_5$ receptor.

Functional Role and Interactions Between Glutamate Receptors

Both NMDA and metabotropic receptors play an important role in long-term adaptive changes (e.g., *synaptic plasticity*) as well as pathological changes (*excitotoxicity*) in the brain. Normal stimulation of glutamate receptor plays a central role in learning and memory (synaptic plasticity) but overstimulation of glutamate receptor, particularly of the NMDA type, results in excitotoxicity in brain (neurodegeneration and apoptosis).

Synaptic plasticity is a term to describe long-term changes that occur during increase in synaptic efficacy; which in turn results by an increase in synaptic proliferation and connectivity at the demand of increased load on memory due to continued learning efforts. These demands are met by a process called *long-term potentiation* (LTP) in which NMDA and metabotropic receptors play a central role. In LTP, there is a long lasting enhancement of synaptic transmission following a short burst of presynaptic stimulation (*conditioning*) *at high frequency*. Adjuvant to LTP is *long-term depression* (LTD) that is produced by *long train of stimuli at lower frequency* mainly in hippocampus, which is involved in learning and memory. The synaptic strength during learning (initiated by LTP and maintained by LDP) involves both the presynaptic and postsynaptic events. It does not occur if the presynaptic action fails to excite the postsynaptic neuron. An enhanced activation of AMPA receptors by glutamate is an essential first step in initiation of LTP.

At normal membrane potential (–70 mV), however, only AMPA receptors are activated by glutamate, while NMDA receptor channels remain blocked by Mg^{2+}. Available glutamate is insufficient to activate metabotropic receptor also (Fig.30.6A). A sustained postsynaptic depolarisation (–40 mV) produced by glutamate acting repeatedly at AMPA receptor, however, overcomes the Mg^{2+} block. NMDA receptor is now activated, which allows Ca^{2+} to enter the cell. The released glutamate is enough to activate metabotropic receptors also, which further potentiates Ca^{2+} release through IP_3 cascade. The resultant rise in Ca^{2+} in postsynaptic cell membrane then activates protein kinase-C (PKC) and nitric oxide synthase (nNOS). PKC also phosphorylates AMPA receptor channels causing facilitation of transmission and maintenance of depolarisation. n-NOS converts L-arginine to nitric oxide (NO), which further facilitates glutamate release (retrograde signalling) and the sequence of receptor activation (Fig. 30.6B). During this maintenance phase (sustained depolarisation) more AMPA receptors are recruited to the post-synaptic membrane. PKC, besides phosphorylating AMPA channels, also phosphorylates signal transduction molecule controlling gene transcription in the postsynaptic cells leading to a permanent increase in the number of synaptic contacts. LTP-like changes have been detected after an increase in learning process. Thus, it is hoped that the drugs capable of enhancing LTP may improve learning and memory.

Excitotoxicity: Ca^{2+} overload is an essential factor in excitotoxicity. Sustained activation of AMPA receptors depolarises the cell and unblocks the NMDA receptor channels permitting Ca^{2+} entry (see above). Simultaneously, metabotropic receptors are also activated causing further release of Ca^{2+} from endoplasmic reticulum. If this Ca^{2+} overload increases, normal feedback control mechanisms fail, which further exaggerate this process to a danger point leading to *excitotoxicity* because of the following events:

(1) Increased glutamate release, **(2)** Activation of proteases and lipases causing membrane damage, **(3)** Formation of reactive oxygen species (ROS), **(4)** Activation of nNOS and production of more NO. Higher concentrations of NO, in presence of ROS, generate peroxynitrite and hydroxy free radicals which cause neurotoxicity. Surprisingly, lower concen-trations of NO are rather neuroprotective, **(5)** Under such pathological conditions, polyamines are dramatically increased which also potentiate excitotoxic mechanisms, and **(6)** There is an increase in arachidonic acid release which favours free radical damage and inhibits glutamate reuptake.

Excitotoxicity is a contributory factor in ischaemic brain damage and in neurodegenerative diseases such as parkinsonism, senile dementia, multiple sclerosis and also in destruction of photoreceptor cells in retina. Inhibitors of nNOS such as ***7-nitroindazole*** protects against ischaemic

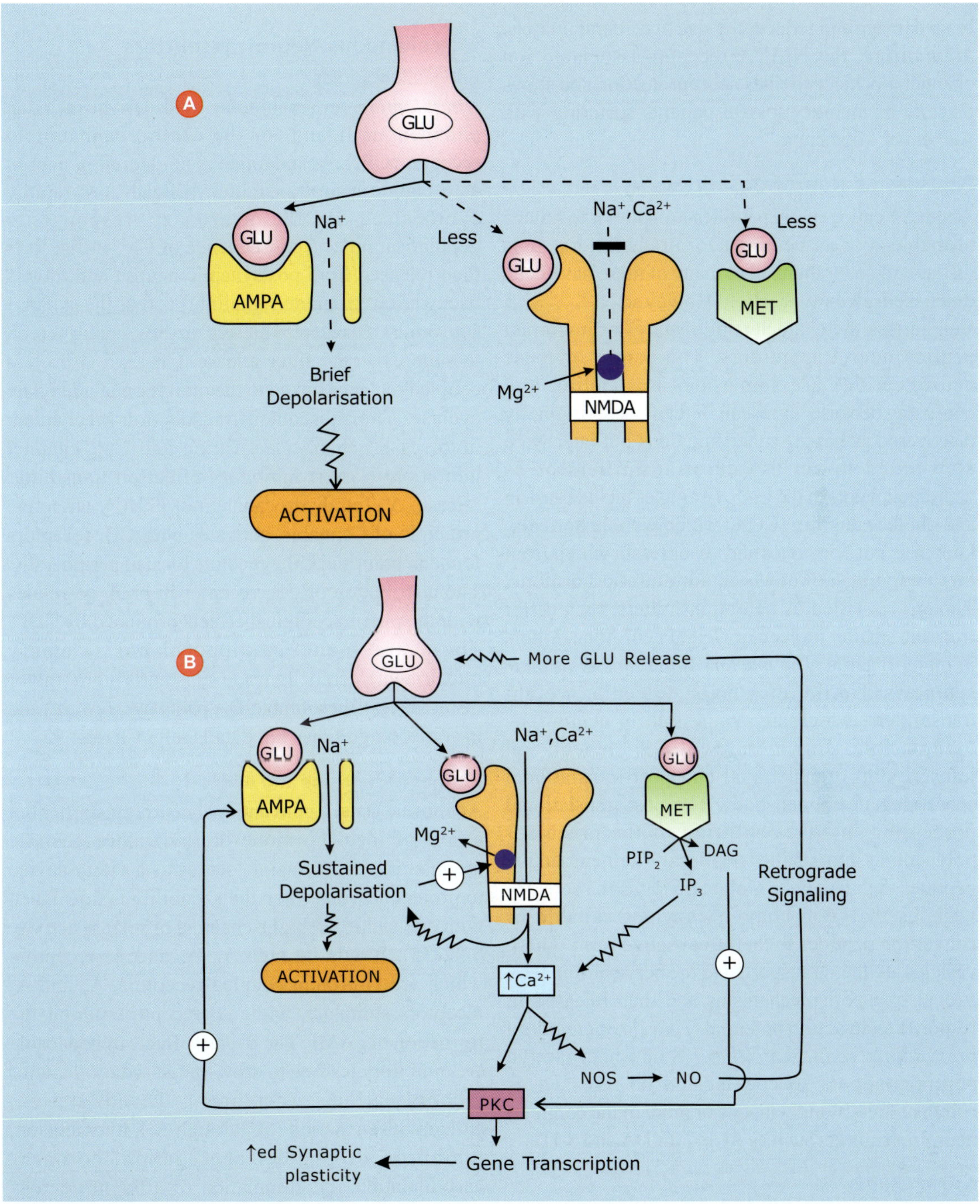

Fig 30.6 (A) At normal membrane potential there is brief depolarisation of AMPA receptors only, due to insufficient glutamate. (B) On sustained depolarisation, enough glutamate is released which then activates AMPA, NMDA as well as metabotropic receptors (MET) with chain of events leading to increased synaptic plasticity

brain damage and reduces the size of cerebral infarcts. ***Memantine***, the NMDA receptor-associated ion channel blocker, provides neuroprotection and slows the rate of memory loss in patients suffering with Alzheimer's dementia.

Peptides as Neurotransmitters

About 24 endogenous peptides are known to have a probable role as central neurotransmitters. It is difficult to cover them all as many of these have been discussed already earlier. However, Table 30.1 summarises the characteristic features of important peptide neurotransmitters. The names of these neuropeptides are sometimes misleading and confusing because almost all of them were originally discovered as having other functions but later were also found to act as neurotransmitters or as neuromodulators in the CNS. Examples include gastrin and cholecystokinin (CCK) which were historically known as gut hormones and vasopressin which from the beginning is known as antidiuretic hormone. Though classified as neurotransmitters, they differ from the smaller molecular weight neurotransmitters in many regards. *The primary difference is in their synthesis.* Unlike the small molecular weight transmitters, which are synthesised in neurons by cytoplasmic enzymes, peptides depend on transcription, translational and post-translational processing in the cell body. The post-translational processing involves splitting of the precursor polypeptide into smaller peptides. The neuroactive peptides then leave the Golgi apparatus in secretory vesicles that also contain enzymes capable of converting peptides to their final active form. These vesicles are then transported to the nerve terminal by axonal transport mechanisms and then released in response to an action potential. *They do not undergo presynaptic reuptake either.* Some neuroactive peptides appear to coexist and be released as cotransmitters along with one or more of the common neurotransmitters such as ACh, NE, DA and 5-HT.

Nitric Oxide

Its role as neurotransmitter in neuroprotection and neurodegeneration has already been discussed along with glutamate receptors (see text) and in Chapter 17.

Miscellaneous Neurotransmitters

Endocannabinoids

Anandamide, an arachidonic acid derivative, is an endogenous ligand for the central cannabinoid receptor (CB_1). Anandamide is not stored in neuron as a classic neurotransmitter. Instead, it is rapidly synthesised by the neuron in response to depolarisation as a consequence of Ca^{2+} influx. It is then released from postsynaptic neuron and travels backward (retrograde signalling) across the synapse activating CB_1 receptor present on presynaptic neuron to suppress transmitter release. CB_1 is a G-protein coupled receptor linked to the inhibition of adenylate cyclase. The subsequent transduction mechanism involves K^+ channel activation and Ca^{2+} channel inhibition to exert inhibitory effect on transmitter release. Δ^9-Tetrahydrocannabinol (THC), an active principle of Cannabis, activates both CB_1 receptors found in brain and CB_2 receptors located peripherally. The distribution of CB_1 receptor in brain co-relates with the pharmacological effects produced by THC. These are found in hippocampus (memory impairment), cerebellum and substantia nigra (motor disturbances), mesolimbic-DA pathways (reward) and in cortex (cognition). For details refer Chapter 35.

Purines (Adenosine and ATP)

Adenosine is not a conventional neurotransmitter but a sort of local hormone or say a "homeostatic modulator", which mainly serves as a safety device to protect neurons when their viability is threatened with crisis like cerebral ischaemia or seizure activity (Ch. 35). It acts through A_1, A_2 and A_3 receptors which are G-protein coupled receptors. A_1 and A_3 receptors stimulate, while A_2 receptors inhibit the formation of cAMP. The overall effects of adenosine are inhibitory leading to drowsiness, sedation, motor incoordination, cerebral vasodilatation, anticonvulsant action (all through A_1); hypotension, inhibition of platelet aggregation, coronary vasodilatation and stimulation of afferent neurons in heart leading to anginal pain (all through A_2) and bronchoconstriction (A_3 receptor action). Methylxanthines antagonise these effects by acting as competitive antagonists at A_1, A_2 and A_3

Table 30.1 Probable Peptide Neurotransmitters

Peptide NT	Chapter No.	Special features
1. **Oxytocin**	41	Inhibitory; involved in mating and parenting behaviour and released during sexual orgasm
2. **Tachykinins**	17	
- Substance-P (agonist at NK_1 receptor)*		Levels reduced in Huntington's chorea
- Neurokinin-A (agonist at NK_2 receptor)		Neurokinins play an important role in pain transmission
- Neruokinin-B (agonist at NK_3 receptor)		
3. **Neurotensin**	17	Lowers body temperature; coexists with DA and NE
4. **Vasoactive intestinal peptide (VIP)**	17	Involved in pain transmission, concentrated in neocortex
5. **Opioid peptides**	37 & 38	
- β-Endorphins		Found in hypothalamus, thalamus, arcuate nucleus and brainstem. Very potent endogenous opioid peptide. Main action on μ and δ receptors
- Enkephalins		Wider distribution in CNS including pain areas of spinal cord. Main action on δ receptors
- Dynorphins		Wider distribution in CNS including dorsal horn of spinal cord. Main action on k receptors
- Endomorphins		Main action on μ receptor; released during stress; decreases pain sensation and increases endurance
- Nociceptin		Endogenous ligand for NOP (ORL-I) receptor; found in hippocampus, cortex and many sensory neurons; involved in modulation of drug reward, reinforcement, learning and memory process
6. **Neuropeptide-Y**	17	Widely distributed in CNS; increases feeding (orexigenic); hypothermia, cerebral vasoconstriction

NT—Neurotransmitter; * Also acts as neuromodulator in nociception

receptors. Adenosine is also considered as an endogenous antiseizure substance (EAS; Ch. 39).

ATP is stored in vesicles and released by exocytosis as cotransmitter along with several neurotransmitters. ATP is present in cytosol in higher concentration and is usually released directly if neuronal viability is threatened (as in stroke, seizures and ischaemia). Released ATP is then rapidly converted to adenosine (Ch. 35).

TYPES OF MENTAL DISORDERS

Based on predominant manifestations, the mental disorders could be categorised as NEUROSES, PSYCHOSES or AFFECTIVE DISORDERS.

I. Neuroses

It is a less serious disorder. The patient's personality is intact, not deranged. There is no loss of contact with realities. Patient knows the causative factor for his anxiety but exhibits emotional disturbances in the form of exaggerated defence or disproportionate anxiety. It could be ***traumatic neurosis***, e.g., when a soldier, with distressing battle experience, is driven back to battlefield. However, in majority of cases it is **PSYCHONEUROSIS** which is an emotional or behavioural disorder arising from an unresolved conflict at subconscious level. Psychoneuroses may be further labelled as:

1. ***Anxiety Neurosis***: It is characterised by a groundless uneasiness, easily provoked irritable behaviour and disproportionate concern and fear for future. It can result due to problems related to examination, to interview, to his performance related to sexual act or to problems at his place of work. Manifestations of such anxiety are sweating, epigastric distress, tremors, dizziness, congestion in chest and hyperventilation etc.
2. ***Phobic Neurosis***: When the cause of anxiety is something else but manifestation of anxiety is just symbolic; for example, patient fears the crowd or there is fear of isolation or fear of unknown.
3. ***Obsessive-Compulsive Neurosis***: It is a state when a person undertakes certain acts repeatedly (e.g., washing hand for 51 times) or performs certain rituals recurrently (e.g., bowing head for 51 times before the deity) just to lessen or relieve the anxiety.
4. ***Hysterical Neurosis (Hysteria)***: It is situational and always in presence of others. The person usually mimics the symptoms of a physical disease dramatically (such as deafness, blindness, loss of speech, amnesia, convulsions and pain) to serve a personal purpose with no awareness of the motives for doing so. For example, a newly-wed bride living in one room with her husband, along with in-laws, may relieve her anxiety (for lack of privacy) by presenting hysterical symptoms.
5. ***Panic Disorders***: These are acute episodic intense attacks of anxiety with overwhelming feelings of dread and sympathetic discharge. Such patients frequently undergo emergency medical evaluation for heart attack, peptic ulcer or hypoglycaemic attack before being diagnosed as a case of panic disorder. If such panic disorder attacks become recurrent the patient gets demoralised, hypochondriacal and depressed.
6. ***Reactive Depression***: It is also called as "neurotic depression" and results due to serious physical illness or bereavement of the dear one or because of some inner guilt which he or she cannot disclose. Manifestations include disproportionate feeling of sadness, guilt or apathy.

II. Psychoses

It is a mental disorder which results either due to some organic disease or due to alterations in the neurotransmitter levels of the brain. The personality of the patient gets deranged and he loses contact with reality. The patient has no insight into the nature of his illness and does incorrect evaluation of his thoughts and feelings and provides incorrect information about the reality even when they are on the contrary. The manifestations are associated with ***delusions*** (i.e., a false belief which cannot be altered with reasoning, e.g., suspecting his wife as adulteress) or ***illusions*** (i.e., mental impression derived from misinterpretation of an actual sensory stimulus, e.g., interpreting flash light as fire and becoming panicky) or ***hallucinations*** (i.e., a false perception occurring without a true sensory stimulus, e.g., *auditory hallucinations*—hearing voices; *visual hallucinations*—seeing bright colours or pictures on wall; *olfactory hallucinations*—complaining of bad smell unnecessarily). Psychoses is of two types: ***organic***, and ***functional***.

A) Organic Psychosis

It occurs due to some organic disease, e.g., cerebral infection by rabies or brain injury due to heavy metal poisoning (e.g., by mercury or lead) or due to chronic alcoholism. It is characterised by dementia, disorientation and disorganised behaviour.

B) Functional Psychosis (Schizophrenia)

Schizophrenia primarily results due to dopaminergic overactivity in limbic area, though the role of other neurotransmitters also cannot be ruled out. Schizophrenics are usually introvert split personalities who show retreat from reality with no coherence between their thought, speech and action. The manifestations of the disease include two types of symptoms—"positive" and "negative".

Positive symptoms include: delusions (often paranoid in nature), illusions, auditory hallucinations (usually in the form of clear voices), thought disorders with irrational conclusions, garbled sentences and stereotyped or at times aggressive behaviour. *Negative symptoms include*: Introvert behaviour, poor socialisation, emotional blunting, lack of motivation and cognitive deficits (lack of attention, loss of memory). The intensity of these symptoms and the disability that they cause, may prevent schizophrenics from enjoying a career, completing an education or enjoying a life that may once have been filled with promise. The rates of employment among such people rarely exceed 20–25 percent. Once a schizophrenic is always a schizophrenic. It is a chronic illness, as less than 15% of patients recover from the first episode of psychoses and return to the lives they enjoyed before. Schizophrenia is of four types.

1. **Simple Schizophrenia**: It is characterised by: **(a)** Early onset, **(b)** General decline in activity, thinking ability and emotions; but it is the family and friends that observe his inactivity and self neglect, not him, **(c)** Conversation is sparse and fragmentary while answers are few and abrupt, and **(d)** Vague delusions with mild hallucinations. Prognosis is very poor. These people end up as long-term patients and at best can perform simple tasks but under supervision.
2. **Hebephrenic (Buffoonish) Schizophrenia**: Its characteristic features are: **(a)** Occurring in adolescence, **(b)** Severely deranged personality distinguished by idiotic/buffoonish euphoria (may act like buffalo or like an emperor), and **(c)** Severe thought disorder, auditory hallucinations with extreme emotional inconsistency.
3. **Paranoid Schizophrenia**: Onset occurs after the age of 30 yrs. Delusions are paranoid and persecutory in nature (e.g., fixed delusions like pride or suspicion). Grandiose ideas are fairly common but the personality is often quite preserved. The patient usually seems to be completely absorbed in his delusions which get fixed and govern his acts accordingly. Many paranoids may conceal their thoughts. Proper treatment can improve their condition.
4. **Catatonic Schizophrenia**: It is uncommon as lot many patients are then finally diagnosed as suffering from organic psychosis when investigated. However, patients with true catatonic schizophrenia may present with acute destructive excitement and may show bizarre acts and postures with persistent stupor. Prognosis is poor.

III. Affective Disorders

In these disorders a particular *mood* of the patient is grossly exaggerated. These disorders may manifest as:

1. Mania

It is characterised by excessive desire, craziness, with pathological ambitions and excitement. There are no delusions. Thought process is coherent but the patient violently opposes any kind of interference with pressured speech.

2. Depression

Characteristic features are morbid feelings, guilt and melancholia. It could be of several types:

- **Neurotic Depression**: See reactive depression discussed above.
- **Endogenous Depression**: It can occur at any time of life. It is exhibited by suicidal or self-destructive thoughts like, "this life is not worth

living". Vegetative signs which usually occur include insomnia, anorexia and weight loss. Depression is related to the deficiency in the levels of 5-HT, NE and DA in the brain.

- **Agitative Depression**: It is characterised by restlessness and apprehensions, which appear after partial recovery from endogenous depression.

3. Manic-Depressive Psychoses (MDP)

It is a *cyclical bipolar* affective disorder in which the mood swings between "extreme excitement" (*manic phase*) and "profound depression" (*depressive phase*).

There is a saying that *neurotics*, being in touch with the realities, build castles in air but do not live in them. *Psychotics*, because of the loss of contact with realities, not only build castles in air but start living in them. *Psychiatrists* are smart owners of these castles as they charge rent from both of them.

CHAPTER 31

General Anaesthetics

COMPETENCY PH1.18

The cardinal features of general anaesthesia include varying degree of analgesia, amnesia, loss of all sensations, reflexes and consciousness. It may also incorporate muscle relaxation with partial loss of homeostatic control of respiratory and cardiovascular functions. An ideal anaesthetic drug should induce the unconsciousness smoothly and rapidly and should provide prompt recovery also, after its discontinuation. No single agent is capable of achieving all these desirable effects without risking the toxicity. Hence, in anaesthetic practice several different categories of drugs are utilised concomitantly to produce a "balanced anaesthesia" by taking advantage of their individual beneficial effects and minimising their individual toxicity. For a classical surgical procedure, the protocol includes the use of preanaesthetic medication (see below) followed by a rapid and smooth induction of anaesthesia with I.V. thiopental or propofol and then the maintenance of anaesthesia with a combination of inhaled and I.V. anaesthetic drugs. Such protocol also includes the use of a neuromuscular blocker (Ch. 14) to facilitate intubation and to suppress muscle tone to the degree required for surgery. For some patients who require minor surgical procedure, a local anaesthetic can be coadministered with low doses of general anaesthetics. This technique, called as "monitored anaesthesia", produces discreet analgesia, does not affect the patency of patient's airway and keeps the patient cooperative for verbal commands.

STAGES OF ANAESTHESIA

The general anaesthesia can be classically divided into four stages of increasing depth of CNS depression. With *diethyl ether* (now obsolete), which produces a slow onset of anaesthesia, all the following four stages are discernible:

STAGE I: *It is the state of analgesia*, because sensory transmission in spinothalamic tract is inhibited. There is no amnesia. Consciousness and sense of touch are present, whereas sense of hearing is enhanced.

STAGE II: *This is the state of excitement and delirium*. The patient shows violent combative behaviour but definitely is amnesic. There is an irregular rise in blood pressure and respiratory rate. To avoid all these undesirable symptoms, a short acting barbiturate, thiopental sodium, is given I.V. before an inhalation anaesthetic is administered.

STAGE III: *It is a state of surgical anaesthesia*. Regular respiration and relaxation of skeletal muscle occurs in this stage. This stage has four planes.

Plane 1: There are roving movements of eyeballs which, later on (while attaining plane 3), get fixed. Respiration and skeletal muscle tone are normal.

Plane 2: Most surgical procedures are performed in this plane. There is progressive loss of corneal, light and laryngeal reflexes. Respiration is slow but regular.

Plane 3: It is a plane of marked muscle relaxation. Respiration is mainly abdominal. Eyeball movement is absent. Pupils are dilated. Light, corneal and laryngeal reflexes are absent.

Plane 4: It is a plane of complete muscle relaxation. Pupils are fully dilated with complete loss of light, corneal and laryngeal reflexes. Respiration is only abdominal.

STAGE IV: *It is a stage of medullary paralysis*. This stage appears due to overdosing. There is severe depression of the respiratory centre as well as of vasomotor center in the medulla. This stage is fatal and death can ensue.

Most surgical procedures are performed under stage III (plane-2) of anaesthesia. However, with *halothane* and other newer general anaesthetics these stages are difficult to be characterised because of the rapid onset of anaesthesia. Secondly, the use of preanaesthetic medication and inducing agents also alter or mask the clinical signs characterising various stages of anaesthesia. Hence the most reliable index for attainment of stage III of anaesthesia, is loss of corneal reflex and establishment of regular respiratory pattern. A fall in BP, cardiac and respiratory depression are the signs of deep anaesthesia. On the contrary, resistance to insertion of endotracheal tube and a reflex increase in respiration and BP after making incision on the skin are the signs of light anaesthesia. Advanced countries, however, use "computer assisted monitoring" of vital signs and cerebral functions to assess the depth of anaesthesia during surgery. Monitoring of vital signs by these techniques reduces the anaesthetic dose requirement, which contributes to a more rapid recovery from general anaesthesia.

TYPES OF GENERAL ANAESTHETICS

General anaesthetics are usually given by inhalation or by intravenous routes.

INHALATION ANAESTHETICS

1) **Gas**: *Nitrous oxide*
2) **Halogenated Liquids**: *Halothane, Methoxyflurane, Enflurane, Isoflurane, Sevoflurane* and *Desflurane*

INTRAVENOUS ANAESTHETICS

1) **Fast Inducers**
   a) ***Barbiturates***: *Thiopental, Methohexital*
   b) ***Non-Barbiturates***: *Propofol, Etomidate*
2) **Slow Inducers**
   Benzodiazepines: *Diazepam, Lorazepam* and *Midazolam*
3) **Dissociative Anaesthetics**: *Ketamine*

PHARMACOKINETIC PRINCIPLES FOR INDUCTION, MAINTENANCE AND RECOVERY FROM ANAESTHESIA

The procedure for producing anaesthesia initially involves smooth and rapid induction followed by its maintenance and thereafter a prompt recovery after the discontinuation of the anaesthetic agent.

Induction

Induction means the time interval between the administration of the anaesthetic drug and the development of the stage of surgical anaesthesia. Fast and smooth induction is always desired to avoid dangerous excitatory phase (stage II) of anaesthesia. Intravenous anaesthetics, such as *thiopental* or *propofol*, are often used for rapid induction, which is then maintained with an appropriate inhalation anaesthetic. As the inducing agents rapidly induce anaesthesia, they must be injected slowly. The unconsciousness results within 25 sec after injection. At this time, additional inhalation (e.g., halothane) or intravenous anaesthetic (e.g., ketamine) may be given to produce the desired depth (stage III, plane-2) of surgical anaesthesia. Skeletal muscle relaxants, such as pancuronium, atracurium or succinyl choline, are also coadministered to facilitate intubation and muscle relaxation.

Lipophilicity is the key factor governing the pharmacokinetics of the inducing drugs. Being highly lipophilic, after a single I.V. bolus injection, these drugs preferentially partition into the highly perfused and lipophilic brain to produce anaesthesia within a single circulation time. Termination of anaesthesia after single boluses of I.V. anaesthetics is primarily by redistribution out of the CNS into muscle, viscera and very lipophilic adipose tissue, rather than by metabolism (see following text and Ch. 6).

Maintenance

Maintenance is the period during which the patient remains in a sustained stage of surgical anaesthesia (stage III, plane-2). Anaesthesia is usually maintained by the administration of the gases or volatile liquid anaesthetics since these agents offer good minute to minute control over the depth of anaesthesia. The anaesthesiologist monitors the patient's vital signs and response to various stimuli throughout the surgical procedure in order to carefully decide about the intermittent concentration to be inhaled or infused looking to the depth of anaesthesia.

The depth of anaesthesia depends upon the concentration of anaesthetic in the CNS. The factors that influence the uptake and distribution of the anaesthetic, govern the rate at which an effective concentration of the anaesthetic would reach the brain. This requires the transfer of the anaesthetic drug from the alveolar air to the blood and then to the brain. Since gases move from one compartment to another within the body according to the gradients of partial pressure, a steady state is achieved only when the partial pressures in each of these compartments is equivalent to that of the inspired anaesthetic mixture. The rate of such transfer, till the attainment of the steady state, depends upon: (a) alveolar wash-in, (b) solubility characteristics of the anaesthetic drug, (c) its concentration in the inspired air, (d) the pulmonary ventilation rate, (e) cardiac output that controls the pulmonary blood flow transferring the anaesthetic gas from the alveoli to the blood flowing through lungs and (f) the partial pressure gradient of the anaesthetic drug between the arterial and the venous blood before its redistribution to all the tissues of the body.

Alveolar Wash-in

It is a process wherein the inspired anaesthetic mixture replaces the normal air inside the lungs. The time required for this process is directly proportional to the functional residual capacity of the lungs and indirectly proportional to the ventilatory rate, and is independent of the physical properties of the anaesthetic gas. Once the partial pressures equalise within the lungs, anaesthetic uptake by the blood from the lungs begins.

Solubility Characteristics of Anaesthetic Drug

Solubility characteristics of an anaesthetic drug are measured by two partition coefficients:

a) *Blood:gas partition coefficient at steady state or equilibrium* (P b/g): The blood:gas partition coefficient is a measure of anaesthetic solubility in the blood. The rank order of blood:gas partition coefficient of various inhalation anaesthetics is: methoxyflurane (12)> halothane (2.3) > enflurane (1.9) > isoflurane (1.4) > sevoflurane (0.6) > desflurane (0.42) = nitrous oxide (0.47). A high blood:gas partition coefficient (e.g., of halothane, 2.3) corresponds to a high degree of solubility in the blood. Hence more time is required to attain its partial pressure in blood for induction. Anaesthetics with low coefficient (e.g., nitrous oxide, 0.47) have a faster induction as they saturate the blood faster with prompt rise in their partial pressure in the blood. Thus P b/g is inversely proportional to rate of induction of anaesthesia; lower the P b/g faster is the induction of anaesthesia.

b) *Oil (lipid):gas partition coefficient at steady state* (P o/g): As the lipid solubility increases, the anaesthetic potency increases, as measured by a decrease in minimum alveolar concentration (MAC). This corroborates with the membrane theory of anaesthesia which predicts that high Po/g means high anaesthetic potency or a decreased MAC value to produce anaesthesia. This suggests that an anaesthetic gas with high blood (lipid) solubility (high P o/g), such as halothane, dissolves heavily in the blood and thus would have a low MAC. However, greater amount of anaesthetic and a longer time would be needed to raise the partial pressure and also for equilibration of partial pressure between the inhaled anaesthetic in the lungs and in the blood (see above). Thus, the disadvantage is that the induction as well as recovery would be slower. However, there would not be any major change in the depth of anaesthesia in response to minor fluctuations in the concentration of the inhaled drug. Thus P o/g is directly proportional to anaesthetic potency (i.e., low MAC value). For MAC value see following text.

Anaesthetic Concentration in the Inspired Air

An advantage is taken of this effect (as discussed above) in anaesthetic practice by selecting the inhaled anaesthetic of moderate blood solubility, such as halothane. Although it has slow onset of effect (slow induction), its concentration can be increased a bit (e.g., 3–4%) initially, to facilitate induction. This is then reduced to 1–2% for maintenance when adequate anaesthesia is achieved. In addition, halothane can be combined with a less soluble agent, such as nitrous oxide, to reduce the time required for induction.

Pulmonary Ventilation and Cardiac Output That Control Pulmonary Blood Flow

The rate of rise of anaesthetic gas partial pressure in arterial blood is directly dependent on pulmonary ventilation and cardiac output which control pulmonary blood flow. For an anaesthetic with low blood solubility (e.g., nitrous oxide), an increase in pulmonary ventilation is accompanied by only a slight increase in its arterial blood partial pressure; but an increase in pulmonary ventilation can significantly increase the partial pressure of the agents with moderate or high blood solubility, e.g., of halothane. This implies that hyperventilation increases the speed of induction of anaesthesia with inhaled anaesthetic that would normally have a slow onset (e.g., of halothane). Respiratory depression, on the contrary, will slow the onset of anaesthesia.

An increased cardiac output, and in turn pulmonary blood flow, results in more effective removal of the anaesthetic drug from alveoli to blood (and *vice versa*) speeding up the induction and recovery from anaesthesia. An opposite effect will be noticed with decreased pulmonary blood flow, as seen in patients with congestive heart failure or with chronic obstructive pulmonary disease.

Arterio-Venous Concentration Gradient

The anaesthetic concentration gradient between the arterial and venous blood depends mainly on the uptake of the anaesthetics by the tissues. After tissue uptake, during arterial circulation, there may be a great difference in the arterial-venous anaesthetic concentration gradient (because venous blood returning to lungs may carry lesser anaesthetic than arterial blood). The greater this difference in anaesthetic partial pressures, the more it has been taken up by viscera, muscle etc., and the more time it will take to achieve equilibrium within brain. The tissue uptake is influenced by factors such as, tissue: blood partition coefficient, rates of blood flow to the tissues and difference in concentration gradient. Organs like brain, heart, liver and kidney, which are highly perfused, significantly influence arterial-venous anaesthetic concentration gradient and rapidly attain a steady state with the partial pressures of the anaesthetic in the arterial blood. The inhaled anaesthetic continues to be distributed in various tissues even during the phase of maintenance but that distribution in other tissues has little impact on the time course of desired anaesthesia. Skeletal muscles, though poorly perfused, have a large mass which prolongs the time needed to achieve the steady state. Bones and cartilages are also poorly perfused with little capacity to store the anaesthetic. Hence these organs have only little impact on the time course of anaesthetic distribution in the body. Fat too is very poorly perfused but has a large capacity to store anaesthetics which by themselves are lipid soluble. This remarkably delays the equilibrium to occur with most anaesthetics at least for the time the anaesthesia is required.

As the venous blood, depleted of anaesthetic, returns to the lungs, more gas moves into the blood from the lungs according to partial pressure gradient. Overtime, when such cycles are repeated, the partial pressure in the alveolar space closely approximates the partial pressure in the inspired mixture and that means the entire system is in equilibrium and that there is no further anaesthetic uptake from the lungs into the blood.

Recovery

When the anaesthetic drug is discontinued, the recovery phase starts, which is reverse of induction. The redistribution of the anaesthetic agent (from its site of action), rather than metabolism underlies the recovery. During this phase the anaesthesiologist has to see that there are no delayed toxic reactions, e.g., ***diffusion hypoxia*** from nitrous oxide. In the recovery phase nitrous oxide, unlike other inhaled anaesthetic, moves out of the blood into the alveoli at a faster rate. This results into significantly lower concentration of oxygen in alveoli. Thus mild diffusion hypoxia occurs, which although transient, may precipitate cardiac arrest in patients with reduced pulmonary and cardiac reserve. Oxygen is, therefore, given during the last few minutes of anaesthesia and in the early post-anaesthetic period. This phenomenon of diffusion hypoxia is more common with gases that are relatively insoluble in blood because just as their induction is faster so is their elimination. Nitrous oxide is still more problematic in this respect because it is used in higher concentration (70%). Highly blood-soluble agents (e.g., halothane) will diffuse out more slowly so that the recovery will be slower just as their induction and with them the risk of diffusion hypoxia is negligible.

Majority of inhaled anaesthetics are primarily removed from the body *via* exhalation, where the same factors that influence the attainment of steady state (with an inhaled anaesthetic) determine the time course of clearance of the drug from the body. Thus nitrous oxide exits the body faster than halothane. However, some of the anaesthetics are metabolised by liver. Thus about 70% of methoxyflurane, 30% of halothane and 5–8% of enflurane are metabolised by liver. Hepatic insufficiency, therefore, can delay the recovery. The rank order for the extent of metabolism of different inhalation anaesthetics by liver is: methoxyflurane >halothane > enflurane > sevoflurane > isoflurane > desflurane > nitrous oxide. The latter is almost totally washed out by exhalation.

POTENCY OF INHALED ANAESTHETICS

The potency of inhaled anaesthetics is quantitated by the ***Minimum Alveolar Concentration*** **(MAC)**, which is the minium concentration of anaesthetic that is required to prevent movement in 50% of patients in response to a standard surgical skin incision. MAC values are expressed as percentage of anaesthetic gas in the inspired mixture. Smaller the MAC value more potent is the anaesthetic. Anaesthetics with higher lipid solubility have lower MAC values.

MAC value of a given anaesthetic decreases with age, hypothermia and by concomitant use of CNS depressant drugs such as sedative-hypnotics, anxiolytics and narcotic analgesics. Sex, species, acid-base balance and arterial blood pressure changes do not influence MAC. The rank order of MAC values (%) of different inhalation anaesthetics is: methoxyflurane (0.16%)< halothane (0.75%) < isoflurane (1.2%) < enflurane (1.7%) < sevoflurane (1.9%) < desflurane (6 %) < nitrous oxide (>100%). The MAC value greater than 100% for nitrous oxide reveals that it is the least potent anaesthetic. It means that at normal atmospheric pressure, even if you give 100% of inspired nitrous oxide, its potency is still not equal to 1 MAC.

MECHANISM OF ACTION

Inhalation anaesthetics are non-selective in their action. The very fact that chemically unrelated drugs produce a state of general anaesthesia argues against a specific anaesthetic receptor.

At molecular level, anaesthetics interact with hydrophobic regions of neuronal membrane proteins that interface with membrane lipids. Inhaled anaesthetics, barbiturates, benzodiazepines, etomidate and propofol facilitate GABA-mediated inhibition at $GABA_A$ receptor sites and thereby increase Cl^- flux through its channel. Ketamine blocks the action of glutamate (an excitatory neurotransmitter) on NMDA receptor. Inhalation anaesthetics (like enflurane and isoflurane) decrease the duration of opening of nicotinic receptor activated Na^+ channels—an action that decreases the excitatory effects of ACh at cholinergic synapses. By affecting neuronal membrane proteins, general anaesthetics disrupt neuronal firing and sensory processing in the thalamus, thereby causing loss of consciousness and analgesic effects. The motor activity is reduced because they also inhibit neuronal output from the internal pyramidal layer of cerebral cortex.

SPECIFIC INHALATION ANAESTHETICS

Each of the inhalation anaesthetics has its own characteristics, advantages and disadvantages. No one is superior to another in all respects.

Nitrous Oxide

Physical Characteristics and Uses: It has a mild sweetish smell. It is neither inflammable nor explosive. It is used to maintain surgical anaesthesia in combination with 30% oxygen and other volatile anaesthetics such as halothane, isoflurane or propofol, and if required, muscle relaxant. For better analgesia a concentration of 50% nitrous oxide with 50% O_2 usually suffices.

Advantages: It has a strong analgesic action. Inhalation of 50% nitrous oxide with 50% O_2 has similar effects to standard doses of morphine. Induction is rapid and recovery time rarely exceeds

4 minutes even after prolonged administration. Nitrous oxide reduces the requirement of other volatile anaesthetics. It has no adverse effects on CVS, respiratory system, kidney and liver (least hepatotoxic). It does not sensitise the heart to catecholamines and has no arrhythmogenic potential. It is, therefore, probably the safest anaesthetic provided that at least 30% O_2 is always administered at the same time.

Disadvantages and Adverse Effects: It is less potent, does not cause bronchodilation and has no muscle relaxant effects. The incidence of post-anaesthetic nausea and vomiting increases with the duration of anaesthesia. Exposure to nitrous oxide for more than 4 hours can cause megaloblastic changes in bone marrow. Because of the prolonged and repeated exposure of operating theatre staff, there is increased risk of abortion and birth defects. Because it swiftly moves into closed body compartments from the blood, it can increase their volume (**pneumothorax**) or increase the pressure inside the sinuses (nasal, eye, middle ear). Continued administration of O_2 may be necessary during recovery especially in elderly patients (to avoid diffusion hypoxia; see above).

Halothane

It is the prototype to which newer agents, in halogenated volatile anaesthetic series, are compared. *Physical Characteristics and Uses*: It is commonly used in all developing countries as it is comparatively inexpensive. It is volatile liquid with mild sweetish odour, non-irritant and non-inflammable. Its deficiencies in terms of poor analgesia and muscle relaxation are compensated by concomitant use of nitrous oxide/opioids and skeletal muscle relaxants. *Advantages*: It is pleasant to breathe and not hepatotoxic to children, which make it the agent of choice for paediatric use. Besides, it is a potent anaesthetic also. It not only abolishes pharyngeal and laryngeal reflexes but is a bronchodilator also; hence preferred for asthmatics. It inhibits intestinal and uterine contractions; hence can be used for assisting external or internal version of foetus during late pregnancy. Recovery from halothane anaesthesia is smooth and, except for shievering, the usual nausea or vomiting are rare.

Disadvantages and Adverse Effects: It has highest blood:gas partition coefficient and hence induction as well as recovery is comparatively slow. It is very poor analgesic or muscle relaxant. Halothane has vagomimetic action and causes bradycardia and transient fall in BP. It reduces cardiac output and sensitises the myocardium to the arrhythmic effects of catecholamines. The latter is especially serious if hypercapnia develops or if the plasma concentration of catecholamines increases due to stress.

Halothane is oxidatively metabolised to tissue toxic trifluoroethanol and bromide ion. This may induce delayed fever (after 2–3 days), anorexia, nausea, vomiting and at times transient hepatitis. However, repeated administration of halothane can cause severe hepatic necrosis (1:50,000). To avoid this risk, halothane anaesthesia is not repeated at intervals of less than 2–3 weeks. Its use during labour can prolong delivery and cause postpartum haemorrhage. Normalisation of mental functions takes several hours after the recovery.

Halothane can trigger malignant hyperthermia in genetically predisposed cases. This life-threatening medical emergency occurs during or immediately after anaesthesia. Succinylcholine, if used as a muscle relaxant (along with halothane), worsens the condition further (Ch. 14). If it happens, *Dantrolene* 1 mg/kg, I.V., is given immediately, with other supportive measures. Further doses of dantrolene are given at 15 min interval, until the patient responds, to a maximum dose of 10 mg/kg (Ch. 14).

Methoxyflurane

Because of slow induction, slow recovery, hepato- and nephrotoxicity, methoxyflurane is not used these days.

Enflurane

Physical Characteristics and Uses: It is nonirritating, noninflammable liquid with mild odour. Its potency lies between halothane and isoflurane. However, after the introduction of isoflurane its use is declining nowadays.

Advantages: Like halothane, it decreases heart rate, cardiac output and BP. Uterine relaxation is also similar to halothane. However, unlike halothane it does not sensitise the heart to catecholamines; hence arrhythmias are rare. Though bronchodilatation is equal, it is a better skeletal muscle relaxant than halothane. It has a rapid induction and rapid recovery than halothane.

Disadvantages and Adverse Effects: Use of enflurane is contraindicated in epileptic patients because it causes CNS excitation. It has greater respiratory depressant action, i.e., assistance is usually needed to prevent acidosis. About 5–8% of enflurane is metabolised to fluoride ions to cause polyuric renal failure (contraindicated in renal failure). There have been a few cases of jaundice and hepatotoxicity but the incidence is much lower than halothane.

Isoflurane

Physical Characteristics and Uses: It is a newer halogenated volatile anaesthetic which is a structural analogue of enflurane. It is 1½ times more potent than enflurane and is noninflammable liquid with pungent odour. It exhibits rapid induction and recovery than halothane. In advanced countries, isoflurane is now the most widely used routine anaesthetic. However, its cost prohibits its use in developing countries.

Advantages: Pupils do not dilate and light reflex is not lost. Isoflurane is a very stable molecule that undergoes minimal metabolism, as a result of which, least fluoride is produced. Hence the chances of organ toxicity (nephrotoxicity, hepatotoxicity) are rare. Unlike halothane, it does not induce cardiac arrhythmias and does not sensitise the myocardium to the actions of catecholamines. Low concentrations of isoflurane do not increase cerebral blood flow or intracranial pressure. It depresses cortical EEG activity and is preferred for neurosurgery. It is also a muscle relaxant. It is a potent coronary vasodilator. Although it irritates upper airway, it is a bronchodilator.

Disadvantages and Adverse Effects: It has a pungent odour and causes bronchial irritation, which makes induction unpleasant. In the patients of coronary artery disease, it may cause redistribution of blood away from the area of inadequate perfusion to one of the normal perfusion. This phenomenon of "coronary steal" (Ch. 20) may precipitate regional myocardial ischaemia. Being a vasodilator it causes hypotension and reflex tachycardia.

Desflurane

Desflurane is structurally similar to isoflurane and has anaesthetic actions similar to halothane as well as to isoflurane.

Physical Characteristics and Uses: It is non-inflammable, non-explosive but irritant volatile halogenated anaesthetic. Because of the lower blood: gas partition coefficient it has a very rapid induction and recovery. Hence in many Western countries it has gained popularity as an anaesthetic for outpatient surgery.

Advantages: Emergence from anaesthesia and recovery from psychomotor and cognitive skills with desflurane are more rapid than any other anaesthetic of this series. This is of advantage for outpatient surgery as the patients can be discharged few hours after surgery. As it undergoes negligible metabolism, there is hardly any release of fluoride ions and hence it carries least risk for organ toxicities. This characteristic favours its use for prolonged anaesthesia. It rarely precipitates malignant hyperthermia and sensitises the myocardium to catecholamines to a lesser extent than halothane or enflurane. Muscle relaxation is equal to isoflurane. Seizure provoking potential is also negligible.

Disadvantages and Adverse Effects: Desflurane is irritant to airways and may provoke breath holding, apnoea, coughing, increased salivation and laryngospasm. Hence it is not suitable for induction in children. Incidence of postoperative nausea and vomiting are greater than propofol (see following text). Depth of anaesthesia fluctuates rapidly with change in inhaled concentration.

Sevoflurane

Physical Characteristics and Uses: It is the latest volatile halogenated anaesthetic with properties intermediate between isoflurane and desflurane. It is non-pungent, non-inflammable. Induction with sevoflurane is rapid (2 min) and smooth because it is non-pungent. Recovery is also faster than halothane.

Advantages: Being non-pungent, it does not cause respiratory irritation. Acceptability is better even by children. Induction and emergence from anaesthesia are as fast as with desflurane. It has good muscle relaxant properties also. Cardiovascular effects are similar to those of isoflurane but it does not produce "coronary steal". It sensitises the myocardium to sympathomimetics to a lesser extent than halothane or enflurane. It makes an excellent choice for inhalation anaesthesia, particularly in children.

Disadvantages and Adverse Effects: It is not a bronchodilator. It may trigger malignant hyperthermia in susceptible patients but risk is much lower than halothane. Although 2% of sevoflurane is metabolised, the concentration of intrarenally generated fluoride ions is low in comparison to methoxyflurane and enflurane. Hence chances of renal toxicity are minimal. It is degraded by contact with CO_2 absorbents such as soda lime. The compound-A (a vinyl ether derivative) thus formed has been shown to be nephrotoxic in rats (not in humans). However, it is best avoided in patients with renal failure. Shivering, nausea and vomiting have been reported in postoperative period. Nevertheless, sevoflurane is considered to be close to an ideal anaesthetic.

INTRAVENOUS ANAESTHETICS

Fast Inducers

Unlike inhaled anaesthetics, intravenous agents do not require specialised vapouriser equipment for their delivery. Intravenous agents like ***thiopental***, ***methohexital***, ***etomidate*** and ***propofol*** are commonly used for induction of anaesthesia because their onset of anaesthetic action is faster than even desflurane or sevoflurane. Recovery also is sufficiently rapid. These are highly lipid-soluble drugs. After a single I.V. injection, their blood concentration rises instantly expediting their faster diffusion into the brain. The recovery occurs quite rapidly as the drug is redistributed in various compartments of the body and the plasma concentration reduces (see Ch. 6). Since it is a single dose, the recovery results due to redistribution and not due to metabolism. In common practice, anaesthesia is initially induced by giving an intravenous anaesthetic and then volatile anaesthetics (with nitrous oxide) are used for maintenance. The anaesthetic potency of these fast inducing I.V. anaesthetics is adequate enough to even use them as sole anaesthetic for short surgical procedures when combined with nitrous oxide and opioid analgesics.

Short-Acting Barbiturates

THIOPENTAL is a ultrashort acting thiobarbiturate (Ch. 32) which induces anaesthesia smoothly within one circulation time (<1 min). Following an I.V. bolus injection it crosses BBB rapidly; as a result the plasma: brain equilibrium is attained swiftly, because of its high lipid solubility. Thereafter, it diffuses rapidly out of brain and is redistributed to body fats, muscles and other tissues (Ch. 6). Consequently its action is terminated and recovery results. It is because of this rapid removal from the brain and its subsequent redistribution that thiopental is so short acting. The typical induction dose is 3–5 mg/kg. Thiopental is metabolised in liver at a rate of 12–15% per hour.

It reduces cerebral metabolic rate of O_2 consumption, which leads to cerebral vaso-constriction with a concomitant reduction in cerebral blood flow and intracranial pressure. This makes it a suitable drug for use in patients with cerebral oedema and brain tumours.

Adverse Effects: Laryngospasm may occur particularly when intubation is attempted while anaesthesia is light. It has no muscle relexant action, hence the use of muscle relaxant is necessary. It has no analgesic activity. Shivering and delirium may occur during recovery. Barbiturates, in general, may precipitate acute intermittent porphyria by inducing the enzyme hepatic ALA synthetase (Ch. 32). Hence it is contraindicated in such susceptible individuals. The pH of I.V. thiopental is 11, hence local tissue damage may result if it extravasates. It also reduces respiratory rate and tidal volume. Other effects are not that serious.

METHOHEXITAL is a thiobarbiturate similar to thiopental but its terminal half-life is considerably shorter (4–5 hrs) and the patient may be road-worthy more quickly. Its use has declined because the recovery is associated with restlessness, coughing and hiccups.

Propofol

Propofol is available as a 1% or 2% emulsion in soyabean oil. Its injection is a bit painful but adding 20 mg of lidocaine to an ampoule of propofol overcomes this drawback. Induction of anaesthesia with 1.5–2.5 mg/kg of propofol occurs within 30 sec and is smooth and pleasant with low incidence of excitatory voluntary movements. The recovery from propofol is also rapid with low incidence of nausea and vomiting because propofol itself has antiemetic action. In contrast to thiopental, recovery from a continuous I.V. infusion of propofol is relatively rapid. On stopping the drug the plasma concentration falls rapidly as a result of both redistribution and metabolism of the drug. Propofol is non-irritant to respiratory airways. However, propofol also has no analgesic or muscle relaxant effects.

Propofol causes dose-dependent cortical depression and has anticonvulsant action. The risk of causing laryngeal spasm is much less compared to barbiturates. In anaesthetic doses, effects on respiration are similar to those of thiopental. Its favourable properties make it particulary suited for outpatient surgery.

Adverse Effects: Apnoea and pain at the site of injection are common adverse effects of bolus administration of propofol. It produces a marked decrease in systemic blood pressure during induction of anaesthesia, primarily because it decreases peripheral resistance. Bradycardia is also frequent.

Etomidate

It has a briefer duration of action (5–10 min) than thiopental and produces much less cardiovascular and respiratory depression. Yet, it has not gained popularity because of the following reasons: It causes pain on injection; excitatory muscle movements are common on induction and incidence of nausea and vomiting are frequent after recovery. It is a poor analgesic and causes adrenocortical suppression by inhibiting 11β- and 17β-hydroxylase (Fig. 42.1). For this reason it is not used for prolonged infusion, because a prolonged decrease in plasma cortisol could be detrimental.

Despite all these disadvantages it is occasionally used for emergency anaesthesia because it causes lesser hypotension than thiopental or propofol.

Slow Inducers

Benzodiazepines (BZDs)

BZDs, of which diazepam is a prototype, are now preferred for endoscopies, cataract operations, cardiac catheterisation, angiographies, fracture settings and ECT etc. In addition to this, they have an important use in preanaesthetic medication and are also frequently used for inducing and maintaining anaesthesia. When injected I.V. (in therapeutic doses) they produce sedation, muscle relaxation and amnesia. ***Diazepam*** (0.2–0.5 mg/kg I.V.), ***lorazepam*** (0.04 mg/kg I.V.) and ***midazolam*** (0.07–0.08 mg/kg I.V.) are generally used in anaesthetic practice. Compared to I.V. barbiturates, BZDs are slow inducers, but they produce a high grade of anterograde amnesia which is clinically beneficial. ***Midazolam*** is the most frequently used BZD because it produces higher degree (>50%) of amnesia. It has a more rapid onset and a shorter elimination half-life (2–4 hrs). In contrast to diazepam and lorazepam, midazolam formulations are water soluble and thus produce lesser irritation. By themselves, BZDs do not depress respiration or cardiac functions. They do not cause postoperative nausea or vomiting. BZDs are poor analgesics. Hence an opioid or N_2O is needed if analgesia is required. Though amnesia is more profound with midazolam and lorazepam, sedation is more with the latter. Hence awakening may be delayed with lorazepam.

Dissociative Anaesthetic – Ketamine

KETAMINE produces *dissociative anaesthesia*, which is characterised by a feeling of dissociation from the surroundings, profound analgesia, immobility and amnesia with light sleep. Its primary site of action is cortex and limbic system and not reticular activating system (site of action of barbiturates). It acts by blocking the action of glutamate (an excitatory aminoacid) at NMDA receptor (Fig. 30.5). It is a highly lipophilic drug. After its fast diffusion into brain it is subsequently redistributed in various body compartments with simultaneous hepatic metabolism followed by urinary and biliary excretion. Its usual induction dose is 1–2 mg/kg I.V.

Ketamine is the only I.V. anaesthetic which possesses significant analgesic properties and produces CNS stimulation. It significantly increases HR, BP and cardiac output, possibly by inhibiting the uptake of norepinephrine at sympathetic nerve terminals. Ketamine markedly increases cerebral blood flow and intracranial pressure. Hence it is contraindicated in the patients of hypertension, ischaemic heart disease, schizophrenia and epilepsy but very suitable for patients of hypovolaemic shock. Recovery is associated with "emergence delirium" characterised by frightening dreams and disorientation. Because of such postoperative psychic phenomena (less in children), associated with its use, ketamine alone is not commonly used. However, use of diazepam (0.2–0.3 mg/kg) or midazolam (0.025–0.05 mg/kg) intravenously, prior to the administration of ketamine, minimises these adverse effects. It is also used with propofol for outpatient anaesthesia and in children for burn dressings. Being a bronchodilator, it is suitable for asthmatics also.

NEUROLEPT-ANALGESIA AND NEUROLEPT-ANAESTHESIA

A fixed dose combination of an opioid analgesic ***fentanyl*** (50 μg/ml) and a neuroleptic ***droperidol*** (2.5 mg/ml) is sometimes used to produce a state of "neurolept-analgesia". It is diluted in a glucose solution and infused intravenously over 10–15 min. Neurolept-analgesia is characterised by a state of calmness, psychic indifference to the surroundings and profound analgesia without any loss of consciousness. The patient though remains drowsy but is cooperative.

Fentanyl is a very potent (80 times more potent than morphine) but a short acting (30–40 min, if given I.M) opioid analgesic while droperidol is a butyrophenone group of short acting neuroleptic which acts by blocking central dopamine (D_2) receptors. It has antiemetic, sedative and anticonvulsant properties, and also potentiates analgesic actions of fentanyl. Other potent and still shorter acting drugs such as ***alfentanil***, ***sufentanil*** or ***remifentanil*** can also be used in place of fentanyl. *Remifentanil* is unique as it is promptly metabolised by plasma as well as tissue esterases and hence respiratory depression can be controlled by regulating its IV infusion.

Neurolept-analgesia is quite suitable for endoscopies, angiographies, burn dressings and for a variety of minor surgical procedures in otherwise poor risk patients. Respiratory depression (due to fentanyl) may be marked, assistance may be needed. Mild postural hypotension (due to α-adrenergic blocking action of droperidol) may occur but the heart is not sensitised to catecholamines. Recovery is slow and psychomotor functions remain depressed for many hours. Neurolept-analgesia can be converted to *"neurolept-anaesthesia"* by concurrent administration of 65% nitrous oxide and 35% oxygen.

Lately dose-dependent cases of QT prolongation and torsade de pointes, including some fatal cases, have been reported with droperidol. A combination of fentanyl and droperidol also causes chest wall rigidity (effect on basal ganglia). Hence both neurolept-analgesia as well as neurolept-anaesthesia have been outmoded. Fentanyl combined with diazepam can obviate the need of neurolept-analgesia for short surgical procedures. Being devoid of cardiotoxicity, fentanyl (I.V) with general anaesthetics, is used in coronary artery by-pass surgery, to provide analgesia.

BALANCED ANAESTHESIA

General anaesthetics are rarely given as sole agents. Rather anaesthetic adjuvants are generally used to augment the specific components of the desired state of surgical anaesthesia, permitting lesser doses of general anaesthetics with fewer side effects. The integral part of general anaesthetic drug regimen to provide balanced anaesthesia includes the following drugs:

Thiopental + Opioid analgesics like pethidine or fentanyl + Skeletal muscle relaxant like pancuronium, and Nitrous oxide along with a inhalation anaesthetic (e.g., halothane).

PREANAESTHETIC MEDICATION

The aim of preanaesthetic medication is to ensure comfort to the patient and to minimise adverse effects of anaesthesia. The drugs given prior to anaesthesia and surgery alleviate anxiety and apprehension, provide analgesia, reduce chances of emesis and autonomic effects during anaesthesia and induce amnesia. Drugs used for preanaesthetic medication are as under:

Antianxiety Drugs: Benzodiazepines such as ***diazepam*** (5–10 mg oral) or ***lorazepam*** (2 mg I.M.) are used to provide relief from apprehension and anxiety and to produce postoperative amnesia. ***Midazolam*** (70–100 μg/kg I.V.) can be given prior to surgery. It provides amnesia and sedation for about 30–40 minutes.

Sedative-Hypnotics: Besides benzodiazepines (as discussed above), ***promethazine*** (25 mg, I.M.) is also widely used because besides being an antihistamine, it has sedative, antiemetic and anticholinergic actions. It causes negligible respiratory depression and has been found very suitable for children (6.25–12.5 mg, I.M.) also.

Opioid Analgesics: ***Morphine*** (8–12 mg I.M.) or ***pethidine*** (50–100 mg, I.M.) is used one hour before surgery. These provide sedation, pre- and postoperative analgesia and reduction in anaesthetic dose. Because of their adverse effects (Ch. 37), use of opioids is now restricted to reduce postoperative pain. When needed, ***fentanyl*** (50–100 mcg, I.M. or I.V.) is preferred just before induction of anaesthesia.

Anticholinergics: ***Atropine*** (0.5 mg I.M.) or ***hyoscine*** (0.5 mg I.M.) or ***glycopyrrolate*** (0.1–0.3 mg I.M.) are given one hour before surgery to reduce salivary, bronchial secretions, vagal bradycardia, hypotension and to prevent laryngospasm. Hyoscine has an additional antiemetic and amnesic effects. Glycopyrrolate acts rapidly and is longer acting. It is a potent antisecretory agent and prevents vagal bradycardia effectively. It is less likely to produce central effects.

Antiemetics: ***Metoclopramide*** (10 mg I.M.) is used as antiemetic and as prokinetic gastric emptying agent prior to emergency surgery. It can be used to prevent postoperative vomiting. Combined use of H_2 blocker (ranitidine or famotidine) with metoclopramide is more effective. ***Domperidone*** (10 mg, oral) is more preferred as it does not produce extrapyramidal side effects like metoclopramide (Ch. 28). ***Ondansetron*** (4–8 mg I.V.), a 5-HT_3 receptor antagonist, has also been found effective in preventing post-anaesthetic nausea and vomiting.

H_2 Receptor Blockers: ***Ranitidine*** (150–300 mg, oral) or ***famotidine*** (20–40 mg, oral) given a night before and in the morning before surgery along with metoclopramide reduces the risk of gastric regurgitation and aspiration pneumonia. Proton pump inhibitor such as ***omeprazole*** (20 mg) with ***domperidone*** (10 mg) is a preferred alternative.

Dexmedetomidine, a centrally active α_2 receptor agonist has been introduced to sedate critically ill patients on ventilator in intensive care units (and even just prior to anaesthesia). It blunts sympathetic response to surgery and stress, does not depress ventilation and reduces anaesthetic as well as opioid requirement (Ch. 12).

CHAPTER 32

Anxiolytics and Hypnotics

COMPETENCY PH1.19

Sedation means decrease in alertness and a decreased responsiveness to any level of stimulation without inducing sleep. ***Hypnosis*** should not be confused with a trance-like state, used in psychiatry, in which the subject becomes passive, highly suggestive and obeys the commands. In medical practice, hypnosis means a state that resembles natural sleep but the person can be aroused by strong stimuli like pin prick or the sound of the alarm clock. ***Anxiety*** is actually an adaptive response which prepares a person to face the challenges of life. Anxiety is characterised by psychologic symptoms (tension, fear, apprehension, lack of concentration etc) as well as by sympathetic plus somatic symptoms (tachycardia, tremors, sweating, GIT distress etc). Fatigue and sleep disturbances are also common. If anxiety presists it impairs person's ability to perform the job and often leads to visceral organ dysfunction and neurological problems. For types of anxiety see Ch. 30.

The difference between an anxiolytic, sedative and hypnotic is generally quantitative. This group of drugs (except benzodiazepines, see below) produces all degrees of non-specific CNS depression starting from relief of anxiety → disinhibition → sedation → hypnosis → anaesthesia → coma and ultimately death. These effects depend upon their dose, their route of administration and their physico-chemical characteristics. A linear dose-response curve, between the increasing doses and intensity of CNS depression, is typical of many of the older sedative-hypnotics like barbiturates. Benzodiazepines and newer anxiolytics, rather have a flatter dose-response curve. These drugs have a greater margin of safety, which leads to their widespread use to treat anxiety states and sleep disorders.

CLASSIFICATION OF ANXIOLYTIC AND HYPNOTIC DRUGS

1. **BENZODIAZEPINES**
   This is the most important group with multifarious uses and may be divided according to their duration of action.
   Short Acting
   Triazolam, Oxazepam , Midazolam, Remimazolam
   Intermediate Acting
   Alprazolam, Estazolam, Temazepam, Lorazepam, Nitrazepam
   Long Acting
   Diazepam, Flurazepam, Clonazepam, Chlordiazepoxide
2. **NON-BENZODIAZEPINE HYPNOTICS**
   Zolpidem, Zaleplon, Zopiclone, Eszopiclone
3. **ATYPICAL ANXIOLYTICS**
   Buspirone, Ipsapirone, Gepirone
4. **β-ADRENOCEPTOR ANTAGONISTS** (non- sedating anxiolytics)
   Propranolol
5. **BARBITURATES**
   As anxiolytic-sedative these are now obsolete, and have been superseded by benzodiazepines. Their use is now confined to anaesthesia and epilepsy. These are broadly classified as follows:
   Long Acting
   Phenobarbital, Mephobarbital
   Short Acting
   Pentobarbital, Amobarbital
   Ultra-Short Acting
   Thiopental, Methohexital
   Long-acting barbiturates are mainly used as anticonvulsants (Ch. 39). Short-acting barbiturates were being used earlier as hypnotics, but are seldom used now. Ultra-short-acting ones are used as inducing agents in general anaesthesia (Ch. 31).

6. **OREXIN RECEPTOR ANTAGONISTS**: *Lemborexant, Daridorexant, Suvorexant*
7. **MISCELLANEOUS GROUP** *Melatonin, Ramelteon, Tasimelteon, Triclophos, Hydroxyzine, Promethazine* and *Pitolisant* are used as sedative-hypnotics.

BENZODIAZEPINES (BZDs)

Benzodiazepines have not only proliferated but superseded barbiturates as hypnotic and sedative as well, because:

1. They do not provide anaesthesia even in high doses and the patient can be aroused. On the contrary, barbiturates provide loss of consciousness and have lower margin of safety.
2. These are not enzyme inducers and hence do not lead to metabolic tolerance. Drug interactions are also less. Barbiturates are potent enzyme inducers, exhibit metabolic tolerance and more drug-drug interactions.
3. BZDs have a very low abuse liability while barbiturates not only exhibit tolerance but cause both psychic and physical dependence.
4. BZDs do not affect REM sleep and cause lesser distortion of normal hypnogram. Barbiturates cause marked suppression of REM sleep, hence there is rebound increase in REM sleep on withdrawal (nightmares). Hangover is also common.
5. BZDs show no hyperalgesia while barbiturates exhibit hyperalgesic action and may even increase the sensitivity to pain.
6. BZDs exhibit amnesia but with no phenomenon of "automatism". Barbiturates are characterised by amnesia with automatism. The latter leads to accidental poisoning; because due to loss of short term memory, the patient forgets whether he has taken the drug or not and takes it again.
7. BZDs can be used as day time anxiolytic-sedative in sub-hypnotic doses. With barbiturates, the accompanied drowsiness is unacceptable.
8. Hypnotic doses of BZDs do not affect respiration or cardiovascular functions, while barbiturates cause respiratory depression and hypotension.
9. There are specific antagonists for BZDs (e.g., *flumazenil*) which can be used in case of poisoning; with barbiturates it is not possible.

Site of Action

BZDs exhibit relatively greater depressant action on limbic system (which regulates thoughts and mental functions) compared to midbrain ascending RAS (which maintains wakefulness). Hence they reduce anxiety at a dose which has little depressant effects on RAS, i.e., they elicit anxiolytic action with less sedative effects. At higher doses, however, they depress RAS and induce sedative-hypnotic action but this property differs qualitatively with individual drug. Muscle relaxation is produced by a medullary site of action, by inhibiting polysynaptic reflexes in the spinal cord. Ataxia is due to their action on cerebellum.

Mechanism of Action

Normally a balance between excitatory inputs (mostly glutamatergic) and the inhibitory inputs (mainly GABAergic) determines the prevailing level of neuronal activity in limbic system and RAS of the brain. If the balance swings in favour of GABA, nervousness and anxiety are reduced while sedation, amnesia, muscle relaxation and ataxia appear. In contrast, a reduction in GABAergic activity elicits arousal, anxiety, insomnia and restlessness. GABA acts on two distinct classes of receptors (Ch. 30):

- $GABA_A$ receptors which are located mainly postsynaptically. These are directly linked with Cl^- ion channels, opening of which causes hyperpolarisation and reduction in membrane excitability.
- $GABA_B$ receptors which are G-protein coupled receptors. Their activation decreases cAMP formation. They cause pre- and postsynaptic inhibition by inhibiting Ca^{2+} channel opening and increasing K^+ conductance.

$GABA_A$ receptor has several different binding sites (Fig. 32.1) which include:

- The neurotransmitter GABA-binding site.
- The modulatory sites to bind benzodiazepines, their antagonists like *flumazenil* and inverse agonists such as β-carbolines.
- The modulatory as well as blocking site at chloride ion channel.

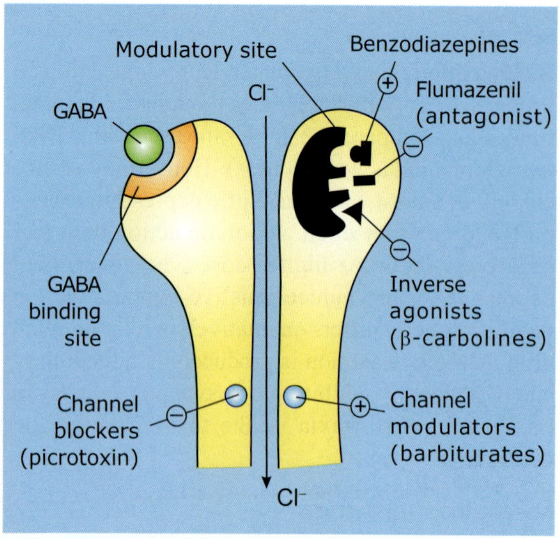

Fig 32.1 Main Sites of Drug Action at $GABA_A$ Receptor

$GABA_A$ receptors are the target for several important centrally acting drugs like benzodiazepines, barbiturates, neurosteroids and picrotoxin. BZDs which have powerful sedative and anxiolytic effects, selectively bind, with high affinity, to the modulatory site on $GABA_A$ receptor in such a way that the binding of GABA to $GABA_A$ receptor is facilitated. This modulatory site of $GABA_A$ receptor is distinct from the GABA binding site and is specific for BZDs; hence it is also referred to as "Benzodiazepine Receptor". BZDs neither substitute for GABA, nor activate $GABA_A$ receptor but rather enhance binding of GABA to the GABA binding site of $GABA_A$ receptor. They appear to increase the *frequency* (*rather than duration*) of GABA gated choride channel opening. A model of hypothetical GABA-BZD-Cl^- ion channel receptor complex with sites of action for agonists, antagonists, inverse agonists, channel blockers and channel modulators is shown in Figure 32.1 (for subtypes of BZD receptor, refer non-benzodiazepine hypnotics discussed below).

BZD Inverse Agonists and Antagonists

Inverse agonists (e.g., β-carboline) exert opposite effects to that of conventional BZDs, producing signs of anxiety and convulsions (see Ch.7). BZD-inverse agonists have no therapeutic utility except as research tools. BZD antagonist *flumazenil* blocks the actions of BZD and BZD agonists and is however used clinically. It undergoes significant first-pass metabolism in liver, hence not used orally. On I.V. injection, the effect starts spontaneously and lasts for 1–2 hrs. Plasma half life is 1–2 hrs. Its main use is to reverse BZD anaesthesia (0.5 mg I.V.) or to treat BZD overdose toxicity (0.2 mg/min; maximum 5 mg; till patient regains consciousness). Side effects are rare except anxiety, tremors and discomfort.

Pharmacokinetic Characteristics

There are marked pharmacokinetic variations among BZDs. Except for midazolam (given I.V. or I.M.), all can be given orally (though absorption varies). Although some of BZDs (diazepam, oxazepam and chlordiazepoxide) are more than 90% protein bound, no significant drug displacement reactions occur because of their marked volume of distribution. They cross placental barrier (caution! pregnancy). Most BZDs are metabolised by phase I metabolic processes and the resultant metabolites are subsequently conjugated (phase II reactions) to form water-soluble metabolites that are excreted in urine. However, many phase I metabolites are pharmacologically active which extend the half-life (and hence duration of action) of the parent drug. These include ***midazolam*** (which acts through its active metabolite, hydroxymethyl midazolam); ***diazepam*** (active metabolite *oxazepam* and nordiazepam also called *clorazepate*); ***flurazepam*** (active metabolite desmethylflurazepam and hydroxymethylflurazepam); ***chlordiazepoxide*** (active metabolite *desmethyldiazepam* and *oxazepam*) and ***alprazolam*** (active metabolite, alfa-hydroxyalprazolam).

Accumulation, with multiple dosing, is not clinically significant with short-acting BZDs but is significant with intermediate-acting and long-acting BZDs. Because of longer t½ , withdrawal effects are milder with long-acting BZDs.

Therapeutic Uses

1. To Treat Anxiety Neuroses

BZDs are currently the most widely used drugs for treating anxiety neuroses. Among these ***alprazolam, lorazepam, oxazepam, diazepam*** and ***chlordiazepoxide*** are commonly used, but the choice of one over the other is largely empirical. *Alprazolam* has anxiolytic-antidepressant effects and, therefore, is useful in anxiety associated with depression (dose 0.25–0.5 mg, BD or TDS) or in panic disorders associated with anxiety (dose maximum up to 6 mg per day in divided doses). It is claimed to produce less drowsiness.

Lorazepam has been preferred for short-lived anxiety states, compulsive-obsessive neuroses and tension-induced psychosomatic symptoms (dose 1–6 mg per day). It is the only BZD which is most suitable for parenteral use also. *Oxazepam* is used for short-lived anxiety states preferably in elderly patients or in those with liver dysfunction because its hepatic metabolism is less and duration of action is short (dose 30–60 mg in three divided doses). *Diazepam* is preferred in acute panic-anxiety states associated with organic disease where sedation is also desired (dose 2–10 mg BD or TDS). *Chlordiazepoxide* is preferred in chronic anxiety states. Its active metabolites prolong its duration of action (dose 20–50 mg per day in 2 or 3 divided doses).

2. To Treat Insomnia

BZDs are the hypnotic drugs of choice for the reasons discussed earlier. A drug with most suitable pharmacokinetic profile is usually selected for individual case. The impaired performance on the following day is largely due to the pharmacokinetic profile of the drug and its dose. The longer acting BZDs end up with hangover or sedation next day while shorter acting drugs precipitate rebound anxiety. Insomnia is divided into three categories:

i) ***Transient insomnia,*** which accounts for approximately 15% of the total cases, generally lasts less than 7 days. Causes of transient insomnia include jet lag, shift work, new place, overnight train journey etc. A rapidly acting, rapidly eliminated BZD like ***triazolam*** (0.125–0.25 mg) or ***temazepam*** (15–30 mg) at bed time is used.

   Triazolam is effective in treating individuals who have difficulty in going to sleep; while *temazepam* is useful for insomnia caused by inability to stay asleep. These drugs are used intermittently rather than daily to avoid residual effects leading to rebound insomnia.

ii) ***Short-term insomnia,*** which lasts for one to three weeks. It is caused by an expected but self-limiting problem such as bereavement, pain and anxiety-provoking occupational problems. The patient may have induction difficulty, frequent nocturnal awakenings and/or early morning awakening. ***Temazepam*** (15–30 mg) or ***flurazepam*** (15–30 mg) or ***estazolam*** (1–2 mg) at bed time are more suited for this type of insomnia.

iii) ***Long-term chronic insomnia***, which lasts longer than three weeks, indicates an underlying disease or a personality disorder. Intermittent use (with a break after every third day) of longer acting BZD like ***flurazepam*** (15–30 mg) or ***nitrazepam*** (5–10 mg) at bed time is preferred because rebound insomnia and withdrawal effects are less marked with these drugs.

However, non-benzodiazepine group of hypnotics are more preferred these days (see below).

3. For Preanaesthetic Medication and Induction of Anaesthesia

Diazepam, lorazepam and ***midazolam*** are generally used for this purpose (Ch. 31). Midazolam (I.V.) is most frequently used as it produces higher degree of amnesia, has a more rapid onset with shorter duration of action.

4. As Skeletal Muscle Relaxants

Diazepam is preferred for relaxant effects in skeletal muscle spasticity of central origin (refer Ch. 14).

5. As Anticonvulsants

Diazepam (slow I.V.) ***lorazepam*** (slow I.V.) and ***clonazepam*** (slow I.V.) are used to treat status epilepticus. Clonazepam may also be used for myoclonic/petit mal seizures. However, tolerance develops (within 3 months) soon to their antiepileptic effects (Ch. 39). Continuous slow I.V. infusion of diazepam can be used to prevent tetanic spasm.

6. Treatment of Alcohol Withdrawal

Diazepam, oxazepam and ***chlordiazepoxide*** are also used to control withdrawal effects of alcohol (Ch. 36).

Remimazolam

Remimazolam is a newer benzodiazepine. It is faster and shorter acting than midazolam. Half-life is 0.5–2 min. It is not effective orally, given intravenously. It is metabolized by hydrolysis due to hepatic carboxylesterase-1 (CES1) to inactive metabolite. It is used for the induction and maintenance of procedural sedation during short procedures (30 min or less).

Adverse Effects

i) BZDs have a high margin of safety. However, they elicit dose-dependent drowsiness, fatigue, disorientation, lethargy and impairment of psychomotor skills. Yet, with them suicidal risk is minimal as these are relatively safe and even 50 times of their therapeutic dose does not endanger life. Nevertheless, a fast I.V. injection can precipitate cardiac arrest.

ii) Tolerance to their sedative effects develops slowly, with only a little tendency to increase the dose. Nevertheless, it may be considered as a drawback. The tolerance occurs to a much lesser extent and does not occur due to induction of hepatic microsomal enzymes as seen with barbiturates. Although the mechanism is unclear, BZDs are reported to be mild "self inducers".

iii) Dependence to BZDs is again mild but the risk factors include continuous use, high doses, the use of BZDs with shorter to medium half-life, use in patients with drug-dependent personality traits and the development of tolerance. Nonetheless, their abuse liability is very low compared to barbiturates. The mechanism of BZD dependence is not clear. Possibly there is gradual decline in the functional GABA activity resulting from down-regulation of GABA receptor after their prolonged use. BZD withdrawal includes anxiety, insomnia, impaired concentration, headache, irritability, tremors, palpitation and vivid dreams (due to an increase in REM sleep) which may persist for some weeks after withdrawal of BZDs.

iv) Advancing age retards the rate of phase I metabolism of BZDs. Thus the effects of long-acting BZDs, if used regularly in elderly people, tends to increase with age resulting in increased confusion and forgetfulness.

v) Paradoxical stimulation may occur, in rare cases, especially with flurazepam.

vi) ***Flunitrazepam*** is one of the tasteless BZDs which has been misused, because of its sedative-amnestic effects, in sexual assaults or so-called "date rapes". It has been misused to obliterate memory of events to escape judicial punishment for the sexual assaults.

Drug Interactions

- BZDs potentiate the effects of other CNS depressants, such as alcohol, hypnotics and neuroleptics.
- Smoking decreases the activity of BZDs.
- Aminophylline antagonises sedative effects of BZDs.
- Enzyme inhibitors like cimetidine and ketoconazole enhance BZD action.

NON-BENZODIAZEPINE HYPNOTICS

Several non-benzodiazepines discussed below are more selective in their central actions as they act as agonist at the modulatory site of $GABA_A$ receptor to which BZDs bind. Two types of BZD receptor have been suggested: ***BZD receptor type I (BZ_1)*** found throughout the brain and in large concentrations in the cerebellum; and ***BZD receptor type II (BZ_2)*** found mainly in the cerebral cortex, hippocampus and spinal cord. It is the BZ_1 receptor that is thought to be responsible for antianxiety, sedative and hypnotic action while BZ_2 receptor appears to be associated with muscle relaxation, anticonvulsant action and amnesia. Most BZDs act on both BZ_1 and BZ_2 receptors. Non-benzodiazepines such as ***zolpidem, zaleplon, zopiclone*** and ***eszopiclone*** act on BZ_1 receptor only; while 1-5-benzodiazepines such as ***clobazam*** act preferably at BZ_2 receptor to elicit muscle relaxant and anticonvulsant actions.

Zolpidem, Zopiclone, Eszopiclone and Zaleplon

These drugs act on BZ_1 receptors and have hypnotic actions. As hypnotic, ***zolpidem*** ($t\frac{1}{2}$ 2–3 hrs) and

zaleplon ($t\frac{1}{2}$ 3–4 hrs) have faster onset of action with shorter duration of hypnotic effects while ***zopiclone*** ($t\frac{1}{2}$ 6–8 hrs) and ***eszopiclone*** ($t\frac{1}{2}$ 6 hrs) are slightly longer acting. In therapeutic doses they hardly alter REM sleep pattern and have minimal daytime residual sedation. The problem of rebound insomnia (after withdrawal of the drug) is also minimal. *Zolpidem* (10–20 mg) and *zaleplon* (10–20 mg) at bed time are used to treat transient insomnia while *zopiclone* (7.5 mg) and *eszopiclone* (1–3 mg) at bed time are used to treat short-term insomnia. Their effects can be blocked by *flumazenil*, which is antagonist at both BZ_1 and BZ_2 receptors.

These drugs have negligible muscle relaxant and anticonvulsant action. The risk of tolerance and dependence is much less after their withdrawal as compared to BZDs. Side effects and safety in overdoses are almost similar to BZDs. Dose reduction is needed in hepatic disease and in elderly patients. Headache, daytime drowsiness and nightmares can occur with higher doses.

ATYPICAL ANXIOLYTICS

Buspirone, Ipsapirone and Gepirone

These drugs act through non-GABAergic systems and have low propensity of side effects compared to BZDs. These drugs exert their anxiolytic effects by acting as a partial agonist primarily at brain $5\text{-}HT_{1A}$ receptors. Hence, by selective activation of the inhibitory presynaptic $5\text{-}HT_{1A}$ receptor, they suppress 5-HT neurotransmission through neuronal system. The drug ***buspirone*** (5–10 mg TDS) is used in anxiety states. However, the useful anxiolytic effects of buspirone are delayed for more than two weeks, which makes it unsuitable for management of acute anxiety states. It has no muscle relaxant, or anticonvulsant or hypnotic action.

Buspirone has minimal abuse liability and elicits no withdrawal reactions like rebound anxiety and insomnia etc., on abrupt discontinuation. Buspirone causes lesser impairment of psychomotor skills and does not potentiate the CNS depressant effects of ethanol (non-sedating anxiolytic drug). However, it can cause tachycardia, nervousness, GIT distress and paresthesias. Although mechanism is unknown, it causes dose-dependent pupillary constriction.

β-ADRENOCEPTOR ANTAGONISTS

Propranolol (Ch. 12)

Worrying situations and apprehensions associated with examinations, job interviews or public address are conducive to palpitation, tremors, GIT upset or even hypertension due to sympathetic overactivity. These symptoms, in turn, reinforce anxiety and thus the vicious cycle continues. *Propranolol* helps to suppress such preformance anxiety by breaking this vicious cycle. Propranolol through its β-blocking action decreases palpitation, tremors, GIT upset, hypertension and blood lactic acid levels. However, at usual dose of 20 mg TDS, the associated CVS effects make it unlikely to be used as potential anxiolytic agent.

BARBITURATES

The barbiturates have the following general formula (Fig. 32.2).

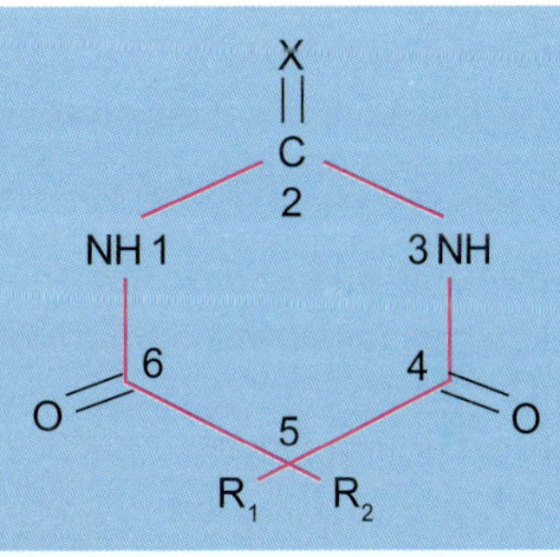

Fig 32.2 General Structural Formula of Barbiturates

British nomenclature ends with "barbitone", e.g., phenobarbitone. American nomenclature ends with "barbital", e.g., phenobarbital. If X = O, the drug is called a "barbiturate" and if X = S then it is called a "thiobarbiturate". If R_1 and R_2 are aliphatic alkyl groups the resultant barbiturate or thiobarbiturate possesses sedative-hypnotic action (e.g., pentothal). If either of R_1/R_2 is phenyl group, the resultant drug has anticonvulsant-sedative action (e.g., phenobarbital). Thiobarbiturates are more lipid soluble than barbiturates, and are ultra-short-acting.

Mechanism of Action

Barbiturates act on the channel modulatory site of $GABA_A$ receptor and potentiate the GABA mediated inhibitory effects by *increasing the duration of chloride channel opening* (Fig. 32.1). At higher concentrations, barbiturates directly increase chloride ion conductance, i.e., they exhibit a GABA mimetic action and not a GABA facilitatory action (as exhibited by BZDs).

Classification

Barbiturates are classified according to their duration of action, which depends on their lipid solubility and pharmacokinetic characteristics (refer earlier text).

Thiopental and ***methohexital*** are ***ultra-short-acting barbiturates*** with duration of action ranging from 15–20 min. These are used by I.V. fast bolus injection to induce general anaesthesia (Ch. 31).

Pentobarbital and ***amobarbital*** are ***Short-acting barbiturates*** and no more in use due to availability of safer alternatives (benzodiazepine).

Phenobarbital and ***mephobarbital*** (duration of action 12–24 hrs) are ***longer-acting barbiturates*** and no more used as sedative and hypnotics but are used as anticonvulsant drugs (Ch. 39).

Pharmacokinetics

i) The rate of absorption of barbiturates depends on their lipid solubility. The pH of solutions of their sodium salts is usually alkaline and therefore cannot be given by I.M. or S.C. routes for fear of necrosis and pain at the site of injection. But these can be given slow I.V., orally and at times rectally. These are weakly acidic drugs. Hence, they remain unionised in acidic pH and fully ionised at alkaline pH.
ii) These are widely distributed depending upon their lipid solubility and the regional blood flow. The action of the ultra-short-acting barbiturates such as thiopental is terminated primarily as a result of redistribution from brain to lean tissues, muscles and then fat and adipose tissue (Ch. 31 and Ch. 6).
iii) These are metabolised by both phase-I (liver microsomal oxidation) and phase-II (glucuronyl conjugation) processes. Their prolonged use leads to an induction of liver microsomal enzymes, which results in the development of metabolic tolerance.
iv) Although excreted through urine, these get readily reabsorbed from renal tubules. Alkalinisation increases their ionisation and therefore increases their renal excretion (Ch. 6).

Pharmacological Effects

i) The ultra-short- and short-acting barbiturates exhibit dose-dependent CNS depressant actions starting from sedation → hypnosis → general anaesthesia to coma and death. The long-acting ones possess primarily sedative-anticonvulsant actions. However, their anticonvulsant action has no relation with their sedative action, because even in sub-sedative doses these drugs retain anticonvulsant actions whereas amphetamine though antagonises the sedative action does not prevent their anticonvulsant actions. They disrupt the balance between REM: NON-REM sleep by decreasing the duration of REM sleep. Hence on withdrawal, there is a rebound increase in REM sleep duration resulting into bad dreams and nightmares with a feeling that "I didn't sleep well".
ii) Barbiturates may show hyperalgesic action, i.e., they may increase the reaction to painful stimuli. Their amnesic action is associated with "drug-automatism" and unintended toxicity (see comparison between BZDs and barbiturates).
iii) Sedative-hypnotic doses have no effect on CVS parameters. Higher doses decrease BP, HR and depresses myocardium.
iv) Sedative-hypnotic doses do not affect respiration. Higher doses depress respiration, cause shallow breathing and Cheyne-Stokes rhythm in breathing. Pulmonary oedema, laryngeal oedema and bronchial pneumonia may also occur.
v) Prolonged use increases the size and weight of smooth endoplasmic reticulum leading to enzyme induction (Ch. 6).

vi) Higher doses have relaxant effects on GIT, bladder and uterus and decrease the urine flow from kidneys (due to decrease in renal blood flow, increase in ADH release and relaxation of bladder).

Therapeutic Uses

i) ***As sedative-hypnotics***, they are seldom used these days, as these have been superseded by BZDs (see earlier text). Short-acting barbiturates such as pentobarbital or secobarbital were being used earlier.
ii) ***In anaesthesia***, ultra-short-acting barbiturates (thiopental) are generally used as intravenous fast inducing agents (Ch. 31).
iii) ***As anticonvulsants***, usually long-acting barbiturates, such as phenobarbital, are used (Ch. 39).
iv) ***To treat hyperbilirubinaemia of neonates***, as they increase the activity of glucuronyl transferase enzyme by enzymatic induction. Hence bilirubin gets conjugated faster and excreted through bile. These drugs also increase the bile flow.

Adverse Effects

i) Repeated use of barbiturates leads to the development of metabolic tolerance due to enzymatic induction. This leads to various drug interactions because of the accelerated metabolism of concomitantly administered drugs along with barbiturates.
ii) Barbiturates have considerable abuse liability and exhibit both psychic as well as physical dependence on withdrawal after prolonged use. Withdrawal symptoms include tremors, insomnia, headache, restlessness and delirium (Ch. 38).
iii) They cause hangover, impairment of judgement and "drug automatism" (see above).
iv) They cause respiratory depression, laryngeal oedema and hypersensitivity reactions (skin rash, swelling of lips and eyelids).

Drug Interactions

Barbiturates reduce the effectiveness of various concomitantly administered drugs due to induction of their metabolism. Such drugs include oral contraceptives, anticoagulants, tolbutamide and theophylline.

Contraindications

i) These are contraindicated in liver dysfunctions, kidney disease and severe pulmonary insufficiency, e.g., emphysema.
ii) Patients having family history of porphyria or in cases of acute intermittent porphyria, because barbiturates cause induction of ALA-synthetase enzyme in mitochondria. This leads to increased synthesis of porphyrins and hence porphyria and neurotoxicity.

Acute Toxicity and Treatment

Barbiturate poisoning is mostly suicidal, rarely accidental. It is characterised by respiratory failure, cardiovascular collapse (due to excessive fall in blood pressure and heart rate), coma and renal failure. Treatment includes gastric lavage, artificial respiration and forced alkaline diuresis with mannitol and sodium bicarbonate. In alkaline urine, barbiturates get ionised and hence their tubular reabsorption is prevented, i.e., their excretion is facilitated (Ch. 6). The use of CNS stimulants is controversial because of the chances of convulsions before and after the recovery.

MISCELLANEOUS GROUP OF SEDATIVE-HYPNOTICS

A number of miscellaneous drugs have been used as alternatives to the benzodiazepines, although there is no convincing evidence of their special value in these conditions. Even their molecular mechanism of anxiolytic and hypnotic effect is not yet clear.

Melatonin and Ramelteon

Melatonin is a hormone produced in the pineal gland from the amino acid tryptophan. Normally it is involved in the protective changes in skin colouration, but it is also secreted during hours of darkness and affects sleep pattern. Usually, the light stimulates the retina and transmits signal through suprachiasmatic nucleus (SCN; of hypothalamus) to pineal gland to inhibit release of melatonin. On the contrary, darkness promotes melatonin secretion from the pineal gland. It then stimulates MT_1 and MT_2 receptor subtypes present in SCN to induce and promote sleep and to maintain the circadian rhythm of the normal "sleep-awake" cycle. ***Melatonin*** is primarily used to alleviate symptoms of jet lag and other disorders resulting from delay of sleep (dose 3 mg, 2 hr before bed time). There are reports that the use of melatonin might enable benzodiazepine therapy for insomnia to be discontinued, without impairing the quality of sleep. However, there is little evidence of its efficacy from large studies, and hence its long-term safety remains to be established. Recently, it has been found useful in elderly hypnotic-dependent insomniacs. It undergoes extensive first-pass metabolism and is excreted mainly by kidney. It decreases serum luteinizing hormone and increases prolactin levels. It is contraindicated in persons taking corticosteroids like dexamethasone or prednisone.

Ramelteon is a selective agonist at the MT_1 and MT_2 receptor subtypes of melatonin. It has recently been approved for the treatment of insomnia in which there is difficulty in falling asleep. There is yet no evidence of its abuse potential, dependence or withdrawal but it can increase prolactin levels. *Adverse effects* include fatigue, dizziness and somnolence.

Triclofos

It is similar to the older agent chloral hydrate as both get converted to trichloroethanol. However, it is more palatable, causes less GIT upset and is better tolerated. Its onset of action is less than 30 min and duration of action is 8–12 hrs. It is used for short-term management of insomnia and in children for sedation during events of recurrent colic. Dose 1 g at bed time.

Hydroxyzine

Some antihistamines, because of their sedative-hypnotic actions are promoted for treating insomnia. But the use of antihistamines, solely for their sedative effect, in anxiety and insomnia is not considered appropriate nowadays. Hydroxyzine (Ch. 24) is an antihistamine having antiemetic, sedative, anticholinergic and local anaesthetic action. It is used for short-term management of anxiety, pre-anaesthetic sedation and pruritus. Its onset of action is 15–30 min and duration of action is 6 hrs. Usual dose is 50–100 mg TDS orally. Its active metabolite is cetirizine.

Promethazine

It is also a sedating antihistamine with antiemetic and anticholinergic properties. It is used for night time sedation (25 mg bed time). Its longer duration of action may cause hangover the next day. It is also popular for use in children as sedative-hypnotic (10 mg orally bed time) but such use is not justified. For adverse effects refer Ch. 24.

Lemborexant

Lemborexant is a *dual orexin receptor antagonist (DORA)*. Orexins are neuropeptides that regulate the sleep-wake cycle. Orexins promote wakefulness by binding G-protein-coupled receptors, OX1R and OX2R. It is indicated for insomnia having difficulties in sleep onset and/or sleep maintenance. *Adverse effects*: Sedation, fatigue, headache, nightmares, sleep paralysis, hallucination and allergic reactions.

Daridorexant

Daridorexant is US-FDA approved *dual orexin antagonist (DORA)*. It is used for insomnia characterized by difficulties with sleep onset and/or sleep maintenance. It is taken orally within 30 min before going to bed. *Adverse effects*: Nausea, vomiting, diarrhoea, headache, fatigue, somnolence and hallucination.

Suvorexant

It is a *dual orexin (OX) receptor antagonist*. It is an inhibitor of OX-1 and OX-2 receptors, approved by the FDA for the treatment of insomnia. Has no rebound insomnia. Less dependence. Effective in chronic insomnia. Suvorexant is FDA-approved for treatment of both sleep-onset and sleep-maintenance insomnia. *Adverse effects*: Weakness, vivid dreams and excessive sleepiness. Others are almorexant and filorexant.

Pitolisant

Pitolisant is a selective histamine (H_3) receptor antagonist or inverse agonist. It is used orally. It is metabolized in liver by CYP2D6 and CYP3A4. It is approved by US-FDA for the treatment of excessive daytime sleepiness (EDS) or cataplexy in adults with narcolepsy. *Adverse effects*: Headache, insomnia, hallucination, anxiety, irritability, cough, muscle pain and allergic reactions.

CHAPTER 33 Antipsychotic Drugs

COMPETENCY PH1.19

Earlier, the antipsychotic drugs were termed as "major tranquillisers". This term has now been discarded as it created confusion with another loose term "minor tranquillisers" (a misnomer for anxiolytic-sedatives). This term also has been abandoned. The present usage, in USA, tends to favour the term "antipsychotic drugs", while that in Europe favours the term "neuroleptic drugs". The antipsychotic drugs are broadly defined as the drugs which are effective in the treatment of schizophrenia and other agitated states. The term is broader and descriptive but is not befitting as all types of psychoses do not respond to this category of drugs. The term neuroleptics incorporates those drugs which produce both antipsychotic and extrapyramidal symptoms at the same dose level. However, after the emergence of drugs like clozapine and its congeners, it has been established that the antipsychotic action and the extrapyramidal effects are not linked to one another. Since these drugs had potent antipsychotic actions with negligible extrapyramidal side effects, these were labeled as "atypical neuroleptics". Again, to call them "anti-schizophrenics" would be too limiting as other types of psychoses (e.g., mania and others) may also respond to them. To avoid any discrepancy, therefore, both the terms *antipsychotics* as well as *neuroleptics* shall be used interchangeably in the following text.

The term schizophrenia (for details refer Ch. 30) is well known but hard to define. It is a type of functional psychoses in which severe personality changes and thought disorders occur with no evidence of organic cerebral damage. The manifestations of the disease include two types of symptoms—"positive" and "negative". *Positive symptoms are characterised by*: delusions (often paranoid in nature), illusions, auditory hallucinations (usually in the form of voices), thought disorders with irrational conclusions, garbled sentences and stereotyped or at times aggressive behaviour. *Negative symptoms include:* introvert behaviour, poor socialisation, emotional blunting, lack of motivation and congnitive deficits (e.g., lack of attention and loss of memory).

PATHOGENESIS OF SCHIZOPHRENIA

The pathogenesis of schizophrenia is unclear. This disorder is far more complex than originally supposed, but it involves a combination of genetic and abnormalities in amine neurotransmitter function (especially that of dopamine).

Genetic Predisposition

Although the pathogenesis is unknown, genetic studies have provided some evidence that inheritance can account for at least some proportion of schizophrenic disorders. In first degree relatives, the risk is about 10 percent. In monozygotic twins, the probability of the other being affected is 50%, compared to 10% for dizygotic twins. Despite evidence for genetic linkage, the results of molecular genetic studies in schizophrenia are inconclusive. Reports of linkage of schizophrenia to loci on chromosomes 1,5,6,8,11 and 22 have been identified, but not yet to any specific genes. However, recently at least one gene which encodes for *neuregulin-1*, has been reported to be associated with schizophrenia, in subsets of some European population only; but whether it applies to other populations also, is yet to be ascertained.

Dopamine (DA) Hypothesis

Circumstantial evidence presented below suggests that an excessive dopaminergic activity underlies this disorder: (1) Positron emission tomography (PET) has shown increased dopamine (DA) receptor density in both the treated as well as untreated schizophrenics compared to normal scans of non-schizophrenic persons; (2) Postmortem studies of the brains of schizophrenics also reveal the presence of increased DA receptor densities; (3) drugs that increase the central DA activity such as levo-dopa (a DA precursor) or amphetamine (a DA releaser) or apomorphine (a DA receptor agonist) either aggravate schizophrenia or precipitate the symptoms of schizophrenia in a normal person; (4) most antipsychotic drugs act by blocking postsynaptic DA receptors (D_2) in CNS especially in mesolimbic-frontal system and (5) levels of homovanillic acid (HVA), a metabolite of DA, in the CSF, plasma and urine increase during early phases of therapy but decline after prolonged use of classical antipsychotic drugs (for reasons, see under mechanism of action). Taken together, the presented evidence strongly favours the hypothesis that DA abnormality is the basis for most of the manifestations of schizophrenia in patients without structural brain changes.

However, if abnormal DA neurotransmitter functions were totally responsible for the pathogenesis of schizophrenia, antipsychotic drugs could have provided absolute cure for schizophrenia—rather than being partially effective for most or ineffective in some of the cases. The recent cloning and characterisation of different DA receptors (particularly D_3 and D_4) may permit more widespread acceptance of this hypothesis if some selective D_3 or D_4 antagonists were available for trials but these are not yet available. The typical antipsychotic drugs like haloperidol and pimozide bind to D_2 receptors more strongly than other DA receptors while atypical neuroleptics like clozapine and olanzapine have little effects on D_2 or D_1 receptors but bind more avidly to 5-HT_2, D_4, α_1 and H_1 receptors. The latter drugs not only possess greater efficacy but exhibit fewer side effects, especially extrapyramidal toxicity. These findings have redirected the research towards the role of other DA and 5-HT receptors in the causation and cure of schizophrenia.

5-HT Hypothesis

The role of 5-HT in schizophrenia is based on the findings that LSD, a central 5-HT_2 receptor agonist, produces hallucinations and sensory disturbances which are similar to those occuring in psychosis and that atypical neuroleptics like clozapine and olanzapine are potent 5-HT_{2A} receptor antagonists. 5HT_{2A} receptors modulate the release of DA in mesolimbic and striatum region. Hence both 5-HT and DA hypotheses for schizophrenia seem to be compatible. This hypothesis too, however, has fallen off because the main psychotic symptoms associated with LSD are *visual hallucinations* while in schizophrenia it is *auditory hallucinations* that predominate. Moreover, there are reports that 5-HT_{2A} receptor blockade, by atypical neuroleptics, merely reduces extrapyramidal toxicity associated with D_2 receptor antagonism.

Glutamate Hypothesis

Another neurotransmitter implicated in the pathophysiology of schizophrenia is glutamate. This hypothesis is based on the findings that glutamate-NMDA receptor antagonists (Ch. 30) such as phencyclidine and ketamine, when administered to normal subjects produce psychotic symptoms, e.g., hallucinations and thought disorders. Moreover, reduced glutamate receptor densities have consistently been reported in postmortem brains of schizophrenics. Glutamate exerts excitatory, while DA exerts inhibitory role over GABAergic striatal neurons which project to the thalamus and serve as a *sensory gate*. Increase in glutamate or decrease in DA activity facilitates GABAergic activity at this "gate" to prevent sensory inputs reaching the cortex. Contrarily, decreased glutamate or increased DA activity will reduce GABAergic activity and will disable the "gate" to allow uninhibited sensory inputs to reach the cortex. Recent reports indicate that underactivity of NMDA receptors is responsible for negative symptoms while over activity of DA receptor results in positive symptoms of schizophrenia (though both reduce GABAergic activity). Hence, novel neuroleptics that enhance NMDA receptor activity may become available in near future.

CLASSIFICATION OF NEUROLEPTIC DRUGS

I. **CLASSICAL or TYPICAL NEUROLEPTICS**

A. Phenothiazines

i) With aliphatic tertiary amine side chain
Chlorpromazine

ii) With piperidine moiety in side chain
Thioridazine

iii) With piperazine moiety in side chain
Trifluoperazine, Perphenazine, Fluphenazine

B. **Thioxanthenes**
Flupenthixol, Thiothixene, Zuclopenthixol

C. **Butyrophenones**
Haloperidol, Benperidol, Droperidol, Domperidone**

D. **Miscellaneous**
*Pimozide, Penfluridol, Molindone, Loxapine, Sulpiride, Amisulpride, Remoxipride, Metoclopramide**

II. **NOVEL or ATYPICAL NEUROLEPTICS**
Clozapine, Olanzapine, Quetiapine, Zotepine, Risperidone, Ziprasidone, Paliperidone, Aripiprazole, Sertindole, Asenapine, Lurasidone
(*These drugs are not used as antipsychotics. They have other uses [see following text]).

MECHANISM OF ACTION

All antipsychotic drugs act as antagonist at D_2 and/ or D_3/D_4 dopamine receptors, but the antipsychotic potency of *classical or typical neuroleptics* generally runs parallel to their blocking action on D_2 receptors. However, the blockade of D_2 receptors in other dopaminergic pathways in brain can not only lead to different neurological and endocrinal side effects but may provide other therapeutic utilities also (see below). *Atypical neuroleptics*, on the other hand, block other monoamine receptors as well, especially 5-HT_{2A} receptors. The distinction between typical and atypical neuroleptics is not clearly defined but rests on their multiple receptor blocking profile, minimal risk of extrapyramidal side effects, their efficacy in refractory cases and against negative symptoms of schizophrenia.

Summarily, there are five important dopaminergic projections or pathways in brain:

1. *Mesolimbic-mesocortical-mesofrontal pathway,* which projects from substantia nigra to limbic system and *controls behaviour*. This is overactive in schizophrenia.
2. *Nigrostriatal pathway,* which projects from substantia nigra to caudate nucleus and putamen. *This controls voluntary movements via extrapyramidal system.*
3. *Tubero-infundibular pathway,* which connects arcuate nuclei and periventricular neurons to hypothalamus and posterior pituitary and *controls prolactin release and other endocrinal consequences.*

   The other two dopaminergic pathways are not clearly defined. These include:
4. *Medullary-periventricular pathway,* which projects from motor nucleus of the vagus and *may be involved in eating behaviour.*
5. *The incerto-hypothalamic pathway*, which connects medial zona incerta to hypothalamus and amygdala. It seems *to control copulatory behaviour in some animal species.*

Typical (Classical) Neuroleptics

The antipsychotic action of typical neuroleptics is now believed to be produced by their competitive blockade of postsynaptic D_2 receptors in mesolimbic system. They also block presynaptic D_2 receptors, but blockade of post-synaptic D_2 receptors is much greater than that of presynaptic D_2 receptors. However, initial period of pre- as well as postsynaptic receptor blockade causes increased synthesis and release of dopamine (DA). This increased turnover of DA results in elevated levels of DA metabolites like HVA and DOPAC in blood and urine. With prolonged use of classical neuroleptics, there is a feedback inhibition of DA release, due to increased concentration of DA in synaptic cleft, which results in the decline of DA turnover and release. Consequently, the HVA and DOPAC levels then return to normal or a bit lower than normal and continue as such following the treatment.

The classical neuroleptics also have a variety of other therapeutically useful and untoward effects which can be traced to the blockade of DA receptors. Thus the competitive blockade of D_2 (also D_1) receptors in nigrostriatal pathway explains the unwanted extrapyramidal effects produced by these drugs. The endocrinal side effects that follow the treatment with these neuroleptics are caused by the blockade of D_2 receptors in the turberoinfundibular pathway that controls prolactin release and other hypothalamic and pituitary functions. The blockade of D_2 receptors in CTZ, empowers them with antiemetic effects. Lastly, many of their autonomic side effects are attributable to their α-adrenergic blocking and anticholinergic properties.

Proper classification of *molindone, loxapine, sulpiride* and *amisulpride* appears to be difficult because these are primarily D_2 antagonists (D_2:5-HT_{2A} ratio is high). Of course, their extrapyramidal side effects are low, yet the incidence is higher than that of atypical neuroleptics. They also increase serum prolactin levels and are not as free of the risk of tardive dyskinesia as are atypical neuroleptics.

Though controversy exists, the differences in the relative receptor binding affinities of various classical neuroleptics can be broadly outlined as follows :

Phenothiazines (*Chlorpromazine*):

$D_2 = \alpha_1 > 5\text{-}HT_2 = D_1 = M_1$

Phenothiazines (*Thioridazine*):

$\alpha_1 > D_2 = 5\text{-}HT_2 = M_1 > D_1$

Thioxanthenes (*Flupenthixol*):

$D_2 = 5\text{-}HT_2 > \alpha_1 = D_1$

Butyrophenones (*Haloperidol*):

$D_2 > \alpha_1 > 5\text{-}HT_2 > D_1$

Miscellaneous (*Sulpiride**): $D_2 > D_3 > D_4$

Miscellaneous (*Pimozide**): $D_2 > 5\text{-}HT_2 > D_4$

Miscellaneous (*Molindone*): $D_2 > 5\text{-}HT_{2A}$

*(*other receptor-blocking effects have no significance)*

Atypical Neuroleptics

The distinction between classical and atypical neuroleptics is not well defined but depends on (a) their unique receptor affinity profile, (b) their more effectiveness against the negative than the positive symptoms of schizophrenia, (c) their effectiveness in patients refractory to typical neuroleptics and (d) their lesser liability for inducing extrapyramidal side effects.

These drugs have a high affinity for 5-HT_{2A} and D_4 receptors which they block competitively. Besides these, they are also antagonist at α_1, M_1, H_1 and D_2 receptors. However, no single receptor action can best predict the antipsychotic efficacy of atypical neuroleptics. Nevertheless, unlike classical neuroleptics whose antipsychotic action primarily depends on their D_2 receptor blockade, the antipsychotic effects of atypical neuroleptics are attributed to a combination of 5-HT_{2A}, D_4 and D_2 receptor blockade. The absence of extrapyramidal side effects appears to correlate with their lower affinity for D_1 and D_2 receptors. Admittedly, the relationship between their receptor specificity and therapeutic use as well as side effects are not yet clearly understood. Had it been clear we might not be using the term "atypical" which reveals our desperation to cover the confusion.

The relative receptor binding affinities of some atypical neuroleptics have been summarised as under:

Clozapine : $5\text{-}HT_{2A} = D_4 > \alpha_1 = D_1 = D_2 = H_1 = M_1$

Olanzapine : $5\text{-}HT_{2A} > D_4 > \alpha_1 = D_1 = D_2 = H_1 = M_1$

Risperidone : $5\text{-}HT_{2A} > D_4 = D_2 = \alpha_1 = H_1 = M_1$

*Quetiapine** : $\alpha_1 > 5\text{-}HT_{2A} = D_2 = M_1$

Aripiprazole : D_2 and $5\text{-}HT_{1A}$ (PA) > $5HT_{2A}$ (ANTA) > $\alpha_1 = H_1$ (ANTA)

Ziprasidone and *Paliperidone*:

$5\text{-}HT_{2A} > D_2 = \alpha_1 = H_1$

Sertindole : $5\text{-}HT_{2A} > D_2 = \alpha_1$

Zotepine : $D_1 = D_2 > 5\text{-}HT_{2A} > \alpha_1 = H_1 = M_1$

Asenapine : $5\text{-}HT_{2A} > D_2 = D_3 = D_4 > \alpha_2 = \alpha_1$

*Lurasidone** : $5\text{-}HT_{2A}$, $5\text{-}HT_7 > D_2$, $5\text{-}HT_{1A}$(PA), No M_1 & H_1 antagonism

*(*lower-potency atypical neuroleptic)*

Aripiprazole is reported to have a novel mechanism of action. It does not block central dopaminergic receptors, but rather is a partial agonist at D_2 and 5-HT_{1A} while antagonist at 5-HT_{2A} receptors. It is vaguely referred to as DA:5-HT stabiliser in CNS. It is not yet clear whether it stabilises the "high affinity form" or the "low affinity form" of DA receptor. The risk of EPS such as acute dystonic reactions and tardive dyskinesia are very low and in some trials equal to placebo.

Paliperidone is an active metabolite of risperidone and shares its pharmacological characteristics. *Sertindole* has a long plasma half-life. Both *sertindole* and *zotepine* can cause cardiac arrhythmias and weight gain. *Asenapine* is an atypical neuroleptic but to be given sublingually (5–10 mg) BD (drawback).

Lurasidone (40–80 mg OD) is FDA approved drug for the treatment of acute decompensation in patients with chronic schizophrenia.

All antipsychotic drugs, in general, exhibit a latent period of 2–3 weeks to attain therapeutic benefits, though their receptor blocking and sedative effects are immediate. This happens because soon after their administration there is transient increase in the activity of dopaminergic neurons (increased DA turnover and/or increase in the number of D_2 receptors in limbic system), which declines after 2–3 weeks of D_2 inhibition.

Majority of neuroleptics are given orally, but their bioavailability increases 10 folds by giving I.M. injection. High molecular weight esters of some depot phenothiazines (e.g., fluphenazine enanthate or decanoate), of thioxanthenes (e.g., flupenthixol enanthate or decanoate) and of butyrophenones (e.g., haloperidol decanoate), dissolved in oil are available as I.M. depot injection. These preparations are longer acting as the plasma/tissue esterases slowly hydrolyse these esters into the free drug.

THERAPEUTIC USES

I. Psychiatric Indications

Neuroleptics are not curative; however, they significantly reduce the symptoms of psychoses and help in managing the patient in socially acceptable limits. These are used preferentially in the following disease sequence.

Schizophrenia

Neuroleptics are presently the mainstay of treatment for schizophrenia. However, some schizophrenics do not respond to drug therapy and virtually none show a complete response. These exceedingly chronic patients are also more prone to develop tardive dyskinesia as a long-term complication of drug therapy.

CHOICE OF THE DRUG: The best guide for selecting a drug for any individual patient should depend on the advantages and disadvantages associated with the neuroleptic drug to be used (see Table 33.1). The American Psychiatric Association (ASA) and the National Institute of Clinical Excellence guidelines (2002) suggest that if the patient is experiencing his or her first psychotic episode of schizophrenia, it is better to initiate therapy with an atypical agent (like olanzapine or risperidone or aripiprazole) because of their better safety profile. However, if the patient has been successfully treated with any typical neuroleptic earlier, which he or she tolerated well, then changeover to an atypical agent is inappropriate. In this regard it may be noted that **(1)** the differences between the groups are greater than the differences within the group and **(2)** the atypical neuroleptics, though carry a reduced risk of adverse effects, are not significantly better than classical neuroleptics in terms of efficacy.

USUAL RANGE OF THERAPEUTIC ORAL DOSES: ***Chlorpromazine*** 25–100 mg TDS (max up to 1 g per day); ***Thioridazine*** 50–100 mg TDS (max up to 800 mg per day); ***Fluphenazine*** 1–3 mg TDS (max up to 20 mg per day); ***Trifluoperazine*** 2–5 mg BD (max up to 40 mg per day); ***Flupenthixol*** 3–9 mg TDS (max up to 18 mg per day); ***Zuclopenthixol*** 20–50 mg daily (or 200 mg I.M. depot inj every 3rd day); ***Haloperidol*** 0.5–5 mg TDS (max up to 60 mg daily); ***Penfluridol*** 20–60 mg once a week (max up to 250 mg once weekly); ***Pimozide*** 2–4 mg once daily (max up to 12 mg per day); ***Loxapine*** 10–25 mg BD (max upto 75 mg per day); ***Sulpiride*** 400–800 mg BD; ***Amisulpride*** 200–400 mg BD (max up to 1 g daily); ***Levosulpride*** 200–300 mg once daily; ***Aripiprazole,*** 10–15 mg once daily (max 30 mg once daily); ***Clozapine*** initially 12.5 mg once or twice daily, slowly increased in increments of 25 mg daily up to a max dose of 300 mg per day; ***Olanzapine*** 5–10 mg once daily (max 20 mg once daily); ***Risperidone*** 1 mg BD, slowly increased in increments of 1 mg per day to a max of 3 mg BD; ***Paliperidone*** 6 mg per day, increased in steps up to 12 mg /day; ***Ziprasidone*** 20 mg BD, increased in steps up to 80 mg BD; ***Quetiapine*** 25 mg BD, increased in steps up to 300 mg BD; Lurasidone 40–80 once daily.

Drug Induced Psychoses

Delusions associated with LSD or amphetamine induced psychoses and delirium ensuing infectious psychoses are combated successfully with neuroleptics.

Schizo-Affective Disorders

The "schizo" component of these disorders may respond to antipsychotics, but the "affective" component, if it is depression, may require concomitant use of an antidepressant drug. If the PATHOGENESIS "affective part" is mania, the use of lithium is not advantageous to begin with, as a monotherapy, because of its slow onset of action. In such cases, concomitant use of neuroleptic (along with lithium) provides better results.

II. Neuro-Psychiatric Indications

Tourette's Syndrome

Tourette's syndrome marked by tics, grunts and vocalisations that are frequently obscene can be preferentially managed by *haloperidol*. *Pimozide* can also be used but carries some risk for prolonging QT interval.

Huntington's Disease

Some progressive choreoathetosis and dementia associated with this disease can be controlled by using *haloperidol* or *chlorpromazine* (Ch.40).

III. Non-Psychiatric Indications

As Antiemetics

Almost all neuroleptics, *except thioridazine, molindone* and *atypical agents*, have antiemetic effect of varying degree. This action is due to D_2 receptor blockade in CTZ as well as in GIT. Some phenothiazine neuroleptics such as *prochlorperazine* are used more as antiemetic than as antipsychotic drugs. Similarly some drugs like *domperidone* (butyrophenone group) and *metoclopramide* (benzamide group-miscellaneous group) have no antipsychotic action as these have very low affinity for D_2 receptors in mesolimbic system. These are rather peripheral dopamine receptor blockers with prokinetic effects and accelerate gastric emptying. They also block D_2 receptors in CTZ and hence used mainly as antiemetic drugs except for motion sickness (Ch. 28). The main side effect of metoclopramide is precipitation of EPS as it also blocks D_2 receptors in nigrostriatal pathway. In motion sickness, a phenothiazine with two C-atom side chain, e.g., *promethazine,* is used as an antiemetic—not because of its D_2 receptor blocking action in CTZ but because of its potent antihistaminic (antiemetic) and anticholinergic (antimotion sickness) effects. Obviously, promethazine carries no risk for EPS, though chemically it is a phenothiazine.

Preanaesthetic Medication

Mainly, *promethazine* is used as preoperative sedative as it has antihistaminic, anticholinergic and antiemetic effects also. A fixed dose combination of a mild neuroleptic *droperidol* (butyrophenone group) plus an opioid analgesic *fentanyl* is sometimes used to produce a state of "neurolept-analgesia".

Droperidol is a short-acting neuroleptic with antiemetic, sedative and anticonvulsant effects (Ch. 31).

Intractable Hiccups

Parenteral *chlorpromazine* or *haloperidol* can control intractable hiccups by some unknown mechanism.

ADVERSE EFFECTS

The atypical neuroleptics have a better safety profile. The adverse effects of classical neuroleptics are mere extensions of their known pharmacological actions. However, some individual drugs have their characteristic allergic or idiosyncratic reactions (see below).

I. CNS Side Effects

Behavioural Effects

These drugs depress the sensory inputs to reticular activating system and hence are liable to cause sedation and psychomotor impairment in high doses. Sedation is more common with phenothiazines, thioxanthenes, clozapine, olanzapine and quetiapine but is less with butyrophenones, pimozide, other atypical agents and suprisingly with fluphenazine decanoate I.M. depot injection. Toxic confusional states may occur with higher doses of neuroleptics that have prominent anticholinergic effects (e.g., phenothiazines, clozapine, olanzapine).

Tolerance and Dependence

Tolerance develops to the sedative and autonomic side effects of neuroleptics but not to their antipsychotic action. Withdrawal symptoms, from abrupt discontinuation, have not been a major problem with most antipsychotics. Sometimes these are manifested as "emergent dyskinesias" but these are neither alarming nor life threatening and hence not the withdrawal reactions in true sense. Physical dependence is almost absent. No drug seeking behaviour is present.

Table 33.1 Selection Criteria for Antipsychotic Drugs

Group/Drug	Advantages*	Disadvantages*
Butyrophenone		
Haloperidol	Fewer anticholinergic side effects; no jaundice; depot injection available; high potency; no weight gain	Severe EPS and tardive dyskinesia
Miscellaneous		
Pimozide	Longer acting; high potency; fewer anticholinergic side effects; good for maintenance	Moderate risk for EPS; prolongation of QT interval; hypokalaemia
Sulpiride	Lesser EPS than haloperidol Lesser sedation, lesser autonomic side effects	Gynaecomastia (↑ prolactin), poor absorption. *Amisulpride* is similar to sulpiride but is long acting, better absorbed and more safe.
Atypical Neuroleptics		
Clozapine	Good for positive and negative symptoms & for resistant cases; high potency; least EPS	Agranulocytosis; weight gain; hypersalivation, risk of diabetes mellitus low seizure threshold
Olanzapine	As above but no agranulocytosis	Weight gain, risk of hyperlipidaemia and new onset diabetes mellitus
Risperidone	High efficacy; no EPS in low doses; same as olanzapine	EPS in high doses; weight gain; gynaecomastia; postural hypotension, cardiac arrhythmia
Quetiapine	Same as for risperidone but less potent	Postural hypotension; dry mouth; weight gain (?); cataract formation (?); priapism(?);shorter half-life-BD dose
Ziprasidone	As for olanzapine; no weight gain; depot injection available	QTc prolongation; diarrhoea or constipation (?), less risk of diabetes m.
Aripiprazole	No EPS; no weight gain; no endo crinal side effect; no ECG changes; longer acting; high efficacy	No data available; unusual D_2 partial agonist action may account for lesser side effects
Zotepine	No EPS, least sedation	Weight gain, cardiac arrhythmias-high dose
Sertindole	Least EPS, longer acting	Weight gain, ventricular arrhythmias, nasal congestion
Asenapine	Least EPS, less weight gain	Sublingual BD dose (5–10 mg), sedation, oral hypoesthesia, postural hypotension, NMS
Lurasidone	Least EPS, less weight gain, less risk of tardive dyskinesia	Less risk of diabetes m.,hyperlipidaemia and QTc prolongation
Phenothiazines		
Chlorpromazine	Inexpensive	Serious autonomic and endocrinal side effects, low potency
Thioridazine	Low incidence of EPS, no jaundice	Cardiotoxicity/cardiac arrhythmia, low potency, no IM depot injection
Fluphenazine	High potency, depot injection available/no jaundice	High incidence of EPS and tardive dyskinesia
Thioxanthenes		
Flupenthixol	Moderate incidence of EPS and tardive dyskinesia; high potency; depot injection available	Not suitable for long-term use; restlessness; gynaecomastia

*(EPS—Extrapyramidal side effects; NMS—Neurolept Malignant Syndrome. * For details see text)*

II. Neurological Side Effects

Six types of neurological side effects are characteristic of classical antipsychotic drugs. Four of these (dystonias, akathisia, parkinsonism and a rare neurolept-malignant syndrome) usually appear early during treatment while the other two (tardive dyskinesia and a rare peri-oral tremors) appear later following prolonged treatment for more than a year. Neurological side effects are more prevalent with classical neuroleptics but are of rare occurrence with atypical agents.

Dystonias

It is characterised by spasm of muscles of tongue, face, neck and back. Exact mechanism is not known but treatment can be made by using antihistaminic-anticholinergic drug such as *diphenhydramine* or *promethazine*.

Akathisia

It is characterised by uncontrollable motor restlessness without any involvement of anxiety. Mechanism is not clear. The use of a non-selective β-blocker such as *propranolol* or drugs like *diphenhydramine* can provide relief.

Parkinsonism

It results due to disturbance in the DA-ACh balance in the basal ganglia because of D_2 receptor blockade. As a result cholinergic influence dominates over dopaminergic, leading to parkinsonian symptoms. Treatment involves restoration of the cholinergic-dopaminergic balance by using centrally acting antimuscarinic drugs like *trihexyphenidyl (benzhexol), procyclidine, benztropine* or *orphenadrine*. However, a DA precursor such as l-dopa is not preferred as it may cure parkinsonism but will precipitate schizophrenia (for details refer Ch. 40).

Neurolept–Malignant Syndrome (NMS)

This life-threatening rare disorder has been observed in patients who are extremely sensitive to the extrapyramidal side effects of neuroleptics. NMS can occur with more potent classical neuroleptics with high EPS liability such as *fluphenazine* and *haloperidol*. With atypical drugs (except for asenapine) it is uncommon. The characteristic features include hyperpyrexia, muscle rigidity, autonomic instability with fluctuating BP, increased myoglobin and increased creatine kinase (reflecting muscle damage). Though exact mechanism of NMS is not clear, the pathogenesis involves central as well as peripheral mechanisms. The central mechanism is the usual DA-receptor blockade by the neuroleptic drug in extrapyramidal and hypothalamic systems, while the peripheral mechanism involves possible effect of neuroleptic on neuromuscular system. The management of NMS includes discontinuation of neuroleptic, supportive therapy for fever and muscle rigidity by giving peripherally acting muscle relaxant, e.g., *dantrolene* or centrally acting muscle relaxant, e.g., *diazepam,* and a DA-agonist like *bromocriptine*.

Perioral Tremors (Rabbit Syndrome)

It is a rare disorder which may occur after long-term use of a potent classical neuroleptic and is characterised by rapid chewing movements made by the patients akin to those made by rabbits. These respond with anticholinergic-antiparkinsonism drugs (See above).

Tardive Dyskinesia

It is a late occurring syndrome characterised by involuntary oro-buccal-lingual dyskinesias (as if the patients were chewing chewing-gum). It has been proposed that to counteract a long-term DA-receptor blockade by a neuroleptic, the striatal nerve cells synthesise newer DA receptors which are supersensitive to even smaller amount of DA (still getting through the neuroleptic block). When dopaminergic activity is increased due to super-sensitivity of DA-receptors in striatum, there is a decrease in the cholinergic activity with an ultimate decrease of GABA release. This decreased release of inhibitory neurotransmitter ends up in an increase in involuntary motor activity. With this background of pathogenesis three pharmacological approaches for its management can be opted: (a) *To decrease the dopaminergic overactivity* – This can be done by raising the dose of the neuroleptic itself. But it may not help as the neuroleptic, by itself, was responsible to produce this supersensitivity state; (b) *To increase cholinergic activity* – To start with, all the antiparkinson drugs/anticholinergic drugs should be withdrawn at once. Thereafter, *choline* or *lecithin* can be used but the doses required are very high and the success rate is poor; (c) *To increase the GABA activity along with "neurolept-holidays"* – It is now logically accepted that for the management of tardive dyskinesia the first step should be to withdraw the neuroleptic as well as antiparkinson-anticholinergic drug, if being used along with neuroleptic. These two steps called "neurolept-holidays" are sufficient enough to bring the improvement within a fortnight. If they do not, one may add *diazepam* (40 mg/day) to enhance GABAergic activity. The substitution of an atypical neuroleptic such as *clozapine* or *olanzapine* could be another option. These drugs do not produce tardive dyskinesia.

III. Autonomic (ANS) Side Effects

α-Adrenergic Blockade

Postural hypotension (peripheral α-receptor blockade) and tachycardia (vagal inhibition) frequently result from the use of the "high dose-low potency" phenothiazines (e.g., chlorpromazine, thioridazine). However, tolerance to these side effects develops later. *Fluphenazine, haloperidol, pimozide, molindone, loxapine, olanzapine* and *ziprasidone* carry lower risk for producing postural hypotension. The α-adrenergic blockade also causes a loss of libido and delayed ejaculation.

Antimuscarinic Effects

Most patients are able to tolerate the antimuscarinic side effects of antipsychotic drugs. These include dryness of mouth, constipation, urinary retention, disturbed accommodation but with no pupillary dilatation (antimuscarinic effects on iris are antagonised by α-adrenergic effects). *Clozapine*, although having potent antimuscarinic blocking effects, produces paradoxical hypersalivation. Anticholinergic side effects are less common with *fluphenazine, thiothixene, haloperidol, pimozide, molindone, risperidone, quetiapine* and *ziprasidone*.

IV. Endocrinal Side Effects

Blockade of DA-receptors in mammotrophs, by neuroleptics, results in hyperprolactinamia which is manifested as galactorrhoea in females and gynaecomastia in males. These drugs also inhibit the release of FSH and LH leading to amenorrhoea and inhibition of ovulation. Blockade of D_2 receptors in medullary-periventricular pathway results in altered eating habits and an increase in appetite which culminate into weight gain. All these endocrinal side effects in women simulate a picture of "pseudo-pregnancy". Hyperprolactinaemia in males is also associated with decreased libido, impotence and infertility. Hyperprolactinaemia is common with phenothiazines, haloperidol, sulpiride and thioxanthene (zuclopenthixol) but is less frequent or absent in atypical neuroleptics. Weight gain is common with phenothiazines, haloperidol, thioxanthenes, clozapine and olanzapine (due to blockade of 5-HT receptors). It is less common with *sulpiride, risperidone, quetiapine, ziprasidone* and absent with *aripiprazole*.

V. Miscellaneous Side Effects

Classical antipsychotics, particularly phenothiazine group, may also be associated with:

- *Jaundice*: It is thought to be hypersensitivity reaction and is of obstructive type with elevated plasma bilirubin but without fever.
- *Photosensitivity*: UV rays in sunlight readily oxidise phenothiazine neuroleptics, forming a pigment that accumulates in melanin-containing tissues of skin.
- *Corneal opacities* and *retinal pigmentation*: Especially with chlorpromazine and thioridazine on long-term use but these are reversible and disappear after discontinuation of the drug.
- *Epileptogenic effects*: Chlorpromazine and thioridazine are especially likely to lower seizure threshold.
- *Poikilothermic effects*: Phenothiazines, in particular, impair the ability of hypothalamic thermoregulatory centre, such that hypothermia (at room temperature) or hyperthermia (at elevated room temperature) may result.

Characteristic Toxicities of Individual Drugs

- ***Clozapine***: It causes *agranulocytosis* in approximately 1–2% of the cases being treated. It usually occurs between sixth and eighteenth weeks of therapy. It is, however, reversible upon discontinuance of the drug. Patients receiving clozapine should have weekly blood counts for the first six

Table 33.2 Drug Interactions with Antipsychotic Drugs

Drug	Effects
Antacids	Decreased absorption of antipsychotic drugs
Anticholinergics	Increased anticholinergic effects
Alcohol	More sedation
Antithyroid drugs	Increased risk of agranulocytosis (with clozapine)
Barbiturates	Decreased antipsychotic effects but more sedation
Carbamazepine and phenytoin	Decreased antipsychotic effects and lowering of seizure threshold (classical neuroleptics)
Chloroquine	May precipitate EPS with phenothiazines
Lithium	Enhancement of neurotoxicity and precipitation of NMS (with haloperidol)
Levodopa	Decreased efficacy of neuroleptics
Oral contraceptives	May potentiate hyperprolactinaemia (with phenothiazines and haloperidol)

Key: EPS—Extrapyramidal side effects; NMS—Neurolept-malignant syndrome

months of the treatment and every month thereafter. It also causes *paradoxical hyper-salivation.*

- ***Thioridazine*** even in therapeutic doses may be associated with minor reversible abnormalities of T-waves. Overdoses of thioridazine are associated with major *ventricular arrhythmias, cardiac conduction block* and *sudden death.*
- ***Pimozide and Ziprasidone***: Both drugs *prolong QT interval* but ziprasidone carries a greater risk. Pimozide also causes hypokalaemia.
- ***Quetiapine***: *Cataract formation* has been reported in patients after long-term therapy with quetiapine. Hence patients should have an eye examination to detect cataract formation before initiating therapy with quetiapine and every six months thereafter. There have been rare reports of *priapism, peripheral oedema* and *hyperventilation* recently, with its use.

DRUG INTERACTIONS

Antipsychotic drug interactions with other drugs and the clinical consequences are summarised in Table 33.2.

Recently Approved Anti-Psychotics

Lumateperone

Lumateperone is approved by US-FDA for the treatment of schizophrenia in adults. It can be used for the treatment of depressive episodes associated with bipolar disorders. Mechanism of action: Antagonist at central serotonin 5-HT_{2A} and dopamine (D_2) receptors. *Adverse effects*: Nausea, vomiting, headache, fatigue, sedation or somnolence, dizziness, dry mouth, increased hepatic transaminases and allergic reactions.

Samidorphan and Olanzapine Combination

Samidorphan, a novel opioid system modulator, acts primarily as a μ-opioid receptor antagonist. It is used with olanzapine. Rationale of combination: Olanzapine has metabolic adverse effects like hyperglycaemia, hyperlipidaemia and weight gain. Addition of samidorphan helps mitigate its metabolic adverse effects. It is used for schizophrenia and bipolar disorder. *Adverse effects*: Nausea, constipation, dizziness, vomiting, somnolence or sedation and fatigue.

Cariprazine

Cariprazine is a partial agonist at central dopamine (D2) and serotonin (5-HT_{1A}) receptors. It is antagonist to 5-HT_2 and histamine H1 receptors. It is used for schizophrenia in adults. It is also indicated for mania and bipolar disorder. *Adverse effects*: Extrapyramidal symptoms like tremors, akathisia, insomnia and weight gain.

CHAPTER 34 Antidepressants & Antimanic Drugs

COMPETENCY PH1.19

Depression is a disorder of mood (not of thought process as in schizophrenia) and hence classified as affective disorder (Ch. 30). There are two major types of depression, namely: ***Unipolar depression*** (about 80% of the depressed cases) in which the mood swings in one direction only (either depression with a feeling of worthlessness or depression with groundless irritability). In such unidirectional swings, the latter type of mood presentation is rare, but may appear during partial recovery from endogenous depression. The other is ***bipolar depression*** (or ***manic depressive psychoses***, MDP) characterised by cyclic manifestations of depression followed by mania (20% of cases, see later). About 60% of the unipolar depressed cases show symptomatology of ***reactive depression*** characterised by disproportionate feeling of sadness, grief and anxiety as a consequence of bereavement of loved one, unemployment, physical illness or social problems. It is self-limiting and usually responds to antianxiety drugs like *alprazolam*. About 25% of the unipolar depressed patients are endogenously depressed with suicidal thoughts. This ***endogenous depression*** may occur at any age and is not self-limiting, unless treated with an appropriate antidepressant drug or by electroconvulsive therapy (ECT). It results either due to genetic causes or due to deranged neurotransmission of NE or 5-HT or both (and possibly of DA) in certain sites of brain.

The monoamine hypothesis of *endogenous depression* suggests that such depression is caused by a functional deficit of NE and/or 5-HT (or of DA) at certain sites in brain; while *mania* results from a functional excess of these neurotransmitters. This theory is based on the ability of the NE and 5-HT uptake inhibiting or monoamine oxidase-A inhibiting drugs to facilitate NE/5-HT neurotransmission and to act as effective antidepressant drugs. Further than that, the drugs like reserpine, which inhibit the storage of 5-HT and NE, also cause depression while tryptophan which increases 5-HT synthesis elevates mood. Therefore, it was reasoned that depression must be associated with a decreased NE/5-HT neurotransmission. Other evidence in support of this hypothesis are: **(1)** CSF levels of 5-hydroxyindole acetic acid (5-HIAA), a metabolite of 5-HT, and urinary levels of 3-methoxy-4-hydroxyphenyl glycol (MHPG), a metabolite of NE, are found to be low in depression, and **(2)** There is lower tryptophan availability in patients of depression.

However, biochemical studies on depressed patients do not entirely support this hypothesis in its simple form. The most obvious inconsistencies in the monoamine hypothesis are: **(1)** Although antidepressant drugs produce a blockade of NE/5-HT reuptake within hours, their clinical benefits typically appear after several weeks of treatment, implicating neuroadaptive changes in receptor regulation and second messenger system as possible mechanism of their action, **(2)** Neither amphetamine nor cocaine are used as antidepressant drugs despite their ability to facilitate NE transmission, and **(3)** Some clinically effective antidepressant drugs have "atypical" actions and seem to lack any NE/5-HT uptake inhibiting action.

Recognising these discrepancies, some authors have suggested other mechanisms for causation of depression. For example:

1. The most consistent adaptive changes seen with different types of antidepressant drugs is the down-regulation of β_1, β_2 and α_2 adrenoceptors as well as of $5\text{-}HT_2$ receptors. Incidentally, ECT also brings about a down-regulation of β_1 and β_2 receptors, which suggests that probably a down-regulation of β-receptors constitutes the primary mode of action of various antidepressant drugs. However, this again necessitates some revision, as β-blockers do not possess antidepressant

action, rather they produce depression in patients after prolonged use.

2. Neuroendocrine abnormalities that reflect the symptoms of endogenous depression include: **(a)** Increase in cortisol level and corticotropin-release hormone (CRH) secretion, **(b)** An increase in adrenal size, **(c)** A failure of exogenously administered dexamethasone to bring a fall in cortisol levels (dexamethasone suppression test), **(d)** A blunted response of thyroid stimulating hormone (TSH) level to induce thyroid-releasing hormone (TRH), **(e)** A reduction in growth hormone concentration, and **(f)** An increase in prolactin levels. *Antidepressant treatment leads to the normalisation of these pituitary-adrenal abnormalities.*
3. The evidence of genetic transmission, however, is not as strong as in bipolar disorder. Monozygotic twins have a higher concordance rate (48%) than the dizygotic twins (20%) with little evidence for any effect of a shared family environment. Studies indicate that, 10–20% of endogenously depressed patients have a first degree relative with depression.

   All these theories are not only complex but imprecise too (except for the consistently observed down-regulation of β_1, β_2, α_2 and 5-HT_2 receptors after antidepressant therapy). The relationship of such findings to the therapeutic effects observed with antidepressant drugs is not consistent either. Hence, the monoamine hypothesis, despite its shortcomings, serves as the best basis for understanding the actions of the majority of antidepressant drugs.
4. Recently, substantial evidence reveal that in depression there is a significant drop in ***brain-derived neurotrophic factor*** (BDNF; a nerve growth factor which regulates neural plasticity and neurogenesis) along with neuronal loss and volume of prefrontal cortex and hippocampus. Conversely, administration of antidepressant increases BDNF levels with an increase in prefrontal cortex and hippocampus volume. The time required for the synthesis of BDNF usually takes 2 weeks which concides with the therapeutic lag observed during the treatment with antidepressants.

Whether there exists any difference in the symptomatology of depression induced by decreased NE transmission or by a deranged serotonin transmission has been a point of debate since long. Yet, the noradrenergic type of depression is associated with psychomotor retardation, decreased libido and weight loss; while 5-HT type of depression is characterised by agitation, sleep disturbances, increased anxiety and weight gain. Other symptoms such as loss of interest, withdrawal from social and pleasurable activities, feeling of guilt and worthlessness, inability to concentrate and unidentifiable somatic complaints are common to both types of depression.

CLASSIFICATION OF ANTIDEPRESSANT DRUGS

- **Drugs Which Block Both NE and 5-HT Reuptake** (Tricyclic Antidepressants; TCAs): *Imipramine, Clomipramine, Amitriptyline, Doxepin*
- **Selective Serotonin-Norepinephrine Reuptake Inhibitors (SNRIs)**: *Duloxetine, Venlafaxine, Milnacipran.* These are just like TCAs but are devoid of the antihistaminic, α-adrenergic blocking and anticholinergic side effects of TCAs.
- **Drugs Which Mainly Block NE Reuptake**: *Desipramine, Nortriptyline, Protriptyline, Maprotiline, Amoxapine, Reboxetine.* The first three are tricyclic antidepressants, while others are recent antidepressants in this group.
- **Selective Serotonin Reuptake Inhibitors (SSRIs)** *Sertraline, Fluoxetine, Fluvoxamine, Paroxetine, Vortioxetine, Citalopram, Escitalopram*
- **Atypical Antidepressants** *Trazodone, Nefazodone, Bupropion, Mirtazapine, Mianserin*
- **Antidepressants of Natural Origin** *St. John's wort* (Active Principle: *Hyperforin*)
- **MAO Inhibitors**
  a) Non-selective (MAO-A and MAO-B inhibitors) *Tranylcypromine*
  b) Selective MAO-A Inhibitors *Moclobemide*
- **NMDA Antagonist**: Esketamine
- **GABA Receptor Modulator**: Brexanolone

MECHANISM OF ACTION

The older term "tricylic antidepressants" is now a misfit as even bicyclic or tetracyclic antidepressants are available for use. To call tricyclics as first generation and tetracyclics as second generation antidepressants is more confusing particularly after the advent of SSRIs and atypical antidepressants which would compel us to extend generations further. Hence a workable classification based on their mechanism of action has been followed in this text.

1. Drugs That Block NE and 5-HT Reuptake

Examples: ***Doxepin, Imipramine, Clomipramine,*** and ***Amitriptyline***.

Chemically these are tricyclic anti-depressants. These drugs block the reuptake of NE and of 5-HT into their respective neuron by inhibiting their respective transporters. Such an action presumably permits more availability and a longer stay of NE and 5-HT at their respective receptor site (Fig. 34.1). They, however, differ in their selectivity of uptake and potency. In addition they bind to α-adrenergic, histaminergic (H_1) and cholinergic (muscarinic) receptors which account for many of their side effects.

2.Selective Serotonin-Norpinephrine Reuptake Inhibitors (SNRIs)

Examples: ***Duloxetine, Venlafaxine*** and ***Milnacipran***.

SNRIs also block NE and 5-HT reuptake like TCAs discussed above; but these differ from TCAs and are more selective in the sense that they lack the α_1-adrenergic, H_1 and cholinergic receptor blocking properties of TCA (hence fewer side effects).

3. Drugs Which Predominantly Block NE Reuptake

Examples: ***Desipramine, Nortriptyline*** and ***Protriptyline*** (these are tricyclic antidepressants); ***Amoxapine, Reboxetine*** and ***Maprotiline*** (these are newer antidepressants).

These drugs predominantly inhibit the NE reuptake, which results in an increased concentration of NE in the synaptic clefts in the CNS (Fig. 34.1). *Amoxapine* blocks postsynaptic D_2 receptors also and hence possesses some antipsychotic action.

4. Selective Serotonin Reuptake Inhibitors (SSRIs)

Examples: ***Sertraline, Fluoxetine, Fluvoxamine, Paroxetine, Vortioxetine, Citalopram*** and ***Escitalopram***

Currently these are the most commonly prescribed antidepressant drugs and are used for some other psychiatric conditions as well. SSRIs selectively increase the levels of serotonin in the synaptic cleft by blocking its uptake by serotoninergic neurons (Fig. 34.1). Escitalopram is 100 times more potent than citalopram.

▪ Features Common to NE and 5-HT Reuptake Inhibitors

All antidepressant drugs, described above, exhibit a biological lag of 2–3 weeks to produce desirable clinical effects, even though their monoamine uptake effects are produced immediately. This suggests that some secondary adaptive changes are important along with their pharmacokinetic characteristics such as their longer plasma half-life. The most consistent adaptive change seen with their long-term use is the down-regulation of postsynaptic β_1, β_2 and 5-HT_2 receptors with simultaneous desensitisation of presynaptic α_2 and 5-HT_1 autoreceptors. The delayed effect of these antidepressant drugs suggests that besides longer t½ and extensive protein binding (see below), the time interval needed to down-regulate and desensitise these receptors is the major contributory factor to the observed biological lag (see earlier text).

5. Atypical Antidepressants

The mode of action of atypical antidepressants is poorly understood and varies from drug to drug.

Trazodone inhibits uptake of 5-HT, blocks 5-HT_{2A} receptor and desensitises presynaptic 5-HT receptor. Blockade of 5-HT_{2A} receptor leads to antianxiety and antidepressant effects (5-HT_{2A} agonists like LSD are CNS stimulants). Desensitisation of presynaptic 5-HT autoreceptor enhances 5-HT release. It also significantly blocks α_1 adrenergic receptors, which is responsible for its sedative side effects, postural hypotension and priapism. ***Nefazodone*** is a congener of trazodone

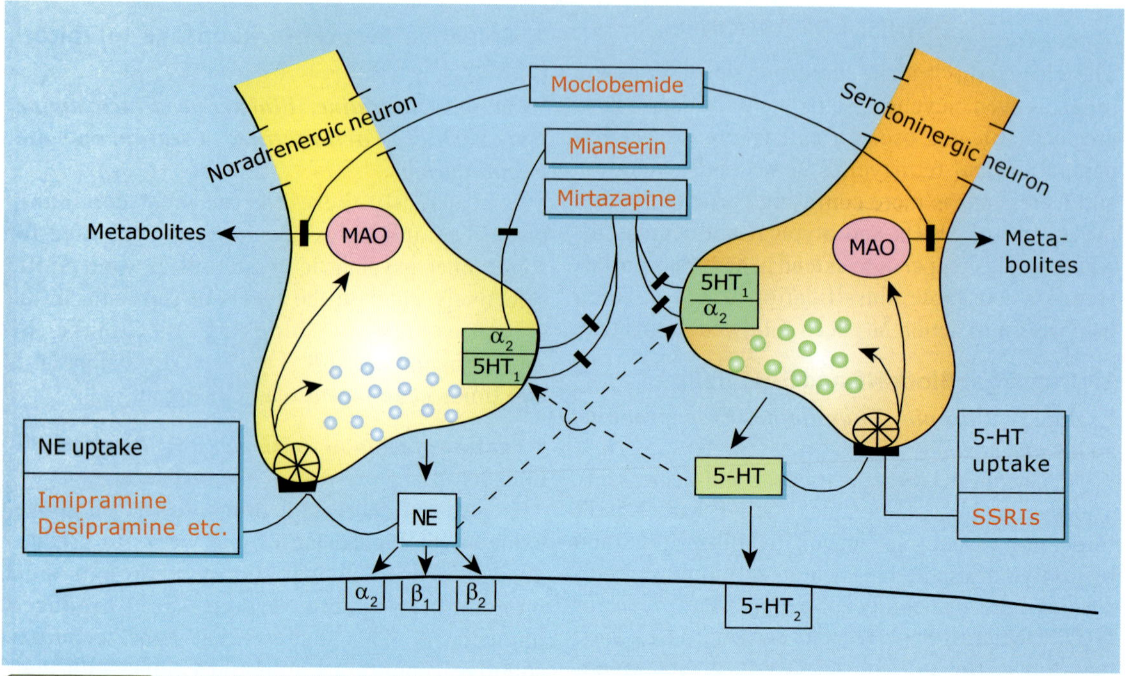

Fig 34.1 Potential Sites of Action of Some Antidepressant Drugs

with lesser side effects and better tolerability. ***Mianserin*** blocks presynaptic α_2 receptors and thus increases the release of NE in brain, which may be responsible for its antidepressant effects. It does not affect NE/5-HT reuptake in CNS. ***Mirtazapine*** acts by blocking presynaptic α_2 autoreceptors and 5-HT_1 heteroreceptors on noradrenergic neurons, as well as 5-HT_1 autoreceptors and α_2 heteroreceptors on 5-HT neurons to enhance both NE and 5-HT release. Unlike SSRIs, mirtazapine has a stronger affinity for 5-HT_1 receptors with no activity on 5-HT_2 and 5-HT_3 receptors. This selectivity helps to diminish the incidence of common side effects associated with SSRIs such as sexual dysfunction, including delayed ejaculation (commonly seen with paroxetine), agitation and insomnia. However, mirtazapine does block H_1 and 5-HT_{2c} receptors which leads to sedation and increased appetite, respectively (Fig. 34.1). ***Bupropion*** is structurally different from all other antidepressant drugs discussed above. Its exact mode of action is not clearly understood. It is a weak inhibitor of neuronal reuptake of 5-HT, NE and DA. Unlike other antidepressants it causes very little sedation and anticholinergic side effects. It rarely produces cardiovascular side effects or sexual dysfunction.

6. Natural Antidepressants

A natural antidepressant, St John's wort (*Hypericum perforatum*), is an OTC drug in many European countries. It contains many active substances, of which *hypericin* and *hyperforin,* are monoamine reuptake inhibitors, mild MAO inhibitors and stimulants at GABA receptors. Its antidepressant (and antianxiety) activity has been confirmed in many trials. It has fewer side effects and is better tolerated than many conventional antidepressants. However, it is a potent enzyme inducer which results in the lowering of plasma concentration and the therapeutic efficacy of warfarin, oral contraceptives, antipsychotics and HIV reverse transcriptase inhibitors such as zidovudine.

7. MAO Inhibitors

The MAO inhibitors increase brain amine levels by inhibiting their metabolism in the nerve endings, resulting in an increase in the vesicular stores of NE and 5-HT. More NE/5-HT is now available for release to enhance the actions of these neurotransmitters. Two isoforms of MAO have been identified (see Ch. 10). MAO-A preferentially metabolises 5-HT and NE and is selectively inhibited by ***clorgyline*** and ***moclobemide***. MAO-B preferentially deaminates phenylethylamine and is selectively inhibited by ***selegiline (deprenyl)***. DA is degraded equally by both MAO-A and MAO-B. ***Tranylcypromine*** is a long acting, nonselective, irreversible inhibitor of MAO allowing NE, 5-HT and DA to accumulate in their respective neurons in brain and periphery. ***Selegiline*** selectively inhibits MAO-B at lower doses (5–10 mg/day) and is not effective in treating depression. In higher doses, it becomes nonselective inhibitor of MAO to exhibit antidepressant and excitant effects but the adverse effects limit its use. However, transdermal patch formulation of ***selegiline*** has been approved for treating depression. ***Moclobemide*** is a selective and reversible inhibitor of MAO-A and is reported to possess moderate antidepressant properties.

As with other antidepressant drugs, MAO inhibitors also show a biological lag of 2–3 weeks to elicit clinical benefits (see above). Incidentally, with the use of MAO inhibitors the tissue and neuronal monoamine levels remain elevated for another 2–3 weeks even after the drug has been largely eliminated and withdrawn. The restoration of normal MAO activity and brain amine metabolism depends on the synthesis of new MAO. Impliedly, a break of about 2–3 weeks is again necessary to switch over to another antidepressant, if desired. This restoration is slow with *phenelzine* (2–3 weeks), moderate with *tranylcypromine* (7–10 days) and faster with *moclobemide* (about 2 days). Nevertheless, for optimal therapeutic benefits a daily dosing schedule is required with MAO inhibitors.

PHARMACOKINETICS

The oral absorption of most of the antidepressant drugs is good, yet the bioavailability is uncertain because of their first-pass metabolism. Bioavailability of citalopram and protriptyline is however > 90%. The plasma half-life of majority of antidepressants is long, hence plasma concentrations build up slowly but once steady state levels are reached, once daily dosing (at bed time) is enough in the maintenance phase. Plasma half-life is less for amoxapine (8 hrs), nefazodone (2–4 hrs), trazodone (4–8 hrs) and venlafaxine (4–9 hrs). The t½ is longer for some of their active metabolites except for fluvoxamine, paroxetine and protriptyline as no active metabolites of these drugs have been identified so far. Among MAO inhibitors, moclobemide is readily absorbed but its first-pass metabolism reduces its bioavailability (t½ 1–3 hrs).

THERAPEUTIC USES

These drugs are primarily used to treat depression but are recommended for some non-psychiatric indications also.

I. Psychiatric Uses

a) Endogenous Depression

There are three types of treatment for depression: psychotherapy, pharmacotherapy and electroconvulsive therapy (ECT). Pharmacotherapy with antidepressants is effective in 60–70% of the depressed patients. It has three treatment phases. The goal of treatment in acute phase is to resolve symptoms; in continuation phase is to prevent relapse; and in maintenance phase is to prevent recurrences in high-risk patients. ECT is used in severe depression where biological lag period of antidepressant drugs can prove to be risky or when the patient has not responded to pharmacotherapy.

Drug Selection: All antidepressant drugs are equally effective, though they have different mechanisms of action and side effects. If the patient has been successfully treated with a particular antidepressant in the past, it is always safer to reinstitute the therapy with the same drug. If the patient has his first episode, it is better to select an antidepressant with side effect profile that suits the patient's requirements. In general, SSRIs, *mirtazapine, nefazodone, duloxetin* and *venlafaxine* are highlighted as the best, fulfilling the needs for tolerability and safety in overdose. Some trials have suggested that *venlafaxine* in slightly higher doses (200 mg/day) has greater efficacy and safety than other antidepressants.

Changing and Stopping Antidepressants: If a drug has to be changed, it should be "cross tapered", i.e., the doses of the new drug should be gradually increased and that of substituted drug must be decreased. On remission, the antidepressants should be continued for another 9 months, at the same dose which provided remission, to prevent relapse. In high-risk patients a 3-year or more continuation of antidepressant drug offers protection from recurrences. When stopping the antidepressant, the dose should be tapered over a period of at least 6 weeks to avoid withdrawal symptoms (anxiety, agitation, nausea). Short-acting drugs, which do not form active metabolites are most likely to cause withdrawal problems after prolonged use.

b) Panic Disorders

SSRIs (e.g., *paroxetine, fluvoxamine* and *fluoxetine*) alone or with *alprazolam* can be used to control panic disorders. However, SSRIs require several weeks to produce full therapeutic effects.

c) Obsessive-Compulsive Disorders (OCDs)

SSRIs, preferably *fluvoxamine*, are quite effective for treating OCDs. *Clomipramine* can also be used as it enhances 5-HT functions. *Citalopram* (10–40 mg/day) is also recommended for use.

d) Attention Deficit Hyperkinetic Disorders (ADHD)

Imipramine and *desipramine* are generally preferred for this purpose. *Atomoxetine,* which is a selective inhibitor of NE uptake, has been introduced as a preferred drug for treating ADHD. It is better tolerated and has lesser side effects. However, this drug should not be used concurrently with SSRIs.

e) School Phobia, Post-Traumatic Stress Disorder and Impulse Control Disorders

For school phobia and social phobia, SSRIs such as *paroxetine* or a reversible MAO-A inhibitor *moclobemide* are preferred. For post-traumatic stress disorder *paroxetine* with *alprazolam* is used. SSRIs are also helpful in preventing autistic thinking (gratification of unfulfilled desire) and impulse control disorders like gambling and kleptomania (uncontrolable desire to steal things).

II. Non-Psychiatric Uses

a) Enuresis and Bed-Wetting in Children

Antidepressants with anticholinergic side effects such as *amitriptyline, desipramine* and *imipramine* are preferred. However in majority of cases, the effect lasts only as long as drug treatment is continued. Unfortunately, the older patients are more sensitive to the anticholinergic side effect of these tricyclic antidepressants.

b) Chronic Pain

Tricyclic antidepressant drugs such as *imipramine, amitriptyline* or *nortriptyline* are usually very effective in treating neuropathic chronic pain by enhancing the activity in noradrenergic pain inhibitory pathway in the spinal cord.

c) Migraine

A tricyclic antidepressant such as *amitriptyline* starting in low doses (10 mg at night) and increasing to 50 mg, in 2–3 weeks, is effective in treating migraine headache.

d) Miscellaneous Uses

- Application of 5% topical *doxepin* cream relieves itching in atopic dermatitis and lichen simplex.
- SSRIs such as *fluvoxamine* and *fluoxetine* are quite effective in treating *bulimia nervosa*, although the doses required are higher, which limits their use for such indication.
- *Bupropion* is used to treat nicotine dependence and smoking cessation. Treatment is initiated with 150 mg once daily for 3 days and then 150 mg twice daily for 6–10 weeks.
- *Citalopram* (or *escitalopram*) is also used to treat ethanol abuse symptoms as it suppresses desire to drink alcohol.

ADVERSE EFFECTS

I. Drugs That Block NE or NE+5-HT Uptake (Tricyclic and newer antidepressants)

The tricyclic antidepressants have lost their place as first line drugs for treating depression because of their bothersome side effects at therapeutic doses and serious toxicity at higher doses. Main adverse effects are as under:

1. CNS Side Effects

- Sedation (primarily due to histamine H_1 receptor blockade). *Imipramine, desipramine, protriptyline* and *lofepramine* cause less sedation. *Amitriptyline, doxepin* and *trimipramine* are more sedating. Other CNS sedative drugs have additive effects.
- Lowering of seizure threshold and precipitation of seizures in patients of epilepsy. *Maprotiline, bupropion* and *clomipramine* are potentially toxic in this regard and are contraindicated in patients with seizure disorder.
- *Amoxapine*, used to treat psychotic depression, also has DA receptor antagonists properties and can induce extrapyramidal effects, gynaeco-mastia (in males) and galactorrhoea (in females).

2. Autonomic Side Effects

a) Anticholinergic Side Effects

Dryness of mouth (predisposing to tooth decay), blurred vision, urinary retention and constipation. These may raise intraocular pressure, i.e., may precipitate glaucoma. Anticholinergic effects are more prominent with *amitriptyline, trimipramine, clomipramine, doxepin* and also with *imipramine.* These are lesser with *desipramine, lofepramine* and *amoxapine.*

b) Peripheral α_1-Receptor Blockade

Manifested as postural hypotension (due to blockade of α_1 adrenoceptors) and tachycardia (also contributed by anticholinergic effects). Postural hypotension is more common with *amitriptyline, imipramine* and also with *trimipramine* but is lesser with *desipramine, nortriptyline, maprotiline* and with *amoxapine.*

3. Endocrinal Side Effects

Characterised by weight gain and sexual disturbances (though less than SSRIs). Weight gain is more commonly seen with *amitriptyline, doxepin, imipramine* and *trimipramine*; moderate gain occurs with *amoxapine* and *maprotiline* and least with *protriptyline, desipramine* and *nortriptyline.*

4. Cardiovascular Effects

Tricyclic antidepressants create cardiac conduction defects that may manifest as T wave flattening or prolongation of QT interval leading to cardiac arrhythmias. This risk is greater with *amitriptyline, imipramine, trimipramine, protriptyline, clomipramine, amoxapine* and *maprotiline.*

II. Selective Serotonin-Norepinephrine Reuptake Inhibitors (SNRIs)

These drugs (see classification) selectively inhibit 5-HT and NE uptake only, but do not block other receptors (e.g., H_1, α_1 and muscarinic receptors) and therefore have a more favourable adverse effect profile. However, they have serotoninergic side effects (e.g., the *discontinuation syndrome* associated with SSRIs). Noradrenergic effects (e.g., insomnia, tachycardia, and anxiety) have also been observed. *Venlafaxine* causes cardiotoxicity in high doses.

III. Selective Serotonin Reuptake Inhibitors (SSRIs)

This class of antidepressants does not exhibit anticholinergic, α_1-adrenoceptor blocking, antihistaminergic and cardiac side effects. These are relatively safe in overdose and presently have a most favourable profile for their use as antidepressants. Yet, important side effects are as follows:

1. On initiation of therapy with SSRI, some patients complain of agitation, anxiety and insomnia. Hence dose should be titrated upward more slowly and may be given in the morning.
2. As many as one-third of the patients may complain of sexual dysfunction including decreased libido, delayed ejaculation and anorgasmia (due to increased serotoninergic tone at the level of spinal cord and above).
3. SSRIs tend to be weight neutral with the exception of *paroxetine* which rather causes weight gain. SSRIs in moderately higher doses may provide weight loss.
4. Nausea and loose stools are also common side effects (due to increased serotoninergic tone in the gut).
5. Sudden withdrawal of SSRIs with shorter t½ (*paroxetine* and *sertraline*) leads to "discontinu-

ation syndrome" (dizzines, paresthesias and headache).

IV. MAO Inhibitors

Main adverse effects include **(a)** postural hypotension, especially seen in elderly, **(b)** inappropriate increase in appetite, causing weight gain, **(c)** dizziness and **(d)** sexual dysfunction. Less common are headache, insomnia, fatigue, dry mouth, constipation, blurred vision, peripheral oedema and restlessness. Compared to *tranylcypromine*, *moclobemide* has a safer clinical profile and is well tolerated.

V. Atypical Antidepressants

Trazodone use is associated with *nausea*, *sedation*, *postural hypotension* and *priapism* leading to impotence. Its α_1 adrenergic blocking property is responsible for the latter two effects. ***Nefazodone*** is more safe and better tolerated. Postural hypotension is less, while priapism is absent. However it can cause hepatotoxicity on prolonged use.

Bupropion, like SSRIs, also causes agitation and insomnia (hence it should not be given at bed time). There is an increased seizure risk associated with its use.

Mirtazapine, being H_1 blocker, causes sedation. It causes weight gain (but lesser than tricyclic antidepressants). ***Mianserin*** is also a H_1 blocker and hence causes sedation. Anticholinergic and cardiac effects are less prominent but seizure risk is associated with high doses. Hepatotoxicity and blood dyscrasias have recently been reported which limit its use.

VI. Antidepressants from Natural Source

St. John's wort has already been discussed earlier.

VII. NMDA Antagonist

Esketamine

Esketamine is an S-enantiomer of racemic ketamine. It is a nonselective, non-competitive antagonist of NMDA receptors. It is approved for the treatment of resistant depression in adults. Intranasal spray is available. Administered twice weekly initially followed by once a week. Adverse effects: Sedation, dissociation, vertigo, lethargy, nausea and vomiting.

VIII. GABA Receptor Modulator

Brexanolone

Brexanolone is a neuroactive steroid that occurs naturally (referred to as natural allopregnanolone) in the body. It is an approved drug for postpartum depression (PPD), a serious complication after child birth. It is proposed that in PPD, endogenous brexanolone levels can quickly drop or fluctuate. Synthetic brexanolone binds with $GABA_A$ receptors, can subsequently facilitate a return of positive allosteric modulator $GABA_A$ modulation and expression gradually return to normal. Adverse effects: Headache, sedation, dizziness, vertigo and dry mouth.

DRUG INTERACTIONS

Tricyclic Antidepressants (TCAs) and Related Drugs

1. TCAs potentiate the effects of directly acting sympathomimetics (causing rise in BP and arrhythmias) but inhibit the effects of indirectly acting sympathomimetics (block their uptake).
2. Anticholinergic drugs aggravate the toxicity of TCAs.
3. T_3 and T_4 potentiate CNS stimulant effects of TCAs.
4. Phenytoin, chlorpromazine and aspirin displace TCAs from protein binding sites. The subsequent rise in their plasma concentration leads to toxicity.
5. MAOIs with TCAs show synergistic actions leading to serious toxicities (hypertension, arrhythmias and seizures).

MAO Inhibitors

1. ***Cheese Reaction***: Various food articles like cheese, beer, red wine, banana, yoghurt and pickled meat contain large quantities of an indirectly acting sympathomimetic called tyramine, which is normally degraded by MAO widely distributed in GIT, liver and in neuronal cytoplasm. But in the presence of a nonselective irreversible inhibitor of MAO it escapes degradation, reaches into systemic circulation, uptaken by the adrenergic neuron and since neuronal MAO is also inhibited, tyramine again escapes metabolic deamination. Ultimately it enters the storage vesicles and displaces large quantities of NE leading to hyperten-

sive crisis. Dietary restrictions are therefore necessary while using tranylcypromine but not with moclobemide as it is a reversible inhibitor of MAO-A and its actions are short-lived.

2. MAOIs along with TCAs or MAOIs along with directly acting or indirectly acting sympathomimetics have synergistic effects leading to hypertension, arrhythmias and seizures (see above).

Selective Serotonin Reuptake Inhibitors (SSRIs)

1. SSRIs inhibit drug metabolising enzymes CYP2D6 and CYP3A4 and hence can elevate plasma levels and toxicity of TCAs, haloperidol, clozapine, warfarin, dextromethorphan, terfenadine, astemizole and cisapride (by retarding their metabolism). Elevated plasma levels of terfenadine, astemizole and cisapride can precipitate arrhythmias.
2. SSRIs with MAOIs (or with triptans, Ch. 24) result in elevated levels of 5-HT in the synaptic cleft leading to "Serotonin Syndrome" characterised by hyperthermia, muscle rigidity, tremors, rapid changes in mental status and cardiovascular collapse.

ANTIMANIC (MOOD STABILISING) DRUGS: LITHIUM CARBONATE

Mania is characterised by an excessive desire and too much of euphoria. It is a sort of pathological excitement with racing thoughts, pressured speech and a little need for sleep. Majority of patients of mania also experience cyclic episodes of mania followed by severe depression with periods of normal mood in between. Thus their mood swings between pathological excitement and profound depression. This is called bipolar manic depressive psychosis. About 15% of the depressed cases suffer from manic-depressive psychosis (MDP). Although the exact pathogenesis of MDP is not known, a genetic predisposition is a strong likelihood. The inheritance rate for monozygotic twin pair approaches 80% and appears to be autosomal dominant transmission.

The exact bioamine disturbance has not been identified either; but a preponderance of NE/DA related activity does seem to exacerbate mania and the drugs that reduce DA or NE activity relieve mania. Balanced neurotransmitter levels help in stabilisation of mood. A manic episode is believed to result from elevated NE levels while depressive phase is associated with a decrease in NE levels.

Lithium is a small monovalent cation like Na^+ or K^+. All these ions appear together in the same group of periodic table. Evidence of Li^+ efficacy for treating MDP was a chance discovery. In 1940, lithium chloride was introduced as a Na^+-free table salt for use by hypertensive patients. Soon, two events occurred: There were reports of severe lithium toxicity and death, while a handful cases of MDP with hypertension showed a definite improvement in their MDP symptoms. It was withdrawn and reintroduced in 1949 but could not gain popularity (as a drug for bipolar depression), because it was being used without monitoring its plasma levels. It was in the period of 1960 to 1970 that the importance of maintaining its therapeutic range of plasma level was realised and an evidence of its therapeutic efficacy was finally established. Over the last two decades, the anticonvulsant drugs such as *carbamazepine* and *valproate* have emerged as alternatives to lithium. An atypical antipsychotic drug *olanzapine* is also being used for its potential mood stabilising actions.

MECHANISM OF ACTION

Normally, IP_3 and DAG serve as second messengers for α-adrenergic and muscarinic neurotransmission. Such an activity is markedly increased in mania. IP_3 and DAG are generated by a Gq protein coupled *phospholipase-C (PLC):inositol phosphate effector system*. The stimulation of PLC hydrolyses PIP_2, a phospholipid component of the membrane, to IP_3 and DAG (Fig. 34.2A). IP_3 being water soluble diffuses through the cytoplasm where it triggers the release of Ca^{2+} from the storage vesicles. DAG remains confined to the membrane and activates Ca^{2+}-sensitive protein kinase-C. These combined effects normally facilitate adrenergic and cholinergic transmission and their effects.

Separate mechanism operates to terminate this second messenger signaling system. IP_3 is inactivated to IP_2, IP_1 and then to inositol. The latter serves as a precursor for PIP, which in turn is a precursor for PIP_2. The latter is recycled to generate IP_3 and DAG if needed. Thus inositol is mainly regenerated from IP_3 and recycled. In mania the neuronal circuits become overactive and start producing more IP_3 and DAG , and in turn inositol, to provide a regular supply of PIP_2 (a precursor for IP_3 and DAG). ***Lithium*** selectively inhibits signal transduction in overactive neurons by blocking the conversion of IP_2 to IP_1 and of IP_1 to inositol. As a result the supply of free inositol to regenerate PIP_2, in the hyperactive neurons, is interrupted and ultimately the release of IP_3 and DAG is also reduced (Fig. 34.2A) which decreases neuronal response to NE (also to DA and 5-HT).

Lithium may also act by some other mechanisms:

1. Several studies suggest that lithium may uncouple receptors from their G-proteins. But this action seems to explain most common side effects observed with lithium (see below).
2. Besides reducing inositol levels in the brain, lithium might be affecting a specific isoform of protein kinase-C (PKC). Alterations of PKC-mediated signaling, alter the gene expression as well as the production of proteins implicated in long-term mood stabilization.

PHARMACOKINETICS

Lithium (given orally) is readily absorbed from the GIT. Distribution occurs throughout the extracellular fluid and body water with no evidence of either protein binding or metabolism. The elimination half-life is 24 hrs but the doses are given at 8 hourly interval. It is excreted primarily through kidney (96%) but through saliva and sweat (4%) as well. Na^+ loading enhances Li^+ clearance while Na^+ depletion promotes Li^+ retention. This important relationship explains the appearance of Li^+ toxicity (see below) associated with diuretics and diarrhoea. Since Li^+ has a low margin of safety and a narrow therapeutic window (0.5– 1.5 mEq/L), the frequent measurements of serum steady state concentration are essential. The therapeutic plasma levels should be between 0.8–1.4 mEq/L, while 0.5–1 mEq/L are optimum for maintenance. Toxicity appears when serum levels exceed 1.5 mEq/L.

THERAPEUTIC USES

Lithium is used as lithium carbonate or as citrate as these are less hygroscopic and less GIT irritant than lithium chloride. However, in stomach it gets converted to lithium chloride. Usual starting dose is 300–600 mg TDS. Such doses produce effective plasma levels of 0.8–1.4 mEq/L. However, the doses must be individualised and adjusted according to the serum levels and clinical response. A maintenance dose is 300 mg TDS, which produces effective serum concentration of 0.5–1.0 mEq/L.

1. Manic Depressive Bipolar Psychoses

Lithium is the first line therapy for the treatment or prevention of bipolar disorders. If an adequate dose is taken consistently, around 65–70% of patients achieve improved control of their illness. The existence of the "rebound effect" on discontinuation of lithium, dictates that a persistent long-term treatment is of great importance particularly if it coincides with a positive family history.

Because the therapeutic actions of lithium take 10–15 days to develop, it is generally used in combination with other drugs. Depending on the clinical presentation, antipsychotics or antidepressants may be added with lithium for treating bipolar depression. Atypical antipsychotic such as *olanzapine* may be used along with lithium during an acute manic episodes particularly if psychotic symptoms are present. Alternatively, *risperidone*, *quetiapine* or *ziprasidone* may be used. Benzodiazepines such as *lorazepam* or *clonazepam* are indicated as adjuvants for short-term management of agitation usually associated with mania. Antidepressants are to be used with caution with lithium although some patients with severe depression may require augmentation with an antidepressant. In such cases of bipolar depression, *bupropion* or *paroxetine* are recommended due to lesser risk for conversion to mania. After control of symptoms, lithium alone is then continued in the maintenance phase.

2. Other Uses

- Leukocyte counts are increased with lithium therapy. This property of lithium is utilised to

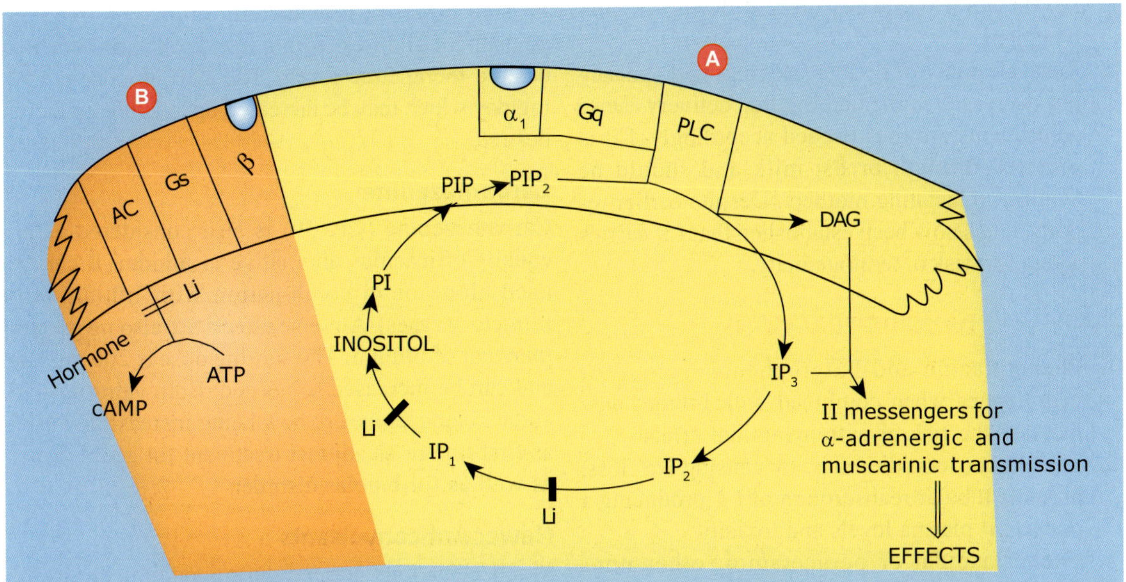

Key: DAG—Diacyl glycerol; IP_3—Inositol triphosphate; PLC—Phospholipase-C; PIP_2—Phosphatidyl inositol-diphosphate; PIP—Phosphatidyl inositol monophosphate; AC—Adenylyl cyclase; Gs and Gq—Coupling G proteins; α_1 and β—α_1-Adrenergic and β-adrenoceptors.

Fig 34.2 (A) Proposed Mechanism of Antimanic Action of Lithium (Li).
(B) Proposed Mechanism of Lithium-Induced Toxic Effects.

treat cancer chemotherapy–induced *leukopenia* and *agranulocytosis*.

- Lithium is occasionally used to treat cluster headache and as an adjuvant to tricyclic antidepressants in *recurrent unipolar depression.*

ADVERSE EFFECTS

Side effects are mild and manageable. Toxicity occurs only at higher plasma levels than desired.

1. Fine tremors (controlled by propranolol), confusion and slurred speech may be seen even at therapeutic concentrations.
2. *Subclinical hypothyroidism* has been reported on long-term use in about 4% of cases. Lithium inhibits TSH-activated adenylate cyclase, and decreases conversion of ATP to cyclic AMP (Fig. 34.2B), which in turn decreases T_3 and T_4 secretion. Administration of liothyroxine reverses these effects.
3. On long-term use some patients develop *nephrogenic diabetes insipidus*, characterised by polyuria and polydipsia. Lithium inhibits ADH stimulated adenylate cyclase and thus decreases conversion of ATP to cAMP (Fig. 34.2B). Collecting ducts, therefore become impermeable to water which is then retained inside the collecting ducts and excreted. Lithium-induced diabetes insipidus is resistant to ADH but responds to the potassium-sparing diuretic amiloride.
4. Lithium causes *diarrhoea* and aggravates diarrhoea of any origin. Diarrhoea causes Na^+ loss which promotes tubular reabsorption of Li^+. An increase in its plasma concentration, further aggravates the diarrhoea.
5. *Oedema* is a frequent adverse effect of Li^+ which is related to the effect of Li^+ on Na^+ retention. *Folliculitis* seems to be a frequent complaint.

Leukocytosis is always present during lithium treatment.

6. Renal clearance of Li^+ increases during pregnancy but decreases immediately after delivery. Dose adjustments are thus needed accordingly. Li^+ is secreted through breast milk and should be avoided in lactating mothers. Despite earlier reports, it has now been established that Li^+ carries a very low risk of teratogenicity.

DRUG INTERACTIONS

1. Phenothiazine and butyrophenone group of neuroleptics when combined with lithium may increase the risk of extrapyramidal effects.
2. Thiazide or loop diuretics, by causing Na^+ loss, promote tubular reabsorption of Li^+ producing a rise in Li^+ plasma levels and toxicity.
3. Except aspirin or paracetamol, other non-steroidal newer anti-inflammatory drugs reduce renal clearance of Li^+.

ALTERNATIVE DRUGS TO LITHIUM

Approximately 50% of patients of mania or bipolar disorder show incomplete or poor response to lithium. Other drugs can also be used as adjuvant or as an alternative to lithium.

Valproic Acid

Valproate (Ch. 39) has been found quite effective in some patients who have failed to respond to Li^+. It can be used alone or in combination with lithium. Its side effect profile favours rapid and frequent adjustment of doses, within few days, to provide the desired therapeutic levels. The starting dose is 750 mg/day which may be increased up to 2000 mg/day if desired.

Carbamazepine

Carbamazepine (Ch. 39) is also considered as an equally efficacious alternative to lithium. It can be used alone or in combination with lithium (for refractory cases). Adverse effects are also no greater than that of lithium. The starting dose is 200 mg BD and can be increased as needed. Both valproic acid and carbamazepine are now being increasingly used as first line or as adjunct treatment for acute mania as well as for bipolar disorder.

Newer Anticonvulsants

Mood elevations noticed during antiepiletic use of *lamotrigine, gabapentin* and *topiramate* (Ch.39) gave rise to the interest of their use as mood stabilizers. Of these, *lamotrigine* has emerged to be especially useful in depressed and rapidly cycling episodes of MDP, as it carries minimal risk of inducing mania.

Atypical Antipsychotics

Olanzapine is now increasingly being used as an adjuvant with lithium for treating acute mania and bipolar disorder as well. Alternatively, *risperidone* or *quetiapine* can also be used (Ch.30).

CHAPTER 35 CNS Stimulants & Psychotomimetic Drugs

COMPETENCY PH1.22

CNS stimulants and psychotomimetics are diverse group of drugs that have little clinical use (except for methylxanthines, see below). These drugs can be broadly classified into three categories:

- Respiratory stimulants and convulsants (analeptic drugs)
- Psychomotor stimulants
- Psychotomimetic drugs

RESPIRATORY STIMULANTS AND CONVULSANTS (ANALEPTIC DRUGS)

Drugs in this category appear to act mainly on brain stem and spinal cord to stimulate respiratory and vasomotor centres. In higher doses they produce convulsions.

Respiratory Stimulants

Examples: DOXAPRAM

The mode of action of these drugs is not properly understood. However, they act by exciting central neurons. At low doses these are more selective for the respiratory centre. These drugs increase the depth of breathing and also blood pressure due to stimulation of the respiratory and vasomotor centers in the medulla.

Doxapram is a short-acting drug with higher margin of safety. It increases tidal volume and the rate of respiration. It is sometimes used **(1)** to counteract post-anaesthetic respiratory depression, **(2)** as an aid to chronic obstructive pulmonary disease, i.e., in hypoxaemic ($\downarrow O_2$ in blood) – hypercapnic ($\uparrow CO_2$ in blood) respiratory failure where these are used along with O_2 inhalation, and **(3)** to abolish episodes of apnoea in premature infants not responding to theophylline. It is given by slow I.V. infusion (2–5 mg/min; max dose 4 mg/kg).

These are contraindicated in the cases of hypoxaemic normocapnic respiratory failure as in asthma; in respiratory failure due to neurological and muscular disease and in epilepsy. *Side effects* include restlessness, tachycardia and in higher doses convulsions and cardiac arrhythmias.

Convulsants

Examples: PICROTOXIN, STRYCHNINE, BICUCULLINE and PENTYLENE TETRAZOLE

These drugs, being convulsants, have no clinical use. However, they are occasionally used as research tools.

Strychnine, a plant alkaloid, is a convulsant poison and is predominantly a spinal cord stimulant. It acts by blocking the receptors for glycine which mediates inhibition of the spinal cord neurons and is intimately involved in the regulation of spinal cord and brainstem reflexes. Strychnine competitively antagonises this inhibition allowing excitatory impulses to be greatly exaggerated. The primary therapeutic consideration in treating the case of strychnine poisoning is to prevent the fatal convulsions by giving *diazepam* or *clonazepam* (slow I.V.). ***Picrotoxin***, another convulsant, blocks the Cl^- ion channel of $GABA_A$ receptor (Fig. 32.1). ***Bicuculline***, a plant alkaloid, also causes convulsions and has no clinical use. It is a $GABA_A$ receptor antagonist. It has no effect on $GABA_B$ receptor and hence can be used as an experimental tool for studying GABA-mediated transmission. ***Pentylene tetrazole*** (*PTZ, Leptazol, Metrazol*) is also a powerful CNS stimulant and a convulsant drug. It causes a direct depolarisation of central neurons. Its convulsant activity in experimental animals provides a useful model for testing anticonvulsant drugs, as it has been noted that the drugs which are effective in petit mal seizures are effective in preventing PTZ-induced clonic convulsions. Again, diazepam or clonazepam which facilitates GABAergic transmission is the drug of choice for picrotoxin, bicuculline and PTZ poisoning.

PSYCHOMOTOR STIMULANTS

Examples:

1. **AMPHETAMINE GROUP**—AMPHETAMINE, DEXAMPHETAMINE, METHAMPHETAMINE, METHYLENEDIOXY METHAMPHETAMINE (MDMA), METHYLPHENIDATE and FENFLURAMINE.
2. **NON-AMPHETAMINE GROUP**—MODAFINIL, ATOMOXETINE, SIBUTRAMINE and PEMOLINE.
3. **COCAINE**
4. **METHYLXANTHINES**—CAFFEINE, THEOPHYLLINE (and derivatives) and THEOBROMINE.

The drugs in this category have a marked influence on mental functions and behaviour to produce excitement, euphoria, increase in motor activity and a reduction in fatigue. Since some of the psychomotor agents from amphetamine group and cocaine produce hallucinations at high doses, many texts classify them under psychotomimetics but these are better considered as related to psychomotor stimulants.

Amphetamine and Non-Amphetamine Group

Mechanism of Action

These drugs enter the nerve ending by active transport and subsequently displace DA (also NE) from storage vesicles by altering their pH. They also have some property to inhibit DA metabolism by inhibiting MAO-B in the nerve ending. As a result the concentration of intraneuronal DA increases. This reverses the direction of the transport mechanism so that DA is now released into the synapse by "reverse transport" rather than by usual exocytosis. This further increases DA concentration in the synaptic cleft.

Pharmacological Effects

The main central effects of amphetamine-like drugs are: **(a)** Increased motor activity, **(b)** Euphoria and excitement, **(c)** Anorexia, and **(d)** Stereotyped and psychotic behaviour with prolonged administration.

In addition, their peripheral sympathomimetic actions include a rise in blood pressure and inhibition of gastrointestinal motility. The pharmacological actions of these drugs have been dealt in Chapter 12.

Amphetamines increase the wakefulness, capacity to work and euphoria. Hence, there is unawareness of fatigue that could be dangerous. With large doses, stereotyped behaviour occurs which consists of characteristic repeated actions. Subjects become confident, talkative and hyperactive. Sex drive is said to be enhanced by amphetamines. Fatigue, both physical and mental, is reduced but the improvement caused by reduction of fatigue can be offset by mistakes committed due to overconfidence. Amphetamine-like drugs (mainly *fenfluramine* and *dexfenfluramine*) cause marked anorexia. However, with continued use, this effect wears off in a few days and the food intake returns to normal. This effect occurs due to their enhancement of 5-HT release.

If amphetamine is taken repeatedly over the course of a few days, a state of amphetamine psychosis can develop which closely resembles schizophrenia; but it is associated with paranoid ideas and auditory and tactile hallucinations rather than visual (unlike LSD). Since higher doses lead to aggressiveness and violent behaviour, death may occur due to violence, accident, murder or even suicide.

Pharmacokinetics

All these agents are well absorbed after oral administration and freely penetrate BBB. A considerable portion of the untransformed (unmetabolised) drug is excreted through urine. Thus, it is possible to ion-trap this weakly basic drug by acidifying the urine, with ascorbic acid or ammonium chloride, thereby reducing its reabsorption from the renal tubules and enhancing its clearance.

Clinical Uses

The therapeutic uses of the amphetamine-like drugs are quite limited. However, some of these are as under:

1. ***Attention Deficit Hyperkinetic Disorder* (ADHD) *with Minimal Brain Dysfunction***: This is generally a childhood disease characterised by hyperactivity, inability to concentrate and impulsive behaviour. Interestingly, none of the mode of actions of amphetamines, discussed above, explains the therapeutic benefits of amphetamines for this indication. Yet, paradoxically ***dexamphetamine***, ***methylphenidate*** and ***atomoxetine*** are quite effective in calming down a good population of these hyperkinetic children. *Pemoline* is no longer used now because of hepatotoxicity.

Atomoxetine is a non-stimulant, non-addicting drug which is NE reuptake inhibitor (instead of DA). It is quite safe except that it is contra-indicated in patients of glaucoma.

2. ***Narcolepsy***: Amphetamines, particularly ***methylphenidate***, are still used for treating *narcolepsy*. This disorder is characterised by sleep attacks particularly during the day time, vivid nightmares that may persist even in the awakening state and sudden loss of muscle tone (cataplexy) which is usually reversible. ***Modafinil*** is a non-amphetamine derivative that has been used successfully in the treatment of narcolepsy. It is devoid of abuse liability (Ch. 12).
3. ***Appetite Suppression***: Earlier, amphetamines, particularly ***fenfluramine*** and ***dexfenfluramine***, were used to treat obesity. Although amphetamines have a significant *anorexic effect*, tolerance to this action develops within few weeks and the food intake returns to normal. In addition, insomnia, pulmonary hypertension and the abuse potentials have discouraged their use in weight control. Hence, their use for this indication is now discarded. A new drug ***sibutramine*** is, however, used for the management of obesity. It blocks the neuronal uptake of mainly NE and 5-HT (but also of DA) at the hypothalamic site that regulates food intake. It can be used in severely obese patients with other risk factors such as diabetes and dyslipidaemia. *Adverse effects* include dry mouth, headache, insomnia, constipation, increase in heart rate and blood pressure (contraindicated in any kind of cardiovascular disease and hence it has been withdrawn from US and Indian market). It should not be taken along with SSRIs (e.g., fluoxetine), serotonin agonists (e.g., sumatriptan) and lithium.

Adverse Effects

1. ***Tolerance*** develops rapidly to the peripheral sympathomimetic and anorexic effects of amphetamines but more slowly to the increased motor activity, euphoria and stereotyped behaviour. The mechanism for the development of tolerance is not clear, yet amphetamine-induced anorexia may play an important role where the patient neglects food but prefers to take the drug for euphoric effects. This leads to ketoacidosis, which facilitates the excretion of the basic drug like amphetamine. Consequently, plasma levels of amphetamine start declining that necessitates further increment in the dose to get the same euphoric effects.
2. These agents produce high ***psychic dependence*** (Ch. 38), and rarely physical dependence (3–5% cases). *Withdrawal symptoms* consist primarily of prolonged sleep, extreme hunger and fatigue with long phases of depression. Dependence is negligible with ***fenfluramine.***
3. ***The acute effects of amphetamine overdose*** include euphoria, dizziness, tremors, hypertension, irritability, anorexia and insomnia. *At higher doses* convulsions, psychotic manifestations, cardiac arrhythmia and coma may ensue. *Treatment of amphetamine toxicity* can be done by using *diazepam* (slow I.V.) or *haloperidol* to treat agitation and psychotic symptoms. Gastric lavage and acidification of urine (see above) can be done to facilitate its excretion. To control hypertension, *nifedipine/labetalol* can be used while cardiac arrhythmias can be controlled with *esmolol.*
4. Sudden deaths have occurred with ***methylenedioxy methamphetamine (MDMA, Ecstasy)*** users even after a single moderate dose. This drug, at times, induces a "heat stroke" like condition which ends up in rhabdomyolysis and renal failure. It also causes inappropriate secretion of antidiuretic hormone leading to water intoxication and hyponatraemia. MDMA possesses hallucinogenic activity similar to mescaline and psychomotor stimulant effects like that of amphetamine. However, hallucinatory effects appear at a higher dose. Besides inducing the release of NE and DA, MDMA also induces the release of endogenous 5-HT, which activates serotonin receptor.
5. ***Methylenedioxy amphetamine (MDA; Love drug)*** is similar to MDMA in its pharmacological profile. However, in a dose of 75 mg it produces psychotomimetic effects with a feeling of closeness to each other, while a dose of 150 mg produces LSD-like effects and a dose of 300 mg produces amphetamine-like psychotic manifestations. *Side effects*, with stimulatory doses,

include tachycardia and hypertension, and with higher doses, arrhythmias.

Cocaine

Cocaine is a natural alkaloid obtained from Coca leaves. It is neither marketed nor used clinically these days because of high abuse liability. Cocaine binds to DA reuptake transporter in the CNS and effectively inhibits the reuptake of DA (also of NE). This leads to an enhancement in the concentration of DA in the synaptic cleft. Consequently, there is an increase in the peripheral sympathomimetic activity and in the psychomotor stimulant effects. The duration of effects of cocaine is much shorter than amphetamine. It is a good surface anaesthetic (Ch. 15) and was earlier used for producing ocular anaesthesia. But, because it causes constriction of conjunctival vessels, leading to dryness and local tissue toxicity to cornea, it is no longer used as a local anaesthetic.

Cocaine is snorted as a powder (nasal insufflation). When cocaine, as a free base, is smoked in a cigarette, its entry through the lungs is almost as fast as by I.V. injection. This method of consuming cocaine is popular in youth as it is not only convenient but carries little social stigma. A cocaine metabolite is deposited in hair follicles and the analysis of its contents has lately revealed the alarming incidence of cocaine abuse, than was obtained through voluntary disclosures.

Tolerance to the actions of cocaine is less marked; rather at times a *reverse tolerance* has been reported (see Ch. 7). *Psychological dependence* with intense drug seeking behaviour is characteristic of cocaine but physical dependence is arguably absent. *Withdrawal effects* include dysphoria, depression, hypersomnia, fatigue, bradycardia and of course, craving for cocaine.

Toxicity of cocaine includes, tachycardia, hypertension and mydriasis which are the consequences of its sympathomimetic action. Besides, it stimulates vomiting centre to produce nausea and vomiting. Since it enhances muscular activity and also stimulates hypothalamic thermostat centre, it produces pyrexia. Overdoses of cocaine are often fatal due to the development of cardiac arrhythmias, convulsions and respiratory depression. Long-term use of cocaine has been reported to induce rhabdomyolysis with acute hepatic and renal failure. There are clear cut deleterious effects on foetus during pregnancy. The incidence of neurological and limb defects were common in the "cocaine babies".

Treatment of toxicity includes the use of *diazepam* (slow I.V.) with *propranolol* (I.V.) or calcium channel blockers to control hypertension, cardiac arrhythmias and convulsions. Psychotic manifestations may require treatment with *haloperidol*. DA agonist like *amantadine* can be used to cure withdrawal effects of cocaine.

Methylxanthines

Since agents belonging to this category possess diverse pharmacological properties, there is always a question as to where these drugs should be discussed appropriately in the pharmacological text. The popularity of xanthine-containing drinks such as coffee, tea and coke appears to be related to their CNS stimulant effects. It is primarily for this reason that xanthines are classified as CNS stimulants in this text.

Examples of xanthine derivatives include: CAFFEINE, THEOBROMINE, THEOPHYLLINE and its derivatives such as AMINOPHYLLINE (Theophylline ethylenediamine), ETOPHYLLINE (Hydroxyethyl theophylline), ACEBROPHYLLINE and ENPROPHYLLINE (3-Propylxanthine).

Theophylline is found in tea, *theobromine* in coca while *caffeine* is found in highest concentration in coffee but is also present in tea and cola drinks.

Mechanism of Action

Several mechanisms have been suggested for their action. Some important ones are as under:

1. Methylxanthines inhibit the enzyme phosphodiesterase (PDE) and hence increase the 3, 5-cAMP levels to cause bronchodilatation. But this inhibition is observed *in vitro* and that too at a higher concentration. Evidently, it is not certain that such a high concentration can be obtained *in vivo* to inhibit PDE. However, lately inhibition of PDE is being believed as an important mode of their action.

2. The most accepted mechanism for methylxanthines is that they inhibit the cell surface receptors for adenosine (A_1, A_2 and A_3). Adenosine is not a conventional transmitter but a sort of local hormone or better say "homeostatic modulator", which mainly serves as a safety mechanism, to protect neurons when their viability is threatened, for example, by ischaemia or seizure activity.

   Adenosine acts through A_1, A_2 and A_3 receptors. These are G-protein coupled receptors linked to the stimulation or inhibition of adenylate cyclase and are widely distributed. The main effects of adenosine mediated through A_1 receptor are: cardiac depression, inhibition of A-V conduction and antiarrhythmic effects and also presynaptic inhibition of transmitter release in CNS and periphery. In the CNS, adenosine generally exerts depressant actions reducing motor activity, depressing respiration, inducing sleep and reducing anxiety (all opposite to those produced by methylxanthines). Neuroprotection in cerebral ischaemia is also mediated through A_1 receptor action. The notable effects of adenosine, mediated through A_2 receptor action are: hypotension, inhibition of platelet aggregation, vasodilatation including of coronaries and stimulation of nociceptive afferent neurons especially in the heart (anginal pain). Bronchoconstriction, probably secondary to the mast cell activation, seems to result from A_3 receptor activation.

   Summarily, the overall effects of adenosine are inhibitory, leading to drowsiness, motor incoordination, cerebral vasodilatation, CNS depression, anticonvulsant action and bronchoconstriction while methylxanthines antagonise these effects by acting as competitive antagonist at A_1, A_2 and A_3 receptors of adenosine. This hypothesis gathers support from two findings: (a) As small as 100 mmol/lit of caffeine concentration in plasma and brain is sufficient to produce appreciable adenosine receptor blockade, but does not produce any significant inhibition of PDE (see above) and (b) Transgenic mice lacking functional A_2 receptors are abnormally active and aggressive; and they fail to show increased motor activity in response to caffeine suggesting that antagonism at A_2 receptor does account for their CNS stimulatory actions.

   Recently, however, this hypothesis has also been questioned on the grounds that *enprophylline*, a thioxanthene derivative, several times more potent than theophylline, does not possess any adenosine receptor antagonist property. It is rather a PDE inhibitor.

3. Methylxanthines also enhance the deacetylation of histones and prevent transcription of inflammatory genes (acetylation of histones activate inflammatory gene transcription). Corticosteroids, partly, also act by the same mechanism and theophylline even in low doses enhances their action.

Pharmacological Actions

CNS Effects

As CNS stimulants, their rank order of potency is: caffeine > theophylline > theobromine. Among adults the average daily consumption of caffeine, from drinking tea or coffee, is about 200 mg. Caffeine about 200 mg taken orally produces mild CNS stimulation causing wakefulness, alertness and increased capacity to do intellectual work with better association of ideas. Performance at motor tasks such as typing and driving is also improved particularly in fatigued subjects but without much improvement in accuracy. Compared to amphetamines, methylxanthines produce equal fatigue reduction, much less locomotor stimulation but produce no euphoria, stereotyped behaviour or psychotic manifestations.

CVS Effects

Methylxanthines produce only a mild increase in heart rate (HR) because increase in HR by direct action is partly antagonised by their vagal stimulation. They produce peripheral vasodilatation, which again is antagonised by their central stimulation of vasomotor centre. Hence the BP is not affected to any noticeable extent. The cardiac output is increased, which is more marked in CHF patients. The coronary blood flow is increased due to coronary vasodilatation, but their use in CHF is debatable. Cranial blood vessels are constricted, O_2 tension in brain is reduced, that serves as the basis for the use of caffeine in migraine.

Renal Effects

Methylxanthines are mild diuretic (specially theophylline), but the action is brief. This action is a consequence of increased filtration pressure at glomerulus (due to dilatation of afferent arterioles of renal tubules) and also due to increased cardiac output.

Miscellaneous Effects

- These agents stimulate medullary respiratory centre.
- All smooth muscles, particularly of bronchi, are relaxed. This leads to bronchodilatation. Biliary spasm is also reduced.
- These facilitate (mainly caffeine) neuromuscular transmission by increasing ACh release, and enhance the contractile power of skeletal muscles. The enhanced diaphragmatic contractility (mainly with theophylline) probably contributes to its beneficial effects in dyspnoea.
- They increase gastric acid and pepsin secretion. Gastric irritation is more with theophylline.
- Theophylline inhibits the release of histamine and other mediators in mast cells, which contributes to its therapeutic benefits in bronchial asthma.

Clinical Uses

1. Caffeine is frequently combined with aspirin for the treatment of *ordinary headache*, and with ergot alkaloids for the treatment of migraine.
2. Oral theophylline can be used in *chronic obstructive pulmonary disease* and in *mild to moderate asthma* as a third line drug, supplemented with inhaled β_2 agonists (e.g., salbutamol). Usual oral dose 5 mg/kg TDS. Intravenous infusion 4–5 mg/kg over 30 min, then 0.5 mg/kg/hr for maintenance.
3. Caffeine (as citrate) or theophylline can be used for the short-term management of *apnoea in premature infants* in the first few weeks of their life.
4. Aminophylline, as an adjuvant with O_2 and morphine, offers some help in relieving the paroxysmal dyspnoea that is often associated with left ventricular failure (see above for reason). When the distinction between cardiac asthma (dyspnoea due to LVF) and bronchial asthma is doubtful, it is safer to use I.V. aminophylline rather than adrenaline (which is contraindicated in LVF) or morphine (which is contraindicated in asthma). Usual oral dose: 225–450 mg BD (oral); for acute dyspnoea: 250–500 mg I.V. infusion over 30 min, then 0.5 mg/kg/hr as maintenance.

Adverse Effects

Theophylline has, however, a narrow margin of safety. The therapeutic plasma levels range from 8–15 µg/ml. As a convulsant, theophylline is more potent than caffeine. The side effects are dose related and with plasma levels above 15 µg/ml, the adverse effects appear in the following sequence: Dyspepsia, headache, insomnia → restlessness, vomiting, palpitations → agitation, tachypnoea, flushing, hypotension → extrasystoles, arrhythmias, delirium, convulsions, coma → death. Children appear to be specially prone to this toxicity.

Drug Interactions

- Agents that decrease theophylline concentration are: Smoking, phenytoin, carbamazepine, rifampin, phenobarbital and charcoal broiled meat. In such situations the dose of theophylline is to be increased.
- Drugs that inhibit theophylline metabolism are: Erythromycin, ciprofloxacin, cimetidine, oral contraceptives and allopurinol. If these are used concomitantly, the dose of theophylline is to be reduced.
- Theophylline enhances the effects of sympathomimetics, digitalis, furosemide, hypoglycaemic agents and oral anticoagulants.

Abuse of Xanthines

Caffeine (or xanthine) containing beverages cause habituation but no dependence. Chronic coffee drinkers who suddenly abstain from taking coffee suffer from headache and a general feeling of fatigue that may last for several days; but these symptoms do not constitute a kind of true abstinence syndrome. Tolerance to the CNS stimulant effects of caffeine is controversial.

PSYCHOTOMIMETIC DRUGS

In layman's terminology, these drugs substitute the present world by an alternative new world, and hence people call them as 'fantasticants'. After the use of these drugs a person feels that no boundary exists between him and the cosmos and that his mind is able to see more than what he can tell and that he can experience more than what he can explain. Hence drug abusers glorify them by the term 'mind expanders'. *Pharmacologically speaking these drugs produce changes in sensory perceptions (visual, auditory and olfactory), thoughts, behaviour and mood. Since their actions mimic psychoses, these are also termed as* ***psychedelics*** *or* ***psychotomimetics****.*

Mood simply means a state of feeling at particular time. *Precepts* are such thoughts or messages which, though originate from outside, have a high degree of agreement with external reality or signals. Those messages which are largely synthesised inside our head but do not have any relationship to external signals or realities are called as '*fantasies*'. If a fantasy is generated during sleep it is called a *dream* and if fantasy occurs during wakeful state it is called as *hallucination*. In short, hallucination is a false perception without a true sensory stimulus. In hallucination, the images are vague and disproportionate.

Drugs commonly assigned to this class include: LYSERGIC ACID DIETHYLAMIDE (LSD), and MESCALINE, PHENCYCLIDINE and CANNABINOIDS. Drugs that should not be included in this category are those that produce alterations in sensory perception in toxic doses only, e.g., atropine, antimalarials and opioids.

Lysergic Acid Diethylamide (LSD)

It is a lysergic acid derivative which occurs in the cereal fungus ergot. Hofmann synthesised and experimented on this drug (1938–1943) and himself experienced its hallucinogenic effects. The drug is capable of producing strong psychedelic effects in doses less than 1 μg/kg. LSD appears to act as an agonist at 5-HT_2 receptors and suppresses electrical activity in serotoninergic raphe neurons which tonically inhibits the visual and sensory inputs. As a result the excitation threshold of retina is decreased and its spontaneous electrical activity increases (i.e., inhibition of inhibition) leading to visual hallucinations. Similarly, the excitation threshold of midbrain RAS is decreased producing a hyper-arousal state. The drug also displays agonist activity at 5-HT_{1A} and 5-HT_{1C} receptors, hence its mode of action is quite complex.

A dose of 25–50 μg produces all the effects of LSD. The onset of effect is fairly rapid but the duration varies from one user to another and also with the dose. Effects normally vanish by 8 hrs. The effects start with *somatic symptoms* such as tremors, blurred vision and tachycardia. After an hour, these are followed by *perceptual symptoms*. *Visual perceptions* are affected by distorted shapes with brilliant colours of changing intensities. Changes in *auditory perceptions* include sharp hearing with difficulties in locating the source of the sound. Thereafter, auditory sense gets fused with visual to provoke a strange feeling where the person starts seeing the sound and hearing the colours. *Olfactory perceptions* (peculiar smell) also get fused with auditory and visual senses. The mood fluctuates (joyous, sad or frightened) and the sense of the time is lost. After about 2 hrs *psychic symptoms* start appearing. These are characterised by dreamy state and *depersonalisation*, as if the soul has come out of the body and looking at it from the ventilator. A sense of union with cosmos is felt. All such experiences may be terrifying (*bad trip*) or hilarious (*good trip*) depending on the user's personality traits. Furthermore, *flashbacks* of the hallucinatory experience can also appear within a week or a month later and it may be precipitated by stress, fatigue or alcohol.

Adverse effects include hyper-reflexia, nausea and muscular weakness. Hallucinatory experience may be accompanied with paranoid delusions, which may lead to homicide or suicide attempts. There is no physical dependence. Even psychic dependence is very mild because "bad trips" and "flashbacks" create panic and discouragement for further use. Higher rate of abortion has been observed in women taking LSD. Teratogenic effects have been reported in some animal species. *Treatment of toxic effects* includes diazepam for sedation and haloperidol for psychotic symptoms.

Mescaline

It is derived from a Mexican cactus and is low potency hallucinogen. Though a phenylalkylamine it does not have marked sympathomimetic effects. It is less active than LSD and is lesser in use.

Phencyclidine (PCP; Angel dust)

It is an anticholinergic with mild hallucinatory effects like disorientation, distorted body images, loss of the sense of time and impairment of the thought processes. Like LSD it also causes occasional bad trips and recurrent psychotic episodes (hence less abused). The mechanism of action of PCP is complex and is still not decided. *Ketamine* is an analogue of PCP, with much lower hallucinogenic potential and is used to produce dissociative anaesthesia (Ch. 31). PCP may be smoked (mixed with tobacco), or snorted, or taken orally or injected intravenously.

Cannabinoids (Δ^9-Tetrahydrocannabinol; Δ^9 THC)

The active principle of the extracts of the hemp plant (*Cannabis sativa* and *Cannabis indica*) is Δ^9-tetrahydrocannabinol (THC). It has been the most popular drug of abuse world over and is used in the following forms:

- The dried leaves are powdered, made a paste and then used as a drink called *Bhang.*
- The dried leaves and flowering tops of the plant are referred to as *marijuana* (grass, pot, weed or reefer) and is smoked in pipes or rolled as cigarettes.
- *Charas* or *hashish* are resinous exudates of flower tops or leaves. It is very potent and is usually smoked in a pipe.

The major psychoactive constituent in marijuana or hashish is THC. The THC content in hashish is more than double that present in marijuana. Its metabolite 11-hydroxy-THC is also highly active.

Pharmacokinetic Aspects

THC is readily absorbed when marijuana is smoked. Pharmacological effects appear within 30 min of the onset of smoking. On oral ingestion THC is absorbed more slowly than by smoking. The terminal half-life of THC in plasma ranges from 18 hrs to 3 days, but the behavioural and the physiological effects return to baseline levels 6 to 8 hours after usage. Being highly lipophilic, THC and its metabolites are sequestered in the body fat and adipose tissue. As a result, excretion continues several days after a single dose.

Pharmacological Actions

Initially, there is CNS stimulation followed by sedation. *During the stimulatory phase* there is euphoria, increased talkativeness, increase in appetite, and a feeling of confidence, relaxation and well-being. Many may laugh uncontrollably while others may become sad and weep. *During the sedative phase* there are mild LSD type effects. Subjects feel that time is passing very slowly. There is retention of fixed unnatural posture. Ability to concentrate is impaired; sleepiness prevails. There is impairment of short-term memory, simple learning tasks and of motor co-ordination. The company of coabusers and the music around, has a great influence on these behavioural effects. *The peripheral effects* of cannabis include: tachycardia, vasodilatation with reddening of conjunctiva (bloodshot appearance), reduction in intraocular pressure and bronchodilatation. *Other central effects* of THC are analgesia and antiemetic action. THC has inhibitory effects on immune functions also.

Mechanism of Action and Clinical Use

Two types of cannabinoid receptors have been identified: CB_1 receptors in the brain and CB_2 receptors in the periphery. Both are G-protein coupled receptors linked to the inhibition of adenylate cyclase. The distribution of CB_1 receptors in specific areas of brain reflects the pharmacological effects produced by THC. These are found in hippocampus (memory impairment), cerebellum and substantia nigra (motor disturbances), mesolimbic DA pathways (reward) and in cortex (cognition). ***Anandamide***, an arachidonic acid derivative, is an endogenous cannabinoid ligand for the CB_1 receptor; although all actions of cannabis are not mimicked by this endogenous cannabinoid.

Dronabinol and ***nabilone*** are the synthetic analogues of THC. These are CB_1 receptor agonists and are used to increase appetite in patients of AIDS who are losing weight. ***Dronabinol*** is also used to prevent emesis caused by cancer therapeutic agent like cisplatin (Ch. 28). ***Rimonabant*** is rather a CB_1 receptor antagonist (it also exhibits some inverse agonist action). It is approved for the treatment of obesity (dose: 20 mg OD before breakfast; see Ch. 72 also). Its use in smoking cessation is an off-labeled indication. *Side effects* include precipitation of anxiety and notable depression in higher doses. However, it has been withdrawn from the market due to development of adverse effects of depression carrying the risk of suicide.

The peripheral cannabinoid receptor (CB_2) is located mainly in the lymphoid system and accounts for the inhibitory effects on the immune system (see above).

Adverse Effects

Cannabis is undoubtedly safer than most abused substances such as opiates and alcohol. Psychological dependence is mild but physical dependence does not occur. There have been no credible reports on fatal overdose. Withdrawal effects are also mild and include irritability, decrease in appetite and insomnia. However, cessation of mild to moderate use of marijuana does not produce withdrawal syndrome. Some degree of tolerance develops to many of the THC effects in heavy marijuana users.

Cannabinoids do impair the cognitive and motor skills needed to complete a complex task, but do not affect the retrieval of previously learned facts. THC causes impairment of short-term memory. Heavy marijuana smokers suffer with bronchitis but definitive evidence of its relationship with the incidence of lung cancer is lacking. Endocrinal side effects include a notable decrease in plasma testosterone and a reduction in sperm count. THC produces teratogenic effects in rats and an increased incidence of chromosomal defects in circulating white cells in human beings but the risk of foetal malformation is negligible.

CHAPTER 36 Ethanol and Other Alcohols

COMPETENCY PH1.20, PH1.21, PH1.23

Ethanol, traditionally referred to as alcohol occupies a place in medicine and pharmacology mainly because of the consequences of its misuse or abuse. About 10% of alcohol users are unable to limit their alcohol consumption and become *alcohol abusers*. Among them, a section of the population who continue to drink alcohol despite the adverse medical consequences suffer from *alcoholism*, a disorder which is difficult to treat. This chapter describes the pharmacological effects of ethanol on a variety of organ systems. Effects of ethanol on foetus and the long-term consequences of prenatal exposure to ethanol are described. Emerging trends in the pharmacotherapy of alcohol dependence and the molecular mechanisms of ethanol action are also reviewed. In addition to ethanol, treatment of methanol and ethylene glycol poisoning is also discussed.

Alcohol is manufactured by fermentation of starch, sugars and other carbohydrates, but the major source of commercial alcohol is molasses, which is the thick mother liquor in the cane sugar industry from which no more sugar can be crystallised, though its sucrose contents are still about 30%.

Anhydrous alcohol is 99.99% w/w of ethanol; absolute alcohol is 99% w/w of ethanol; rectified spirit is 90% w/w of ethanol, while denatured alcohol is the ethanol to which some substances (e.g., methanol, camphor, terpineol, aniline dyes or diethylphthalate) have been added. Denatured alcohol, therefore, is unfit for consumption as a drink. It is then made available for industrial use or for adding in varnishes and paints. Earlier alcohol contents were assessed by proof strengths and 100% proof spirit was the one which contained 49.29% w/w or 57.1% v/v of ethanol. There are a large variety of alcoholic beverages. In 'Light Beers' the alcohol content is 5–6%; in 'Strong Beers' it is up to 10%. Rum, gin, whiskey, vodka and brandy are the "spirits" which are obtained after distillation of the fermented liquor. The alcohol content of these liquors varies from 40–45%. 'Wines' are undistilled. 'Sweet Wines' contain some unfermented sugar. 'Champagne' (12–15% alcohol) is an effervescent wine. It is bottled prior to the completion of fermentation process and hence becomes aerated.

MECHANISM OF ACTION

The mechanism of action of alcohol is poorly understood. However, no specific receptors for ethanol have been identified. Ethanol enhances the action of GABA at $GABA_A$ receptor similar to the actions of benzodiazepines. The latter also intensifies many of the acute effects of alcohol. The benzodiazepine antagonist *flumazenil*, on the other hand, reverses the central depressant actions of alcohol; but the use of flumazenil to reverse ethanol intoxication and to treat the dependence could not become popular as it paradoxically carries a risk for seizures and thus can increase its long-term toxic manifestations. Ethanol also inhibits the ability of glutamate to activate NMDA receptor and thus inhibits the opening of Ca^{2+} channel linked to NMDA receptor.

PHARMACOKINETICS

Ethanol is absorbed rapidly from the GIT. Food, specially milk, delays its absorption by slowing gastric emptying. Distribution is rapid with volume of distribution (aVd) approximating total body water (0.5–0.7 L/kg). It crosses BBB as well as placental barrier but the concentration in brain is very close to the concentration of ethanol in blood, because the brain receives a larger proportion of blood flow.

About 95% of the absorbed alcohol is metabolised, the remaining 5% is excreted through breath, urine and sweat. Although this fraction is pharmacokinetically insignificant, it provides the basis for estimating blood-ethanol concentration from measurements in breath. The blood concentration of alcohol has great medicolegal importance. Alcohol in alveolar air is in equilibrium with that in pulmonary capillary blood and this ratio is relatively constant (80 mg/100 ml of ethanol in blood is equivalent to 35 μg/100 ml of ethanol in expired air) which forms the basis of the breath analyser test.

A substantial fraction of ethanol is cleared by first-pass hepatic metabolism before it undergoes regular metabolism. Hepatic metabolism of alcohol follows zero-order kinetics, i.e., a fixed amount of 8–12 ml or 7–10 g of alcohol is metabolised per hour, irrespective of its blood concentration. Therefore when alcohol absorption is slow, more is removed by first-pass metabolism, whereas if ethanol absorption is rapid (i.e., portal vein concentration is high), most of the ethanol passes into the systemic circulation. That is why drinking alcohol on empty stomach produces much greater pharmacological effects.

Ethanol is metabolised first to acetaldehyde and then to acetic acid. Two major pathways of alcohol metabolism to acetaldehyde, which take place entirely in liver, have been identified (Fig. 36.1).

A) Metabolism of Alcohol to Acetaldehyde

1) Alcohol Dehydrogenase Pathway (Responsible for 75 % of its metabolism)

Alcohol dehydrogenase (ADH) enzyme found mainly in liver, stomach and intestine oxidises about 75% of ethanol to acetaldehyde (Fig. 36.1). Since there is only a limited supply of the coenzyme NAD^+, the metabolism of ethanol to acetaldehye by ADH follows zero-order kinetics (see above). Gastrointestinal metabolism of ethanol is lower in women than in men because women have lower levels of gastric ADH enzyme.

2) Mixed Function Oxidase (cytochrome P-450) System (Responsible for remaining 25% of its metabolism)

As the concentration of ethanol increases above 100 mg/dL, the ADH system gets saturated owing to the depletion of NAD^+. In such situations the body does not depend upon the ADH-NAD^+ system to oxidise ethanol but rather increases the activity of mixed function oxidase system which uses NADPH as a cofactor instead of NAD^+. During chronic alcohol use there is an induction of this enzyme system and therefore the metabolism of other drugs (steroids, oral anticoagulants and paracetamol; see Ch. 26)), which are metabolised by this system, also increases. However, the reverse is not true, i.e., the enzyme-inducers such as barbiturates do not increase the metabolism of alcohol as the mixed function oxidase system is not the main system involved in the oxidation of alcohol and this system operates only when the levels of alcohol go beyond 100 mg/dL.

B) Metabolism of Acetaldehyde to Acetic Acid

About 75–80% of the acetaldehyde produced is converted to the acetate in the liver by aldehyde

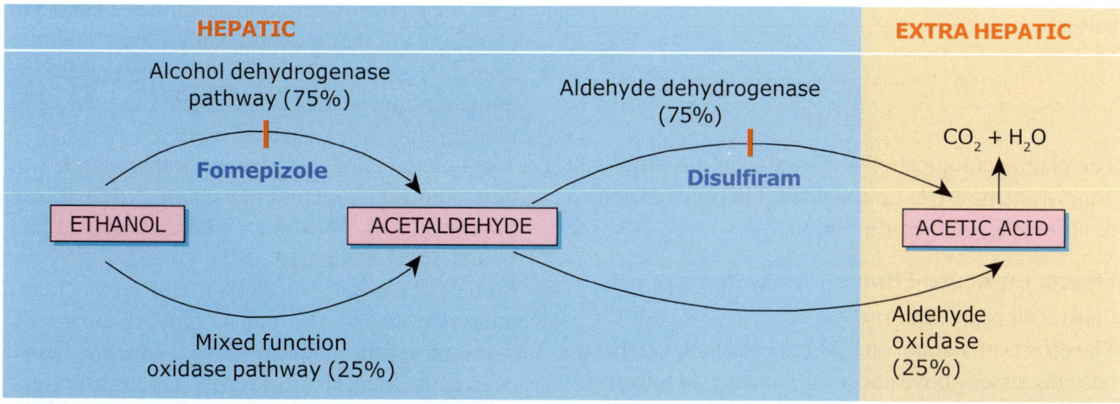

Fig 36.1 Metabolism of Ethanol

dehydrogenase (ALDH). Only 20–25% of acetaldehyde is converted to acetic acid extrahepatically by an enzyme aldehyde oxidase. The product of this reaction is also acetate, which can be further metabolised to CO_2 and water (Fig. 36.1).

Alcohol Dehydrogenase and Aldehyde Dehydrogenase Inhibitors

The aldehyde dehydrogenase enzyme (ALDH) is inhibited by ***disulfiram*** and by other drugs including *metronidazole, oral hypoglycaemics*, certain cephalosporins like *cifotetan* and *cefoperazone* and urinary antiseptics like *nitrofurantoin*. When alcohol is consumed in presence of disulfiram, conversion of acetaldehyde to acetic acid is stopped. Hence acetaldehyde accumulates to cause distressful effects comprising facial flushing, nausea, vomiting, dizziness and headache. Other drugs cited above can also cause a disulfiram-like reaction if combined with ethanol. This type of reaction is extremely unpleasant, but not life-threatening, and hence disulfiram can be used as an aversion therapy to discourage people from consuming alcohol. Even then, for the risk of severe reaction, disulfiram is seldom used as an aversion therapy of alcohol dependence. *Side effects* of disulfiram include rashes, metallic taste and abdominal upset. ***Daidzin,*** an active principle of a Chinese herbal drug, is also a specific inhibitor of aldehyde dehydrogenase. This drug is traditionally being used to treat alcoholics in China.

Fomepizole is an inhibitor of alcohol dehydrogenase enzyme and is used for the treatment of methyl alcohol or ethylene glycol poisoning (see below).

PHARMACOLOGICAL EFFECTS OF ALCOHOL

The pharmacological effects of alcohol on different organ systems are to be considered in terms of acute or chronic alcohol consumption.

Effects on Acute Ethanol Consumption

Central Nervous System

The effects of alcohol on CNS, at cellular level, have been discussed above under the heading "Mechanism of action". The acute effects of alcohol on CNS comprise sedation, relief from anxiety, loss of inhibitions and impaired judgement and driving skills. These symptoms and impairment of driving ability occur at alcohol blood levels between 50–100 mg/dL. Blood levels of 120–160 mg/dL are usually assigned for "gross drunkenness", which is characterised by ataxia, slurred speech, mental clouding and grossly impaired motor functions (drunken gait). Levels between 200–300 mg/dL produce emesis and stupor, whereas levels greater than 300 mg/dL generally lead to coma, respiratory and cardiovascular depression. Levels higher than 500 mg/dL are usually lethal. Additive CNS depression occurs with concomitant administration of benzodiazepines, phenothiazines, tricyclic antidepressants and opiates.

Heart

At blood concentration of approximately 100 mg/dL, ethanol significantly decreases myocardial contractility. Acetaldehyde may cause cardiac abnormalities by altering myocardial stores of catecholamines. Large doses depress vasomotor centre also leading to a fall in BP.

Smooth Muscles and Other Effects

- Ethanol causes cutaneous vasodilatation, which leads to feeling of warmth, but actually increases heat loss.
- Ethanol produces relaxation of uterus but the dose needed is large enough to cause drunkenness in the mother. The use of alcohol to prevent premature labour, evidently has serious disadvantages.
- Diuresis is often associated after alcohol intake. It is caused by inhibition of antidiuretic hormone secretion and partly due to water intake with the drinks. However, tolerance develops rapidly, so diuresis is not sustained on chronic use. Alcohol intake rarely impairs renal function.
- Alcohol is believed to have an aphrodisiac action. Aggressive sexual behaviour is due to loss of inhibitions. However, performance of the sexual act is hampered.
- Moderate amounts of alcohol cause catecholamine release and also reduce glucose uptake by the tissues; this results in hyperglycaemia. However, acute intake causes NAD^+ depletion and inhibits gluconeogenesis leading to hypoglycaemia.

- Alcohol requires no digestion and is rapidly absorbed to instantly supply 7 calories of energy per gram as compared with 9 g from fat and 4 g from carbohydrate and protein. But this energy cannot be stored or utilised for body building; chronic use rather leads to nutritional deficiencies. Thus alcohol serves as an expensive as well as nutritionally worthless food.

Effects of Chronic Alcohol Consumption

Chronic ethanol intake adversely affects the functions of several vital organs, as discussed below.

Nervous System

Tolerance and Physical Dependence

On chronic consumption of ethanol, tolerance develops to the subjective and behavioural effects of alcohol. Chronic alcoholics may function almost normally at much high blood levels (above 180 mg/dL) than occasional drinkers. It is both the cellular adaptive as well pharmacokinetic type of tolerance. The reduced rate of absorption due to induration of gastric mucosa and faster metabolism due to induction of mixed function oxidases are responsible for the development of pharmacokinetic tolerance.

Chronic alcohol drinkers, when forced to abstain from alcohol, experience distressing withdrawal symptoms with physical dependence. These withdrawal effects comprise hyperexcitability, toxic psychosis, delirium tremens and seizures. The physical dependence, at times, is so alarming that merely reducing the rate of consumption may lead to the signs of withdrawal. The withdrawal effects develop after about 8 hours of abstinence from alcohol. In the first stage, which lasts for about 24 hours, the main symptoms are tremors, nausea and sweating. Fever and hallucinations may also ensue. This phase is followed by seizures and in next 3 days 'delirium tremens' develops, which is characterised by confusion, agitation, aggressiveness and hallucination. Psychological dependence upon alcohol is characterised by a compulsive desire to experience the rewarding effects of alcohol drinking (see above).

Neurotoxicity

Neurological deficits occur in chronic heavy drinkers causing ataxia, dementia and peripheral neuropathies. Wernicke-Korsakoff syndrome, through rare, is important as it is rarely seen in absence of alcoholism. It is associated with thiamine deficiency occurring due to consumption of large amounts of alcohol over extended periods. This syndrome is characterised by ataxia, confusion and paralysis of the extraocular muscles. Prompt treatment with I.V. or I.M. thiamine is essential to prevent permanent brain damage. Alcohol also impairs visual acuity with painless blurring of the vision on chronic consumption.

Liver and GIT

A long-term excessive ethanol consumption causes fatty liver which progresses to hepatitis (inflammation of liver) and eventually to irreversible hepatic necrosis, fibrosis and failure. Subsequently, the bleeding oesophageal varices may develop if the portal blood flow is diverted around the fibrotic liver. Another factor contributing to liver damage is malnutrition, because heavy intake of alcohol daily, though provides sufficient calories, yet unlike normal diet it does not provide vitamins and amino acids. Cellular toxicity *per se* of ethanol also promotes inflammatory changes in liver. Women appear to be more susceptible to alcohol hepatotoxicity than men. Chronic alcohol consumption is by far the most common cause of chronic pancreatitis. It occurs due to direct cellular toxicity of ethanol on pancreatic acinar cells and due to alterations in the permeability of pancreatic epithelial cells due to ethanol, which promotes the formation of protein plugs and calcium carbonate–containing stones. Irritation, inflammation, bleeding, scarring or even induration of the gut mucosa occur after chronic heavy use of ethanol and may hamper absorption process to exacerbate nutritional deficiencies particularly of water-soluble vitamins.

Cardiovascular System

Long-term heavy alcohol consumption leads to dilated cardiomyopathy with ventricular hypertrophy and fibrosis. Alcohol also interferes with the therapeutic benefits of β-blockers and ACE inhibitors. Heavy drinking is associated with atrial as well as ventricular arrhythmias. Syncope during alcohol withdrawal may be due to these arrhythmias. Heavy chronic use of alcohol is an important cause of hypertension which should always be considered in both diagnosis and management.

Blood Lipoproteins and Platelet Functions

Moderate intake of alcohol (one or two normal drinks per day) increases high-density lipoproteins (HDL) and decreases low-density lipoproteins (LDL), which may account for the observed protective effect against ischaemic heart disease. Ethanol may also protect against ischaemic heart disease by inhibiting platelet aggregation. This effect is observed by moderate–normal drinking of alcohol (10–20 mmol/L) and results from inhibition of arachidonic acid formation from phospholipids. However, it is not yet established definitely as to how these two effects are important clinically.

Megaloblastic anaemia has been observed in chronic alcoholism due to alcohol-related folic acid deficiency. Iron deficiency anaemia also may result from gastrointestinal bleeding.

Endocrine Effects and Electrolyte Balance

Chronic alcoholism can produce testicular atrophy, gynaecomastia and impotence. A "pseudo-Cushing's syndrome" is usually observed in chronic alcoholics, which partly results due to an increase in plasma hydrocortisone levels because ethanol inhibits hydrocortisone metabolism in the cirrhotic liver. Alcoholics with cirrhotic liver may exhibit ascites, oedema and effusions due to decreased protein synthesis and portal hypertension. Secondary aldosteronism in chronic alcoholism can cause hypokalaemia which contributes to muscle weakness. Some alcoholics may develop ketosis, caused by increased lipolytic factors such as cortisol or growth hormone.

Effects on Foetal Development

Severely alcoholic women usually suffer from amenorrhoea secondary to liver damage. Hence pregnancy is unlikely to occur; even spontaneous miscarriage rate in the second trimester is doubled if 1–2 units of alcohol is consumed per day. However, consumption of about 6–10 units of alcohol per day during pregnancy causes *foetal alcohol syndrome* which occurs in about 3 per 1000 live births born to such alcoholic mothers. This syndrome is characterised by microcephaly, mental retardation, flattened face, retarded growth and other major (cardiac) or minor (malformation of eyes and ears) congenital abnormalities.

A lesser degree of impairment, called "*alcohol-related neurodevelopmental disorder*" may also occur and its incidence is about three times more than foetal alcohol syndrome. It is characterised by behavioural as well as cognitive and motor deficits. It may occur in pregnant women consuming 3–5 units of alcohol per day. The mechanisms that underlie ethanol's teratogenic effects are unknown. However, foetal liver has negligible alcohol dehydrogenase while concentrations of alcohol in foetus are equal to its concentration in maternal blood (alcohol easily crosses placental barrier). This ethanol then triggers apoptotic neurodegeneration in CNS. Alcohol is easily secreted through breast milk which may delay motor development in the child.

Miscellaneous Effects

- The effects of alcohol on immune system are complex. Chronic alcoholics are predisposed to lung infections which increases the mortality risk of patients suffering from pneumonia.
- Ethanol is not a primary carcinogen, but its chronic use is associated with an increased incidence of neoplastic disease like breast and liver carcinoma.
- Ethanol alters uric acid metabolism both by increasing uric acid production and by decreasing renal uric acid excretion. Hence due to hyperuricaemia, gout may be precipitated.

TREATMENT OF ACUTE AND CHRONIC ALCOHOLISM

A) Management of Acute Alcohol Toxicity

Intoxication due to acute intake of ethanol is managed by maintenance of vital signs and prevention of aspiration of vomitus. Treatment of hypoglycaemia and ketosis can be made by giving I.V. glucose. Thiamine (I.V. or I.M.) and correction of electrolytes may also be required.

B) Mechanism for Development of Physical Dependence

Chronic ethanol administration produces various adaptive changes in the CNS neurons to antagonise the acute cellular effects that it produces. As a result, there is an up-regulation of NMDA receptors and proliferation of L-type Ca^{2+} channels associated with these receptors. There is a small reduction in the density of $GABA_A$ receptors also. During chronic exposure to ethanol, Ca^{2+} entry tries to recover (owing to proliferation of Ca^{2+} channels); and on ethanol withdrawal, the Ca^{2+} entry and the neurotransmitter release are increased above normal, which is possibly linked to physical withdrawal symptoms such as CNS hyper-excitability and neurotoxicity.

The neurotransmission events involved in the sensation of the reward are also important. Alcohol affects the local concentrations of NE, 5-HT, DA and opioids—neurotransmitters involved in the brain reward circuits. The turnover of NE and DA in brain is enhanced by alcohol through an opioid receptor dependent mechanism which is probably responsible for the pleasurable effects of alcohol and the genesis of alcohol dependence. Though the effects of alcohol are purely depressant, it increases the impulse activity by disinhibiting the dopaminergic reward pathway in the mesolimbic dopaminergic neurons. The neurobiological basis of the switch-over from the willing and the controlled alcohol intake to compulsive and uncontrolled addiction is not clear. Impairment of the dopaminergic reward system (due to development of tolerance) and the resultant increase in the alcohol consumption can be one of the possibilities for alcohol-seeking behaviour.

C) Management of Withdrawal Syndrome

The characteristic features of alcohol withdrawal syndrome have been described above. This abstinence syndrome is usually managed by administration of a long acting sedative-hypnotic (e.g., *chlordiazepoxide* or *diazepam*). The intensity of withdrawal syndrome may be reduced by *clonidine* and *propranolol*. Clonidine, an α_2-adrenoceptor agonist, acts by inhibiting the exaggerated transmitter release that occurs during withdrawal, while propranolol, being a β-blocker, antagonises the effects of excessive sympathetic effects. Once the withdrawal phase is over, the benzodiazepines may be withdrawn with gradual dose tapering. Complete detoxification is not achieved with just a few days of alcohol abstinence. Several months may be needed for restoration of normal sleep, and decrease of tremors and anxiety.

D) Management of Alcohol Dependence

Alcohol dependence (alcoholism) is seen with 4–5% of the population and is difficult to treat, because of high relapse rate. The main pharma-cological approaches are as under:

i) The first approach to pharmacotherapy is to render ethanol consumption unpleasant (aversion therapy). This is accomplished by giving *disulfiram* as discussed above (but rarely used now). Dose: 1 g on 1st day; reduce by 250 mg daily; keep 250 mg for maintenance once daily.
ii) Another approach is to use such a drug which reduces the craving for alcohol or which blunts the pleasurable "high" that comes with renewed drinking. *Naltrexone*, an opioid receptor antagonist, in a dose of 50 mg once a day is used to treat alcohol dependence. It has been demonstrated that opioid antagonists inhibit craving for alcohol while opioids increase craving for alcohol.
iii) It has been shown that the anticonvulsant drug, *topiramate,* is also effective in reducing craving in chronic alcoholics. The drug potentiates the inhibitory effects of GABA (like benzodiazepines) but acts at a site different from benzodiazepines or barbiturates.
iv) The selective serotonin reuptake inhibitors (SSRIs), such as *fluoxetine*, which can increase serotoninergic activity in CNS may also be helpful in this regard. *Ondansetron*, a 5-HT_3 antagonist, has also been successfully used.
v) To reduce craving for alcohol, *acamprosate* is being used. It reduces the effects of excitatory amino acids such as glutamate on NMDA receptor and at the same time facilitates GABA

neurotransmission. It also possesses some opioid antagonist activity and increase serotonin levels in synapses. *Acamprosate* may cause GIT upset and skin eruptions as side effects.

Rimonabant: It is a CB_1 cannabinoid receptor antagonist has been found to be useful in alcohol withdrawal syndrome.

Psychotherapy and counselling are also very helpful.

DRUG INTERACTIONS

- Chronic consumption of alcohol increases the risk of hepatotoxicity due to *paracetamol*. This is probably due to increased cytochrome P-450 (CYP2E1) mediated conversion of paracetamol to a reactive hepatotoxic metabolite N-acetyl-p-benzoquinoneimine (Ch. 26).
- *All cerebral depressants* (hypnotics, sedatives, phenothiazine group of neuroleptics and antihistamines) can synergise with ethanol. This can be serious even at therapeutic doses in relation to car driving.
- Chronic alcoholics are relatively tolerant of general anaesthetics like *halothane*.
- *A disulfiram-type reaction* occurs with metronidazole, tinidazole, chlorpropamide, cefoperazone, cefamandole and cifotetan (see above).
- Alcohol enhances the hypoglycaemic effects of *insulin* and *sulfonylureas*.
- Some alcoholic drinks, like beer and wine, contain tyramine which is sufficient to cause hypertensive crisis in a patient taking *monoamine oxidase inhibitors* (Ch. 34).

CLINICAL USES OF ETHANOL

- As skin antiseptic (76% v/v) is most effective.
- Alcohol has astringent action (precipitates proteins) and is used to harden the skin to prevent bed sores.
- To treat methanol poisoning (see below).

METHANOL

Methanol is used as an industrial solvent and to adulterate ethanol in order to make it unfit to drink. Methanol poisoning is quite common either because of unscrupulous mixing of methanol with alcoholic beverages or because of its ingestion accidentally.

PHARMACOKINETICS

Methanol is metabolised in the same way as ethanol (Fig. 36.2) first to formaldehyde by alcohol dehydrogenase and then to formic acid by aldehyde dehydrogenase.

Like ethanol, the metabolism of methanol follows zero-order kinetics but the rate of metabolism is 1/7th that of ethanol. Formaldehyde is much more reactive than acetaldehyde and reacts rapidly with proteins of the retina causing retinal damage. Formic acid, unlike acetic acid, cannot be utilised in tricarboxylic acid cycle and is liable to cause acidosis and tissue damage. The formic acid itself promotes lactic acidosis by enhancing pH dependent hepatic lactate production. Majority of the toxic symptoms are largely due to formic acid, since its further metabolism is slow and folate dependent. The clinical features of methyl alcohol poisoning comprise severe malaise, vomiting, abdominal pain, loss of visual

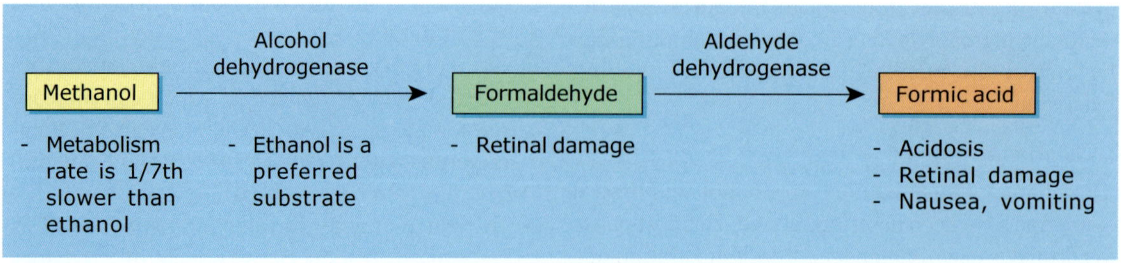

Fig 36.2 Metabolism of Methanol

acuity, and if pupils are dilated and non-reactive total blindness is probable. Vomiting, hypotension and tachypnoea (due to acidosis) are common. This is followed by respiratory and circulatory collapse, coma and death. Therapy is directed at :

- *Inhibiting methanol metabolism to prevent formation of toxic metabolites*: Ethanol has higher affinity than methanol for alcohol dehydrogenase, an enzyme responsible for methanol oxidation to formaldehyde in the liver. Ethanol 100 mg/dL in blood saturates alcohol dehydrogenase and retards methanol metabolism ultimately to formic acid. Ethanol (10% v/v) is administered through a nasogastric tube in a loading dose of 0.7 ml/kg followed by 0.15 ml/kg/hour drip. Treatment has to be continued for several days until no methanol is detectable in the blood. However, this is often done in conjunction with haemodialysis to remove unchanged alcohol which has a small volume of distribution (0.5–0.7 L/kg). ***Fomepizole,*** a competitive inhibitor of alcohol dehydrogenase, has also proved effective in severe methanol poisoning and is less likely to cause cerebral de pression.
- *Eliminating methanol and its toxic metabolites by dialysis*: In this regard haemodialysis is 2–3 times more effective than peritoneal dialysis. Folinic acid 30 mg I.V. 6–8 hourly may protect against retinal damage by enhancing formic acid metabolism.
- *Combating acidosis*: Sodium bicarbonate is given by I.V. infusion to correct acidosis and to prevent retinal damage. Its infusion should continue till acidosis is corrected because the patient may show relapse if bicarbonate administration is discontinued soon.
- *Other measures*: Gastric lavage, support for respiration, and protection of eyes from light.

ETHYLENE GLYCOL

It is a constituent of antifreeze formulation for car radiators. It is clandestinely used to provide sweetness to white table-wines. It is oxidised in the body by alcohol dehydrogenase to glycoaldehyde and then by aldehyde dehydrogenase to oxylic acid, which causes acidosis, cardiopulmonary complications, renal pain and tubular necrosis because of the formation of oxalate crystals in nephrons, which is the key to the diagnosis of ethylene glycol poisoning. Acidosis is corrected with I.V. sodium carbonate infusion; hypocalcaemia with calcium gluconate; and ethanol administration to retard degradation of ethylene glycol to toxic metabolites (like methanol).

Fomepizole is used in the same manner as for methanol poisoning, to competitively inhibit the metabolism of ethylene glycol by alcohol dehydrogenase. Though very effective, the drug enjoys the "orphan drug" status because ethylene glycol poisoning is relatively uncommon. Haemodialysis is finally used to eliminate ethylene glycol and its toxic metabolites.

- Drugs that can precipitate disulfiram like reaction: Metronidazole, Sulfonylureas, Griseofulvin, Phenylbutazone, Nitrofurantoin.

CHAPTER 37 Opioid Analgesics & Opioid Antagonists

COMPETENCY PH1.19

Pain is an ill-defined, disabling accompaniment of many medical conditions. It is often evoked by an external or internal noxious stimulus. *Analgesics* are the drugs which possess significant pain-relieving properties by acting in the CNS or on peripheral pain receptors without significantly affecting consciousness. Analgesics are divided into two groups:

I. Narcotic/Opioid/Morphine like analgesics
II. Non-narcotic/Nonsteroidal anti-inflammatory-analgesic-antipyretic agents (see Ch. 26).

This chapter starts with a discussion on pathophysiology of pain. This is then followed by a discussion on endogenous opioid peptides with a focus on opioid receptors, because opioid analgesics exert their therapeutic effects by mimicking the actions of these endogenous opioid peptides at these receptors. Opioid analgesics act primiarily at the level of spinal cord and brain while NSAIDs (Ch.26) act primarily at peripheral sites to inhibit the synthesis or activity of pain-sensitising substances like prostaglandins.

PATHOPHYSIOLOGY OF PAIN

There are classically two components in pain perception: **(1)** ***The nociceptive component***, which is a disabling, unpleasant sensation evoked by noxious stimuli and conveyed to CNS by ascending pathways; and **(2)** ***The affective component***, which is the psychological response towards the pain and conveyed from CNS to dorsal horn by descending pathways.

The ***ascending pain pathways*** (Fig. 37.1A) transmit pain impulses from the dorsal horn of the spinal cord to medulla, midbrain, thalamus, limbic structures and the cortex. The pain activates the terminals of primary afferent neuron (PAN) fibers (Aδ & C) which enter the spinal cord, where they synapse onto spinothalamic tract (STT) neurons. The Aδ (fast conducting) fibers constitute the neo-STT pathway which projects to somatosensory cortex (SSC) and alerts the person about the presence and location of the intense, sharp somatic (integumentary pain). He may use withdrawal reflexes to avoid the noxious stimuli or use NSAIDs if pain is due to tissue injury. This functional projection is also called ***sensory-discriminative component.*** The C-fibers (slow conducting) constitute the paleo-STT pathway which project to the limbic structures and mediate the ***motivational-affective (mood) response*** towards dull aching visceral pain (e.g., pain related to myocardial infarction) or burning neuropathic pain (e.g., of trigeminal neuralgia, post-herpetic neuralgia and diabetic neuropathy). The function of this component is to enable the person to bear the pain, experience the discomfort and modify his emotional reaction to the pain.

The ***descending pathways*** from the midbrain (Fig. 37.1A) exert rather inhibitory effects on dorsal horn transmission and play an important role in the regulatory feedback loop to control the pain transmission through the dorsal horn (see "gate-control mechanisms" discussed below). The descending neuronal tracts from the periaqueductal gray (PAG) matter activate rostroventral medulla (RVM) and nucleus raphe magnus (NRM). From NRM, 5-HT and enkephalin are released at substantia gelatinosa of the dorsal horn to inhibit ascending pain transmission (Fig. 37.2) through STT neurons. From loculus ceruleus (LC), there is release of NE which also has a similar inhibitory effects on pain transmission from dorsal horn.

The pain transmission through substantia gelatinosa (SG) *via* STT is modulated, or **gated**, by the descending inhibitory pathways and by the sensory Aβ fibers arising in peripheral tissues. The interneurons in the SG of dorsal horn are inhibitory as they release met-enkephalin. The peripheral Aβ

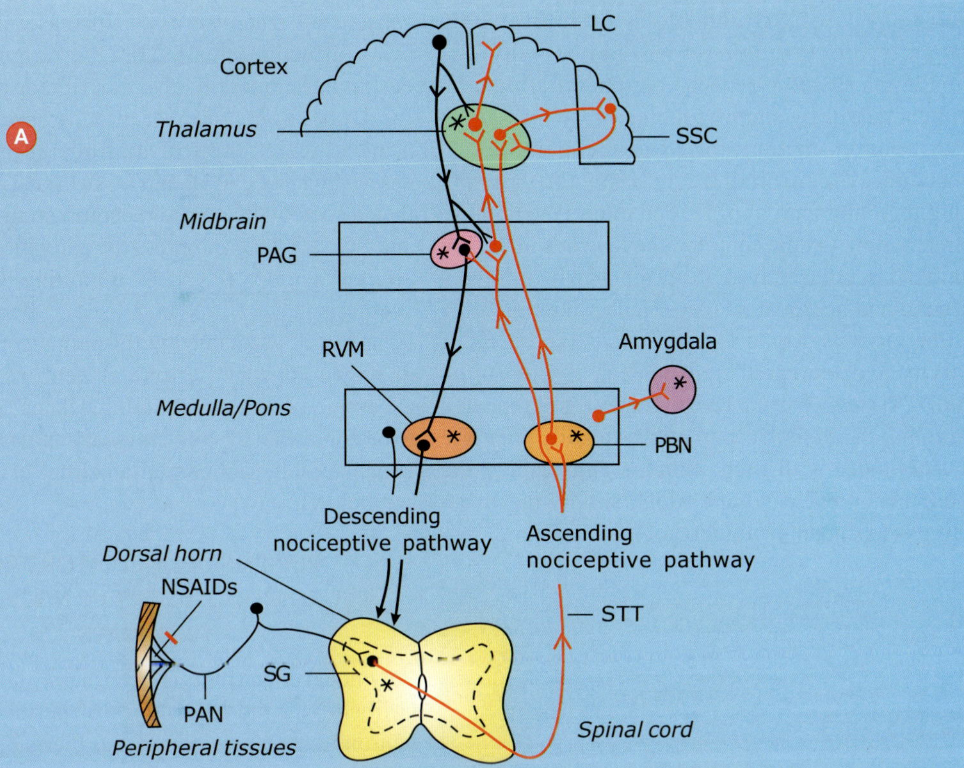

Key: SG—Substantia gelatinosa; PAG—Periaqueductal grey; RVM—Rostroventral medulla; PBN—Parabrachial nuclei; SSC—Somatosensory cortex; LC—Limbic cortex; STT—Spinothalamic tract; PAN—Primary afferent neuron; *Sites of opioid action.

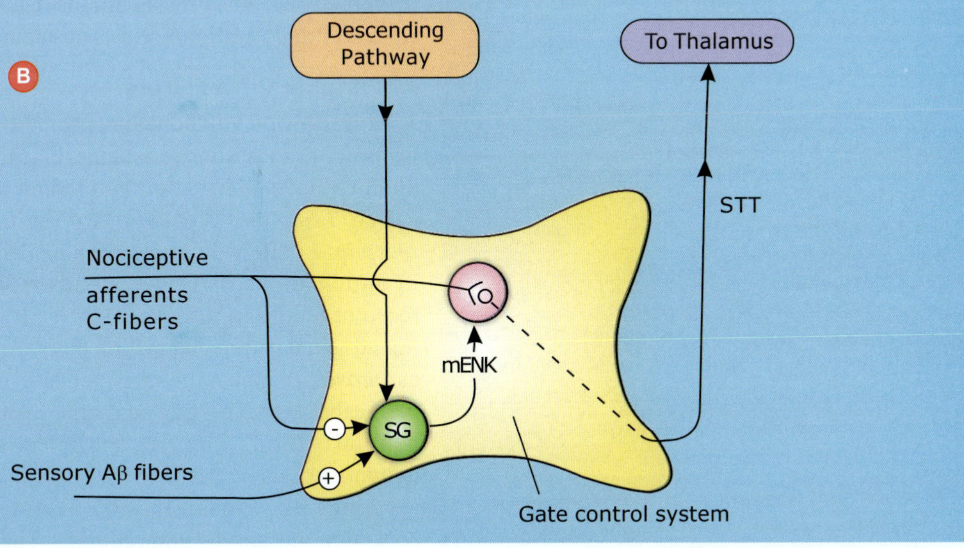

Fig 37.1 (A) Ascending and Descending Nociceptive Pathways, (B) Gate Control System

fibers stimulate the release of met-enkephalin from interneurons of SG and block or inhibit pain transmission through STT. That is why the stimulation of these sensory peripheral fibers by acupuncture or by simply rubbing or by massaging with counter-irritants provide the pain relief. Descending neuronal tracts also activate the inhibitory interneurons of SG and inhibit the impulse transmission. On the contrary, the neurons in SG are inhibited by nociceptive C-fiber inputs which convey visceral and neuropathic pain. Hence, the repetitive C-fiber activity would lead to successive bursts of activity and increased transmission through ***gate control system*** (Fig. 37.1B). In the event of repeated stimulus, the synaptic potentials steadily increase in amplitude with each stimulus and display the phenomenon of "wind up" which simply means an activity-dependent facilitation of transmission.

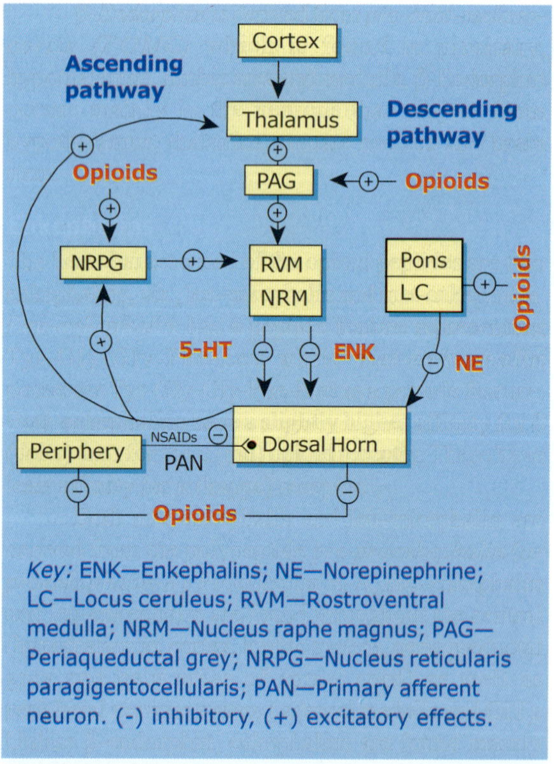

Key: ENK—Enkephalins; NE—Norepinephrine; LC—Locus ceruleus; RVM—Rostroventral medulla; NRM—Nucleus raphe magnus; PAG—Periaqueductal grey; NRPG—Nucleus reticularis paragigentocellularis; PAN—Primary afferent neuron. (-) inhibitory, (+) excitatory effects.

Fig 37.2 Descending Inhibitory Neuro-transmission Control of Nociceptive Pathways.

In dorsal horn, this facilitation is provoked by NMDA, substance-P and nitric oxide. Increased production of nerve growth factor (NGF), by peripheral tissues during inflammation, also contributes to the central facilitation of pain transmission leading to hyperalgesia. Opioid analgesics activate the descending PAG, NMR and LC neuronal pathways and they also activate opioid receptors in the spinal cord and SG . NSAIDs suppress the activation of primary afferent neurons (PAN) by inhibiting prostaglandin synthesis (Fig. 37.1A and 37.2). Neuropathic pain is, however, associated with spontaneous activity in damaged sensory peripheral neurons rather than excessive peripheral stimulus. Hence, it is difficult to be controlled by conventional analgesic drugs (but treated by some anticonvulsant drugs or by capsaicin; see below).

PERIPHERAL MEDIATORS AND NEUROMODULATORS IN NOCICEPTIVE PATHWAYS

Polymodal nociceptors (PMN; mainly nonmyelinated C-fibers) are the main types of peripheral sensory neurons that respond to noxious thermal, chemical or mechanical stimuli. The chemical stimuli acting on PMN to cause pain, include substance-P, neurokinin-A and B (Ch. 17), bradykinin (Ch. 24), 5-HT and histamine (Ch. 24), prostaglandins (Ch. 25), protons (H^+), ATP and vanilloids (e.g., capsaicin).

A) Peripheral Mediators

1. Capsaicin and Vanilloid Receptor (TRPV-1)

Capsaicin, an active substance in chilli peppers, produces intense irritation by binding to a receptor called ***T****ransient* ***R****eceptor* ***P****otential* ***V****anilloid receptor-****1*** (TRPV-1). It has been named as TRPV-1 in anticipation of further members of vanilloid receptor family (if discovered later). It is a multiple ligand-gated cation channel receptor. Agonists such as ***capsaicin*** open the channel and increase the permeability to Na^+, Ca^{2+} and other cations causing depolarisation. This receptor has an unusual polymodal characteristic in the sense that it not only responds to capsaicin but also to heat, H^+ concentration and to ***anandamide***. The latter is an endogenous cannabinoid receptor agonist (Ch.35) but is an agonist at TRPV-1 also (though less potent than capsaicin).

TRPV-1, like any other ionotropic receptor, is modulated by phosphorylation. The pain-producing mediator ***bradykinin***, which acts through the G-protein coupled bradykinin receptor (B_2) phosphorylates TRPV-1 and facilitates the opening of the ion channels linked to TRPV-1.

TRPV-1 knockout mice show reduced responsiveness to noxious heat stimulus and fail to show thermal hyperalgesia in response to inflammation. TRPV-1 expression is also known to be increased in inflammation. Hence lately it is believed that TRPV-1 receptor mechanism may be playing a key role in producing hyperalgesia.

Interesting Features of Capsaicin

i) Avian TRPV-1 receptor differs from mammalian TRPV-1; that is why birds do not respond to capsaicin and rather relish chilli peppers.
ii) The large influx of Ca^{2+} into nerve terminals, that capsaicin produces, may be enough to cause nerve terminal degeneration which takes weeks to recover. Hence capsaicin products are used topically to relieve neuropathic pain but its strong irritant initial action is a major drawback.
iii) Capsaicin when applied to bladder causes degeneration of C-fiber afferent nerve terminals and hence has also been used to treat urinary incontinence associated with bladder hyperactivity in patients of spinal injury.

2. Other Peripheral Mediators

Although both histamine and 5-HT are known to be released locally in inflammation, these have only a minor role in causing pain. H^+ (low pH) and ATP stimulate nociceptive afferent neurons partly by opening acid-sensitive ion channels (ASICs) and partly through activation of TRPV-1 receptors. Prostaglandins (Ch. 25) and bradykinins (Ch. 24) have already been discussed earlier.

B) Main Neuromodulators in Nociception

There are three endogenous tachykinins—substance-P, neurokinin-A and neurokinin-B—which are widely distributed centrally as well as peripherally (Ch. 17). There is evidence to suggest that substance-P is released not only in the periphery and in the dorsal horn, in the nociceptive pathway, but also in inflammatory conditions such as arthritis and inflammatory bowel disease. Its release in the periphery contributes to neurogenic inflammation while in the dorsal horn contributes to the "wind up" phenomenon (see above). Substance-P produces a slow depolarising response in the postsynaptic cells, which builds up during repetitive stimulation, and is supposed to facilitate NMDA-receptor mediated transmission.

There are three tachykinin receptors NK_1, NK_2 and NK_3 which have substance-P, neurokinin-A and neurokinin-B respectively as their agonist. Nociceptive transmission and neurogenic inflammation are mediated mainly through NK_1 receptors but surprisingly NK_1 receptor antagonists are not effective as analgesics, which further precipitates the existing confusion.

ENDOGENOUS OPIOID PEPTIDES

Until 1970s, the existence of endogenous opioid-like system in the brain remained unproven. Morphine group of drugs were believed to exert their analgesic effects through the interactions with other neurotransmitter systems or by binding to the "opiate receptor". Initial findings about naloxone, an opioid receptors antagonist, were also misleading. Although it was effective in antagonising the effects of opiates given exogenously, it had no effect on normal persons if given alone. Later it was noticed that naloxone reversed the electrical stimulation induced analgesia in certain brain regions. It was therefore suspected and questioned as to why the nature should put an "opioid receptor" in the brain in anticipation of the discovery of morphine by the pharmacologists and why an emotionally charged soldier feels no pain even when he sustains severe injuries in the battle-field. Such inquisitiveness and subsequent research led to the discovery of an "endogenous opioid peptide system" operating in the brain and that morphine and other opioids apparently mimic the actions of these "endogenous opioid peptides" by binding to various types of opioid receptors (for their details, see below).

Subsequently, a number of endogenous opioid peptides having morphine-like actions were isolated from brain, pituitary, spinal cord and GIT. There are three distinct families of opioid peptides: the ***endorphins, enkephalins*** and ***dynorphins.*** All of them share a common terminal amino acid sequence of 5 amino acids : Tyr^1-Gly^2-Gly^3-Phe^4-(joined to Met^5 or Leu^5). This amino acid sequence may be considered as "opioid peptide feature". These peptides are derived from their three precursor polypeptides: ***Pro-opiomelanocortin (POMC), Preproenkephalin (or Proenkephalin-A)*** & ***Preprodynorphin,*** respectively.

β-Endorphin

β-Endorphin posseses a Tyr-Gly-Gly-Phe-Met opioid peptide feature plus a chain of other 26 amino acids, i.e., a peptide chain of total 31 (26 + 5) amino acids. It has greater affinity for μ (mu) opioid receptor than for δ (delta) and κ (kappa) receptor.

β-Endorphin is derived from *pro-opio-melano-cortin (POMC)* which is found in pituitary, hypothalamus, limbic area and medulla. β-Endorphin occurs mainly in the neurons that project from hypothalamus, thalamus, arcuate nucleus and brain stem.

Enkephalins

The best characterised of the opioid peptides are two enkephalins, *viz*., leu-enkephalin and met-enkephalin. ***Leu-enkephalin*** has a peptide feature representing Tyr-Gly-Gly-Phe-Leu while ***met-enkephalin*** possesses Tyr-Gly-Gly-Phe-Met as a peptide feature. Both enkephalins have a slightly higher affinity for δ (delta) than for the μ (mu) opioid receptor. These have least affinity for κ (kappa) receptor.

Both met-enkephalin and leu-enkephalin are derived from the polypeptide *pre-proenkephalin* (*or proenkephalin-A*). Proenkephalin-A, met-enkephalin and leu-enkephalin are found throughout the central (hypothalamus, cortex, limbic system, periaqueductal grey and pain areas of spinal cord) as well as peripheral nervous system (adrenal medulla and GIT). Unlike β-endorphin, enkephalins are found mainly in shorter interneurons in many brain areas.

Dynorphins

All dynorphins have a common Tyr -Gly-Gly-Phe-Leu terminal amino acid sequence feature. But *dynorphin-A, dynorphin-B, α-neoendorphin* and *β-neoendorphin* possess an extension of additional amino acids. These have greater affinity for κ (kappa) than for μ (mu) or δ (delta) opioid receptors. These are derived from *preprodynorphin* which has a wider distribution like enkephalins.

Dynorphin is also found in the dorsal horn of the spinal cord where it plays a critical role of sensitising the nociceptive transmission. This pronociceptive action of dynorphin-A in the spinal cord appears to be independent of the opioid receptor action. Rather dynorphin-A binds to and activates NMDA receptor. Hence its mode of action and effects in nociception can go either way in both directions.

Endomorphins

Recently two endogenous opioid peptides, viz., *endomorphin-1* and *endomorphin-2* have been found in the brain which are released during stress and in anticipation of pain to diminish the sensation of pain and to increase the endurance. These bind with higher affinities to μ (mu) receptors. These have shortest and unique amino acid sequence features: Tyr-Pro-Trp-Phe (for endomorphin-1) and Tyr-Pro-Phe-Phe (for endomorphin-2). The precursors of these two endogenous opioid peptides are not known.

Nociceptin

More recently discovered 4th opioid receptor added new dimension to opioid research as none of the above endogenous opioid peptides recognise this receptor. As a result, it was classified as "orphan receptor". Soon after, a new endogenous peptide, ***nociceptin*** (also called *orphanin-FQ*), was derived from its precursor ***pro-orphanin*** found in hippocampus, cortex and many sensory neurons. It has a total 17 amino acid sequence like that of dynorphin-A, except that its terminal amino acid sequence feature is Phe-Gly-Gly-Phe-Thr instead of Tyr-Gly-Gly-Phe-Leu as in dynorphin-A (see above). Since nociceptin (orphanin-FQ) has finally been identified as an endogenous ligand for this receptor, it is no longer considered as orphan now.

It is now termed as ***orphanin opioid-receptor-like, type-I*** (ORL-1) or ***a nociceptin/orphanin-FQ receptor*** (N/OFQ Receptor). The Committee on Receptor Nomenclature and Drug Classification of the International Union of Pharmacology has recently recommended the term **"NOP" (nociceptin opioid peptide) receptor** instead of N/OFQ or ORL-1 receptor.

The nociceptin opioid peptide, by activating NOP receptor, modulates drug reward, reinforcement, learning and memory processes. The name nociceptin was coined because it paradoxically causes hyperalgesia, when injected into brain, an effect opposite to other endogenous peptides (opposing classical μ [mu] receptor mediated analgesia). Hence, its effects on nociception are more complex and can go in either direction depending upon the underlying behavioural state of the subject. To aggravate the confusion further are the reports that nociceptin (orphanin-FQ) precursor ***pro-orphanin*** also provides another peptide called ***nocistatin*** whose pharmacological effects are opposite to that of ***nociceptin.***

The affinity of different endogenous opioid peptides to the opioid receptor subtypes is summarised below:

μ-Receptor: Endomorphins = Endorphin > Enkephalins = Dynorphins

δ-Receptor: Enkephalins = Endorphin > Dynorphins

κ-Receptor: Dynorphins = Endorphin > Enkephalins

OPIOID RECEPTOR TYPES

With such a large number of endogenous peptide ligands discovered, it is not surprising that multiple classes of opioid receptors have also been found. Three opioid receptors have been cloned: **mu (μ), kappa (κ)** and **delta (δ).** Their functional characteristics, endogenous ligands, selective agonists and antagonists and their distribution in CNS, ANS, peripheral nervous system and GIT have been detailed in Table 37.1.

A fourth receptor **NOP (nociceptin opioid receptor),** with high sequence homology to these three opioid receptors has also been identified. Despite its structural similarity with opioid receptors, opioids *do not* bind to NOP receptor with high affinity. An endogenous peptide *nociceptin* (orphanin-FQ), which is structurally similar to dynorphin, appears to be an endogenous ligand for NOP receptor. Nociceptin, however, does not act at any of the three opioid receptors and, instead, the *nociceptin-NOP receptor complex* may produce a biphasic hyperalgesic-analgesic response (see above). The NOP receptor is also involved along with other receptors in causing opioid reward and reinforcement. Another endogenous peptide *nocistatin,* is also derived from the same gene that gives rise to nociceptin. Nocistatin is reported to block the effects of nociceptin; but interestingly it does not displace nociceptin from its NOP-receptor indicating that the opposing effects of nocistatin are produced through a yet unknown receptor.

Morphine and other pure agonists have greatest affinity for **μ receptors** in CNS and peripheral nervous system but have lower affinity for κ and δ receptors. Among the endogenous opioid peptides, endomorphin-1 and endomorphin-2 have the highest affinity for μ receptors. Two subtypes of μ receptors have been characterised: μ_1 receptor, which is associated with supraspinal analgesia, euphoria and physical dependence and selectively blocked by ***naloxonazine***; and μ_2 receptors, which mediate spinal analgesia, respiratory depression and constipation. Dynorphin-A, an endogenous opioid peptide, is thought to be the natural ligand for the **κ receptor,** of which three subtypes have been identified. Two κ receptors mediate spinal (κ_1) and supraspinal (κ_3) analgesia and are also responsible for the peripheral analgesic effects of the mixed agonist-antagonist group of opioid analgesics (see below). The exact role of κ_2 receptor is not established yet.

Similarly two sub-types of **δ receptors** have also been identified, at which enkephalins act as prototypic agonists. Again, the precise role of these subtypes is not clearly understood. The δ receptor is also involved in spinal analgesia, as well as in causing opioid reinforcement and reward (along with μ receptors). Thus although morphine and other pure agonists preferentially bind to μ receptors they also produce effects at δ and κ-opioid receptors also, particularly at high doses.

In contrast to the traditional view that opioid analgesia is mediated exclusively through central action, ***peripheral opioid receptors*** have recently been discovered and shown to mediate analgesic effects when activated by locally applied opioid agonists. Opioid receptors (mainly μ) are present on peripheral sensory nerves and are up-regulated during the process of inflammation. Their endogenous ligands—the opioid peptides—are expressed in the immune cells present within the peripheral inflammed tissue. These endogenous opioid peptides are secreted from the immunocytes, occupy opioid receptors on sensory nerves and produce analgesia by inhibiting either the excitability of these nerves or the release of the excitatory pro-inflammatory neuropeptides (e.g., substance-P, etc.). The peripheral administration of opioids, e.g., into the knees of the patients undergoing arthroscopic knee surgery has shown promising clinical benefits. The local application of exogenous opioids or of enzyme inhibitors, which prevent the degradation of endogenous opioid peptides, therefore, may provide a new approach to pain management by producing analgesia without central side effects (Table 37.1).

Opioid Receptor Transducer Mechanisms

At molecular level all opioid receptors (including NOP receptor) are linked to G-protein. Action commonly produced at these opioid receptors include:

a) Inhibition of adenylyl cyclase leading to decrease in intracellular cAMP with consequent decrease in cell-excitability (mainly through μ and δ receptors)
b) Activation of K^+ channels and subsequent increase in K^+ conductance to produce hyperpolarisation of neurons and a decrease in their excitability (mainly through μ and δ receptors), and
c) Inhibition of Ca^{2+} conductance by suppressing voltage-gated N-type Ca^{2+} channels (mainly through κ- receptor).

Because Ca^{2+} influx is needed for the stimulus-induced neurotransmitter release, opioids decrease the release of neurotransmitters like substance-P and glutamate from nociceptive terminals. Thus the neuronal hyperpolarisation coupled with decreased neuro-transmitter release in CNS and myenteric neurons, hamper the transmission of the nociceptive information at the first central synapse (Fig. 37.3).

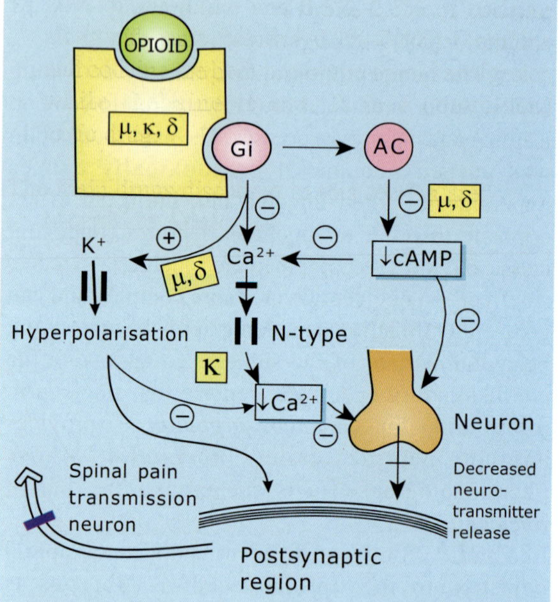

Key: Gi—Coupling protein; AC—Adenylyl cyclase; μ (mu), δ (delta), κ (kappa) receptors.

Fig 37.3 Opioid Receptor Transducer Mechanisms

PHARMACOLOGY OF OPIOID ANALGESICS

Opioid analgesics were earlier termed as *narcotic analgesics*; but this term is lesser in use nowadays, because several narcotic analgesics do not cause narcosis while many drugs which cause narcosis (e.g., barbiturates, ethanol and some general anaesthetics) are not analgesics. The term *narcotics*, these days, is reserved only for legal aspects and covers only those drugs whose manufacture, distribution and prescribing comes under *Narcotic Drug Act*. The term *opiate analgesics*, though frequently used, is not satisfactory either. Opiate means "from opium"; but several analgesics

Table 37.1 Functional Characteristics of Opioid Receptors

Parameters	μ (mu)	κ (kappa)	δ (delta)	NOP receptor
Distribution[1]	Periaqueductal gray, thalamus, nucleus tractus solitarious, area postrema, dorsal horn	Cerebral cortex, striatum, midbrain, hippocampus, dorsal horn. medulla	Same areas as for kappa receptor; trigeminal nucleus, myenteric plexus	Hippocampus, cerebral cortex, sensory neurons, descending pain control cricuit
ANALGESIA Supraspinal Spinal Peripheral	 + + + (μ_1) + + (μ_2) + +	 + (κ_3) + (κ_1) + +	 — + + –	 +/– (Biphasic)[2] +/– (Biphasic)[2] +/– (Biphasic)[2]
Respiratory depression	+ + + (μ_2)	+	+ +	–
Euphoria	+ + + (μ_1)	–	–	–
Motivational effects/reward	+ +	–	+ +	+ +
Dysphoria	–	+ + +	–	–
Miosis	+ +	+	–	–
Constipation	+ + (μ_2)	+	+ +	–
Sedation	+ +	+ +	–	–
Physical dependence	+ + + (μ_1)	+	–	–
Agonist	Methadone* Endorphin Endomorphin 1 and 2	Dynorphin-A	Enkephalins	Nociceptin*
Antagonist	β-Funaltrexamine Naloxonazine* (μ_1)	Norbinaltorphimine*	Naltrindole*	Nocistatin*

1. Opioid receptors are also present in the ANS, peripheral nerves and GIT, where they affect blood pressure, nociception & GIT motility
2. Regulates basal pain sensitivity depending on the pre-existing state of pain, leading to biphasic hyperalgesic or analgesic activity.
* Selective action. Naloxone and Naltrexone are opioid antagonists at all the three types of opioid receptors ($\mu > \kappa > \delta$)

belonging to this group are not obtained from opium, as these are synthetic. The term *opioid analgesics* means "opium-like analgesics" and is grammatically as well as scientifically more correct. Hence throughout the text, the term "opioid" shall be used.

Opium is an extract of the juice of the poppy *Papaver somniferum.* The unripe seed capsules of the poppy plant are incised and the milky exudate is collected, dried and powdered. This is called opium powder. It contains two major groups of alkaloids.

i) ***Benzyl-isoquinoline group of alkaloids***: It contains two major alkaloids: ***Papaverine*** (1%) and ***Noscapine*** (6%). Papaverine has no analgesic properties. It is a directly acting smooth muscle relaxant and is occasionally used as vasodilator or to treat erectile dysfunction (Ch. 44). Noscapine is also not an analgesic but a cough suppressant (antitussive; Ch.49).

ii) ***Phenanthrene group of alkaloids***: Depending upon the source, the opium powder contains 8%–20% of ***morphine*** and 0.5%–2.5% of ***codeine*** along with some ***thebaine*** (0.2%–0.4%). Morphine and codeine are both prototype opioid analgesics while thebaine is not. It is a convulsant toxic drug.

The main drugs discussed in this section are:

- **Morphine Analogues**

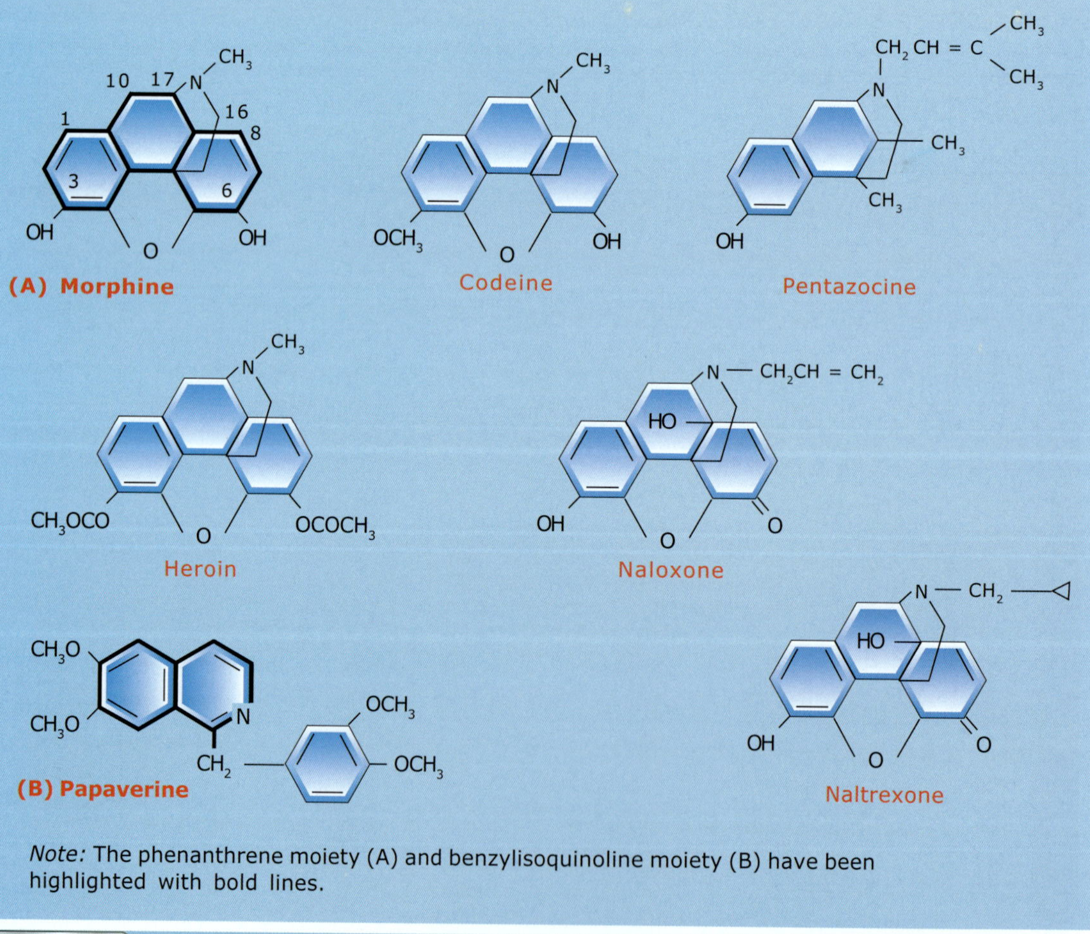

Note: The phenanthrene moiety (A) and benzylisoquinoline moiety (B) have been highlighted with bold lines.

Fig 37.4 Some Alkaloids Derived from Opium, and Structural Formulae of Opioid Agonists, Partial Agonists and Antagonists.

- *Agonists*: Morphine, Diamorphine (Heroin), Codeine, Pholcodeine, Levorphanol
- *Partial agonists*: Nalorphine, Levallorphan
- *Antagonists*: Naloxone, Naltrexone, Nalmefene

■ **Synthetic Derivatives Unrelated to Morphine**

- *Agonists*: Pethidine (Meperidine), Fentanyl, Sufentanil, Alfentanil, Remifentanil, Methadone, Oxycodone, Etorphine, Dextropropoxyphene
- *Partial agonists*: Pentazocine, Nalbuphine, Butorphanol, Buprenorphine.
- *μ (mu) Receptor agonist with other mode of action*: Tramadol,Tapentadol
- *Those lacking analgesic activity and having other uses*: Loperamide, Noscapine, Diphenoxylate, Dextromethorphan.

The structural formulae of morphine, some other agonists, partial agonists and antagonists have been depicted in Figure 37.4. The pharmacological actions described below for the prototype opioid agonist, *morphine*, can also be shared with other opioid agonists with some variations between individual drugs. Their characteristic features, compared to morphine, are listed in Table 37.2.

MORPHINE (PROTOTYPE OPIOID AGONIST)

Morphine is the prototype opioid analgesic (pure agonist) which is widely used for pain control. Therefore morphine is discussed in greater detail than other opioid analgesics and what is stated for morphine applies in general for other pure agonists as well. Significant differences that do exist between morphine and other opioid agonists have been summarised in Table 37.2.

A) Central Pharmacological Effects

1. Analgesia

Morphine increases pain threshold. The sites of opioid analgesia include periphery (μ) and both spinal (μ_2) and supraspinal (μ_1) brain areas, particularly limbic system. Opioid analgesics reduce both the sensory as well as the affective (emotional) components of pain (especially the affective component). Patient reports that pain is still there but is not hurting him much. Further, the opioids are generally more effective against dull, continuous pain such as deep seated visceral pain than a sharp intermittent integumentary pain. Neuropathic pain (e.g., trigeminal or peripheral nerve injury) is less responsive to opioids than is nociceptive pain (see earlier text). Elimination half-life of morphine increases with age and thus the pain relief provided by morphine increases with old age.

2. Euphoria, Dysphoria and Convulsions

Morphine causes an appreciable sense of well-being (μ_1). The distress and anxiety associated with pain are reduced. In patients who are distressed, *euphoria* is pronounced but in those who are accustomed to chronic dull pain, there is little or no euphoria. Some patients, however, complain of *dysphoria* (κ) characterised by restlessness and malaise. Although opioids usually depress polysynaptic responses but, in high doses, they can increase monosynaptic responses through supraspinal stimulation which can lead to *convulsions*.

3. Sedation

Drowsiness and clouding of judgement are frequently associated with opioid-induced analgesia. Sleep is induced more commonly in the elderly than in young. However, opioids disrupt the normal REM sleep pattern.

4. Respiratory Depression

Both analgesia (μ_1 and μ_2) and respiratory depression (μ_2) are mediated by μ receptors and, therefore, morphine-induced analgesia is directly proportional to respiratory depression in a dose-related fashion. Opioids depress respiration at the level of medulla controlling respiratory centre. In addition, they produce indifference towards breathing, but the patient starts breathing if commanded. However, the respiratory depression by opioids is not accompanied by depression of the medullary centers controlling CVS functions (in contrast to general anaesthetics and barbiturates). As a result, the respiratory depression produced by opioids is far better tolerated than a similar degree of depression caused by general anaesthetics and barbiturates. Nonetheless, the respiratory depression caused by opioids is a major undesirable effect as it occurs at therapeutic doses and it is the commonest cause

Table 37.2 Characteristics and Comparison of Opioid Analgesics

Drug	Receptor activity			Dose (mg) Parenteral*	Route	Use	Dependence liability	Remarks
	μ	κ	δ					
Morphine (prototype)	+++	+	+	10–15	IV, IM, SC	See text	See text	See text
Codeine	++	+	+	60	Oral, IM (mainly oral)	Mild analgesic Mainly cough suppressant	Much less than morphine Less euphoria	Less first-pass. Acts as a prodrug to morphine. Other substitutes: *Pholcodeine, dihydrocodeine*
Dextropropoxyphene	++	+	+	60–100	Oral only	Mild analgesic, usually combined with paracetamol	Very low Less euphoria	Less constipating than codeine. *Ethoheptazine* has similar features
Fentanyl	+++	–	+	0.05–0.1	IV, IM	Acute pain Neurolept-analgesia with droperidol	High, but shorter duration of action (1–1.5 hr) discourages its use	High potency allows even transdermal administration. Other substitutes. *Alfentanil* (0.5 hr) and *Sufentanil* (0.5–1 hr) have shorter duration of action and are more potent
Heroin (Diamorphine)	+++	+	+	3–5	IM	Banned drug. Use for chronic pain is irrational	High with euphoria (+++) and orgastic pleasure (++)	Rapid onset. High lipid solubility, better BBB penetration
Methadone	+++	–	–	5–10	IM, SC, oral	Chronic pain. Treatment of opioid withdrawal	Low; longer t ½ (40 hrs), hence less severe and gradual withdrawal effects (see text)	Less first-pass, less constipation. Less euphoria. Less sedation
Meperidine (Pethidine)	+++	+	+	50–100	IM, SC	Acute pain (less in use). Preanaesthetic medication. Postanaesthetic shivering	High. Least miosis as miosis due to morphine moiety is antagonised by mydriasis due to atropine moiety. Hence a favourite addicting drug among medical staff (no miosis; escape detection)	The metabolite norpethidine is toxic - risk of convulsions. Part structure related to atropine. No anti-tussive action, less histamine release, less constipation
Tramadol	+	–	–	50–100	Oral, IV	Postoperative or chronic neuropathic pain, labour pain	Low	Inhibit uptake of NE & 5-HT. Lesser resp. depression. Metabolite of trazodone. Lowers seizure threshold
Tapentadol	+	–	–	50–100	Oral	Postoperative and neuropathic pain	Low	Should be avoided in hepatic and renal failure, may precipitate seizure

* Only parenteral doses are given, although these can be administered by other routes.

of death in acute opioid poisoning. Tolerance to respiratory depression also develops more slowly compared to analgesic and euphoric effects.

5. Cough Suppression

Morphine and other agonists (e.g., codeine) are effective antitussives. Their cough suppressant effect, surprisingly, does not correlate proportionately with their analgesic and respiratory depressant effects, because several non-analgesic and non-respiratory depressant opioids (e.g. dextromethorphan and noscapine) are effective antitussives (see following text). In addition, suppression of cough reflex occurs at doses lower than those required to produce analgesia or to depress respiration. Tolerance, however, develops later to the antitussive actions of opioid analgesics.

6. Miosis

Miosis due to morphine is a centrally mediated effect caused by μ and κ receptor induced stimulation of III cranial nerve nucleus. There is no direct action on the circular or radial muscles of iris because there is no miosis if morphine solution is instilled in the eye. Tolerance to this effect does not develop and therefore opioid addicts continue to have pin-point pupil although they develop tolerance to other opioid effects. Pin-point pupil is also an important diagnostic sign in opioid toxicity because most other cases of poisoning, presented with coma and respiratory depression, have pupillary dilatation.

7. Nausea and Vomiting

Initially, opioids directly stimulate the CTZ and produce emesis; later they depress the vomiting centre. Hence, if vomiting occurs it would occur soon after the administration of morphine and would disappear with its repeated administration. There is some vestibular component to the nausea also, as vomiting occurs more frequently in ambulatory than in recumbent patients after giving morphine.

B) Peripheral Pharmacological Effects

1. Peripheral Analgesia

As discussed earlier in this chapter, opioid receptors are located both centrally as well as peripherally.

During inflammation, peripheral opioid receptors are up-regulated. The endogenous opioid peptides contained in monocytic cells or lymphocytes are then attracted to the site of inflammation and released to combat pain associated with tissue injury. Hence exogenously administered opioid agonist, directly to the site of inflammation (e.g., intra-articular injection of morphine in knee joints), can provide an effective peripheral analgesia.

2. Gastrointestinal Tract: Morphine and most opioid pure agonists produce uncomfortable constipation (μ_2) by increasing the sphincter tone and reducing the motility by producing spasm all along the GIT. They also delay the gastric emptying. Opioids also decrease the awareness for the necessity to defecate, which also partly contributes towards constipation. Through an action on delta receptors, morphine and endogenous peptides (enkephalins and beta-endorphins) also reduce secretion of Na^+, K^+Cl^- from the intestinal mucosa. Tolerance to the constipative and anti-secretory effects of opioids does not occur. The GIT actions form the basis for their use in the management of diarrhoea, specially due to decreased secretion of water and electrolytes from the entric mucosa. Rats and mice, after administration of morphine, exhibit a characteristic "*Straub tail reaction*", which is presented with raising and stiffening of the tail caused by the spasm and increased tone of the muscle at the base of the tail.

3. Biliary Tract: Pressure in the biliary tract increases as opioids cause contraction of gall bladder and constriction of the sphincter of Oddi. Consequently, opioids should be avoided in patient suffering from biliary colic caused by gall stone. Morphine holds back pancreatic juice and increases serum amylase concentration. Hence it should also be avoided in pancreatitis.

4. Urinary Bladder: Constriction of the urinary sphincter can cause difficulty in urination, while contraction of detrusor muscle makes urgency to urinate, which often is very troublesome to the patient. Consequently, catheterisation becomes necessary in such situations.

5. Other Smooth Muscles

Opioids in therapeutic doses do not produce significant bronchoconstriction *per se* but may aggravate an asthmatic attack resulting in part from histamine release. Increased uterine tone may significantly prolong labour and may increase neonatal morbidity due to bronchoconstriction and foetal respiratory depression.

6. Cardiovascular Effects

The vasomotor center of medulla is relatively unaffected by opioid analgesics and hence CVS actions are usually minor at analgesic doses. Postural hypotension and bradycardia seen with larger doses of opioids occur partly due to histamine release and partly due to inhibition of adrenergic tone centrally. Increased Pco_2 levels lead to cerebral vasodilatation and an increase in intracranial pressure.

C) Tolerance

Tolerance develops over days with continued use of morphine. Tolerance does not develop uniformly to all opioid effects. In general, tolerance develops to the depressant effects of opioids but not to the stimulant effects. Thus, tolerance develops to opioid induced analgesia, euphoria, sedation and respiratory depression, but not to **m**iosis, **c**onstipation and **c**onvulsions (to remember: MCC). Consequently, the addicts can tolerate 50 times the normal analgesic dose of morphine with relatively little discomfort due to respiratory depression but have marked symptoms of constipation and miosis. The tolerance to respiratory effects develops rather slowly compared to analgesic effects. As a result, for any addict, there is always an opioid dose capable of producing death by respiratory depression till tolerance develops. *Cross tolerance* occurs between opioids acting at the same receptor but not between opioids acting on different receptors. Partial agonists induce tolerance to the agonist actions only, not to the antagonist effects. The antagonists, such as naloxone, do not induce tolerance to their own actions.

The tolerance to opioids is a **cellular adaptive type of tolerance,** as it does not result due to their increased metabolic degradation, or due to inhibition of the release of endogenous opioid peptides. Two mechanisms are, however, suggested: **(a)** tolerance may develop due to long-term desensitisation or down-regulation of receptor-effector coupling mechanisms that are not properly understood; **(b)** there may be some intracellular mechanism which involves a compensatory increase in Ca^{2+} levels in the cells, increased production of cAMP, decreased efflux of K^+ and the resultant return of the release of neurotransmitters and neuromodulators to normal levels (see Ch.38).

D) Dependence

Morphine produces pronounced ***physical dependence,*** as its abuse potential is high and its cessation is characterised by life-threatening withdrawal (abstinence) syndrome which are opposite to its pharmacological effects. The withdrawal symptoms, therefore, include pain, hyperventilation, coughing, mydriasis, hypertension, diarrhoea, dysphoria, agitation and piloerection (cold turkey). However, emesis remains common as a withdrawal effect as well as a pharmacological action.

There is some *psychological dependence* also which contributes more to drug-seeking behaviour than does physical dependence. Opioids facilitate DA transmission in mesocortical or mesolimbic pathways and thus activate endogenous reward pathways in the brain (Ch. 38). Babies born to opioid-addicted women also exhibit withdrawal signs but because of slower metabolism of opioids in newborn, these symptoms are mild. Abrupt withdrawal rebound is usually considered as "nor-adrenergic storm". The rate of firing of locus ceruleus neurons is reduced by opioids and is increased during withdrawal. The treatment of opioid withdrawal has been discussed in Chapter 38.

E) Miscellaneous Effects

- Opioids induce the release of histamine which leads to itching sensation and bronchoconstriction associated with its use.
- There is evidence in humans that the long-term use of opioids depresses the immune system (T-helper and T-suppressor cells) leading to increased susceptibility to infection.
- Opioid analgesics, through stimulation of μ and δ receptors in hypothalamic nuclei, decrease the release of DA and thus increase the release of prolactin. Opioids also bind in the supraoptic nuclei of hypothalamus and increase the release of ADH.

Pharmacokinetics

Oral morphine is subject to extensive first-pass metabolism—mainly glucuronide conjugation in the gut wall and liver. As a result only about 20% of the dose reaches the systemic circulation. Its preferred routes of administration are I.V., I.M. or S.C. Yet, morphine is now available for *oral use* in *controlled release tablet* to produce longer lasting analgesia in patient suffering from chronic cancer pain. Anaesthetists sometimes prefer to administer morphine intrathecally, the advantage being that it provides very effective analgesia, avoiding undesirable respiratory depressant effects.

Morphine crosses BBB less readily than heroin, but easily crosses placental barrier causing respiratory distress to foetus at birth. Further, glucuronidation by the foetus is slow, which may lengthen its t½.

The conjugated metabolites are usually inactive with an exception of morphine-6-glucuronide which has high affinity for μ receptors and is a potent analgesic. Excretion of the metabolites requires adequate renal function, as their main route of excretion is renal; other routes are of minor importance. Glucuronides also reach the gut *via* biliary secretion where these are deconjugated and hydrolysed. Most of the morphine is then reabsorbed and undergoes enterohepatic circulation.

Clinical Uses of Morphine and Other Opioids (Remember ALAAD)

1. As Analgesic

Opioids are used for relief of moderate to severe deep- seated visceral pain such as pain associated with MI, renal colic, traumatic, postoperative and cancer pain. *Controlled release morphine* or oxycodone tablets are available for *oral administration* to treat continuous pain in cancer patients. I.M. or S.C. route is preferred to control postoperative pain. *Transdermal patch* is a good alternative for patients with chronic pain who are unable to take opioids orally. A controlled-release transdermal patch is available for fentanyl. *Buccal transmucosal* fentanyl can be used for episodes of breakthrough pain. *Nasal preparation* of strong opioids have recently been approved and introduced. *Intra-articular injection* of morphine in knee joints can produce an efficacious peripheral analgesia. Combinations of codeine or dextropropoxyphene with NSAIDs are supra-additive and are used to treat milder pain such as headache and neuralgias. ***Patient Controlled Analgesia (PCA)*** is a new alternative method of self-administration of an opioid agonist by parenteral route (usually I.V.). The use of an indwelling catheter allows the patient to administer the drug (usually fentanyl) at frequent intervals for relief of severe pain. *PCA system* allows the patients the freedom to self-assess the need to push a tailored dose of an opioid. *Paradoxically, dependence is rarely observed in patients using PCA for acute pain management.* However, the patient has to be trained for such administration.

2. Acute Left-Ventricular Failure (LVF)

Morphine (I.V.) is the most commonly used drug for the treatment of dyspnoea associated with LVF. Morphine reduces anxiety associated with shortness of breath in these patients, and also decreases cardiac preload (reduced venous tone) and afterload (reduced peripheral resistance).

3. Cough Suppressant (Antitussive)

Codeine and its analogues suppress cough in sub-analgesic doses. Some non-analgesic, non-addictive opioid derivatives are used primarily as antitussives (see following text).

4. In Anaesthetic Practice

Pethidine is used for preanaesthetic medication for its sedative and analgesic properties (Ch. 31). Fentanyl and its analogues are the primary components of neurolept-analgesia, neurolept-anaesthesia and balanced anaesthesia (Ch. 31). Fentanyl (I.V. or epidural) is used to provide anaesthesia during coronary bypass grafting because it has no cardiovascular toxicity. *Intrathecal or epidural injection* of morphine (or fentanyl) produces long-lasting and effective segmental anaesthesia, which may be useful for critically ill patients at risk for respiratory depression and other autonomic side effects.

5. Diarrhoea

Some synthetic non-analgesic, non-addictive opioid derivatives like diphenoxylate and loperamide are used primarily to control non-infectious acute diarrhoea (see following text).

Adverse Effects

From the on-going discussion, the adverse effects and contraindications of opioids become self evident. Given S.C. or I.M., morphine 10 mg is usually adequate to provide an effective analgesia. With 15 mg I.M., adverse effects appear. The toxic effects of morphine are obviously an extension of its pharmaclogical effects and include: **(a)** respiratory depression, **(b)** constipation, **(c)** bronchospasm (due to histamine release), **(d)** postural hypotension (see above), **(e)** urinary retention, **(f)** nausea and vomiting, **(g)** urticaria and itching (due to histamine release), **(h)** tolerance (on prolonged use) and **(i)** dependence (on prolonged use; see above).

Acute (overdose) Poisoning

Opioid poisoning may be accidental or suicidal or seen in drug addicts due to overdosing. In a normal adult, 50 mg of morphine (I.M.) produces acute toxicity, which is presented by coma, severe respiratory depression, pin-point pupils, occasional jerks, convulsions and cyanosis. Pulmonary oedema occurs at terminal stage and finally respiratory failure leads to death.

Treatment consists of: **(a)** Supportive measures like maintenance of blood pressure and respiratory support, **(b)** gastric lavage with potassium permanganate to remove unabsorbed drug and that coming through enterohepatic circulation, and **(c)** use of the ***specific antidote***: ***naloxone*** 0.4–0.8 mg I.V. repeatedly after every five minutes till respiration recovers and then repeated every 1–3 hrs later, till morphine is cleared out of the body.

Contraindications

Morphine is contraindicated in **5H** and **3B** conditions noted below:

1. **H**ypotension (itself causes postural hypotension).
2. **H**epatic damage (itself metabolised by liver).
3. **H**ypertrophy of prostate (due to urinary retention).
4. **H**ead injury (elevated Pco_2 will worsen raised intracranial pressure. Pin point pupils will also mask the prognosis).
5. **H**ypothyroidism (prolonged and exaggerated response to opioids).

1. **B**ronchial asthma (worsening due to histamine release; also builds up mucus in lungs due to antitussive action).
2. **B**iliary colic (itself causes spasm of sphincter of Oddi).
3. **B**abies (infants are more susceptible to respiratory depression due to morphine).

Drug Interactions

1. If opioids are given by epidural route, the use of corticosteroids should be stopped 2 weeks prior to the insertion of catheter to prevent chances of infection, as opioids increase immunosuppressive effects of steroids.
2. Any opioid partial agonist should not be given to the patients receiving pure opioid agonist as there is a risk of precipitating severe and abrupt withdrawal symptoms besides decreasing analgesia.
3. MAO inhibitors potentiate the effects of morphine by slowing its metabolism.
4. Morphine and other opioids exhibit intense sedation when combined with other sedatives such as alcohol, barbiturates and antipsychotics.

Recently Approved Opioid

Oliceridine

Oliceridine is a recently approved opioid drug by the US-FDA. It acts as a selective μ-opioid receptor agonist. It is not effective orally, given intravenously. Oliceridine exerts significant analgesic effects within 5–20 min following administration but dissipates quickly due to short half-life (1–3 hrs). Oliceridine is used for the management of acute severe pain, if inadequate treatment or require i.v. opioid analgesic. *Adverse effects*: Nausea, vomiting, sedation, headache, respiratory depression, tolerance and dependence.

MIXED AGONIST-ANTAGONISTS AND PARTIAL AGONISTS

These were developed with a hope that such drugs would be potent analgesics devoid of dependence and abuse liability. However, it was soon realised that neither these are free from tolerance and dependence nor they are useful analgesics because of their dysphoric effects. Mixed agonist-antagonists differ from morphine in that **(1)** They lack full agonist activity at μ-receptors—hence lesser risk of respiratory depression, constipation, tolerance and dependence but with lesser efficacy than morphine as analgesics; **(2)** They exhibit moderate agonist activity at κ-receptors—hence dysphoric, psychotomimetic or even hallucinatory (at high dose) effects; **(3)** Facilitate NE release—hence ↑in HR, force of contraction and even BP (in high doses) and **(4)** Precipitate withdrawal syndrome, because of some antagonist (partial agonist) actions at μ receptors (if administered along with pure agonists).

Pentazocine

Receptor action: μ (weak antagonist); κ (moderate agonist); δ (weak agonist).

Pentazocine is effective orally, though it has a high first-pass effect (Dose: 50–100 mg QID orally). It is indicated for postoperative moderately severe pain such as burns and trauma. Its dysphoric and psychotomimetic effects limit its use in chronic cancer pain. It is contraindicated in **(1)** patients of MI (as it increases HR and cardiac workload), **(2)** epileptic cases (as it decreases seizure threshold), **(3)** psychoses (because of its psychotomimetic effects) and **(4)** head injury (as it increases intracranial pressure). Because of such unpleasant effects the abuse potential is low. Nevertheless, tolerance and physical dependence do develop on repeated use. It can precipitate abstinence syndrome in morphine addicts (see above). Pentazocine with tripelennamine (antihistamine) produces euphoric effects equal to heroin. Hence heroin addicts use this combination in absence of heroin and not pentazocine alone.

Nalbuphine

Receptor action: μ (moderate antagonist); κ (moderate partial agonist); δ (weak agonist ?).

It is a pentazocine analogue which is equipotent to morphine and 5 times more potent than pentazocine when administered parenterally. However, its efficacy is less than morphine. It produces less dysphoria and fewer psychotomimetic side effects (may be because of no δ action). It does not cause cardiovascular stimulation either. It precipitates withdrawal in morphine addicts. Abuse potential is low. It is used for moderate to severe pain and for obstetrical analgesia (Dose: 10 mg I.V. or I.M. QID).

Butorphanol

Receptor action: μ (partial agonist); κ (strong agonist); δ (no action).

Though more potent than pentazocine, it has lesser efficacy than morphine, i.e., higher doses do not proportionately induce respiratory depression or analgesia. Dysphoric and psychotomimetic effects are less marked. Blood pressure is not affected. Abuse potential is low, withdrawal effects are mild. It is less likely to precipitate withdrawal symptoms in an opioid-dependent person. It is usually given parenterally as its oral bioavailability is low. Nasal spray formulation is also available. It is used for postoperative and other short-lasting pain. Paradoxically, butorphanol produces significantly greater analgesia in women than men (Dose: 0.5–2 mg I.V. QID).

Buprenorphine

Receptor action: μ (strong partial agonist); κ (moderate antagonist); δ (mild antagonist ?); NOP receptor (agonist).

It is 25–35 times more potent than morphine. Being a strong partial agonist at μ receptor it is more liable to cause respiratory depression along with analgesia but with least dysphoria. It binds to μ receptors with high affinity and dissociates very slowly. Consequently, (a) its respiratory depressant effects are not readily reversed by *naloxone* which makes its unsuitable for obstetric use and (b) makes it an attractive alternative to *methadone* for management of opioid withdrawal (Ch. 38). Like pentazocine it is used for controlling moderate to severe pain. Sublingual preparations are also available. Abuse potential is less than morphine (Dose: 0.3–0.6 mg I.M or slow I.V., QID).

Nalorphine

Receptor action: μ (moderate antagonist); κ (moderate agonist); δ (no action). Its use is now obsolete.

MU (μ) RECEPTOR AGONIST WITH OTHER MODE OF ACTION

Tramadol

It is a synthetic opioid with unique dual-action analgesic that acts by activating μ receptor weakly as compared to morphine and inhibiting the reuptake of serotonin and noradrenaline (NA) similar to tricyclic antidepressant drugs in the CNS. It has been suggested that the weak μ receptor agonistic activity is reinforced by activating the monoaminergic pain inhibitory pathways in the spinal cord. It appear to be 10-time less potent than morphine. The drug is administered orally or parenterally in the dose of 50–100 mg daily to treat acute mild to moderate (labour pain) and chronic neuropathic pain (Table 37.2). Tramadol has been reported to lower the seizure threshold and may produce increased risk of suicidal ideation and behaviour. Therefore, this analgesic should not be given with antidepressant drugs which have similar potential for such adverse reactions.

Tapentadol

Like tramadol, tapentadol acts as analgesic by dual mechanism of action mediated by μ receptor agonist and inhibition of the uptake of noradrenaline (NA) in the CNS. It is effective in moderate to severe pain and in a dose dependent (50,75,100 mg) manner when administered orally every 4–6 hr intervals. After single oral dose serum concentration peaks at 1.25 hrs and terminal t½ is 4 hrs. This drug is not recommended in people with severe hepatic and renal failure or a history of seizure. As tapentadol inhibits NA reuptake, it should not be given with MAO inhibitors. CNS depression can occur if tapentadol taken with other centrally acting drugs, including alcohol.

OPIOID ANTAGONISTS

The substitution of N-methyl by a bulkier N-allyl group at piperidine nitrogen changes an agonist to an antagonist (Fig. 37.4). ***Naloxone, naltrexone*** and ***nalmefene*** are pure opioid competitive antagonists at all the three types (μ, κ, δ) of opioid receptors. However, they block μ receptors at lower doses than those required to block κ and δ receptors. Given alone to non-addicts or opioid-free person, these antagonists exhibit no pharmacological effects. No tolerance, dependence or withdrawal effects have been noticed.

Naloxone

Receptor action: μ (strong antagonist); κ (moderate antagonist); δ (weak antagonist).

Naloxone has a fast onset of action (minutes) with a plasma half life of 1–2 hrs. It has an extensive first-pass metabolism which considerably reduces its oral bioavailability. Naloxone is primarily used for the treatment of opioid overdose. When given I.V. to such patient, naloxone will dramatically reverse the opioid effects within minutes and would effectively normalise respiration, level of consciousness, pupil size, bowel activity and awareness of pain. However, because of its shorter duration of action the patient who promptly recovers after a single dose of naloxone swiftly proceeds to respiratory depression and coma, after 1–2 hrs. Hence, naloxone should be given in a dose of 0.4–0.8 mg I.V. every 5 min till the desired parameters become normal. Thereafter, additional doses may be given I.V. or I.M. every 30–60 min till all the opioid is cleared off the body, to prevent the relapse. Naloxone can also be used to reverse the agonist actions of mixed agonist-antagonists overdose (e.g., of pentazocine). It also inhibits acupuncture analgesia because the latter is associated with the release of endogenous opioid peptides. The lack of response to naloxone in a case of respiratory depression of unknown cause is highly suggestive of a non-opioid drug intoxication.

It can also be used as a diagnostic test for a case of opioid addiction as naloxone in such cases will almost instantaneously precipitate an opioid withdrawal syndrome. It is also used to revert neonatal respiratory depression, due to opioid use during labour. Side effects of naloxone are only minor.

Naltrexone

Receptor action: μ (strong antagonist); κ (strong antagonist); δ (weak antagonist).

Naltrexone is 3–5 times as potent as naloxone and has a longer duration of action (t½ 10–12 hrs). It exhibits significant first-pass metabolism in liver, but its major metabolite is also equally active and hence it can be administered orally. Its pharmacokinetic parameters suggest that it can be used for treatment of opioid dependence in an opioid detoxified, formerly addict patient. It is a good maintenance drug for treating addicts, but before initiating the treatment an opioid-free period of 10 days is essential. For this a great deal of motivation is needed. Doubts can be verified by performing a naloxone challenge test. Naltrexone is also reported to decrease craving for alcohol in chronic alcoholics. Side effects are minor but high doses are hepatotoxic.

Methylnaltrexone

It is a quarternary derivate of naltrexone. When administered orally it acts locally as powerful μ receptor antagonist in the intestine and relieves the GI spasm in patients of opioid toxicity and dependence. It has been approved by the FDA in 2016 for the treatment of opioid induced GI spasmodic pain, and constipation in terminally ill patients who take high doses of morphine to relieve metastatic cancer pain.

Nalmefene

It is a naltrexone derivative but can be used only intravenously. It can be used like naloxone to treat opioid overdose. It lacks hepatotoxicity of naltrexone. It has been approved for the treatment of cholestatic pruritus (20 mg BD) also.

Alvimopan

It predominantly blocks peripheral μ receptor in the gut (μ_2) and does not cross BBB. Hence, it has been approved for relieving constipation of an opium addict without risking the precipitation of opiate withdrawal. (μ_1). It is also used to treat postoperative paralytic ileus following bowel resection.

OPIOIDS HAVING LEAST ANALGESIC, LEAST DEPENDENCE BUT SELECTIVE ACTIONS

Antitussives

The larger the substituent at the phenolic-OH group at C-3, the greater is the antitussive action of the opioid drug. Such antitussive drugs in opioid series are ***dextromethorphan, noscapine*** and ***benzonatate.*** These drugs act centrally on the medullary cough centre, exhibit no analgesia and possess negligible abuse liability. Their side effects are minimal at therapeutic doses. *Benzonatate*, besides depressing central cough mechanisms, also acts by inhibiting stretch receptors of respiratory mucosa.

Antidiarrhoeals

Diphenoxylate (active metabolite *difenoxin*) and ***loperamide*** are used as antidiarrhoeals and not as analgesics. The likelihood of their abuse is remote as they have a very limited access to the brain and mainly acts on opioid μ receptors in the intestine.

CHAPTER 38

Drug Dependence and Drug Abuse

COMPETENCY PH1.22, PH1.23

DEFINITIONS AND TERMINOLOGY

The professionals in the field of drug abuse and drug addiction have so much diverse background, that adopting a common definition for terms such as drug abuse, misuse, habituation, addiction and dependence becomes very difficult if not impossible. *Polydrug abuse* further complicates the conclusions drawn from epidemiology and clinical studies, because users often attempt to modify the selected drug effects by coabusing drugs with opposite pharmacological effects.

Indiscriminate use of any drug, other than a CNS stimulant or depressant drug, is called its MISUSE, e.g., misuse of laxatives, purgatives or of antibiotics etc., while the misuse of any CNS stimulant or a depressant drug is called its ABUSE. The term abuse also, unfortunately, has different meanings for different people. It also means any use of a drug for nonmedical purposes, not only for altering consciousness or mood but also for body building. Till 1964, DEPENDENCE was considered as biological phenomenon often associated with 'drug abuse', but its precise scientific meaning was not clear. For example, if someone is occasionally taking alprazolam, as self-medication, to relieve anxiety, then it may be a drug abuse without dependence, whereas if a diabetic person is taking insulin every day, he is dependent on insulin without any drug abuse or misuse. Similarly there could be misuse of laxatives/purgatives leading to dependence. The problem was that the term dependence was being used indiscriminately with no demarcations between its literal and scientific meaning. These discrepancies were resolved later (see below).

Almost all abused substances or drugs produce an effect on the brain that is perceived as desirable and will initiate a ***"drug seeking behaviour"***. The properties of the drug that are responsible for drug seeking behaviour are often referred to as ***"reinforcing properties"***. These drugs produce effects that are so desirable that the user is compelled to get more of the drug. The primary reinforcing property of the drug is the "*positive affective state*" called EUPHORIA that it produces. This term indicates anything from pleasantness or a sense of well-being to an excitement resembling orgastic pleasure. Euphoria is considered to be a "*positive reinforcing*" property of the drug that an individual would desire or would like to seek. In addition, the drug can also function as "*negative reinforcer*" in that it offers relief from a negative affective state, e.g., DYSPHORIA.

Chronic exposure to reinforcing drugs can lead to *drug addiction* (again an imprecise term, see following text) which is characterised by an increase in drug seeking behaviour called CRAVING. The evaluation of drugs for their craving or reinforcing property forms the basis for assessing their ABUSE POTENTIAL. The abuse potential of a drug can be qualitatively assessed (strong, moderate or mild) on a rodent model by implanting a cannula in the reward area (mesolimbic area) of the brain. In an animal cage, a bar is placed in such a way that pressing the bar automatically delivers a fixed dose of the trial drug to the animal. If the animal eventually and repeatedly presses the bar or tries to overcome the intentionally placed obstacles, to press the bar, it can be concluded that the drug has a positive reinforcing behaviour, i.e., abuse potential.

The older terms, HABITUATION and ADDICTION are not scientifically defined but surprisingly have not been completely abolished yet from the textbooks. The term ***habituation*** can be used if **(a)** *the detrimental effects of the abused drug* are restricted to the person himself and *not to the society*, **(b)** there is *no intense craving for seeking the drug*, **(c)** there is *no development of tolerance* and **(d)** *there are no distressful withdrawal effects*, i.e., there is *no necessity or physical need to continue with the drug* for the fear of abstinence syndrome. Examples include taking tea or coffee. *Addiction* involved the recurrent abuse of a drug where the individual becomes so obsessed to procure and use the drug that it becomes his primary aim, which in turn disrupts his abilities to adjust in the family, the society or at his place of work. ***Addiction*** included the following features: **(a)** *the detrimental effects of the drug* not only *harm* the individual but *the society as well*, **(b)** there is always *an intense craving to procure the drug by any means*, **(c)** there is *development of tolerance* and hence a need to increase the dose to get the same rewarding experience, and **(d)** *there are life-threatening or alarming withdrawal effects* after cessation of the drug and hence there is a *physical need to continue with the use of the drug for the fear of abstinence syndrome.* However, as it may be noticed, the features of habituation and addiction might also overlap and the terminology may become misleading. Consider a person who was a regular user of marijuana and *only once he had such intense craving* (due to environmental settings) that he committed a crime to procure this drug. On the contrary, consider a medical professional but an opioid (pethidine) addict who regularly had an intense craving for the drug but never committed any crime as his operation theatre staff and doctor friends were regularly obliging him for his requirements. In first case the craving was caught while in second case it remained unnoticed. Hence in 1974–75, WHO deleted all such terms (like habituation and addiction) and introduced another term called DRUG DEPENDENCE which meant: **a)** a state arising from *repeated, periodic* or *continuous use of a drug*, **(b)** a state which includes *all types of detrimental effects,* whether to himself, to the family, to the society or to the career, **(c)** a state that includes *all grades of craving* to procure the drug, and **(d)** a state which includes *all types of psychological and physical needs* to continue with the use of the drug for the *fear of getting distressful withdrawal effects*. Thus WHO provided a wider canvas for presenting the picture by using the terms such as "all grades of craving", "all types of psychological or physical needs" and "all sorts of detrimental effects" etc.

Besides drug abuse, many self-gratifying drug seekers also inhale different types of volatile substances that may affect CNS. These may include lacquer-paint solvents, petrol, nail polish remover or any pressurised aerosol or liquid petroleum gas. This type of abuse was earlier classified separately as *substance abuse*. Later on the Diagnostic and Statistical Manual of Mental Disorders 4Ed, (DSM-IV, 1994), and the one published by American Psychiatric Association (DSM-IV TR2000) recommended the use of a single term "SUBSTANCE ABUSE" to include *all sorts of drug abuse* including even those used for body building and inhalation of different types of volatile substances. Similarly, the manual suggests the use of a single term "SUBSTANCE DEPENDENCE" in place of so many confusing terms, like habituation, addiction and drug dependence.

Substance dependence requires at least 3 (even more) of the following symptoms to be present for diagnosis: **(1)** development of tolerance, **(2)** distressful abstinence syndrome after cessation of the drug, **(3)** persistent desire to use the drug (craving) or failure to cut down its use, **(4)** substance use in larger amounts than intended, **(5)** withdrawal from social, occupational or recreational activities, **(6)** considerable time spent for obtaining the drug which becomes his life-style, e.g., visiting multiple doctors, quacks or his contacts in illicit drug trade, and **(7)** continued use despite health, social, economic, family and legal problems resulting from substance use.

The DSM-IV TR criteria for ***substance abuse*** requires at least one (or more) of the following symptoms to be present for diagnosis: **(1)** recurrent substance use resulting in a failure to fulfill his/her major obligations at work, school or home (e.g., repeated absence or poor performance at work; expulsion from school), **(2)** recurrent substance use even in situations where it should not be used, e.g., during driving; operating a machine or operating upon the patient, **(3)** recurrent substance-use despite punitive action, e.g., punishment for disorderly conduct, and **(4)** recurrent substance-use despite having interpersonal and family problems, e.g., arguments or physical fight with spouse about the consequences of abuse. The "substance abuse" discards all other terms like misuse, abuse or habituation. Substance abuse does not apply on taking tea, coffee or smoking 10 cigarettes a day without inhalation.

TOLERANCE, DEPENDENCE, REBOUND, RELAPSE, WITHDRAWAL AND DETOXIFICATION

Tolerance develops if, after repeated administration, a given dose of a drug produces a decreased effect than expected, or conversely, when larger doses are needed to obtain the effects obtained with previous dose. It may be classified as *pharmacokinetic* (as with barbiturates) or *pharmacodynamic* (as with opioids) or as *reverse tolerance* (*sensitisation*, as with cocaine). For details refer Chapter 7. Related to this is ***cross tolerance*** where, once tolerance to primary drug develops, the individual also exhibits cross tolerance to related classes of drugs. For instance, individuals tolerant to morphine are also tolerant to other opioids and chronic alcoholics are also tolerant to benzodiazepines or even general anaesthetics. ***Dependence*** is a physiological state of neuroadaptation (see below) resulting from repeated administration of the drug, necessitating its continued use to prevent the appearance of distressing withdrawal (abstinence) syndrome which is manifested as opposite to the pharmacological effects of the drug. ***Cross dependence*** means the ability of a drug to suppress the manifestations of withdrawal (or physical dependence, see below) produced by another drug. ***Withdrawal*** or ***abstinence syndrome*** is a term used for the adverse (sometimes life threatening) psychologic and physiologic reactions to an abrupt discontinuation of a dependence-producing drug.

The ***substance dependence*** may be of two types: PSYCHOLOGICAL (PSYCHIC) DEPENDENCE which is characterised by **(a)** moderate compulsive drug seeking behaviour (craving) for personal satisfaction, e.g., cigarette smoking, **(b)** tolerance may or may not be present and if present it is usually either of pharmacokinetic type or tachyphylaxis but rarely pharmacodynamic (cellular adaptive), and **(c)** withdrawal effects are less frequent and mild which can be tolerated as these are never life threatening. PHYSICAL DEPENDENCE is characterised by **(a)** intense craving for the drug, e.g., alcohol, opioid use, **(b)** tolerance is invariably present (mainly pharmacodynamic type), and **(c)** withdrawal effects are severe and distressing manifested by symptoms that are frequently opposite to those sought by the abuser. *Psychological (psychic) dependence* appears prior to *physical (physiological) dependence* but inevitably does not lead to it. Agents having physical dependence do possess psychic dependence as well, but reverse may not be true. Physical dependence is closely associated with the phenomenon of tolerance but the reverse may not be true.

Rebound means an exaggerated manifestation of the original disease symptoms experienced immediately after discontinuation of the drug providing the clinical benefits, e.g., *rebound hypertension* occurring after sudden discontinuation of clonidine or β-blockers. Rebound phenomenon should not be confused with withdrawal syndrome as there is no craving or dysphoria after the cessation of the drug. ***Relapse*** refers to re-occurrence of the same disease symptoms, from which the patient suffered, after discontinuation of the treating drug, e.g., if a diabetic person suddenly stops taking insulin, there would be *relapse* of diabetes (not rebound or withdrawal syndrome). ***Detoxification*** (in drug abuse terminology) means slow tapering of the drug that has caused dependence and would cause withdrawal if stopped suddenly. It can be accomplished either by slowly withdrawing the dependence producing drug or by substituting the cross-dependent drug (see below) so that the neuroadaptive mechanisms can slowly become normal without causing withdrawal symptoms. Tapering of the doses of β-blockers or clonidine, to prevent rebound hypertension, is not called detoxification but *tapered-dose discontinuation.*

WHY PEOPLE GO FOR DRUGS

The "drive(s)" that induce a person to resort to drugs are outlined below along with neuropharmacological aspects of drug reinforcement and reward

(Fig. 38.1). The "drives" include: **(a)** to get relief from tension and anxiety, **(b)** to satisfy their curiosity about the "*kicks and pleasure*" the drugs provide, **(c)** to show their identity by exhibiting hostility towards the society, **(d)** a notion of being accepted by the Hi-Fi modern society, and also **(e)** a notion that drugs provide new ideas for creativity.

The "drive(s)" cited above bring a normal person to a "drive state" and to cope with this situation, he has two options: (a) either to fight with the situation and circumstances with full determination or to become an escapist or to try other resorts to allay the anxiety or (b) to obtain "chemical vacation" from intolerable drives with the help of drugs. The choice of the drug would depend on his personality traits, e.g., an extrovert person would prefer stimulant drugs like amphetamine while an introvert person would like to go for opioids or barbiturates. If the drug provides a quick and better relief, the tendency to reinforce increases. That means whenever a "drive state" arises next time, the desire to seek the drug will be reinforced. The *reinforcement power* of the commonly abused drugs is given below (Fig. 38.2).

DRUGS OF ABUSE THAT ENGENDER DEPENDENCE

- ***Agents having only mild psychological (psychic) dependence (low withdrawal, no physical dependence)***

  Coffee, Tea, Cigarette smoking (up to 10 cigarettes a day, without inhalation).

- ***Agents with moderate to severe psychological dependence (low withdrawal, slight physical dependence).***

  Marijuana, Hashish (psychic dependence mild; physical dependence doubtful; tolerance may develop). **LSD** (psychic dependence mild, physical dependence nil, tolerance ±). **Amphetamines, Cocaine** (psychic dependence severe, physical dependence mild, tolerance mild).

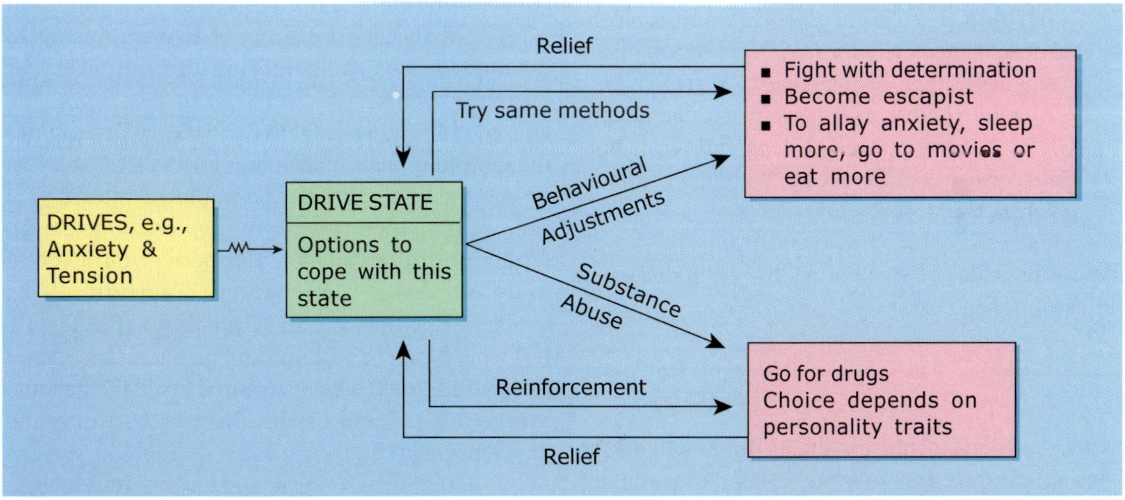

Fig 38.1 Interplay Between the Drives, Drive-state and Restoration to Drugs

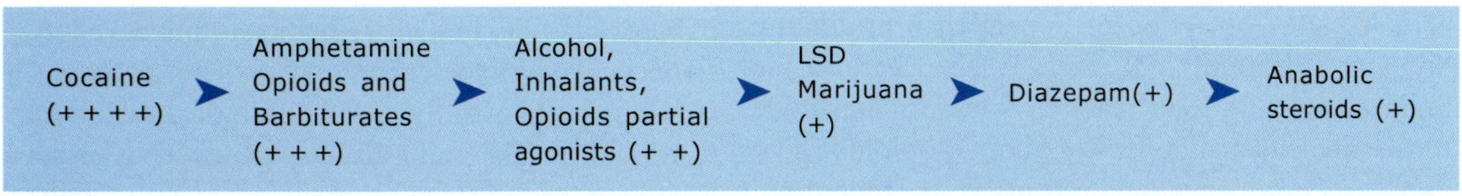

Fig 38.2 The Reinforcement Power of Commonly Abused Drugs

Nicotine (20 cigarettes or more a day with inhalation) (psychological dependence severe, physical dependence mild, withdrawal effects low). **Inhalants** (psychic dependence moderate, physical dependence nil, withdrawal effects low, tolerance ±).

- ***Agents having moderate to severe psychological dependence with mild physical dependence***

  Benzodiazepines (moderate psychic dependence, mild physical dependence on moderate and prolonged use, withdrawal effects mild, tolerance occurs, mechanism uncertain – self induction?)

  Alcohol (moderate use) (severe psychic dependence, mild physical dependence, mild withdrawal effects, tolerance develops).

- ***Agents having severe psychological and physical dependence***

  Opioids (severe psychic as well as physical dependence, pharmacodynamic tolerance marked, withdrawal effects severe and precipitated by naloxone).

  Barbiturates (severe psychic as well as physical dependence, withdrawal effects severe, pharmacokinetic type of tolerance)

  Alcohol (heavy use) (severe psychic dependence, moderate physical dependence on prolonged use, tolerance occurs, withdrawal effects severe).

Abuse potential of these drugs has been discussed in earlier chapters.

NEUROPHARMACOLOGY OF THE REWARD AND REINFORCEMENT

Almost all dependence-producing drugs activate the "reward-reinforcement pathway" called the mesolimbic dopaminergic pathway. Some even consider this to be the "pleasure centre" of the brain and dopamine as a "pleasure neurotransmitter". Even though the primary sites of action of dependence producing drugs are different and generally elsewhere in the brain, all these drugs increase the release of dopamine in the nucleus accumbens. Although opioids (μ, κ and δ receptors), cannabinoids (CB_1 receptor), amphetamine, cocaine (dopamine transporters), barbiturates (Cl^- channel of GABA receptor), nicotine (Na^+ channel linked to nicotinic receptor) and ethanol (Ca^{2+} channel linked to NMDA receptor) elicit their acute behavioural effects by different mechanisms, the ultimate drug actions at these targets lead to an elevation of extracellular DA levels in nucleus accumbens.

D_2 receptor antagonists injected into the mesolimbic area of the brain reduce the self-administration of the drug in rodents. Similarly, removal of D_2 receptors in a transgenic mouse strain, eliminated the reward and reinforcement properties of morphine administration, without eliminating other opioid effects including withdrawal effects.

MECHANISMS FOR THE DEVELOPMENT OF TOLERANCE, DEPENDENCE AND WITHDRAWAL EFFECTS

In the major areas of brain, usually there is a balance between an excitatory (E) and inhibitory (I) neurotransmitter (Fig. 38.3, state-1) and the body tries to counteract the stimulant or depressant effects of the abused drug, if it is subjected to prolonged use, by increasing the inhibitory or excitatory activity, respectively. In this figure, the abused drug shown is inhibitory (ID), which mimics the inhibitory neurotransmitter (I). As a result of its primary action, the balance would be altered to a state of inhibition (I + ID) or depression (state 2). After its prolonged use, the body would try to increase the excitatory activity (as counteradaptation, E + E). The balance (E + E = I + ID) would then be restored and the increasing doses of the drug would now be required to obtain the same inhibitory effects of the drug (i.e., tolerance develops, state 3).

If this drug (ID) is suddenly withdrawn, a disbalance would occur which must obviously produce effects and symptoms opposite to those of the drug (withdrawal effects, state 4). The latent hyperexcitability in such a situation is unmasked (E + E) because physiological restoration of normal balance would take its own time. The biological restoration to normal levels could also be achieved by proper treatment (state 5) (see below). However, the state of inhibition (I + ID), to which the addict was used

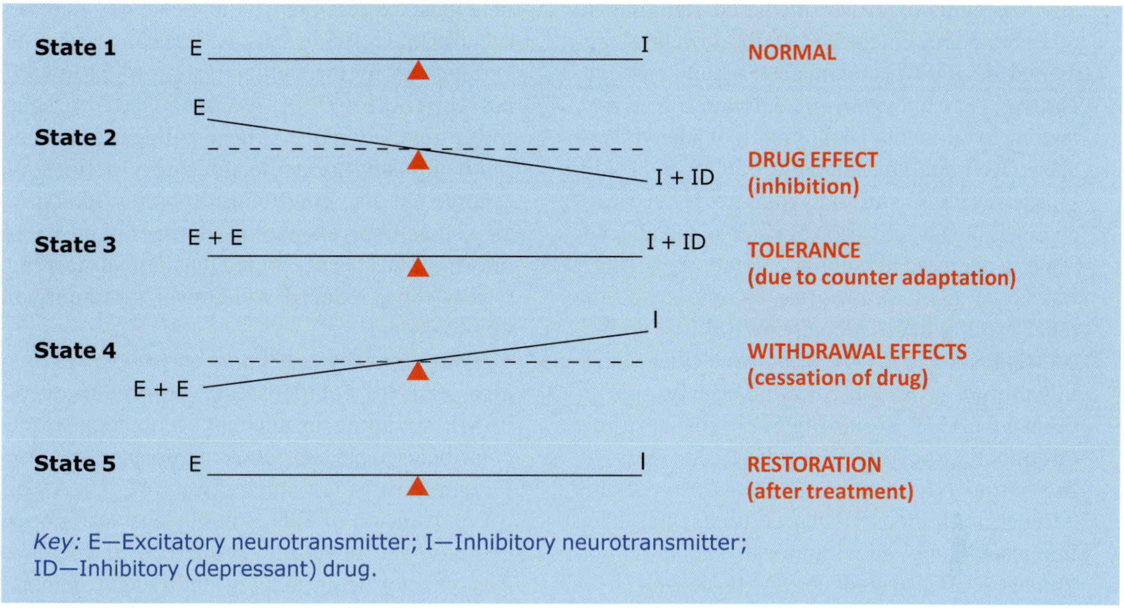

Fig 38.3 A Model of CNS Counteradaptation After Drug Abuse

to, could be obtained by providing him the same drug (ID). The very fact that the discontinuance of an abused drug may precipitate withdrawal symptoms provides an incentive to continue its use. If a physically dependent addict oscillates between feelings of euphoria and thereafter dysphoria, related to withdrawal, he would exhibit drug seeking behaviour to negate the unpleasant feelings.

Dependence is more commonly associated with abuse of short to intermediate acting drugs such as *secobarbital, pentobarbital, lorazepam, alprazolam, pethidine, morphine* and *heroin* etc. Dependence on longer acting agents such as *phenobarbital, chordiazepoxide, flurazepam* or *methadone* is less common because drugs with longer half-lives produce a less severe withdrawal syndrome, that too of longer duration. Dependence is rarely associated with intravenously administered ultra-short acting drugs like *pentothal, methohexital, midazolam* and *fentanyl* derivatives because these agents cannot be taken frequently enough to maintain adequate plasma concentrations needed to avoid withdrawal effects.

NEUROPHARMACOLOGICAL ADAPTATIONS DURING DEPENDENCE

For each class of abused drugs (benzodiazepines and barbiturates Ch. 32; amphetamines, cocaine and cannabinoids Ch. 35; alcohol Ch. 36 and opioids Ch. 37), the neuropharmacological mechanisms involved in the development of tolerance, dependence and withdrawal have already been described. We, hereby, summarise as to how chronic exposure to drugs of abuse induces adaptive changes in neuronal signal transduction pathways.

- *Chronic exposure to ethanol* leads to compensatory increase in the density of NMDA receptors and L-type voltage-gated Ca^{2+} channels in the brain. This leads to neuronal hyperactivity observed during alcohol withdrawal. NMDA and L-type channel antagonists, therefore, decrease withdrawal effects of alcohol in rodents. Chronic exposure to ethanol also down-regulates the $GABA_A$ receptor activity. This also contributes to alcohol withdrawal. Benzodiazepines, therefore, due to their GABAergic properties are useful in reducing alcohol withdrawal symptoms. Ethanol also up-regulates cAMP-mediated signaling in other brain areas including midbrain ventral tegmental area (VTA) and nucleus accumbens.

- *Opioids, on brief exposure*, activate μ receptors leading to Gi-mediated inhibition of adenylyl cyclase (AC) and consequently of cAMP, protein kinase-A (PKA) and voltage-gated N-type Ca^{2+} channels but an activation of K^+ channel, all leading to a decrease in cellular excitability (Ch. 37, Fig. 37.3). *Chronic exposure of opioids*, on the other hand, induces a compensatory rise in AC, cAMP, PKA and cAMP response element binding protein (CREB). Simultaneously, the increased cAMP signaling in locus ceruleus enhances functioning of Na^+ channels by promoting NE release. Hyperactivity of this adrenergic nucleus (locus ceruleus) has been implicated in opioid withdrawal. The up-regulation of CREB also mediates cAMP-dependent gene expression. All these changes increase the intrinsic firing rate of neurons in locus ceruleus partly through activation of an inward Na^+ current (Fig. 38.4; see also Fig. 37.2). Thus the up-regulation of cAMP signaling cascade not only opposes the acute inhibitory actions of opioids but also contributes to opioid tolerance as well as hyperexcitability during opioid withdrawal. It has been reported that animals lacking CREB show reduced withdrawal symptoms of opioid drugs.

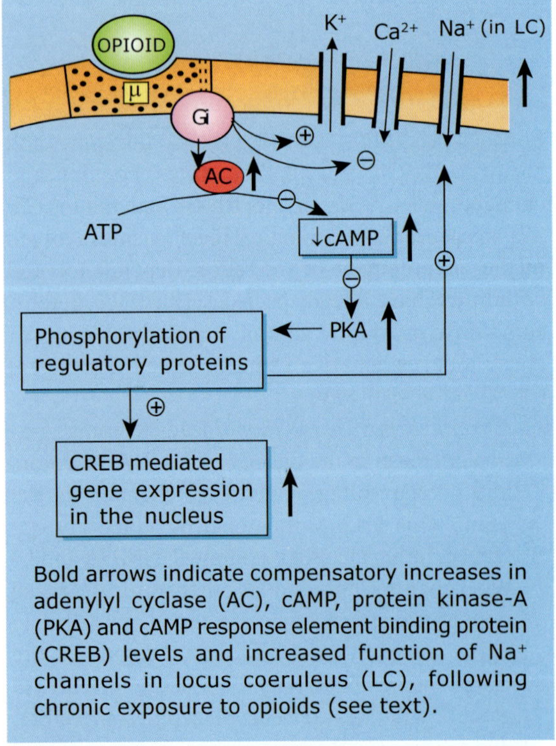

Bold arrows indicate compensatory increases in adenylyl cyclase (AC), cAMP, protein kinase-A (PKA) and cAMP response element binding protein (CREB) levels and increased function of Na^+ channels in locus coeruleus (LC), following chronic exposure to opioids (see text).

Fig 38.4 Opioid Signaling in Brain After Brief and Chronic Exposure

- *Chronic exposure to cocaine and amphetamines* also leads to compensatory up-regulation of cAMP signaling in nucleus accumbens which contributes to psychostimulant tolerance, because pharmacological activation of PKA or overexpression of CREB in nucleus accumbens decrease the rewarding properties of cocaine. The receptor neuroimaging studies have demonstrated that chronic abuse of cocaine down-regulates D_2 receptors and up-regulates dopamine transporters. Normally, *on brief exposure, cocaine* binds to dopamine transporters and inhibits dopamine reuptake; while amphetamine causes intracellular release of dopamine from its vesicles and then reverse transports this dopamine through dopamine transporters. These actions serve to elevate the extracellular levels of dopamine in the synaptic cleft (Ch. 35).
- At a cellular level *nicotine* acts on nicotinic-acetylcholine receptors (N_N) to produce neuronal excitation. *Its reinforcing properties* are associated with increased activity in the mesolimbic dopaminergic pathway as discussed above. Effects of nicotine are mediated by enhancing the permeability of Na^+ through nicotinic-cholinergic receptor gated Na^+ channels. *Chronic exposure of nicotine* desensitises these receptors, but simultaneously also leads to a substantial increase in the number of these receptors (an effect opposite to that produced by chronic administration of most dependence-producing drugs). It may represent an adaptive response to prolonged receptor desensitisation.

The overall effect of nicotine may reflect a balance between the activation of neuronal nicotinic receptors (causing normal excitation) and the desensitisation (causing synaptic block). However, as the cellular effects of nicotine get diminished, after chronic exposure, it is also possible that the additional binding sites represent the desensitised rather than functional receptors.

- *Cannabinoids* and opioids share common signaling pathways in the brain for reward and reinforcement but as there is hardly any physical dependence or withdrawal syndrome developing with the use of cannabinoid, the associated neuroadaptive mechanisms have little relevance if any.

DESIGNER DRUGS

Designer drugs are synthetic substances, prepared in clandestine laboratories, that are inexpensive to produce and difficult to detect. Such molecular manipulations of the widely abused drugs are done by some chemists to avoid Drugs and Narcotic Act regulations and to make huge profits. These include the amphetamine analogue, 3,4-methylenedioxymethamphetamine (MDMA), known as "Ecstasy" on the streets. Another is "China White" which is a synthetic analogue of fentanyl with 1000–1500 times of its potency. The consequences of "designer drug abuse" are, however, unpredictable and in some instances lethal. For example, efforts to make pethidine substitute resulted in an end product, methyl-phenyl-tetrahydropyridine (MPTP) which unfortunately causes nigrostriatal lesions and produces parkinsonism. It is now used as pharmacological tool to produce parkinsonism. One can easily imagine what kind of future holds to individuals and for the society with such clandestine activities around.

TREATMENT OF DRUG DEPENDENCE

The ultimate goal of treatment program is to achieve a "drug free status" as early as possible and to prevent the relapse of drug abuse. The drug free status is achieved with the help of pharmacotherapy while "relapse prevention strategies" involve rehabilitation and psychosocial interventions. The pharmacological approaches to treat drug dependence and withdrawal include: **(a)** short-term or long-term substitution of the abused drug by a similar drug having longer plasma half-life, **(b)** an aversive therapy by using a drug which produces unpleasant response after an intake of the abused drug, **(c)** use of a proper antagonist, to prevent relapse, once the drug free status is achieved, **(d)** use of such drugs which reduce craving for the abused drug and **(e)** rehabilitation and psychosocial interventions. Withdrawal effects of benzodiazepines and barbiturates (Ch. 32), amphetamines, cocaine and cannabinoids (Ch. 35); alcohol (Ch.36) and opioids (Ch. 37) have already been discussed earlier, hence treatment of their withdrawal effects is discussed below.

Treatment of Opioid Dependence

Substitution Therapy

The most commonly used strategy is to switch the patient from a short-acting opioid, such as heroin, to a long-acting agonist such as ***methadone***. With such a substitution, the addict is spared from the undesirable effects of withdrawal because the opioid receptors remain occupied for a longer duration. Thereafter, methadone can be withdrawn in tapering doses over a period of weeks. The pharmacological basis of using *methadone* depends on its oral effectiveness (once daily dosing), longer duration of action and development of cross tolerance between it and other opioids. An even longer acting analogue ***levo-alfa-acetyl methadol*** **(LAAM)**, with alternate day oral dosing and reduced abuse potential can also be used, but with a caution as it prolongs QT interval and may lead to life-threatening arrhythmias. Another option is ***buprenorphine*,** a partial opioid agonist, that can be given orally once daily.

Use of an Opioid Antagonist

A long-acting, orally active opioid antagonist ***naltrexone*** provides another treatment option in that the addicts who are completely withdrawn from opioid (after methadone therapy) can be maintained in such a state further, to block pleasurable effects leading to relapse. It can be given three times a week in doses of 100–150 mg (or 50 mg OD) or in the form of depot injection on monthly basis. However, the therapy is successful only if the patient is already detoxified and is "opioid free" for the past 10 days; otherwise, the opioid withdrawal effects would be precipitated.

Use of Clonidine or Lofexidine

To detoxify the patient and to prevent relapse, ***clonidine,*** a centrally acting sympatholytic agent, can also be used. By reducing the central NE outflow from locus ceruleus, clonidine reduces the severity of distressful withdrawal effects of opioids such as hypertension, anxiety, headache, tremors, intestinal cramps and diarrhoea. ***Lofexidine*** causes lesser hypotension compared to clonidine. Both have no narcotic action and are not addictive.

Rehabilitation and Other Aspects

The pharmacotherapy is more rewarding if combined with rehabilitation program which includes proper education and counselling. Besides treating withdrawal and dependence, all possible efforts should be made to prevent AIDS, hepatitis, bacterial endocarditis and other consequences of contaminated needle exchange between I.V. opioid dependent addicts.

Treatment of Alcoholism

The treatment of both acute and chronic alcoholism has already been discussed in detail in Chapter 36.

Treatment of Barbiturates and Benzodiazepines Dependence

If short-acting barbiturates such as *pentobarbital* or *secobarbital* have been abused, a long-acting barbiturate such as ***phenobarbital*** may be substituted as a pharmacologically equivalent drug and then gradually withdrawn with tapering doses. If a long-acting barbiturate is abused, the same drug is allowed to continue but it is gradually withdrawn at a rate of 10% of the daily requirement. Complete detoxification may be achieved in 2–3 weeks duration.

For detoxification of barbiturates, an osmotic diuretic with sodium bicarbonate can also be used to alkalinise the urine and to hasten the elimination of the drug. During this period the abused barbiturate may also be substituted with a antihistamine (***diphenhydramine***) for symptomatic treatment of withdrawal effects. The latter may then be withdrawn after successful detoxification. Seizures represent a medical emergency during withdrawal and can be treated by parenteral administration of ***diazepam*** or ***carbamazepine.***

With *benzodiazepines* (BZDs) the physical dependence is rare, but may occur following long-term treatment with doses of 40 mg/day or more of diazepam. Nonetheless, if an intermediate to short acting BZD has been abused, a long acting BZD such as ***chlordiazepoxide*** can be substituted as the pharmacologically equivalent drug which can be subsequently withdrawn in tapering doses. The BZD receptor antagonist ***flumazenil*** can be used to specifically block the toxicity of BZDs overdose or to prevent relapse after detoxification.

Treatment of Nicotine Dependence

Nicotine dependence has already been discussed in detail in Ch. 13.

Treatment of Withdrawal From Stimulants and Psychotomimetics

The pharmacological approach towards the management of withdrawal from amphetamines, phencyclidine, cocaine, LSD and marijuana have already been dealt in Chapter 35.

Treatment of Withdrawal From Inhalants

There is little evidence that the signs of abstinence occur in individuals when inhalants are withdrawn, suggesting that physical dependence is not the part of the experience of these abusers. Since abusers are still taking these agents repeatedly there seems to be some psychic dependence on them. No specific treatment is available because the toxic effects of inhaled solvents and aerosols may be caused by more than one substance and also because solvents typically contain more than one volatile compound. These may be tainted also with heavy metals such as lead, mercury, nickel and cadmium. Rehabilitation and education of such patients is more rewarding.

Withdrawal From Anabolic Steroids

Patients abusing anabolic steroids, e.g., ***stanozolol*** for body building, are seldom covered by deaddiction programs. Yet, they may come to deaddiction centres if they suffer from excessive aggression, sexual dysfunction or mood fluctuations. Again, mere counseling may suffice, with gradual withdrawal of the anabolic steroid. Such patients may also be advised to avoid going to gyms as these are the favourable sites for acquisition of steroids.

CHAPTER 39 Antiepileptic Drugs

COMPETENCY PH1.19

Epilepsy is a common neurological abnormality affecting about 1% of the world population. A *seizure* means a paroxysmal abnormal discharge at high frequency, from an aggregate of neurons in cerebral cortex. The term seizure needs to be carefully distinguished from convulsions and epilepsy. *Epilepsy* is a condition characterised by recurrent episodes of such seizures. That means, a patient should not be described as having epilepsy until a few episodes of "non-febrile" seizures have appeared. The site of the origin of discharge is called "epileptic focus". From here the discharge spreads to the surrounding areas of the brain. The word *fit* is often used colloquially to describe an epileptic seizure. *Convulsions* are involuntary, violent and spasmodic or prolonged contractions of skeletal muscle. That means, a patient may have epilepsy without convulsions and *vice versa.*

CLASSIFICATION OF SEIZURES

At present there are two systems of classification of seizure disorders. The first system is based on seizure types and their characteristic features. This system is more useful in selecting the appropriate drug for treating a particular type of seizure. The second system is based on epilepsy syndrome which includes aetiological factors, frequency of attacks, age at the onset and clinical manifestation of epilepsy. The "Syndrome Classification" is more useful in assessing the long-term prognosis after deciding the therapeutic strategy. Since syndrome classification is more complex, because of too many variables, a simplified approach based on classification of "seizure types" is more suited to our discussion on antiepileptic drugs. Broadly speaking, the seizure activity is either ***generalised*** or ***partial.***

Generalised Seizures

These seizures arise from both cerebral hemispheres and diencephalon simultaneously, involving the entire body, and have characteristic bilateral pattern in EEG recording. These are of following types.

Grand Mal or Tonic-Clonic Seizures

These are *usually* associated with an *aura* prior to seizures. The patient falls to the ground in stiff tonic phase (legs extended) with an *epileptic cry*, caused by tonic contraction of laryngeal muscles. This is followed by *clonic convulsions* (repetitive bilateral muscle jerking) and then to *coma* which may last for about 15–30 min. Recovery is associated with stupor, amnesia, mental confusion, postictal (post seizure) depression, incontinence and exhaustion. EEG shows a bilateral diffused pattern of high-voltage polyspikes of 10–30 Hz/sec in tonic-clonic phase. Almost 10% of total epileptic cases suffer from grand mal epilepsy but fortunately respond well to pharmacotherapy. In some cases, grand mal seizures occur repeatedly with no recovery of consciousness in between the attacks. These type of seizures are called as ***status epilepticus,*** which represent a state of clinical emergency.

Petit Mal or Absence Seizures

There is *no aura* associated with this disorder and attack appears without warning. There is usually *no loss of consciousness*. The seizure typically lasts for few seconds, so if there is a lapse of consciousness, it is hardly for 5 sec with no loss of postural control. There is no postictal confusion or amnesia. Absence seizures are characterised by subtle bilateral motor symptoms such as rapid blinking of eyelids, chewing movements or small amplitude clonic jerks of the hands for a few seconds. The EEG hallmark of typical absence seizures is a generalised symmetric 3 Hz spikes and wave pattern of discharge per second that begins and ends suddenly. These are the main seizure types in 15–20% of epileptic children. These children may experience absence seizures hundred times per day.

About 60–70% of such patients will have spontaneous remission during adolescence. These seizures too, are responsive to pharmacotherapy.

Atypical absence seizures are of slower onset and of longer duration. These are less responsive to pharmacotherapy as these are associated with other neurologic complications like mental retardation.

Myoclonic Seizures

These are bilateral epileptic myoclonus characterised by sudden and brief skeletal muscle contraction that may involve the entire body or one part of the body. Most commonly the patient complains of sudden jerking movements appearing during sleep. EEG shows 2 Hz spikes and wave pattern per second.

Akinetic (Atonic) Seizures

These are characterised by sudden loss of postural tone. The head may sag to one side or the patient may fall all of a sudden. The consciousness may be impaired for a brief period but there is no postictal confusion. The EEG shows brief generalised spike and wave discharge followed by diffused slow waves that correlate with loss of muscle tone.

Clonic Seizures

These are characterised by repetitive muscle jerks. EEG shows fast activity (10 Hz or more) slow waves.

Tonic Seizures

These are characterised by rigid violent muscular contraction with stiff and fixed extended limbs. EEG shows low-voltage fast-activity waves.

Partial Seizures (Localised/Focal)

These are the most common seizure types occurring in approximately 80% of epileptic patients. The seizure activity is restricted to a discreet area belonging to one cerebral hemisphere only. These are of three types:

Simple Partial Seizures (Jacksonian Seizures)

These are characterised by unilateral clonic movements that begin in one group of muscles and spread gradually to adjacent group reflecting the march of epileptic activity (e.g., mouth, thumb, great toe). Such type of Jacksonian seizures are called *Jacksonian motor seizures*. Alternatively, the patient may have somatosensory symptoms such as auditory, visual or olfactory hallucinations or at times "pins and needle" sensations with no reason (*Jacksonian sensory seizures*). There is no loss of consciousness in simple partial seizures.

Complex Partial Seizures (Psychomotor Epilepsy)

These usually originate in the temporal or the frontal lobe and are accompanied by partial loss of consciousness. It is a dreamy state of psychic seizures where the patient behaves as partially conscious with *automatism*. He may get up, put on his clothes, start walking or even drive his car but does not follow your commands and does not even recollect the events after the attack is over. The attack is usually associated with auditory, visual or olfactory aura. Sometimes patient shows other types of *automatisms* like lip smacking, fumbling and scratching of which the patient has no memory.

Partial Seizures Evolving to Secondary Generalised Seizures

These are the type when partial seizures progress to generalised/tonic/clonic/tonic-clonic seizures. Patients usually report aura beforehand.

Unclassified Seizures

It covers undetermined epilepsies and epileptic syndromes such as: **(a)** ***Febrile seizures*** wherein young children frequently develop seizures with illness accompanied by hyperpyrexia, **(b)** ***Infantile spasm*** with progressive mental retardation. These are generalised tonic-clonic convulsions of short duration which may appear frightening but are usually benign. These have not yet been classified because of insufficient data or atypical pattern of the seizures.

CLASSIFICATION BASED ON EPILEPSY SYNDROMES

To satisfy the need for a more accurate description of a seizure disorder the above classification, based on seizure types, have been remodulated into different epilepsy syndromes. Each syndrome attempts to incorporate the aspects such as type of seizure, aetiology, anatomy, precipitating factors, age of onset, severity and chronicity of attacks as well as prognosis. One major advantage of the "syndrome classification" is to recognise that a simple partial seizure can later progress to complex partial seizure and then to a secondary generalised seizure. In doing so, this classification does not require that a seizure should be classified into one specific seizure category. There are at present more than 40 distinct epilepsy syndromes and more may follow. All of them fall into three categories:

1. IDIOPATHIC, in which no cause could be identified *except for genetic linkage*. Examples include: *Juvenile myoclonic epilepsy syndrome, mesial temporal lobe epilepsy syndrome* and *juvenile absence epilepsy syndrome.*
2. SYMPTOMATIC, in which the *seizures are associated with some identifiable underlying disorders*. Examples include *Lennox-Gastaut epilepsy syndrome* (impaired cognitive functions) and *chronic progressive epilepsia partialis continua of childhood* (developmental abnormalities in brain).
3. CRYPTOGENIC, in which the epilepsy appears to be symptomatic but *the exact cause is not known*. Examples include: *West's syndrome* (infantile spasm), *neonatal seizures* and *febrile convulsions.*

Since the classification based on "epilepsy syndrome" has more impact on guiding clinical assessment and the prognosis of epilepsy, than on proper selection of an antiepileptic drug, our discussion would utilise the classification based on the types of epileptic seizure as described earlier.

AETIOLOGY OF SEIZURES AND EPILEPSY

Epilepsy has several causes which are presented below:

1. *Genetic or heredity*: It is apparent that hereditary factors do play a role in the etiology of human epilepsies and that epilepsy genes do exist and may be quite important in the aetiology of at least some forms of epilepsies such as juvenile myoclonic epilepsy syndrome, childhood absence epilepsy syndrome, juvenile absence epilepsy syndrome and progressive myoclonic epilepsy syndrome. Most of these result from the cumulative effect of more than one mutant gene (polygenic).
2. Brain lesions, mainly due to birth trauma.
3. Infections like cerebral meningitis and brain abscess.
4. Metabolic disorders like lack of oxygen, alkalosis, hypoglycaemia, hypocalcaemia, hyperpyrexia and vitamin B_6 deficiency.
5. Sudden withdrawal of many drugs of abuse such as barbiturates and alcohol.
6. Viewing television, disco flashes and listening full blast Pop music (Musicogenic temporal lobe seizures).

ENDOGENOUS ANTISEIZURE SUBSTANCES (EAS)

It seems, some sort of regulatory mechanism must be existing within the body, otherwise why, without outside drug intervention, there should be a spontaneous arrest of seizure activity after an attack and why the brain could remain seizure free for sometime between the two intervening attacks (postictal refractory period). The available reports are strongly in favour of an involvement of the purine nucleoside ***adenosine***—as an endogenous **a**ntiseizure **s**ubstance (EAS) in epilepsy. Adenosine has been shown to inhibit spontaneous firing of cells in virtually all areas of brain including cerebral cortex. It has been identified endogenously, causes hyperpolarisation and exhibits A_1 receptor mediated anticonvulsant effects in animal models when administered exogenously. Since it is released postictally and itself is not tonically active, A_1 receptor antagonists *per se* do not exhibit any convulsant activity. Elevated adenosine levels have been reported immediately after the seizure activity both in animal models as well as in patients. *Adenosine*, therefore, seems to fulfil all the criteria for an EAS and may open altogether new vistas in the development of newer antiepileptic drugs.

MECHANISMS OF ACTION OF ANTIEPILEPTIC DRUGS IN GENERAL

Anticonvulsant drugs act by different mechanisms to suppress repetitive firing action potentials by an epileptic focus in the brain. These are briefly discussed below. However, some drugs act by multiple mechanisms which are discussed with individual drugs.

A) Mechanisms of Drugs Used in Grand Mal and Partial Seizures

1. Inhibition of Use-Dependent Na^+ Channels (Fig. 39.1B)

Many drugs (e.g., ***phenytoin***, ***carbamazepine***, ***valproate***, ***lacosamide***, ***rufinamide*** and ***lamotrigine***) preferentially block the voltage-gated (VG) Na^+ channels that remain open due to repetitive neuronal firing. The higher the frequency of the firing the greater is the block. These drugs, prolong the duration of 'inactivated phase' of VG-Na^+ channel and delay its reversion to the 'resting phase'. This reduces their chances of becoming available again for activation (for details refer Ch. 15). Inhibition of VG-Na^+ channels ultimately diminish glutamate release from the glutamatergic neurons.

2. Enhancement of GABAergic Action (Fig. 39.1 A)

Some of the antiepileptic drugs (e.g., ***phenobarbital*** and ***benzodiazepines***) activate $GABA_A$ receptors to facilitate GABA-mediated opening of Cl^- channels. Benzodiazepines increase the frequency while phenobarbital increases the duration of the opening of Cl^- channel (Ch. 32). Some drugs (e.g., ***vigabatrin***) inhibit the enzyme GABA-transaminase, which is responsible to metabolise GABA, and thus increase the neuronal concentration of GABA. ***Tiagabine*** and ***valproate*** rather inhibit GABA uptake by inhibiting the GABA uptake transporter (GAT) in neurons as well as in glia. It enhances the availability as well as the inhibitory actions of GABA at postsynaptic $GABA_A$ receptors. ***Valproic acid,*** also activates glutamic acid decarboxylase (GAD) and thus increases the synthesis of GABA (Fig. 30.2).

3. Blockade of NMDA or AMPA Receptors (Fig. 39.1B)

Activation of NMDA and AMPA receptors by glutamate produces depolarising responses (Ch. 30) and initiates seizure activity. The anticonvulsant action of ***felbamate*** involves blockade of NMDA receptors. ***Rufinamide*** is known to inhibit metabotropic glutamate subtype 5 receptor (mGluR5). ***Phenobarbital, topiramate, lamotrigine*** and ***perampanel*** block AMPA receptors. ***Valproate*** possibily inhibits glutamate synthesis.

4. Blockade of Voltage-gated N-Type Ca^{2+} Channels (Fig. 39.1B)

Some drugs (***lamotrigine*** and ***gabapentin***) act by inhibiting VG-Ca^{2+} channels (N-type) which ultimately decrease the synaptic release of glutamate.

5. Selective Binding to Synaptic Vesicular Protein (SV_2A)

Levetiracetam selectively binds to SV_2A protein of synaptic vesicles in glutamatergic and GABAergic neurons (Fig. 39.1 A & B) and decrease the synaptic release of glutamate while increase the release of GABA (modulates the release).

6. By Blocking the Effects of Neurotrophic Factors (Fig. 39.1B)

Lacosamide inhibits **C**ollapsin-**R**esponse **M**ediator **P**rotein (CRMP-2). This protein is involved in the production and release of **B**rain-**D**erived **N**eurotrophic **F**actor (BDNF) and other neurotrophins (NT-3). BDNF and NT-3 play on important role in epileptogenesis by provoking membrane excitability and by promoting synaptic plasticity.

B) Mechanisms of Drugs Used in Petit Mal (Absence Seizures)

1. Inhibition of T-type Ca^{2+} Channels (Fig. 39.1B)

Ethosuximide is a major drug used for the treatment of absence seizures. It inhibits the low threshold Ca^{2+} currents carried by T-type Ca^{2+} channels (see Ch. 20). T-type Ca^{2+} currents are responsible for generating the thalamic cortical pacemaker currents, in the form of 3 Hz spikes and waves, seen in petit mal attack. Inhibition or reduction of the low-threshold T-type Ca^{2+} channels also account for the anti-seizure activity of ***valproic acid*** against absence seizures.

ANTICONVULSANT DRUG THERAPY: GENERAL CONSIDERATIONS

- Antiepileptic drugs can control but do not cure epilepsy. The primary objective of anticonvulsant therapy is to suppress seizures and provide neuroprotection by minimising deleterious

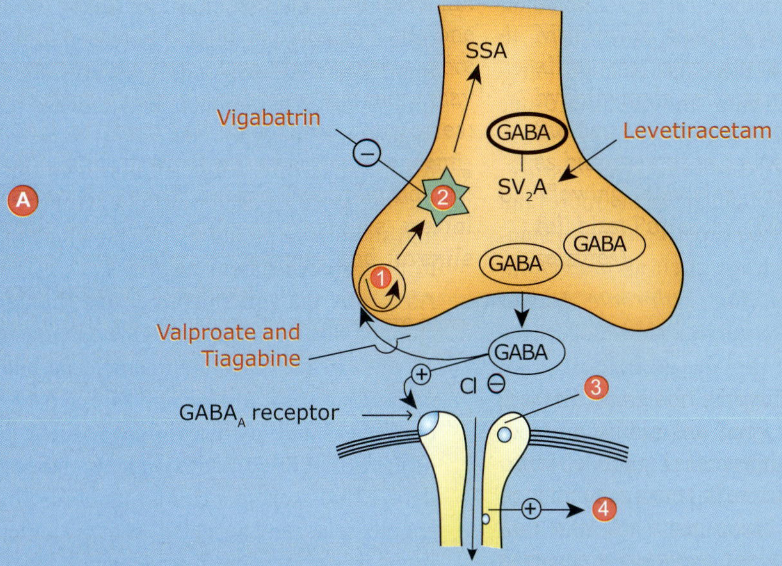

Key: (1) GABA uptake transporter; (2) GABA transaminase; (3) Modulatory site for *benzo-diazepines*; (4) Site for channel modulators, e.g., *phenobarbital*; SSA, Succinic Semialdehyde (metabolite of GABA)

(A) Sites of Action of Various Anticonvulsant Drugs Acting by Enhancement of $GABA_A$ Receptor Activity

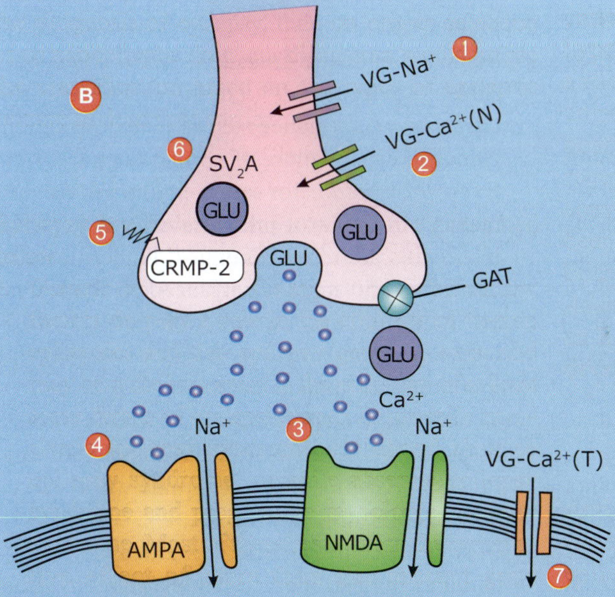

Key: (1) Drugs that Block Voltage-gated Na^+ Channel (Phenytoin, Carbama-zepine, Valproate, Lamotrigine and Lacosamide). (2) Drugs that Block Voltage-gated N-Type Ca^{2+} Channels (Lamotrigine, Gabapentin and Pregabalin). (3) Drugs that Block NMDA Receptors (Felbamate). (4) Drugs that Block AMPA Receptors (Phenobarbital, Topiramate and Lamotrigine). (5) Drugs that Inhibit CRMP-2 (Lacosamide, see text). (6) Drugs that Inhibit SV_2A Protein (Levetiracetam). (7) Drugs that Block T-Type Ca^{2+} Channels (Ethosuximide and Valproate). GAT—GABA uptake transporter (see text)

(B) Sites of Action of Various Anticonvulsant Drugs Which Decrease Glutamatergic Activity.

Fig 39.1 Summarizing Mechanism of Action of Various Anticonvulsant Drugs

effects from seizure attacks. Many patients with epilepsy have to take medication throughout their life to ensure control of seizures.

- Over the past 15 years there has been an introduction of at least 30 new antiepileptic drugs (*vigabatrin, gabapentin, lamotrigine, topiramate, levetiracetam, felbamate, oxcarbazepine, lacosamide* and many more) but none has been found to be superior to major standard anticonvulsant drugs such as *phenytoin, carbamazepine* and *sodium valproate*. Newer additions are merely serving as "add-on" drugs.
- Broadly speaking, the drugs effective in generalised tonic-clonic seizures (grand mal) are usually effective in partial seizures (more specifically complex partial seizures). Sudden withdrawal of these drugs carries a greater risk of precipitating withdrawal seizures. These drugs are not effective in, rather can aggravate, absence (petit mal) and myoclonic seizures.
- On the contrary, the drugs effective in petit mal (absence) seizures can be used for treating myoclonic seizures but not grand mal or partial seizures. A sudden withdrawal of drugs belonging to this category, carries a lower risk of precipitating withdrawal seizures. Nevertheless, it is generally recommended that the antiepileptic drug should always be withdrawn slowly over a period of six months.
- Among the currently available antiepileptic drugs, ***phenytoin, phenobarbital, primidone, carbamazepine*** and ***oxcarbazepine*** are ***enzyme inducers. Oxcarbazepine*** appears to induce hepatic enzymes to a lesser extent than ***carbamazepine*** which minimises its drug interactions. On the other hand, ***valproic acid*** is a potent ***enzyme inhibitor.***
- Many clinicians no longer undertake routine monitoring of plasma concentration for most anticonvulsant drugs because plasma concentrations hardly serve as a useful guideline to change the dose. It is not a substitute for clinical assessment. *The exception is phenytoin* which follows mixed-order elimination kinetics. As a result, a monitoring of its plasma concentration becomes essential because its therapeutic window is also smaller (see text). With other drugs, usually the dose is increased to the maximum tolerated level and, if seizures do not stop, it is replaced by another. Newer drugs may also be added, if desired.
- Most antiseizure drugs are not highly bound to plasma proteins except for phenytoin (90–92%) and sodium valproate (93–95%) which may lead to drug displacement reactions.
- As a rule, the antiepileptic drugs should not be stopped during pregnancy. One can use the lowest dose of the least teratogenic drug but maternal seizures should not be allowed to go unchecked as they are harmful to the foetus because of the possibility of anoxia and metabolic disorders. Minor seizures can be ignored. Folic acid supplements may be added, as many antiepileptic drugs (see text) cause folic acid deficiency which is reponsible for neural tube defects (spina bifida and anencephaly). Antiepileptic drugs which are enzyme inducers (see above) lower the maternal plasma levels of vitamin K, leading to postpartum haemorrhage. Hence oral vitamin K, may also be supplemented during the last two weeks of the pregnancy.
- Some antiepileptic drugs (*phenytoin, phenobarbital, primidone, carbamazepine* and *oxcarbazepine*) induce steroid metabolising enzymes to cause failure of normal contraception. Even *topiramate* for some unknown reasons makes birth control pills less effective. Hence if the pills are to be continued, higher doses of oestrogen (50 mg/day) are needed. Such dose adjustments are not needed with *sodium valproate* or *lamotrigine* as these are enzyme inhibitors not inducers.

  Though antiepilepsy drugs are secreted through breast milk to some extent, the risk:benefit ratio favours breast feeding to continue whilst taking antiepileptic drugs.
- In spite of controversies, it is at least clear that children born to mothers taking anticonvulsant drugs have an increased risk of teratogenicity leading to congenital malformations. Available

literature shows teratogenic rank order of various antiseizure drugs as follows:
Trimethadione > valproic acid > phenytoin > phenobarbital = primidone > carbamazepine > oxcarbazepine > topiramate > lamotrigine = ethosuximide.

With current information, among the standard drugs, *carbamazepine, oxcarbazepine, lamotrigine* and *ethosuximide* seem to be the safest drugs during pregnancy.

INDIVIDUAL DRUGS

Therapeutic spectra of various antiepileptic drugs discussed below has been summarised in Fig. 39.2.

Phenytoin

Phenytoin is an oldest non-sedative antiepilepsy drug. Chemically it is diphenylhydantoin. ***Fosphenytoin*** is a prodrug which is rapidly converted to phenytoin in the plasma. It is better tolerated than phenytoin on parenteral administration. Phenytoin provides a good example of the application of pharmacokinetics for successful prescribing (see below).

Mechanism of Action

Phenytoin, at therapeutic plasma levels (10–20 μg/ml), blocks the use-dependent Na^+ channels and thus inhibits the generation of repetitive action potentials (see above; Mech. A-1). At higher doses it also reduces the influx of Ca^{2+} (during depolarisation) and suppresses repetitive firing of neurons (Mech. A-4). Both these actions decrease glutamate release.

Therapeutic Uses and Plasma Levels

1. ANTIEPILEPTIC USE: To treat partial seizures (specially psychomotor), generalised tonic-clonic and status epilepticus (*fosphenytoin*, slow I.V.). Both phynytoin or fosphenytoin provide a longer duration of seizure control than is provided by a benzodiazepine in the treatment of status epilepticus. For psychomotor seizures, this drug is the drug of first choice. For generalised tonic-clonic and status epilepticus it serves as a second choice. Phenytoin is *contraindicated* in petit mal (absence) and in myoclonic seizure (Fig. 39.2).
2. NON-ANTIEPILEPTIC USE: **(a)** To treat trigeminal neuralgia where it is second choice (carbamazepine serves as first choice), **(b)** to treat ventricular arrhythmias due to digitalis toxicity (see Ch. 22), and **(c)** to enhance wound healing as recent reports suggest that phenytoin holds promise in healing of wounds (see below).
3. THERAPEUTIC PLASMA LEVEL for most of the epileptic patients is between 10–20 μg/ml. In usual practice, oral therapy is started with a dosage of 300 mg/day which keeps the patient seizure free with minimal side effects. If seizures are not controlled, doses may be increased in smaller increments of 25–30 mg giving ample time for attainment of steady state levels before further increasing the dose. Plasma levels above 20 μg/ml lead to toxicity.

Pharmacokinetics

Oral absorption is slow but is complete (80–90%). Changing from one dosage form of a particular brand to another can lead to suboptimal or toxic plasma levels, due to differences in bioavailability. Phenytoin is not given by I.M. or I.V. route (except for fosphenytoin). I.M. injection of phenytoin gets precipitated in muscle and causes pain, while I.V. injection can produce thrombophlebitis and hypotension. Even fast I.V. injection of fosphenytoin can lead to cardiovascular collapse and hence should be administered slowly.

Phenytoin is 90–92% protein bound. It is a potent enzyme inducer both for CYP3A4 and glucuronyl transferase enzymes. Metabolites are eliminated through urine. Phenytoin, as free drug, is also excreted through saliva. Its elimination is dose dependent and follows saturation (mixed order) kinetics. Up to plasma levels of 10–20 μg/ml, its elimination obeys I order kinetics. Hence its half-life remains constant and plasma levels do not fluctuate. Beyond 20 μg/ml, the elimination follows zero-order kinetics and hence a slight increase in its dose results into larger increase in plasma concentration leading to toxicity.

Periodic assessment of plasma concentration and subsequent dose adjustments are therefore needed particularly in neonates and in patients suffering from uraemia, liver disease and hypoproteinaemia. Its plasma half-life is about 24 hrs; hence five days are needed to attain steady state plasma levels. This time lag can be shortened by giving a loading dose (if required) followed by a maintenance dose.

Adverse Effects

- **Overdose Toxicity** (Plasma levels beyond 30 µg/ml): It is manifested by nystagmus, ataxia, CNS depression, lethargy, and blurred vision. If the dose is very high or if I.V. injection is administered faster, it can lead to cardiovascular collapse and coma.
- **Chronic Toxicity** (after prolonged use) is manifested as follows:

a) ***Gingival hyperplasia and coarsening of facial features***: Phenytoin after being secreted through saliva, inhibits the enzyme collagenase which is responsible for the breakdown of collagen of connective tissues. It has been reported that phenytoin increases platelet-derived growth factors-B (PDGF-B) and its mRNA from macrophages that are thought to enhance wound healing, induce gingival fibroblast and promote local angiogenesis.

b) ***Megaloblastic anaemia***: Phenytoin induces hydroxylating enzyme activity for which folates are the cofactors. As serum folic acid levels go down, the body's demand for folic acid increases. This leads to megaloblastic anaemia, which is responsive to folic acid supplements.

c) ***Vitamin K deficiency***: caused by phenytoin, leads to hypoprothrombinaemia and consequently haemorrhage in the newborn if the mother had received phenytoin during pregnancy. Vitamin K supplements can therefore be used either for treatment or as prophylaxis.

d) Phenytoin increases the metabolism of calciferol and ***produces vitamin-D deficiency.*** Phenytoin also increases the metabolism of vitamin K and reduces the concentration of vitamin K-dependent proteins which are necessary for normal Ca^{2+} metabolism in bone. *This leads to rickets in malnourished children and osteomalacia in adults.* These conditions can be prevented by administering both vitamin D and vitamin K.

e) ***Hirsutism*** (in females) and ***acne*** may appear due to increased secretion of androgens.

f) Phenytoin inhibits insulin secretion and may cause ***hyperglycaemia.*** It also ***decreases ADH release.***

g) Use of phenytoin during pregnancy increases the risk of ***congenital malformation (cleft lip, cleft palate and congenital heart disease).*** These are associated with the formation of a toxic epoxide metabolite and also with the impaired DNA synthesis due to folate deficiency.

h) Other adverse effects include ***hypersensitivity reactions*** like skin rashes, fever, hepatitis and some CNS effects such as vertigo, nausea, tremors and confusion.

i) Phenytoin should not be discontinued suddenly as it ***may precipitate withdrawal seizures.***

Drug Interactions

1. Phenytoin, being enzyme inducer, increases the metabolism of corticosteroids, oral contraceptives (see above), doxycycline, rifampicin, theophylline, levodopa, vit. D and vit. K. The therapeutic efficacy of these drugs is, therefore, impaired by phenytoin.
2. Enzyme inhibitors like disulfiram, cimetidine, isoniazid, chloramphenicol decrease the metabolism of phenytoin (increase its plasma concentration).
3. Carbamazepine and phenytoin or phenobarbital and phenytoin increase each other's metabolism.
4. Sodium valproate displaces protein bound phenytoin and inhibits its metabolism also. Hence plasma level of free phenytoin increases.

Phenobarbital and Primidone

Barbiturates having an aromatic (phenyl) ring at position-5, exhibit anticonvulsant action (Fig. 39.3). Primidone is a deoxyphenobarbital (one oxygen less). It is metabolised to phenobarbital and phenylethyl malonamide and all these three agents are anticonvulsants. Since both phenobarbital and primidone are similar chemically and pharmacologically, both will be discussed together.

Mechanism of Action

Phenobarbital binds to the channel modulatory site on the GABA receptor and enhances the GABA

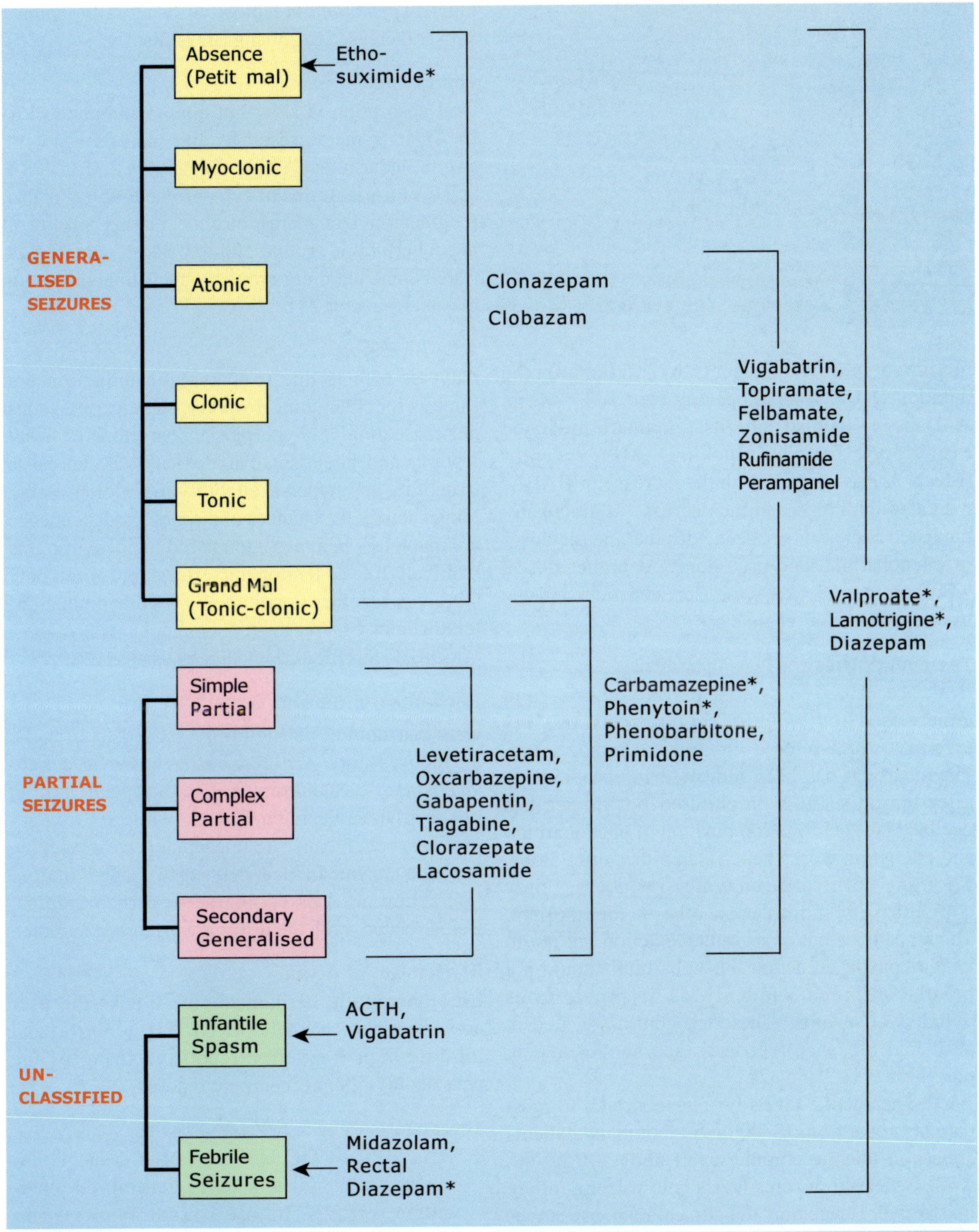

Fig 39.2 Therapeutic Spectra of Various Antiepileptic Drugs. *Drugs of first choice; rest are "add-on" drugs

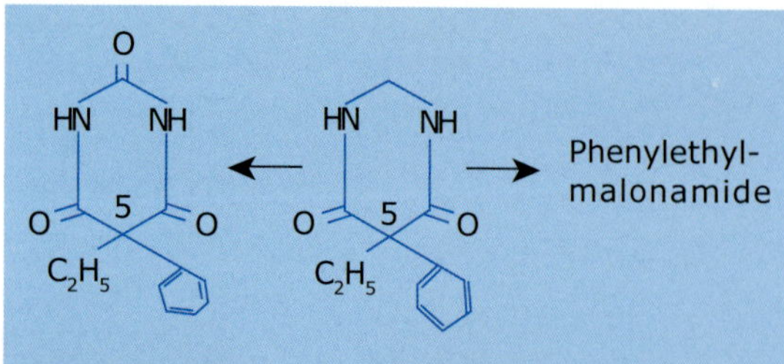

Fig 39.3 Structural Relationship Between Primidone and Phenobarbital

mediated inhibitory effects by increasing the duration of Cl^- channel opening (Fig. 39.1; Mech. A-2 above). It also inhibits glutamate mediated excitatory effects by blocking AMPA receptor (Mech. A-3 as above). Both the increase in GABA-mediated inhibition and the decrease in glutamate-mediated excitation are seen with therapeutic doses of phenobarbital and primidone. At higher doses, however, they block L-type Ca^{2+} channels and the use-dependent Na^+ channels.

Therapeutic Uses and Plasma Levels

Both are effective against partial seizures and generalised tonic-clonic seizures but are less effective than phenytoin and carbamazepine. Phenobarbital has been indicated for prophylaxis after febrile seizures in children but its use has declined (see below). Combination of phenobarbital and phenytoin works better than either drug alone. Though both are enzyme inducers, they competitively inhibit each other's metabolism. Tolerance develops to its sedative action but not to its anticonvulsant action. Phenobarbital should not be discontinued suddenly as it precipitates withdrawal seizures. These are contraindicated in petit mal (absence) seizures (see above) and in porphyria (Ch. 7 and 32).

Therapeutic levels for phenobarbital in most patients range from 10–40 μg/ml; but many patients appear to tolerate chronic levels above 40 μg/ml, while in febrile seizures levels below 15 μg/ml are ineffective. Hence only the clinical response serves as a guildeline for dose adjustments. Usual doses for *phenobarbital* are 60–180 mg daily orally at night; of *primidone* are initially 125 mg daily at night, slowly increased to 250 mg BD orally.

Pharmacokinetics

Oral absorption is slow but almost complete (85–90%). It is metabolised by liver and is a potent enzyme inducer for CYP2A, CYP2B, CYP2C, CYP3A and CYP6A isoforms of cytochrome P-450 and also for glucuronyl transferase enzyme. Plasma half-life of phenobarbital is around 100 hrs; hence once steady state is reached there are very small fluctuations in plasma levels for 24 hrs.

Adverse Effects

Adverse effects due to enzymatic induction are same as for phenytoin. However, phenobarbital does not cause gingival hyperplasia, coarsening of facial features and hirsutism. Paradoxically, it can cause irritability and hyper-excitability in children. Being longer acting, the chances of developing dependence are much less (Ch. 38). Compared to phenytoin it is relatively free of teratogenic effects; but when both are given together (a commonly used combination) teratogenicity increases for some unknown reasons. For DRUG INTERACTIONS refer Chapter 32.

Carbamazepine and Oxcarbazepine

Carbamazepine is structurally related to tricyclic antidepressants while oxcarbazepine is a keto analogue of carbamazepine. The therapeutic profile of oxcarbazepine is similar to, while its toxicity profile is better than, carbamazepine. Oxcarbazepine is a mild enzyme inducer and hence chances of drug interaction are less compared to carbamazepine. Being related, both the drugs are discussed together.

Mechanism of Action

Like phenytoin, carbamazepine blocks the use-dependent Na^+ channels (Mech. A-1 as above) and inhibits high-frequency repetitive firing of the neurons in brain, at therapeutic doses.

Therapeutic Uses and Plasma Levels

- ANTIEPILEPTIC USE: It is the drug of first choice for partial as well as generalised tonic-clonic seizures. Its use is contraindicated in absence seizures.

- NON-ANTICONVULSANT USE: It is a drug of first choice for **(a)** trigeminal neuralgia and in other neuropathic pain such as glossopharyngeal neuralgia and post-herpetic neuralgia. However, it is not an analgesic as it is ineffective in other types of pain such as headache or backache. It seems to interrupt temporal summation of high-frequency afferent nerve impulses; **(b)** carbamazepine is also effective in treating manic depressive psychosis (Ch. 34).
- THE THERAPEUTIC PLASMA LEVELS are 4–8 μg/ml, but these barely correlate with the clinical response as some patients report diplopia even at plasma levels of 6–7 μg/ml while others can tolerate levels above 10 μg/ml. The usual adult dose, given orally, is 100–200 mg twice or thrice daily increasing slowly to a maximum of 200-400 mg twice or thrice daily. For ***oxcarbazepine*** the usual oral dose is 300 mg BD daily which can be slowly increased to 450 mg BD daily.

Pharmacokinetics

Oral absorption of carbamazepine is slow. Giving the drug after meals helps the patients to tolerate. It is distributed mainly in brain, liver and kidneys. Carbamazepine is metabolised by CYP3A4, a cytochrome P-450 isoform which it induces along with glucuronyl transferase leading to various drug interactions. Its metabolites are excreted through urine. ***Oxcarbazepine*** is, however, a poor enzyme inducer. It is rapidly converted to 10-hydroxy metabolite which itself has anticonvulsant effects.

Adverse Effects

(a) The dose-related adverse effects of carbamazepine start with drowsiness followed by dizziness, headache, slurred speech, vertigo, ataxia and diplopia. For drowsiness and headache, the tolerance develops over a period of few weeks; **(b)** The drug can cause allergic reaction such as rashes and fever. Other idiosyncratic reactions include blood dyscrasias, aplastic anaemia, leukopenia, hepatitis and systemic lupus erythematosus but these are seen in patients being treated for trigeminal neuralgia; **(c)** Since carbamazepine stimulates ADH secretion (Ch. 17) it can cause water retention and hyponatraemia, **(d)** Risk of teratogenicity with carbamazepine is low but can induce finger nail hypoplasia, craniofacial defects and delayed development of foetus. However, its combination with valproic acid increases the risk of teratogenicity. Nonetheless, the overall incidence of toxicity of carbamazepine seems to be fairly low at usual therapeutic doses.

Oxcarbazepine shows lesser hypersensitivity reactions and has milder side effect profile compared to carbamazepine.

Drug Interactions

- Erythromycin, fluoxetine and isoniazid inhibit the metabolism of carbamazepine and precipitate toxicity.
- Carbamazepine and phenytoin increase each other's metabolism.
- Being enzyme inducer, it reduces the plasma concentration of haloperidol and oral contraceptives.
- No clinically significant drug displacement reactions occur with carbamazepine.

Ethosuximide

Ethosuximide belongs to the succinimide group of anticonvulsants. Being the drug of first choice for absence (petit mal) seizures it is also called "pure petit mal drug". Earlier, another drug *trimethadione* was used to treat absence seizures, but it is now no longer employed because of its toxicity and teratogenicity.

Mechanism of Action

It inhibits the low-threshold T-type Ca^{2+} channels (Mech. B-1, as above).

Therapeutic Uses and Plasma Levels

It is used as a pure petit mal drug. The therapeutic plasma levels are 60–100 μg/ml. These can be achieved by an oral dose of 20–30 mg/kg/day. Some patients can tolerate plasma concentrations up to 120 μg/ml without any complaints of side effects. Salivary titres also reflect plasma concentrations accurately, and may be useful to monitor blood levels.

Pharmacokinetics

Absorption is almost complete after oral administration. It is metabolised in liver and its metabolites are excreted through urine. The drug obeys first-order elimination kinetics.

Adverse Effects

It commonly causes GIT distress, headache, dizziness, hiccups, lethargy and euphoria. Serious reactions with ethosuximide are rare; yet non-dose related idiosyncratic adverse effects may include skin rashes, fever, eosinophilia and bone marrow depression. Ethosuximide is lesser teratogenic compared to other drugs and hence is preferred in pregnancy.

Drug Interactions

Valproic acid inhibits ethosuximide metabolism and clearance and increases its plasma levels.

Trimethadione

Though no longer used these days, it can still be used in patients not responding to any other drug. Its mechanism of action and therapeutic uses are similar to ethosuximide. Oral doses for adults are 30 mg/kg/day. The drug is much more toxic than ethosuximide. *Adverse effects* include *sedation* and *reversible hemeralopia* (glare effect and photophobia due to drug effects on neural layers of retina). If it occurs, there is no need to withdraw the drug but the patient should be advised to wear coloured glasses. The drug has *serious teratogenic effects* and if it is to be used during pregnancy, a medical termination of pregnancy should be advised.

Valproic Acid (Sodium Valproate)

Whether it is used as valproic acid or as sodium valproate or as valproate semisodium (divalproex), it is the valproate ion $(C_3H_7)_2.CHCOO^-$ which is the active form and is absorbed from GIT. The latter is also available as enteric-coated tablet and in extended release form.

Mechanism of Action

The drug probably owes its broad spectrum of activity to more than one molecular activity. It has been shown to **(1)** block use-dependent Na^+ channels (Mech. A-1); **(2)** increase GABA activity by activating glutamic acid decarboxylase (GAD) and by inhibiting GABA transaminase (Mech. A-2 above); **(3)** decrease the release of excitatory neurotransmitter glutamate in the brain and **(4)** blocks T-type Ca^{2+} channels (Mech. B-1 as above).

Therapeutic Use and Plasma Levels

- ANTIEPILEPTIC USE: Valproate has a broader spectrum of antiepileptic activity. It is very effective against absence seizures (mechanism B-1). It is usually preferred if the patient has concomitant generalised tonic-clonic attacks and myoclonic seizures. In combination with clonazepam it can be used to treat cortical myoclonus. A few patients of atonic attacks and many cases of partial seizures also respond with valproic acid. It is also a drug of choice for Lennox-Gastaut syndrome and for infantile spasm because of its wider therapeutic spectrum. As discussed above the withdrawal of valproate should be gradual to avoid precipitation of withdrawal seizures.
- THE THERAPEUTIC PLASMA LEVELS of valproate range from 50–100 μg/ml which may be attained by giving an oral dose of sod. valproate as 300 mg BD orally, slowly increased to 500 mg - 1 g BD. For valproate semisodium (Divalproex sod.) the dose is 500 mg BD, slowly increased to 1 g BD. Some patients can tolerate levels in excess of 100 μg/ml or a dose of 60 mg/kg/day, so the clinical assessment is a better index than plasma levels.
- NON-ANTIEPILEPTIC USE: **(1)** As discussed in Chapter 34, enteric-coated tablet of valproate semisodium (divalproex sodium) is used to treat manic depressive bipolar disorder; **(2)** Divalporex is also used for the prophylaxis of migraine and tension type cluster headache in a dose equivalent to 250 mg of valproic acid twice daily; **(3)** Valproate has been used with metyrapone to reduce cortisol secretion in the management of Cushing's syndrome; **(4)** Valproate due to its GABAergic action has been tried with encouraging results in the management of tardive dyskinesia and **(5)** It can also be used as an alternative drug to carbamazepine to treat trigeminal neuralgia.

Pharmacokinetics

Valproate is well absorbed (80%) following an oral dose. Food delays absorption, but the toxicity is reduced if the drug is given after meals. It is 90–95% bound to plasma proteins. It is potent enzyme inhibitor and can inhibit its own metabolism and that of other drugs like phenobarbital. The protein binding property and its enzyme inhibiting action can contribute to many drug interactions. An enteric-coated tablet as well as slow release preparation of divalproex sodium is also available.

Adverse Effects

Dose related side effects include weight gain, increase in appetite, GIT distress, tremors and reversible alopecia. Idiosyncratic toxicity is limited to hepatotoxicity which may be fatal. The risk is greater in children below 3 years and in those taking a combination of valproate with phenobarbital. Other idiosyncratic toxicities include pancreatitis and thrombocytopenia (but rarely). Valproic acid is associated with neural tube defects and its use during pregnancy results in a higher risk of spina bifida.

Drug Interactions

- It is not a CNS depressant but potentiates the CNS depressant effects of phenobarbitone and benzodiazepines.
- Valproic acid increases the plasma concentration of phenobarbital.
- It decreases the metabolism as well as displaces phenytoin from protein binding sites which results in increased phenytoin toxicity.

Benzodiazepines

The remarkable antiseizure potency of benzodiazepines has two prominent drawbacks which limit their usefulness as antiepileptic drugs. The first is their pronounced sedative effects and second is the development of tolerance to their anticonvulsant effects. Several benzodiazepines are used in the management of epileptic seizures. All of them share a common mechanism and pharmacological actions. Hence they will be discussed here as a class and individual members will be mentioned for specific indication. Their pharmacokinetics, other uses, adverse effects and drug interactions have been discussed in Chapter 32.

Mechanism of Action

They enhance the frequency of GABA-mediated Cl^- channel opening (Mech. A-2, as above). At higher doses they also block use-dependent Na^+ channels which contributes to their effectiveness in treating generalised status epilepticus.

Individual Drugs and Their Use

Lorazepam when injected in the dose of 4 mg I.V. (0.1mg/kg I.V. in children) at the rate of 2 mg/min repeated as per need every 10 min is the first choice of drug for the treatment of status epilepticus. It exerts a robust and sustained anti-seizure effect lasting for 6–12 hrs because of its high water solubility and slow distribution in the body. The incidence of thrombophlebitis in the injected blood vessel is quite low as compared to diazepam which is also used as an alternative drug for the same indication by the I.V. route.

Diazepam given in the dose of 10–30 mg (0.2–0.3 mg/kg in children) by slow I.V. administration is highly effective for terminating generalised tonic-clonic status epilepticus. It is also used (I.V.) for treating local anaesthetic induced seizures. For children at high risk of developing recurrent febrile seizures, rectally administered diazepam, at the time of fever, may prevent recurrent seizures. *Diazepam nasal spray* is recently approved for short-term management of epilepsy.

Clonazepam is more potent and longer acting than diazepam. It has greater efficacy against absence seizures and is also useful *as an adjuvant* in myoclonic and akinetic epilepsy.

Clorazepate is used *as an adjunct* drug for the treatment of complex partial seizures, in childhood myoclonic epilepsy and in complex partial seizures.

Clobazam is less sedative and longer acting than diazepam. It is active against partial and generalised seizures in the patients of all ages but is usually indicated for *adjunctive therapy.*

NEWER ANTIEPILEPTIC DRUGS

Newer agents are mostly "add-on" drugs that are expected to have more favourable safety profile in terms of toxicity, teratogenicity and drug interactions. The promising drugs among them are discussed below:

Vigabatrin

It is an irreversible inhibitor of GABA transaminase and thus elevates GABA levels in the brain (Mech. A-2; Fig 39.1A). The primary indication for vigabatrin is in the treatment of simple and complex partial seizures but it can also be used for generalised seizures. It can also be used as an adjunct drug for treating drug-refractory epilepsy and infantile spasm. It should not be used in cases of absence epilepsy or myoclonic seizures. The usual dose is 2 g/day orally, to be taken in equally divided doses. *Side effects* include behavioural changes (caution for psychic or elderly patients), sedation, amnesia and weight gain. Vigabatrin in 1% of cases causes irreversible visual field defects due to peripheral retinal atrophy. Hence, it should not be used in patients with pre-existing visual field defects and in children suffering from infantile spasm, in whom visual field monitoring is not possible.

Tiagabine

It inhibits GABA uptake by neurons and glia and thus increases the GABA content of brain (Mech. A-2; Fig. 39.1A). It is primarily used for the treatment of partial complex seizures, and as an adjunctive drug for refractory complex epilepsy. *Side effects* include dizziness, fatigue, sedation, tremors and confusion. Usual doses for adults are 20–60 mg/day in three to four equally divided doses.

Gabapentin and Pregabalin

Both are GABA analogues which readily cross BBB, and increase the synthesis and release of GABA to increase the GABA concentration in the brain. They also inhibit N-type Ca^{2+} channels and decrease the synaptic release of glutamate (Mech. A-4 as above) in therapeutic doses. Recent evidence suggests that they also function as $GABA_B$ receptor agonists.

The absorption of gabapentin from intestine depends on the carrier system and shows the property of saturation. Therefore increasing the dose does not proportionately increase the amount of drug absorbed which makes it relatively safe drug even after over-dosing. It is neither metabolised, nor bound to plasma proteins and is excreted unchanged by kidneys. Drug interactions are also minimal.

As an adjunct, it is effective in treating drug resistant partial seizures and generalised tonic-clonic seizures. Usual adult dose is 200–300 mg orally TDS. During chronic nerve injury, the $\alpha 2\delta$ subunits of L-type Ca^{2+} channels, in peripheral nerves, get up-regulated resulting in various types of neuropathies. Gabapentin binds tightly to $\alpha 2\delta$ type subunits and therefore has been found useful in treating diabetic neuropathy, post-herpetic neuralgia, trigeminal neuralgia and pain associated with multiple selerosis, albeit in higher doses (1800 mg/day orally in divided doses). *Side effects* include drowsiness, fatigue, dizziness, weight gain and ataxia. Dose of ***pregabalin*** is 200–600 mg orally TDS. Uses and effects are similar to gabapentin.

Topiramate

It is a broad-spectrum anticonvulsant drug acting by multiple mechanisms such as **(1)** blockade of use-dependent Na^+ channels (Mech. A-1), **(2)** activation of $GABA_A$ receptor and **(3)** inhibition of AMPA receptors for glutamate (Mech. A-3). It is most useful for generalised tonic-clonic, partial and absence seizures as well as for Lennox-Gastaut syndrome. Usual adult dose ranges from 300–600 mg/day orally in divided doses. *Side effects* include sedation, somnolence, amnesia, urolithiasis (as it also inhibits carbonic anhydrase enzyme) and teratogenic risk (hypospadias in male infants).

Zonisamide

This is also a broad-spectrum anticonvulsant drug having multiple modes of action which include **(1)** blockade of use-dependent Na^+ channels (Mech. A-1 in Fig.39.1) and inhibition of T-type Ca^{2+} channels (Mech. B-1 in Fig.39.1). It has a good bioavilability, linear elimination kinetics, negligible protein binding and renal excretion. The drug is effective against partial, generalised tonic-clonic and myoclonic seizures. It is also useful against infantile spasm and Lennox-Gastaut syndrome. Usual dose for adults ranges from 100–600 mg/day orally in two or three equally divided doses. *Side effects* include drowsiness, amnesia, skin rash and kidney stones (due to carbonic anhydrase inhibition).

Lamotrigine

It also has a broad spectrum of antiepileptic action. It directly blocks voltage-gated Na^+ channels (Mech. A-1) as well as N-type Ca^+ channels (Mech. A-4) and ultimately inhibits the release of excitatory neurotransmitter glutamate. It is quite effective in treating partial, generalised tonic-clonic, secondary generalised, absence and atonic seizures. It also appears to be effective in myoclonic seizures in children. The drug in a dose of 100–200 mg/day orally is also effective in treating bipolar disorder as an "add-on" drug (Ch. 34). *Side effects* include dizziness, ataxia, diplopia and skin rash (more common and severe in children below 16 yrs).

Felbamate

It blocks voltage-gated Na^+ channels, yet blockade of NMDA receptors that express NR2B subunit by antagonism at glycine site of the receptor seems to be a more plausible mechanism of its action (Mech. A 3 in Fig.39.1). It is useful in drug refractory epilepsies such as Lennox-Gastaut syndrome. Other indications include atonic seizures, atypical absence seizures, partial seizures and generalised tonic-clonic seizures. Usual *side effects* are insomnia, nausea, dizziness and ataxia. Unfortunately, felbamate is associated with unpredictable incidence of fatal aplastic anaemia and hepatotoxicity, hence its use is not popular. It has been withdrawn from market in some countries or available with restrictions.

Rufinamide

The drug is not structurally related to other anti-epileptic drugs, yet blocks neuronal sodium channel activation. In high doses it may have an inhibitory effect on metabotropic glutamate subtype 5 receptor (mGluR5). For the treatment of focal seizures and drop attacks of Lennox-Gastaut type epileptic syndrome in children above 4-yr. Like felbamate, rufinamide does not show serious adverse effects, and can be an alternative option for treating refractory epilepsy.

Perampanel

Perampanel is a non-competitive antagonist of postsynaptic AMPA receptor and thought to reduce the glutamate-induced generation and spread of seizurogenic neurotransmission in the brain. The drug has been approved for adjunct therapy in patients with partial epilepsy with or without secondary generalized seizures. Common ADR observed with the drug are: weight gain, dizzness, fatigue, somnolence, provocation of psychiatric problems like hostility, aggression and suicidal ideation. High doses ($\geq$ 120 mg/day) may produce altered gait, ataxia and balance disorder, therefore the drug should be given cautiously in elderly patients.

Levetiracetam

It is a piracetam derivative whose mechanism of action is uncertain. However, it binds selectively to SV_2A protein of synaptic vesicles in glutamatergic and GABAergic neurons (Mech. A-5). The drug is used specifically for treating partial seizures. Its elimination kinetics is linear and hence drug interactions are minimal. Usual oral adult dose is 500 mg twice daily. *Side effects* include somnolence, asthenia and dizziness.

Lacosamide

This drug has been approved by FDA for the treatment of partial seizures. It acts by inhibiting **(1)** VG-Na^+ channels (Mech. A-1) and **(2)** Collapsin-Response Mediator Protein-2 (CRMP-2) (see Mech. A-6 above). Usual doses start with 50 mg BD orally and increasing by 100 mg every week till 300 mg BD. *Side effects* are mild, e.g., headache, nausea and dizziness. Oral bioavailability is 100%. No clinically important drug interactions have been reported. It is neither an enzyme inducer nor inhibitor.

Cenobamate

It is approved by US-FDA for the treatment of partial onset seizures. It blocks neuronal voltage-gated sodium channels. Cenobamate also acts as a positive allosteric modulator of GABAA receptors independently from the benzodiazepine binding site. It is absorbed orally and metabolized in the liver by cytochrome P450 enzymes. It induces CYP3A4 and 2B6 metabolic enzymes. Hence, it has many drug interactions with phenytoin, lamotrigine and carbamazepine. *Adverse effects*: Somnolence, dizziness, diplopia, and disturbances in gait and coordination.

Stiripentol

Stiripentol is an aromatic alcohol which is unrelated to the structure of other antiepileptics. It increases GABAergic neurotransmission in CNS. It is used in Dravet syndrome which is a severe myoclonic epilepsy in infancy. It is approved as an adjunctive treatment for infants with GTCS and clonic seizures not controlled by other drugs. *Adverse effects*: Drowsiness, agitation, hypotonia, irritability and weight loss.

Brivaracetam

Brivaracetam is another drug that binds to synaptic vesicular protein 'SV2A' in synaptic vesicle. It is used in refractory partial seizures and GTCS. *Adverse effects*: Sleepiness, behavioural changes, ataxia and dizziness.

Cannabidiol

Cannabidiol is a constituent of the marijuana plant Cannabis sativa but does not cause psychoactive effects like euphoria. The mechanism is not clear exactly, but it is thought to affect transmission of electrical signals by modulating movement of calcium in neurons. It also affects signalling mediated by adenosine which has important role in seizure suppression. It is used in seizures associated with Lennox-Gastaut syndrome and Dravet syndrome. *Adverse effects*: Fever, weight loss, fatigue, somnolence, rash and elevated transaminases.

GUIDELINES FOR ANTIEPILEPTIC DRUG USAGE

Select a drug depends on type of seizure, toxicity profile of drug, convenience of administration, cost, age, sex etc. Monitor liver functions, if patient is taking valproate. *Educate patient*: Do not withdraw drug suddenly as it precipitates seizures. Educate about specific adverse effects of drug and do not take any other drug without consultation of doctor. *Avoid polypharmacy*: As antiepileptic drugs have more drug interactions: Do not use FDCs of antiepileptic drugs.

Epilepsy in Pregnancy

Antiepileptics should be continued during pregnancy, as abrupt withdrawal may precipitate status epilepticus. Lowest possible dose should be given. Avoid valproate, phenytoin. Carbamazepine; these are teratogenic drugs associated with major malformations. *Newer antiepileptics* (Lamotrigine , levetiracetam, topiramate) are considered to be safer in pregnancy. *Folic acid supplementation* (0.5 mg/day) should be given to prevent neural tube defect. *Prophylactic vitamin K_1* should be administered (10 mg/day) to prevent hemorrhage in the neonate.

Table 39.1 Choice of antiseizure drugs

Types of seizure	Preferred drugs	Alternative drugs
GTCS, SPS	Lamotrigine, Valproate, Carbamazepine	Phenytoin, Clobazam, Phenobarbitone
CPS	Lamotrigine, Valproate, Carbamazepine	Gabapentin, Phenytoin, Levetiracetam
Absence	Valproate (>2 years), Ethosuximide (< 2 years)	Clonazepam, Clobazam, Lamotrigine
Myoclonic	Valproate	Levetiracetam, topiramate
Atonic	Valproate	Lamotrigine
Febrile seizure	Diazepam (rectal)	Lorazepam
Infantile spasm	Valproate, Clonazepam, Vigabatrin	–
Eclampsia	Magnesium sulphate	–

CHAPTER 40 Drug Therapy for Neurodegenerative Disorders

COMPETENCY PH1.19

Relative to its size, the brain experiences a higher quantum of oxidative stress, excitotoxicity, protein deposition (amyloidosis) and apoptosis. All such events cause devastating damage to the brain cells and neurons leading to a variety of neurodegenerative disorders. Some of these include:

1. **Alzheimer's dementia** in which the neuronal injury is primarily in the hippocampus and cortex;
2. **Parkinson's disease,** a disabling motor impairment due to loss of nigrostriatal dopaminergic neurons;
3. **Huntington's chorea** in which GABAergic striatonigral pathway is impaired;
4. **Amyotrophic lateral sclerosis** (ALS or Lou Gehrig disease) in which there is degeneration of spinal, bulbar and cortical neurons, and
5. **Multiple sclerosis,** which is an autoimmune disorder resulting in the impairment of nerve conduction due to demyelination of neurons.

Millions of brain cells are non-replicable. This means that once they are damaged they would remain, most likely, dysfunctional for rest of the life. The neurodegenerative disorders cited above, therefore, are merely the part of progression that begins with the aging of the brain due to oxidative damage and excitotoxicity. When eventually enough brain cells are damaged, in some specified area, the respective neurodegenerative disease is manifested. People don't just wake up one day and have Alzheimer's or Parkinson's diseases as these diseases rather represent the end stages of free radical induced damage to the brain. Consequently, the drug therapy has little to offer in such situations as it provides merely symptomatic relief and does not cure or prevent the progression of the disease satisfactorily. However, the pharmocological intervention in most of these diseases either allows protection or provides compensation for the neuronal loss.

PARKINSON'S DISEASE

Parkinson's disease is a slowly progressive neurodegenerative disease characterised by:

Pill rolling tremors, **A**kathisia (inability to sit still), **R**igidity, **K**inesias (akinesia, bradykinesia), **I**nstable (stooped) posture, **N**o arm swinging in rhythm with legs, **S**ialorrhea, **O**culogyric crisis (eyes are held fixed for a variable length of time), **N**ervous depression, **I**nvoluntary tremors, **S**eborrhea and **M**asked facial expression. The term ***parkinsonism*** applies for a disease state having such common characteristics while ***Parkinson's disease (paralysis agitans)*** is restricted to the primary or idiopathic parkinsonism. Most patients suffer from this type of parkinsonism and intriguingly the causes remain unknown or are multifactorial, e.g., genetic predisposition and aging of brain due to free radical damage to dopaminergic neurons in basal ganglia. The clinical symptoms of Parkinson's disease appear at about 80% loss in dopaminergic neurotransmission which gradually worsens with the age of the patient. Prognosis, even after drug therapy is, therefore, poor.

Secondary parkinsonism occurs from known cause and many of these are curable. It may result after prolonged use of antipsychotic drugs (D_2 receptor antagonists). Unlike idiopathic parkinsonism (Parkinson's disease), the striatal contents of DA are not reduced by administration of these drugs. They rather decrease the dopaminergic activity by blocking the postsynaptic D_2 receptors. Parkinsonism may also result by poisoning due to manganese, carbon monoxide or MPTP (Ch. 38)—a side product formed during faulty synthesis of pethidine. MPTP is a protoxin which is converted to a reactive methylphenyl pyridinium (MPP^+) by MAO-B enzyme. MPP^+ free radical is then selectively taken up by cells in the substantia nigra through DA reuptake transporters.

Once inside the cell, MPP^+ inhibits mitochondrial complex-1 resulting into inhibition of oxidative phosphorylation (involved in neural mitochondrial respiratory processes) and ultimately cell death. The progressive degeneration of striatal dopaminergic neurons that follows leads to parkinsonism. Incidentally no such toxin has yet been identified in the environment. Hence, the incidence of such type of parkinsonism is restricted to pethidine abusers only. However, MPTP-induced parkinsonism in experimental animals now provides a pharmacological model for evaluating antiparkinsonism drugs on non-human primates.

Genetic and Neuropathological Features

Parkinsonism usually afflicts 1–2% of individuals over the age of 65 years. A small subset of patients has familial form of parkinsonism with an autosomal dominant pattern of inheritance. Genetic mutations in at least three proteins have been identified so far. These genes encode for α-synuclein and carboxy terminal hydroxylase of parkin and ubiquitin.

The most prominent pathological findings in Parkinson's disease are: (1) degeneration of darkly pigmented dopaminergic neurons in the substantia nigra. This results due to accumulation of neuromelanin which is possibly derived from oxidised dopamine, (2) loss of DA in the neostriatum and (3) the presence of intracellular inclusion bodies known as Lewy bodies. However, whether these inclusions contribute to neuronal degeneration or they are simply the byproducts of degenerated neurons is not clear. In addition to cell death in substantia nigra, patients with Parkinson's disease may exhibit neuronal amyloid-like protein deposition.

Neurotransmitter Role in Parkinsonism

The input unit of basal ganglia is neostriatum (corpus striatum) while the output unit is substantia nigra pars reticulata (SNPR) and globus pallidus medialis (GPM). The excitatory inputs to neostriatum from cerebral cortex involve glutamatergic neurons. The neostriatum in turn projects to SNPR and GPM *via* two pathways: The *direct* and the *indirect* pathways (Fig. 40.1A). The *direct pathway* from the striatum to SNPR and GPM involves inhibitory GABAergic neurons. The *indirect pathway* involves two other nuclei in between: the globus pallidus lateralis (GPL) and subthalamic nucleus (STN). The primary projection from the neostriatum to GPL and secondary projection from GPL to STN involve GABAergic neurons and both are inhibitory; while the third projection from STN to SNPR and GPM is *via* excitatory glutamatergic neurons. The output from SNPR and GPM to thalamus is *via* inhibitory GABAergic neurons while from thalamus to cerebral cortex is *via* glutamatergic excitatory neurons.

The dopaminergic neurons from substantia nigra pars compacta (SNPC) also project to the neostriatum leading to excitation of striatal neurons belonging to direct pathway, by acting on excitatory D_1 receptors. To counterbalance the activity of the direct pathway, these dopaminergic neurons, from SNPC, also inhibit the striatal neurons of the indirect pathway, by acting on inhibitory D_2 receptors. The large cholinergic striatal interneurons tend to oppose the actions of dopaminergic neurons in both the pathways.

In short, a functional balance between dopaminergic and cholinergic system in neostriatum maintains the optimal tone and movement of voluntary muscles by keeping a balanced regulation of the direct and the indirect pathway. *The direct pathway*, generally inhibits SNPR and GPM and thus disinhibits the thalamic drive and increases the motor activity (i.e., by inhibiting the inhibitory GABAergic neurons projecting from SNPR and GPM to thalamus). *The indirect pathway* which involves excitatory inputs from STN to SNPR and GPM inhibits thalamic activity and decreases the cerebral control on voluntary movements (due to excitation of GABAergic neurons projecting from SNPR and GPM to thalamus).

In Parkinson's disease (PD), there is a loss of dopaminergic neurons (Fig. 40.1A) projecting from SNPC to neostriatum, which leads to the neuronal imbalance in the dopaminergic and cholinergic levels (Fig. 40.1B). The lack of dopamine (DA) due to degeneration of DA neurons, indirectly leads to hyperactivity of cholinergic neurons, as the cholinergic system *per se* is not primarily affected. This imbalance alters the neostriatal outflow pathways. *The direct pathway* from neostriatum to SNPR becomes suppressed whereas the indirect pathway from neostriatum to GPL to SNPR, through

STN becomes overactive. This results in an enhanced activation of SNPR outflow to thalamus through GABAergic neurons which ultimately exerts an overall suppression of the thalamic-cortical pathway and inhibition of the voluntary movements (bradykinesia or akinesia). Tremors associated with Parkinson's disease have been more difficult to explain. Some reports suggest a role of thalamus in tremor generation. The redressing of balance between dopaminergic and cholinergic systems by drugs (see below) prove beneficial in the management of Parkinson's disease. However, no clinically useful drugs for Parkinsonism are presently available based on GABA or glutamate role in the circuitry of the basal ganglia (Fig. 40.1).

DRUG THERAPY FOR PARKINSON'S DISEASE

Since there is no cure for Parkinson's disease, the aim of drug therapy is to provide symptomatic relief by the use of drugs that can restore the dopaminergic and cholinergic balance that is disturbed due to degeneration of dopaminergic neurons in the nigrostriatal pathway (Fig. 40.1B). Such drugs belong to following categories:

I. Drugs Which Increase Dopamine Levels

a) Levodopa with Carbidopa

DA itself does not cross BBB, and its peripheral effects provide no benefits in parkinsonism. On the contrary, ***levodopa***, the precursor of DA (Fig. 12.2), can cross BBB where it is decarboxylated to DA. If administered alone, unfortunately, only about 1–3% of levodopa actually enters the brain unaltered, which provides insufficient levels of DA in the brain. About 97–99% of levodopa gets metabolised in GIT and pripheral tissues by dopa decarboxylase enzyme to DA (which now cannot penetrate BBB). This means that levodopa must be given in larger amounts if it is used alone. To prevent its peripheral degradation, *levodopa* is usually coadministered with either ***carbidopa*** or ***benserazide***, a peripheral dopa decarboxylase inhibitor. The combination of levodopa with benserazide or carbidopa lowers the dose requirement of levodopa and reduces the incidence of peripheral side effects associated with its use (Fig. 40.2). Two types of such fixed dose formulations (Sinemet®) are available (1:4 or 1:10, i.e., carbidopa 25 mg + levodopa 100 mg or carbidopa 25 mg + levodopa 250 mg).

Levodopa is widely used for treatment of all types of parkinsonism, except the one associated with antipsychotic drug therapy because it can cure the parkinsonism but will precipitate schizophrenia for which antipsychotic therapy was instituted. A beneficial response to levodopa is obtained in nearly 75% cases of idiopathic parkinsonism. All clinical manifestations of parkinsonism respond to some extent to ***levodopa*** + ***carbidopa*** therapy. However, tremors are less responsive to this therapy, than is rigidity or bradykinesia, but abnormalities of posture, locomotion and other symptoms all improve with such treatment. The therapy is started with a smaller dose, i.e., carbidopa 25 mg + levodopa 100 mg (1:4 ratio) three times a day to be taken one hour before meals. It is ultimately increased to 1:10 ratio, i.e., carbidopa 25 mg + levodopa 250 mg thrice a day. If need arises, a dopamine agonist is added to increase dopaminergic activity (See below) (Fig. 40.2).

Adverse Effects

Fluctuations in Response

Patients receiving long-term levodopa therapy commonly experience a "*wearing-off effect*", which means that the duration of benefit usually shortens from each dose of levodopa as the therapy progresses. Patients can also develop sudden, unpredictable fluctuations between mobility and immobility characterised by "*on-off phenomenon*". In the "*on state*" the patient enjoys normal mobility, which is followed by the "*off-state*" wherein the patient may be unable to rise from the chair on which he had sat down a few minutes ago. Levodopa has a very short half-life (1–2 hrs), and the rapid fluctuations in its plasma levels seem to be responsible for this "*on-off phenomenon*". The concomitant use of COMT inhibitors such as *tolcapone* or *entacapone* (see below) helps in counteracting the fluctuations in the plasma levels of levodopa.

Dyskinesias

These are excessive and abnormal choreiform movements of limbs, trunk, face and tongue. These symptoms occur in majority (50–90%) of cases receiving long-term high dosage levodopa therapy.

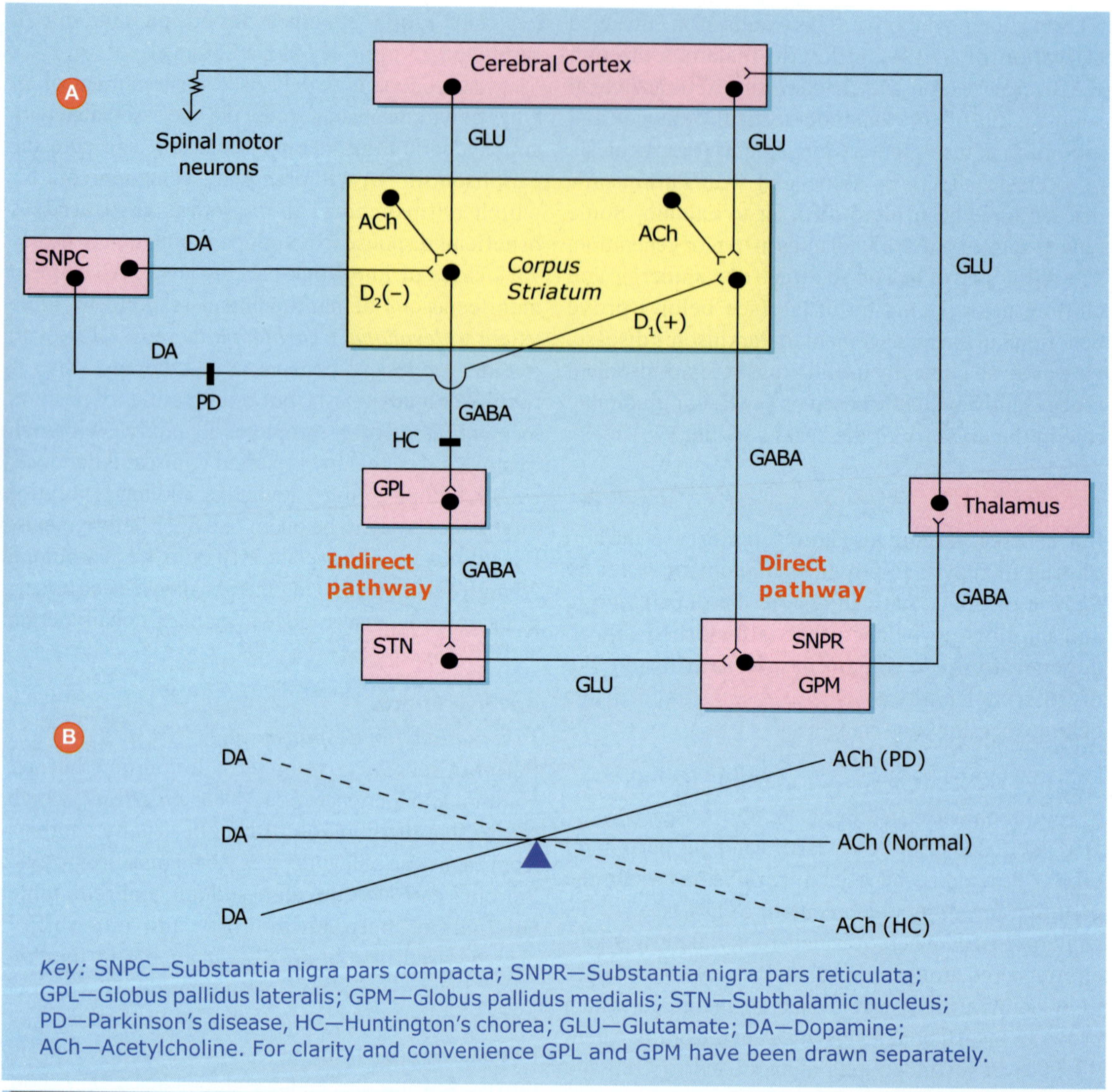

Fig 40.1 The Functional Circuitry Between the Cortex, Basal Ganglia and Thalamus with Neurotransmitter Role in Motor Neurons.

Dyskinesias disappear if the dose of levodopa is reduced, but this causes rigidity to return. Therefore, the margin between the beneficial effects and the toxicity becomes progressively narrower, as the therapy with levodopa advances. The mechanism underlying these abnormal movements is unclear, but probably relates to fluctuating plasma levels of levodopa and to the development of supersensitive DA receptors.

Other Central Side Effects

These include vivid dreams, delusions, hallucinations, confusion and sleep disturbances, especially in the elderly. Prolonged therapy with levodopa and carbidopa, by increasing DA activity in brain, can precipitate schizophrenia-like syndrome in elderly, which can be controlled by giving olanzapine, quetiapine or risperidone.

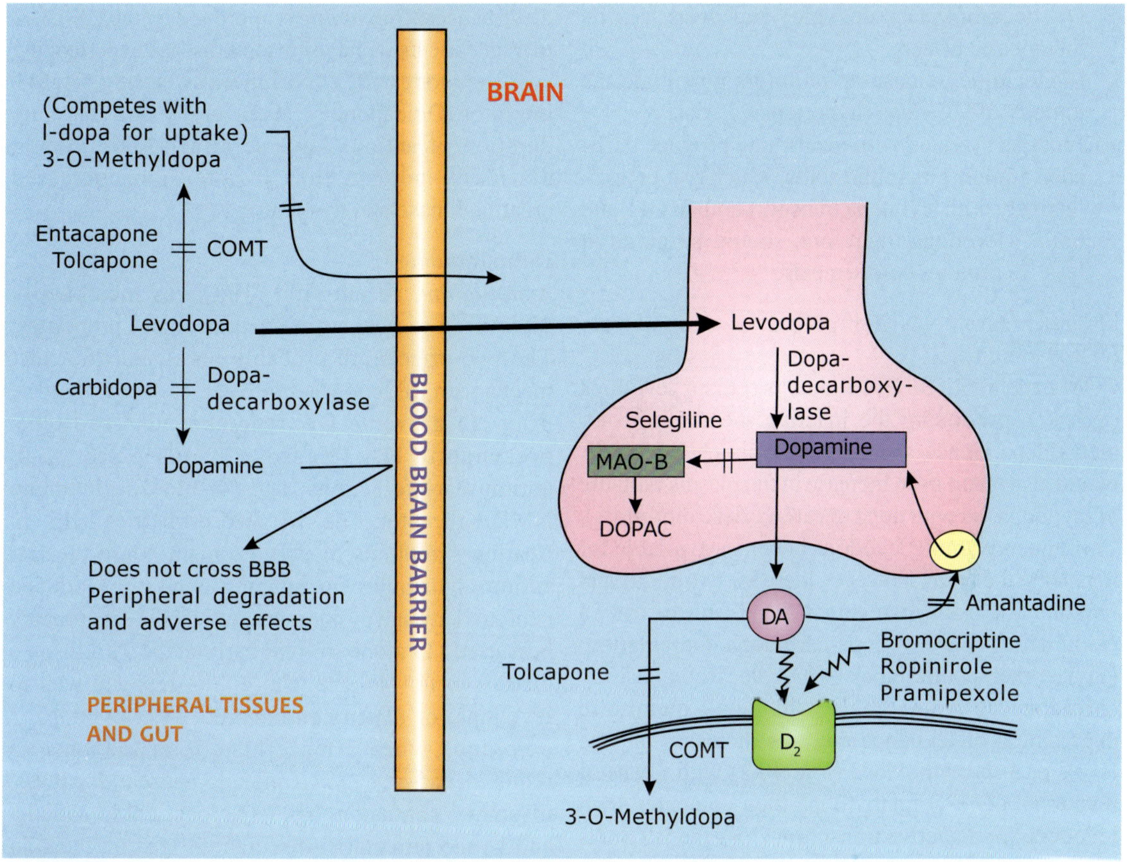

Fig 40.2 Mechanism of Action of Various Dopaminergic Drugs Used in the Treatment of Parkinson's Disease

Cardiovascular Side Effects

Postural hypotension may occur as a result of the release of DA into the circulation, after some peripheral decarboxylation of levodopa, but tolerance develops later. Cardiac arrhythmias may at times occur in some patients and are attributed to the stimulation of cardiac α_1 and β_1 adrenoceptors by DA.

Peripheral Side Effects

Anorexia, nausea and vomiting (due to stimulation of CTZ by DA) can occur in 80% of patients taking levodopa alone. Nausea-vomiting is much less with the combination of levodopa with carbidopa. Tolerance also develops to these effects at a later stage. However, if need arises, domperidone (Ch. 28) may be used to prevent nausea and vomiting.

Miscellaneous Side Effects

- Levodopa may cause mydriasis and may precipitate an attack of glaucoma in some patients.
- Abnormalities in smell or taste; hot flushes and precipitation of gout.
- Mild but transient increase in blood urea, serum transaminases, alkaline phosphatase and bilirubin.

Contraindications

(a) Psychoses, (b) Narrow angle glaucoma, (c) Cardiac arrhythmias and (d) Melanoma (as levodopa is a precursor of skin melanin).

Drug Interactions

- Pyridoxine (vit. B_6) enhances the extracerebral metabolism of levodopa (as it is a cofactor for

DA-decarboxylase enzyme) and decreases its therapeutic effects.

- Monoamine oxidase-A inhibitors potentiate the toxicity of levodopa (hypertensive crisis).
- Proteins ingested with meals may produce sufficient amounts of amino acids, which compete effectively with levodopa transport both in GIT and brain. Levodopa, therefore, should be given at least 30 minutes before meals.

b) Catecholamine-O-Methyl Transferase Inhibitors (COMT Inhibitors)

COMT metabolises DA and its precursor levodopa (Ch. 12), producing the inactive metabolite 3-O-methyldopa. Hence, an inhibition of peripheral COMT would also result in an increase in the plasma half-life of levodopa (as with dopa decarboxylase inhibitors). Consequently, more levodopa becomes available for transfer to the brain. However, there are two additional reasons for administering COMT inhibitors in conjunction with levodopa-carbidopa combination: **(1)** The therapeutic block of DA decarboxylase by carbidopa activates COMT-mediated metabolic degradation of levodopa and this increases plasma levels of 3-O-methyldopa (Fig. 40.2) with a loss of levodopa. **(2)** 3-O-methyldopa then competes with levodopa for an active transport across the BBB. As a result, the therapeutic effectiveness of levodopa is reduced. Selective COMT inhibitors such as ***tolcapone*** and ***entacapone*** not only diminish the peripheral metabolism of levodopa (by COMT) but also increase its bioavailability in the brain (by reducing the concentration of 3-O methyldopa and its competition with levodopa for active transport to BBB). The levodopa dose can be reduced further and its effects are enhanced or extended in patients who have developed response fluctuations—leading to smoother "on-off" with more prolonged "on state." The pharmacological effects of ***tolcapone*** and ***entacapone*** are similar. However, tolcapone has both central and peripheral effects while entacapone is a peripheral blocker of COMT. Tolcapone has been occasionally associated with severe hepatotoxicity and death and hence entacapone is generally preferred as it is devoid of hepatotoxicity. The *side effects* common to both drugs include dyskinesias, nausea, diarrhoea, postural hypotension and sleep disturbances. ***Opicapone*** is approved by the US-FDA to treat patients with Parkinson's disease experiencing "off" episodes. It is peripherally acting COMT inhibitor. Opicapone is given orally and has long duration of action. Adverse effects: Dry mouth, dizziness, hallucination, hypotension, increased creatine kinase and dyskinesia.

c) Amantadine

Amantadine, an antiviral drug, was incidentally discovered to possess antiparkinsonism properties. The two effects are probably unrelated. Its exact mechanism of action is not clear. It seems that the drug **(1)** prevents DA reuptake; **(2)** facilitates presynaptic DA release; **(3)** possesses weak antimuscarinic actions; and **(4)** blocks glutamate NMDA receptor. The first two properties help in treating symptoms of parkinsonism while the last action contributes in reducing excitation-induced neurotoxicity and dyskinesias. Amantadine is probably best used **(1)** alone to treat early-stage Parkinson's disease or for patients who do not respond well to levodopa, or **(2)** in combination with levodopa + carbidopa when a more beneficial response is required. *Adverse effects* include nausea, dizziness, insomnia, confusion, hallucinations, ankle oedema and livedo reticularis (discoloured area on the skin due to passive congestion). Amantadine and antimuscarinic drugs exert additive CNS side effects.

II. Drugs Which Prevent Dopamine Degradation

MAO-B Inhibitors (Selegiline, Safinamide, Rasagiline)

Selegiline (deprenyl) is an irreversible inhibitor of MAO-B, a principal enzyme in dopaminergic neurons, responsible for metabolism of dopamine (Ch. 12). This makes more DA available for stimulation of its receptors (Fig. 40.2). Selegiline, as a monotherapy, is useful in early stage Parkinson's disease, but in late-stage parkinsonism it is used in conjunction with levodopa + carbidopa to reduce the requirements of levodopa and to minimise the problem of dyskinesias associated with long-term use of levodopa. A neuroprotective effect of selegiline in parkinsonian patients has also been proposed. Though controversial in human beings, selegiline may retard the progression of Parkinson's disease by reducing the oxidative damage due to the formation of free radicals produced during the metabolism of dopamine (Fig. 40.3). It has been suggested that the neuroprotective and antiapoptotic effects of selegiline are related to its metabolite desmethyl selegiline.

Selegiline may cause insomnia and hence the standard dose schedule is 5 mg with breakfast and 5 mg with lunch. Selegiline has little effect on MAO-A and therefore usually does not cause the hypertension associated with the ingestion of tyramine-enriched food, except in high doses (Ch. 34). Selegiline should not be co-administered with tricyclic antidepressants and selective serotonin reuptake inhibitors for the risk of acute toxic reactions such as hyperpyrexia, agitation, delirium and coma.

Rasagiline is similar to selegiline, but is more potent. It prevents the formation of neurotoxin MPP^+ from MPTP and thus provides neuroprotective effects in patients of Parkinson's disease. Antioxidants + tocopherol (vit. E) are reported to increase the effectiveness of rasagiline or selegiline but large scale multicentered trials are needed to confirm the claims.

Safinamide is given orally, metabolized in liver by hydrolytic oxidation to the primary metabolite safinamide acid. *Adverse effects*: Nausea, insomnia, anxiety, cough, dyskinesia, hypertension and allergic reactions.

III. Drugs Which Stimulate Dopamine Receptors

Dopamine Agonists

These drugs directly stimulate DA receptors and do not depend on the formation of DA from levodopa. Besides complementing levodopa, these drugs offer several advantages: they **(1)** do not require their metabolic conversion to DA; **(2)** do not depend on the functional integrity of nigrostriatal dopaminergic neurons; **(3)** have longer duration of action than levodopa with lesser dyskinesias and 'on-off' phenomenon; **(4)** are more selective than levodopa on specific subpopulations of DA receptors and **(5)** are less likely to generate damaging free radicals.

Bromocriptine and ***cabergoline*** are amine ergot derivatives which share a common DA like structure, while ***ropinirole*** and ***pramipexole*** are new non-ergot derived DA receptor agonists (Fig. 40.2). There is no evidence that one agonist is superior to another. *Adverse effects*: Anorexia, nausea, vomiting, vertigo, postural hypotension, painless peripheral or digital vasospasm, peripheral oedema, pleural fibrosis and erythromelalgia are the side effects associated

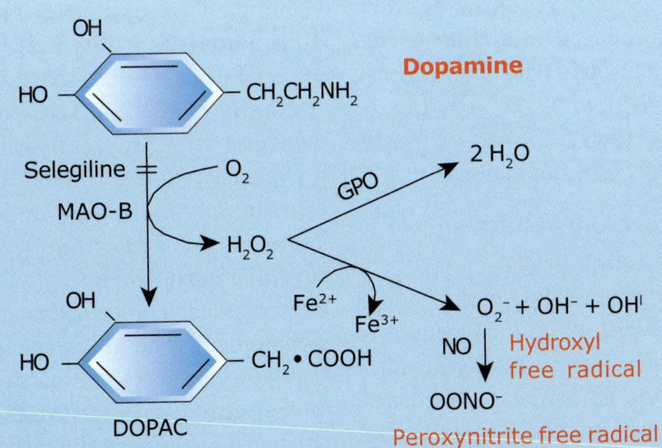

Key: DOPAC—Dihydroxyphenylalanine; GPO—Glutathione peroxidase. It has been found that Fe^{2+} is pathologically elevated in the substantia nigra of the patients with Parkinson's disease.

Fig 40.3 Dopamine Metabolism and Oxidative Damage to Substantia Nigra.

with ergot-derived DA agonists which generally limit their use. Erythromelalgia consists of red, tender, painful swollen joints of feet and hands. These symptoms are less frequent and less severe with ***pramipexole*** and ***ropinirole***. They provide rapid achievement of therapeutic response and are better tolerated, and therefore are increasingly used as monotherapy. *Pramipexole* (0.125–0.75 mg OD) or *ropinirole* (0.25 mg OD) are also used to treat "restless legs syndrome" particularly in diabetic patients with neuropathy. Though rarely, an uncontrollable tendency to fall asleep at unusual times and a development of compulsive behaviour has been observed in patients receiving pramipexole and ropinirole.

Bromocriptine is a potent D_2 receptor agonist and a weak D_1 antagonist. ***Cabergoline*** is like bromocriptine but longer acting ($t_{1/2}$>80 hrs). ***Ropinirole*** and ***pramipexole*** are D_2, D_3 and D_4 receptor agonists with more selectivity for D_2 receptor. The agents are most commonly used either as inital monotherapy (reduced risk of dyskinesia compared to levodopa) or as an adjunct to levodopa + carbidopa treatment to smooth out its 'on-off' phenomenon. *Pramipexole* is excreted mainly (96–98%) by kidney, while *ropinirole* is metabolised mainly by CYP1A2. Hence, ciprofloxacin which inhibits CYP1A2 can significantly increase ropinirole plasma concentration. Lately, a new non-ergot DA receptor agonist, ***Rotigotine,*** has been introduced in a ***transdermal patch formulation***. It is a D_2 and D_3 receptor agonist. D_3 agonist action is linked with slowing of neurodegenerative process. *Side effects:* somnolence. *Drug interactions:* not major.

IV. Drugs Which Restore DA-ACh Balance

Centrally Acting Antimuscarinic Drugs

The efficacy of these drugs in treating parkinsonism is due to their ability to block muscarinic receptors in the striatum. In the absence of the inhibitory control of DA, the activity of the intrastriatal cholinergic interneurons becomes dominant. Blockade of central muscarinic receptors by these drugs reduces striatal cholinergic activity (Fig. 40.1B). The muscarinic antagonists are most commonly used to treat **(1)** early-stages of the disease; **(2)** late-stage parkinsonism as an adjunct to levodopa + carbidopa therapy; and **(3)** neuroleptic-induced extrapyramidal side effects (Ch. 33). The drugs in this category include: ***trihexyphenidyl (benzhexol), procyclidine, orphenadrine*** and ***benztropine***. Interestingly, these drugs correct tremors and rigidity of parkinsonism more efficiently than other symptoms. The *adverse effects* are related to their anticholinergic actions and include: dry mouth, blurred vision, urinary retention, constipation and in high doses confusion, delirium and hallucinations. For drug interactions and contraindications see Chapter 11.

Trihexyphenidyl has been reported to have some abuse potential and parkinsonian patients may display "fake" parkinsonian signs to obtain the drug. The antihistamine ***diphenhydramine***, because of its anticholinergic effects can also be used to treat milder parkinsonism.

Istradefylline is a selective adenosine A_{2A} receptor inhibitor. These receptors are found in the basal ganglia, a region of the brain degeneration in Parkinson's disease, and are also significantly involved in motor control. It is approved for Parkinson's disease 'Off' period due to levodopa therapy. *Adverse effects*: Nausea, vomiting, dyskinesia, hallucination, insomnia, dizziness and allergic reactions.

HUNTINGTON'S CHOREA

Huntington's disease (HD) is an inherited (autosomal dominant) disorder characterised by choreic hyperkinesias (dance-like movements of limbs and rhythmic movements of tongue and face) and dementia with progressive brain degeneration. Its prevalence rate is 1:10,000. It is caused by a genetic error in *huntingtin gene* and subsequent abnormal synthesis of a *huntingtin protein* that contains several repeats of polyglutamine. The larger the number of such repeats, the earlier the appearance of symptoms. The huntingtin gene interacts with various regulatory proteins that participate in excitotoxicity and apoptosis. Some of these interactions are enhanced by the polyglutamine repeats in the mutant huntingtin protein, which may account for the neuronal loss in cortex and striatum resulting in progressive severe involuntary jerky (choreiform) movements.

The neuropharmacological change in HD is the degeneration of GABAergic neurons in the striatum (Fig. 40.1A). There is 75% reduction in the activity of glutamic acid decarboxylase (an enzyme responsible for GABA synthesis). It is believed that loss of GABA-mediated inhibition in the basal ganglia produces hyperactivity of dopaminergic neurons. There is also a significant decline in the concentration of choline acetyl transferase (an enzyme responsible for the synthesis of ACh) in the basal ganglia of such patients.

The treatment strategy followed in parkinsonism of "replacing" the missing neurotransmitter has not proved clinically effective in HD because GABA receptor agonists or even inhibitors of GABA catabolism have not provided any clinical benefits. Administration of choline chloride to compensate cholinergic underactivity is not therapeutically useful either. Surprisingly, adjusting the DA/ACh balance (Fig. 40.1B) by antagonising DA overactivity has proved more effective, in reducing the involuntary movements while drugs such as levodopa or bromocriptine make them worse. Thus the antipsychotic drugs such as ***chlorpromazine, haloperidol*** which are potent DA receptor antagonist and even an atypical neuroleptic ***olanzapine*** (Ch. 33) are useful in HD. A dopamine depleting drug ***tetrabenazine*** has also been found useful in HD.

ALZHEIMER'S DISEASE (AD)

Alzheimer's disease (AD) is the most prevalent form of dementia which does not have any previous cause such as stroke, brain trauma or alcohol toxicity. It is also distinct from vascular dementia, which is associated with brain infarction. The cardinal features of AD are progressive loss of memory and disordered cognitive functions, with loss of short-term memory that usually precedes the loss of long-term memory. Alzheimer's patients not only do not know what day it is, they do not even recognise their own families. Other signs of AD include reduced verbal fluency and impairment of speech due to failure of arranging words in proper sequence. Ultimately, with progression of brain degeneration, patient may fall into a vegetative state. Death is usually associated with complications of immobility (e.g., pneumonia or pulmonary embolism).

The main pathological features of AD comprise:

1. Amyloid plaque, consisting of extracellular deposits of β-amyloid protein (Aβ) in selective areas of brain such as cortex, hippocampus, amygdala and subcortical nuclei etc. Neurotoxicity in AD results from excessive formation of Aβ protein. Familial AD (rare) results from mutations in the genes for amyloid precursor protein (APP) which causes an increase in Aβ formation.
2. Intraneuronal neurofibrillary tangles which comprise of the aggregates of highly phosphorylated form of normal neuronal protein (Tau). The relationship of these neurofibrillary tangles to neurodegeneration is not known. It is still not clear whether the neuritic plaques and/or the tangles are causative factors or the byproduct of free radical damage leading to brain degeneration. However, major evidence suggests that both the processes are responsible for neuronal cell death and disruption in synaptic signaling.
3. Marked decrease in choline acetyltransferase and loss of cholinergic neurons in the brain. The cholinergic neurons, destroyed in AD, originate from nucleus basalis in the forebrain and project to the frontal cortex and hippocampus and play a critical role in learning, memory and cognition.

The loss of cholinergic activity in brain of Alzheimer's patients led to the use of cholinesterase inhibitors that can cross BBB. These drugs block the degradation of ACh and increase the availability of ACh in synaptic clefts. ***Tacrine***, a longer acting reversible anticholinesterase, can be used for palliative treatment of mild to moderate form of AD. It is orally active and provides improvements in memory, cognition and in general well-being soon after the initiation of the therapy. Long-term administration or using this drug for the middle or late stages of AD provides mixed results. Tacrine facilitates the release of ACh from cholinergic nerve endings as well. However, it produces significant, although reversible, hepatotoxicity in therapeutic doses; hence its use has declined. ***Donepezil, rivastigmine*** and ***galantamine*** are reversible anticholinesterases having better penetration into CNS. These are less toxic and better tolerated than tacrine, but clinical results are only modest and temporary. Usual dosage are: ***Donepezil,*** initially 5 mg once daily in the evening increased maximum up to 10 mg once daily after 4 weeks; ***Rivastigmine***, initially 1.5 mg orally BD increased up to 3 mg BD after 2 weeks; ***Galantamine,*** initially 4 mg BD orally, increased up to 8 mg BD after one to two weeks. Lately, ***transdermal rivastigmine patch*** has been introduced (applied every 24 hrs) to improve patient compliance. Use of these drugs is not associated with hepatotoxicity except for peripheral cholinergic side effects, e.g., diarrhoea, nausea, vomiting and increased urination.

Recently, ***acetyl-L-carnitine,*** a structural analogue of ACh has shown promise in decreasing signs and symptoms of dementia in AD. Besides increasing cholinergic transmission, ***acetyl-L-carnitine*** also has some antioxidant properties and thus slows down the progression of the disease.

4. It is also postulated that excitotoxicity due to enhanced glutamate transmission via NMDA receptors, also contributes to pathophysiology of AD. ***Memantine*** (5 mg once daily, slowly increased to 10–20 mg /day which can also be given in divided doses as 10 mg BD) is a non-competitive antagonist of NMDA receptor. It is better tolerated and less toxic than cholinesterase inhibitors.
5. Nootropic drugs such as ***piracetam***, and ***aniracetam***, though effective in animal models, are probably ineffective in AD. Recent studies have shown that high doses of ***vitamin E*** (1000 IU BD) plus ***antioxidants*** containing ***vitamin C, vitamin A, zinc, selenium*** and ***bioflavanoids*** or ***spirulina*** significantly decrease the progression of AD even in middle stage.
6. Some evidence reveal that ***Rosiglitazone*** (Ch. 47), the ***Statins*** (Ch. 23) and ***Ibuprofen*** (Ch. 26) have beneficial effects in AD.
7. Recent trials with antiamyloid monoclonal antibody ***Bapineuzumab*** have provided very encouraging results but its approval is awaited.
8. **Aducanumab** is recently approved by US-FDA for the treatment of Alzheimer's disease. It is a monoclonal IgG1 antibody that targets extracellular amyloid-β plaques in the brain. Aducanumab treatment is associated with slowing the rate of progression of Alzheimer's disease and decreases p-tau proteins in cerebrospinal fluid. Given intravenously 10 mg/kg. *Adverse effects:* Nausea, headache, confusion, delirium, disorientation, dizziness, vision abnormality and allergic reactions.

MULTIPLE SCLEROSIS (MS)

This common neurologic disorder, which probably has an autoimmune basis, has its greatest incidence in young adults. Pathologically, scattered focal areas of demyelination are found in brain, spinal cord and in optic nerves. It is characterised by weakness, numbness and tingling in limbs, spastic paraparesis, diplopia and sphincter disturbances leading to urinary urgency. MRI of brain or cervical cord is often helpful in demonstrating the presence of a multiplicity of lesions. There are no means to prevent the progression of this disorder and some disability is likely to result eventually.

In patients with relapsing-remitting MS (RRMS) or secondary progressive MS (SPMS), treatment with ***interferon beta-1b*** (INF-b; 6 mIU, I.M. once a week) or with ***glatiramer acetate*** (20 mg S.C. daily) reduces the frequency of relapses. Side effects of INF-b include flu-like symptoms which usually resolve in 2–3 months or can be managed by paracetamol. However, the high cost per patient treated in relation to the benefit gained has discouraged the widespread use of INF-b. *Glatiramer acetate* is a synthetic polypeptide which resembles myelin basic protein. Its side effects include episodes of flushing, chest tightness and palpitation after the injection. However, these are self-limiting. A monoclonal antibody called ***natalizumab*** (I.V.) has also been approved lately. The presence of lymphocytes around neuronal fibers is implicated in the immune proccesses that contribute to the pathogenesis of MS. *Natalizumab* blocks the process of cell adhesion to lymphocytes in the CNS (See chapter 69). ***Fingolimod*** is an orally effective (0.5–1.25 mg OD) immunomodulator, recently approved to treat MS. It suppresses the release of lymphocytes from lymphoid tissue and protects myelin sheaths of CNS from their attack. ***Mitoxantrone*** is an anticancer drug which has also been recently approved for MS. It suppresses T-cells, B-cells and macrophages attack on the myelin sheath. Spasticity associated with MS can be treated by giving ***baclofen*** or by administering ***tizanidine*** with ***diazepam***.

Excessive fatigue associated with MS can be reduced by taking rest or by giving ***fluoxetine*** 20 mg once a day.

Ocrelizumab is a humanized monoclonal antibody designed to selectively target CD20, a cell surface antigen present on B lymphocytes. It causes antibody-dependent cellular cytolysis and complement-mediated lysis. It is diluted and then slowly infused intravenously. It is used for adults with relapsing or primary progressive forms of multiple sclerosis. *Adverse effects* are respiratory tract infections, infusion-related reactions, rash, skin infections, neutropenia and depression.

Nabiximols is derived from *Cannabis sativa* plant. It is given as spray for multiple sclerosis (MS). It improves symptoms of MS like spasticity and pain when administered as an add-on therapy with standard therapy. Common *side effects* are dizziness, fatigue, depression, disorientation and euphoria.

Ozanimod is a sphingosine 1-phosphate (S1P) receptor modulator. It is used orally for relapsing forms of multiple sclerosis (MS), including relapsing-remitting disease and active secondary progressive disease. *Adverse effects* are abdominal pain, upper respiratory tract infection, elevated hepatic transaminase and hypotension.

Siponimod is a sphingosine-1-phosphate (S1P) receptor modulator. It prevents entry of T lymphocytes into the central nervous system. This reduces inflammation and progression of multiple sclerosis. It is used for relapsing forms of multiple sclerosis (MS). *Adverse effects* are abnormal liver function, hypertension, peripheral oedema, bradycardia and convulsions.

WILSON'S DISEASE

Wilson's disease is caused by a genetic failure to eliminate copper absorbed from food so that it accumulates in brain, kidney, liver and cornea. It is characterised by hepatolenticular degeneration with a variety of motor disturbances such as rigidity, akinesia and dystonia. Treatment is done by chelating excess copper with ***d-penicillamine*** (500 mg BD or TDS orally) or with ***trientine*** (1 g orally per day). *Adverse effects* of d-penicillamine include nausea, lupus-like syndrome, optic neuropathy and blood dyscrasias. Trientine is safer but may cause mild iron deficiency anaemia. ***Potassium disulfide*** (20 mg TDS) reduces the intestinal absorption of copper and acts synergistically if prescribed in conjunction with d-penicillamine.

Zinc sulfate (200 mg/day) decreases copper absorption from GIT. It is much safer than other drugs and can be used singly for maintenance therapy or jointly with d-penicillamine. However, these drugs may not control the neurological symptoms if treatment is started late in the course of disease. To control neurological symptoms, at this stage, *levodopa* + *trihexyphenidyl* combination can be used.

AMYOTROPHIC LATERAL SCLEROSIS (ALS)

ALS (also called Lou Gehrig's disease) is a progressive, and devastating neurodegenerative disease of motor neurons characterised by muscle wasting and atrophy (hence the term *amyotrophic*). It starts with spontaneous twitching of motor units, difficulty with chewing and swallowing, respiratory failure leading to death within 2–5 years. ALS is currently untreatable. The cause is unknown but some evidence suggest **(i)** a defect in the functioning of ***superoxide dismutase***, an enzyme that scavenges superoxide free radicals, and **(ii)** a decreased uptake of glutamate by astroglial glutamate transporters. This leads to overactivity of NMDA receptors and ***excitotoxicity due to glutamate.*** One cellular defense against this excitotoxicity is the enzyme superoxide dismutase.

One drug ***Riluzole*** (50 mg BD; see page 215) has lately been approved for treating ALS. It diminishes glutamate release and thus decreases excitotoxicity. It is well tolerated except nausea, dizziness and weight loss. But, the drug is more effective in bulbar onset disease, rather than with limb onset disease. The decline in muscle strength may also be slowed by using ***gabapentin*** (Ch. 39). Surprisingly, ***ceftriaxone*** (a III generation cephalosporin, Ch. 55) has been found to facilitate astroglial glutamate uptake and thereby possesses good anti-excitotoxic properties. It is undergoing trials for ALS.

CHAPTER 41

SECTION 8—HORMONES AND HORMONE ANTAGONISTS

Pituitary Hormones, Hypothalamic Releasing Factors & Drugs Affecting Uterus

COMPETENCY PH1.37, PH1.40, PH1.41

Endocrinology involves an understanding of hormone secretion, hormone actions, their feedback control mechanisms and treatment of endocrine disorders. The term ***endocrine*** differentiates the action of hormones secreted internally (e.g., insulin from pancreas) from those secreted externally (*exocrine*, e.g., pancreatin or pancrelipase enzymes from pancreas). ***Hormones*** are chemical substances which are synthesised by specific endogenous glands and secreted internally, directly into the blood stream, to act far away from the site of their production and release, on the specific target organs. This definition does not include non-hormonal substances like glucose (though it is synthesised and secreted by the liver) and autacoids which are synthesised in specific tissues and released locally to act at the site of their release (e.g., histamine, bradykinin and prostaglandins).

Chemically, hormones can be divided into seven major classes: **(1)** ***amino acid derivatives*** such as dopamine, catecholamines and thyroid hormones; **(2)** ***neuropeptides*** such as gonadotropin-releasing hormone, thyrotropin-releasing hormone and somatostatin; **(3)** ***simple proteins*** like corticotropin (ACTH); **(4)** ***large proteins*** such as insulin, luteinising hormone (LH) and parathyroid hormone (PTH); **(5)** ***glycoproteins*** like thyroid stimulating hormone (TSH); **(6)** ***steroids*** such as cortisol, estrogens, progesterons and glucocorticoids and **(7)** ***vitamins*** such as vit. D. Some newly discovered hormones such as *inhibin, ghrelin* and *leptin* have also become part of medical science on the basis of their functional role as hormones rather than through their structural resemblance or mechanism of action.

FUNCTIONS OF HORMONES

Subsequent chapters describe the details of the functions of different hormones. However, the physiological functions of hormones, in totality, can be divided into three major areas: **(1)** growth and differentiation, **(2)** maintenance of homeostasis and **(3)** reproduction.

Growth and Differentiation

Many hormones play vital role in the complex phenomenon of growth and development of secondary sexual characteristics. For example, short stature may be caused by growth hormone deficiency or due to hypothyroidism while development of secondary sexual characteristics takes place under the influence of ovarian and testicular hormones.

Maintenance of Homeostasis

Though virtually all hormones affect homeostasis, the most important among them are: **(1)** regulation of glucose levels by insulin; **(2)** regulation of Na^+ and K^+ concentration by aldosterone; **(3)** regulation of Ca^{2+} and phosphorous levels by parathyroid hormone and **(4)** regulation of serum osmolality by vasopressin.

Reproduction and Functional Integration

The stages of reproduction include: **(1)** sex determination during foetal development; **(2)** sexual maturity during puberty; **(3)** conception, pregnancy, lactation, maternal behaviour and **(4)** ultimately cessation of reproductive capability at menopause (females) or old age (males). All these stages involve an interplay of sex hormones (Ch. 43 & 44). In addition to sex hormones, prolactin is involved in lactation and oxytocin mediates the suckling response and milk release (see following text).

HORMONE RECEPTORS AND MECHANISMS OF HORMONE ACTIONS

Receptors for hormones are divided into three major classes: **(1)** ***membrane receptors,*** which primarily bind neuropeptide hormones and catecholamines.

The membrane receptors are of several types: **(i)** *G-protein coupled receptors* working through adenylase-cAMP system (as for NE, E, DA, TSH, FSH, LH, PTH and ACTH) or through phospholipase-C-inositol system (as for oxytocin, vasopressin); **(ii)** *Tyrosine-kinase receptors* like for insulin, growth hormones and growth factors; **(iii)** *Cytokine receptor* as for prolactin and some growth factors and **(iv)** *Serine-kinase receptors* as for activin, transforming growth factor-β and bone morphogenic proteins. **(2)** ***cytosolic receptors***, as for steroidal hormones such as glucocorticiods, mineralocorticoids, estrogens, progestins and androgens and **(3)** ***nuclear receptors,*** as for thyroid hormones (T_3 and T_4). Receptor numbers, for hormones, vary greatly in different target tissues. For example, ACTH receptors are located almost exclusively in the adrenal cortex and FSH receptors are found exclusively in gonads. Contrarily, insulin and thyroid receptors are widely distributed reflecting the need for hormone-induced metabolic responses in all organs. For details of these receptors refer Ch. 7 and the related figures.

HYPOTHALAMIC-PITUITARY RELATIONSHIP

Though the pituitary gland is often referred to as "Master of Endocrine Orchestra", its functions are primarily controlled by the hypothalamus. The pituitary gland consists of an *anterior lobe* (*adenohypophysis*), the *intermediate lobe* and *posterior lobe* (*neurohypophysis*). It is connected to hypothalamus, which lies above it, by the stalk that contains neurosecretory fibers, capillaries and the hypophyseal portal venous system that drains the hypothalamus and perfuses the anterior pituitary by a number of releasing factors (RF) or releasing hormones (RH). The factors are also blood-borne messengers and are undoubtedly hormones as such. Nevertheless, the term "factor", though irrational, is in use simply to demarcate that their structure is not known. These hypothalamic releasing factors/ hormones stimulate the anterior pituitary to produce and secrete a number of tropic hormones, that in turn stimulate target glands to secrete hormones which finally act on the cells of target organs far away from the site of their release (Fig 41.1 & 41.2). Each ***anterior pituitary*** hormone is produced by separate group of cells, which are named according to the hormones they secrete. For example: *somatotrophs* (secrete growth hormone, GH); *lactotrophs* (secrete prolactin, PRL); *gonadotrophs* (secrete follicular stimulating hormone, FSH; and luteinising hormone, LH); *thyrotrophs* (secrete thyroid stimulating hormone, TSH) and *corticotrophs* (secrete adreno-corticotrophic hormone, ACTH). ***The intermediate lobe*** of the pituitary gland secretes mainly melanocyte stimulatory hormone (MSH) and γ-lipotropin hormones but these are probably not that important, as hormones, in human beings. The ***posterior lobe*** of the pituitary secretes two peptide hormones called vasopressin and oxytocin. However, both these hormones are synthesised in the hypothalamus and simply transported *via* the neurosecretory fibers of the hypothalamic stalk to the posterior pituitary where these are mainly stored and then released.

Pituitary hormone secretions are regulated by *negative* (*rarely positive*) *feedback mechanisms*. Thus, broadly speaking, the secretions of the releasing factors/hormones from the hypothalamus get decreased when the concentrations of the target gland hormone get increased and *vice versa.* These negative feedback pathways are "long" as well as "short" negative feedback pathways. If the hormone secreted from the peripheral glands affects both the hypothalamus and the anterior pituitary, then it makes a *long negative feedback loop*; and if they affect only the anterior pituitary to decrease its secretion of tropic hormone then it constitutes a *short negative feedback loop* (Fig. 41.2).

HYPOTHALAMIC AND ANTERIOR PITUITARY HORMONES

There are, at present, seven sets of release hormones (RH) or release inhibiting hormones (RIH; some referred to as factors) that originate in the hypothalamus and regulate the secretions of anterior pituitary. Some hormones from anterior pituitary act directly on target organs. These include growth hormone (GH) and prolactin (PRL). Others regulate

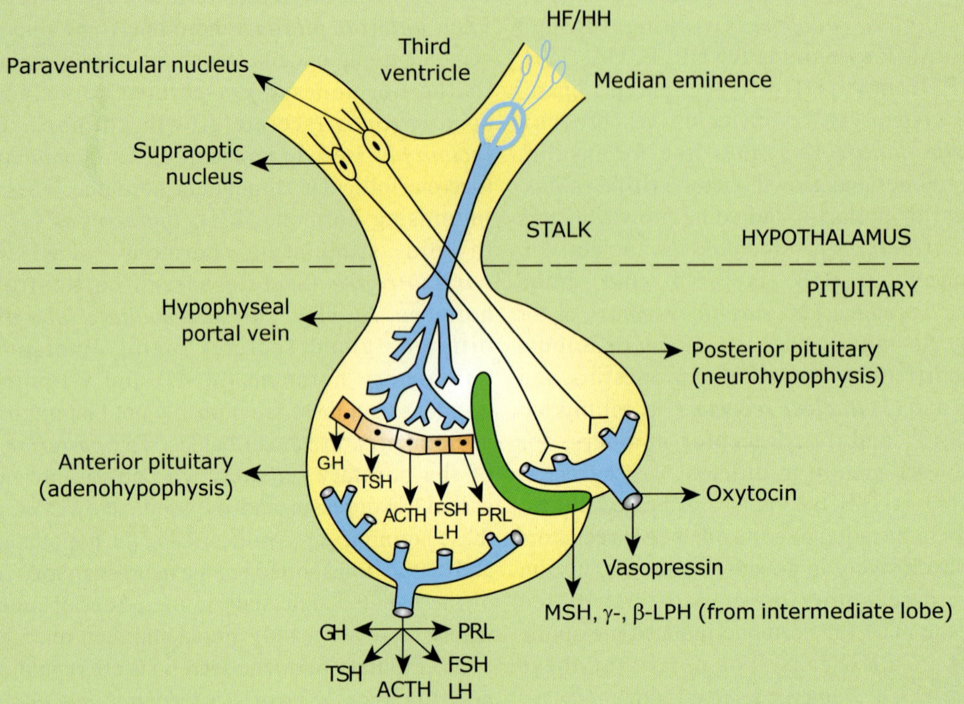

Key: HF—Hypothalamic factors; HH—Hypothalamic hormones; GH—Growth hormone; TSH—Thyroid stimulating hormone; ACTH—Adrenocorticotropic hormone; FSH—Follicle stimulating hormone; LH—Luteinising hormone; PRL—Prolactin; MSH—Melanocyte stimulating hormone; γ-, β-LPH—γ and β-lipotropin hormones.

Fig 41.1 Functional Anatomy, Vascular and Neuronal Relationship Between Hypothalamus and Pituitary

the functions of related endocrine glands such as thyroid stimulating hormone (TSH), which controls the secretions from thyroid gland; adrenocorticotrophic hormone (ACTH), which influences the functions of adrenal cortex, and gonadotropins (follicular stimulating hormone—FSH; and luteinising hormone—LH), which control the functions of gonads (Fig. 41.2). These are discussed below.

Growth Hormone (GH)

Secretion of GH is regulated by the action of ***growth hormone-releasing hormone (GHRH)*** released from hypothalamus. If given I.V., S.C. or intranasally, GH-RH causes secretion of GH instantly from somatotrophs with peak concentration being achieved in one hour. However, relative potencies by these three routes are 300:10:1, respectively.

Sermorelin, a synthetic analogue of GHRH, is used as diagnostic agent for testing the capacity and rate of pituitary GH secretion in suspected cases of childhood short stature. A rise in the serum GH levels demonstrates the somatotrophs' ability to produce GH and considered as a favourable response to GH-RH or *sermorelin* therapy. *Unwanted effects* include flushing, injection site pain, dizziness, hyperactivity and urticaria.

Somatostatin is rather a ***growth hormone release-inhibiting hormone (GHRIH)***. It primarily inhibits the secretion of GH, but also of thyroid stimulating hormone (TSH, thyrotropin) from

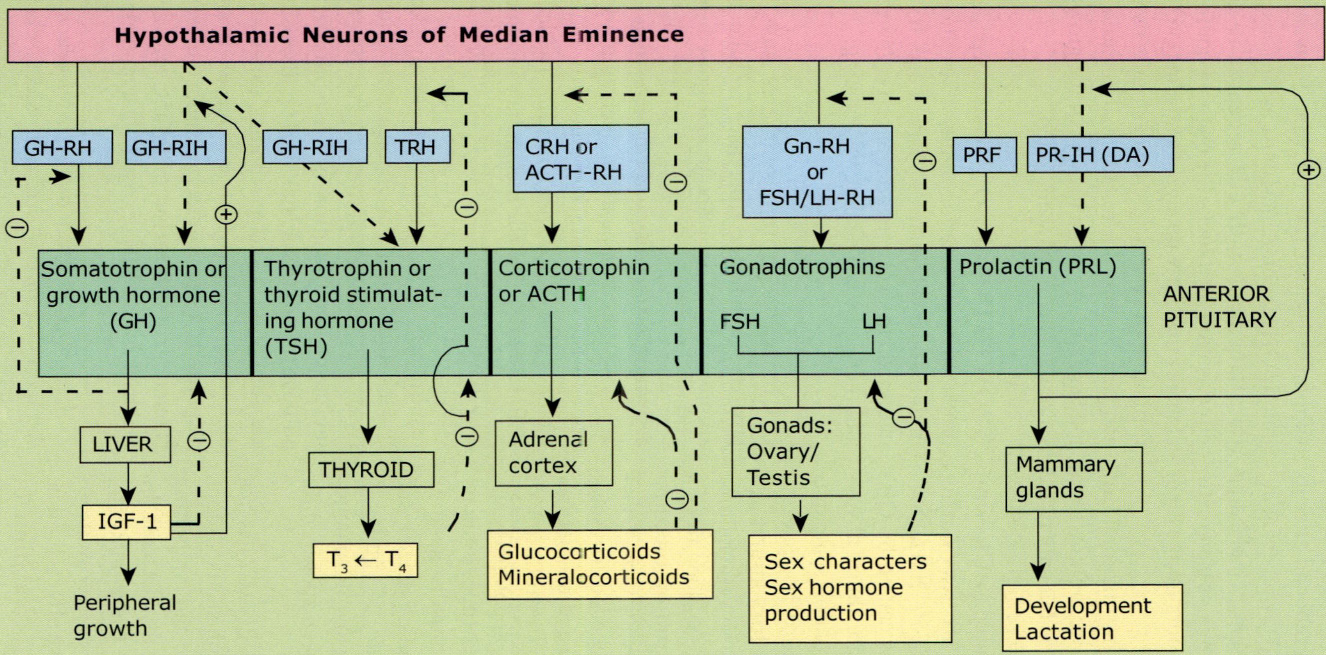

Key: GHRH—Growth hormone releasing hormone; GH-RIH—Growth hormone release inhibiting hormone or Somatostatin; TRH—Thyrotropin releasing hormone; Gn-RH—Gonadotropin releasing hormone; PRF—Prolactin releasing factor; PR-IH—Proloctin release inhibiting hormone (dopamine); FSH—Follicle stimulating hormone; LH—Luteinising hormone; IGF-1—Insulin-like growth factor-1; Broken lines—Inhibition

Fig 41.2 Links Between Hypothalamus, Pituitary, Target Gland Hormones, Target Organs and Feedback Mechanism in Operation.

anterior pituitary; of insulin from pancreas and of gastrin from GIT. Use of somatostatin, is very limited due to: **(a)** its very short half-life; **(b)** lack of specificity for inhibiting only GH and **(c)** GH rebound after its discontinuation. Currently, it is used to prevent acute bleeding from oesophageal varices, upper GI bleeding from haemorrhagic gastritis, intestinal or pancreatic fistula or from hypersecretory tumours of intestinal tract.

Octreotide is a long-acting analogue of somatostatin. It is 45 times more potent than somatostatin in inhibiting GH release but only twice as potent in reducing insulin secretion. Hence, compared to somatostatin, chances of having hyperglycaemia as side effect are less during treatment with octreotide. In doses of 50–200 μg S.C. TDS, octreotide reduces symptoms caused by GH-secreting pituitary tumours, which are almost always associated with acromegaly. It also controls symptoms in patients of carcinoid syndrome, VIP-secreting tumours, gastrinoma and secretory diarrhoea associated with diabetes and irritable bowel syndrome (Ch. 28 and 29). It decreases mucosal blood flow, a property that is utilised for controlling bleeding oesophageal varices and bleeding peptic ulcer. Other uses include treatment of AIDS-associated diarrhoea, breast cancer, Cushing's syndrome and insulinoma. ***Sandostatin*** is a slow- release formulation of octreotide. *Adverse effects* include, abdominal pain, nausea, steatorrhoea, and gallstones (due to biliary stasis but usually occurs after six months therapy). Long-term use may lead to conduction defects and vitamin B_{12} deficiency. ***Lanreotide*** is similar to octreotide but is also used in treating thyroid tumours. Its longer-acting formulation has been approved for treating acromegaly.

TREATMENT OF ACROMEGALY has met with limited success. Dopamine agonists like l-dopa or bromocriptine, though increase the circulating levels of GH (see above), paradoxically, decrease the levels of GH in cases of acromegaly. ***Octreotide*** (50–100 μg S.C. TDS) can be used but its route of administration, high cost and adverse effects limit its use. However, longer acting formulation of ***lanreotide*** can be used (see above). Surgical intervention is more preferred.

Pegvisomant (S.C.) is a new GH-receptor antagonist that has been approved for treating acromegaly. It prevents peripheral GH-binding to its receptor and suppresses serum IGF-1 levels. Pegvisomant is a unique GH receptor antagonist in the sense that after its attachment with GH receptor it allows its dimerisation but blocks the ongoing conformational changes that activate signal transduction. However, formation of specific antibodies limits its long-term efficacy. Finally, due to failure of negative feedback mechanisms, some incidences of the growth of GH-secreting adenomas were noted.

GROWTH HORMONE (GH) is a peptide hormone produced by the anterior pituitary. Secretion of GH is high in the newborn till 4 years of age. It remains at intermediate level until after puberty (25 years of age) and then there is a decline with ageing.

Pharmacological Actions

GH increases protein synthesis and promotes positive N_2 balance (increases cellular uptake of amino acids). The anabolic and growth-promoting effects of GH are indirect and are mediated by activating *insulin-like growth factor type-1* (IGF-1; Fig. 41.2), predominantly at open epiphyses of long bones—thus causing bone growth. This growth factor is also called ***somatomedins*** (which includes IGF-1 and IGF-2). The metabolic consequences of a pharmacologic dose of GH is an initial insulin-like effect followed by an effect antagonistic to that of insulin, i.e., a decrease in glucose uptake into the tissues and an increased release of glucose from liver, i.e., diabetogenic effects. There is also increased mobilisation of free fatty acids from adipose tissues (lipolysis), thus predisposing toward the formation of ketone bodies especially among diabetics. IGF-1 (which is released from liver in response to GH) also has inhibitory effects on GH release from anterior pituitary and a positive feedback to GH-RIH release from hypothalamus (Fig. 41.2).

Factors other than GHRH which stimulate the secretion of GH are: deep sleep, exercise and hypoglycaemia. Some drugs such as d-amphetamine and l-dopa also stimulate release of GHRH. Activation of β-adrenoceptors facilitate the release of GHRIH.

Hence, propranolol being β-blocker indirectly promotes the secretion of GHRH.

Factors other than GHRIH that suppress the secretion of GH are: hyperglycaemia and use of corticosteroids. Activation of α-adrenoceptors increases the release of GHRH; consequently, α-blockers indirectly decrease the release of GHRH.

Excess/Deficiency of Growth Hormone

Excess of GH production, before puberty, leads to "gigantism", while after puberty leads to "acromegaly" which is characterised by enlargement of legs and arms, and protrusion of lower jaw. Deficiency of GH leads to dwarfism (short stature).

Preparations and Uses of GH

Human pituitary GH (*Somatotropin*; t½ 25 min) is no longer used. Recombinant human GH (rhGH) is most commonly used. Two such longer-acting preparations are now available: ***Somatropin*** and ***Somatrem***. Both of them are equipotent to somatotropin. Therapy with ***somatropin*** (1.5 mg/kg, S.C., monthly) permits many children with short stature to achieve normal adult height. Adult-onset GH deficiency is usually due to damage to hypothalamus or pituitary caused by tumour, infection or radiation therapy. ***Somatropin*** can be given subcutaneously to an adult in doses of 0.2–0.4 mg/kg every two weeks. Somatropin can also be used for increasing height of girls with Turner's syndrome (failure of ovaries to respond to pituitary hormones). It is now also approved by FDA for AIDS related wasting of muscles. It is a potent anabolic agent approved for management of burn injuries. It is at times abused by athletes and used for its anti-aging effects but it does not reverse the manifestations of normal aging.

Adverse effects include precipitation of type-2 diabetes; induction of insulin resistance; arthralgia in hand and wrist; pain at injection site; lipodystrophy; fluid retention and headache (due to a possibility of intracranial hypertension). Patients with Turner's syndrome have an increased risk of otitis media.

Mecasermin: Many short-statured children have IGF-1 deficiency that is non-responsive to somatropin treatment. *Mecasermin* is a combination of recombinant human IGF-1 with recombinant human IGFBP-3. Such a combination maintains the desired half-life of IGF-1. It is given initially in a dose of 0.04–0.08 mg/kg, S.C. twice daily, increasing weekly up to a maximum of 0.12 mg/kg S.C. twice daily. *Adverse effects* include hypoglycaemia (given with food), reversible rise in liver enzymes and intracranial hypertension.

Somapacitan

Somapacitan is a recently approved growth hormone preparation. It binds and stimulates the growth hormone receptors. It induces intracellular signalling to up-regulate insulin-like growth factor I (IGF-1). Somapacitan is used as a replacement for growth hormone in adults having growth hormone deficiency.

Lonapegsomatropin

Lonapegsomatropin undergoes autocleavage to release active somatropin from the methoxypolyethylene glycol carrier. Somatropin binds to the growth hormone receptors leading to direct effects and IGF-1 mediated indirect effects. It is given subcutaneously to treat short stature due to inadequate secretion of endogenous growth hormone.

Thyroid Stimulating Hormone (TSH)

Thyroid stimulating hormone (TSH, *thyrotropin*) is a glycoprotein hormone. Its secretions are pulsatile and follow a biological rhythm with levels of TSH being highest during sleep at night. However, because of relatively low amplitude of pulses and longer half-life of TSH, its single determination provides reasonable assessment of its circulating levels. TSH stimulates the thyroid to synthesise thyroglobulin and the thyroid hormones: triiodothyronine (T_3) and thyroxine (T_4). It also promotes trapping of iodide by thyroid (for more details refer Ch. 45). *Somatostatin* (GHRIH) and *lanreotide*, the longer acting somatostatin analogues, effectively suppress TSH release (Fig. 41.2).

TSH has very limited therapeutic use. Still it is used for diagnostic purposes and to stimulate ^{131}I uptake in patients with thyroid cancer. ***Thyrotropin alpha*** (rhTSH) is a recombinant human TSH (half life 22–24 hrs). It is now commercially available. It is being used to help in detection of metastatic differentiated thyroid carcinoma. Usually, the management of thyroid carcinoma requires a total thyroidectomy, postoperative ^{131}I therapy followed by the replacement therapy with T_3 (triiodothy-ronine) or T_4 (levothyroxine). To check and evaluate for recurrences of such thyroid carcinomas, thyroxine replacement is withdrawn for 4–6 weeks so that there is hypothyroidism and a rise in serum TSH levels. These elevated TSH levels stimulate any remaining tumour cell to resume its uptake of ^{131}I. Administration of ***thyrotropin alpha*** (0.9 mg/day I.M. for 2 days) can provide comparable TSH elevation without any need to discontinue thyroxine and risk for causing hypothyroidism. If after administration of ^{131}I, in presence of recombinant human TSH, there is a rise in serum thyroglobin or a positive ^{131}I scan, there has been a recurrence of the thyroid cancer. *Side effects* of TSH include nausea, headache and asthenia. TSH can also cause neurologic deterioration in patients with brain metastases.

TSH secretion is controlled by ***thyrotropin releasing hormone*** **(TRH, *protirelin*)**, which in turn is inhibited by T_3 and T_4 negative feedback mechanism (Fig. 41.2). An increase in the concentration of free T_3 and T_4 in circulation results in decreased TSH gene transcription and decreased TSH secretion. In myxoedema, TSH levels are found elevated because of the lack of feedback inhibition (due to low T_3 and T_4 levels). In hyperthyroidism, thyroid stimulating immunoglobulins get attached to the thyroid cells and stimulate them in the same way as TSH. As a result, TSH levels are low. **TRH (protirelin)** is a tripeptide hormone found in paraventricular nuclei of the hypothalamus. TRH is then secreted into the hypothalamic-hypophyseal portal venous system to stimulate pituitary to produce TSH. Not only TSH, TRH also stimulates lactotrophs to secrete prolactin (PRL). TRH has a short plasma half-life of 4–5 min. It is now no more used to diagnose hyper- or hypothyroidism. *Adverse effects* also last for a few minutes and include an urge to urinate, nausea, flushing, metallic taste and marked but transient blood pressure fluctuations. ***Protirelin*** is a synthetic analogue of TRH.

Prolactin (PRL)

Prolactin is a peptide hormone produced by anterior pituitary. Its structure is similar to GH. PRL secretion is under tonic inhibitory control of hypothalamus. PRL release inhibitory hormone (PRIH) is dopamine (DA) which inhibits PRL release (Fig. 41.2) by acting on D_2 receptors of lactotrophs. The factor causing PRL release (PRF) from the hypothalamus has not been characterised yet. The potential candidates could be oxytocin, TRH or even endogenous opioid peptides. However, the main stimulus for PRL release is suckling of breast nipples by an infant during breast-feeding. Blood PRL levels are higher in adult females than the males. Progressive increase occurs during pregnancy, peaking at delivery if breast-feeding is initiated soon. Thereafter, high PRL levels are maintained by suckling and then decline if breast-feeding is discontinued.

PRL has mammotropic (growth of milk secreting epithelium) as well as lactogenic (milk producing) effects. There is some evidence that PRL also plays a role in regulating immune mechanisms and in stimulating mitogenesis in lymphocytes. *A deficiency of PRL* is manifested by failure to lactate or by luteal phase defect. *An excess secretion of PRL* leads to hyperprolactinaemia, which is characterised by galactorrhoea, amenorrhoea and infertility in females because high PRL levels inhibit the secretion of gonadotropin (see following text), which leads to a decrease in ovarian functions and lack of ovulation. That is how suckling reflexes provide natural contraception to the lactating mother till the child is on breast-feeding. Galactorrhoea from excess PRL, results due to induction of milk secretion as the inhibitory influence of estrogen and progesterone levels is physiologically curtailed. Hyperpro-lactinaemia is also associated with enhanced risk for osteoporosis. PRL receptors are abundant in osteoblasts of developing bones and the accompanying low estrogen levels contribute to accelerated bone loss in hyperprolactinaemic women. In males hyperprolactinaemia can lead to gynaecomastia, hypogonadism, loss of libido and impotence for obvious reasons as discussed above. *Factors which stimulate PRL secretions* include suckling, sleep, orgasm, stress, hypoglycaemia, vasoactive intestinal peptide (VIP) and hypothyroidism (probably because enhanced TRH secretion stimulates PRL release). Chronic renal failure also elevates PRL levels by decreasing peripheral PRL clearance. Because dopamine is a PRL release inhibiting hormone, D_2 receptor antagonists such as chlorpromazine, haloperidol and metoclopramide as well as dopamine depleters such as reserpine and α-methyldopa can facilitate PRL secretion (galactorrhoea and gynaecomastia as side effects).

Factors which decrease PRL secretion include dopamine, dopamine agonists such as l-dopa, bromocriptine, cabergoline, pergolide and quinagolide. No drug is available for use in prolactin deficient patients. PRL itself is not used clinically.

Treatment of hyperprolactinaemia: Inhibition of prolactin secretion can be achieved with DA agonist drugs such as ***bromocriptine, cabergoline, pergolide*** and ***quinagolide.*** The latter is a non-ergot drug, others are ergot derivatives with high affinity to D_2 receptors of the pituitary. These drugs lower circulating PRL levels and reduce the size of pituitary-prolactinomas. Treatment with ***cabergoline*** is initiated at 0.25 mg orally twice a week. The dose is then increased gradually up to a maximum of 1 mg twice weekly depending on the values of serum PRL levels. ***Quinagolide*** in doses of 0.2–0.6 mg/day orally suppresses PRL release and shrinks prolactinomas. It has a longer t½ and is better tolerated than ergot derivatives. Its use in parkinsonism has been discussed in Chapter 40. ***Bromocriptine*** (2.5 mg once daily orally for 3 days, increased gradually to 2.5 mg BD for 15 days) can also be used to suppress lactation. For preparations see Ch. 40.

Common adverse effects of DA agonists used to treat hyperprolactinaemia are, syncope, nausea, vomiting, constipation and hallucinations. High doses of ergot derivatives may cause cold-induced peripheral digital vasospasm.

Adrenocorticotropic Hormone (ACTH; Adrenocorticotropin; Corticotropin)

ACTH is a peptide hormone produced by the anterior pituitary whose primary function is to stimulate synthesis and release of *cortisol* by the adrenal cortex (for details refer Ch. 42). Hypothalamus regulates ACTH release from anterior pituitary through ***corticotropin releasing hormone*** (CRH; Fig. 41.2). ACTH, then stimulates adrenal cortex to produce glucocorticoids, mineralocorticoids and androgens. ACTH has only a minor stimulatory effect on the secretion of aldosterone whose release is primarily controlled by angiotensin II on adrenal cortex. In turn, circulating levels of corticosteroids act on both hypothalamus and the anterior pituitary to suppress the release of ACTH, completing the negative feedback loop (Fig. 41.2). By these negative feedback mechanisms, the prolonged use of glucocorticoids, in non-endocrine disease, leads to iatrogenic suppression of pituitary-adrenal axis and of ACTH secretion.

Secretion of ACTH has a characteristic circadian rhythm, peaking at 6 a.m., decreasing during afternoon and reaching lowest at midnight. Superimposed on this endogenous rhythm, *ACTH secretion is stimulated by* a variety of stimuli, e.g., trauma and severe stress (like surgery, anxiety, fear, severe pain, exposure to severe cold and hypoglycaemia). When given chronically, ACTH also causes hyperpigmentation of skin because its terminal amino acid sequence (1–13) is identical to melanocyte stimulating hormone (α-MSH). Hence, there is always a α-MSH activity intrinsic to ACTH. In high doses ACTH activates MSH receptors also.

Excess production of ACTH leads to adrenal hypertrophy and pituitary hyperplasia and disease situations like Cushing's syndrome characterised by moon face, acne, centripetal obesity, hypertension, osteoporosis, hyperglycaemia, virilism, peptic ulcer and poor wound healing.

Absence or deficiency of ACTH results in adrenal atrophy, pituitary insufficiency and diseases like Simmond's disease and hypopituitary cachexia leading to decrease in BMR, loss of pubic hair, impotence in man, amenorrhoea in women and a decrease in 17-ketosteroids.

ACTH therapy is no more preferred these days primarily because it stimulates secretions of mineralocorticoids and androgens besides glucocorticoids. It also causes Na^+ and water retention and hypokalaemia. Glucocorticoids are more preferred for therapeutic purposes, because there are no such benefits that ACTH can achieve but corticosteroids cannot.

Cosyntropin is a synthetic human ACTH, used for the diagnosis of pituitary-adrenal axis disorders. If after giving *cosyntropin* (25 IU, I.V.) there is an increase in plasma cortisol levels, the adrenal functions are normal and it is not a case of primary adrenal insufficiency. If there is no increase in plasma cortisol levels, there is primary adrenal insufficiency. Cosyntropin, sometimes can be used for treating adrenocortical insufficiency in children as it does not suppress their growth and its withdrawal is no problem (compared to glucocorticoids).

Adverse effects: There are virtually no adverse effects from diagnostic doses of cosyntropin. However, ACTH shares all adverse effects of corticosteroids except suppression of adrenal cortex. It also causes hyperandrogenism in women. Acne, Na^+ retention, hypokalaemia and allergy are more common with ACTH than with glucocorticoids. Thinning of skin is less severe with ACTH. Cosyntropin is less allergic than natural ACTH.

Gonadotropins

The hypothalamic neurons of the median eminence, under the influence of dopamine, secrete a ***gonadotropin-releasing hormone*** (GnRH or FSH/LHRH) in discrete pulses every 60–120 min. GnRH is then transported to the anterior pituitary by hypothalamic-hypophyseal portal venous system. Gn-RH is a decapeptide glycoprotein. Under its pulsatile influence, anterior pituitary secretes two gonadotropic hormones: The ***follicle stimulating hormone*** (FSH) and ***luteinising hormone*** (LH). The latter in males, is also known as *interstitial cell stimulating hormone* (ICSH). Both FSH and LH control the activity of gonads. It is not very clear how hypothalamus achieves a divergent pattern of FSH and LH secretion in menstruating women through a single GnRH. It has been suggested that the lower pulse frequency favours FSH secretion, whereas higher pulse frequency favours LH secretion. Though GnRH is the main regulator of LH and FSH secretion, FSH synthesis is also under a separate control of gonadal peptides 'inhibin' and 'activin', which are members of transforming growth factor-β (TGF-β) family. ***Inhibin*** selectively suppresses FSH whereas ***activin*** stimulates FSH synthesis (Fig. 43.2 and 44.1). *It has also been observed that pulsatile mode of Gn-RH input promotes gonadotroph responsiveness whereas continuous GnRH exposure leads to their desensitisation* (Fig. 41.3).

Functions of FSH in females include: **(1)** gametogenesis; **(2)** follicular development; **(3)** production of estrogen and to some extent progesterone and **(4)** regulation of menstrual cycle.

Functions of FSH in males include: the stimulation and maintenance of spermatogenesis in the seminiferous (Sertoli) cells of testis.

Functions of LH in females incorporate: **(1)** induction of ovulation; **(2)** formation and maintenance of corpus luteum; **(3)** promotion of estrogen and progesterone production and **(4)** regulation of menstrual cycle.

Function of LH (ICSH) in males involves biosynthesis of androgens and testosterone by interstitial (Leydig) cells of testis.

Feedback mechanisms in regulation of FSH and LH are as under (Fig. 41.2 and 41.3).

- Higher blood levels of testosterone, estrogen and progesterone provide a negative feedback to reduce the release of GnRH from the hypothalamus (long loop). Higher blood levels of these hormones also provide a negative feedback to reduce the release of FSH and LH from pituitary (short loop). Testosterone is weaker than estrogen in inhibiting FSH and LH secretion.
- A unique but a transient positive feedback also operates to promote the FSH and LH release above the 'set-point' in pubertal and adult females as is usually seen preceding ovulation (LH surge).

An altered physiology of hypothalamic-pituitary-gonadal axis leads to following consequences:

- Premature activation of hypothalamic-pituitary system leads to "precocious puberty" both in boys and girls. In boys it is characterised by premature virilism, spermatogenesis and develop ment of sexual characteristics before 9 years of age. In girls it is evident as breast budding and

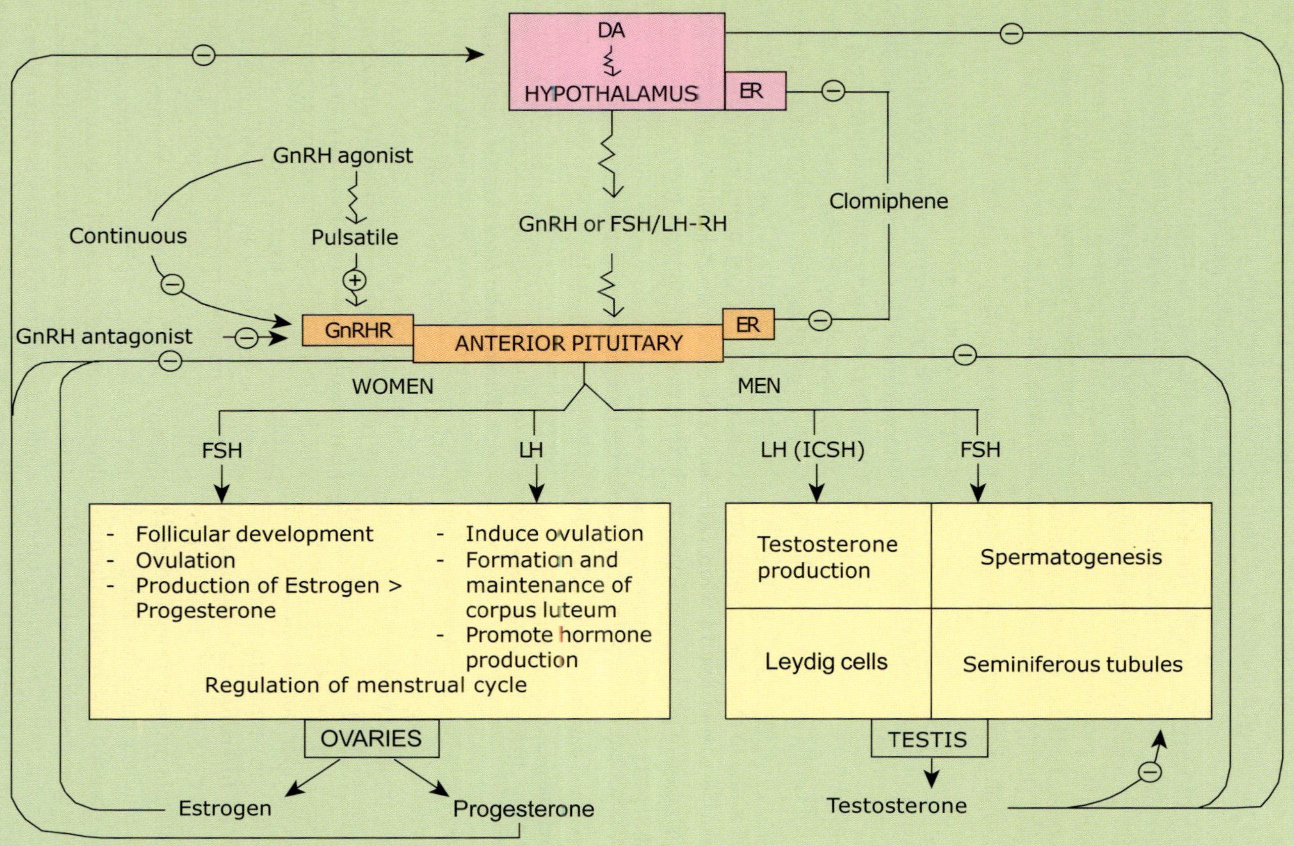

Key: ER—Estrogen receptor; GnRHR—GnRH receptor.

Fig 41.3 Regulation of Gonadotropin Release from Anterior Pituitary by Hypothalamic Gonadotropin-Releasing Hormone (GnRH), and Feedback Mechanisms.

occurrence of menstrual cycle before the age of 9 years.

- Conversely, the derangement of hypothalamic-pituitary system (i.e., hypogonadotropic-hypogonadism) can lead to "delayed puberty" in both boys and girls.
- Excess production of FSH/LH in adult females causes polycystic ovaries, ovarian enlargement and rupture while younger boys and girls may suffer from precocious puberty.
- Contrarily, inadequate FSH/LH secretion results in amenorrhoea and sterility in women while in man it may lead to oligozoospermia, impotence and infertility.

Preparations and Uses of GnRH, GnRH Agonists, GnRH Antagonists and Gonadotropins

I. Gonadorelin (GnRH)

It is a synthetic human GnRH. It has a short plasma half life (4–6 min) due to rapid metabolic degradation. It binds avidly to receptors on pituitary gonadotrophs and can be administered I.V. or S.C. Pulsatile I.V. administration of gonadorelin every 1–4 hours stimulates FSH/LH secretion. However, as discussed above, continuous therapy desensitises pituitary gonadotrophs and causes a fall in FSH/LH by inhibiting their release.

Therapeutic Uses: It has been used for the following:

A) ***Diagnostic Use***: To determine whether hypogonadism (in cases of delayed puberty) is due to a defect in anterior pituitary release of LH or in the hypothalamic release of LHRH (GnRH). If gonadorelin (100 μg S.C. or I.V.) evokes a rise in LH levels, the defect lies at hypothalamic level and if it does not, the defect lies at pituitary level.

B) ***Treatment of Infertility***: **(a)** ***in females***: Gonadorelin (5 μg I.V., every 90 min) when administered in a pulsatile manner, from a portable pump, can stimulate pituitary functions and is used to treat infertility caused by hypothalamic-hypogonadotropic hypogonadism in females. During follow-up, when ovarian follicles get matured, ovulation is induced by giving hCG (5000 IU, S.C.). Thereafter luteal phase is maintained with 1500 IU (S.C.) of hCG every third day for remaining 12 days (see following text). **(b)** ***In males***: Initially, 4000 I.U. of hCG (S.C.) is administered per week for six months to one year to achieve masculinity (i.e., to attain adequate testosterone levels and secondary sex characters due to its LH action). Thereafter, a pulsatile infusion of gonadorelin (I.V.) is done every 90 min to induce and maintain spermatogenesis. However, as 3–6 months of bolus infusions are required before significant number of matured sperms are seen, this procedure is not preferred. Instead, the preparatory hCG treatment is followed by a combined therapy with hMG and hCG (see following text).

II. GnRH Agonists

These include ***leuprolide, nafarelin, buserelin, deslorelin, goserelin, triptorelin*** and ***histrelin***. These are more potent and longer acting than GnRH (gonadorelin). These can be administered I.M., S.C. or *via* nasal spray. These have higher affinity for GnRH receptors and reduced susceptibility to metabolic degradation. As discussed above, these GnRH analogues, if administered as I.M. depot injection for 1–2 weeks, inhibit gonadotropin (FSH/LH) release and suppress gonadal functions, due to down-regulation and desensitisation of GnRH receptors. Spermatogenesis/ovulation ceases while testosterone/estradiol levels decline drastically. These effects are, however, reversible and recovery occurs after two months of stopping the treatment.

Therapeutic Uses: GnRH agonists are rarely used for stimulation of gonadotropin production (infertility). These are usually given S.C. or I.M. depot or by nasal spray route for suppression of FSH/LH release. These agents virtually induce reversible pharmacological oophorectomy or orchiectomy, which can be utilised to treat precocious puberty, polycystic ovarian disease and prostatic carcinoma. Analogously, these can be used against estrogen receptor positive (premenopausal) breast cancer. Such treatments are called androgen deprivation therapy (ADT) or androgen suppression therapy (AST) when used for prostate cancer and estrogen deprivation therapy (EDT) when used for estrogen-dependent breast or genital cancers. Their use as contraceptive for both sexes is under investigation. These are also used as an adjunct in *in vitro* fertilisation (IVF) technology (see below).

Since these agonists do not quickly dissociate from the GnRH receptor, they intially increase the

FSH and LH secretion and consequently “flare-up” the symptoms of prostatic/breast carcinoma during first two weeks. The concurrent use of an antiandrogen (flutamide) prevents this reversible flare-up; but as down-regulation of receptors develops, the adverse effects gradually decline. The dosage schedules of some of these analogues for different indications are given below:

Leuprolide: Endometriosis (3.75 mg/month I.M. depot); Uterine fibroids (3.75 mg/month, I.M. depot); Prostate cancer (7.5 mg/month, I.M. depot); Precocious puberty (0.05 mg/kg/day, S.C.).

Nafarelin: Endometriosis (0.2 mg BD, nasal spray in alternate nostril); Uterine fibroids (50–400 μg BD, nasal spray, for 3–6 months, in alternate nostril); Precocious puberty (1.6 mg/day or 0.8 mg BD nasal spray in alternate nostril).

Goserelin: Endometriosis (3.6 mg S.C. implant every 28 days); Uterine fibroids (same as above); Prostate carcinoma (10.8 mg S.C. implant every 12 weeks).

Buserelin: Endometriosis (150 μg TDS nasal spray in alternate nostril); Prostate carcinoma (100 μg QID, nasal spray in alternate nostril. In advanced stage 500 μg).

Histrelin: Administered S.C. as histrelin acetate in usual doses equivalent to 10 μg of histrelin/kg/day, for majority of indications.

Triptorelin: Prostate cancer (3.75 mg/month or 11.25 mg/3-month formulation as I.M. depot injection)

Adverse Effects: The side effects of GnRH agonists are just the manifestations of hypoestrogenism and include hot flushes, headache, nausea, osteoporosis, breast atrophy, vaginal dryness and loss of libido. There may be local swelling at the site of injection and sometimes allergic manifestations such as bronchospasm and anaphylaxis (due to histamine release). *Nafarelin* nasal spray may cause sinusitis. There are reports that GnRH agonists used in the treatment of advanced prostate cancer may increase the risk of heart problems by 30%.

III. GnRH Antagonists

Cetrorelix, ganirelix, abarelix and ***degarelix*** are the four currently available GnRH receptor antagonists for clinical use. They competitively block the GnRH receptor in the pituitary and inhibit the release of FSH and LH (Fig. 41.3). Reduction of LH in men subsequently leads to a rapid decrease of testosterone release from the testes whereas in women it leads to a suppression of estrogen release from the ovaries and the endogenous LH surge.

Therapeutic Uses

a) ***Advanced Prostate Cancer***: These are preferred over GnRH agonists because they do not cause an initial increase (flare-up) in gonadotropin secretion and do not cause histamine release. Hence, they do not exacerbate the cancer symptoms initially (see above) and do not cause anaphylactoid reaction either. *Abarelix* (I.M.) and *degarelix* (S.C.) are being currently used in men suffering from advanced prostate cancer. *Abarelix* was withdrawn from the U.S. market in 2005 but is marketed in Europe. Degarelix is approved and marketed in USA as well as in Europe.
b) ***Uterine Fibroids*** **and** ***Endometriosis***: GnRH antagonists are also used to treat uterine fibroids and endometriosis in women. *Cetrorelix* in a dose of 3 mg S.C. depot injection, once weekly, for 2 months can be used to treat endometriosis. For uterine fibroids it is used in a dose of 3 mg S.C. every 4th day before surgery (presurgical short-term treatment). The therapy is started from the first day of the menstrual cycle. A new GnRH antagonist **JV-1-36**, in recent clinical trials (2009) has been shown to markedly inhibit endometriotic cell proliferation and survival.
c) ***As an Adjunct During in Vitro Fertilisation (IVF)***: *In vitro* fertilisation is a technique enabling pregnancy in infertile woman when all measures fail. Following a drug-induced follicle maturation, a sample of matured ova with follicular fluid is collected and fertilised with male partner's sperm and incubated. The resulting zygote is then introduced into the woman's uterus for implantation.

When exogenous gonadotropin (hMG) is used to activate follicular development (usually from the 3rd day of menses), there is risk of premature ovulation caused by a premature endogenous surge in LH secretion. To prevent this and to provide a controlled ovarian stimulation, hMG is always administered along with a GnRH antagonist (to block the effects of endogenous FSH and LH) or with a continuous (daily) administration of GnRH agonist (to desensitise and down-regulate GnRH receptors). After an appropriate follicular maturation, the hMG and GnRH agonist or Gn RH antagonist are discontinued and final oocyte maturation is induced by giving hCG (I.M.). The ovas are then harvested laparoscopically and retrieved for IVF. GnRH antagonists offer several advantages over continuous treatment with GnRH agonists: **(i)** Since they provide immediate antagonist effects, their duration of administration is shorter. GnRH agonist is started midway through the preceding luteal phase while a GnRH antagonist can be administered 6–8 days after the menses. **(ii)** These have a lower risk of ovarian hyperstimulation syndrome and multiple pregnancies and **(iii)** They produce a better suppression of gonadotropin secretion than agonists. Commonly used GnRH agonists are ***buserelin*** (200–500 μg S.C. once daily) or ***nafarelin*** (200–400 μg BD nasal application). Among GnRH antagonists, ***cetrorelix*** (250 μg S.C. once daily) or ***ganirelix*** (250 μg S.C. once daily) are commonly used.

IV. Natural Gonadotropins and Gonadotropin Preparations

Natural gonadotropins, FSH and LH, are glycoproteins secreted and produced by anterior pituitary (also from chorion and placenta). Large amounts of gonadotropins are present in the urine of women following menopause in whom estrogen no longer exerts feedback inhibition on the pituitary. The latter consequently secretes large amounts of FSH and LH. The functions of FSH and LH in females as well as in males have been described above. FSH and LH have a very short plasma half-life (>5 min) and are difficult to obtain in large quantities in purified form. Hence, these are usually obtained from other sources as described below. All these preparations are used intramuscularly:

1. **From the Urine of Postmenopausal Women**: Two different preparations of urinary gonadotropins have been obtained:
   a) ***Menotropins or Human Menopausal Gonadotropins (hMG)***: It contains FSH+LH activity. Although it is a more purified preparation, it contains a number of other urinary proteins. It is therefore administered intramuscularly to avoid incidence of hypersensitivity reactions.
   b) ***Urofollitropin or Urinary FSH (uFSH)***: It is a highly purified preparation of human FSH from which most of the LH has been removed by immunodepletion. It has only FSH activity.
2. **Recombinant FSH (rFSH)**: At present two rFSH preparations are available—**follitropin α** and **follitropin β**—which differ slightly in their carbohydrate side chains. Since these are considerably purer, both can be administered subcutaneously.
3. **From the Urine of Pregnant women or Human Chorionic Gonadotropin (hCG)**: The foetal placenta secretes this gonadotropin (hCG) which is identical to LH in chemical structure and pharmacological actions. hCG is then absorbed in the maternal circulation and maintains corpus luteum of pregnancy, before placenta is able to produce its own estrogen and progesterone to maintain endometrium of uterus. Although hCG is of placental origin, it is excreted in the urine by the mother, from which it is extracted commercially. hCG binds to LH receptor with equal affinity and efficacy but being more stable than LH, it is used as luteinising hormone substitute and is given intramuscularly. ***Choriogonadotropin alfa*** (r hCG) is a recombinant from of hCG and is given S.C.

Therapeutic Uses: These preparations are primarily used to treat infertility in males and females, though they have other related uses also.

A) ***To Treat Infertility in Females***: Ovarian follicular growth and maturation requires uFSH or hMG treatment for a gonadotropin deficient woman. Once adequate follicular development has occurred, ovulation requires administration of chorionic gonadotropin (hCG).
   Hence, initially 75 IU of hMG (menotropin) or uFSH (urofollitropin) are administered intra-

muscularly daily for 9–12 days until evidence of adequate follicular maturation is established. hMG or uFSH is then discontinued and 5000–10000 IU of hCG are administered (I.M.) from the next day to induce ovulation. As ovulation occurs within the next 24–48 hrs, 75% of women may conceive. Purified FSH (urofollitropin, uFSH) is more preferred to treat infertility in women with polycystic ovarian disease. In this disease LH and androgen production may already be elevated.

B) ***To Treat Infertility in Males***: As a first step, external sexual maturation is attained by pretreatment with chorionic gonadotropin (hCG) in a man with pituitary insufficiency. hMG is then added (along with hCG) to stimulate spermatogenesis.

Hence, a pre-treatment is done with 5000 IU (I.M.) of hCG three times a week for up to one year to achieve masculinisation and normal serum testosterone levels. After completion of this regimen, a combination of menotropin (hMG) 75 IU (I.M.) thrice a week and hCG 2000 IU (I.M.) twice a week is administered for at least 4 months. Success rate is 65%. However, if there is no response, the menotropin dose may be increased but not of hCG to avoid hyperandrogenism.

C) ***Cryptorchism***: In prepubertal boys up to 8 yrs of age, descent of testes can be induced by androgens whose production is stimulated by LH. Hence 1000–2000 IU of hCG can be administered intramuscularly 2–3 times a week till testes descend. If 2–6 weeks treatment brings no results a surgical intervention is imperative because undescended testes can cause infertility and predispose to testicular cancer.

D) ***To Aid in vitro Fertilisation***: Menotropin (hMG) has been used to induce maturation of ova and their timely ovulation to facilitate their harvesting for *in vitro* fertilisation (see above). Nowadays, purified FSH (urofollitropin, uFSH) is preferably used to prepare follicles for *in vitro* fertilisation because LH activity in hMG may cause premature ovulation.

E) ***To Regress AIDS-Related Kaposi's Sarcoma***: Injection of hCG (LH action) into the lesions of such sarcomas has been reported to cause regression. However, higher doses are required for obtaining such benefits.

F) ***Diagnostic Use***: I.M. injection of hCG given three–four times repeatedly produces a rise in testosterone levels (in male) and estradiol levels (in female) in patients suffering from constitutional delay in onset of puberty. Such a rise is not seen in patients where delayed puberty is due to hypogonadotropic-hypogonadism.

Adverse Effects: The adverse effects of hMG include polycystic ovaries, multiple birth (due to stimulation of too many follicles), ovarian enlargement-ascites and rupture, spontaneous abortions and gynaecomastia in man.

The side effects related to hCG are precocious puberty, abdominal pain, nausea, headache, oedema and gynaecomastia in males (due to hCG-induced estradiol secretion).

POSTERIOR PITUITARY HORMONES

The two hormones—oxytocin and antidiuretic hormone (ADH, vasopressin)—that are released from posterior pituitary are actually synthesised in hypothalamic cells. **ADH (*vasopressin*)** is chiefly a product of supraoptic nucleus while ***oxytocin*** is derived primarily from paraventricular nucleus. Ironically, therefore, the term "posterior pituitary hormones" seems to be a misnomer because these hormones are actually synthesised in hypothalamus and then simply emptied into posterior pituitary capillaries from where these are drained into systemic circulation.

Out of these two hormones, *vasopressin* (and its antagonists) has been dealt extensively in Chapter 17. Here we limit our discussion to *oxytocin* only.

Oxytocin

The name *oxytocin* is derived from the term 'OXYS' meaning "quick" and "TOKOS" meaning 'childbirth'. Hence, from the term oxytocin it appears that the essential role of oxytocin should be in parturition (child birth) but it is not. Its essential role is in milk ejection. Incidentally again the name oxytocin does not match to its principal physiological action (in the same way as the term vasopressin is still being used in place of antidiuretic hormone).

Oxytocin is a peptide hormone secreted from the posterior pituitary, whose primary role is in milk ejection in a lactating mother. It also has a facilitatory role in initiation of labour and parturition. The inter-relationship between the pharmacological actions of oxytocin and the factors controlling oxytocin release are summarised in Figure 41.4. Oxytocin has a circulating half-life of 5 minutes. It is not bound to plasma proteins and is metabolised by the liver and excreted through kidneys. 2 mg = 1 IU of oxytocin.

Pharmacological Actions

Breast

Oxytocin causes contractions of myoepithelial cells surrounding the mammary alveoli leading to milk ejection. Suckling by the infant stimulates nipple mechanoreceptors, which in turn convey impluses to hypothalamus. This promotes the release of oxytocin through posterior pituitary, which further provokes milk ejection.

Uterus

Estrogen sensitises the uterus to oxytocin action while progesterone decreases. Non-pregnant uterus and that during early pregnancy are resistant to oxytocin (only 8% sensitivity). Pregnant uterus is most sensitive. The sensitivity increases rapidly during the last trimester and is maximum at the onset of labour. During threatened or actual abortion, the myometrium of uterus is very sensitive to oxytocin. At the onset of labour or during abortion, oxytocin increases the magnitude as well as rate of contractions of the upper segment of the body of the uterus (fundus). This further facilitates relaxation of cervix because due to the pressure from foetus head, the lower segment of the uterus (body) and the cervix are already in the process of relaxation. Thus, oxytocin facilitates and coordinates the already existing uterine contractions, in the benefit of childbirth, by preparing the birth canal. Sensory nerves of the vagina, stimulated by the pressure generated by foetus head propagate reflexes and send impulses to hypothalamus, which further promotes release of oxytocin from posterior pituitary. Local prostaglandin release also increases oxytocin, which further stimulates uterine contractions during labour. The cycle goes on till the childbirth takes place. Oxytocin level then quickly falls during puerperium.

Miscellaneous

- In high doses oxytocin causes vasodilatation, a decrease in BP and reflex tachycardia. Oxytocin helps in the closure of umbilical vessels at the time of birth.

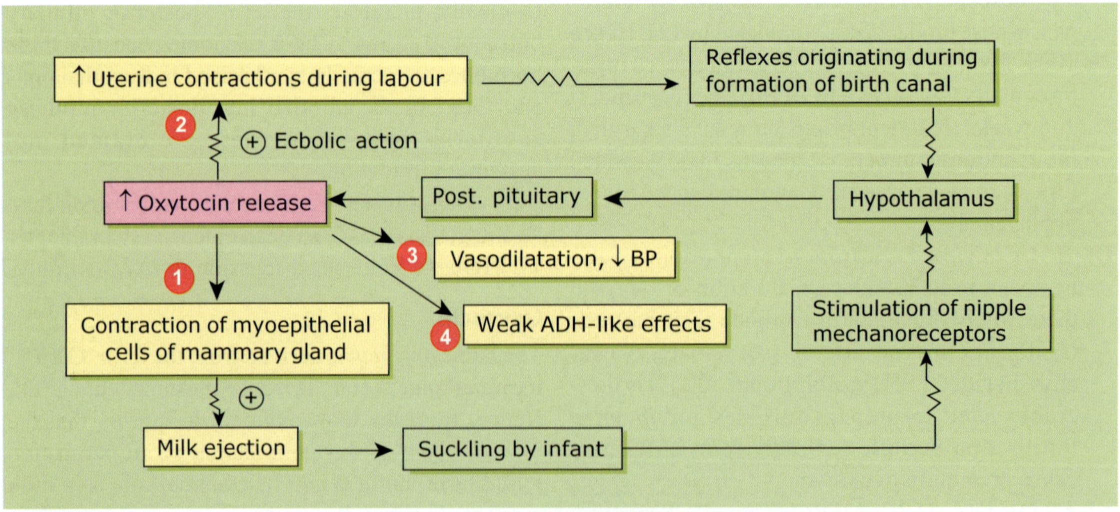

Fig 41.4 Inter-relationship Between Pharmacological Actions (1–4) and Factors Stimulating Oxytocin Release. (The pharmacological actions [1–4] have been shown in yellow boxes.)

- Oxytocin in high doses exerts weak ADH-like action and has mild antidiuretic effects.
- Oxytocin receptors are found not only on the uterus but also in the limbic system. Animal model reveals that oxytocin plays an important role in the mating and parenting behaviour. Oxytocin is also released during sexual orgasm.

Oxytocin Receptor and Antagonists

Oxytocin receptors are G-protein coupled receptors which when stimulated lead to the generation of IP_3 and subsequent mobilisation of Ca^{2+} from intracellular stores and depolarisation-induced activation of voltage-sensitive Ca^{2+} channels. The number of oxytocin receptors differs at various stages of pregnancy and increases significantly late in gestation, which parallels the marked increase in myometrial sensitivity to oxytocin. An oxytocin receptor antagonist, ***atosiban,*** has recently been approved (not in USA) to inhibit premature labour (preterm labour). It is administered as I.V. bolus followed by continuous I.V. infusion for not more than 48 hrs. *Adverse effects* include nausea, vomiting, vasodilatation, hyperglycaemia and rash.

Therapeutic Uses

1. *To Promote Milk Ejection and Resultant Breast Engorgement*

Intranasal spray of oxytocin (25–30 IU) is made into each nostril, in sitting position, 2–3 minutes before nursing. It is also used in milk-yielding cows to facilitate "milk let down". However, it does not increase milk production.

2. *Initiation and Augmentation of Labour*

Oxytocin is used to induce labour in following conditions: **(a) Situations Requiring Early Vaginal Delivery**: Such conditions include Rh problems, maternal diabetes, pre-eclampsia, erythroblastosis and placental insufficiency. For this purpose, oxytocin is given by slow I.V. infusion containing 5 IU of oxytocin in 500 ml glucose-normal saline. The infusion may be accelerated according to the response. The drug is discontinued if uterine contractions become very strong. **(b) Uterine Inertia**: Oxytocin (2–5 IU in 500 ml of normal saline) can be infused (slow I.V.) to augment contractions if uterine contractions are feeble.

Oxytocin should not be used to accelerate normally progressing labour.

3. *Control of Postpartum Bleeding*

Oxytocin 5 IU, I.M. or by I.V. infusion provides immediate response. I.M. injection of oxytocin, after placenta is expelled, causes tetanic contractions of uterus and arrests postpartum haemorrhage.

Desamino oxytocin: It is a buccal formulation of oxytocin, which is convenient to administer, but is less potent. Its dose schedules and uses are as under:

- *Induction of labour*—50 IU buccal tablets repeated 30 min till the desired effects are obtained. Maximum dose is 10 tablets (or 500 IU).
- *Uterine inertia*—25 IU every 30 min till the desired effects are obtained.
- *Breast engorgement and milk let down*—25–50 IU just before breast-feeding.

Adverse Effects and Contraindications

Non-judicious use of oxytocin can lead to foetal/maternal soft tissue injury, rupture of uterus and foetal asphyxia. It has a weak antidiuretic effect. Hence if larger doses are used along with normal saline, water intoxication may result, which may be serious in cases of pre-eclampsia.

Contraindications include cephalo-pelvic disproportion, breech presentation, placenta praevia, and foetal distress due to any reason. In such situations, delivery by caesarean section is preferred.

UTERINE STIMULANT (OXYTOCIC) AND UTERINE RELAXANT (TOCOLYTIC) DRUGS

Oxytocic Drugs (Uterine Stimulants)

Drugs and hormones used clinically to enhance uterine contractions, are primarily employed either to induce or to augment contractions during delivery or at various stages of labour. These are particularly useful in restricting an extended pregnancy, preventing the early rupture of membranes or aiding placental insufficiency. Many of them are also useful in minimising postpartum haemorrhage. In the category of oxytocic drugs are included *oxytocin* (as discussed above), ergot alkaloids (Ch. 24) and prostaglandins (Ch. 25).

Ergot Alkaloids (Ergonovine and its Analogues)

Effect on Uterus: ***Ergometrine (ergonovine)*** and its synthetic analogues, viz., ***methylergonovine*** and ***dihydroergonovine,*** are used clinically. The latter has a selective and more potent effect on the uterus. Ergometrine and its analogues increase myometrial contractions involving the fundus, the body and the cervical segments of the uterus. In therapeutic doses, the contractions tend to be sustained with intervening relaxations; but in higher doses there is no relaxation in between two tonic contractions. The uterus is more sensitive to ergometrine at term. These are partial agonist-antagonist at 5-HT_2 and α-adrenergic receptors present on uterine myometrium.

Therapeutic Uses: Ergometrine derivatives are used for following conditions:

a) ***Management of Third Stage of Labour***: Ergometrine (0.2–0.5 mg) is injected intramuscularly after the appearance of the anterior shoulder of the foetus. Contractions occur within 2–3 min. Oxytocin 5 IU may also be added if necessary. Ergonovine should not be used to induce labour or to accelerate normally progressing labour unless there is uterine atony. Since the cervical segment is also contracted, there is a risk of foetal distress, compression, asphyxia and death.

b) ***To Treat Postpartum Haemorrhage (PPH)***: Ergonovine (0.2–0.5 mg I.M.) can be administered to prevent PPH after normal or caesarean delivery. Contractions of myometrial meshwork compress the bleeding arteries, which stops the bleeding.

c) ***To Ensure Normal Involution***: In multipara and other cases where uterus may not involute rapidly, 0.125 mg of ergometrine can be given TDS for 7 days.

Adverse Effects: The drug in the stipulated doses is quite safe. However, it may produce nausea, vomiting, headache and a decrease in milk secretion (due to dopaminergic action—inhibition of prolactin release). It is contraindicated in angina pectoris, myocardial infarction, history of cerebrovascular disease, transient ischaemic attacks or hypertension.

Prostaglandins

PGE_2, its synthetic analogue ***dinoprostone***; $PGF_{2\alpha}$, its synthetic analogue ***carboprost*** and PGE_1 analogue ***misoprostol*** are used as potent uterine stimulants specially in the latter part of pregnancy and to cause ripening of the cervix. Their pharmacological actions, use in obstetrics and side effects have already been described in detail earlier (Ch. 25).

Recent clinical trials have shown that *misoprostol* (Ch. 27) is also an effective agent for both cervical ripening and induction of labour. It has been found to be as efficacious as *dinoprostone*, produces lesser side effects and is much less expensive (see also Ch. 43). Recently it has also been observed that *carboprost tromethamine* can be successfully used to control postpartum bleeding, that was secondary to loss of uterine tone and in cases where myometrium was unresponsive to oxytocin, ergonovine or methylergonovine. Given intramuscularly, carboprost (0.25 mg every hour) causes immediate and sustained uterine contractions. Clinical data have revealed that its use has saved many women from operative interventions to control PPH (including hysterectomy). The prostaglandins are not used concomitantly with oxytocin because of the possibility of uterine rupture.

Tocolytic Drugs (Uterine Relaxants)

The primary use of uterine relaxants is in the prevention of premature labour, i.e., labour that starts before the end of 37th week of gestation. Premature labour can develop spontaneously or may follow genetically predisposed early rupture of foetal membrane. Tocolytic agents act either directly to suppress myometrial smooth muscle contractions by decreasing intracellular Ca^{2+} concentration and reducing the effect of Ca^{2+} on muscle contraction; or they may act indirectly by inhibiting synthesis/release/receptor actions of prostaglandins or oxytocin. These drugs have been used to delay labour, arrest threatened abortion or to treat dysmenorrhoea. Suppression of labour may be needed to allow the foetus to mature, to initiate glucocorticoid therapy to the mother so that the lungs of newborn get sufficient time for maturation and that the neonatal respiratory distress is reduced. By delaying labour, logistics can be optimised so that the baby is born at a centre which has facilities for neonatal intensive care. Tocolytic agents used for this purpose include β_2-adrenoceptor agonists, magnesium sulfate, and Ca^{2+} channel blockers.

β_2-Adrenoceptor Agonists

Selective β_2 receptor agonists such as ***ritodrine, salbutamol, terbutaline, orciprenaline*** and ***isoxsuprine*** are known to relax uterine myometrium (Ch. 12 & 48). These drugs act by binding to β_2 receptors on myometrium and activating adenylyl cyclase. This in turn increases cAMP levels which activate cAMP dependent protein kinase. Hence intracellular Ca^{2+} concentration is decreased leading to muscle relaxation. Among several β_2 receptor agonists only ritodrine holds some promise; with others the uterine relaxant effects are unpredictable. For desirable effects, ***ritodrine*** is started as 50 mcg/min I.V. infusion. The rate is then increased every 10 min till uterine contractions cease or maternal heart rate rises maximum up to 120/min (β_1 side effect). Contractions are then kept suppressed by giving it (10 mg, I.M. QID) for 2 days. Preterm labour from these drugs can be arrested up to 72 hours. Efficacy of β_2 agonists beyond this time frame is in dispute but even this delay is desirable as it can bring 20% increase in the survival rate for the foetus. *Side effects* result both from their residual β_1 effects and from their ability to stimulate β_2 receptors elsewhere in the body. Such effects include palpitation, tremors, nausea, vomiting, shortness of breath, hyperglycaemia, hypokalaemia and hypotension. Serious complications in higher doses include pulmonary oedema, cardiac insufficiency, arrhythmias and myocardial ischaemia.

Magnesium Sulfate

It is neither a specific antihypertensive nor an anticonvulsant, yet when given by I.V. infusion (I.V. bolus 2–4 g over 15 min followed by I.V. infusion of 1–2 g/hr) it controls convulsions and reduces blood pressure in patients of pre-eclampsia. It directly uncouples excitation-contraction in myometrial cells and inhibits cellular action potentials. Magnesium sulphate is usually preferred over β_2 agonists in patients having cardiac problems, diabetes, hyperthyroidism and hypertension. For effective inhibition of uterine activity, the plasma levels of magnesium sulphate should range from 6 mEq/L to 7.5 mEq/L. Below these levels tocolysis may be hard to achieve; above these levels patients initially lose patellar reflexes. Above 10–12 mEq/L there is respiratory depression and arrest both in mother as well as in neonate. Higher than these levels, cause cardiac arrhythmias and cardiac arrest. In therapeutic doses, side effects observed are feeling of warmth, sweating, flushing, dry mouth, nausea, headache and palpitation.

Ca^{2+} Channel Blockers

Calcium channel blocker, e.g., ***nifedipine*** (Ch. 19 & 20), is one of the recent drugs examined for tocolytic actions. It acts by impairing the Ca^{2+} entry into myometrial cells *via* voltage-dependent L-type channels to inhibit uterine contractility. At present the use of nifedipine is restricted to prophylaxis of recurrent premature labour. Oral nifedipine 10 mg every ½ hr till uterine contractions subside followed by 10 mg oral QID has been used for tocolytic purposes. However, at this dose tachycardia and hypotension appear as prominent side effects. More studies are needed before its usefulness can be fully ascertained.

CHAPTER 42 Adrenocortical Steroids and their Analogues

COMPETENCY PH1.38

The medullary portion of adrenal gland secretes predominantly epinephrine (also norepinephrine) on sympathetic stimulation (Ch. 10 & 12), while the three zones of adrenal cortex (see below), using cholesterol as a substrate, produce a large number of steroid hormones collectively called ***corticosteroids***. Precisely speaking, the term *corticosteroid* refers to both glucocorticoids as well as mineralocorticoids (as both hormones are produced by adrenal cortex), but it is often used as a synonym for ***glucocorticoids***. The name glucocorticoid has been assigned because they play an important role in glucose metabolism, are synthesised in adrenal cortex and have a steroidal structure (**Gluco**se + **Cort**ex + Ster**oid**).

STEROID BIOSYNTHESIS

The mammalian adrenal cortex is divided into three concentric zones: the *zona glomerulosa, zona fasciculata* and *zona reticularis* (Fig. 42.1B). The *zona glomerulosa* produces mineralocorticoids, such as aldosterone, which regulates salt and water metabolism. *Zona fasciculata* predominantly produces glucocorticoids, such as hydrocortisone (cortisol) and corticosterone, which regulate carbohydrate and protein metabolism. *Zona reticularis* is, however, primarily involved in the biosynthesis of androgens, which serve as the principal source of estrogens in men and in postmenopausal women (Fig. 42.1A).

While secretions by the two inner zones (zona fasciculata and reticularis) is controlled by ACTH from anterior pituitary, aldosterone produced by zona glomerulosa is principally under control of renin-angiotensin system. 11-Deoxycorticosterone (see below), a mineralocorticoid produced from zona fasciculata is, however, under the control of ACTH.

Cholesterol is an obligatory building block in the biosynthesis of adrenocorticoids. Cholesterol is transported into mitochondria of steroidogenic tissue, where its side chain is cleaved by desmolase to produce pregnenolone. This step is the rate limiting step in the steroid biosynthesis.

The pregnenolone, then leaves the mitochondria and becomes an obligatory precursor of glucocorticoids, mineralocorticoids as well as for androgens. The biosynthetic pathway next branches into 3 different routes (Fig. 42.1A). One route passes through progesterone → 11-deoxycorticosterone → corticosterone to aldosterone; the other proceeds from 17-α-hydroxypregnenolone → 17-α-hydroxyprogesterone → 11-deoxycortisol to hydroxycortisone (cortisol); the third route goes ahead with 17-α-hydroxypregnenolone → dehydroepiandrosterone → androstenedione to testosterone, oestradiol and oestrone.

The glucocorticoid and mineralocorticoid actions and their secretions from zona glomerulosa and zona fasciculata are not completely or specifically separated in human steroidogenesis. For example, 11-deoxycorticosterone is a mineralocorticoid but is secreted from zona fasciculata; hydrocortisone (cortisol) is a glucocorticoid while corticosterone possesses combined gluco+mineralocorticoid activity but both are secreted from zona fasciculata. Various steps in the steroidogenesis depend upon the enzymes involved and the site of their expression. Aldosterone synthase is normally expressed only in the zona glomerulosa (outer layer). It is the site of aldosterone biosynthesis. 11-β, 17-α and 21-β-Hydroxylase are expressed in the inner two layers (zona fasciculata and zona reticularis). These are the sites for cortisol, corticosterone and androgen biosynthesis (Fig. 42.1).

STEROID NOMENCLATURE

All corticosteroids possess a cyclopentano-

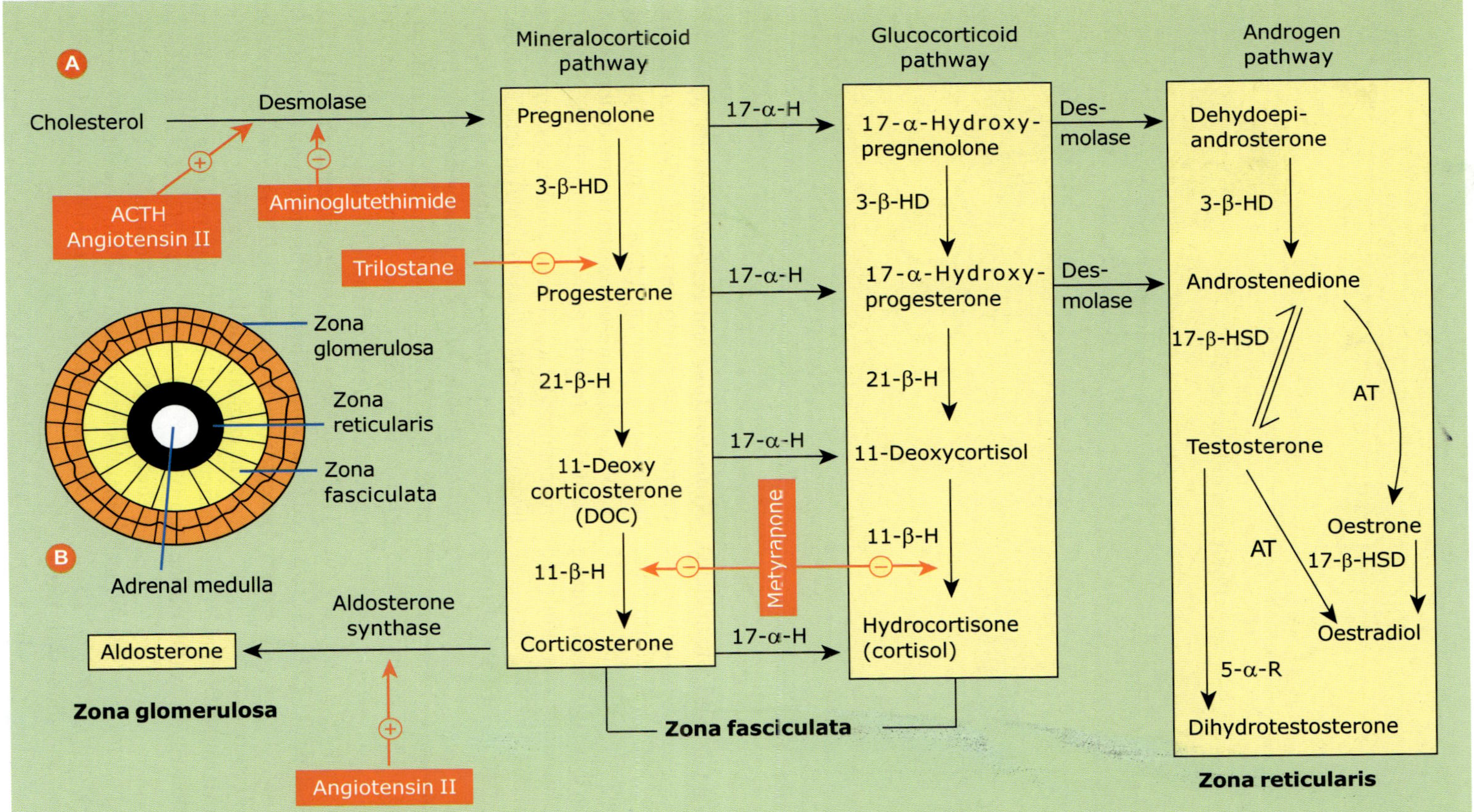

Key: 3-β-HD—3-β-Hydroxydehydrogenase; 11-β-H—11-β-Hydroxylase; 17-α-H—17-α-Hydroxylase; 21-β-H—21-β-Hydroxylase; AT—Aromatase; 5-α-R—5-α-Reductase; 17-HSD—17-Hydroxy steroid dehydrogenase.

Fig 42.1 (A) Adrenocorticosteroids Biosynthesis. (B) Adrenal Cortex and Its Zones. Site of actions of drugs has been indicated by **red**.

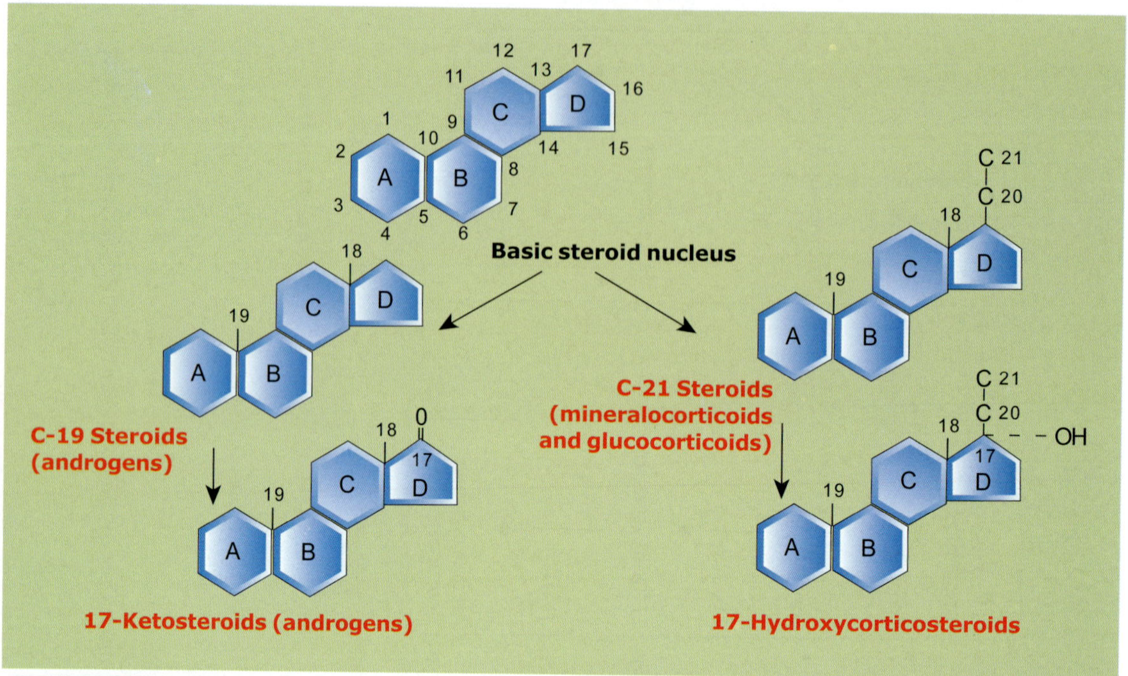

Fig 42.2 Basic Steroid Structure and Nomenclature

perhydro-phenanthrene ring (steroid basic nucleus) from which various adrenocorticosteroids are derived (Fig. 42.2). The letters A–D indicate cyclopen-tane+phenanthrene rings. Numbers 1–17 refer to C-atom positions on these four rings. During steroidogenesis, this basic nucleus is modified during subsequent conversions (Fig. 42.2).

C-19 steroids have CH_3 groups at C-18 and C-19 positions.

C-17 ketosteroids are like C-19 steroids but with a ketone (C=O) group at C-17 position. These are usually androgens.

C-21 steroids are also like C-19 steroids but with two carbon atom side chain (C-20 & C-21) at C-17 position of ring D. These are either glucocorticoids or mineralocorticoids.

17-Hydroxy corticosteroids are similar to C-21 steroids but with an additional hydroxy (OH) group at position 17 of ring D.

At times, confusion prevails over the similar sounding names like *hydrocortisone, cortisol, cortisone* and *corticosterone*, and about their inter-relationship.

Hydrocortisone and ***cortisol*** mean the same. It is primarily a glucocorticoid. ***Cortico-sterone*** possesses a combined gluco+ mineralocorticoid activity and is biosynthesised *via* mineralocorticoid pathway. It gets converted to aldosterone (a mineralocorticoid) in zona glomerulosa and also to hydrocortisone (the glucocorticoid) in zona fasciculata (Fig. 42.1). ***Cortisone*** is a biologically *inert form* of hydrocortisone. Though hydrocortisone (cortisol) is primarily a glucocorticoid, it has some mineralo-corticoid actions also. However, in mineral-ocorticoid sensitive tissue like kidney, the action of 11-β-hydroxy steroid dehydrogenase (11-β HSD) enzyme converts hydrocortisone to mineralocorticoid receptor inactive *cortisone*. The latter is only seldom used in clinical practice. In patients having genetic deficiency of 11-β-HSD enzyme, cortisol cannot be converted to cortisone. Hence, it binds to mineralocorticoid receptor to exhibit mineralocorticoid activity. This condition is termed as *apparent mineralocorticoid excess syndrome,* which is characterised by hypokalaemia and hypertension.

STEROID TRANSPORT IN BLOOD AND MECHANISM OF ACTION

Glucocorticoids in systemic circulation are reversibly bound to *transcortin* (a corticosteroid binding α-globulin). About 80% of the normal cortisol content in human plasma is bound to transcortin, while only 10% is bound to the regular serum albumin; the remaining 10% is the biologically active free hormone.

Glucocorticoid Receptor

The glucocorticoid receptor has been dealt in detail under cytosolic receptor functioning (Ch. 7). Briefly, glucocorticoids exert their physiological actions by binding to the cytsolic glucocorticoid receptor. The glucocorticoid receptor forms a homodimer (GR+GR) complex with glucocorticoids (Fig. 7.10) which translocates to the nucleus and binds to glucocorticoid response elements (GREs) in the promoter region of specific genes, either upregulating (transactivating) or down-regulating (transrepressing) the gene expression.

The ***transactivation*** involves the formation of the resultant specific or edited mRNA, which is transported out to the cytoplasm for the production of the desired proteins that bring about the final hormone response (Fig. 7.10). Besides inducing the enzymes involved in their metabolic actions (e.g., cAMP dependent kinase), glucocorticoids also induce the formation of *annexin*-1 (*lipocortin*-1), which inhibits phospholipase-A_2, and contributes to the anti-inflammatory action of the steroids (Fig. 25.1). However, the synthesis of annexin-1 (after its induction) is slow and hence as predicted the anti-inflammatory effects of glucocorticoids take several hours to become evident.

The ***transrepression*** is brought about by inhibition of the activity of various transcription factors (e.g., AP-1 and NF-kB). These transcription factors are enhancers of transcription. The inhibition of the transcription of the genes for COX-2, cytokines and inducible form of nitric oxide synthase is again contributory for their anti-inflammatory and immunosuppresive action. In contrast to these genomic effects, some actions of corticosteroids may be immediate (see below) and are mediated by membrane-bound receptors (non-genomic effects).

Regulation of gene expression and protein synthesis by glucocorticoids takes time. Hence, there is a biological lag of several hours before their effects are manifested. However, the duration of various responses continues even after steroid levels fall. Thus, there is evidence that side effects elicited by corticosteroids can be minimised and effects can be sustained by alternate day therapy.

Mineralocorticoid Receptor (MR)

Two genes for the corticoid receptor have been identified; one encoding the classic *glucocorticoid receptor* and the other for *mineralocorticoid receptor*. Although much less studied than the glucocorticoid receptor, the basic principles of its action and binding domains appear to be similar. MR also binds to a very similar, if not identical, mineralocorticoid responsive element (MRE). In addition, unlike glucocorticoid receptor, the MR has a restricted expression. These are expressed mainly in kidney but also in colon, salivary glands, sweat glands and hippocampus.

Aldosterone exerts its effects on Na^+ and K^+ homeostasis primarily by acting on MR, expressed in distal renal tubules and collecting ducts. Some of the effects of glucocorticoids can be attributed to their binding to MR. Indeed MRs bind aldosterone and hydrocortisone (cortisol) with equal affinity. Hydrocortisone is primarily a glucocorticoid but has some mineralocorticoid action also. Cortisol on binding to MRs in the kidney, is inactivated by 11-β-hydroxy steroid dehydrogenase (11-β-HSD) to receptor inactive cortisone (see above). Aldosterone escapes degradation by 11-β-HSD because, in physiological settings, it exists as "hemiacetyl" derivative which is resistant to such degradation. This explains why the specificity of MRs for aldosterone action on kidney is maintained, in the face of much higher levels of , round the clock, circulating cortisol.

PHARMACOLOGICAL ACTIONS

General Considerations

- Actions of corticoids are divided into: (a) *Glucocorticoid actions,* which govern carbohydrate, protein and fat metabolism and other therapeutically useful effects like anti-inflammatory and immunosuppressant actions; (b) *Mineralocorticoid actions,* which govern Na^+, K^+ and fluid homeostasis.

- Several synthetic steroids have been developed in which it has been possible to separate the glucocorticoid from the mineralocorticoid action (Table 42.1); but it has not been possible to separate the anti-inflammatory actions of glucocorticoid from their other actions like effects on carbohydrate, protein and fat metabolism. More potent the glucocorticoid more powerful are its anti-inflammatory effects. However, recently some "selective Glucocorticoid Receptor Agonists" have been developed (see below).
- Corticoids have *direct* as well as *permissive actions*. By permissive action is meant that in absence of which certain normal functions get derailed. For example, in absence of glucocorticoids there is down-regulation of adrenergic and AT_1 receptors, which markedly blunts the normal physiological response of adrenaline (causing a fall in BP and bronchoconstriction). Glucocorticoids permissively enhance the actions of adrenaline on these tissues by increasing the expression of adrenoceptors.
- Administration of exogenous glucocorticoid depresses the secretions of CRH and ACTH by negative feedback mechanisms (Ch. 41). The physiological secretion of endogenous glucocorticoids, therefore declines or gets inhibited causing atrophy of the adrenal cortex. Sudden withdrawal of exogenously administered glucocorticoid, after prolonged therapy, may precipitate acute adrenal insufficiency and it may take several months before hypothalamic-pituitary-adrenal cortex axis resumes its normal functions.
- A deficiency in corticosteroid production from adrenals is called *Addison's disease,* which is characterised by either *acute adrenal crisis* (severe hypotension, hyperkalaemia and hyponatraemia) or *chronic adrenal crisis* (weight loss, weakness, anorexia, nausea, pigmentation and generalised hair loss). It may have an autoimmune aetiology or may result after sudden withdrawal of glucocorticoids after prolonged use. A related condition is called ***Simmond's disease*** in which there is atrophy of pituitary—not of adrenals.
- If corticosteroids are produced in excess, the clinical condition is called *Cushing's syndrome*. The clinical manifestations would depend on which type of steroid is in excess. The predominance of glucocorticoid is manifested as moon face, red cheeks, increased abdominal fat, buffalo hump, muscle wasting, thinning of skin and osteoporosis. An excess production of mineralocorticoid results in disturbances of Na^+ and K^+ balance. This may be a consequence of *primary hyperaldosteronism* (due to adrenal tumour or Conn's syndrome—an important cause of hypertension) or of *secondary hyper-aldosteronism* (due to overactive renin-angiotensin system that occurs in extra-adrenal stimulation of aldosterone secretion as occurs in nephrotic syndrome, congestive cardiac failure and cirrhosis of liver).
- The pharmacological effects of exogenously administered corticosteroids are largely the exaggerations of the physiological functions of the endogenous corticoids. A review of their physiological features is helpful in understanding the pharmacological and toxic actions of corticoids (see below).

Glucocorticoid Actions

A) Carbohydrate and Protein Metabolism

Glucocorticoids exert prominent anti-insulin effects (hyperglycaemia) through various mechanisms summarised below:

1. They decrease the peripheral utilisation of glucose by decreasing its cellular uptake.
2. They enhance the expression of the hepatic enzymes involved in gluconeogenesis and stimulate glucose synthesis from amino acids.
3. For gluconeogenesis to happen, they mobilise amino acids by inhibiting protein synthesis in muscle, connective tissue and skin (antianabolic effect).

Glucocorticoids also promote deposition of glycogen in the liver by inducing hepatic glycogen synthetase. This probably is a consequence of insulin secretion in response to hyperglycaemia. The net result of glucocorticoid administration is the increases in blood sugar, liver glycogen and excretion of urinary nitrogen. As a result, the prolonged high-dose therapy with glucocorticoids causes the clinical manifestations of diabetes-like state and protein wasting.

The physiological role of glucocorticoid seems to provide natural protection to glucose-dependent vital organs, such as brain and heart, during starvation and malnourishment.

B) Fat Metabolism

In adipose tissues, glucocorticoids permissibly enhance the lipolytic effects of growth hormone, adrenaline and thyroxine. The mobilisation of free fatty acids is increased. But, as discussed above, the glucose utilisation by both adipose tissue and muscle is inhibited. The resulting hyperglycaemia leads to some release of insulin. Consequently, the net result of increased glucocorticoid levels is an increase in the deposition of fats. Long-term administration of high doses of glucocorticoid causes redistribution of fat from peripheral stores toward central locations such as back of the neck and shoulders (***buffalo hump***), abdomen and face (***moon face***)—the result termed as ***centripetal obesity***—and ***cuta striae*** on the areas of the trunk, where the skin gets stretched by the accumulation of the fat. The pattern of redistribution of fat sounds quite intriguing; nevertheless, it has been suggested that adipocytes in the trunk region are very sensitive to the elevated levels of insulin (resulting from steroid-induced hyperglycaemia), which promotes preferential deposition of fats over centripetal region. The peripheral adipocytes, on the other hand, are much less sensitive to insulin and therefore respond instead to the glucocorticoid facilitated effects of adrenaline, growth hormone and thyroxine, etc.

C) Anti-inflammatory Effects

The endogenous glucocorticoids prevent an "excessive response" of the body's powerful defence mechanisms during stress, infection and inflammation, which otherwise would have been hazardous. Hence, exogenously administered glucocorticoids are very useful in treating conditions of unwanted inflammation and immune response but on prolonged therapy also carry the hazard of suppressing the necessary protective response to inflammation and infection (wound healing and repair). Glucocorticoids inhibit inflammation irrespective of its cause. Both the early components (e.g., oedema, pain, heat, fibrin deposition, etc.) and late components (collagen synthesis and wound healing, etc.) are retarded. The anti-inflammatory actions of glucocorticoids are mediated by the following mechanisms:

1) In Macrophages, Monocytes, Endothelium and Fibroblasts

In these cell types, glucocorticoids induce the production of lipocortin (transactivation of annexin-1) which inhibits phospholipase A_2 (Ch. 25). The resultant decrease in the production of arachidonic acid leads to a reduction in the synthesis of prostaglandins, leukotrienes and platelet activating factor, which are important mediators of inflammation. They also block the production and release of cytokines (IL-1, IL-4, IL-6 and TNF-α) with concomitant reduction in the activation of T-cells and suppression of fibroblast proliferation. This reduces the process of chemotaxis. They also inhibit the synthesis of adhesion molecules (e.g., edothelial leukocyte adhesion molecule-1 and intracellular adhesion molecule-1) in the endothelial cells. As a result they promote leukocyte localisation and impair their recruitment to the sites of inflammation.

2) Transrepression of Proinflammatory Transcription Factors

Glucocorticoids inhibit proinflammatory transcription factors such as nuclear factor-kB (NF-kB) and activatory protein (AP-1). These factors are actually enhancers of transcription of genes for COX-2, various cytokines, and for inducible nitric oxide synthase (iNOS).

3) Lymphocytes

They reduce the release of cytokines (IL-1, IL-2, IL-4, IL-6) from lymphocytes leading to reduced tissue damage. Glucocorticoids also decrease the number of lymphocytes (T and B cells), monocytes, eosinophils and basophils in circulation.

4) Miscellaneous Effects

i) ***Basophils and Mast Cells***: Glucocorticoids decrease IgE-dependent release of histamine and leukotriene C-4 from basophils and hence decrease the capillary permeability. They also cause vasoconstriction when applied directly to the skin possibly by suppressing mast cell degranulation.

ii) ***Acute Phase Reactant***: Glucocorticoids decrease the production of acute phase reactant from macrophages and endothelial cells.

iii) They decrease the production of collagenase and stromelysin and thus prevent collagen degradation and hinder tissue damage. After prolonged therapy they decrease the production of collagen and thus obstruct healing and repair.

D) Immune Response

Glucocorticoids suppress the cell-mediated immunity. They act by inhibiting genes that code for the cytokines IL-1, IL-2, IL-3, IL-4, IL-5, IL-6, IL-8, and IFN-γ, the most important of which is IL-2. Lesser cytokine production reduces the T cell proliferation. Glucocorticoids also suppress the humoral immunity, causing B cells to express smaller amounts of IL-2 and of IL-2 receptor. This diminishes both B cell clone expansion and antibody synthesis. The diminished amounts of IL-2 also cause fewer T lymphocyte cells to be activated. Glucocorticoids also down-regulate the expression of Fc receptors on macrophages, so there is a decreased phagocytosis of opsonised cells. The efficacy of glucocorticoids in controlling graft rejection is due to their ability to (a) reduce antigen expression from the grafted tissue, (b) delay revascularisation and (c) decrease sensitisation of cytotoxic T-lymphocytes.

E) Calcium and Other Electrolyte Metabolism

The steroid binding specificity of glucocorticoid and mineralocorticoid receptors overlap in the distal and collecting tubules so that glucocorticoids may mediate mineralocorticoid-like effects (see below). Glucocorticoids also decrease the intestinal transport of Ca^{2+} by antagonising the action of 1,25-dihydroxy vitamin D_3 and promote Ca^{2+} excretion through kidney. There is also loss of Ca^{2+} from bones due to loss of osteoid. Vertebrae and ribs show increased resorption. Glucocorticoids also amplify the actions of parathyroid hormone. All these effects precipitate osteoporosis.

F) Cardiovascular Effects

Glucocorticoids directly stimulate cardiac output and permissibly potentiate the response of vascular smooth muscles to the pressor effects of catecholamines and angiotensin II. Steroids retard the metabolism of circulating catecholamines by inhibiting their extraneuronal uptake. The resulting hypertension may predispose the patients to coronary heart disease, if prolonged therapy is employed.

G) Haematopoietic System

Glucocorticoids increase the number of RBC, platelets and neutrophils in circulation, but decrease lymphocytes, eosinophils and basophils. Though the normal lymphoid tissue is not affected, glucocorticoids show marked lytic effects on malignant lymphatic cells, which explains their use in treating lymphomas.

H) Central Nervous System

Therapeutic doses of steroids cause mild euphoria which is independent of their other pharmacological actions. Subsequently insomnia, anxiety or depression may ensue. Higher doses lower the seizure threshold and may precipitate seizures in epileptic patients. This action is again independent of electrolyte changes in brain as aldosterone does not lower seizure threshold.

I) Miscellaneous Effects

1. Normal physiological amounts of cortisol are needed for maintaining normal glomerular filtration.
2. Glucocorticoids play an important physiological role in the development of foetal lungs. The production of pulmonary surface active material (surfactant), required for proper air breathing, is stimulated by glucocorticoids.
3. Large doses of glucocorticoids are associated with the development of peptic ulcer. They possibly suppress the immune response against *Helicobacter pylori*. They also increase the secretion of pepsin and gastric acid.

4. Renal excretion of uric acid is increased by glucocorticoids.
5. They inhibit the thyroid stimulating hormone pulsatility and the nocturnal surge of this hormone by depressing thyrotropin-releasing hormone secretion at hypothalamic level. They also depress growth hormone secretion.

Mineralocorticoid Actions

Aldosterone is the most important mineralocorticoid in humans. Mineralocorticoids promote Na^+ reabsorption from the distal convoluted and cortical collecting renal tubules with concomitant increased excretion of K^+ and H^+ (Ch. 16 and 18).

Three types of mechanisms operate for aldosterone-promoted Na^+ reabsorption. First is the rapid non-genomic effect through stimulation of Na^+/H^+ exchanger in the apical membrane. Second is a delayed effect by binding to the mineralocorticoid receptor within the cell and directing the synthesis of specific mediator proteins (aldosterone-induced proteins; AIP), that activate Na^+ channels in apical membrane. Third is by increasing the number of Na^+/K^+ ATPase molecules (Na^+ pumps) in the basolateral membrane. The latter is a long-term effect exerted by aldosterone. The concomitant increased excretion of K^+ results from influx of K^+ into the tubular cell (from the blood) by the action of Na^+/K^+ ATPase in the basolateral membrane. This is followed by an efflux of K^+, from the cell into the lumen, through apical K^+ channels (Ch. 16).

The specificity of mineralocorticoid receptor, expressed on kidneys, is conferred at least in part by the presence of the enzyme 11-β-HSD, which converts cortisol to receptor inactive cortisone (see above), thus ensuring that the renal cells should respond only to bonafide mineralocorticoids.

STEROID PREPARATIONS AND THEIR RELATIVE POTENCIES

Chemical modifications of cortisol have generated several synthetic glucocorticoids, with primarily glucocorticoid rather than mineralocorticoid activity with longer duration of action. Some of these agents are listed and compared with cortisol in Table 42.1. The intermediate (12–36 hrs) and long-acting (36–72 hrs) glucocorticoids have a greater ratio of glucocorticoid: mineralocorticoid activity. Consequently these agents are preferred for long-term use in the treatment of chronic inflammatory disorders because they cause less disturbances in electrolyte and fluid balance than does hydrocortisone. Normally, these synthetic analogues do not effectively distinguish between anti-inflammatory effects, metabolic effects and their suppressive effects on HPA axis. However, many of them have an advantage that their Na^+ retention effects are not as marked as of hydrocortisone in equipotent anti-inflammatory doses. A vast range of different glucocorticoid preparations are available for oral, parenteral, inhalational, topical and ophthalmic use (Table 42.1 and 42.2).

THERAPEUTIC USES

A) Endocrinal Uses

1) Replacement Therapy

Treatment of adrenal insufficiency, regardless of any cause, requires replacement therapy with corticosteroid.

Acute Adrenal Insufficiency (Addisonian Crisis)

It is characterised by severe hypotension, hyponatraemia and hyperkalaemia, extreme weakness, GIT distress and dehydration. It is a life-threatening emergency (caused by stress, trauma or surgery) and requires immediate institution of corticosteroid therapy. In addition to large amounts of parenteral hydrocortisone (100 mg I.V. TDS with I.V. infusion of normal saline, until the patient is stable), there is always a need to correct fluid and electrolyte imbalance. The dose of cortisol is gradually reduced to a maintenance dose of 50 mg/day. A mineralo-corticoid (fludrocortisone) can now be added in a dose of 0.1 to 0.2 mg/day orally. The hyponatraemia and hyperkalaemia of Addisonian crisis responds to this treatment.

Chronic-Primary Adrenocortical Insufficiency (Addison's Disease)

Its clinical features are similar to but milder than those of acute state and is characterised by weakness,

Table 42.1 Comparative Steroid Potencies, Duration of Action and Preparations Available

Steroid	Duration of action	Gluco-corticoid activity	Mineralo-corticoid activity	Equivalent dose (mg)	Preparation available
GLUCOCORTICOIDS				(Anti-inflammatory)	
Hydrocortisone (cortisol)	8–12 hrs SHORT	1	1	20	O/I/T
Cortisone	8 hrs	0.8	0.8	25	O/I/T
Prednisone		4	0.5–0.8	5	O
Prednisolone*	12–36 hrs	5	0.5–0.8	5	O/I/T
Methylprednisolone	Intermediate	5	0–0.5	4	O/I/T
Triamcinolone		5	0	4	O/I/T
Deflazacort		5–6	0	6	O
Paramethasone	36–72 hrs	10	0	2	O/I
Betamethasone	Long acting	25	0	0.65	O/I/T
Dexamethasone*		30	0	0.75	O/I/T
MINERALOCORTICOIDS			(Na^+ Retaining dose)		
Aldosterone	30 min	0.3	3000	Not used	Endogenous
Fludrocortisone	18–30 hrs	10	200	0.2	O
Desoxycortico-sterone	70–80 min	0	20	2.5	SL/IM

Key: O—Oral; I—Injectable; T—Topical; SL—Sublingual; IM—Intramuscular. * These are also used in ophthalmic preparations. Hydrocortisone (cortisol) is the standard drug for comparing glucocorticoid activity.

Table 42.2 Synthetic Glucocorticoids Available for Topical, Inhalation and Ophthalmic Use

Steroid	Preparation	Steroid	Preparation
Alclometasone	Topical	Dexsoximetasone	Topical
Amcinonide	Topical	Flucinolone	Topical
Beclomethasone	Topical/Inhalation*	Flunisolide	Inhalation
Budesonide	Inhalation*	Fluoromethalone	Ophthalmic
Clobetasol	Topical	Fluticasone	Topical/Inhalation
Clocortolone	Topical	Halcinonide	Topical
Desonide	Topical	Medrysone	Ophthalmic

* 8 puffs QID equals to 14 mg of oral prednisone OD

fatigue, anorexia, weight loss, hypotension, hyperpigmentation, loss of body hair and inability to maintain blood glucose levels during fasting. There is deficiency of cortisol as well as aldosterone due to nonfunctional adrenal cortex. In such patients any infection, trauma or shock may provide a stimulus to produce acute adrenal insufficiency which could be life threatening. Treatment requires 20–30 mg of hydrocortisone orally daily. Usually, two-third of the dose is given in the morning and one-third in the evening to mimic the normal diurnal rhythm of cortisol secretion. This may also be supplemented with 0.1–0.2 mg/day of fludrocortisone orally.

Chronic-Secondary Adrenocortical Insufficiency

This occurs due to suppression of hypothalamic-pituitary-adrenal axis and is characterised by low levels of cortisol but normal levels of aldosterone. Treatment requires hydrocortisone, 20–30 mg orally once daily, as described above. There is no need to add any mineralocorticoid as in such cases the function of zona glomerulosa (which synthesises aldosterone) is normal.

Congenital Adrenal Hyperplasia

Congenital enzymatic defects in adrenal biosynthetic pathways (Fig. 42.1) lead to diminished cortisol and aldosterone production. As a result the bulk of progesterone and pregnenolone is diverted toward the synthesis of androgens. This triggers the compensatory hypersecretion of ACTH leading to enlargement of the adrenal cortex.

The most common defect is a *deficiency or lack of 21-β-hydroxylase enzyme.* In the *simple virilising form* of adrenal hyperplasia, the enzyme deficiency is partial but the overproduction of androgens causes virilisation and accelerated growth ending with early epiphyseal fusion. In *salt wasting form* the deficiency of this enzyme is complete. Hence the hypersecretion of ACTH cannot bring the cortisol and aldosterone production rate back to normal. These patients may develop potentially fatal salt wasting if not treated. Treatment is to give hydrocortisone 0.6 mg/kg oral daily, in divided doses round the clock, to maintain feedback inhibition to pituitary. If salt wasting persists, fludrocortisone 0.1–0.2 mg/day orally may be added. In *the hypertensive form* of adrenal hyperplasia, the enzymatic *defect is at the level of 11-β-hydroxylase.* This results in increased production of 11-deoxycorticosterone which has mineral-ocorticoid activity and hence hypertension with or without hypokalaemic alkalosis ensues; and because increased androgen production also continues (under the production of ACTH) virilism is similar to that described above. *Hirsutism* in females, besides other reasons, could also be a result of mild atypical form of congenital adrenal hyperplasia with only a *mild deficiency of either 21-β- or 11-β-hydroxylase enzyme.* However, the enzymatic defect is too mild to be detected in childhood but becomes evident only at puberty. The treatment of all these conditions requires the administration of a glucocorticoid (see above) in amounts adequate to suppress adrenal-androgen secretion but insufficient to compromise bone growth and mineralisation.

Maintenance Therapy in Cushing's Syndrome (After Surgical Removal of Pituitary/Adrenal Tumour)

Cushing's syndrome is usually a result of bilateral adrenal hyperplasia secondary to an ACTH-secreting pituitary adenoma or due to tumour of the adrenal gland. The manifestations are as if there is chronic presence of excessive glucocorticoids (see above text and Ch. 41). This disorder is treated by surgical removal of the tumour producing ACTH or cortisol. Such patients must receive large doses of cortisol (300 mg as I.V. infusion) during and following the surgical removal of the tumour. Thereafter, the doses are tapered slowly to normal replacement levels (20–30 mg/day). Rapid reduction should be avoided to prevent withdrawal effects. After adrenalectomy, the long-term maintenance is similar to that outlined above for adrenal insufficiency.

2) Diagnostic Use

The dexamethasone suppression test is used for the diagnosis of Cushing's syndrome. Dexamethasone acts on the hypothalamus (like cortisol) to reduce the output of corticotrophin releasing hormone (CRH). But it does not interfere with measurement of endogenous corticoids in blood or urine (e.g., of cortisol). A normal suppression of cortisol production, after administering dexamethasone indicates that HPA axis is intact. Failure of suppression implies a pathological hypersecretion of ACTH by the pituitary tumour or of cortisol by adrenal tumour. As a screening test, dexamethasone 1 mg is given orally at 11 PM and a plasma sample is obtained in the following morning at 8 AM. In normal individuals the morning cortisol levels are usually less than 3 mg/dL, whereas in Cushing's syndrome it is greater than 5 mg/dL.

B) Non-Endocrinal Uses

In addition to replacement therapy, the glucocorticoids are used in a large number of non-adrenal disorders. In none of these conditions, do the corticoids have specific actions on the basic disease process despite their ability to produce dramatic improvement on signs and symptoms. For example, in patients of rheumatoid arthritis, glucocorticoids can effectively relieve the distressing inflammation and pain but the affected joints continue to deteriorate. Hence the use of glucocorticoids in situations other than replacement therapy is only palliative.

Glucocorticoid therapy for periods up to one week usually does not cause significant suppression of HPA axis. If the therapy has continued for more than 2 weeks the dose of glucocorticoid should not be decreased or stopped abruptly, as it may precipitate suppression of HPA axis (see above). Single dose (even higher) or short courses of 5 to 7 days are not likely to harm and can be used to overcome the crisis. When corticoids are used on a long-term basis, their administration on alternate days should be preferred to minimise the suppression of HPA axis as there is a recovery period between each dose. Giving a glucocorticoid every other day between 6 to 9 a.m. mimics the normal diurnal rhythm of cortisol secretion. Some of the non-endocrinal uses are as under:

1) Anti-inflammatory Therapy

Long-term use of corticosteroids to treat inflammatory disorders should always be viewed with caution. Systemic corticoids should be used cautiously in *rheumatoid arthritis* (see above). If these are to be used as a last resort, these should be used in small doses for short period of time. NSAIDs are more preferred in *rheumatoid arthritis*, *osteoarthritis* and *ankylosing spondylitis*. However, intra-articular injection of glucocorticoid may be used to control exacerbations. In *acute gouty arthritis* too, these are the last resort when NSAIDs and other drugs have failed. In *ulcerative colitis* and *Crohn's disease*, these are indicated only during acute phase if the disease is not responding to 5-amino salicylic acid (Ch. 29). In such cases these may be used orally or as retention enema. Topical instillation as eye drops or as ointments is effective in large number of *inflammatory eye diseases* such as *allergic conjuctivitis, iritis* and *iridocyclitis*. These should not be used in infective conditions, unless there is associated inflammation where these can be applied along with an effective antibiotic. These are also administered by retrobulbar injections to avoid systemic side effects. Generally, hydrocortisone, prednisolone, dexamethasone, fluorometholone or medrysone are used in various ophthalmic preparations. For systemic use, prednisolone or daflazocort, which have mainly glucocorticoid activity are chosen, so as to avoid mineralocorticoid side effects. Large doses of dexamethasone or betamethasone, given on early symptoms and for brief period are helpful to reduce oedema/inflammation in *acute spinal cord injury*. Dexamethasone 10 mg I.M. initially, then 4 mg QID orally/I.M. for 2–4 days and then withdrawing over 7 days reduces *cerebral oedema* due to cerebral tumours, encephalitis or meningitis. Topical steroids are highly effective in several *inflammatory/allergic* and in *eczematous skin disease*. In serious conditions like exfoliative dermatitis, pemphigus vulgaris and Stevens-Johnson syndrome glucocorticoids may be used systemically.

2) Immunosuppressive Therapy (See Ch. 69 also)

a) Collagen Vascular Disease

Most cases of systemic lupus erythematosus (SLE), polymyositis, cranial gaint cell arteritis (to save eyesight), polyarteritis nodosa, sarcoidosis and mixed connective tissue disease syndrome need corticoids for saving the life. Initially, high doses are used and then tapered to maintenance dose after the remission.

b) Skin Graft and Organ Transplant

High doses of corticosteroids are used along with other immunosuppressant drugs (e.g., azathioprine) to prevent rejection. The doses are then tapered to maintenance dose.

c) Nephrotic Syndrome

Patients with nephrotic syndrome secondary to minimal lesion nephropathy, which is normally immunologically mediated, respond well to steroid therapy. Initial daily dose of prednisolone 60 mg/day for 6 weeks is sufficient to provide remission in 95% of cases within 3 months. However, cessation of steroid therapy results in relapse (evidenced by recurrent proteinuria) which necessitates an addition of other immunosuppresant drug (e.g., azathioprine).

d) Autoimmune Diseases

Autoimmune haemolytic anaemia, thrombocytopenia, and active chronic hepatitis usually respond to corticosteroids. However, long-term therapy is needed as relapses occur on withdrawal of drug.

e) Chronic Demyelinating Polyneuropathies

In such cases glucocorticoids suppress the immune reaction but may not retard the progression of the disease. However, in Guillain-Barre syndrome, glucocorticoids reduce the inflammation and improve the final outcome.

3) Bronchial Asthma

Inhaled/systemic glucocorticoids are the mainstay of the therapy for moderate to severe asthma. Inhaled steroids (beclomethasone, budesonide, flunisolide, fluticasone, mometasone and triamcinolone) are particularly effective and are preferred for long-term use because they minimise systemic uptake and side effects. This therapy is often combined with an inhaled bronchodilator such as salbutamol. The concomitant use of β-adrenergic agonists or theophylline enables the use of a lower dose of glucocorticoid besides reducing the chances of developing resistance to the steroid therapy (see Ch. 48 also).

4) Severe Allergic Reaction

Corticoids are used for the treatment of anaphylaxis reactions due to penicillins and radiocontrast media or by any other reason. Alone, they are not able to control acute manifestations of anaphylactic shock as they have a slow onset of action. Hence, these are used along with adrenaline (I.M. or S.C.) and antihistamines (I.M.).

5) Stimulation of Lung Maturation in the Foetus

Foetal secretion of cortisol governs lung maturation in the foetus (see above). Treatment of the mother with large doses of betamethasone (12 mg I.M. followed by 12 mg I.M. the next day) reduces the incidence of respiratory distress in infants delivered prematurely. Betamethasone has a better permeability through placenta because its placental metabolism as well as maternal protein binding is less than cortisol or prednisolone.

6) Malignancies

Glucocorticoids are important components in the treatment of haematopoietic malignancies, Hodgkin's and other lymphomas because of their marked lympholytic effects to reduce cell proliferation, to promote cell cycle arrest and to induce cell death by apoptosis. However, the development of resistance may limit the effectiveness of steroid therapy.

7) Hypercalcaemia

Hyperparathyroid hypercalcaemia does not respond to steroid therapy. Nonetheless, hypercalcaemia of sarcoidosis and of vitamin D intoxication respond to prednisolone 30 mg/day for 10 days. Hypercalcaemia of malignancies responds poorly.

8) Myasthenia Gravis

The fact that ACh receptor antibodies are responsible for neuromuscular transmission defect and that glucocorticoids also exert a facilitatory action on neuromuscular transmission, provide a rationale for their use in myasthenia gravis.

9) Infective Disease

These are also used in the treatment of a number of HIV-related disorders including *Pneumocystis carinii* pneumonia and *Mycobacterium avium complex*. However, these are used as an adjuvant drug only to decrease the inflammatory reaction and to allow time for antimicrobial agents to exert their effects. They are not much useful in severely immunocompromised HIV patients. As they activate latent tuberculosis, these should be used under a suitable cover of antitubercular drugs while treating tubercular meningitis or pulmonary tuberculosis.

10) Shock

The combination of glucocorticoid and dopamine therapy preserves renal blood flow during shock. A massive infusion of glucocorticoid can restore cardiac output and reverse hypotension by sensitising the response of adrenoceptors in heart and blood vessels to the stimulant action of catecholamines.

ADVERSE EFFECTS

Although glucocorticoids are valuable agents in the situations described above, they have considerable potential to cause greater harm than good. The adverse effects of corticosteroids are extension of their pharmacological actions (see above) occurring with prolonged therapy, which is a great limitation for their use in chronic diseases. Major adverse effects of glucocorticoid therapy are as under:

1) Altered Distribution of Fat

Long-term use of glucocorticoids results in classic "Cushingoid appearance", which is characterised by moon-like face, accumulation of fat in the back of the neck (buffalo hump), in the supraclavicular region and on upper abdomen. The obese trunk may markedly contrast with thin limbs. The enhanced lipolysis seen with glucocorticoids leads to such changes (see above).

2) Oedema, Hypokalaemia and Hypertension

Na^+ and water retention, hypertension and hypokalaemic alkalosis are rare complications with the use of highly selective synthetic glucocorticoid with dietary salt restrictions. However, prolonged use of even these glucocorticoids can produce a gradual rise in BP and oedema.

3) Suppression of HPA Axis

As discussed above, prolonged administration of high doses of glucocorticoids results in suppression of adrenal corticosteroid production and adrenal insufficiency (if used for a long time and stopped suddenly without tapering the dose).

4) Osteoporosis and Osteonecrosis

Osteoporosis is a common adverse effect of the long-term glucocorticoid therapy and can make the patient prone to traumatic fractures. In post-menopausal women, this complication may be especially serious. Glucocorticoids reduce Ca^{2+} absorption from the intestine and also increase the renal excretion of Ca^{2+} (see above). Resorption of bones occurs through an increase in parathyroid hormone release and due to direct inhibitory effects of glucocorticoids on osteoblasts (see Ch. 46).

5) Hyperglycaemia and Glycosuria

A diabetic-like state can be precipitated due to increased gluconeogenesis, insulin resistance and impaired glucose tolerance (caution: diabetes).

6) Peptic Ulcer

There is increased incidence of gastric ulcers in patients treated with glucocorticoids. When they occur there is a high incidence of associated complications such as haemorrhage and perforation. This is related to the decreased synthesis of PGE_2 and PGI_2, which provide protection to gastric mucosa (Ch. 27). Concomitant use of NSAIDs increases the risk of gastric ulceration.

7) Ocular Effects

Posterior subcapsular cataract and glaucoma can be precipitated from either topical or systemic use of glucocorticoids for longer duration. Children, diabetic persons and patients of rheumatoid arthritis are more susceptible to such adverse ocular effects.

8) Myopathy and Muscle Wasting

Large doses of glucocorticoids especially the fluorinated synthetic analogues (e.g., betamethasone and triamcinolone) can cause muscle wasting particularly of limbs. A negative nitrogen balance results from imbalance between protein synthesis and proteolysis. It reflects the antianabolic effects of glucocorticoids in cutaneous and musculoskeletal tissues.

9) Susceptibility to Infections

It results due to immunosuppressive effects of glucocorticoids. Latent tuberculosis may be reactivated after initiation of glucocorticoid therapy. Poor wound healing may occur during long-term glucocorticoid therapy. Thus it is mandatory to administer suitable antibiotics in proper dosage along with steroids especially when there is a history of chronic infection.

10) CNS Side Effects

Mild psychologic disturbances (euphoria, early morning insomnia and nervousness) to pronounced psychiatric effects (schizophrenic and manic depressive psychosis) can occur during glucocorticoid therapy; but such reactions are usually reversible and disappear after discontinuation of the therapy.

11) Miscellaneous

Acne, thinning of skin, purple striae on thighs and lower abdomen, hirsutism, anovulation, menstrual irregularities, weight gain, pancreatitis, hyperlipidaemia and hepatomegaly may occur during long-term glucocorticoid therapy. Topical administration may produce local skin atrophy. In patients of AIDS who are treated with glucocorticoids, Kaposi's sarcoma becomes activated.

A newly introduced glucocorticoid, ***deflazacort***, has similar efficacy to prednisolone (Table 42.1) but is claimed to have lower incidence of side effects such as bone loss, growth suppression in children, glucose intolerance and Cushing's syndrome.

CONTRAINDICATIONS

Since corticosteroids may have to be used as a life saving measure, the following relative contraindications should be taken into consideration: Peptic ulcer; diabetes mellitus; hypertension; osteoporosis; tuberculosis and other infections (unless there is suitable cover of antibiotics in proper dosage); psychosis; epilepsy; cataract; congestive heart failure; renal failure and herpes simplex keratitis. Long-term use of corticosteroids may be avoided during pregnancy for the risk of foetal defects.

The absolute contraindications are Cushing's syndrome and herpes ocular infection.

SELECTIVE GLUCOCORTICOID RECEPTOR AGONISTS (SEGRAs)/MODULATORS (SEGRMs)

The glucocorticoids, in clinical use till date, do not distinguish among transactivation and transrepression. The "wanted" anti-inflammatory and immunosuppressive effects of glucocorticoids result from both transactivation and transrepression, while their metabolic adverse effects (e.g.diabetes, osteoporosis, skin atrophy, etc.) are manifested through transactivation. Genetically modified mice expressed with a modified GR, which is unable to dimerise and incapable to bind DNA (see Fig. 7.10), were still responsive to the anti- inflammatory effects of glucocorticoids while the metabolic side effects were practically nonexistent. This revealed that the selective glucocorticoids receptor agonists (SEGRAs), so called "dissociated GR ligands" which are able to transrepress without transactivation, can provide desirable anti-inflammatory effects avoiding undesired metabolic side effects. In other words SEGRA, like glucocorticoids, bind to and activate GR; but in contrast to them, SEGRAs selectively activate the GR in such a way that they more strongly transrepress than transactivate (resulting in lesser side effects). Some of the SEGRAs, which are currently undergoing clinical trials from June -2009 are Mapracorat (BOL- 303242-X or ZK 245186), ZK 216348 and 55 D1E1. Interestingly all these have nonsteroidal structure. Oral SEGRAs can revolutionize the therapy with glucocorticoids in chronic inflammatory diseases of skin and eyes or in conditions where long-term immunosuppression or treatment of systemic inflammatory conditions are desired. However, SEGRAs are likely to be less effective in hyperproliferative diseases like psoriasis where atrophic effects of conventional glucocorticoids would be more beneficial.

GLUCOCORTICOID SYNTHESIS INHIBITORS

Metyrapone

It inhibits the steroid 11-β-hydroxylase enzyme that converts 11-deoxy precursors to corticosterone, hydrocortisone (cortisol) and aldosterone (Fig. 42.1). However, there may not be mineralocorticoid deficiency because of the compensatory increase in the production of 11-desoxycorticosterone which is also a mineralocorticoid. Therefore, the net result of 11-β-hydroxylase inhibition is the diminished production and release of cortisol. In response to falling cortisol levels there is compensatory rise in ACTH secretion (from pituitary) and in the secretions of the precursor 11-deoxysteroids (from adrenal cortex).

a) *Diagnostic Use*: It is used to test responsiveness of pituitary and its ACTH-secreting capacity when the adrenals are functioning in the normal manner. If the defect lies at pituitary level, the metyrapone administration cannot cause a compensatory increase in the urinary excretion of 17-hydroxy or 11-hydroxy corticosteroids. On the other hand, if pituitary functions and ACTH secretions are normal (as occurs in adrenal hyperplasia), the inhibition of cortisol secretion, after administering metyrapone, will stimulate ACTH secretion with an increase in the urinary excretion of precursor steroids such as 17-hydroxy and 11-deoxycorticosteroids. Metyrapone is now seldom used in the differential diagnosis of Cushing's syndrome because direct measurement of plasma corticotrophin provides good results.
b) *Clinical Use*: The steroid inhibiting properties of metyrapone have been used in the treatment of Cushing's syndrome. It is the only adrenal inhibiting medication which can be administered to pregnant women with Cushing's syndrome.
c) *Side Effects*: Transient dizziness, GIT distress, salt and water retention and hirsutism which results from diversion of 11-deoxycortisol precursor to 11-deoxycorticosterone and androgen synthesis (Fig. 42.1).

Aminoglutethimide

This drug blocks the conversion of cholesterol to pregnenolone (Fig. 42.1) and causes a reduction in the synthesis of all types of corticosteroids. It also reduces estrogen production by inhibiting aromatase enzyme in the peripheral and the steroid target tissues. Such a drug-induced adrenalectomy is an efficacious treatment for metastatic breast and prostate cancer (as it diminishes the levels of circulating sex hormones also). Glucocorticoids are also administered concomitantly to suppress enhanced ACTH release. For this, cortisol is preferred over dexamethasone because aminoglutethimide markedly enhances the hepatic microsomal metabolism of dexamethasone. It is also used in Cushing's syndrome that results from adrenal carcinoma. It can also be used in congenital adrenal hyperplasia in which it protects the patient from excessive secretion of endogenous androgens. Since aminoglutethimide therapy is frequently associated with mineralocorticoid deficiency, mineralocorticoid supplements are also administered usually. *Side effects* include ataxia, lethargy, dizziness and rashes, though tolerance to these effects develops later. It has been withdrawn by the manufacturer becuase of its hepatotoxicity and endocrinal side effects.

Mitotane

It is an adrenocorticolytic agent and produces selective atrophy of the zona fasciculata and zona reticularis. This results in a rapid reduction in the levels of adrenocorticosteroids and their metabolites in blood and urine. It is used in treating Cushing's syndrome resulting from an inoperable adrenal carcinoma or adrenal hyperplasia. *Adverse effects* include GIT distress, lethargy, confusion, skin rashes and altered hepatic functions.

Trilostane

It is 3-β-hydroxysteroid dehydrogenase inhibitor and therefore interferes with the synthesis of adrenal and gonadal hormones (Fig. 42.1). Trilostane, like aminoglutethimide, also inhibits the conversion of androgens to estrogens and has largely replaced surgical adrenalectomy for treating cancer. It is also useful in postmenopausal women with breast cancer. Concurrent glucocorticoid replacement therapy is however essential (see above). *Side effects* include flushing, nausea, diarrhoea, oedema of palate, skin rashes and hepatic dysfunctions.

Ketoconazole

It is an effective antifungal agent. In man it inhibits steroid synthesis in adrenal cortex and gonads. The drug inhibits the activity of CYP17 (17 α-hydroxylase) and also blocks 3-β-hydroxy steroid dehydrogenase enzyme activity. It can be used for the treatment of Cushing's syndrome in patients undergoing surgery or receiving pituitary radiotherapy. In such cases and in elderly people it serves as valuable alternative for the control of hypercortisolism. Common *side effects* include pruritus, GIT distress and liver dysfunction.

Abiraterone

It is an orally active steroidal prodrug undergoing clinical trials for the treatment of refractory prostate cancer with encouraging results. It blocks 17-α-hydroxylase (CYP17) and 17, 20-lyase enzyme activity and drastically reduces the synthesis of cortisol. To prevent compensatory release of ACTH from pituitary, a glucocorticoid can be used concomitantly.

GLUCOCORTICOID ANTAGONISTS

Mifepristone

It is pure competitive antagonist not only on progesterone but on glucocorticoid receptors as well. Its use in termination of pregnancy and as progesterone antagonist is discussed in Chapter 43. Higher doses of mifepristone inhibit glucocorticoid receptor and thus block the feedback regulation of the HPA axis, thereby increasing the endogenous ACTH and cortisol levels which tend to reverse its glucocorticoid receptor blocking action. Today, the application of mifepristone is limited to inoperable patients with ectopic ACTH secretion or adrenal carcinoma who have failed to respond to other therapeutic manipulations. Mifepristone is not an antagonist at mineralocorticoid receptor; hence cortisol can elicit some mineralocorticoid action leading to K^+ depletion and Na^+ retention. Thus an administration of a mineralocorticoid receptor antagonist such as spironolactone may be necessary. Hypoadrenalism, nausea, drowsiness, abdominal and pelvic pain have been reported as *side effects* with mifepristone.

MINERALOCORTICOID ANTAGONISTS

These agents compete with aldosterone for mineralocorticoid receptor binding sites and decrease its peripheral effects.

Spironolactone

It is used in the treatment of primary aldosteronism as it reverses its manifestations. It has also been useful in establishing the diagnosis and in reducing the signs and symptoms when surgical removal of adenoma is not possible or delayed. When used diagnostically, administration of 500 mg/day of spironolactone for 7 days can reverse hypokalaemia. To treat primary aldosteronism it is given in the doses of 50–100 mg/day. It is also an androgen antagonist and is used in the treatment of hirsutism in women. The use of spironolactone as diuretic (Ch. 16) and in hypertension (Ch. 19) has been discussed earlier. *Adverse effects* include hyperkalaemia, cardiac arrhythmias, gynaecomastia, menstrual abnormalities, skin rash and GIT distress.

Eplerenone

It is a new and more selective aldosterone antagonist. It has no effects on androgen receptors and hence does not produce gynaecomastia. Hyperkalaemia produced is also mild. It has been approved for the treatment of hypertension (50–100 mg/day; see also Ch. 16). *Adverse effects*—mild hyperkalaemia.

Drospirenone

It is a new progestogen with antimineralocorticoid and antiandrogenic properties. At present it is being used as a progestogenic component of a combined oral contraceptive (Ch. 43). *Adverse effects*—hyperkalaemia.

Finerenone is a nonsteroidal mineralocorticoid receptor antagonist. It is approved by US-FDA for heart failure in chronic kidney disease associated with type 2 diabetes to lower the risk of decline in glomerular filtration rate and end stage kidney disease. *Adverse effects*: Electrolyte disturbances like hyperkalaemia, hypotension and hyponatraemia. Others are nausea, vomiting, diarrhoea, abdominal pain, chest pain, fainting and muscle cramps.

CHAPTER 43

Estrogens, Progestins & Contraception

COMPETENCY PH1.37, PH1.39, PH1.40

The natural estrogens and progestogens (or progestins) are called sex hormones with steroidal chemical characteristics. However, "estrogens" and "progestogens" are the generic terms as their activity is shared by many synthetic steroidal and nonsteroidal agents also. Biologically important natural estrogens include *estradiol, estrone* and *estriol*. Estradiol (17-β-estradiol) is the most potent estrogen that is secreted by the ovaries. Estrone is 1/10th as biologically active as estradiol and is formed by extraglandular conversion of androstenedione in peripheral tissues. In liver it is produced by oxidation of estradiol. Estriol is a conjugated metabolite of estrone and estradiol, excreted in urine, and is the weakest of these 3 estrogens. The distinguishing chemical features of estrogens are that these have an aromatic ring A with phenolic OH at position-3. The distinguishing chemical features of progesterone are that it is a C-21 steroid with a ketone group at C-3 (Fig. 43.1).

The principal pathways of estradiol and progesterone biosynthesis are shown in Figure 42.1 and 43.1. Ovary is the major site of estrogen and progesterone biosynthesis in non-pregnant premenopausal women. The most abundant physiologic estrogen in premenopausal women is estradiol while in man and postmenopausal women, the most abundant estrogen in plasma is estrone. In pregnant women the foetoplacental unit is the major source of estrogens and progesterone. Peripheral sites of estrogen synthesis include liver, kidney, brain, adipose tissues, skeletal muscle and testes. Progesterone is the principal hormone secreted by the corpus luteum and placenta (see below). It is also secreted by testes and adrenal glands in small amounts. The combined estrogen and progesterone production by all peripheral sites is only 10% of that produced by ovaries in normal premenopausal women. However, in postmenopausal women, the ovarian steroidal hormone synthesis declines while the peripheral estrogen biosynthesis accounts for all the estrogen produced in the body.

MECHANISM OF ACTION

Estrogens bind strongly (90%) to sex hormone-binding α_2 globulin (SHBG) and to serum albumin with low affinity. The free fraction of estrogens enters the cell and binds to estrogen receptor. Progesterone in plasma is 89% protein bound to corticosteroid-binding α-globulin and also to serum albumin. It is not bound to sex steroid-binding α_2 globulin (SHBG). It is the free progesterone that enters the cell and binds to progesterone receptors.

There are two types of estrogen receptors—ER-α and ER-β—and two forms of progesterone receptors—PR-α and PR-β. Most tissues express both subtypes of estrogen receptors. However, ER-α predominates in uterus, vagina, breast, hypothalamus, pituitary and blood vessels whereas ER-β receptors have a wider distribution in prostate gland. Estradiol has equal affinity for ER-α and ER-β. Unlike estrogen receptors, the progesterone receptors are confined mostly to the female genital tract, breast, pituitary and CNS. All agonists and antagonists display similar binding properties to both PR-α and PR-β receptors. Reports are, however, forthcoming on the tissue selective modulations of progesterone receptors as has been in the case of ER (see below).

The estrogen and progesterone receptors (like glucocorticoid receptor) are cytosolic receptors which are bound to heat shock proteins (Hsp90) that stabilises them (see Ch. 7 and Fig. 7.10). Binding of the sex hormone (estrogen/progesterone) to its receptor (ER/PR, respectively) release it from the stabilising protein. The homodimers of the receptor-hormone complex then bind to the respective hormone response elements (estrogen response or progesterone response elements, in the nucleus) to activate gene transcription. Like corticosteroids, the

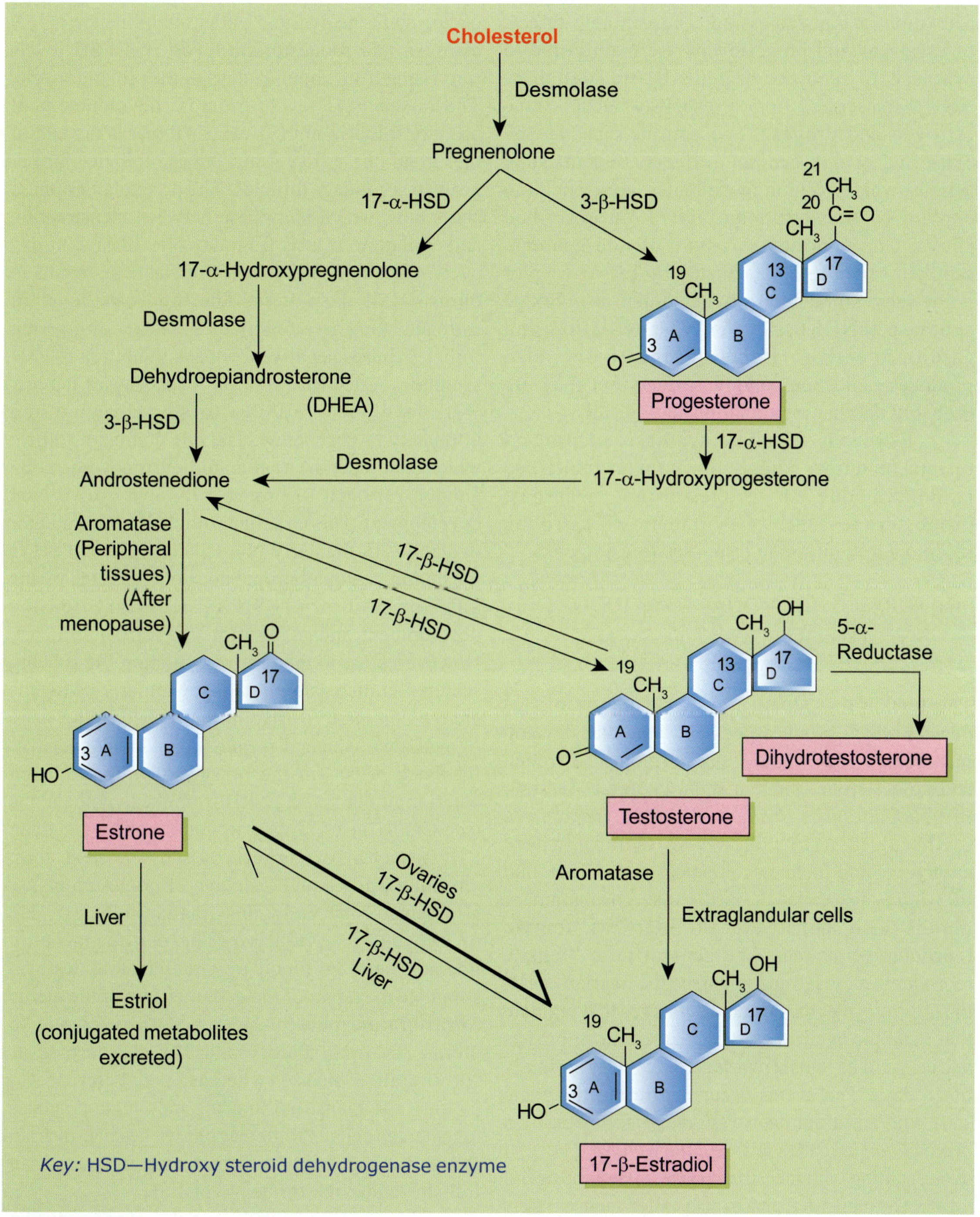

Fig 43.1 Principal Pathways of Estradiol and Progesterone Biosynthesis

gene transcription is promoted through trans-activation or transrepression. The genomic effects of estrogens and progestogens are mainly due to synthesis of requisite proteins by translation of mRNA transcribed from a responsive gene. Some estrogen and progesterone actions can also be classified as non-genomic effects. Several such actions, which occur in few minutes, are difficult to explain by transcriptional activation described above. One important example of non-genomic estrogen action that is mediated by ER-α receptor is the rapid stimulation of endothelial nitric oxide synthase (eNOS) to provide vasodilation and cardioprotective effects. Progesterone also produces rapid non-genomic effects but they are probably not that important physiologically.

Estrogens stimulate synthesis of progesterone receptors and potentiate target tissue responses due to progesterone; whereas, progesterone inhibits synthesis of estrogen receptors to limit tissue responses to estrogens.

INTEGRATED HORMONAL CONTROL OF THE FEMALE REPRODUCTIVE SYSTEM

(Fig. 43.2)

The female reproductive system consists of: (a) *ovaries* which produce oocytes (cells that develop into mature ova), female sex hormones (estrogen and progesterone), inhibin and relaxin (see below); (b) *fallopian tubes (oviducts),* which transport ova to the uterus; (c) *uterus* (the womb), where embryonic and foetal development takes place, and (d) *vagina,* also called the birth canal. The mammary glands also constitute the part of female reproductive system. The general term "female reproductive cycle" encompasses the ovarian cycle, the uterine cycle, the hormonal changes that regulate them and the cyclical changes that occur in breasts and cervix. The female reproductive cycle is normally of 28 days. The events occurring during the cycle start with an initial *menstrual phase* followed by a *preovulatory* and then *postovulatory phase*. The next cycle, starting with menstrual phase, then starts again.

The menstrual phase (also called menses) lasts roughly for the first five days of the 28 days cycle. During the menstrual phase, the changes start occurring in the ovaries. Under the influence of low estrogen and progesterone levels, the FSH levels start rising from about 25 days of the previous cycle. The raised FSH levels promote development of primary follicles in the ovaries. Towards the end of menstrual phase (day 4 to 5), these follicles further grow to secondary follicles. The preovulatory phase starts now, which is a phase between menstruation and ovulation. It lasts from day 6 to 13 in a 28-day cycle. Out of about 20 such follicles, one begins to outgrow all the others. The moderate level of estrogen being secreted by these cluster of growing follicles causes negative feedback inhibition of FSH secretion. A decrease in FSH levels causes the less well developed follicles to stop growing and ultimately to degenerate. The one dominant follicle which matured into Graafian follicle is now secreting enough estrogen to promote its own growth and development. This Graafian follicle is now ready for ovulation. In the early preovulatory phase, FSH is the dominant gonadotropic hormone secreted by the anterior pituitary. FSH is necessary for the development and maturation of ovarian follicles. However, close to the time of ovulation LH is being secreted in increasing quantity. Similarly estrogens are the dominant ovarian hormone before the stage of ovulation, which also exert a paradoxical positive feedback effect on the release of both LH from anterior pituitary and GnRH from the hypothalamus (see Ch. 41 also). This estrogen-stimulated sudden LH surge also triggers ovulation. Less than physiologically active amounts of progesterone are also being produced by the Graafian follicles a day or two before ovulation. The estrogens being liberated into the blood by Graafian follicles also stimulate the repair of the endometrium of the uterus (proliferative phase). Hence, with reference to uterus, the preovulatory phase is also termed as "proliferative phase", whereas, with reference to ovaries, the menstrual and the preovulatory phase together are called "follicular phase" because ovarian follicles are growing and maturing into Graafian follicles under the influence of FSH.

At ovulation, there is rupture of the Graafian follicle with the release of secondary oocyte into the pelvic cavity. It occurs on the 14th day in a 28-day cycle. The movements of fimbriae and the ciliary action inside the fallopian tube mucosa, carry this ovum through the fallopian tube. After ovulation, the Graafian follicle collapses and the remaining follicular cells enlarge to form corpus luteum under the influence of LH (Corpus = main part of any organ; Luteum = a sort of gland formed in ovary performing endocrine functions. Also named because it contains a yellow pigment lutein). Stimulated by LH, the corpus luteum secretes estrogen, progesterone, relaxin and inhibin.

The "post-ovulatory phase" is more constant in duration and lasts for next 14 days from day 15th to day 28th in a 28-day cycle. It is an interval between ovulation and the onset of next menses. During this phase the corpus luteum formed under the influence of LH starts secreting increasing quantities of estrogens and progesterone. Interestingly, the paradoxical positive feedback effect of high levels of estrogens on hypothalamus and anterior pituitary does not occur in presence of progesterone (see above). With reference to ovaries, the post-ovulatory phase is also called "luteal phase". Progesterone produced by corpus luteum is responsible for converting the estrogen-primed uterine endometrium into secretory phase to receive a fertilised ovum (Pro=favour, Gestin=gestation). Hence with reference to uterus, the luteal phase of an ovarian cycle is also called the "secretory phase" because in this phase the secretory activity of the endometrial glands is increased. If the fertilisation of the ovum and subsequent implantation of the zygote does not occur, the simultaneously rising levels of estrogen and progesterone (secreted by corpus luteum) inhibit GnRH and LH release. When LH levels decline, the corpus luteum degenerates and becomes corpus albicans (white body). After degeneration of corpus luteum, secretion of estrogen and progesterone declines to initiate another menstrual cycle. The stratum functionalis portion of the uterine endometrium becomes detached and is discharged along with small amounts of blood through vagina during menstruation. Side by side, the decreasing levels of estrogen and progesterone during menstruation period provide a positive feedback for the release of GnRH and subsequently of FSH for the start of the next follicular phase of the ovarian cycle. A summary of all such hormonal interactions with correlation of ovarian and uterine cycles is presented in Figure 43.2.

Implantation

About 6 days after fertilisation, implantation takes place. At this time the endometrium is in its secretory phase. During the first 3 to 4 months of pregnancy, the corpus luteum is maintained to continue the secretion of estrogen and progesterone until placenta takes over the charge of hormone-producing functions. During this interval chorion starts producing human chorionic gonadotropin (hCG), which mimics LH action and stimulates continued production of estrogen and progesterone from the corpus luteum. This is necessary for the continued attachment of the embryo and the foetus to the lining of the uterus. The presence of hCG is therefore an indication of pregnancy. The chorion later develops into the placenta by the 3rd month of pregnancy. It is formed by the chorion of the embryo and a portion of endometrium of the mother. Thus from 3rd to 9th month the placenta supplies the levels of estrogen and progesterone needed to maintain the pregnancy and to develop and prepare the mammary glands for lactation. The placental hormone production from 3rd to 9th month not only maintains pregnancy but takes over management of the mother's body in preparation for parturition (birth) and lactation. The hCG levels then decrease sharply over the 4th and 5th month and finally levels off until childbirth. After the delivery, estrogens and progesterone in blood decrease to normal levels.

Relaxin is a hormone produced by the placenta and corpus luteum. Its physiological role is to relax pubic symphysis and to help dilate the uterine cervix toward the end of pregnancy. Both these actions assist in delivery. ***Inhibin*** is a hormone produced by ovaries (corpus luteum) and testes. It is also secreted by human placenta at term. Its role is to inhibit secretion of FSH (once follicular phase is over) and to regulate the secretion of hCG from the chorion. The other physiological functions of estrogen and progesterone are summarised in Tables 43.1 and 43.2 respectively.

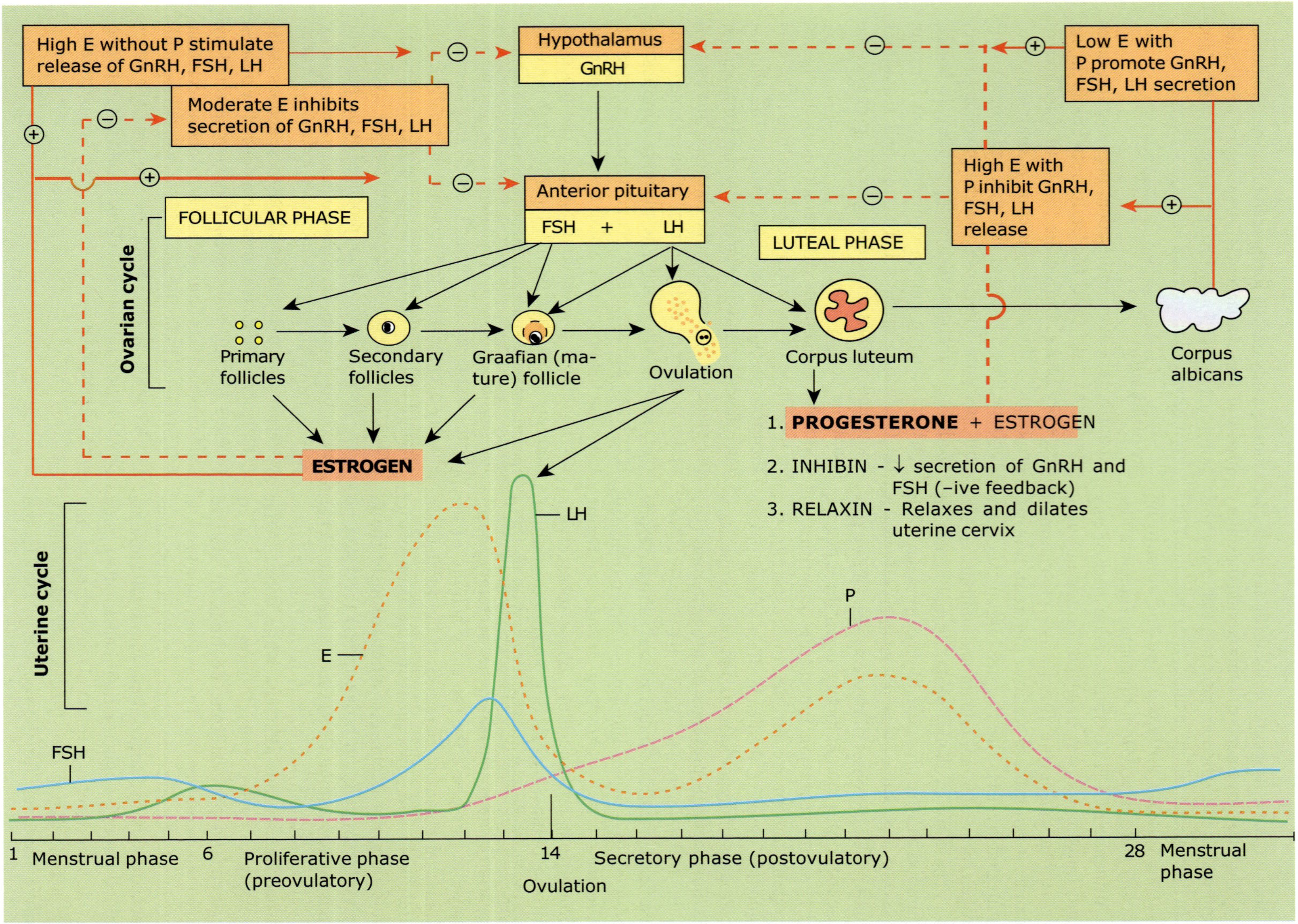

Fig 43.2 Correlation of Ovarian and Uterine Cycles With Hormonal Secretions (*Key:* E—Estrogen; P—Progesterone)

Table 43.1 Physiological Effects of Estrogens

System affected	Effects observed
1. **Female reproductive system**	
a) Fallopian tubes, uterus and vagina	Pubertal growth and development. Thickening and cornification of vaginal epithelium
b) Mammary glands	Proliferation of ducts and stroma. Pubertal growth
c) Uterine endometrium	Proliferation
d) Cervix	Watery secretion to facilitate sperm penetration
2. **Central Nervous System**	
a) Libido	Role not established
b) FSH/LH secretion	Feedback control (see text)
3. **Chemoreceptor trigger zone**	Nausea-vomiting
4. **Blood**	
a) Coagulation factors	Decreased antithrombin III, increased circulating levels of factors II, VII, IX and X; thromboembolic predisposition
b) Lipid profile	Increase in HDL-C, decrease in LDL-C, increase in triglycerides
5. **Metabolic effects**	
a) General	Anabolic effects
b) Carbohydrate metabolism	Weak diabetogenic action, glucose intolerance
c) Fluids	Sodium and water retention (increased angiotensinogen synthesis in liver)
d) Bones	Maintain bone mass and decrease in bone resorption by antagonising the osteoclastogenic effects of parathyroid hormone and interleukin-6
6. **Other effects**	
a) Axillary, pubic hair, fat and skin	Growth of hair as per female pattern, distribution of fat as per female contours; pigmentation particularly on nipples and on genital organs
b) Gall bladder	Gall bladder stones, cholestatic jaundice (increased cholestrol excretion in bile)
c) Liver	Increased circulating levels of proteins: sex hormone binding globulin, thyroxine binding globulin, transcortin and transferrin etc. Hepatic adenoma on prolonged use

Table 43.2 Physiological Effects of Progesterone

System affected	Effects observed
1. Reproductive system	
a) Fallopian tubes, uterus and vagina	Growth and development. Inhibition of uterine contraction during pregnancy and of immunological rejection of the foetus
b) Uterine endometrium	Induction of secretory phase in the estrogen-primed endometrium
c) Mammary glands	Development of alveo-lobular secretory system of breast for lactation
d) Cervix	Viscous, scanty mucus secretion as barrier to sperm penetration
2. Central nervous system	
a) FSH/LH secretion	Feedback control (see text)
b) Libido	Role not established
c) Body temperature	Thermogenic
d) Mood	Depressant effects
3. Metabolic effects	
a) Carbohydrate metabolism	Increases basal insulin levels and insulin response to glucose
b) Fat deposition	Increased. Appetite increased
c) Lipid profile	Decrease in HDL-C and increase in LDL-C levels
d) Respiration	Stimulation
e) General	Catabolic actions

ESTROGENS: PHARMACOKINETICS

Natural estrogens are orally inactive due to first-pass effect. Synthetic ones are orally active. The hepatic side effects of estrogens can be minimised by routes that avoid first-pass exposure, i.e., vaginal, transdermal or by injection. Estradiol is converted by the liver and other tissues to weaker estrogens, *viz.*, estrone and estriol. Their 2-hydroxy derivatives and the conjugated metabolites are then excreted through bile. The conjugated metabolites are hydrolysed in the intestine to active estrogens and reabsorbed. The resulting enterohepatic circulation of the orally administered estrogens therefore exhibit high ratio of hepatic to peripheral effects. Their hepatic effects are thought to be responsible for some undesirable side effects such as thromboembolic disorders and hepatic adenomas on prolonged use.

ESTROGEN PREPARATIONS

1. **Natural Steroidal Estrogen**
   - ESTRADIOL benzoate/cypionate/enanthate/valarate; available as I.M. injection/I.M. depot injection/transdermal patch/vaginal cream; ESTRONE and ESTRIOL (weaker estrogens).
2. **Synthetic Steroidal Estrogens**
   - ETHINYL ESTRADIOL (orally active); MESTRANOL (prodrug for ethinyl estradiol); QUINESTEROL and TIBOLONE
3. **Synthetic Nonsteroidal Estrogens**
   - DIETHYLSTILBESTEROL (stilboesterol), orally active; DIENESTROL (only topical use as vaginal cream; suspected carcinogenic if used parenterally); CHLOROTRIANISENE and METHALLENESTRIL – Oral, but lesser in use.

4. **Conjugated Estrogens**
   - It is a mixture of 52.5–61.5% of sodium estrone sulfate and 22.5–30.5% of sodium equiline sulfate (a natural estrogen derived from pregnant mare). The total of the two combined estrogens should be 79.5 to 88% of the labelled content of conjugated estrogens.

Equivalent parenteral doses of different commonly used estrogens are: Estradiol 0.1 mg = Ethinylestradiol 0.1 mg = Conjugated estrogens 0.65 mg = Mestranol 0.15 mg = Diethylstilbesterol 10 mg.

ESTROGENS: THERAPEUTIC USES

The chief therapeutic uses of estrogens are as a component of oral contraceptives (covered in the following section) and for hormone replacement therapy in postmenopausal women. In addition, they are used for a variety of other purposes as discussed below:

Postmenopausal Hormone Replacement Therapy

Menopause starts after menstruation has ceased. This is the result of declining ovarian functions. There is no progesterone synthesis in postmenopausal women, while estrogen production is only about 10% of that in premenopausal women. Menopausal symptoms are more severe after oophorectomy than with natural menopause. Hormone replacement therapy (HRT) generally includes the administration of estrogen + progestin combinations. The five common symptoms associated with menopause are osteoporosis, vasomotor disorders (hot flushes), cardiovascular problems, urogenital atrophy and psychological disturbances.

Osteoporosis: Osteoporosis leads to a decrease in bone mass and constitutes the most serious consequence of the menopause. As a result, about 25% of the women, in the age of 70–80 years, may have hip fractures. Conjugated equine estrogens (0.625 mg/day) or a transdermal patch of estradiol serves as a most effective therapy for osteoporosis as it can prevent bone loss and even increases bone density in postmenopausal women. However, it should be noted that estrogens can prevent further bone loss but cannot restore the bone loss which has already occurred. Estrogen alone replacement therapy (ERT) in a woman with intact uterus carries a risk of endometrial cancer, but it is not a concern in a woman who had undergone hysterectomy. Alternatively, estrogens should be given in cyclic manner followed by 7 to 10 days of treatment with progestins (norethindrone acetate) alone to control the endometrial proliferation. Alternatives to HRT for osteoporosis include *raloxifene,* a selective estrogen receptor modulator (SERM), which is specifically approved for the prevention and treatment of osteoporosis (see below). Other alternatives are discussed in Ch. 46.

Vasomotor Symptoms: Vasomotor symptoms (hot flushes) are common, affecting 70 to 80% of postmenopausal women. These symptoms appear because of the release of LH in absence of estrogen, the levels of which have declined. Short-term *conjugated equine estrogen therapy* (2–3 years) is recommended for two reasons; first, because short-term therapy is not associated with cancer risk and secondly because the vasomotor symptoms are troublesome only for initial 2–3 years. *Medroxyprogesterone acetate* is also effective in suppressing these symptoms.

Cardiovascular Symptoms/Disease: Protective effects of estrogens on lipid profile are well recognised. The incidence of coronary artery disease is low in premenopausal women, rises after menopause and is reduced after estrogen therapy (transdermal patch of *estradiol*, esterified estrogens like *sodium estrone sulfate* or *conjugated estrogens*). However, the use of HRT for prevention of cardiovascular disease has not been supported by recent trials. It was concluded that the use of estrogen+ progestin combination in postmenopausal women was associated with no change in the incidence of MI despite a 11–12% reduction of LDL-C; rather thromboembolic as well as gall bladder disease and risk of breast cancer were increased.

Urogenital Atrophy: Postmenopausal atrophy of the tissues of distal vagina may result in painful sexual intercourse and frequent genitourinary infection. These symptoms do not improve unless treated with a combination of minimally effective doses of an estrogen and a progestin. Estrogen can be administered orally or topically (as vaginal cream) while progestin is given orally. Topical application is also preferred in cases suffering primarily with vulvitis or senile vaginitis.

Neuroprotective and CNS Effects: Insomnia and fatigue in postmenopausal women are related to low levels of estrogens. HRT with estrogen alone usually lessens these symptoms. There is some evidence that ERT improves cognitive abilities in postmenopausal women suffering from Alzheimer's disease. However, large scale studies are needed to assess the neurological benefits of estrogens. ERT has also been found to prevent the occurrence of migraine headaches in postmenopausal women.

Another popular alternative to HRT is the drug ***tibolone***, which is a synthetic 19-norsteroid derivative with estrogenic, progestogenic and weak androgenic properties. In a dose of 2.5 mg per day it suppresses the menopausal symptoms including osteoporosis. As no endometrial stimulation has been noted it can be used continuously without cyclical progesterone, avoiding withdrawal bleeding (usually seen with combined preparations). *Side effects* include occasional vaginal spotting, weight gain and growth of facial hair. However, it is contraindicated in suspected cases of hormone dependent breast or uterus carcinoma.

ERT in Primary Ovarian Failure

Primary ovarian failure may be due to ovarian dysgenesis or due to hypopituitarism. In both cases treatment is started at the age of 13–14 years with small doses of estrogens in cyclic pattern (ethinyl estradiol 0.01 mg for 3 weeks every month for 4 months and then 0.02 mg for 3 weeks every month for one year). When pubertal and sexual characteristics develop, progesterone is added during the last week of every month to induce regular menstrual bleeding. Androgens (Ch. 44) or growth hormones (Ch. 41) may then be included in the treatment regimen to promote height and normal growth. Menopause is considered as secondary ovarian failure.

Dysfunctional Uterine Bleeding

This unpredictable and painless uterine bleeding is not due to abnormalities of uterus but rather due to chronic anovulatory cycles. This occurs when the normal sequence of follicular and luteal phase, which is maintained by corpus luteum, is disrupted. A progestin given cyclically can stop the episode of prolonged bleeding. Estrogens have only adjuvant role. Recurrences may be prevented by giving cyclic oral contraceptive for 2–3 months.

Dysmenorrhoea

In dysmenorrhoea, menstrual bleeding is frequently associated with discomfort and pain. There is usually an increased prostaglandin synthesis in the endometrium of such patients and hence NSAIDs like flufenamic acid or aspirin are the first line drugs to be used. However, cyclic estrogen therapy (with added progestin) provides benefits to some patients.

Acne and Hirsutism

Acne occurs at puberty due to increased androgen secretion. Cyclic treatment with estrogens (with added progestins) provide relief by suppressing ovarian production of androgens by inhibiting gonadotropin release from the pituitary. Such therapy is not suitable for boys. Even in girls, topical therapy (e.g., antibiotics and tretinoin) is more preferred nowadays. Estrogens also suppress ovarian androgen production by inhibiting LH secretion, which may help in reducing hirsutism but such therapy is rarely used nowadays.

Carcinoma Prostate

It is a testosterone dependent tumour. Use of estrogens for such condition has become outdated. GnRH agonists with or without androgen antagonists or Gn RH antagonists are more preferred because of lesser side effects (Ch. 41).

ESTROGENS: ADVERSE EFFECTS

The major concerns about the use of estrogens are as under (for related discussion see above):

In Males: Gynaecomastia, feminisation and decreased libido, when given to treat carcinoma prostate.

In Females: Breast tenderness, migraine headache, nausea, withdrawal bleeding, amenorrhoea, endometrial hyperplasia, risk of breast cancer and increased incidence of vaginal and cervical adenocarcinoma in female offspring of mother taking synthetic estrogen in first trimester of pregnancy.

In Both Sexes: Gallstones and gall bladder disease, hepatic dysfunction, predisposition to thromboembolic disorders, precipitation of diabetes and fluid retention.

ESTROGENS: CONTRAINDICATIONS

Pregnancy; thromboembolic disorders; diabetes; hepatic failure; estrogen dependent carcinoma of breast; endometrial carcinoma; endometriosis and undiagnosed genital bleeding as it may be mistaken for fibroid bleeding or bleeding from endometrial carcinoma.

ESTROGENS: DRUG INTERACTIONS

1. Most antibiotics reduce the microbial flora of GIT, which retards the enterohepatic circulation of estrogens. Higher doses of estrogens are thus required to maintain the plasma levels.
2. Enzyme inducers like rifampicin, phenytoin, carbamazepine and barbiturates increase their metabolism and decrease their effectiveness.
3. The dose of insulin or oral hypoglycaemic agents have to be increased in presence of estrogens.

SELECTIVE ESTROGEN RECEPTOR MODULATORS (SERMs)

SERMs are nonsteroidal synthetic agents whose agonist or antagonist activities on estrogen receptor (ER) are tissue selective. They produce beneficial estrogenic effects in certain organs/tissues (bone, brain and liver) and prevent certain deleterious estrogenic effects in some organs or tissues (breast and endometrium) by exhibiting antagonistic or no activity on ER. Examples include ***clomiphene, tamoxifen, doloxifen, toremifen, fulvestrant, raloxifene*** and ***ormeloxifen***. Earlier clomiphene and tamoxifen were classified as estrogen antagonists. Later it was realised that their action differs in different tissues: agonists in some while antagonist in others. Hence, all such drugs were later grouped as SERMs.

Clomiphene

Clomiphene is orally active SERM with both agonist and antagonist properties. Its estrogen agonist activities have been demonstrated in other animal species. In humans, it acts as a competitive antagonist of ER in hypothalamus; and thus fails estrogen's negative feedback effects on the release of GnRH. After clomiphene administration, the pulse frequency of GnRH release is enhanced leading to increased FSH and LH secretion. The drug therefore facilitates ovulation and is used to treat infertility due to anovulation. It is of no use in patients with primary ovarian or pituitary failure. Concurrent use of menotropins or hCG improves the success rate. It can also be used to treat male infertility due to oligozoospermia because increased gonadotropin secretions promote testosterone secretion and spermatogenesis. However, success rate is low. It is also used as an adjunct drug along with gonadotropins to improve maturation and harvesting of ova for *in vitro fertilisation*.

Adverse effects include twins or even multiple pregnancy; ovarian enlargement and polycystic ovaries (overstimulation may lead to rupture and internal haemorrhage); hot flushes (due to antagonism of peripheral ER); weight gain; reversible alopecia and vertigo.

Tamoxifen, Doloxifen, Toremifen and Fulvestrant

Tamoxifen acts as potent ER antagonist in breast cells, blood vessels and some peripheral sites but has agonistic actions in uterus, bone, liver and pituitary. Because of its antagonistic action in breast, tamoxifen is the first choice hormonal treatment of breast carcinoma in both pre- and postmenopausal women. Tamoxifen upregulates transforming growth factor-β (TGF-β) (down-regulation of TGF-β has been reported to be associated with progression of malignancy). Tamoxifen also provides improvement in bone density and prevents postmenopausal osteoporosis. This may also be related to upregulation of TGF-β since this cytokine keeps a balance between bone-producing osteoblasts and bone-resorbing osteoclasts. Improvement in lipid profile and thus lowering of coronary artery disease risk is another advantage of tamoxifen therapy (ER agonist actions on liver). However, its ER agonist effects on uterus and blood coagulation factors increase the risk of endometrial cancer and deep vein thrombosis. *Adverse effects* include hot flushes, vomiting, menstrual irregularities, anorexia, mild leucopenia and mild ocular effects. ***Doloxifen*** and ***toremifene*** are structurally related to tamoxifen with similar pharmacological properties, indications and toxicity.

Fulvestrant, although a pure antiestrogen, is paradoxically a Selective Estrogen Receptor Down-regulator (ESRD). It has no agonist action on ER in human beings either. It down-regulates ERs by promoting degradation of ERs by proteasomal enzymes. It is used to treat tamoxifen-resistant breast cancer.

Raloxifene and Ormeloxifen

Raloxifene has antiestrogenic effects on breast and endometrial tissue but estrogenic effects on bone, lipid metabolism and blood coagulation. It produces dose-dependent increase in osteoblast activity and decrease in osteoclast action and hence has been marketed for treatment and prevention of osteoporosis in postmenopausal women. In these women, raloxifene provides and maintains a favourable lipid profile also. Its use reduces the risk of breast cancer by 65–70% in ER positive breast cancer. It does not stimulate endometrial proliferation and hence there is no risk for endometrial carcinoma either. *Adverse effects* include hot flushes, leg cramps, increased risk for deep vein thrombosis and pulmonary embolism (estrogenic effects on blood coagulation).

Ormeloxifen (centchroman) is also a SERM which is estrogen antagonist in breast and uterus. It has been approved for treatment of dysfunctional uterine bleeding associated with anovular cycles occurring near menopause. Since it has antiestrogenic as well as antiprogestogenic actions, it is used as nonhormonal oral contraceptive also (see following section). It is being investigated for the management of osteoporosis, breast and endometrial carcinoma. *Side effects* are mild such as nausea, headache, fluid retention and weight gain.

Bazedoxifene and Conjugated Estrogen

Bazedoxifeneis a Selective Estrogen Receptor Modulator (SERM) having estrogen-like effects on bone (increase bone density) and lipids (decrease LDL) while antiestrogenic in uterus and breast (reduces risk of endometrial hyperplasia). It is combined with conjugated estrogen. It is used for vasomotor symptoms associated with menopause. *Adverse effects*: Nausea, diarrhoea, dyspepsia and muscle spasm.

ESTROGEN SYNTHESIS INHIBITORS

The estrogen synthesis inhibitors, in therapeutic use, involve the inhibition of aromatase, an enzyme responsible for converting testosterone to estradiol. Examples of aromatase inhibitors include the first generation drug ***aminoglutethimide*** (Ch. 42) and the new generation drugs such as ***anastrozole, letrozole, fadrozole*** and ***vorozole,*** which are nonsteroidal agents (Ch. 67). ***Formestane*** and ***exemestane*** are potent, selective steroidal agents that are aromatase inactivators. All of them have been used for "estrogen receptor expressing breast carcinoma", resistant to tamoxifen. These have also been successfully employed as adjuncts to androgen antagonists (Ch. 44) in the treatment of precocious (premature) puberty and as primary treatment of excessive aromatase syndrome. Common *side effects* include hot flushes, joint pain and thromboembolic disease (delayed toxicity).

PROGESTINS: PHARMACOKINETICS

Progesterone is not effective if administered orally because of considerable first-pass metabolism in liver. Its plasma half-life is very short (5–7 min). It is metabolised to pregnanediol and is excreted through urine as pregnanediol glucuronide. However, a high dose oral micronised progesterone formulation has been developed which provides progestational effect for adequate duration. Most of the synthetic progestins are orally active and are metabolised slowly. Though their plasma half-life ranges from 10–24 hrs, the duration of their effect persists for 1–3 days.

PROGESTIN PREPARATIONS

These are not a uniform group of compounds. All of them differ from progesterone in chemical and pharmacological aspects. Yet these can be broadly classified as under:

I. **Progesterone Analogues** (C-21 steroid structure) ***Hydroxyprogesterone Acetate*** (I.M.); ***Medroxyprogesterone Acetate*** (I.M., Oral); ***Megestrol Acetate*** (Oral); ***Dihydrogesterone*** (Oral) and ***Nomegestrol*** (Oral); ***Micronised Natural Progesterone***.

These are pure progestins with weak androgenic and antiovulatory activity. These are used as adjuvants to estrogens for **(a)** HRT in postmenopausal women, **(b)** threatened abortion and **(c)** endometriosis, i.e., for selective progestational effects. ***Nomegestrol*** is also a 17-norprogesterone derivative. It has anti-androgenic property with weak antiovulatory effects. However, it has stronger effects on endometrium and is used to treat endometriosis.

II. **19-Nortestosterone Derivatives** (C-19 steroid structure)

Norethindrone (*Norethisterone*, oral); ***Norethynodrel*** (oral); ***Lynestrenol*** (***Ethinyl estrenol***, oral); ***Allylestrenol*** (oral); ***Norgestrel*** (oral) and ***Levonorgestrel*** (oral). These are 19-nortestosterone derivatives (Fig. 42.2 and 43.1) and are devoid of 19-CH_3 in testosterone molecule. 19-nortestosterone derivatives have primarily progestogenic activity, with weak estrogenic, weak androgenic activity; but these have potent antiovulatory effects. Hence these are mainly used for contraception in combination with estrogens.

III. **Other 19-Nortestosterone Derivatives**

Desogestrel (oral); ***Norgestimate*** (oral); ***Gestodene*** (oral)

These are very potent pure progestins with no androgenic effects. They exhibit strong anti-ovulatory action. Hence these are used as contraceptives in combination with estrogens. Compared to older 19-nortestosterone derivatives, they do not antagonise the beneficial effects of estrogens on lipid profile and are suitable for women with hyperandrogenemia.

PROGESTINS: THERAPEUTIC USES

- The major use of progestins are for ***HRT*** (discussed above) and for ***hormonal contraception*** (discussed below). For HRT, a progestin lacking androgenic activity is preferred and given in combination with estrogens.
- In addition, these are used to treat ***dysfunctional uterine bleeding*** (see above). Norethindrone 20–40 mg/day promptly stops bleeding. Subsequent cyclic treatment, along with estrogen, regularises and normalises the menstrual flow.
- Progestin therapy for ***endometriosis*** is effective, cheap and generally well tolerated. ***Danazol*** is another effective alternative (Ch. 44). Endometriosis results from the presence of ectopic endometrial cells outside the uterus. These cells continue to respond to estrogen and progesterone but may show subtle differences in estrogen receptors and progesterone receptor function and concentration. Manifestations are dysmenorrhoea, painful pelvic swelling and infertility. The goal of the therapy is to induce estrogen-poor environment to inhibit the proliferation of these ectopic endometrial cells. Continued administration of progestins induces an anovulatory, estrogenic-poor state by suppressing the synthesis of estrogen receptors and by inhibiting gonadotropin release.
- Progestins are palliative in 50–60% cases of ***inoperable endometrial carcinoma*** as they regress metastatic endometrial mass in high doses.
- Progestins alone or in combination with estrogens have been used to treat ***premenstrual tension*** characterised by headache, backache, irritability, fluid retention and breast tenderness a few days before menstruation. Relatively higher doses are required to suppress ovulation. Suppression of ovulation by cyclic treatment with combined estrogen+progesterone is also very effective, as it decreases the release of $PGF_{2\alpha}$ during ovulatory cycle.
- Progestins can also be used ***diagnostically to test for estrogen secretion and for endometrial responsiveness***. If medroxyprogesterone (10 mg/day oral) is given for 5–7 days, it is followed by withdrawal bleeding in amenorrhoeic women

only (when the endometrium had been primed by estrogen). A combination of estrogen+progestin can also be used to test endometrial responsiveness in patients with amenorrhoea.

- Recent reports suggest that progestins can also be used in treating ***premature labour and infertility*** (luteal support in cases of luteal phase dysfunction).

PROGESTINS: ADVERSE EFFECTS

Breast engorgement, rise in body temperature, headache, fluid retention, depression and irritability, acne, weight gain, decreased libido, irregular menstrual cycle and breakthrough bleeding, and increased incidence of thromboembolism. 19-Nortestosterone derivatives lower HDL-C levels and exhibit atherogenicity.

Contraindications include depression and pregnancy. Progestins can cause virilisation of foetus and even congenital abnormalities. ***Drug interactions*** are not that significant except that enzyme inducers like rifampicin, barbiturates, phenytoin, carbamazepine and topiramate tend to decrease the effects of progestins by promoting their liver metabolism.

ANTIPROGESTINS

Mifepristone

It is a synthetic steroid derivative, which competitively binds to peripheral progesterone receptors blocking the effects of progesterone. It is a potent anti-progestin that acts as contra-gestational agent when taken within 50 days of last menses. It causes termination of pregnancy directly, by blocking progesterone support to endometrium leading to endometrial shedding and release of prostaglandins to induce uterine contractions. Mifepristone also sensitises myometrium to prostaglandin action to facilitate menstruation. The conceptus is then detached from the uterine wall and hCG levels decline resulting in luteolysis. Progesterone secretion then decreases and cervix is softened to make conditions favourable for abortion. Mifepristone is orally active. It also has antiandrogenic as well as antiglucocorticoid activity and has been used in the treatment of Cushing's syndrome also (Ch. 42).

The uses of mifepristone are as follows:

1. ***Termination of pregnancy*** *(of up to 50 days)*: Mifepristone (600 mg, orally) followed 36–48 hours later by administering PGE_1 (*misoprostol* 400 mg oral or *gemeprost* 1 mg as intravaginal pessary).

   For midtrimester medical abortion (13–24 weeks): Mifepristone (600 mg oral) followed 36–48 hours later by *gemeprost* (1 mg intravaginally every 3–4 hrs to a maximum of 5 mg). However, success rate in this case is low (25–30%). In the event of failure, surgical termination of pregnancy should be performed. Usually, mifepristone has decreased effectiveness after 7 weeks of pregnancy, because the placenta starts producing enough progesterone to overcome the antiprogestin effects of mifepristone.
2. ***As contraceptive***: Mifepristone (600 mg orally) taken within 72 hours of unprotected coitus interferes with implantation and is a highly effective method of emergency contraception. Similarly, mifepristone (200 mg single dose orally) taken 2 days after the mid cycle every month also prevents conception (see following section).
3. ***For softening of cervix***: Mifepristone (600 mg single oral dose, 36–48 hrs prior to procedure) may also be used for softening and dilatation of cervix prior to surgical termination of pregnancy.
4. ***For induction of labour***: Mifepristone (600 mg daily for 2–3 days) can be used for induction of labour following intrauterine foetal death.
5. It has also been investigated with encouraging results in ***endometriosis, uterine fibroids (leiomyomas), for progesterone dependent brain neoplasm (meningioma)*** and for ***breast cancer.***

Side effects include failed abortion, prolonged bleeding (which stops spontaneously), abdominal cramps, vomiting, diarrhoea and anorexia.

Onapristone is similar to mifepristone but is pure progesterone receptor antagonist. ***Gestinone*** is an antiprogestin which is more efficacious in treating endometriosis. *Side effects*: hirsutism and fluid retention.

SELECTIVE PROGESTERONE RECEPTOR MODULATORS (SPRMs)

The features that distinguish SPRMs from receptor full agonists (such as progesterone) and full antagonists (such as mifepristone and onapristone) is that their action differs in different organs or tissues (agonist activity in tissues where coactivators predominate and antagonist activity where corepressors are in excess—see glucocorticoid mechanism of action in general). This provides selective stimulation or inhibition of progesterone-like action in different tissues and increases the possibility of dissociation of desirable therapeutic effects and undesirable side effects of progesterone derivatives. Examples include: ***Ulipristal acetate, asoprisnil*** and **CDB-4124 (*Proellex*).** Among these, ***Ulipristal*** has been approved and marketed for emergency contraception (see below). ***Proellex*** **(CDB -4124)** is under clinical trials to treat uterine leiomyoma, endometriosis, fibroid tumours and breast cancer. ***Asoprisnil*** is under investigation for treating uterine leiomyoma. While CDB 4124 and asoprisnil were found effective for the treatment of uterine fibroids and endometriosis, the undesirable endometrial thickening (a side effect) may limit their use for not more than 3 to 4 months.

CONTRACEPTION

Contraception means interception in the birth process at any stage ranging from ovulation to ovum implantation. An ideal contraceptive agent should not only be safe but provide reversible suppression of fertility.

Contraceptives in current use are:

A. **ORAL CONTRACEPTIVES (OCs)**
   - i) COMBINATION PILLS: Containing a combination of estrogen+progestins in varying amounts or in phased regimens (MONOPHASIC, BIPHASIC or TRIPHASIC).
   - ii) MINI PILLS (PROGESTIN-ONLY PILLS): Containing progesterone preparation alone.
   - iii) POST COITAL (MORNING AFTER) PILLS or Emergency contraceptive pill
   - iv) CENTCHROMAN: Non-hormonal estrogen receptor antagonist.

B. **INJECTABLE CONTRACEPTIVES**
   - i) DEPOT MEDROXYPROGESTERONE ACETATE (DMPA)
   - ii) ESTRADIOL VALARATE + 17-HYDROXYPROGESTERONE CAPROATE
   - iii) ESTRADIOL CYPIONATE + MEDROXYPROGESTERONE ACETATE

C. **RECENT CONTRACEPTIVE METHODS**
   - i) LEVONORGESTREL subcutaneous implant
   - ii) LEVONORGESTREL intrauterine inserts

D. **HORMONAL CONTRACEPTION IN MALES**
   - i) TESTOSTERONE UNDECANOATE
   - ii) TESTOSTERONE UNDECANOATE + DEPOT MEDROXYPROGESTERONE ACETATE (DMPA)
   - iii) GOSSYPOL

Oral Contraceptives (OCs)

Combination Pills

It is the most popular and effective method for contraception with 99–99.5% success rate. These preparations contain judiciously balanced formulation with low doses of estrogens and progestins so that side effects are minimised without affecting contraceptive efficacy. Although most of the formulations are balanced, yet a more estrogenic preparation can be preferred for women having acne and hirsutism while a more progestogenic preparation can be selected for women having a history of heavy menstrual bleeding. The following are some popular combinations:

ESTROGEN		PROGESTIN
1. Ethinyl estradiol (30 μg)	+	Norgestrel (300 μg)
2. Ethinyl estradiol (30 μg)	+	Levonorgestrel (150 μg)
3. Ethinyl estradiol (50 μg)	+	Norgestrel (0.5 mg)
4. Mestranol (50 μg)	+	Norethindrone (1 mg)
5. Ethinyl estradiol (30 μg)	+	Desogestrel (150 μg)

These are called ***"Monophasic Combination Pills"*** as there is no phasic increase or decrease in the estrogen/progestin content during 21 days of pill administration. The first pill is taken on the 5th day after the start of menses. Thereafter, one pill is to be taken each day consecutively for 21 days. Then, next 7 days are "pill free period" and the next course starts again after the 5th day of menses. On repeating this schedule, the cycle becomes anovulatory (due to estrogenic effect) with a regular cyclic menstrual bleeding on withdrawal of the pill (due to progestogenic effect). Most branded preparations provide a packet of 21 tablets only; others provide a packet of 21+7 extra pills, which contain either lactose or some iron preparation. In the latter case the women should be advised to take one pill a day for all through 28 days as numbered on the strip of the tablets. If the woman misses one pill some day, she should take 2 pills next day and then continue one pill a day as usual. If the pills have been missed for 2–3 days or at frequent days, then the course should be stopped, mechanical barriers like condoms, diaphragm or jelly should be used and the next course should start from the 5th day of menses as usual.

Biphasic and ***triphasic pills*** mimic the hormonal changes during the menstrual cycle as physiologically as possible. ***Biphasic pills*** have a fixed dose of estrogen for 21 days but with increasing doses of progesterone during two successive phases, i.e., from the day 1–10 and 11–21. Next 7 days are pill- free days.

For example: Ethinyl estradiol (35 μg) + Norethindrone (0.5 mg). A pack of ten tablets from day 1 to day 10. Then, Ethinyl estradiol (35 μg) + Norethindrone (1 mg). A pack of 11 tablets from day 11 to day 21. These are not marketed in India.

Triphasic pills provide a bit higher dose of estrogen at near midcycle but increasing doses of progesterone for three successive phases, i.e., for days 1 to 6, 7 to 11 and 12–21 days. This is then followed by a gap of 7 days as pill-free period. For example:

Ethinyl estradiol 30 μg + Norgestrel 0.05 mg (6 Tabs from day 1–6)
Ethinyl estradiol 40 μg + Norgestrel 0.075 mg (5 Tabs from day 7 to 11)
Ethinyl estradiol 30 μg + Norgestrel 0.125 mg (10 Tabs from day 12–21)

Mechanism of Action: The combination pills suppress the ovulation by inhibiting the release of FSH and LH (mainly estrogenic effect). High doses of estrogen also inhibit LH surge. The role of progesterone is to ensure withdrawal bleeding after stopping the medication. Combined estrogens + progestins effects, therefore, disrupt the proliferative and secretory phases of endometrium, reducing the chances of nidation of the ovum. Progestogenic effects increase the viscosity of the cervical mucus rendering the environment hostile for sperm penetration. Normal ovulatory cycle is regained within 1–3 months of stopping the OC.

Side Effects: Certain side effects are acceptable; others warrant discontinuation of the OC.

Mild (no need to withdraw OC): These are *estrogenic effects* which include nausea, migraine, breast tenderness, mild oedema, withdrawal bleeding which at times fail to occur (not with biphasic or triphasic pills). *Progestogenic effects* include increase in appetite, weight gain, acne, hirsutism (mild), decrease in libido, increase in body temperature.

Moderate (may warrant discontinuation of OC): *Estrogenic effects* which include vertigo, leg and uterine cramps, precipitation of diabetes. *Progestogenic effects* which include breakthrough (spotting) bleeding (not with biphasic or triphasic pills); monilial vaginitis (urethral dilatation and bacteriuria); amenorrhoea (even after stopping OC).

Serious (needs stoppage of OC): Mainly *estrogenic effects* which include thromboembolism (incidence 3:1000); women with blood group A, B and AB are more prone than those with blood group 'O' probably because those with blood group A, B and AB have genetically low levels of antithrombin III as compared to those with blood group 'O'. Other effects include cholestatic jaundice, cholelithiasis and hepatic adenoma. OCs *with higher progestin contents* carry a risk for MI and cerebrothrombosis (incidence 1.5:1000). Risk for cancer with OCs is controversial (see below).

Contraindications: Pregnancy, as there is risk of congenital limb deformities; genital carcinoma, masculinisation of female while cryptorchism in male offspring. Thromboembolic disorders; hepatic, renal and gall bladder disease; breast carcinoma; undiagnosed vaginal bleeding; diabetes, obesity, hypertension, porphyria and epilepsy (OCs decrease seizure threshold).

Drug Interactions: Enzyme inducers and antibiotics (as discussed above).

Minipills (Progestin-only Pills)

The "progestin-only pills" are given to those cases where estrogens are contraindicated. Pills are prescribed soon after delivery and continued without interruption. However, success rate is lower compared to combination or phasic pills (98.3%). Examples: Norethindrone 350 µg or Norgestrel 75. These are not marketed in India.

Mechanism of Action: Progestins place the endometrium prematurely to the secretory phase and increase the viscosity of cervical mucus making the environment unfavourable to sperm penetration.

Side Effects: These are less effective. Side effects include acne, hirsutism and amenorrhoea. However, if there is amenorrhoea for more than 45 to 60 days, minipills should be stopped and pregnancy test performed to avoid confusion between the side effect of "minipill" or therapeutic failure of OC.

Post-coital "Morning After Pill"

High dose estrogen and/or high dose progestin are quite effective in emergency contraception when given immediately after unprotected coitus (rape or condom rupture). The following four regimens are available:

a) Two tablets of the progestin levonorgestrel (0.75 mg each). The first tablet must be taken as soon as possible (within 48 hrs of the coitus) and the second tablet is taken after 12 hrs. Alternatively, 1.5 mg (as single tab.) can be taken once within 48 hrs of the unprotected coitus. This is more effective (98.75%) and better tolerated than high dose estrogen + progesterone combination (see below).
b) Ethinyl estradiol (50 µg each tablet) + Levonorgestrel (250 µg each tablet). Two such tablets are to be taken within 72 hrs of the unprotected coitus and then next 2 tablets after 12 hours. However, success rate is low (90–91%) and incidence of severe nausea and vomiting is more.
c) Mifepristone 600 mg single dose taken within 72 hrs of unprotected intercourse is an effective method to prevent pregnancy with lesser side effects (see earlier text).
d) ***Ulipristal*** (a SPRM; see above) in a single oral dose of 30 mg is more effective than levonorgestrel in avoiding pregnancy if taken within 120 hrs/5 days) after an un-protected intercourse. However, the drug is embryotoxic in animal studies; hence a pregnancy must be excluded. Common side effects are abdominal pain and menstrual disorder.

If these measures fail and pregnancy occurs, medical termination of pregnancy is advised to avoid teratogenic deformities of the foetus.

Centchroman (Ormeloxifen)

It is a nonsteroidal estrogen antagonist or SERM (see previous text) developed at CDRI India and introduced in the National Family Welfare Programme to be distributed as an oral contraceptive under the brand name "SAHELI". It is available as tablets containing 30 mg of *centchroman* in each tablet. Unlike hormonal OCs which are taken daily for 21 days followed by 7 days of pill-free period, *centchroman* is taken twice in a week for first three months and then once a week subsequently to be continued irrespective of the following menstrual cycles, as long as contraception is desired. The first tablet should be taken on the first day of menstrual cycle (e.g., Sunday). Then, the second tablet should be taken on 4th day of the cycle (i.e., Wednesday). Subsequent tablets are to be taken on every Sunday and Wednesday for first 3 months, followed by once a week on the same day every week, i.e. Sunday or Wednesday as the case may be. The missed tablet should be taken as soon as possible and the normal schedule should then be adhered to. If the dose is missed by 2 to 7 days, the normal dose schedule is maintained, but mechanical barrier contraception (e.g. condoms) are used as preventive measure additionally, till the next menstrual period. If the dose is missed for more than 7 days, reinitiate the biweekly schedule for 3 months and weekly schedule thereafter. Contraceptive effect of centchroman is readily reversible within 6 months and subsequent pregnancy is normal. Newborns present normal milestones and have no congenital abnormalities.

Centchroman is a potent competitive antagonist at peripheral estrogen receptors and suppresses proliferative stage of endometrium. It also accelerates ovum transport, without affecting ovulation. Summarily, it desynchronises the event of ovum transport with endometrial phases of development.

Centchroman does not cause nausea, vomiting, vertigo, weight gain, hypertension and breakthrough bleeding as seen with steroidal OCs. Likewise, unlike hormonal OCs it causes no thrombotic episodes, no risk of cancer and no adverse effects on lipid profile. It does not exhibit androgenic, antiandrogenic or progestational properties; similarly, it does not affect the secretions of pituitary, thyroid or adrenal hormones in its OC doses. Occasionally, the menstrual cycle is likely to be prolonged in about 8% of the users which is of no consequence if tablets have not been missed. However, if it is prolonged for more than 15 days, pregnancy should be ruled out. If pregnancy occurs, the treatment should be discontinued and pregnancy should follow the natural course as there is no risk of teratogenesis with centchroman.

Contraindications for the use of centchroman are: jaundice or hepatic dysfunction, polycystic ovarian disease, cervical hyperplasia, tuberculosis, renal disease or hypersensitivity with centchroman.

Injectable Contraceptives

a) ***Depot medroxyprogesterone acetate (DMPA; Depot Provera)***: It is a longer-acting progesterone derivative to be injected intramuscularly in a dose of 150 mg every third month starting just after parturition or during first five days of menstrual cycle. It is useful in patients where compliance is a problem or in patients having heavy menstrual bleeding or in those for whom estrogens are contraindicated, e.g., those suffering from migraine, thromboembolism, oedema, hypertension or diabetes. *Mode of action* is same as for minipills. *Side effects* include irregular bleeding ending up in amenorrhoea and anovulation. Osteoporosis may occur on prolonged use as Gn suppression may cause low estrogen levels. There may be weight gain and increased risk of breast cancer. If pregnancy occurs, it should be terminated to avoid the risk of congenital deformities.

b) ***Combined estrogen-progestin injectable contraceptives***: **(i)** The most widely used formulation is "*Number-1*" developed in China. This contains ***estradiol valerate*** *5 mg* + ***17-hydroxy progesterone caproate*** *250 mg* to be given I.M. every month. **(ii)** The other combination contains ***estradiol cypionate*** *5 mg* + ***DMPA*** *25 mg* to be given intramuscularly once in 2 months. The advantages of such long-acting injectable contraceptives are that they provide a single defined and predictable bleeding every month and have high contraceptive efficacy. The mechanism of action and side effects resemble combination pills.

Recent Contraceptive Methods

NORPLANTS: It contains a set of 6 capsules each filled with 36 mg of ***levonorgestrel*** (total 216 mg) for subcutaneous implantation on the inside of the upper arm. If kept implanted, one set of 6 tubes remains effective up to 5 years but the contraceptive effects are readily reversible with removal of implants. The mechanism of action and side effects are like that of minipills.

INTRAUTERINE INSERTS: A relatively new intrauterine contraceptive device releases ***levonorgestrel*** at a rate of 20 μg per day into the uterine cavity for a period of 5 years. The progestin preparation acts locally on the endometrium and hence systemic side effects are minimal. The return of fertility is immediate after removal of these progestaserts.

Hormonal Contraception for Men

Oral contraception for men remains elusive, but the efforts in this direction are optimistic. Recent WHO-sponsored clinical trials revealed that initial dose of 1000 mg (I.M.) of ***testosterone undecanoate*** followed by 500 mg maintenance doses after every six weeks produced reversible azoospermia in majority of men and no pregnancy was caused by any of these men in the 6 months efficacy phase of the study. In another study ***DMPA*** was combined with ***testosterone undecanoate***. 97 percent of male volunteers revealed reversible azoospermia within 3 months of initiating the study with minimum side effects. This shows that a suitable hormonal regimen could be developed to induce azoospermia with minimum side effects.

GOSSYPOL: It is an orally effective nonsteroidal drug obtained from cotton seed and used in China. The suggested dose is 20 mg/day for initial 2–3 months followed by 50–60 mg/week as a maintenance dose for *not more* than 2 years at a stretch. It decreases sperm counts and reduces sperm motility drastically within 3 months. It destroys elements of the seminiferous epithelium but does not alter the endocrine function of the testis significantly. Infertility develops after a couple of months but recovery is restored several months after discontinuation. However, recovery is possible if sperm count has not gone too low or the drug has not been continued for over 2 years. Hence at times it is not a safe as a reversible method for contraception. It has got no hormonal or hormonal antagonist activity but its mechanism of action is not clearly defined. *Side effects* include hypokalaemia with muscle weakness and transient paralysis. Diarrhoea and breathlessness may also occur but libido is not affected. It has also been tried as intravaginal spermicidal contraceptive with encouraging results.

Non-contraceptive Health Benefits of Oral Contraceptives

Described below are some pleasant aspects of contraceptive use:

a) The estrogen-progesterone pill is associated with "reduced risk" of functional ovarian cysts, ovarian cancer, endometrial cancer, fibrocystic breast disease and bleeding uterine fibroids.
b) The menses becomes more regular, with reduced blood loss, less premenstrual tension and dysmenorrhoea.
c) There is lower incidence of ectopic pregnancy, endometriosis and pelvic inflammatory disease.
d) Iron deficiency anaemia and rheumatoid arthritis are less common.
e) Combination pills with newer progestins, e.g., with ***desogestrel*** are more safe for women who suffer from weight gain, acne, hirsutism or raised LDL-C because *desogestrel* lacks androgenic side effects. A combined pill of ***estrogen*** with an antiandrogen ***cyproterone acetate*** (Ch. 44) has recently been found useful for treating acne and hirsutism.

CHAPTER 44 Androgens and Drug Treatment of Erectile Dysfunction

COMPETENCY PH1.37

Androgens is a generic term which includes all natural as well as synthetic steroidal drugs having masculinising properties. They possess some anabolic actions also that are manifested as increased protein synthesis, increased bone remodeling and growth and stimulation of bone marrow. But the ratio of their androgenic:anabolic activity differs from compound to compound. The natural androgens are testosterone and 5-α-dihydrotestosterone (DHT). These are secreted primarily by testes and are responsible for development of sex organs and secondary sex characters in a boy at puberty. The testes produce sperms and steroid hormones that regulate male sexual functions. Both processes are under complex feedback control of the hypothalamic-pituitary-testicular axis.

PHYSIOLOGICAL REGULATION OF TESTICULAR FUNCTIONS

The testis consists of two components: (a) clusters of interstitial cells (or Leydig cells) where androgenic steroids are synthesised and (b) a system of seminiferous tubules (or Sertoli cells) for spermatogenesis. Gonadotropin releasing hormone (GnRH) released from hypothalamus regulates the production of gonadotropins—LH (ICSH) and FSH—from pituitary.

LH in turn stimulates Leydig cell functions (i.e., synthesis of testosterone) while FSH controls Sertoli cell's functions and spermatogenesis (Fig. 44.1). Because hypothalamic GnRH is secreted in discrete pulses, the plasma concentration of LH, FSH and testosterone are also secreted in a pulsatile manner that corresponds to the secretions of GnRH. However, in contrast to women, in whom the frequency and amplitude of LH pulses vary (e.g., during LH surge), the frequency of LH pulses, in adult men, is relatively constant.

Testosterone secretion is regulated primarily by pituitary LH and an increase in its concentration causes a negative feedback, i.e., it decreases GnRH pulse frequency and diminishes pituitary release of LH. However, prolonged elevation of plasma LH (as in testicular deficiency) renders the pituitary less sensitive to negative feedback control by testosterone. The physiological plasma level of testosterone in adult male ranges from 3 to 13 μg/L. In females it is 10% of that of males.

Spermatogenesis is dependent on both pituitary FSH and testosterone production by the adjacent Leydig cells. The major site of FSH action is Sertoli cells which regulate germ cell proliferation and maturation in seminiferous tubules. Testosterone appears to be essential for viability and maturation of sperms and acts through testosterone receptors located in seminiferous tubules. The normal adult testes produce >100 million sperms per day. Though the Sertoli cells do not synthesise testosterone they can convert it to estradiol and dihydrotestosterone after it diffuses from the adjacent Leydig cells. The Sertoli cells also produce two gonadal peptides, ***inhibin-B*** and ***activin,*** which regulate FSH release from pituitary by feedback control mechanism. *Inhibin-A and B* are heterodimeric while *activins* are homodimeric proteins. *Inhibin-B* is the major form of inhibin in males, produced by Sertoli cells and has a negative feedback control over FSH release *without affecting LH* release (Fig. 44.1). *Activins* are produced in pituitary as well as in gonads and stimulate (positive feedback) FSH production. It sounds interesting that secretions of FSH are not governed by testosterone as it has been observed that: (a) increased testosterone levels have no effect on plasma FSH concentration and (b) atrophy or damage of seminiferous tubules reduces inhibin-B production and leads to a selective increase in plasma FSH levels irrespective of testosterone and LH levels. This means that inhibin-B and activin, as discussed above, are regulating FSH secretions from the pituitary.

Inhibin, however, does not affect the hypothalamic secretion of GnRH.

STEROIDOGENESIS

The pathways of synthesis of testosterone in the testes are similar to those described earlier for the adrenals (Fig. 42.1) and ovary (Fig. 43.1). Testosterone, a 19-carbon steroid hormone is synthesised from cholesterol primarily in the Leydig cells of testis, but also by adrenal cortex and the theca cells of the ovary following the pathway shown in Figure 43.1.

The mitochondrial oxidation and cleavage of cholesterol side chain by desmolase enzyme results in the production of pregnenolone. This reaction is rate limiting step in the biosynthesis of testosterone. Pregnenolone is then returned to the cytoplasm where it serves as the principal precursor of testosterone.

Further biosynthesis of testosterone from pregnenolone can occur along two distinct pathways (Fig 43.1). One pathway is through 17-α-hydroxy-pregnenolone to dehydroepiandrosterone (DHEA) to androstenedione. In human testes, this pathway is the major pathway used for the biosynthesis of

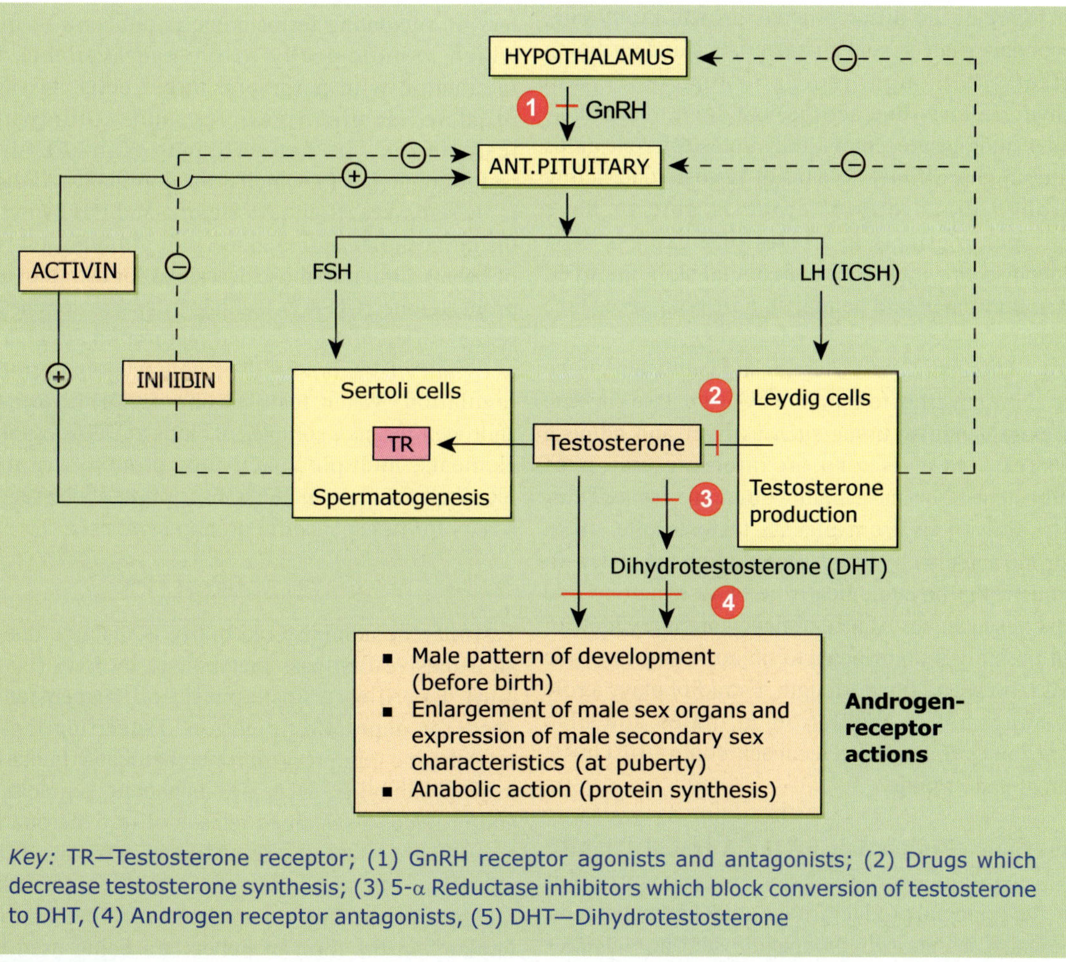

Key: TR—Testosterone receptor; (1) GnRH receptor agonists and antagonists; (2) Drugs which decrease testosterone synthesis; (3) 5-α Reductase inhibitors which block conversion of testosterone to DHT, (4) Androgen receptor antagonists, (5) DHT—Dihydrotestosterone

Fig 44.1 Hormonal Control of Testicular Functions and Inter-relationship of Hypothalamus-Pituitary-Testicular Axis and Sites of Action of Antiandrogens (numbers in **red**).

testosterone. The second pathway is through progesterone to 17-α-hydroxyprogesterone to androstenedione. The microsomal enzyme 17-β-hydroxy steroid dehydrogenase (17-β-HSD), then catalyses the conversion of androstenedione to testosterone.

Peripheral Conversion of Testosterone: Testosterone serves as prohormone for the formation of two other hormones—dihydro-testosterone (DHT) and estradiol. Some effects of testosterone appear to be mediated by testosterone itself, some by dihydrotestosterone and some by estradiol. Testosterone is reduced by 5-α reductase enzyme to dihydrotestosterone (Fig. 43.1), which is responsible for many of the differentiative, growth promoting, secondary male sexual characteristics and virilising effect. Although both testosterone and dihydrotestosterone act through same receptor—called androgen receptor—dihydrotestosterone binds with a higher affinity. As a result, testosterone, acting through dihydrotestosterone is able to have androgenic effects in tissues that express 5-α-reductase enzymes, e.g., non-genital skin, the liver, prostate in men and genital skin of both sexes (see below).

Circulating testosterone and androstenedione are also converted to estradiol by aromatase enzyme in extraglandular tissue such as liver and adipose tissues. There is also an interconversion of androstenedione and estradiol through estrone. Thus, estradiol arises from plasma testosterone, from estrone and also by direct secretion by the testes. In women, the physiological role of testosterone and the consequences of its deficiency are not yet clear, but possibly it contributes to libido, energy, muscle mass, body and bone strength. Estradiol plays a role in bone matrix regulation in males and also contributes to negative feedback control of GnRH and gonadotropins.

Androgen Production by the Adrenal Glands: Although glucocorticoids and mineralocorticoids are the principal products of the adult adrenal glands, they also secrete dehydroepiandrosterone (DHEA), androstenedione and testosterone. The concentration of DHEA and androstenedione in circulation increases between 7 to 10 years of age. The secretion of adrenal androgens declines in the elderly and during severe illness. DHEA and androstenedione, from adrenals, support other androgen-dependent pubertal changes in humans. Recent studies suggest that DHEA may have other CNS and metabolic effects and may prolong the life span in rabbits. In men it seems to improve the quality of life and prevent atherosclerosis.

MECHANISM OF ACTION

Testosterone in circulation is reversibly bound to two major proteins: albumin (40%) and a **s**ex **h**ormone **b**inding gamma **g**lobulin (SHBG; 58%). Thus 2% or less of circulating testosterone is unbound or free, which is biologically active and available for interaction with peripheral target cells. In skin, prostate, seminal vesicles and epididymis, testosterone is converted to 5-α-dihydro-testosterone (DHT), which is the dominant androgen in these tissues. Both testosterone and DHT bind to the intracellular androgen receptor initiating a series of events similar to those described for estradiol and progesterone (Ch. 43) leading to spermatogenesis, sexual differentiation, sexual maturation at puberty, external virilisation and of course gonadotropin regulation. When testosterone or DHT forms a androgen-receptor complex, it binds to DNA response elements; multiple coactivator proteins are then recruited resulting in the transcription of messenger RNAs for tissue specific protein synthesis.

PHARMACOKINETICS

Testosterone administered orally is inactive due to an extensive first-pass metabolism by liver ($t_{1/2}$ 15 min). Esterified testosterone in oil suspension is used for depot IM injection. Esterification of testosterone (e.g., testosterone enanthate) increases its lipid solubility, decreases its hepatic degradation and provides a sustained release of testosterone for a period of 1–2 weeks. Transdermal patches are also available but are reported to cause some skin reaction at the site of application. Testosterone implants in the form of pellets are being used but with limited success. Recently buccal tablets and biodegradable microspheres, containing testosterone, for IM injection have also become available but their acceptability is being tested.

Testosterone, DHEA and androstenedione are metabolised in the liver primarily to 17-ketosteroid metabolites which are inactive. All such metabolites are conjugated to glucuronic acid or sulfuric acid and excreted through urine and bile.

PHYSIOLOGICAL ACTIONS AND PHARMACOLOGICAL EFFECTS

Androgens produce both virilising and protein anabolic actions which are summarised below (mainly of testosterone and DHT):

1. MALE REPRODUCTIVE SYSTEM: Sexual differentiation in foetus; penile and scrotal growth in male child (adult penis does not grow even with high doses of androgens); growth of prostate and seminal vesicles; spermatogenesis and maintenance of sexual functions in men.
2. SECONDARY SEX CHARACTERS: Govern changes that occur at puberty: appearance of pubic, axillary and beard hair; male pattern baldness; growth of larynx and thickening of vocal cords leading to deepening of voice; masculinity.
3. CENTRAL NERVOUS SYSTEM: Feedback control of LH and FSH in conjunction with inhibin-B and activin (refer text); increase in libido; aggressiveness.
4. ANABOLIC ACTIONS: Reduced excretion of nitrogen in urine indicating an increase in protein synthesis and decrease in protein breakdown within the body; Na^+ and water retention; increase in bone density, muscle mass & haeme synthesis.
5. METABOLIC EFFECTS: Increased liver synthesis of clotting factors, triglyceride lipase, α-antitrypsin and haptoglobin; decrease in HDL; accelerated erythropoiesis by increasing erythropoietin production and haemoglobin synthesis.
6. OTHER EFFECTS: *Bones*: Increase in linear skeletal growth and closure of epiphyses (on prolonged use); increase in bone density at puberty but osteoporosis in old age when levels decline. *Skin*: Increase in the activity of sebaceous glands, hence thicker and oilier skin; acne.
7. IN FEMALES: Hirsutism; deepening of voice; frontal baldness; enlargement of clitoris; prominent musculature; suppression of ovulation and irregular menstruation.

THERAPEUTIC USES OF ANDROGENS AND SYNTHETIC ANABOLIC STEROIDS

The primary therapeutic use of androgens is as replacement therapy in testicular deficiency (hypogonadism) but these are also used for other indications and abused for their protein anabolic effects (specially the synthetic anabolic steroids). Drugs with a high ratio of androgenic to anabolic effects are preferred for androgen replacement therapy (e.g., treating hypogonadism) whereas drugs with a reduced androgenic:anabolic ratio are used for treating anaemia and protein loss etc.

1. Replacement Therapy in Hypogonadism

Male Hypogonadism: It can be testicular as occurs in *primary hypogonadism* or it may result from abnormalities of the hypothalamic-pituitary axis as occurs in *secondary hypogonadism*. Primary hypogonadism is associated with elevated levels of LH and FSH while secondary hypogonadism is associated with inappropriately low levels of LH and FSH with little impact of GnRH stimulation. Androgen replacement in these individuals usually restores secondary male sexual characteristics such as libido and potency. However, androgen replacement therapy is successful only if the end organs are sensitive to androgens. Hence, these may be useful in primary or secondary hypogonadism, cryptorchism and in delayed puberty but not in eunuchoid phenotypes or in cases of pseudohermaphroditism. The compounds most effective in bringing about masculinisation are the longer acting IM depot injection of testosterone enanthate or cypionate (Table 44.1).

Androgen replacement therapy has been found to be moderately useful in increasing libido and sexual performance in men who have true testicular failure. However, it is wise to avoid such indiscriminate use of androgens in the elderly age group because of high incidence of prostate carcinoma. DHEA has been claimed to retard aging process, but larger studies are needed to assess the usefulness of this therapy.

Female Hypogonadism: The virilising side effects of androgens have limited their use in women, yet these can be used in certain clinical situations. In prepubertal females with hypopituitarism, in whom all other hormonal deficiencies have been corrected (e.g., estrogens, progesterone, thyroid, adrenal and growth hormone), normal sexual development and growth of body stature are not complete without small amounts of androgen hormone replacement. A combination of methyl testosterone plus diethylstilbesterol has been demonstrated to be very useful in inducing complete secondary sex characters in these females.

- Low doses of androgens have also been used to improve libido in postmenopausal women when combined with estrogen replacement therapy.
- These have been used, in conjunction with estrogens, to reduce breast engorgement during postpartum period.

2. Treatment of Anaemia

Natural androgens stimulate erythrocyte production and earlier were used to treat refractory anaemia such as aplastic anaemia, haemolytic anaemia, sickle cell anaemia or in certain anaemias secondary to endocrine hypofunction or myeloid hypoplasia. However, recombinant erythropoietin has largely replaced the androgens for this purpose.

3. For Osteoporosis

Ca^{2+} ion excretion is sharply reduced by androgens and hence were once being used to treat osteoporosis. Bisphosphonates (Ch. 46), however, have largely replaced androgens for this purpose.

4. As Growth Stimulators

Androgens promote linear growth and if used carefully, children will probably achieve their expected adult height. However, if treatment is too vigorous, epiphyseal closure takes place and further growth ceases after initial benefits. Unfortunately the action of androgens on epiphyseal centers continues for several months even after the discontinuation of therapy which limits their utility for this purpose.

5. Attacks of hereditary angioneurotic oedema

can be prevented with methyltestosterone or stanozolol. They probably act by increasing the synthesis of complement C-1 inhibitor (see danazol).

6. Use as Protein Anabolic Agents

Drugs like ***methandienone, nandrolone, oxymetholone*** and ***stanozolol*** are synthetic 19-nortestosterone derivatives, which possess a higher degree of anabolic activity compared to their inherent androgenic activity. The ratio of androgenic:anabolic activity of testosterone is 1:1; but the anabolic steroids have ratios between 1:3 to 1:10 (Table 44.1). The anabolic steroids were developed with an idea of avoiding virilising side effects of androgens while retaining mainly their anabolic effects; but the efforts have met with only limited success because their anabolic effects are mediated through the same androgenic receptor. The anabolic steroids increase protein synthesis, enhance muscle mass, improve appetite resulting in weight gain and a sense of well being.

- Androgens with anabolic activity can be used in an attempt to recover protein loss after trauma, surgery and in patients of hormone dependent metastatic mammary cancer.
- Testosterone therapy improves weakness and muscle wasting in AIDS patients with low testosterone levels.

ADVERSE EFFECTS

Though relatively safe, their use can lead to significant toxicity if used in inappropriate doses or for inappropriate indications or reasons.

1. Toxicity in Men

a) Androgen administration to normal males inhibits the release of LH and FSH due to negative feedback mechanism. As a result, endogenous testicular production of testosterone is reduced. If the administration is continued, spermatogenesis is hampered causing oligozoospermia and infertility.

Table 44.1 Androgen Preparations with Relative Androgenic: Anabolic Activity

Drug	Route	Dose (for adults)	Androgenic: Anabolic activity
1. Testosterone propionate	IM	10–15 mg on alternate day	1:1
	Buccal	5–20 mg/day	
2. Testosterone enanthate	IM	200 mg fortnightly	1:1
3. Testosterone cypionate	IM	200 mg fortnightly	1:1
4. Methyl testosterone	Oral,	25–50 mg/day	1:1
	Buccal	5–10 mg/day	
5. Mesterolone	Oral	25 mg TDS	1:1
6. Fluoxymesterone	Oral	2–10 mg/day	1:2
7. Methandrostenolone (Methandienone)	Oral	2–5 mg/day	1:3
8. Oxymetholone	Oral	1–2 mg/kg/day for at least 3–6 months	1:3
9. Nandrolone	IM	25–50 mg/week	1:2.5 to 1:4
10. Stanozolol	Oral	2–6 mg/day	1:4 to 1:5
11. Oxandrolone	Oral	2.5–5 mg TDS	1:3 to 1:10

b) Peripheral conversion of testosterone to estrogen can cause gynaecomastia, specially if the patient is having liver disease.

c) In elderly men, androgen can stimulate the growth of prostatic neoplasm.

2. Toxicity in Women

Masculinisation, virilisation, hirsutism, frontal baldness, shrunken breasts and deepening of voice which are quite distressing to women. In addition, clitoral hypertrophy and menstrual irregularities may develop. Anabolic steroids taken by women during pregnancy may cause pseudohermaphroditism in the genetically female foetus.

3. Toxicity in Either Sex

Androgen administration to male or female adults at high dosages results in fluid retention (oedema), erthrocytosis and polycythaemia, cirrhosis of liver, acne, a decrease in HDL-C and an increase in LDL-C. Methyltestosterone and fluoxymesterone can cause cholestatic jaundice and even benign liver tumours. Children receiving vigorous treatment with anabolic steroids can develop precocious puberty with shortening of stature due to closure of epiphyses.

4. Anabolic Steroid Abuse in Sports

Anabolic steroids are most commonly abused by athletes to increase muscle mass, strength and their performance. Such abuse by athletes has attracted worldwide attention. An anabolic steroid abuser usually takes up to 26–30 times the therapeutic dose to improve the competitive performance but at such a dose the adverse effects outweigh the benefits derived, which by themselves are doubtful. Serious unwanted effects include testicular atrophy, sterility and gynaecomastia in males. In women athletes, there is inhibition of ovulation, hirsutism, deepening of voice, frontal alopecia and acne. Increased aggressiveness, psychotic symptoms and increased risk of coronary heart disease have been noted in both sexes. 17-α-Alkyl substituted anabolic steroids (oxymetholone and stanozolol) can produce cholestatic jaundice and worsen lipid profile in both sexes. The anabolic steroids are included in the "Dope Test" performed on athletes before the start of world famous games competition.

CONTRAINDICATIONS

Pregnancy (see above), carcinoma of prostate or breast, liver and kidney dysfunction. These should be used cautiously in patients of hypertension, congestive heart failure, nephrotic syndrome, in lactating mother, in elderly people, and in patients suffering from migraine and diabetes.

SELECTIVE ANDROGEN RECEPTOR MODULATORS (SARMs)

SARMs are, recently developed, novel class of androgen receptor ligands which provide customized response, i.e., selective anabolic effects in muscles or bones without producing androgenic effects on prostate and testes in males. In females these may increase bone mass and libido without causing virilisation. These are claimed not to affect lipid profile adversely and are devoid of hepatotoxicity.

Unfortunately the first generation SARMs, developed till date, are not truly selective as they still possess a ratio of anabolic to androgenic effects up to 10:1. However, these are orally active and are devoid of hepatotoxicity (most anabolic steroids in use are to be injected and cause hepatotoxicity on prolonged use). These are being developed since 2003 and are undergoing clinical trials. Notable among them is ***ostarine*** which is intended mainly for osteoporosis but also for andropause. Another in trials is S-4503 which has shown promising results in treating osteoporosis in women with least risk for virilisation. The commonly used protocol for determining androgenic:anabolic ratio uses the relative weights of ventral prostate (VP) and levator ani (LA) muscle of male rats. The VP weight is an indicator of androgenic effects while LA weight reflects anabolic effects. In early 2000s this procedure was standardized and is known as Hershberger assay.

ANTIANDROGENS (IMPEDED ANDROGENS)

Potential sites of action of antiandrogens include: (1) gonadotrophin suppression, (2) inhibition of testosterone synthesis, (3) inhibition of conversion of testosterone to DHT and (4) androgen receptor blockade (Fig. 44.1). Obviously, the potential uses of antiandrogens include suppression of androgen excess and its effects (such as precocious puberty, hirsutism and acne etc.) as well as treatment of androgen-dependent tumours (such as testicular and prostatic tumours).

GnRH Analogues

GnRH agonists such as ***leuprolide, nafarelin, buserelin, deslorelin*** and ***goserelin*** virtually induce reversible pharmacological oophorectomy or orchiectomy which can be utilised to treat precocious puberty, polycystic ovarian disease and prostatic or breast carcinoma. These can be administered IM, SC or *via* nasal spray. When used continuously (rather than pulsatile) they inhibit LH and FSH release due to down-regulation and desensitisation of GnRH receptors leading to a drastic decline in testosterone levels. The combination of these GnRH agonists with an androgen antagonist *flutamide* (see below) can prevent the initial flare up of the disease symptoms by providing an effective inhibition of androgenic activity. GnRH antagonists such as ***cetrorelix*** and ***ganirelix*** can also be used to treat prostatic carcinoma as they do not cause initial increase in FSH/LH secretion and do not exacerbate the cancer symptoms initially. For details refer Ch. 41.

Androgen Synthesis Inhibitors

Ketoconazole is a broad-spectrum antifungal drug (Ch. 60), which also inhibits biosynthesis of testosterone in both the adrenals and testis, but in high doses (800–1600 mg/day, orally; Ch. 42). This drug is sometimes used for large virilising adrenal tumours that cannot be surgically removed. It can also be used to treat prostatic carcinoma, but the need for higher doses limits its usefulness.

5-α-Reductase Inhibitors

Finasteride is a 5-α-reductase inhibitor that blocks the conversion of testosterone to DHT in target tissues (Fig. 43.1 and 44.1). Since DHT is the main intracellular androgen in the prostate, finasteride (5 mg/day, orally) is effective in suppressing DHT-mediated prostatic tumour growth and in benign prostatic hyperplasia. However, clinical response may take from 6–12 months; hence if there is obstructive urine flow, it can be used concomitantly with α_1-adrenoceptor antagonist such as *terazosin*. Finasteride in lower doses of 1 mg/day orally, is also approved to treat male pattern baldness. After one year therapy, the success rate is about 50%. ***Dutasteride*** is a competitive inhibitor of both types of 5-α-reductase (type I and II). With this inhibitor there is no need to add a α_1-adrenoceptor antagonist because the clinical response comes faster than finasteride. The principal *adverse effects* of *finasteride* and *dutasteride* include decreased libido and decreased volume of ejaculate on prolonged use. Other recently 5-α reductase inhibitors under investigation are ***turosteride, bexlosteride*** and ***izonsteride***.

Androgen Receptor Antagonists

Flutamide is a nonsteroidal androgen receptor antagonist that inhibits testosterone and DHT binding to the adrogen receptor (Fig. 44.1). It is primarily used for the treatment of prostatic carcinoma (250 mg TDS, orally). For maximal clinical effectiveness, it has to be used in combination with GnRH analogue *leuprolide acetate* (to reduce tumour flare-up symptoms). It is also used to treat hirsutism and frontal baldness in women, but its hepatotoxicity on prolonged use limits its utility. In men it causes mild gynaecomastia probably by increasing testicular estrogen production. ***Bicalutamide*** (150 mg/day, orally) and ***nilutamide*** (150 mg/day, orally) are potent orally active androgen receptor antagonists, which can be administered as a single daily dose in patients with metastatic prostate carcinoma. However, in combination with *leuprolide*, the dose of these drugs may be reduced to as low as 50 mg/day, orally.

Cyproterone acetate is a synthetic steroidal derivative, which is also a competitive antagonist at androgen receptor. It also has a marked progestational effect at hypothalamic receptors and thus decreases FSH/LH release due to negative feedback, which further increases its antiandrogenic effects. It can be used to decrease sexual drive in sex maniacs, to prevent precocious puberty in boys, to suppress acne, to antagonise hirsutism and virilism in females and to treat prostatic hyperplasia. It has an orphan drug status and rarely used.

Spironolactone is a competitive inhibitor of aldosterone (Ch. 42) and a potassium-sparing diuretic (Ch. 16). However, it also competes with DHT for the androgen receptors in the target tissues. It is used in a dose of 50–200 mg per day orally, for the treatment of hirsutism in women but rarely. Hyperkalaemia may be watched periodically.

Danazol

It suppresses gonadotropin release from pituitary in both sexes leading to an inhibition of testicular and ovarian functions. It has a mild androgenic, anabolic and progestational activity. It has been used (200 mg/day, orally) for the treatment of endometriosis, fibrocystic disease of the breast and premenstrual tension syndrome. Surprisingly, it is also used to prevent the attacks of hereditary angioneurotic oedema, a disorder characterised by recurrent oedema of skin and larynx. These patients lack the endogenous inhibitor of the activated first component of the complement (C-1; see above). *Danazol* increases serum concentration of this inhibitor protein. Interestingly, it is also used to treat infertility in women as it has been observed that if danazol is withdrawn suddenly after 3–4 months of use, there is rebound fertility in women. It is also used to prevent bleeding episodes in haemophilics as it increases procoagulant factor VIII. *Side effects* include hot flushes, loss of libido, muscle cramps and amenorrhoea (in higher doses). It has virilising action in females. Being teratogenic it should not be used during pregnancy.

DRUG TREATMENT OF ERECTILE DYSFUNCTION

The term Erectile Dysfunction (ED) means an inability of the man to attain and maintain the erection of penis, for sufficient duration, to permit satisfactory sexual intercourse. ED has long been the subject of research both by quacks and medical professionals practising allopathy and herbal medicines. Over the centuries, quacks are engaged in a huge trade of animal parts that unfortunately bear some resemblance to penis (e.g., nose horn of rhinoceros) with a false belief that consuming extracts or ashes of these substances will restore their virility. Substances currently favoured by practitioners of herbal medicine include *ginseng* and *kava*. ED is frequently assumed to be a normal physiological event associated with aging, but that is not entirely true unless the man is above 70 years of age. ED contributes to psychological stress that affects marital and social relationship.

ED can be due to vascular, neurological, hormonal and psychological factors. The process of ED is governed by nitric oxide-cGMP biochemical pathway (see below and Ch. 17 and 20). Most cases of secondary ED are related to arteriosclerosis, hypertension, diabetes and Peyronie's disease of penis. About 25% of ED cases are drug related (Table 44.2). Other risk factors associated with ED include chronic illness, cigarette smoking, heavy alcohol consumption, sedentary life with obesity.

Table 44.2 Drugs Associated With Erectile Dysfunction

Therapeutic class	Drug class/Drug
Antihypertensives	β-Blockers, clonidine, α-methyldopa, thiazide diuretics
Antipsychotics	Phenothiazines, thioxanthenes
Antidepressants	Selective serotonin reuptake inhibitors*, MAO inhibitors
Anxiolytics	Benzodiazepines
Hormones	Antiandrogens, estrogens
Miscellaneous	Alcohol, metoclopramide, opioids, nicotine

*Paradoxically SSRIs are used for the treatment of premature ejaculation (see text).

Physiology of Penile Erection

Penile erection is the result of a complex interaction between CNS, ANS, physical as well as psychological factors. Erection requires relaxation of nonvascular smooth muscle of corpora cavernosa. This relaxation permits inflow of blood, at nearly arterial pressure,
into the sinuses of cavernosa leading to erection.

Nitric oxide (NO) is the principal modulator of penile erection. The physiological erection occurs in response to the release of NO from nonadrenergic-noncholinergic (NANC) nerves (Ch. 10) associated with parasympathetic discharge (S_2–S_4). Thus the parasympathetic innervation as well as NO synthesis and release process should be intact and active for erection to occur. As discussed earlier (Ch. 17 and 20), NO release during sexual stimulation activates guanylate cyclase, resulting in increased levels of cGMP. The latter activates specific protein kinases, reduces cytosolic Ca^{2+} and produces relaxation of smooth muscles by dephosphorylation of myosin light chains (Fig. 20.3). Following an erection or the return to the flaccid state the resultant cGMP is hydrolysed to GMP by phosphodiesterase-5 (PD-5) enzyme. Although other types of phosphodiesterases are also present in the corpus cavernosum, they do not seem to play a significant role in erection.

Individual Drugs

Earlier measures often employed to promote penile rigidity included insertion of penile prosthetic devices or surgery or intracavernosal injection of drugs. Recently, the introduction of ***sildenafil (Viagra)*** and its analogues, which are orally active, transformed the treatment scenario of ED and these are now the drugs of choice for most men suffering from ED.

1. Oral Therapy

Phosphodiesterase-5 Inhibitors

Sildenafil and Congeners

As discussed above, NO activates guanylyl cyclase, which forms cGMP from GTP. cGMP produces smooth muscle relaxation leading to erection. The duration of action of cGMP depends on its degradation by phosphodiesterase-5 (PD-5) enzyme. Sildenafil inhibits PD-5 selectively and thus increases cGMP levels by inhibiting its breakdown (Fig. 44.2). Sildenafil (25–50 mg) is indicated for the treatment of ED in men due to organic or psychogenic causes. At recommended doses, it has no effect in the absence of sexual stimulation. It should be taken approximately one hour prior to the anticipated sexual activity although its beneficial effects last for about four hours after administration. However, it should not be used more than once per day.

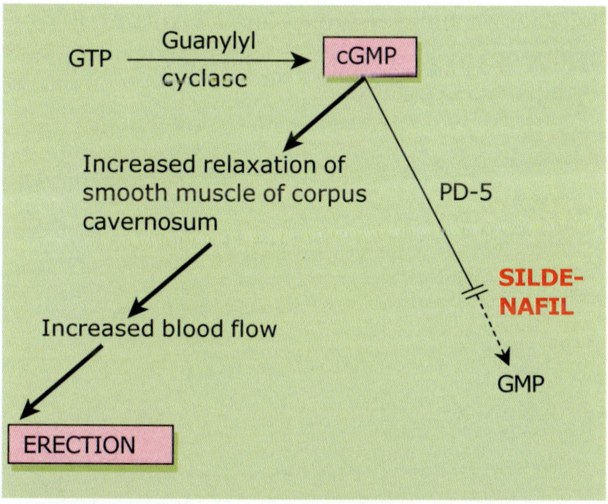

Fig 44.2 Mechanism of Action of Sildenafil. PD-5—Phosphodiesterase-5

Its oral bioavailability is 40%. It is 95% bound to plasma proteins. The major metabolite N-desmethyl sildenafil is about 50% as potent as sildenafil. The major route of its elimination is biliary.

Adverse effects include headache, nasal congestion, flushing and mild decrease in BP. Disturbances in colour vision (loss of blue/green discrimination) are also reported probably because of inhibition of PD-6, which is present in retina and is important in colour vision (contraindicated in patients of retinitis pigmentosa). Because of its ability to potentiate the activity of NO, concurrent use of organic nitrates for angina, hypertension or MI is absolutely contraindicated (unless there has been a gap of at least 6 hrs between their use).

Cytochrome CYP3A4 enzyme inhibitors such as *ketoconazole, itraconazole, cimetidine* and *erythromycin* significantly increase sildenafil plasma concentrations, while enzyme inducers like *carbamazepine* and *rifampicin* significantly decrease its plasma levels. Since other vascular beds are also affected by sildenafil, it has other possible uses also. Pulmonary vasoconstriction in response to hypoxia is almost completely averted by sildenafil. Hence it is therapeutically used to treat *pulmonary hypertension,* which is a serious and poorly treated condition particularly in children (PD-5 is present in the smooth muscle of lungs also).

Two similar, orally active, PD-5 inhibitors, *viz,* ***tadalafil*** (5–20 mg) and ***vardenafil*** (5–20 mg) have also been marketed. However, these have no significant advantage over sildenafil. Fatty meals decrease the oral bioavailability of sildenafil and vardenafil but not of tadalafil. ***Avanafil** (50–100 mg)*: It is recently approved phosphodiesterase-5 inhibitor. It is used in erectile dysfunction.

2. Intracavernosal Injection Therapy

Until the advent of sildenafil, intracavernosal injection therapy was the most useful pharmacological method for treating ED. The major disadvantage of this method is the need for repeated self injection into the penis which is not only painful but causes fibrosis. As a result the long-term drop-out rates are high. However, it is still a valuable option in men unresponsive to or unable to take oral therapy.

Alprostadil

Alprostadil is a PGE_1 analogue (Ch. 25) that can be injected directly into the cavernosa or placed inside the urethra as a minisuppository from which it diffuses into cavernosal tissue. It is useful in most men not responding to sildenafil. Its use is associated with low incidence of priapism and fibrosis. Erection is, however, painful. Triple therapy involving the combination of *alprostadil, papaverine* and *phentolamine* has been reported to be effective and to have a relatively low incidence of side effects. *Ketanserin* (Ch.24) combined with *alprostadil* and given intracavernosally also provides efficacious results.

3. Transcutaneous Application Therapy

A number of studies have also investigated transcutaneous delivery of ***glyceryl trinitrate, papaverine, minoxidil*** or ***alprostadil*** from creams, gels or pastes and their usefulness in ED. However, their clinical usefulness has not been fully established.

4. Herbal Agents

Herbal drugs are claimed to exhibit varying degrees of effectiveness although most of them are associated with anecdotal reports. As a result, these are not widely used among mainstream therapeutic options for ED. Natural sex stimulants of herbal origin include ***Ginseng, Kava*** and ***Ginkgo biloba***. Their use in folk medicine in some countries is likely due to their claimed aphrodisiac effects which are difficult to verify clinically.

5. Drugs for Premature Ejaculation

Dapoxetine

Dapoxetine is a short acting selective serotonin reuptake inhibitor (SSRI) used to treat premature ejaculation in men. It modulates the sympathetic ejaculatory reflexes causing an increase in pudendal motor neuron reflex discharge latency. Oral bioavailability is 42%. Usual oral dose is 30–60 mg, 2 hr prior to sexual act, preferably only once in a day. It is *contraindicated* in cardiac disease like heart failure, ischaemic and valvular heart disease, AV block or sick sinus syndrome. *Adverse effects* include dizziness, headache, nausea, insomnia and decrease in libido (1 in 100 cases). *Drug interactions* include MAOIs and SSRIs (risk of serotonin syndrome), alcohol (risk of syncope), α_1-adrenergic blockers (e.g., doxazosin) or PDE-5 inhibitors (e.g., sildenafil) which may precipitate orthostatic hypotension.

CHAPTER 45

Thyroid and Antithyroid Drugs

COMPETENCY PH1.36

To begin with, we briefly outline the structure, regulation and physiology of thyroid gland and the abnormalities in thyroid functioning. We then proceed to consider the drugs which can be used for thyroid hormone replacement when there is hypothyroidism and the drugs that decrease the thyroid functions when there is hyperthyroidism.

The basic unit of thyroid is a *follicle,* which is a sphere of the epithelial follicular cells surrounding a semifluid material called *colloid* (Fig. 45.1). The follicular cells, under the influence of TSH, secrete two thyroid hormones, thyroxine (T_4) and tri-iodothyronine (T_3), which are iodine-containing amino acid derivatives. The optimal circulating levels of T_3 and T_4 are constantly required for normal body functions. The colloid contains thyroglobulin (TGB) which is a high molecular weight glycoprotein containing about 115 tyrosine residues. Iodination of these tyrosine residues plays an important role in the biosynthesis of T_3 and T_4. A few cells lie embeded between the follicles. These are called *parafollicular cells* or *C (clear)-cells*. They produce calcitonin, a hormone that influences Ca^{2+} homeostasis.

BIOSYNTHETIC PATHWAYS, SECRETION, TRANSPORT AND METABOLISM OF THYROID HORMONE

The thyroid is the only gland in the endocrine system that not only synthesises and releases its secretory products (T_3 and T_4) but stores them in large amounts that are sufficient for nearly 100 days supply. Other hormones are synthesised on demand and released.

Iodide Trapping By Follicular Cells (Step 1)

The thyroid follicular cells trap iodide (I^-) by actively transporting it from the blood into the cytosol

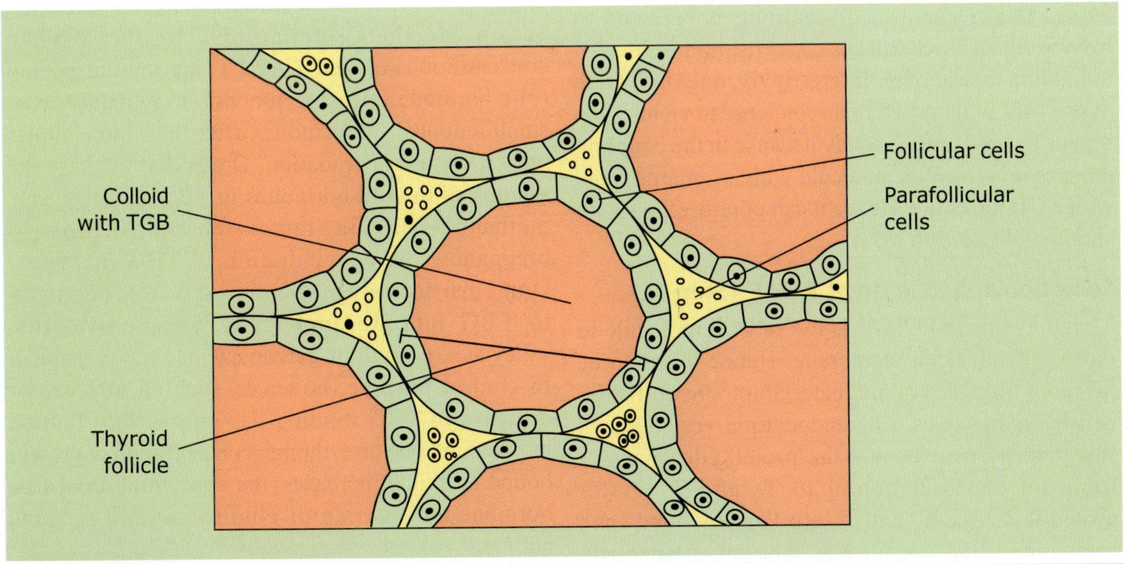

Fig 45.1 Simplified Histology of Thyroid Gland. TGB—Thyroglobulin

(Fig. 45.2). Iodide is taken up by Na^+/I^- symporter (NIS). A minimum of 60 μg of elemental iodine is required each day for thyroid hormone synthesis. The iodide uptake is competitively inhibited by thiocynate and perchlorate ions.

Synthesis of Thyroglobulin (TGB) and Oxidation of Iodides (Step 2)

Negatively charged I^- (from ion trapping) cannot bind to tyrosine of thyroglobulin (TGB; see below step-3). Rather, these anions must first undergo oxidation to iodine ($2I^- \rightarrow I_2$) under the catalytic influence of an enzyme thyroperoxidase. As I^- ions are being oxidised to I_2 they pass through the apical membrane into the colloid.

Iodination of Tyrosine (Step 3)

As soon as iodine is formed, it attaches to tyrosine (Tr) residues of TGB molecules in the colloid. Binding of one iodine at position-3 of the ring yields monoiodotyrosine (MIT or T_1) and a second iodination at position-5 of the ring gives diiodotyrosine (DIT or T_2). This process is also called "organification of iodine".

Coupling of MIT or DIT (Step 4)

Two DIT (T_2) molecules now join to form T_4, while one MIT (T_1) and one DIT (T_2) join to form T_3 (Fig. 45.2). The mechanism of coupling is believed to involve again a peroxidase system similar to that of iodination (see above). Interestingly, only two DITs or one MIT with one DIT can condense to yield TGB-bound T_4 and T_3 respectively because in the coupling process it is the DIT molecule which remains fixed with TGB molecule. Hence it can couple either with another DIT or with MIT.

Secretion and Release of T_3 & T_4 (Step 5)

T_3 and T_4 bound to TGB is too large a molecule to cross follicular cell membrane. Hence it has to be taken up from the colloid material into the follicular cell by endocytosis. The endocytotic vesicles then fuse with lysosomes and the proteolytic enzymes then act on TGB bound to T_3 and T_4. After proteolysis, free T_3 and T_4 are then secreted and transported into the plasma. The simultaneously released MIT and DIT are either recycled or metabolised within the cell. In recycling they undergo deiodination enzymatically and the iodine, thus removed, is then reused.

Transportation of T_3 and T_4 Into Plasma and Their Protein Binding (Step 6)

The T_4 and T_3 that are released from the thyroid gland are strongly but reversible bound to three types of plasma proteins. Thyroxine-binding globulin (TBG) is the major binding protein which binds about 75% of the circulating T_3 and T_4. However, T_4 binds more avidly to this protein than T_3. Thyroxine-binding prealbumin (TBPA) binds approximately 15–20% the hormones while thyroxine-binding albumin (TBA) binds only 12–15% of these hormones. More than 99% of T_3 and T_4 remains protein bound with only very little free T_3 (0.5%) or free T_4 (0.05%) available to enter the cells (Fig. 45.2). Higher protein binding of T_4 contributes for its longer plasma half-life (6–8 days) compared to T_3 (1 day). It is the concentrations of free T_3 and T_4 in the plasma that are regulated by hypothalamic-pituitary-thyroid axis.

The total amount of thyroid hormone bound to plasma proteins is about three times that is secreted and metabolised in 24 hours. Such an extensive protein binding serves three functions: (a) extrathyroidal storage of hormone, (b) a buffering action so that fluctuations in the plasma concentrations of free T_3 and T_4 are minimised and (c) a hormone releasing function to replenish even small amounts of hormones after their intracellular utilisation and degradation. Drugs that increase the binding of thyroid hormones to TBG are estrogens, methadone, heroin, tamoxifen and SERMs. In pregnancy, the concentration of TBG increases. Drugs that decrease the binding of thyroid hormones to TBG include androgens, glucocorticoids, salicylates, phenytoin, carbamazepine and frusemide. In clinical practice, however, such an increase or decrease in TBG binding has only a very limited implication; because, though concentration of protein bound hormone increases, the concentration of free hormone and its rate of elimination still remains normal.

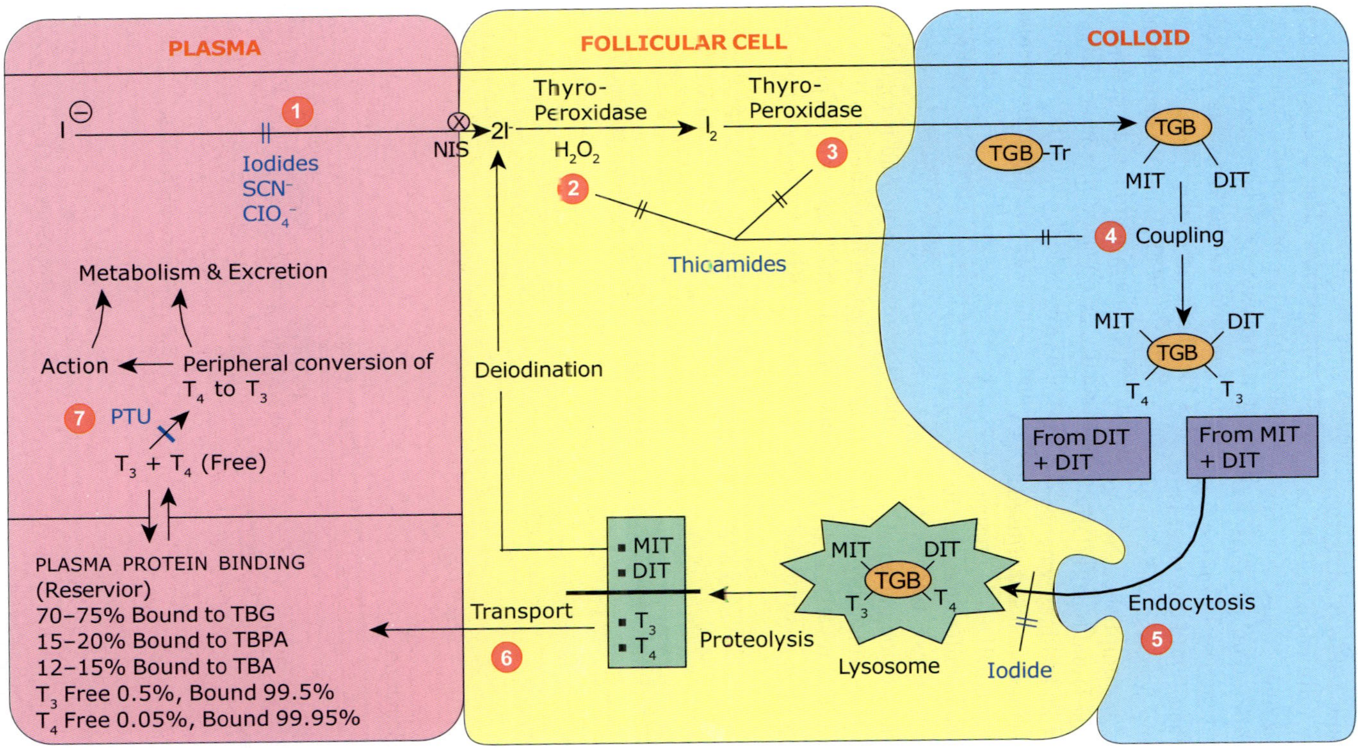

Key: TGB—Thyroglobulin, Tr—Tyrosine residues; TBG—Thyroxine binding globulin; TBPA—Thyroxine binding prealbumin; TBA—Thyroxine binding albumin; PTU—Propylthiouracil; NIS—Na^+/I^- Symporter.

Fig 45.2 Biosynthetic Steps For T_3 and T_4. Steps are shown by encircled numerals (see text). Sites of action of antithyroid drugs have been shown in **blue**.

Peripheral Activation of T_4 to T_3 and Metabolism of Thyroid Hormones (Step 7)

In humans, the major metabolic pathway of thyroid hormones consists of deiodination by three isoforms of 5'-deiodinase enzymes (Fig.45.3). The major pathway for the metabolism of T_4 is its monodeiodination to highly active hormone T_3 (about 5 times more potent than T_4). In this process, there is removal of an iodine from the outer ring (B) of thyroxine (T_4). It is accomplished by 5'-deiodinase enzyme type I (DID-I) and type II (DID-II). DID-I is found in liver and kidney where it generates T_3 which goes into circulation and utilised by most peripheral target tissues. DID-II is present in brain, pituitary, skeletal and cardiac muscle. It supplies intracellular T_3 to these tissues by deiodination of T_4. There is also deiodination of T_4 involving removal of iodine from inner ring (A) to yield an inactive metabolite called reverse T_3 (rT_3) (Fig. 45.3). It is DID-III which is involved in deiodination of inner ring (A) of T_4. DID-III is present in placenta, skin and to some extent in brain. Foetus does not depend on maternal T_3 and T_4 for his/her requirements. The reverse T_3 of the foetus is usually found in the amniotic fluid or in the foetal blood. Its presence is indicative of the fact that the thyroid functions of the foetus are normal (because it is a metabolic product of foetal T_4).

Both T_3 and rT_3 (also T_4) undergo subsequent deiodination, deamination and decarboxylation to yield totally deiodinated thyronine (To). These are excreted as glucuronyl and sulfate conjugates. Part of T_3 and T_4 undergo enterohepatic circulation also.

REGULATION OF THYROID HORMONE SECRETION

T_3 and T_4 synthesis in thyroid is regulated by TSH (Fig. 45.4) released from pituitary. If the circulating levels of free T_3 and T_4 are high, the pituitary reduces its sensitivity to TRH secreted by hypothalamus. This

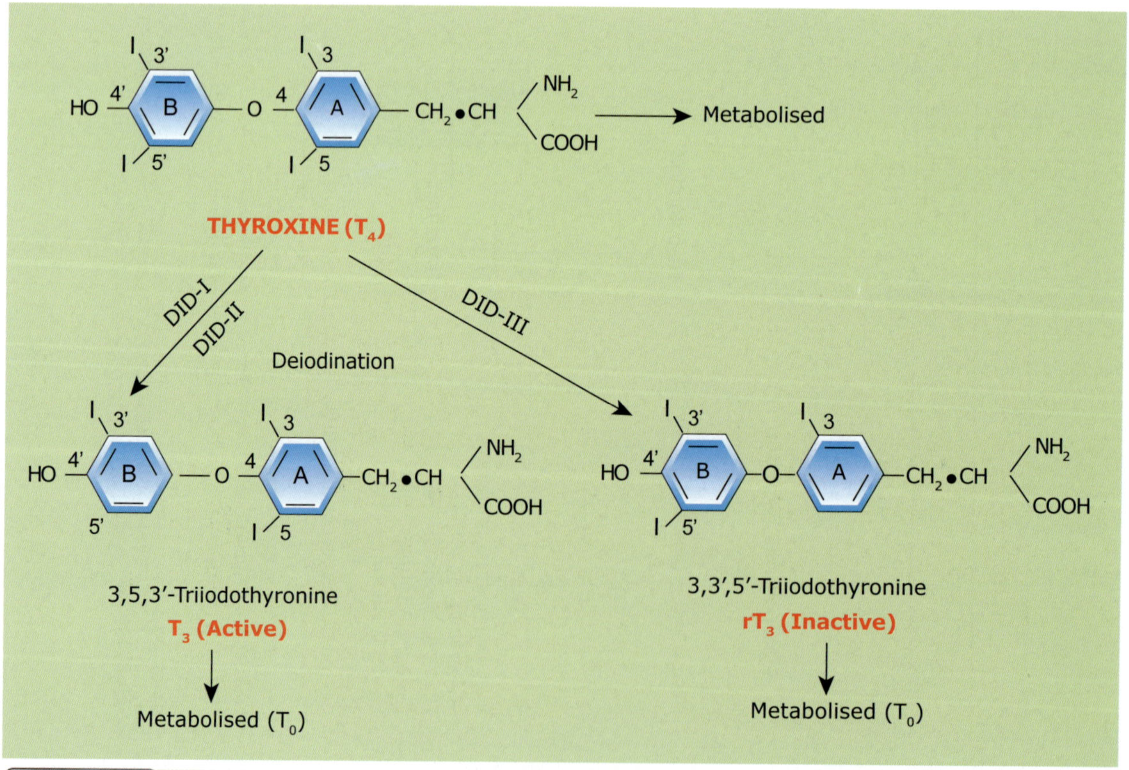

Fig 45.3 Metabolism of Thyroxine (T_4). DID = 5'-deiodinase enzyme

results in decreased synthesis and release of TSH (for details refer Ch. 41), by negative feedback mechanisms. Counter-regulatory substances from the hypothalamus, such as somatostatin and dopamine, also inhibit TSH release. If the circulating levels of free T_3 and T_4 are low, the pituitary becomes more sensitive to TRH, from the hypothalamus. This stimulates TSH secretion with subsequent release of more thyroid hormone. A synthetic tripeptide ***protirelin*** also acts like TRH and stimulates TSH secretion.

Acute psychosis or longer exposure to cold activate TRH release. Severe stress has opposite effects. Physiological amounts of iodide are necessary for thyroid hormone production. Higher amounts have inhibitory effect. TSH by acting on thyroid receptors controls all aspects of thyroid hormone synthesis (Step 1 to 7; Fig. 45.2).

MECHANISM OF ACTION OF THYROID HORMONES

Both T_3 and T_4, in their free form, diffuse across the cell membrane and bind to intracellular thyroid receptor in target tissues. They act by a mechanism rather similar to that of corticoids. After they enter the cell, T_4 is converted to T_3 and consequently T_4 can be regarded as prohormone for T_3. The latter has greater affinity than T_4 for the thyroid receptor. When T_3 is bound, the receptors change conformation, the co-repressor complex is suppressed while a co-activator complex is recruited. This stimulates transcription, resulting in synthesis of proteins that produce various physiological actions of T_3. However, in anterior pituitary, T_3 and T_4 suppress transcription of genes related to the synthesis of TSH (during negative feedback).

PHYSIOLOGICAL ACTIONS OF THYROID HORMONES

Since most body cells have thyroid hormone receptors, T_3 and T_4 exhibit widespread effects throughout the body; **(a) Effects on Metabolism**: T_3 and T_4 ***increase basal metabolic rate (BMR)*** by promoting the consumption of cellular O_2 to produce ATP. Increase in BMR, increases cellular metabolism

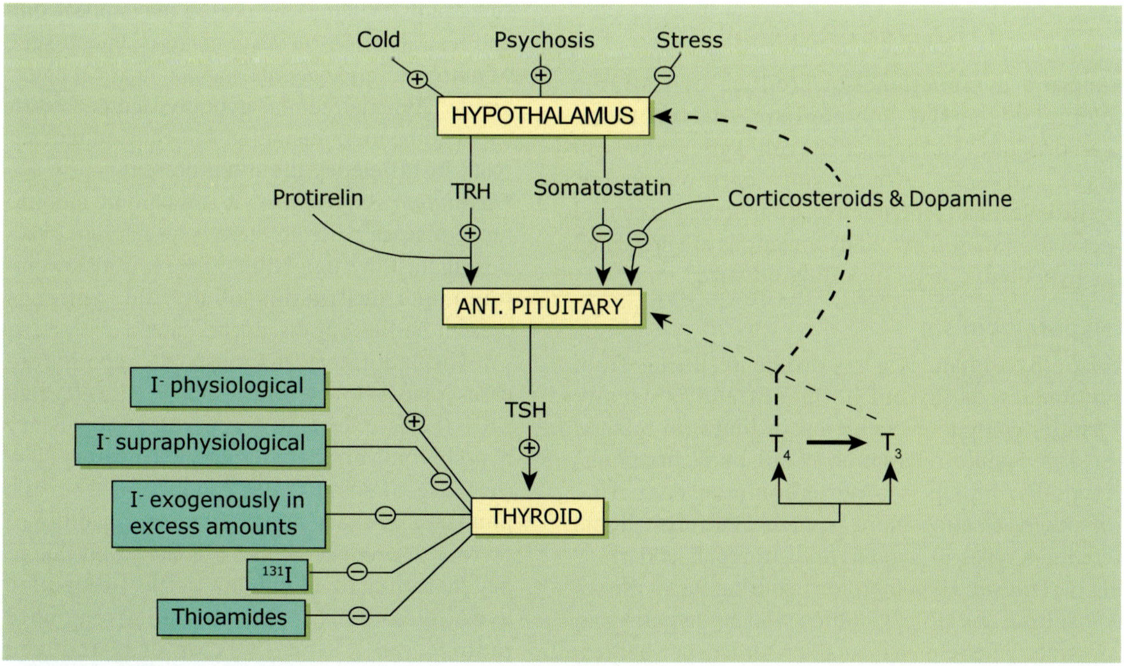

Fig 45.4 Regulation of Thyroid Hormone Secretion

of carbohydrates, proteins and lipids. In the regulation of metabolism, the thyroid hormones stimulate protein synthesis and increase the use of glucose and fatty acids for ATP production. Lipolysis is also increased which enhances cholesterol excretion (reduces blood cholesterol levels).

Thyroid hormones also play an important role in the maintenance of normal body temperature by producing ***calorigenic effects.*** They synthesise and recruit additional Na^+/K^+ ATPase pumps which utilise the ATP (see above) to efflux Na^+ from the cytosol to extracellular fluid and influx K^+ from the extracellular fluid into the cytosol. The utilisation of ATP liberates heat to raise the body temperature. Normal mammals, therefore, can survive in even extreme cold conditions. Thyroid hormones also ***up-regulate β-receptors*** and therefore, enhance the sensitivity of heart to catecholamines; **(b) Growth and Development**: Together with growth hormone and insulin, T_3 and T_4 ***accelerate body growth*** mainly the ***development*** and ***growth of central nervous system*** and ***skeletal system.***Deficiency of these hormones during childhood causes severe mental retardation and stunned bone growth.

THYROID DISORDERS

Thyroid dysfunction can produce undesirable changes in the metabolism of proteins, carbohydrates and lipids at the cellular level that can have adverse effects on cardiovascular, gastrointestinal, reproductive, peripheral and central nervous system. Thyroid dysfunctions are presented as hypothyroid or as hyperthyroid state.

Hypothyroidism

Hypothyroidism is a syndrome resulting from deficiency of thyroid hormones and is usually manifested by a reversible but at times (in infants) an irreversible retardation of all body functions. Hypothyroidism is a more common endocrine disorder affecting more women than men. Some common types of hypothyroidism are as under:

1. ***Cretinism***: Hypothyroidism during foetal life results in *cretinism*. Children who are hypothyroid since birth remain mentally retarded, pot-bellied, yellow-skined dwarfs and are called *cretins*. In cretins, the degree of hypothyroidism is severe but goiter may or may not be present. Cretinism results either due to iodine deficiency or due to the presence of ectopic thyroid or due to the presence of TSH receptor-blocking antibodies. If dectected early it can be prevented by giving oral thyroid hormones.
2. ***Myxoedema***: Hypothyroidism during the adult years produces myxoedema. A hallmark of this disorder is an oedema (accumulation of interstitial fluid rich in proteoglycan contents) that causes the facial tissues to swell and look puffy. Patients of myxoedema have a low BMR, deep hoarse voice, bradycardia, decreased cardiac output (low output cardiac failure), constipation, low body temperature, sensitivity to cold, dry hair including loss of outer third of eyebrows, muscular weakness, general lethargy, decreased libido, infertility, increased triglycerides and LDL-C and a tendency to gain weight. They are usually sensitive to certain drugs like opioids, barbiturates and general anaesthetics. The brain has already reached maturation by this age, so mental functions are not altered. However, in severe myxoedema, the person may appear dull and less alert. *Myxoedema coma* is an end state of untreated myxoedema and is a medical emergency. Hyponatraemia, hypoglycaemia, hypercapnia, impaired mentation and concomitant adrenal insufficiency are often present.
3. ***Hashimoto's thyroiditis***: It is a chronic autoimmune disease wherein there is an immune reaction against thyroglobulin. Since it is a slow autoimmune destruction of thyroid, goiter is present earlier but disappears later.

The laboratory diagnosis of hypothyroid cases, reveals low serum T_3 and T_4 with elevated TSH levels except in the cases of secondary hypothyroidism where serum TSH levels are low (because of insufficient production from the pituitary). Primary hypothyroidism (inability of thyroid to produce T_3 and T_4) can result due to degeneration of glandular tissue (idiopathic hypothyroidism), thyroid ablation with radioactive iodine (^{131}I) or drug-induced hypothyroidism as seen with drugs like lithium, thioamides, iodides and amiodarone etc. Hypothyroidism resulting from thyroidectomy or with ^{131}I is always severe but goiter is absent. Drug-induced hypo-thyroidism is mild but goiter is present.

Management of Hypothyroidism

The management of hypothyroidism can be made by replacement therapy of thyroid hormones, except in cases of drug-induced hypothyroidism where the causative drug should be withheld. Preparations commonly used are as under:

Levothyroxine (T_4) Sodium

The aim of the replacement therapy is to establish euthyroidism with T_3, T_4 and TSH levels remaining in normal range. Since most of T_4 is easily deiodinated to T_3, it is normally unnecessary to use more expensive T_3 preparation. Moreover, excellent oral bioavailability of T_4 with longer plasma half-life, allows for a convenient once-daily administration. Since it also prevents the stimulant effects of TSH on the thyroid gland (negative feedback), it is also useful in the management of simple nonendemic goiter (see below), chronic thyroiditis and TSH-dependent thyroid carcinoma. It is administered initially in a dose of 50–100 µg orally daily, increased by 25–50 µg at 2 weeks interval unless patient does not complain of adverse effects such as palpitation, tremors or sweating or until the serum TSH levels become normal and the patient is euthyroid. For infant (cretinism) the dose is 10–15 µg/kg/day; for a child of 6–12 months 6–8 µg/kg/day; for 1–5 years 5–6 µg/kg/day; and for 6–12 years 3–5 µg/kg/day. The drug is then continued for life with periodic TSH evaluation and subsequent dosage adjustments.

Liothyronine (T_3) Sodium

It is costlier and has a shorter half-life than T_4 and hence not preferred. However, it can be used in special situations such as in severe myxoedema, myxoedema coma, for short-term suppression of TSH in patients undergoing surgery of thyroid cancer and in such cases of 5'-deiodinase deficiency which cannot convert T_4 to T_3.

Management of Other Hypothyroidism Conditions

Myxoedema Coma

Because it is an emergency, ***liothyronine*** (T_3) is preferred over l-thyroxine (T_4). Liothyronine in a loading dose of 100 µg is given I.V. followed by 25 µg every six hourly I.V. daily. Hydrocortisone 100 mg I.V. followed by 25–50 mg 8 hourly may also be given to prevent concomitant adrenal insufficiency. Other supportive measures may also be necessary.

Hypothyroidism During Pregnancy

Because of the elevated maternal TBG during pregnancy (see above), the free serum T_4 levels should be assessed to decide the dose. The daily dose of thyroxine should be sufficient to meet the demands for foetal brain development. Usually 20% higher than usual doses are needed.

Subclinical Hypothyroidism

This condition is associated with a small rise in LDL with slight lowering of HDL, with risk of developing atherosclerosis and coronary artery disease. It is characterised by euthyroid status with raised TSH levels. The treatment can be ignored, unless there are clinical symptoms of hypothyroidism, presence of a goiter and detectable thyroid antibodies or raised LDL.

Endemic Goiter

It occurs in persons living in areas having low levels of I_2 in food and water. In such cases the thyroid gland increases in size to produce and compensate the desired amounts of T_3 and T_4. The condition can be controlled by ensuring adequate iodine intake (in the form of KI) through salt and bread. However, if due to severe iodine deficiency, hypothyroidism has supervened, use of levothyroxine is indicated and withdrawn once euthyroid status is attained and adequate iodine intake has started.

Endemic Cretinism

It occurs due to damage caused to CNS of the foetus *if the mother is living in the iodine deficient area and is having endemic goiter*. Iodine is needed for myelination of CNS neurons of the foetus. Hence in the first trimester, till foetal thyroid gland develops and works independently, the foetus is entirely dependent on maternal T_3 and T_4. To prevent mental retardation of the foetus, because of endemic cretinism, the mother should be treated with levothyroxine as described above under hypothyroidism during pregnancy.

Adverse Effects

These include tachycardia, palpitation, cardiac arrhythmias, tremors, weight loss, headache, diarrhoea, insomnia and heat intolerance. In patients of ischaemic heart disease, rapid correction of hypothyroidism may precipitate angina. These symptoms subside if medication is withheld for couple of days.

Drug Interactions

- Thyroid hormone therapy may increase the requirement of insulin in diabetic patients.
- With thyroid hormone therapy, larger dose of digoxin may be needed for digitalisation.
- During concomitant therapy, the doses of anticoagulants have to be reduced as thyroid hormone increases the metabolism of vitamin K-dependent clotting factors.

Hyperthyroidism

The term *hyperthyroidism* means the disorders resulting from the overproduction of T_3 and T_4 by the thyroid itself, while *thyrotoxicosis* results from ingestion of excessive quantities of thyroid hormones (e.g., while treating hypothyroidism) rather than from overactivity of thyroid gland. However, both terms are being used interchangeably. It is hyperthyroidism which responds to the drug treatment or by radioactive iodine or by surgical ablation of the gland. For treating thyrotoxicosis, the dose of thyroid hormone is to be reduced or withheld for several days. Of the various types of hyperthyroidism, the following are more common:

1. ***Graves Disease***: It is an autoimmune disorder and is the most common type of hyperthyroidism. The patient produces the TSH receptor stimulating antibodies [TSH-R Ab (stim)], also called as thyroid stimulating immunoglobulins (TSI). These antibodies mimic the actions of TSH on the thyroid gland but are not regulated by the normal negative feedback control through the overproduction of T_3 and T_4. As a result the thyroid gland is continually bombarded with TSI to produce T_3 and T_4. In these patients the serum concentration of T_3, T_4 and TSH-R Abs (stim) are elevated while TSH levels are low. The primary sign is an enlargement of thyroid gland (diffused goiter) with exophthalmos (protrusion of eyes). Exophthalmos results due to increased periorbital oedema with retraction of upper eyelid (due to increased tone of its superior palpebral muscle). Newborns have an increased risk of transient thyrotoxicosis, called *neonatal Graves' disease* due to transplacental transfer of TSH-R Abs (stim).
2. ***Toxic Uninodular or Multinodular Goiter***: Autonomous toxic adenomas of thyroid may be single (Plummer's disease) or multiple (toxic multinodular goiter). These adenomas are not associated with infiltrative ophthalmology or dermopathy (pretibial myxoedema). Antithyroid antibodies are usually absent and the test for TSH-R Abs (stim) is negative. Functional autonomy of the nodules develops over time and the disease progresses from nontoxic to toxic phase. Symptoms are usually milder than Graves disease. Continued autonomous growth of this nodular or multinodular adenomas results in excessive secretion of T_4 and T_3 and thyrotoxicosis.
3. ***Subacute Thyroiditis***: It usually results due to viral infection and is characterised by a moderately enlarged and tender thyroid. If the gland is nontender, it is called *silent thyroiditis*. T_3 and T_4 are transiently increased resulting in transient thyrotoxicosis. Hyperthyroidism is then followed by hypothyroidism.

Clinical Manifestations of Hyperthyroidism

The signs and symptoms of hyperthyroidism, *regardless of the cause*, may include: Increased BMR, heat intolerance, tachycardia, increased cardiac output (high output cardiac failure), cardiac arrhythmias, menstrual irregularities, warm moist skin, hyperglycaemia, skeletal muscle weakness with muscle wasting, fine tremors, diarrhoea, weight loss (despite an increased appetite), insomnia, hyperreflexia and nervousness. In addition, exophthalmos and dermopathy (pretibial myxoedema) are characteristic features of Graves' disease, but may not be present in other forms of thyrotoxicosis (see above).

Thyroid Storm

It is an extreme manifestation of thyrotoxicosis. It is invariably fatal and usually occurs in association with Graves disease or with toxic multinodular goiter. Thyroid storm is usually abrupt and occurs in patients whose pre-existing thyrotoxicosis has been treated either incompletely or not at all. This crisis is related to cytokine release and also to acute immunological disturbances precipitated by trauma, surgery, diabetic ketoacidosis and toxaemia of pregnancy. A patient, who has not been rendered euthyroid with antithyroid drugs prior to surgery, is at more risk for having thyroid storm. In such case general anaesthesia *per se* or the stress of the procedure may serve as the precipitating factor. The clinical manifestation of thyroid storm includes severe hypermetabolism with fever, profuse sweating, tachycardia, arrhythmias, diarrhoea, and marked delirium. Pulmonary oedema and high output congestive heart failure may also develop. If the crisis is not managed properly, stupor and coma may supervene followed by death.

Management of Hyperthyroidism

Hyperthyroidism may be treated surgically or pharmacologically. The major drugs used to inhibit production of T_3 and T_4 are thioamides, radioactive iodine (^{131}I) and iodide. The classification of drugs used in the treatment of hyperthyroidism is given below:

A. THIOAMIDE DERIVATIVES
   Propylthiouracil, Carbimazole and Methimazole
B. RADIOACTIVE IODINE
   ^{131}Iodine
C. IODIDES
   Aqueous potassium iodide solution; Lugol's iodine (Collosal iodine solution 0.16%)
D. IODINATED CONTRAST MEDIA
   Oral Ipodate and Ipanoic acid; Diatrizoate (I.V.)

Thioamides

Propylthiouracil, carbimazole and ***methimazole*** are the major drugs belonging to this group. Methimazole (methylthiouracil) is the active metabolite of carbimazole and is about 10 times more potent than propylthiouracil. All of these drugs have a shorter plasma half-life (2–6 hrs), yet it has little influence on the duration of their antithyroid action and on their dosing schedule because all of them get selectively accumulated in the thyroid gland. All the three drugs have a thiocarbamide group in common that is essential for their antithyroid activity. The usual oral dose schedule for ***propylthiouracil*** is 50–150 mg TDS followed by maintenance dose of 25–50 mg BD; ***carbimazole*** 5–15 mg TDS initially followed by maintenance dose of 2.5–10 mg BD and ***methimazole*** 5–15 mg TDS initially followed by maintenance dose of 5–10 mg BD or OD.

Mechanism of Action: These drugs inhibit thyroid hormone production by : **(a)** inhibiting thyroid peroxidase which is required for intrathyroidal oxidation of I^- (Fig. 45.2, step 2), **(b)** by inhibiting the iodination of tyrosine (step 3) and **(c)** by inhibiting the coupling of MIT or DIT to form thyroid hormones (step 4). As a result there is decrease in thyroid hormone production. Since the synthesis rather than release of T_3 and T_4 is affected, their onset of action is slow often requiring 3–4 weeks before the pre-existing glandular stores of T_3 and T_4 are depleted. ***Propylthiouracil*** also inhibits peripheral conversion of T_4 to T_3 (step 7) by inhibiting DID-I enzyme.

Therapeutic Uses: Antithyroid drug therapy is more useful in young patients with small glands and moderate disease. This is the only therapy which leaves the thyroid gland intact but the treatment period lasts for 1–2 years and relapse rate is high. The dose schedules have been described above. These drugs are used for the management of hyperthyroidism, thyrotoxic crisis and for the preparation of patients for surgical subtotal thyroidectomy. Since in hyperthyroidism there is upregulation of β_1 receptors in the myocardium and the sensitivity of the heart to catecholamines increases, a β-blocking drug like propranolol is generally used with these drugs adjunctively. Besides preventing the thyrotoxicosis-induced tachycardia, tremors, sweating and anxiety it has an additional advantage of inhibiting peripheral conversion of T_4 to T_3. However, its use is contraindicated in cases having congestive heart failure, heart block and bronchial asthma. Except for propylthiouracil which is highly protein bound and therefore crosses placenta less readily, carbimazole and methimazole cross the placental barrier more easily. Caution must therefore be employed when using these drugs in pregnancy. Propylthiouracil is not secreted through breast milk either, hence there is no need to avoid breast-feeding.

Adverse Effects: These include pruritic or urticarial rash which is controlled by antihistamines. There may be vasculitis, arthralgia, cholestatic jaundice and lupus-like reaction. The most serious adverse effect is agranulocytosis (incidence 1:500). However, the reaction is reversible as the drug is discontinued. Periodic leukocyte counts, during the therapy, are therefore essential and patient's complaints for sore throat and fever should not be ignored.

Radioactive Iodine

Microcurie amounts (25–100 microcurie tracer doses) of ^{131}I have diagnostic use for evaluating thyroid functions, while 5–15 millicurie of ^{131}I is used for nonsurgical thyroid ablation in the cases of hyperthyroidism. The ^{131}I isotope has a half-life of 8 days and emits γ-rays and β-particles. Given orally, it gets accumulated in the thyroid gland where the β-particles destroy the thyroid parenchyma. Symptoms of hyperthyroidism completely subside within 2–3 months. Hypothyroidism may occur later as a delayed side effect. Although dangers of thyroid carcinoma,with such dose are rare, yet ^{131}I should not be given to children and to pregnant women.

Iodides

It is an oldest remedy for thyroid disorders. Commonly used preparations are Lugol's iodine (collosal iodine 0.16% , oral) or aqueous KI solution. Though iodides are required for thyroid hormone synthesis, higher concentration of iodide limits its own transport (step 1) and also thyroid hormone release (step 5; Fig. 45.2 and 45.4). In addition, high iodide concentration reduces thyroid blood flow to a moderate extent. These effects make KI an ideal agent to **(1)** prepare the patient preoperatively for thyroidectomy because it makes the gland less vascular and more compact and **(2)** treat severe thyrotoxicosis when a rapid decrease in circulating levels of T_3 and T_4 are desired (dose > 6 mg/day). As the thyroid gland escapes from the iodide block (within 4–8 weeks), I^- accumulates within the thyroid gland and hormone synthesis resumes. For this reason iodides alone are not used for treatment of hyperthyroidism. KI is used in combination with propylthiouracil in the management of thyroid storm (see below) to promptly inhibit T_3, T_4 secretion. KI can also protect the thyroid gland from subsequent damage if administered immediately or before any radiation hazard (e.g., accident/radiation leakage in nuclear power plant as occured in Japan) because KI would inhibit the uptake and incorporation of radioactive iodine into thyroglobulin.

Hypersensitivity to iodides is the major adverse effect. Iodism is a chronic iodine toxicity which is reversible upon discontinuance. These include acneiform rash, swollen salivary glands, stomatitis, metallic taste, bleeding disorders and conjunctivitis. Iodides are partly excreted through saliva.

Iodinated Contrast Media

The iodinated radio-contrast media—***oral ipodate*** and ***ipanoic acid*** and I.V. ***diatrizoate***—are also used for the treatment of hyperthyroidism. These are richly iodinated compounds which inhibit 5'-deiodinase (DID-I and DID-II) enzymes and therefore prevent the conversion of T_4 to T_3 in the liver, kidney, pituitary gland and brain. This accounts for the dramatic improvement in both subjective and objective symptoms of hyperthyroidism particularly when they are used as an adjunctive therapy with thioamides. These are fortunately less toxic as iodine is covalently bound in these compounds. Moreover, contrast media used for this purpose, are administered at a lower dose than that used for cholecystography and pyelography. Their toxicity is similar to iodides discussed above. Since the combination of contrast agents with antithyroid drugs develops resistance with time, such combination is reserved for short-term treatment of patients with severe thyrotoxicosis and significant morbidity (e.g., myocardial infarction, or stroke) for rapid control of elevated plasma T_3 concentrations.

Management of Thyroid Storm

When thyroid storm is strongly suspected, vigorous and prompt management is mandatory. It is directed at decreasing both the synthesis and release of thyroid hormones, as well as blocking the increased adrenergic activity along with supportive measures. Hormone synthesis is blocked by giving ***propylthiouracil*** 250 mg orally QID. It is preferred because it also blocks the peripheral conversion of T_4 to T_3. The release of thyroid hormone from the gland is reduced by giving ***collosal iodine*** (saturated KI solution) >6 mg daily orally or radiocontrast media as discussed above (e.g., ***sodium ipodate*** 1 g orally daily). The latter also blocks peripheral conversion of T_4 to T_3. To control the increased sympathetic activity and associated CVS manifestations, ***propranolol*** should be administered in a dose of 40–80 mg orally QID (or 1–2 mg slow I.V.). It also blocks peripheral conversion of T_4 to T_3.

Alternatively, if the patient is having associated complications like asthma or heart failure, ***diltiazem*** may be used in a dose of 90–120 mg orally TDS or QID. ***Hydrocortisone*** (50 mg I.V. QID) may also be added in the treatment regimen to protect the patient against shock. It also blocks conversion of T_4 to T_3.

Supportive measures are also essential to control fever (wet sponging, paracetamol), heart failure and electrolyte disturbances. If these measure fail, *plasmapheresis* can be done to remove large amounts of protein-bound thyroid hormones which promptly lower the circulating T_3 and T_4.

CHAPTER 46 Parathyroid Hormone, Vitamin D, Calcitonin and Drugs Affecting Calcium Balance

COMPETENCY PH1.36

The principal hormone-regulators of bone mineral homeostasis (Ca^{2+} metabolism and bone remodeling) are: ***Parathyroid hormone*** (PTH; a polypeptide), ***Vitamin D*** (a secosteroid), ***Calcitonin*** (CT; a polypeptide) and ***Fibroblast Growth Factor-23*** (FGF-23; a long chain polypeptide). Other hormones such as thyroid hormones, insulin, growth hormones, androgens, estrogens and glucocorticoids also influence Ca^{2+} and PO_4^{3-} homeostasis and bone metabolism, but these are considered as secondary regulators. The three primary target tissues for these regulators are bone, kidney and intestines. Therefore, the maintenance of serum Ca^{2+} levels and bone integrity is the net result of a complex but coordinated interplay between these four regulators and their target tissue effects. Figure 46.1 depicts the interrelationship between the actions of parathyroid hormone (PTH), vitamin D, calcitonin (CT) and fibroblast growth factor-23 (FGF-23) on bone, kidney and intestine; and outlines the events that increase blood calcium levels in response to hypocalcaemia and the events that decrease the blood calcium levels in response to hypercalcaemia.

The level of Ca^{2+} in plasma is regulated principally by PTH and CT (Fig. 46.1). A low plasma Ca^{2+} levels (***hypocalcaemia***) activates PTH release which increases bone resorption by stimulating osteoclasts in bone tissues to release Ca^{2+} and PO_4^{3-} from bone matrix into the blood. PTH also enhances reabsorption of Ca^{2+}, from glomerular filtrate, through renal tubules back into the blood (with associated PO_4^{3-} diuresis). Another effect of PTH on kidney is to promote formation of the hormone *calcitriol* (1,25-dihydroxy cholecalciferol or 1,25-dihydroxy vitamin D_3) which is the active form of vitamin D_3. Calcitriol induces enterocyte differentiation in the intestine, which in turn promotes more absorption of Ca^{2+}. The synthesis of calcitriol is also regulated by PTH. The net result is an increase in the serum Ca^{2+} levels (counteraction of hypocalcaemia) and decrease in serum PO_4^{3-} levels.

Hypocalcaemia may result due to increased Ca^{2+} loss, reduced Ca^{2+} intake, elevated levels of PO_4^{3-} (as one goes up, the other goes down) or because of its altered regulation as occurs in hypoparathyroidism. Hypocalcaemia is characterised by numbness and tingling of the fingers, hyperactive reflexes, muscle cramps, tetany, convulsion and bone fractures.

In contrast, ***hypercalcaemia*** results in CT synthesis and release with concomitant inhibition of PTH secretion. CT decreases blood Ca^{2+} levels by inhibiting osteoclast and stimulating osteoblast activity. In other words, in the presence of CT, osteoblasts remove Ca^{2+} and PO_4^{3-} from the blood and deposit it in bone matrix as calcium phosphate salts (↓ in bone resorption). CT also increases renal excretion of Ca^{2+} and PO_4^{3-}. The net result, therefore, is lowering of serum level of Ca^{2+} and PO_4^{3-} by accelerating their absorption into the bone from the blood (counteraction of hypercalcaemia).

The characteristics of hypercalcaemia include lethargy, weakness, paraesthesia, anorexia, nausea, vomiting, polyuria, itching, pain in bones, depression, confusion and ultimately stupor and coma.

PARATHYROID HORMONE

Biosynthesis, Storage and Release

The four parathyroid glands are located posterior to the thyroid gland. Its principal cells secrete parathyroid hormone. PTH is initially synthesised as a larger molecule—*preproparathyroid hormone*—which is then cleaved to smaller unit called *proparathyroid hormone*. The proPTH polypeptide is then transported into the cisternal space where another proteolytic enzyme cleaves it into PTH (84 amino acids), which is now ready for release from storage granules.

Hypocalcaemia is the principal factor regulating PTH synthesis and release. It is believed to be mediated through activation of adenylate cyclase (present in parathyroid gland) and subsequent increase in the intracellular cAMP. PTH is rapidly metabolised in liver and kidney. Its plasma half-life is very short (2–5 min).

Parathyroid Hormone Related Peptide

Hyperparathyroidism characterised by excess production of PTH is a common cause of hypercalcaemia and usually results from autonomously functioning adenomas or hyperplasia. Hypercalcaemia of malignancy is also common and is usually due to overproduction of parathyroid hormone related peptide (PTHrP) by cancer cells. Both PTH and PTHrP act through the same G-protein coupled PTH/PTHrP receptor. PTHrP has recently been isolated, its structure identified and has been synthesised also (for uses see below).

PTH Actions on Target Tissues

PTH, as discussed above, regulates Ca^{2+} and PO_4^{3-} flux across the cellular membranes in bones, kidney and intestine (see under vit. D_3) resulting in increased serum Ca^{2+} and decreased serum PO_4^{3-}.

Effects on Bones

PTH has multiple effects on bone to influence Ca^{2+} and PO_4^{3-} metabolism (Fig. 46.1). Firstly, PTH increases the activity and number of osteoclasts, i.e., the cells that are responsible for bone resorption. However, this stimulation of osteoclasts is neither a direct effect nor as simple process as it seems. Interestingly, both resorption and bone formation are enhanced by PTH, but the net effects of excess of PTH is to increase bone resorption. Actually, PTH in low to physiological levels and in intermittent doses increases bone formation without stimulating bone resorption. This finding has led to the recent trials of recombinant PTH (rPTH) and of PTHrP (see above) for the treatment of osteoporosis. However, in conditions that result in prolonged hypocalcaemia (e.g., vit. D deficiency or malabsorption syndrome), PTH stimulates release of Ca^{2+} from the bones.

In bones the target cells appear to be the osteoblasts, because the PTH receptors are not expressed on the surface of osteoclasts. PTH acts on PTH receptor present on osteoblasts (bone forming cells) and induces the synthesis of **R**eceptor **A**ctivator of **N**uclear factor for **KB L**igand (RANK-L). The latter interacts with **R**eceptor **A**ctivator of **N**uclear factor-**KB** receptors (RANK receptors) present on osteoclasts and osteoclast precursors to increase both the numbers and activity of osteoclasts. Active osteoclasts then secrete acid and proteolytic enzymes which resorb the bone matrix (Fig. 46.2).

Effects on Kidney

PTH acts directly to increase renal tubular reabsorption of Ca^{2+} and to increase renal tubular excretion of PO_4^{3-} resulting in decreased serum phosphate and increased serum calcium concentrations (Fig. 46.1). PTH in the kidney also stimulates the conversion of 25 (OH) D_3 (calcifediol) into 1,25 $(OH)_2$ D_3 (calcitriol). Intrarenal calcitriol also amplifies PTH-induced Ca^{2+} reabsorption and PO_4^{3-} diuresis.

Effects on Intestine

PTH does not directly affect intestinal calcium absorption but it increases Ca^{2+} and PO_4^{3-} absorption from intestine indirectly through induction of calcitriol synthesis and enhanced absorption from enterocytes.

Other Effects

PTH decreases Ca^{2+} levels in ocular lens which may be responsible for development of cataract in patients of hypoparathyroidism. PTH also decreases Ca^{2+} levels in breast milk and saliva. PTH increases the ability of nephron to reabsorb Mg^{2+} but promotes the excretion of amino acids, sodium bicarbonate and chloride.

Therapeutic Uses

PTH is not used therapeutically. It is short acting and is to be given parenterally. Vitamin D is cheaper and can be given orally (see below). Recently human recombinant PTH (rPTH or ***Teriparatide***) has been synthesised and approved for the treatment of osteoporosis. It is given S.C. in a dose of 20 IU/day cyclically for 12–18 mths to increase the bone density in individuals with a history of fractures, osteopenia and osteoporosis. PTHrP (see above) has also been synthesised and is undergoing clinical trials for use in osteoporosis.

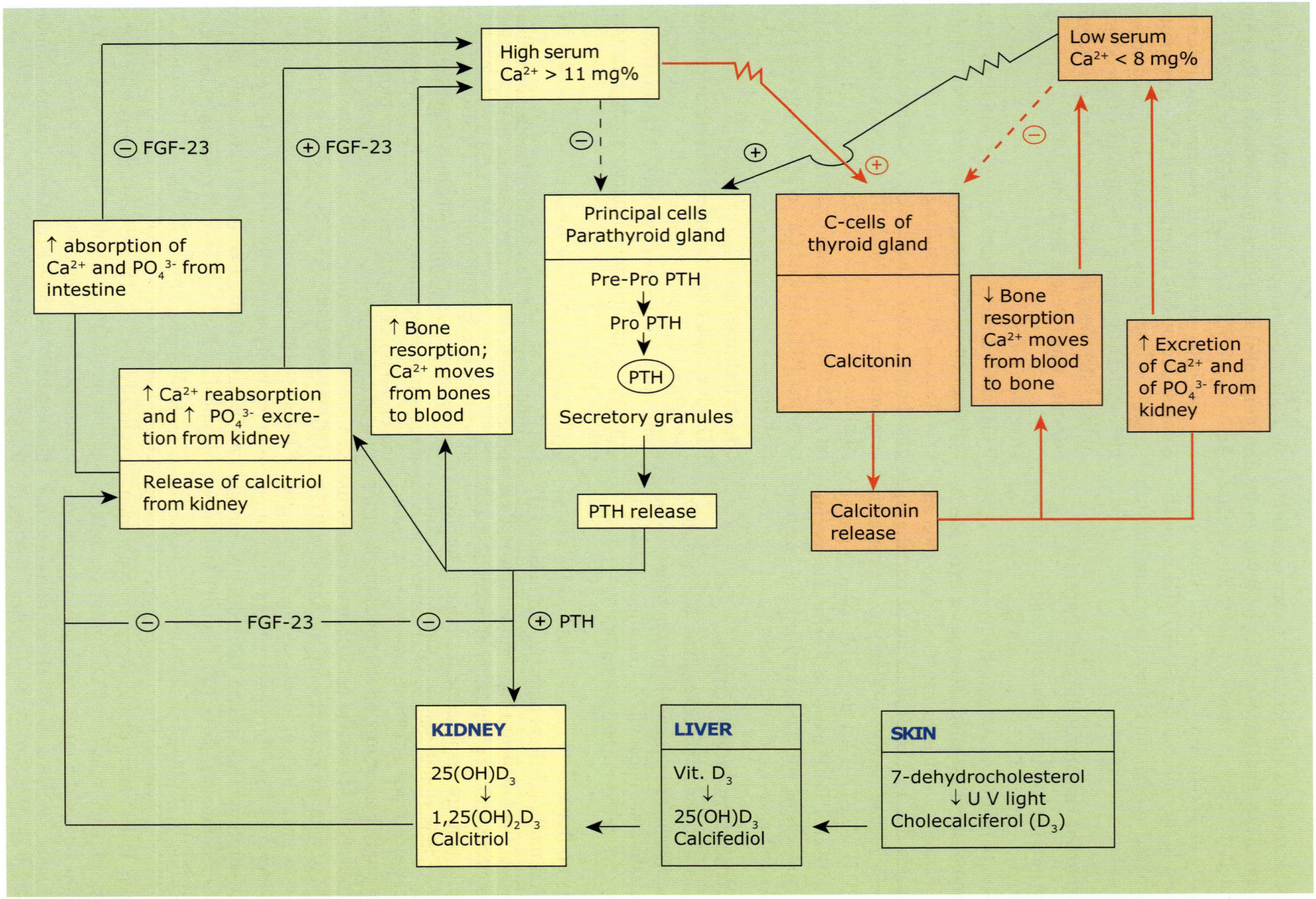

Fig 46.1 Hormonal interactions controlling calcium homeostasis. For abbreviations refer text.

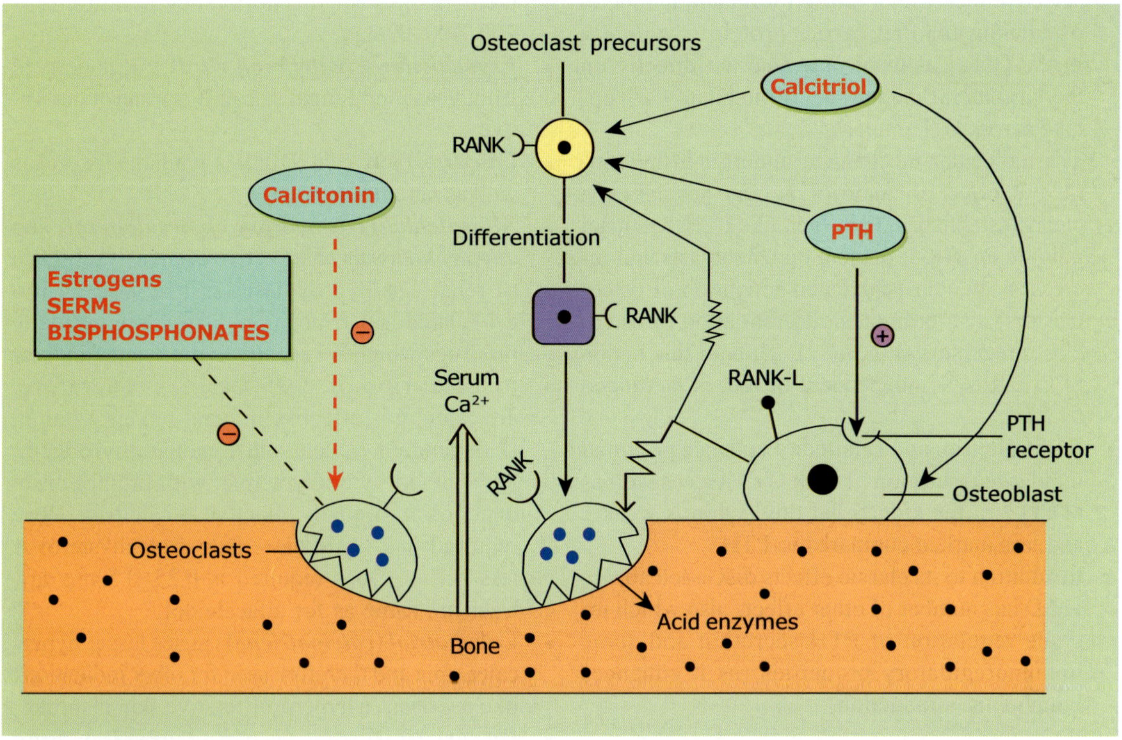

Fig 46.2 Effects of Calcitriol, PTH and Calcitonin on Osteoblast and Osteoclast Activity

VITAMIN D

Vitamin D is the name given to two related substances called ***cholecalciferol*** (vit. D_3) and ***ergocalciferol*** (vit. D_2). Cholecalciferol (D_3) is produced in the skin from 7-dehydrocholesterol by the action of UV light from the sun rays (Fig. 46.1), while ergocalciferol (D_2, also called calciferol) is derived from vegetable source. The primary source of vitamin D_3 in humans is not dietary but is from UV photoconversion to vit. D_3 in skin as stated above. Though cholecalciferol and ergocalciferol differ slightly in their chemical structure, but in humans this difference is of little physiological significance. Ergocalciferol is the form used in commercial vitamin formulations and in dairy products as it can act as substrate for both 25-hydroxylase and α-hydroxylase enzyme system of liver and kidney to form 25 (OH) D_3 and 1,25 $(OH)_2D_3$ respectively. Vitamin D_3 is a prohormone and is not biologically active but is metabolised to active derivatives by liver and kidney. Vitamin D_3 ***(cholecalciferol)*** produced in skin is first hydroxylated in the endoplasmic reticulum of liver to form 25(OH)D_3 ***(calcifediol)*** which is active. This metabolite is further α-hydroxylated by the mitochondrial P-450 in the kidney to the major active metabolite called 1,25$(OH)_2D_3$ ***(calcitriol)***. This conversion step is modulated by PTH. Both calcifediol and calcitriol are available for oral use, while calcitriol can also be used parenterally.

Vitamin D_3 and its active metabolites circulate in plasma tightly bound to a vitamin D binding α-globulin. Liver appears to be the major site of vit. D metabolism. Excess vit. D is stored in fat and adipose tissues.

Vitamin D Actions on Target Tissues

1. Calcitriol appears to act on the intestine and stimulates Ca^{2+} and PO_4^{3-} absorption. Though mechanism is not yet clear, calcitriol binds to its receptor present on gut and leads to a

selective increase in transcription and induction of calcium binding carrier protein (*calbindin*) in the GIT. Calcitriol may also act directly on the basolateral membrane to modulate Ca^{2+} uptake across GIT mucosa.

2. The molecular mechanism underlying the antirachitic effect of calcitriol on bone has not been clearly established. However, like PTH, calcitriol induces RANK-L present on osteoblasts and increases osteoblast-mediated activation of osteoclasts. It also promotes differentiation of osteoclast precursors (Fig. 46.2). Though this action of calcitriol is independent of, but is facilitated by PTH.
3. Both calcitriol and calcifediol enhance proximal tubular reabsorption of both Ca^{2+} ions as well as of PO_4^{3-} in the kidney but this action is weaker and less marked compared to PTH.
4. In addition to its classic effects discussed above, vit. D has number of other effects also which include regulation of PTH secretion and some immunoregulatory properties (as it enhances lymphokine production).

Thus, in contrast to PTH, which raises the serum Ca^{2+} and reduces serum PO_4^{3-} levels, the net effects of vit. D_3 is to raise both of these levels. High levels of Ca^{2+} and PO_4^{3-} reduce the rate of production of calcitriol by the kidney. Calcitriol itself directly inhibits PTH secretion also, independently of its effects on serum Ca^{2+}, by direct action on PTH receptors. These actions provide important negative feedback loops controlling secretions of calcitriol and PTH.

Vitamin D Preparations

Vitamin D comes in many formulations, e.g., in multivitamin preparations, in combination with calcium salts and as vitamin D granules alone. Many dairy products like milk, butter, cheese and oils are also fortified with vitamin D. Various vitamin D preparations are listed below:

- ***Cholecalciferol*** is vit. D_3 derived from UV conversion of 7-dehydrocholesterol in skin. It is available as granules for oral ingestion and as oily solution for I.M. injection. One microgram of cholecalciferol = 40 IU of vit. D. Daily requirement to prevent the deficiency symptoms is 200–400 IU/day.
- ***Ergocalciferol* (*calciferol, vit.* D_2)**: It is derived from yeast and fungal sterol. It is a sterol derivative.
- ***Calcitriol*** (active vit. D_3): It is available for oral as well as parenteral use.
- ***Alfacalcidol* (*1-α-hydroxy cholecalciferol*)** and ***dihydrotachysterol*** are active even in the absence of renal 1-α-hydroxylase (as it is already hydroxylated at 1-α position). These are synthetic prodrugs which are rapidly hydroxylated in liver to calcitriol or $1,25(OH)_2D_3$. Therefore, alfacalcidol is effective in renal rickets, vitamin D dependent rickets and hypoparathyroidism. Alfacalcidol is orally active, with prompt onset of action and equally effective as calcitriol. Dose required is 1–2 μg/day. Dihydrotachysterol is less active. Dose required is 0.25–0.5 mg/day. Uses are same as for alfacalcidol.
- ***Calcipotriol* (*calcipotriene*)** causes lesser hypercalcaemia and therefore used for other indications like psoriasis, a hyperproliferative skin disorder.
- ***Doxercalciferol* (*1-α-hydroxy-*D_2)** and ***paricalcitol*** (*19-nor-1,25-dihydroxy-*D_2) have been recently introduced for treating secondary hyperparathyroidism with chronic renal disease. They can lower plasma PTH levels without significantly raising plasma Ca^{2+} levels.

The last three compounds are calcitriol analogues which bind poorly with vitamin D binding α-globulin. As a result their clearance is faster. Such analogues carry lesser risk of causing hypercalcaemia and hypercalciuria (compared to calcitriol) and therefore these can be used for other therapeutic indications where hypercalcaemia can be avoided.

Vitamin D Deficiency Symptoms

These include fall in plasma Ca^{2+} and PO_4^{3-} levels due to inadequate intestinal absorption. As a result PTH secretion is stimulated and to restore serum calcium, bone resorption occurs. In children, the deficient calcification of osteoid tissue results in bony deformities like bow legs, enlarged skull, spinal curvature, chest deformities and hepatosplenomegaly—the characteristic features of rickets. In adults decalcification and demineralisation of bones leads to osteomalacia, which is characterised by bone tenderness with pain and loss of bone density.

Hypervitaminosis D

It is characterised by elevated plasma Ca^{2+} levels and its ectopic deposition in various other tissues such as blood vessels, parenchymal organs and soft tissues. Weakness, fatigue, vomiting, diarrhoea, polyuria, renal stones, hypertension and growth retardation (in children) can occur. However, hypervitaminosis D occurs after chronic ingestion of more than 50,000 IU/day of vit. D_3. Recovery may not be complete and may take longer time even after stopping vit. D intake and keeping the patient on low calcium diet.

Drug Interactions

- Liquid paraffin reduces vitamin D absorption—causes deficiency.
- Phenytoin and phenobarbitone on prolonged use enhance the metabolism of vit. D by enzymatic induction and also decrease the responsiveness of target tissues to vit. D. This leads to rickets in children and osteomalacia in adults.

CALCITONIN (CT)

- Calcitonin is a single chain polypeptide having 32 amino acid residues and molecular weight of 3600. A disulfide bridge (S=S) between position 1 and 7 is essential for biological activity. CT is synthesised and released from the parafollicular C-cells of the thyroid gland. Within the C-cells of thyroid, CT is processed from a CT precursor (MW 15,000) which serves as prohormone. From the precursor molecule calcitonin gene related peptide (CGRP; Ch. 17) is also generated. However, it has no role in Ca^{2+} homeostasis. It is rather a powerful vasodilator.
- Rising serum Ca^{2+} levels are the principal stimulus for CT synthesis and release. CT has been isolated from other tissues also (such as thymus, pancreas and adrenals) and its release is also stimulated by other hormones such as glucagon, gastrin, cholecystokinin and serotonin but its physiological significance is not clear. However, recently it has been postulated that gastrin-induced CT release may help regulate postmeal Ca^{2+} deposition in the bone. Although blood CT level is usually low, it gets elevated in cases having medullary carcinoma of thyroid which may serve as its diagnostic test.
- The metabolic degradation of CT occurs fast (plasma half-life 10 min) in both liver and kidney. However, its action lasts for several hours.
- The actions of CT are probably mediated through increase in cAMP formation *via* adenylate cyclase activation. CT release is stimulated by hypercalcaemia but suppressed by hypocalcaemia (Fig. 46.1). Its actions are usually opposite to that of PTH. CT inhibits the process of bone resorption by direct inhibitory action on osteoclast (Fig. 46.2). It promotes deposition of postprandial Ca^{2+} into the bone. CT also inhibits proximal tubular Ca^{2+} and PO_4^{3-} reabsorption by acting directly on the kidney.
- The ability of CT to block bone resorption and lower Ca^{2+} levels makes it a useful drug for the treatment of Paget's disease, hypercalcaemia and osteoporosis.
- The most commonly used CT preparation is ***synthetic salmon calcitonin***. It is more potent and longer acting due to slower metabolism. It is administered S.C. or I.M. one IU = 4 mg of standard CT. Its nasal spray formulation is also available, but the absorption is slower.
- *Adverse effects* include nausea, flushing, tingling sensation in fingers, altered taste and allergic reactions. CT may interfere with actions of digoxin, due to lowering of plasma Ca^{2+} levels.

FIBROBLAST GROWTH FACTOR-23 (FGF-23)

(and its interactions with PTH and vitamin D)

The net effect of PTH is to raise serum calcium and to reduce serum phosphate. It is the concentration of free Ca^{2+} that is detected by parathyroid gland and which serves as a stimulus for PTH release. Physiological role of calcitriol (vit. D_3), on the other hand, is to increase serum calcium as well as serum phosphate levels. Increases in the serum phosphate levels (by vit. D_3) reduce the concentration of free ionised Ca^{2+} (by forming calcium phosphate) which leads to enhanced PTH secretion; while reduction in serum phosphate levels maintains the ↑ed concentration of free Ca^{2+} ions once the hypocalcaemia is corrected. Here comes the role of yet another long chain polypeptide regulator of calcium homeostasis called ***Fibroblast Growth Factor-23*** (FGF-23) which is produced in osteoblasts and osteocytes in the bone. Its role is to inhibit the undue synthesis of calcitriol so as to decrease Ca^{2+} and PO_4^{3-} absorption from the intestine as well as to increase phosphate excretion from the kidney (Fig. 46.1). The net result being to keep the serum PO_4^{3-} levels low so that PTH can maintain physiological levels of serum Ca^{2+} once the hypocalcaemia is corrected. However, excess production of FGF-23 can lead to osteomalacia by inhibiting calcitriol production. Calcium homeostasis in the body, therefore, is finely regulated with a critical check and balance effects of PTH, Vit. D_3, calcitonin and FGF-23.

OTHER HORMONAL AGENTS AFFECTING CALCIUM HOMEOSTASIS

Glucocorticoids

Prolonged administration of glucocorticoids is a common cause of osteoporosis in adults. In post-menopausal women this complication may be serious while in growing children, glucocorticoids can suppress skeletal growth and maturation. However, glucocorticoids have proved useful in reversing the hypercalcaemia associated with sarcoidosis (wherein the production of $1,25(OH)_2D_3$ is increased) or in the cases of hypervitaminosis D. However, hyperparathyroid hypercalcaemia does not respond, while hypercalcaemia of malignancies responds poorly. For details refer Ch. 42.

Estrogens

Estrogens can prevent accelerated bone loss and can increase bone density in postmenopausal women. However, it should be noted that estrogen can prevent further bone loss but cannot restore the bone loss which has already occurred. Estrogens (1) reduce the bone resorbing actions of PTH, (2) increase the levels of calcitriol in the blood and (3) have direct favourable effects on bone remodeling by causing apoptosis of osteoclasts (Fig. 46.2). The observed increase in blood calcitriol levels are not due to its increased synthesis but results as a consequence of increased PTH and decreased serum Ca^{2+} and PO_4^{3-} levels. Estrogens are mainly used to treat postmenopausal osteoporosis. For details refer Ch. 43.

Androgens

Ca^{2+} excretion is sharply reduced by androgens and hence were once being used to treat osteoporosis. Bisphosphonate (see below), however, have largely replaced androgens for this purpose.

NONHORMONAL AGENTS AFFECTING CALCIUM HOMEOSTASIS

Bisphosphonates (BPNs)

- Bisphosphonates are synthetic pyrophosphate derivatives that inhibit osteoclasts-mediated bone resorption. In BPNs, the " phosphorus-oxygen-phosphorus" moiety of pyrophosphate (found in bone hydroxyapatite) is substituted with a more stable "phosphorus-carbon-phosphorus" moiety. The BPNs analogues in clinical practice, have different substitutions on the central C-atom.
- The BPNs inhibit osteoclastic resorption of bones by binding to the hydroxyapatite crystals of bone. When osteoclasts attach to the bone matrix, during resorption process, BPNs are released from the bone which are then internalised by endocytosis into the osteoclasts to accelerate their apoptosis. The number of osteoclasts is therefore reduced. In addition, BPNs also inhibit the release of interleukins (IL-6) to suppress differentiation of osteoclast precursors. The net effect therefore is the inhibition of osteoclast-mediated resorption and promotion of bone remodeling by an increase in bone density. Only amino-bisphosphonates (e.g., ***risedronate*** and ***alendronate***) have lately been found to block mevalonate synthesis that appears to be critical for osteoclast survival. Statins (Ch. 23) also block mevalonate synthesis and are reported to promote bone formation, indicating that inhibition of mevalonate synthesis may constitute another approach towards management of osteoporosis.

The first generation BPNs include ***etidronate, clodronate*** and ***tiludronate.*** These are less potent than other BPNs. *Etidronate* is least preferrred BPN nowadays for osteoporosis as its long-term use leads to osteomalacia. It is more preferred (oral/IV) for treating Paget's disease and for treating ectopic ossification. *Tiludronate* orally can be used to treat osteoporosis and Paget's disease.

The second generation drugs are about 100 times more potent than first generation. These include amino BPNs, e.g., ***alendronate, pamidronate*** and ***ibandronate. Alendronate*** can be given in a dose of 10 mg/day or 70 mg/week orally on empty stomach (see below) while ***ibandronate*** is given in a dose of 2.5 mg /day or 150 mg/month orally. For patients who can not tolerate oral BPN or for whom oral BPN are contraindicated, I.V. BPNs are available. For such patients ***Pamidronate*** is given I.V. in doses of 30–60 mg by slow infusion in 0.9% slaline every 2–6 months. Alternatively ***zolendronate*** can also be given I.V. in doses of 2.5 mg/kg.

The third generation BPNs include ***risedronate*** (oral, I.V.), ***zolendronate*** (I.V.), ***neridronate*** (an amino BPN, oral, I.V.) and ***oxidronate*** (I.V.). These are 1000 to 10,000 times more potent than first generation BPNs. ***Risedronate*** can be given orally in a dose of 5 mg/day or 35 mg/week.

BPNs are commonly used to treat osteoporosis, to reduce fracture rates and to treat hypercalcaemia due to malignancy. A combination of BPN with calcitonin is more effective in treating osteoporosis and Paget's disease. In addition, adequate intake of calcium with vit. D should also be maintained. The oral BPNs are better tolerated once weekly or monthly without costing their efficacy. Oral bioavailability is poor; food further decreases their absorption. Hence, these should be taken on empty stomach with full glass of water (see adverse effects).

- Adverse reactions: commonly oral BPNs can cause gastric irritation, nausea, chest pain, hoarseness of voice, erosive oesophagitis, particularly in patients with hiatus hernia and gastro-oesophageal reflux.

Decreased renal function, gastro-oesophageal reflux and peptic ulcer are main contraindications for their use. Irritation due to gastro-oesophageal reflux can be minimised by taking the drug with a glass of water and remaining either upright or in ambulatory condition for 1/2 hour (60 min for *ibandronate*). Flu-like symptoms are common with I.V. infusion of and *pamidronate*. Patients receiving higer doses of BPNs for longer periods or those receiving high I.V. doses of *zolendronate* for hypercalcaemia of malignancy may develop osteonecrosis of jaws (but not with therapeutic doses of BPNs).

OTHER NONHORMONAL AGENTS AFFECTING CALCIUM HOMEOSTASIS

- **SELECTIVE ESTROGEN RECEPTOR MODULATORS (SERMs)**: These are nonsteroidal synthetic agents whose activities on estrogen receptors are tissue selective (Ch. 43). They produce beneficial estrogenic effects in bone, brain and liver but prevent certain deleterious estrogenic effects in some organs/tissues such as breast and endometrium. ***Raloxifene*** is currently being used for the treatment of postmenopausal osteoporosis. *Raloxifene*, is a better estrogenic agent in bone and reduces the risk of vertebral fractures of 30–50%. The drug produces dose-dependent increase in osteoblast activity and reduction in osteoclast action.

- **CALCIMIMETICS**: Recently calcium sensing receptors (CaSR) have been identified on parathyroid gland which seem to regulate PTH secretion. Higher calcium levels activate CaSR and block PTH secretion. ***Cinacalcet*** is a calcimimetic which blocks PTH secretion by this mechanism and is approved for the treatment of secondary hyperparathyroidism in chronic renal failure (dose: 30 mg once daily, titrated upward to 180 mg once daily) and for the treatment of PTH releasing parathyroid carcinoma (dose: 30 mg BD titrated upward to 90 mg TDS orally).
  Adverse effects: hypocalcaemia.

- **STRONTIUM RANELATE**: It is a ranelic acid salt of strontium. It blocks differentiation of osteoclasts and also promotes their apoptosis and thus prevents bone resorption. It also promotes bone formation (i.e., increases bone forming markers). It is being used in European Countries to treat osteoporosis as it significantly reduces the risk of spine and hip fractures. Side effects in therapeutic doses are rare or mild. Dose: 2 g/day orally.

- **SEVELAMER HYDROCHLORIDE**: Hyperphosphataemia results due to hypoparathyroidism, hypervitaminosis-D and is a common complication of renal failure. Emergency treatment of hyperphosphataemia needs dialysis but routine management requires the use of phosphate binding gel, e.g., *Sevelamer* (800 mg TDS with meals) plus calcium supplements. *Adverse effects*: Constipation, epigastric distress and headache.

- **THIAZIDE DIURETICS**: These have been discussed in detail in Chapter 16. Thiazide diuretics reduce renal calcium excretion and are used for reducing hypercalciuria and incidence of calcium oxalate stone formation (as they also decrease urinary oxalate excretion). Thiazides increase the effectiveness of PTH in stimulating calcium reabsorption by renal tubules. Moreover, lowering of the intracellular Na^+ (due to its excretion by thiazides) enhances Na^+/Ca^{2+} exchange in basolateral membrane of the distal tubules, which in turn promotes overall reabsorption of Ca^{2+}. Thiazides are more useful in prevention rather than treatment of osteoporosis.

- **FLUORIDES**: Though well known for prophylaxis of dental caries, its efficacy to prevent osteoporosis is debatable, because of its toxicity and dose-dependent effects on bone. In high doses fluoride rather increases the risk of all kinds of fractures. Fluoride gets incorporated into bone matrix and forms fluoroapatite in place of hydroxyapatite. Hence, initially it makes bone denser but at a later stage, if the process continues, the bone loses its biomechanical strength.

CHAPTER 47 Insulin and Other Antidiabetic Drugs

COMPETENCY PH1.36

The pancreas has both endocrine and exocrine functions. The *exocrine secretions* are mostly the digestive enzymes such as pancreatic amylase (a carbohydrate digesting enzyme), trypsin and chymotrypsin (protein digesting enzymes) and pancreatic lipase (a triglyceride digesting enzyme). Scattered among the exocrine portion of the pancreas are millions of tiny clusters of endocrine tissue called *pancreatic islets* or *islets of Langerhans,* which contains four types of cells secreting different hormones:

1. ***Alpha cells*** **(A-cells)** which constitute about 17% of islet mass, and secrete ***glucagon*** that raises blood sugar levels.
2. ***Beta cells*** **(β-cells)** which constitute about 70% of islet mass, and secrete ***insulin*** that lowers blood sugar levels.
3. ***Delta cells*** **(D-cells)** which constitute about 7% of the islet mass and secrete *growth hormone release-inhibiting hormone* or ***somatostatin***. In pancreas it inhibits the secretions of glucagon and insulin. In hypothalamus it inhibits the synthesis and release of growth hormone while in GIT it inhibits the release of gastrin.
4) ***The F-cells*** which constitute the remainder of the islet mass, secrete ***pancreatic polypeptide*** which regulates the release of *pancreatic digestive enzymes and contraction of gall bladder*.

Glucagon and insulin are two most important endocrine hormones that maintain the glucose homeostasis.

GLUCAGON

Decreased blood levels of glucose, sympathetic stimulation (as in exercise) and high protein diet (rich in amino acids) stimulate glucagon release; while hyperglycaemia and somatostatin inhibit glucagon secretion. If, however, the blood glucose-dependent negative feedback mechanism fails, the A-cells will secrete glucagon continuously and hyperglycaemia would result.

Glucagon raises blood glucose levels by accelerating breakdown of glycogen into glucose (glycogenolysis) and conversion of lactates and amino acids into glucose in the liver (gluconeogenesis), releasing glucose into blood.

GIT effects of glucagon include relaxation of the gut and inhibition of gastric acid secretion. It has potent inotropic and chronotropic effects on heart. These effects are similar to that produced by β_1-adrenoceptor agonists without involving the role of β_1-receptors. It has a very short t½ (3–5 min).

THERAPEUTIC USES include: (1) to treat severe hypoglycaemia (1 mg I.M.) or hypoglycaemic coma (1 mg I.V.) due to insulin in the patients of type I diabetes (see text) and (2) as an aid to X-ray examination and Magnetic Resonance Imaging (MRI) of the GIT (as it relaxes intestine).

Adverse effects are rare but may include transient nausea and vomiting.

INSULIN

Unless insulin is present to facilitate the uptake of glucose, it penetrates most tissues only slowly. Glucose plays the dominant role in the regulation of insulin secretion. Maintenance of blood glucose levels within the normal physiological limits is primarily accomplished by insulin and glucagon. Any excess in the regulation of insulin or glucagon can lead to hypoglycaemia or hyperglycaemia, respectively.

Chemistry, Biosynthesis and Secretion

Biosynthesis of insulin involves a precursor molecule called ***preproinsulin.*** The subsequent proteolytic cleavage of preproinsulin, by endopeptidases, gives rise to ***proinsulin***. In proinsulin (Fig. 47.1), there are two polypeptide chains—A and B—which are connected to each other by ***C (connecting) peptide chain.*** The proteolytic degradation of proinsulin, in Golgi apparatus by proteases, results in the formation of ***insulin*** along with ***C-peptide*** in equimolar concentrations, which are then stored in the pancreatic β-cells granules. When proinsulin is converted to insulin, the C-peptide part is knocked off. The C-peptide of proinsulin facilitates the correct folding of A and B chains of insulin and also maintains the alignment of disulfide bridges in the insulin molecule before its own removal. Both insulin and C-peptide are liberated together during insulin release. The role of C-peptide during insulin release is not clear. ***Insulin*** is a polypeptide containing 51 amino acids (MW 5800). It is composed of two chains (chain-A of 21 and chain-B of 30 amino acids) that are joined together by two disulfide cross-bridges (Fig. 47.1). Granules within β-pancreatic cells store insulin in a form of complex containing 2 atoms of zinc with 6 molecules of insulin. Human pancreas contains up to 8 mg of insulin which is equivalent to approximately 220 units of insulin (1 mg = 28 units of insulin approximately).

Glucose levels > 70 mg/dL stimulate insulin synthesis and release. Glucose stimulates insulin secretion through a series of regulatory steps that begin with its transport into the β-cells by the GLUT-2 glucose transporter (present on β-cells of pancreas). Further metabolism of glucose *via* glucose-6-phosphate and pyruvate generates ATP which inhibits the activity of ATP-sensitive K^+ channels. The inhibition of this K^+ channel decreases β-cell membrane K^+ outward conductance and thereby induces β-cell membrane depolarisation, opening of voltage-dependent Ca^{2+} channels (which leads to an influx of Ca^{2+}) and stimulation of insulin secretion. The ATP -sensitive K^+ channel has receptors for certain oral hypoglycaemic agents also, such as for sulfonylureas and therefore named SUR, i.e. sulfonylurea receptor and meglitinides. These agents too, block the ATP-sensitive/dependent K^+ channel, thereby depolarising the membrane (as in muscles and nerves) and causing the insulin release by the same mechanism (Fig. 47.2). In the resting cell, the normal ATP levels are low and K^+ diffuses down its concentration gradient through these ATP-regulated channels and maintains the intracellular potential at a negative (fully polarised)

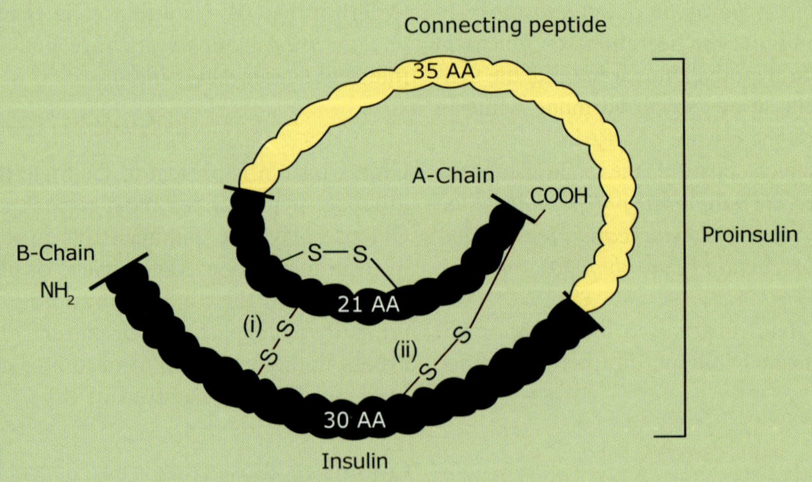

Fig 47.1 Structure of Proinsulin and Insulin. When C-peptide (**yellow**) is removed, insulin (**black**) is formed. Insulin has two chains of amino acids (AA) joined by disulfide (-S-S-) bonds (i and ii). 'A' chain consists of 21, while 'B' chain consists of 30 amino acids (AA).

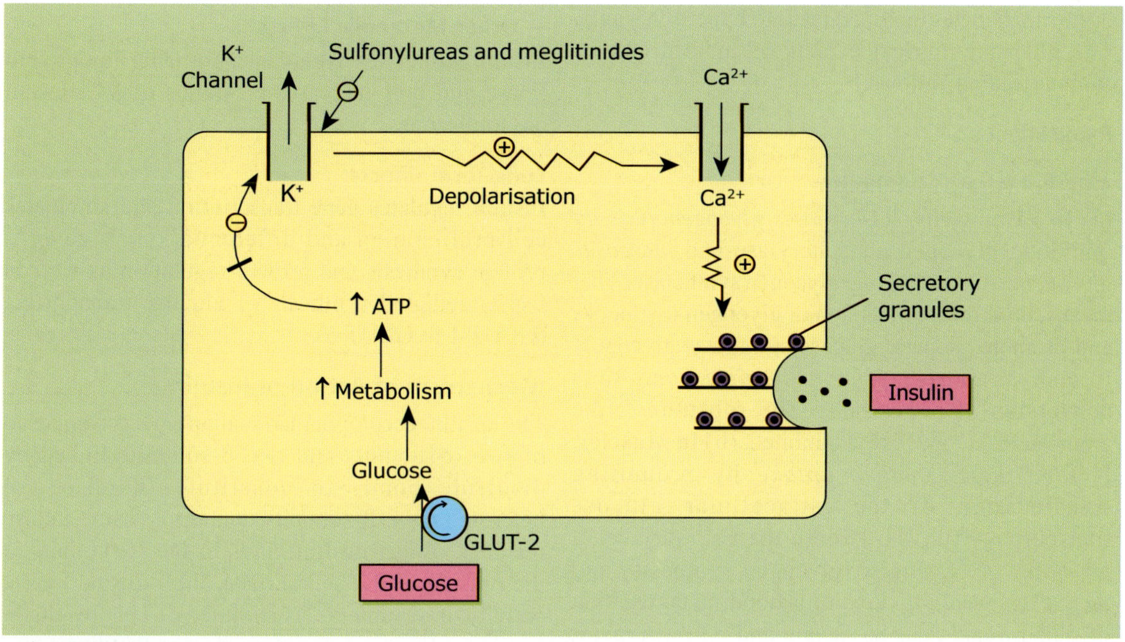

Fig 47.2 Control of Insulin Release From the Pancreatic β-Cells by Glucose and Certain Oral Hypoglycaemic Agents. GLUT-2—Glucose Transporter-2

level. Hence, insulin release from resting cell is minimal.

Other stimulants for insulin release include amino acids (mainly arginine and leucine) and fatty acids. Acetylcholine (vagal stimulation of pancreatic islets) stimulates insulin release; while adrenaline increases blood glucose by inhibiting insulin release (*via* α_2-adrenoceptors) and by promoting glycogenolysis (*via* β_2-adrenoceptors) in striated muscles and liver (Ch. 10 and 12). As discussed above somatostatin inhibits insulin release. Meals induce even larger bursts of insulin secretion that usually last for 2–3 hrs before returning to base level. Derangements in insulin secretion are one of the earliest signs of β-cells dysfunction in diabetes mellitus (see below).

Insulin and Insulin-like Growth Factors (IGFs): Inter-Relationship

In response to growth hormone, cells in liver and other tissues secrete small protein hormones called ***insulin-like growth factors (IGFs)*** which may enter the blood stream from the liver or act locally in other tissues. IGFs cause cells to grow and multiply by increasing uptake of amino acids into cells and accelerating protein synthesis. Growth hormone and IGFs together, therefore, help maintain mass of muscles and bone and promote muscle reapir. IGFs also enhance lipolysis in adipose tissues so that released fatty acids can be utilised for ATP production by body cells. Besides influencing protein and lipid metabolism, IGFs also affect glucose metabolism by decreasing glucose uptake and increasing glycogenolysis in liver to release glucose into blood. That means high levels of growth hormone and IGFs cause hyperglycaemia while low levels do just the opposite.

Pharmacological Actions of Insulin

Insulin promotes the uptake and storage of glucose, fats and proteins through effects on liver, muscles and adipose tissues (also referred to as storage hormone). It also influences the cell growth and metabolic functions of various tissues. Excess secretion of insulin (as in insulinoma) leads to hypoglycaemia, while lack of insulin release (as occurs in diabetes mellitus) leads to hyperglycaemia. The pharmacological effects of insulin can be summarised as follows:

Rapid Effects

- **Carbohydrate Metabolism**

(a) In Liver Cells: It *decreases glycogenolysis* by inhibiting glycogen phosphorylase and *increases glycogenesis* by activating glycogen synthetase. That means, it inhibits conversion of glycogen to glucose and promotes hepatic glucose storage as glycogen. It also *decreases gluconeogenesis* and thus conversion of noncarbohydrate substrates (like amino acids) to glucose is inhibited, **(b) In Muscles**: It *facilitates glucose uptake* by promoting translocation of the intracellular glucose transporter-4 (GLUT-4) onto the cell surface. It *promotes glycogenesis* (glycogen synthesis) and *increases glycolysis* (i.e., mitochondrial conversion of glucose and ADP to lactate and ATP—a major source of energy for voluntary and cardiac muscle) and **(c) In Adipose Tissues**: It *facilitates glucose uptake* (through GLUT-4). It *increases* intracellular *glucose oxidative metabolism*. Glycerol, thus produced, is esterified with fatty acids to form triglycerides (i.e., it *increases the synthesis of TGs*).

- **Protein Metabolism**

(a) In Liver Cells: It *decreases protein breakdown* and *inhibits oxidation of amino acids to ketoacids* and **(b) In Muscles**: It *increases protein synthesis* and *increases amino acid uptake* by muscle cells to produce a net positive nitrogen balance.

- **Fat Metabolism**

(a) In Liver Cells: It *increases lipogenesis* (i.e., conversion of glucose and other nutrients to fatty acids) and **(b) In Adipose Tissues** : It *increases fatty acid synthesis* and *triglycerides formation and storage*; *decreases lipolysis* (hydrolysis or breakdown of fats) and blunts lipolytic action of adrenaline, growth hormone and glucagon.

Thus insulin lowers the blood glucose levels by promoting the glucose utilisation and suppressing its production.

- **Other Metabolic Effects**

Insulin stimulates vascular endothelial lipoprotein lipase and thus increases clearance of VLDL and chylomicrons.

Long-Term Effects

Insulin regulates gene transcription and stimulates cell proliferation and differentiation. It governs protein synthesis and growth regulation as well as DNA-mediated synthesis of glucose transporters (GLUT-1 to GLUT-5).

Mechanism of Action of Insulin

The insulin receptor in mammalian cells is composed of two α-subunits and two β-subunits linked by disulfide bonds to constitute the β-α-α-β heterotetramer. β-subunits contain tyrosine kinase residues. When insulin binds to the α-subunits at the outside of the cell surface, the tyrosine kinase activity, in β subunits, is stimulated. This results in autophosphorylation of the adjacent β-subunit and phosphorylation of the tyrosine residues present on cytoplasmic protein called *insulin receptor substrate* (IRS). This initiates a series of events that culminate into a cascade of phosphorylation and dephosphorylation reactions. Certain second messengers such as inositolphosphatidylglycans (IPGs) and DAG are also generated by phosphorylation of IRS and subsequent activation of specific phospholipase-C. These are believed to mediate the ***rapid actions of insulin*** on different metabolising enzymes.

Insulin also stimulates the glucose transport across cell membrane by ***ATP-dependent translocation of glucose transporter-4 (GLUT-4) to the plasma membrane,*** an event that is crucial for glucose uptake by skeletal muscle and fat cells. GLUT-4 is predominantly present on skeletal muscles and adipose tissue.

Over a period of time, phosphorylation of IRS also results in activation of transcription factors that enhance DNA synthesis and proliferation and differentiation of several cell types ***(long-term effects of insulin).***

Finally, the insulin receptor complex is internalised by endocytosis, which is followed by

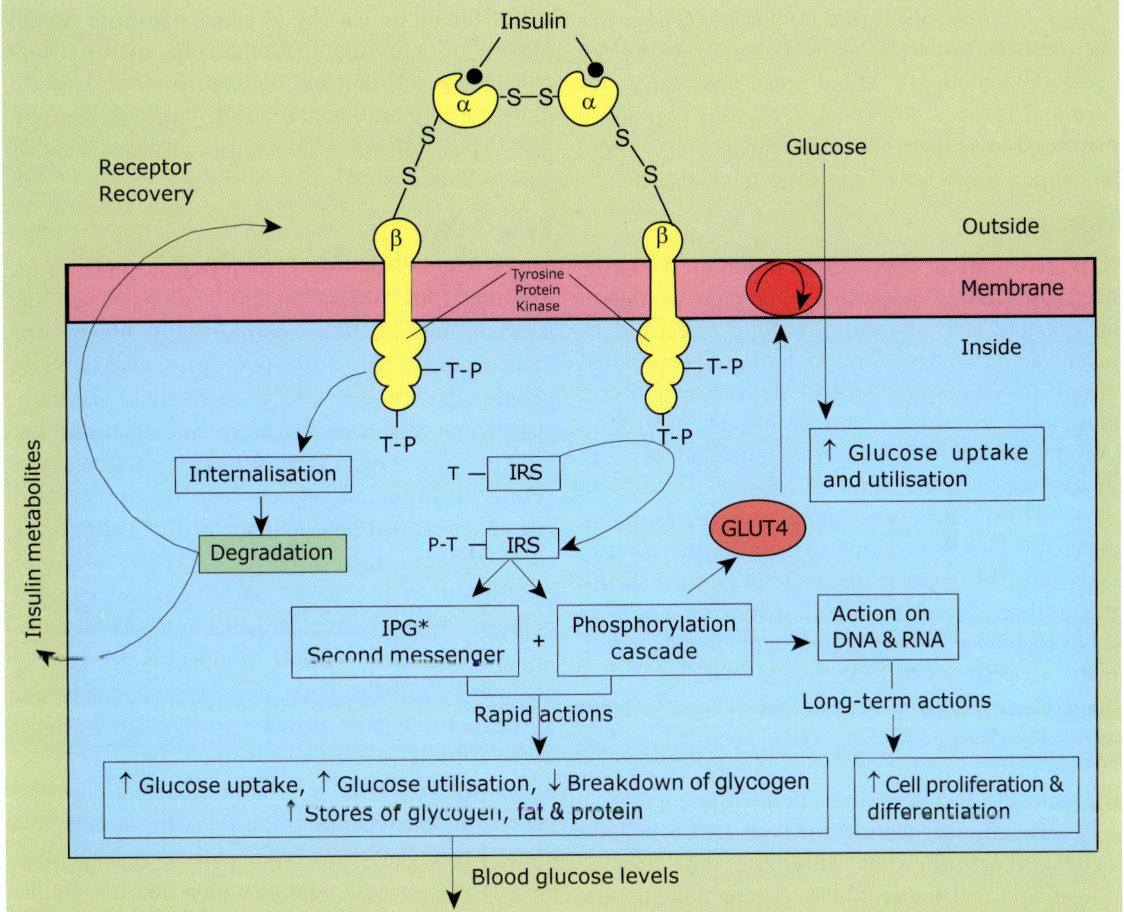

GLUT-4—Glucose transporter-4; IRS—Insulin receptor substrate; T—Tyrosine; P—Phosphate; *Inositolphosphoglycans (IPGs) are released outside of the cell but then transported back into the cell

Fig 47.3 Insulin Signaling Pathways

degradation of insulin and recycling of the receptor to the cell surface. These events are shown schematically in the Figure 47.3.

DIABETES MELLITUS (DM)

Diabetes mellitus (meli=honey) is a group of heterogeneous disorders in which carbohydrate metabolism is reduced while that of proteins and lipids are increased. Hyperglycaemia is a common end point for all types of DM and is an important parameter to evaluate the efficacy of antidiabetic drugs. As hyperglycaemia increases, there is a loss of glucose through urine (*glucosuria*). Virtually all forms of DM are due to either a decrease in the circulating levels of insulin (*insulin deficiency*) or a decrease in the response of target tissues to insulin (*insulin resistance*). Although insulin treatment has largely increased the life expectancy of diabetic patients, diabetes remains the third leading cause of death, the second leading cause of blindness as well as of renal failure. The hallmarks of DM are three "polys": an excessive urine production (*Polyuria*), an excessive thirst (*Polydipsia*) and an excessive eating (*Polyphagia*). The disease has two major forms: Type-1 and Type-2 DM; but two more diabetes disease states have also been included. These are: Type 3 (other) and Type 4 (gestational DM).

Type-1 DM

It is also called "**I**nsulin **D**ependent **D**iabetes **M**ellitus" (IDDM) because in such patients, due to an absolute lack of insulin, regular injections of insulin are needed to save life. Earlier, it was called "*juvenile-onset diabetes*" because it most commonly develops either before puberty or in youngsters below 20 years of age and persists throughout their life.

IDDM is mainly an autoimmune disease of the pancreatic β-cells resulting in their degeneration in over 95% of cases (type-1A). It could also be idiopathic (type1B). Viral infection such as echovirus can also damage pancreatic β-cells in less than 5% cases (type 1B). Approximately 10% of diabetics suffer from type-1 DM. These patients have a low degree of genetic predisposition, yet 15–20% of patients reveal a positive family history and the incidence in homozygous twins is about 50%.

The clinical features of type-1 DM include hyperglycaemia with polyuria, polydipsia, polyphagia and **ketoacidosis**. These patients are generally not obese. *Diabetic ketoacidosis is the end result of insulin deficiency in uncontrolled type-1 diabetes.* Since insulin is not present to aid the entry of glucose in skeletal muscles and body cells, most cells now use fatty acids to produce ATP to compensate and to provide calories. This accelerated fat breakdown generates acetyl-CoA. But, due to DM, this acetyl CoA cannot be removed by Krebs cycle (to H_2O_2 and CO_2) and therefore gets accumulated. In absence of aerobic carbohydrate metabolism, two acetyl-CoA molecules join to form acetoacetic acid, and β-hydroxybutyric acid, which are collectively called ***ketone bodies*** and excreted in urine (ketonuria). The acetoacetate (ketone body) is converted in liver to acetone which is excreted through lungs and provides ***a fruity odour to the breath of these patients.*** These metabolic products cause metabolic acidosis or ***diabetic ketoacidosis,*** which decreases glucose utilisation in brain and decreases pH of the blood leading to coma and death. Renal losses of glucose (glycosuria), nitrogenous substances and ketone bodies promote osmotic diuresis (polyuria) that can result in dehydration and thirst (polydipsia). Ketoacidosis means a state of ketosis with acidosis.

Type-2 DM

This is also called "**N**on-**I**nsulin **D**ependent **D**iabetes **M**ellitus" (NIDDM) or "maturity onset diabetes" (as it occurs late in life). Approximately, 90–95% of diabetics have type-2 diabetes. It usually occurs in people who are over 40 and overweight. For these people diabetes arises not from lack of insulin but because their target cells have either become relatively insensitive to insulin (peripheral resistance to insulin) or their insulin secretion is less but is not totally lacking. Genetic predisposition, in type-2 DM, is important as there is greater than 95% concordance in identical twins.

Classical clinical symptoms of type-2 diabetes are almost same as for type-1, but type-2 diabetics are less prone to develop diabetic ketoacidosis. Instead, they may develop hyperosmolar coma, a condition characterised by severe hyperglycaemia and dehydration. It is a clinical emergency that requires faster management with prompt insulin administration and I.V. fluids. ***In type-2 DM, some endogenous insulin is always available which prevents the breakdown of fats with lesser likelihood for ketoacidosis.***

Various complications often develop as a consequence of the metabolic derangements in DM (type-1 and type-2) over many years (particularly if there is poor glycaemic control). As a result there may be ***microvascular complications*** (e.g., retinopathy, nephropathy and neuropathy) as well as ***macrovascular complications*** such as atherosclerosis and diabetic dyslipidaemia (elevated TGs and LDL). Diabetic neuropathy results due to demyelination of axons. Diabetic retinopathy and nephropathy result due to accumulation of sorbitol produced by glucose reduction by aldose reductase. Sorbitol causes thickening of the basement membrane of capillary endothelium, which leads to the narrowing of the microvessels and deficiency in tissue perfusion. A major complication of diabetes is the formation of cataract because excess glucose gets deposited on lens to make it cloudy. Brain is the last organ to be affected in diabetes because it can utilise blood glucose in the absence of insulin (fortunately!).

Type-3 DM

In this type, there are secondary causes of hyperglycaemia, e.g., chronic pancreatitis or chronic drug therapy with glucocorticoids, thiazide diuretics, diazoxide, growth hormone or with some protease inhibitors used to treat human immunodeficiency virus infections (e.g., saquinavir).

Type-4 DM

It is also called "**G**estational **D**iabetes **M**ellitus" (GDM). It is observed in approximately 4–5% of all pregnancies. Elevated blood sugar levels are usually observed in second or last trimester of pregnancy and usually resolved during the postpartum period. There is no genetic predisposition. The most plausible cause is that during pregnancy, the placental hormones promote insulin resistance.

Diabetic Control and Measurement of Glycosylated Haemoglobin

Diabetic control is not easily estimated by just determination of blood glucose, as these values may vary on day-to-day basis. Instead, glycosylated haemoglobin (HbA_{1C}) can be measured which provides an integrated measure of glycaemic control over the life span of the red-cell (approximately 120 days). Sustained elevation of blood glucose as occurs in both type-1 and type-2 DM is damaging to the microvasculature. The damage is believed to result from the non-enzymatic glycosylation of proteins in blood vessel wall and generation of the reactive products as a result of the abnormal metabolism of glucose and lipids. Haemoglobin is also glycosylated on its valine amino acid terminal to form glycosyl valine adduct called ***glycosylated haemoglobin*** (**HbA_{1C}**). The rate of glycosylation in RBC is directly proportional to glucose concentration. Because the half-life of HbA_{1C} is the same as that of RBC, the concentration of HbA_{1C} in circulation can be used to assess the control of the glycaemic state over a period of 120 days prior to sampling. HbA_{1C} values of 6% are equal to 110 mg/dL of blood glucose. The goal for having tight glycaemic control in diabetes is to maintain HbA_{1C} values below 7%, as the values less than this have been shown to reduce the risk of microvascular complications such as retinopathy, nephropathy and neuropathy. HbA_{1C} values of more than 8% means there has been a poor control of blood glucose in patients of DM.

TREATMENT OF DIABETES MELLITUS

Dietary restriction, exercise and ***insulin therapy*** are the cornerstones of the management of **type-1 diabetes.** There is usually less insulin resistance in type-1 diabetics. However, if resistance develops, glitazones (see below) may also be added.

Weight reduction, dietary restrictions and exercise are also proven ways to increase insulin sensitivity in **type-2 diabetes** and many patients can be effectively treated by such approaches. However, optimal control of blood glucose levels are not achieved sometimes even when patients adhere to weight reduction program, which necessitates drug therapy. The oral (or S.C.) agents that are used to treat type-2 diabetes can be divided into the following two categories:

- Oral hypoglycaemic agents which include ***sulfonylureas*** and ***meglitinide*** group of drugs.
- Antihyperglycaemic agents which include ***metformin, α-glucosidase inhibitors, thiazolidinediones (glitazones), incretin mimetics, DPP-4 inhibitors, sodium-glucose cotransporter-2 inhibitor*** and ***amylin receptor agonists.***

For individuals unable to achieve glycaemic control with oral (or S.C.) drug therapy, insulin has to be added and if insulin resistance develops later, addition of glitazones should be considered.

INSULINS: USE AND CHARACTERISTICS

Sources of Insulins

Beef insulin differs by three amino acids from human insulin, whereas only one amino acid distinguishes pork and human insulin. Thus, pork insulin being more homologous to human insulin is less immunogenic than beef insulin (risk of transmission of mad cow disease also). Although pork insulin is derived directly from pigs, mass production of human insulin is done by recombinant DNA techniques wherein a human proinsulin gene is inserted into *E.coli* or yeast. When *E.coli* grow or yeast cells multiply, lots of proinsulin is synthesised which is then extracted and processed to form *human insulin*. It is called human insulin because its structure is same as that of normal human insulin, but it is not obtained from human pancreas. *Human insulin* is more water soluble and has more rapid S.C. absorption. Some insulins have been modified through genetic engineering to produce insulin analogues that possess novel pharmacokinetic properties (e.g., insulin glargine and insulin detemir; see below). Insulin obtained from pancreas is complexed with zinc and therefore is extracted in the form of zinc-insulin complex which is not water soluble at neutral pH. This can also be converted to sodium salt, which is water soluble at neutral pH. For therapeutic purpose, dosages and concentration of insulin are expressed in units.

Pharmacokinetics

Being a high molecular weight polypeptide, insulin is rapidly inactivated if administered orally. Intravenous injections of rapid acting soluble insulin can be given, but in emergency such as in diabetic coma. Intramuscular injections of insulin are also used but less often because absorption is more rapid. Hence insulin is usually administered subcutaneously. Depending on the type of insulin, the rate of its absorption can be modulated by altering the polymerisation of insulin molecule, e.g., *monomers are absorbed faster compared to dimers or hexamers* (see below).

Liver and kidney are the principal sites of hormone uptake and degradation. Hepatic insulinase destroys about 60% of insulin. In the kidney it is metabolised within the proximal convoluted tubules of the nephron. Plasma half-life of insulin is less than 10 min.

Insulin Preparations

Insulin preparations are classified according to their duration of action as ***ultrashort- (or Rapid/Fast-), short-, intermediate-*** and ***long-acting*** preparations. Their characteristic features are shown in Table 47.1 and Box 47.1.

1. ***Ultrashort-acting Insulins*** **(Rapid-/Fast-acting insulins**: **Insulin Lispro, Insulin Aspart** and **Insulin Glulisine)** have been designed to promote rapid absorption from the subcutaneous tissue. Their action starts within 15–30 min and lasts for 3–4 hrs. These are absorbed as monomers which promotes their rapid uptake and absorption from subscutaneous tissue. These are soluble insulins, dispensed as clear solutions at neutral pH and **Insulin Aspart** can be administered I.V. also. These are useful in controlling the hyperglycaemia that occurs immediately after meals. These are mostly used in combination with one of the basal or long acting insulins to provide immediate insulin following a meal and to maintain a baseline level of insulin between the two meals.
2. ***Short-acting Insulin*** **(Regular Insulin)**: Its effect starts within 60 min and lasts for 6–8 hrs (approx). It is soluble human crystalline insulin made by recombinant DNA techniques and have added Zn ions to promote stability and hexamerization. In solutions, it exists as hexamer but as the drug is diluted by interstitial fluid the hexamers breakdown into dimers and finally as monomers which have a faster absorption. **Regular insulin** is designed to control post-meal hyperglycaemia and is also a preparation of choice for the management of diabetic ketoacidosis for which it is used intravenously.
3. ***Intermediate-acting Insulin*** **(NPH** or **Isophane Insulin)**: NPH insulin has a slower onset (about 2 hrs) but a longer duration of action (16–20 hrs). **NPH insulin** is a cloudy complex in which the insulin is conjugated with modifier arginine-rich protein—protamine obtained from fish sperm. NPH insulin has a **N**eutral pH, conjugated with **P**rotamine and was developed by **H**agedorn. **Isophane insulin** is that NPH insulin which has 6 molecules of insulin per molecule of protamine. After the S.C. injection, proteolytic tissue

Table 47.1 Pharmacokinetic Characteristics of Different Insulin Preparations[1]

Types of Insulin	Source	Onset[2] (min)	Peak[2] (hrs	Duration[2] (hrs)	Comments
I. PRANDIAL/BOLUS INSULINS[3]					
Ultrashort (Rapid/Fast) - acting Insulins					
1. *Insulin lispro*[1]	Human modified analogue	15–30	1–1.5	3–4	Clear solutions (pH 7.4); given S.C.; can be mixed with NPH insulin
2. *Insulin aspart*[1]	– do –	– do –	– do –	– do –	Clear solution (pH 7.4); given S.C.; can be given I.V.; can be mixed with NPH insulin
3. *Insulin glulisine*[1]	– do –	– do –	– do –	– do –	Clear solution (pH 7.4); given S.C.; can be mixed with NPH insulin
Inhaled Insulin[4]					
Human insulin (Liquid formulation)	Human	5–10	1	3–5	Liquid or solid powdered human insulin filled cartridges are available for loading on the electronic inhalation device
Short-acting Insulin					
1. *Regular insulin (crystalline Zn-insulin)*	Human or pork	30–60	2–3	6–8	Clear sol.; given S.C. or I.V.; can be mixed with all types of insulins; except long acting insulin analogues
II. BASAL INSULINS[5]					
Intermediate-acting Insulin					
1. *Neutral Protamine Hagedorn (NPH) or Isophane insulin (Zn-suspension)*	Human or pork modified by Protaimine	90–120	5–10	16–20	Cloudy solution; given S.C. only (**not I.V.**); can be mixed with ultrashort-acting and regular insulin
Long-acting Insulins					
1. *Insulin glargine*[1] *(Lantus)*	Human modified analouge	120–240	Peak-less/Flat	16–24	Clear solution at pH 4; given S.C. only (**not I.V.**); should not be mixed with other insulins
2. *Insulin detemir*[1] *(Levemir)*	-do-	-do-	-do-	20–24	Clear solution at pH 4; given S.C. only; should not be mixed with other insulins; lower risk of nocturnal hypoglycaemia
3. *Insulin degludec*[1] *(Tresiba)*	-do-	-do-	-do-	> 24 (upto 42)	Clear solution at pH 7.4; given S.C.; should not be mixed with other insulins; nocturnal hypoglycaemia is reported to be less as compared to Lantus

[1] Inhaled insulin, short-acting insulin and NPH insulin are insulin preparations and all rest are insulin analogues. What chemical modifications are made in the two chains (A & B) of native insulin molecule to create different analogues are described in Box No. 47.1

contd.

[2] All time periods are applicable in relation to when the insulin preparation is administered by S.C. route. However, there are a lot of variations from patient to patient depending on a variety of factors such as the solubility of insulin preparation/analogue, local blood and lymphatic flow at the site of injection and potential circulatory factors (lipotrophy or lipohypertrophy), etc.

[3] **Prandial/Bolus Insulins** are used to mimic pancreatic beta-cell release of insulin in response to meal (*prand* in latin) load and act rapidly (with 10–20 min), peak at 1 hr and have a duration of 3–4 hrs. These are called bolus because all are administered (whether by S.C. or by inhalation route) 30min prior to the first bolus of the meal to check the post-prandial hyperglycaemia.

[4] US Food and Drug Administration (FDA) in 2014 has approved an inhaled liquid/solid powder human insulin preparation with an electronic device that senses patient's inhalation velocity and delivers the insulin when inhalation velocity is maximum. The device can administer the desired dose in 1-unit increments. Studies have shown that inhaled insulin is as effective as injectable formulations and is well tolerated.

[5] **Basal Insulins** include both Long-acting and Intermediate-acting (i.e. NPH insulin, the latter is considered in some text books of Pharmacology as long-acting insulin as its duration is more than 12–16 hrs). Insulins which are administered once or twice daily and provide more consistent low (peakless or flat) level release of insulin that plateau for many hours to provide basal coverage of blood glucose level with lower risk of nocturnal hypoglycaemia. In type-1 diabetes mellitus where insulin is the only treatment for controlling the blood glucose is typical basal/bolus (prandial) regimen consists of a long-acting insulin once (or twice daily) with boluses of fast-acting insulin before meals. Pre- mixed insulin preparations are consisting of 25–30% fast-acting and 70–75% long acting analogues are administered twice daily (30 min before lunch and dinner, respectively).

Box 47.1 Differences in Amino Acid Composition in Chain 'A' or 'B' in the Native Human Insulin Molecules to make Ultrashort (Rapid/Fast-acting) - or Long-acting Analogues

Type of Human Insulin Analogue	Position in Chain 'A' or 'B'				
	A-21	**B-3**	**B-28**	**B-29**	**B-30**
Ultrashort (Rapid/Fast-acting) Analogues					
Native Human Insulin	Aspargine	Aspargine	Proline	Lysine	Threonine
Insulin lispro	Aspargine	Aspargine	Lysine	Proline	Threonine
Insulin aspart	Aspargine	Aspargine	Aspartate	Lysine	Threonine
Insulin glulisine	Aspargine	Lysine	Proline	Glutamate	Threonine
Long-acting Analogues					
Insulin glargine	Glycine	Aspargine	Proline	Lysine	Threonine[a]
Insulin detemir	Aspargine	Aspargine	Proline	Lysine[b]	None (threonine removed)
Insulin degludec	Aspargine	Aspargine	Proline	Lysine[c]	None (threonine removed)

[a] Two additional arginine residues are conjugated to threonine at B-30

[b] A 14-Carbon fatty acid (myristic acid) chain is conjugated to lysine at B-29 and threonine is removed from B-30

[c] A 16-Carbon fatty diacid (hexadecandioic acid) is conjugated to lysine at B-29 via a carboxy-L-glutamic acid linker and threonine is removed from B-30

enzymes degrade the protamine slowly to permit sustained absorption of insulin. NPH is more prone to erratic absorption and shows an intra-patient variability than the long-acting/basal insulin analogues. It must be gently rolled/shaked or inverted to resuspend the solution prior to administration to avoid wide variability in its absorption and action profile. Intermediate-acting insulins are usually given S.C. (not I.V.) and are used to control diabetes in a variety of situations, *except for diabetic ketoacidosis.*

4. ***Longer-acting Insulins*** **(Insulin Glargine, Insulin Detemir and Inslulin Degludec)**: **Insulin glargine** (Lantus) is a long-acting insulin analogue that has two extra (arginine) amino acids added onto (threonine at B30 of) human insulin and one amino acid that is different (glycine at A21 instead of arginine) from human insulin (Box 47.1). These chemical changes create a molecule that is (1) soluble at pH 4 but (2) become less soluble and more stable in subcutaneous tissue at physiological pH as it now can form dimers or hexamers at this pH. Injection of insulin glargine forms the microfined precipitate in subcutaneous tissue, as the pH of the drug solution rises from 4 to 7.4. As a result, a steady and a sustained (peakless) release of insulin takes place from the site of injection (no peak or trough in its levels). Because it is necessary to keep it in solution prior to injection, its pH has to be maintained acidic (pH 4). Hence, insulin glargine *must not be mixed* with any other form of insulin for injection. Insulin glargine causes lesser hypoglycaemia at night. **Insulin detemir** (Levemir) has a fatty acid side chain (myristic acid) which enhances its binding to albumin. Slow dissociation from albumin results in slow and sustained release. Like insulin glargine, it should not be mixed with any other preparation. **Insulin degludec** (Tresiba), like Insulin detemir, has a fatty acid side chain (hexadecanedioic acid) attached via gamma-L-glutamyl spacer to the amino acid lysine at position B-29. This chain in insulin structure allows for the formation of multi-hexamers to form a subcutaneous depot that results in slow and sustained insulin release into the systemic circulation. It has a duration that lasts for more than 24 hrs, making it an ultra-long acting insulin analogue. Thus a three-times weekly S.C. regimen appears to meet the basal insulin need with fewer episodes of nocturnal hypoglycaemia.
5. ***Inhaled Insulins:*** Inhaled insulins marketed earlier were later withdrawn as they used to get deposited in pharynx causing pharyngitits and pulmonary fibrosis. Antibody formation was another drawback. Currently, two inhaled recombinant human regular insulins (1) EXUBERA prepared by using Nektar Therapeutics Proprietary Technology and (2) AFREZZA prepared by Technosphere Technology has been approved by the FDA. Both are indicated for type-1 as well as type-2 DM. EXUBERA inhalation alone is sufficient for type-2 DM patients but type-1 DM cases still need other type of insulin injection (S.C.) daily in addition to EXUBERA. AFREZZA works like ultra-short acting insulins but inhaled at meal time to control rapid rise in blood glucose levels (Table 47.1). It carries lower risk of causing hypoglycaemia and weight gain. EXUBERA has been withdrawn from the market by its promoter due its less demand by the patient.

Therapeutic Uses

1. For patients with type-1 diabetes (see above): usually NPH insulin is often combined with short-acting regular insulin and is administered S.C. before meals.
2. Many patients with type-2 diabetes ultimately require insulin therapy.
3. For gestational diabetes (if not controlled by diet).
4. ***For emergency treatment of diabetic ketoacidosis (diabetic coma)*:** This emergency is usually faced in the patients suffering from type-1 diabetes. The patients are usually dehydrated, hyperventilating with loss of consciousness. The treatment regimen is as follows:
   - A bolus dose of 0.1 U/kg I.V. of short-acting regular insulin is followed by 0.1 U/kg/hr I.V. infusion till glucose level falls to 300 mg/dL. Then its rate is reduced to 2–3 U/hr (not per kg per hr) till the patient regains consciousness.

- I.V. normal saline to correct dehydration and 5% glucose if the patient shows hypo-glycaemia.
- When insulin is infused and ketoacidosis subsides, K^+ channels open and K^+ is driven intracellularly. This leads to hypokalaemia. Hence 20 mEq/hr I.V. drip of KCl or K_3PO_4 may be given to correct hypokalaemia.
- During ketoacidosis and due to hyperventilation, plasma pH comes down to 6.8 from 7.4. Hence 50 mEq of sodium bicarbonate is added to the I.V. drip. However, it is not routinely needed.
- Other supportive measures if necessary.

5. ***Non-ketonic hyperglycaemic (hyperosmolar) coma***: This usually occurs in elderly type-2 diabetic cases and is characterised by dehydration and haemoconcentration and is usually fatal if untreated. The general principles of treatment are same as for diabetic ketoacidosis except that fluid replacement should be faster along with prophylactic heparin therapy.
6. For emergency treatment of hyperkalaemia, insulin is given with glucose to lower extracellular K^+ *via* redistribution into cells (rare indication).

Adverse Effects

1. ***Hypoglycaemia***: This can occur in any diabetic patient following intensive insulin therapy, or by missing a meal or by performing vigorous exercise. Symptoms include sweating, tremor, palpitation, piloerection, anxiety (due to counter-regulatory sympathetic drive), headache, dizziness, hunger, fatigue and finally coma (due to deprivation of brain of its glucose and essential nutrients). Treatment needs glucose orally or I.V. (in severe cases) or glucagon 0.5 to 1 mg I.V. Normally, a sweet drink or chocolate would suffice.
2. ***Lipodystrophy*** can occur at the site of S.C. injection. It is not a problem with newer preparations. It can be avoided by changing the injection site.
3. ***Allergic manifestations*** (urticaria, angioedema) may be observed with beef or pork insulin but rarely with human insulins.
4. ***Insulin resistance*** seems to have developed if the insulin requirements seem to exceed 100 U/day. It is usually seen with beef/pork insulins and to a lesser degree with human insulins. The mechanism involves development of antibodies to homologous contaminating proteins which also bind insulin.

ORAL HYPOGLYCAEMIC AGENTS

Oral hypoglycaemic agents are used to treat type-2 DM and as their name implies they have the potential to decrease blood glucose to subnormal levels and also promote insulin release from pancreatic β-cells. There are two classes of oral hypoglycaemic agents: The *sulfonylureas* and the *meglitinides*.

Sulfonylureas

Numerous sulfonylureas are now available. ***Tolbutamide*** and ***chlorpropamide*** belong to first generation sulfonylureas but in current clinical practice they have been laid to rest. Their characteristic features have been specified in Table 47.2 along with second generation drugs such as ***glibenclamide (glyburide)***, ***glipizide, gliclazide*** and ***glimepiride***.

Mechanism of Action

1. The main action of sulfonylureas is on β-cells, stimulating insulin secretion and thus reducing blood glucose levels. These drugs reduce the outward K^+ conductance by binding to the sulfonylurea receptors present on ATP-sensitive K^+ channels, causing depolarisation, followed by Ca^{2+} entry and insulin secretion (Fig. 47.2). Thus these drugs are effective only in patients having properly functioning pancreatic β-cells.
2. They also suppress glucagon levels which again indirectly contributes to their hypoglycaemic effects.
3. They also bind to sulfonylurea receptors on the K^+ channels *in extrapancreatic cells* and are believed to increase the number of insulin receptors on target cells particularly in liver. However, the significance and validity of these findings are debatable.

4) *Glimepiride, gliclazide* and *glipizide* have an additional effect, that is, they increase the sensitivity of peripheral tissues to insulin.

Table 47.2 Important Features of Sulfonylureas

Drug (dose)	Onset	Duration	Comments*
I Generation			
Tolbutamide	1 hr	6–12 hrs	Weaker, short acting, less likely to cause hypoglycaemia
Chlorpropamide	1 hr	24–60 hrs	More potent, longest acting, can cause prolonged hypoglycaemia; also potentiates ADH action
II Generation			
Glibenclamide or Glyburide (5–15 mg OD or BD)	1–4 hrs	10–24 hrs	150 times more potent than tolbutamide; may cause severe hypoglycaemia
Glipizide (5–20 mg OD or BD)	1–3 hrs	10–24 hrs	100 times more potent than tolbutamide; may cause prolonged hypoglycaemia. Less weight gain
Gliclazide (40–250 mg OD or BD)	1–3 hrs	10–24 hrs	12 times more potent than tolbutamide; has antioxidant action; less weight gain; has antiplatelet action also
Glimepiride (1–6 mg OD)	1–3 hrs	10–24 hrs	Same as glipizide but more potent and less hypoglycaemia

* For other effects see text

Glimepiride and *gliclazide* have antioxidant action also.

Pharmacokinetics

Sulfonylureas are well absorbed after oral administration. Glipizide absorption is delayed by food. All sulfonylureas are highly protein bound (90–98%). Plasma protein binding is highest for glimepiride (98%). These are metabolised in liver and/or kidney and excreted in urine. The duration of action for II generation sulfonylureas is 24 hrs.

Adverse Effects

Side effects with second generation drugs are less often compared to first generation drugs. The most important adverse effect is hypoglycaemia which, if severe, can lead to coma. Hypoglycaemia is a particular problem in elderly patients with impaired hepatic and renal functions who are taking longer-acting sulfonylureas. These drugs are less effective in severely obese type-2 diabetics possibly because of the insulin resistance that often accompanies obesity. Sulfonylureas also tend to cause weight gain due to fluid retention and oedema. These cross placental barrier and may cause foetal hypoglycaemia or hypoglycaemia at birth. Hence, these are not used in gestational diabetes and contraindicated in pregnancy. Sulfonylureas (particularly chlorpro-pamide) inhibit aldehyde dehydrogenase and exhibit a disulfiram-like effect with alcohol. Rare side effects include photosensitivity, skin rash, blood dyscrasias and cholestatic jaundice.

Drug Interactions

1. Drugs that potentiate the effects of sulfonylureas are:
   - Oral anticoagulants, ketoconazole, chloramphenicol and MAOIs inhibit their metabolism;

while probenecid and allopurinol decrease their urinary excretion.
- Salicylates, sulfonamides and clofibrate (these agents displace them from protein binding sites).
- Non-selective β-blockers, e.g., propranolol (which masks the symptoms of sulfonylureas induced hypoglycaemia and also synergise their action; for details refer Ch. 12).

2. Drugs that decrease the effects of sulfonylureas are:
   - Phenobarbitone, phenytoin and rifampicin (these agents induce the metabolism of sulfonylureas).
   - Corticosteroids, diazoxide, thiazides, estrogens and thyroid hormones (they suppress insulin release or antagonise its effects).

Meglitinide Analogues

These are quick and short-acting *insulin secretion enhancers* (*insulin secretagogues*). Their mode of action is similar to sulfonylureas, that is, they stimulate insulin release from pancreatic β-cells.

Because of their rapid onset of action, these drugs are administered shortly before a meal to reduce the postprandial glucose rise in type-2 diabetic patients, inadequately controlled with diet and exercise. Hence, ***hypoglycaemia is a great risk*** if the meal is delayed or skipped. These drugs usually cause less weight gain and are less allergenic than sulfonylureas. Later in the course of disease, they can be combined with metformin or glitazones (see below). Two drugs which belong to this series are:

Repaglinide: Onset of action 1 hr; duration of action 4–5 hrs; dose 0.25–4 mg orally before each meal.

Nateglinide: It is a D-phenylalanine derivative; onset of action 1 hr; duration of action 4–5 hrs; dose 60–120 mg orally before each meal. Lower risk for hypoglycaemia.

ANTIHYPERGLYCAEMIC AGENTS

Antihyperglycaemic agents refer to a category of drugs that are capable of lowering elevated levels of blood glucose but which have relatively little potential to produce hypoglycaemia. None of them promote insulin release as discussed above.

Biguanides

Phenformin and ***metformin*** are two drugs which belong to the group biguanides. Out of these, phenformin has been discontinued as it causes lactoacidosis and is devoid of any long-term benefits. ***Metformin*** is the only drug in this class that is being currently used.

The currently proposed mechanisms of metformin action include: **(1)** increased uptake and utilisation of glucose by skeletal muscles, which reduces insulin resistance, **(2)** inhibition of hepatic as well as renal gluconeogenesis, which decreases hepatic glucose output, **(3)** slowing of glucose absorption from GIT, which increases availability of glucose for its conversion to lactate by enterocytes and **(4)** promotion of insulin binding to its receptor. Unlike sulfonylureas it does not lower blood glucose levels in normal persons, does not stimulate insulin release, i.e., it does not depend on functional pancreatic β-cells for its action and can be given to obese patients as it does not cause weight gain. Besides lowering elevated blood glucose levels, it also lowers LDL, VLDL and elevates HDL levels. When used as monotherapy, metformin rarely causes hypoglycaemia.

It has a plasma half-life of 2–3 hrs and duration of action of about 6–10 hrs. It is not bound to plasma proteins, not metabolised and is excreted unchanged by the kidneys.

Clinical use of metformin is in the patients with type-2 diabetes. Instead of stimulating appetite it causes anorexia and for this reason metformin is often the first choice drug in the treatment of obese type-2 diabetic cases. It can be combined with sulfonylureas, meglitinides and with glitazones to treat insulin resistance syndrome. Metformin therapy decreases the risk of macrovascular as well as microvascular disease. A most common drug treatment schedule is to give 500 mg metformin tablet with breakfast and a second 500 mg tablet with evening meal. *Adverse effects* of metformin are nausea, metallic taste, anorexia, flatulence and diarrhoea (which in 3–5% cases may be persistent). Long-term use may decrease absorption of vitamin B_{12} (additional supplements may be needed). Lactic acidosis normally is a rare problem, yet patients of renal or hepatic disease, hypoxic pulmonary disease or heart failure are predisposed to lactic acidosis because of reduced drug elimination or reduced tissue oxygenation. Alcohol ingestion can also precipitate severe lactic acidosis because alcohol potentiates the effects of metformin on lactate metabolism. ***Non-diabetic use***: Metformin has also been used to treat hirsutism in individuals with polycystic ovarian syndrome and may enhance fertility in these women perhaps by decreasing androgen levels and enhancing insulin sensitivity.

α-Glucosidase Inhibitors

Acarbose, ***miglitol*** and ***voglibose*** are the three drugs which belong to this group. The α-glucosidase enzyme facilitates digestion of complex starches, oligosaccharides and disaccharides into monosaccharides so that these are absorbed from the small intestine. This digestion is also facilitated by pancreatic α-amylase. The α-glucosidase inhibitors are competitive inhibitors of intestinal α-glucosidases as well as of α-amylase. Thus, these drugs reduce postprandial digestion and absorption of carbohydrates and thus lower postmeal hyperglycaemia. Regular use also tends to lower HbA_{1C}, body weight and serum triglycerides. Acarbose is usually taken in a dose of 50–100 mg TDS at the beginning of each major meal. They do not directly affect insulin secretion. Acarbose is minimally absorbed but miglitol is, however, absorbed. Some part of acarbose is excreted as such through faeces while a part is metabolised by intestinal bacterial flora.

Adverse effects include flatulence, diarrhoea and abdominal pain due to fermentation of undigested carbohydrates in the lower GIT. They do not cause hypoglycaemia by themselves but may cause when used with sulfonylureas. If that occurs, it should be corrected by giving glucose, not sucrose, because its breakdown by these drugs is already blocked. Miglitol has mild lactase inhibitory action but somehow does not lead to lactose intolerance. These drugs are contraindicated in inflammatory bowel disease and intestinal obstruction. These drugs are used as monotherapy in early type-2 diabetes and with sulfonylureas in obese type-2 patients.

Thiazolidinediones (Glitazones)

Glitazones are a newer class of antihyperglycaemic agents. Two drugs in this class, ***rosiglitazone*** and ***pioglitazone***, are in current use.

Mechanism of action: **(1)** glitazones act as agonist to a nuclear receptor called **P**eroxisome **P**roliferator-**A**ctivated **R**eceptor-gamma (PPAR-γ), which is expressed mainly in adipose tissue, skeletal muscle and liver. Activation of PPAR-γ promotes transcription of insulin responsive genes which control glucose and lipid metabolism (see Ch. 7 also). This increases insulin sensitivity and decreases insulin resistance in patients of type-2 DM. **(2)** Glitazones also increase the number of GLUT-4 glucose transporters (Fig. 47.3) in cell membranes of skeletal muscle and adipose tissues, which promotes peripheral uptake and utilisation of glucose. **(3)** They also decrease hepatic glucose output by inhibiting gluconeogenesis. **(4)** They decrease HbA_{1C} levels. **(5)** They increase HDL-C and lower triglyceride levels. Rosiglitazone increases LDL-C but pioglitazone has variable effects.

The patients who would benefit the most from the glitazones are of type-2 diabetes exhibiting substantial amount of insulin resistance, i.e., who require high doses of insulin (>100 U/day).

Pioglitazone is administered in a dose of 11–45 mg once daily orally; duration of effect lasts for more than 24 hrs. ***Rosiglitazone*** is given in a dose of 4–8 mg once daily; duration of action is same as for pioglitazone. However,the insulin sensitising action of glitazones takes several weeks to develop. Secondly, if a glitazone is to be added to the diabetic regimen, the dosage of sulfonylureas or of insulin should be decreased to compensate for any enhanced insulin sensitivity. These are also used in combination with metformin.

Adverse effects include weight gain, which is attributable to fluid retention and oedema. There is also an increase in the extravascular fluid, increased deposition of subcutaneous fat and haemodilution leading to a concomitant reduction in haemoglobin concentration. Hepatotoxicity with pioglitazone and rosiglitazone is rare, yet regular liver function tests are advisable. Glitazones are contraindicated in hepatic failure, pregnancy, lactating mother, in children and in heart failure (cause fluid retention). It is quite possible that these drugs could cause ovulation to resume in women who are anovulatory because they decrease insulin resistance (e.g., in polycystic ovary syndrome). Recent clinical trials cast doubts on their future role in treating diabetes because they increase the risk of heart failure and myocardial infarction. Rosiglitazone has been withdrawn from Indian market.

Incretin-mimetics

Incretins are a group of metabolic hormones that include **G**lucagon-**L**ike **P**eptide-**1** (GLP-1) and **G**lucose-dependent **I**nsulinotropic **P**olypeptide (GIP) that are released after meals from the upper and lower bowel and augment glucose-dependent insulin release, during the phase of nutrient absorption from the GIT. The GLP-1 has a very short half-life (1–2 min) and is metabolised quickly by **Dip**eptidyl **P**eptidase **IV** (DPP-IV) enzyme.

Exenatide is a long acting analogue (resistant to DPP-IV degradation) obtained from the salivary gland venom of Gila monster. It is a potent agonist at GLP-1 receptor (incretin mimetic). It is orally inactive and hence given S.C. 30–60 min before meals. Being GLP-1 receptor agonist it **(1)** stimulates insulin secretion from β-cells of pancreas, **(2)** decreases glucagon release, **(3)** slows the rate of nutrient absorption by slowing gastric emptying and **(4)** decreases appetite by acting at the level of hypothalamus (induces weight loss). It is used along with metformin and/or sulfonylureas particularly in resistant type-2 DM patients. *Adverse effects:* nausea, anorexia, diarrhoea and necrotising pancreatitis (rarely).

Liraglutide, ***albiglutide***, ***dulaglutide semaglutide*** are recently developed long acting GLP-1 agonists given once weekly by SC injection in type-II DM (see Ch. 72 for detailed description).

Dipeptidyl Peptidase-4 (DPP-4) Inhibitors

Sitagliptin, ***vildagliptin***, ***saxagliptin***, ***linagliptin***, and ***alogliptin***, are orally active selective inhibitors of DPP-4 enzyme that inactivates GLP-1. As a result GLP-1 levels are increased to more than double and its actions prolonged. Consequently these drugs **(1)** increase insulin secretion, **(2)** decrease glucagon release, **(3)** delay gastric emptying and **(4)** suppress appetite and weight (as discussed above). These have a longer t½. They are also used along with metformin and/or sulfonylureas for resistant type-2 DM patients. *Adverse effects:* Nasopharyngitis (because substance-P is also a substrate for DPP-4 whose levels get elevated); GIT distress and diarrhoea. As discussed above it rarely produces hypoglycaemia unless used with sulfonylureas. Successful sitagliptin therapy requires adequate levels of GLP-1 which may not be feasible in patients taking strict carbohydrate-free diet. Secondly, DPP-4 metabolises several other peptides as well (e.g., substance-P, GHRH and neuropeptide-Y).

Amylin-mimetic Drugs

Amylin is a neuroendocrine peptide hormone co-secreted with insulin from pancreatic B-cells. Its role is to **(1)** inhibit glucagon secretion, **(2)** delay gastric emptying and **(3)** suppress appetite. ***Pramlintide*** is a modified amylin peptide which is an agonist at amylin receptor (a G-protein coupled receptor). It is used as an adjunct to insulin in type-1 DM cases and insulin requiring type-2 DM patients. *Adverse effects:* nausea, diarrhoea and headache.

Sodium-Glucose Cotransporter-2 (SGLT-2) Inhibitors

SGLT-2 inhibitors [(e.g., ***dapagliflozin*** (2.5–10 mg/day), ***canagliflozin, empagliflozin*** (10–25 mg/day)], are newer, orally effective, antidiabetic drugs that have been approved, whereas ***sergliflozin*** and ***remogliflozin*** are undergoing phase III clinical trials. The kidney continuously filters glucose through glomerulus and nearly all of this glucose is reabsorbed back from the proximal tubule by a transporter called sodium-glucose cotransporter-2 (SGLT-2). Inhibiting SGLT-2 decreases the amount of glucose reabsorption from the proximal tubule and increases its excretion in urine. SGLT-2 is exclusively distributed on the proximal tubule of the kidney. These drugs have greater efficacy in the diabetic kidney to excrete excess glucose from the blood. ***Ertugliflozin***: It is a selective sodium-glucose transporter-2 (SGLT2) inhibitor. It decreases renal reabsorption of glucose and increases its excretion. It can be given orally as monotherapy or incombination with other drugs. ***Advantages:*** SGLT-2 inhibitors cause **(1)** weight loss, **(2)** no hypoglycaemia as they are excreting only the excess of glucose from the blood and not inducing insulin secretion, **(3)** improve insulin resistance by depleting toxic levels of glucose and **(4)** beneficial effects in patients of DM with hypertension because of their diuretic effects. ***Disadvantages:*** **(1)** Because of polyuria (glucosuria) there would be more polydipsia, **(2)** Increased risk of urinary bacterial/fungal infection in presence of glucosuria and **(3)** Risk of Na^{2+} loss also, as sodium-glucose cotransporter has been inhibited.

NEW ORAL DRUGS FOR DIABETES MELLITUS

1. Dopamine Receptor Agonist: *Bromocriptine*

Bromocriptine reduces HbA1c levels by less than or equal to 0.5% in poorly controlled diabetic patients, who are treated with diet alone or with one or the other antidiabetic oral drug. The drug may cause nausea, dizziness, headache and vomiting. A suppression of hepatic glucose production by a dopamine-induced modulation of hepatic-hypothalamic circuitary as bromocriptine has no effect on insulin secretion or insulin sensitivity in peripheral tissues.

2. Bile Acid Sequestrant Resin: *Colesevelam*

The drug, ***colesevelam***, is a bile acid binding and cholesterol lowering agent (see Ch. 23), which has recently been approved as an antihyperglycaemic agent for persons with type 2 diabetes who are taking other medications or have not achieved adequate control with diet and exercise. It involves an interruption of entero-hepatic circulation of bile, leading to a decrease in the farnesoid X-receptor (FXR) activation. Bile acids are natural ligands of FXR and the latter is a nuclear receptor, which affects bile acid cholesterol and glucose metabolism. Indirectly it may be related to altered G protein-coupled membrane receptor, **TGR 5** [**T**akeda **G** protein **R**eceptor **5**, which is also known as **G P**rotein-coupled **B**ile **A**cid **R**eceptor-**1 (GP-BAR-1)** or **M**embrane **B**ile **A**cid **R**eceptor **(M-BAR)**] present on the intestinal mucosal surface, resulting in an increased secretion of GLP-1 or other incretins and an inhibition of hepatic glycogenolysis.

3. Dual PPAR-alpha and PPAR-gamma Receptor Agonist: Saroglitazar (affinity for PPAR-α > PPAR-γ).

Recently a novel class of agents have been developed, which act as balanced agonist on both the **P**eroxisome **P**roliferator-**A**ctivated **R**eceptors-alpha and gamma **(PPAR-α/γ)**. Agonistic action at PPAR-alpha (like fibrates) targets lipid levels, which improves dyslipidaemia and agonistic action at PPAR-gamma (like glitazones) targets glucose level, which improves peripheral glucose sensitivity and glycaemic index in diabetes. One such agent, ***saroglitazar*** is a predominantly PPAR-α agonist with moderate PPAR-γ agonist activity. When administered in oral doses of 2–4 mg per day, demonstrated dose-related and clinically meaningful effects in glycaemic parameters (reduction in HbA1c by about 0.6–0.8% compared to placebo). However, weight gain, concern for heart failure and bone fractures are some adverse effects noted in clinical studies.

4. Teplizumab

Type 1 diabetes (T1D) is an autoimmune disorder in which T cell-mediated destruction of pancreatic β cells occur. The T cell receptor (TCR) comprises TCR α and β chains together with six CD3 molecules, including two CD3 ε chains. It is responsible for recognizing antigens on the MHC complex to elicit an immune response. Teplizumab, a humanized IgG1 antibody, specific for the ε chain of CD3 and inhibits T cell activation through steric inhibition of antigen recognition. Recently, teplizumab has shown efficacy in delaying the time to diagnosis in patients at high risk of developing T1D. It is injected i.v. as the first and only recently approved treatment by US-FDA to delay the onset of type 1 diabetes (T1D) in adults and paediatric patients aged 8 years and older. Adverse effects are lymphopenia, leukopenia, anaemia, serious infections, headache and cytokine release syndrome.

Tirzepatide

It is a recently approved dual glucose-dependent insulinotropic polypeptide (GIP) and glucagon-like peptide-1 (GLP-1) receptor agonist. Pharmacodynamic effects observed include lower fasting and postprandial glucose concentration, decreased food intake and reduced body weight. It is given subcutaneously every week injection. It is used as an adjunct to diet and exercise to improve glycaemic control in adults with type 2 diabetes mellitus. *Adverse effects* are nausea diarrhaea, decreased appetite, abdominal pain, injection site reaction and allergic reactions.

CHAPTER 48

SECTION 9—DRUGS ACTING ON RESPIRATORY SYSTEM

Drug Therapy of Bronchial Asthma

COMPETENCY PH1.32

The term asthma is derived from the Greek word meaning "to stay awake in order to breathe" or "difficulty in breathing". Asthma is a chronic inflammatory disease in which the patient suffers from reversible episodes of airways obstruction due to bronchial hyper-responsiveness. However, chronic inflammation can lead to irreversible airways obstruction later. In the early acute phase, besides smooth muscle spasm, there is excessive secretion of mucus that may clog the bronchi and bronchioles and worsen the attack. In the late (chronic or delayed) phase, inflammation continues, accompanied by fibrosis, oedema and necrosis (death) of bronchial epithelial cells. Though the world-wide incidence is up to 5% of adult population and up to 10% of children, yet there is a growing concern about its pharmacotherapy as fatalities usually occur and mortality rates are reported to be increasing day by day.

The cardinal symptoms of asthma are breathlessness, wheezing, cough and chest tightness with worsening of these symptoms at night. In an acute attack, the respiratory rate is rapid and tachycardia is common. The peak expiratory flow (PEF), forced expiratory volume per second (FEV_1) and maximal mid-expiratory flow (MMEF), all get decreased in asthma. In acute attack, PEF and FEV_1 are usually less than 50% of normal value with MMEF of about 20% of the predicted value. The increased resistance to air flow results due to multiple factors (see below) including bronchoconstriction, bronchial secretions with shedding of epithelium and thickening of the airway smooth muscle.

Asthma may be described as *extrinsic* when it is associated with exposure to specific allergen (pollen or house dust mite). This may be *atopic* or *non-atopic extrinsic asthma.* Majority of patients suffer from atopic extrinsic asthma. Sensitisation with specific vaccine may help such patients. In others, the attack may be stimulated by some non-specific stimulus, e.g., chemical irritants. In such cases, IgG and IgM antibodies circulate in the blood but are not attached to mast cells or basophils. Neutrophils ingest these antigen-antibody complexes and destroy them. As a result, lysosomal enzymes are liberated which digest the remaining mucoproteins. Drugs which can stabilise the lysosomal membrane, e.g., glucocorticoids (see below), provide relief to these patients. This is termed as *non-atopic extrinsic asthma.* In contrast, a large number of patients (specially those who acquire asthma after the age of 40 yrs) have no identifiable external precipitating factor or immunological basis for asthmatic attack. This is termed as *intrinsic asthma.* Many patients may have both extrinsic and intrinsic forms of asthma. *Extrinsic asthma* is episodic and less prone to develop into *status asthmaticus,* while *intrinsic asthma* is perennial and is more prone to develop into *status asthmaticus. Status asthmaticus* is a severe acute asthma, which is life-threatening condition involving exhaustion, cyanosis, bradycardia, hypotension, dehydration and metabolic acidosis. *Cardiac asthma* is a bronchospasm precipitated by uncompensated congestive heart failure (Ch. 22).

PATHOPHYSIOLOGY OF ASTHMA AND NEUROHUMORAL CONTROL OF AIRWAYS

In a conceptual model of asthma (Fig. 48.1), antigens (pollen or house-dust mites) sensitise individuals by eliciting the production of IgE type of antibodies which remain either circulating in the blood or become attached to the mast cells (of nasal/bronchial tissues) and basophils. On re-exposure to the same antigen, the resulting antigen-antibody reaction on the surface of lung mast cells causes their degranulation releasing spasmogens such as histamine, serotonin, PGD_2 and cysteinyl leukotrienes (LTC_4 and LTD_4). Both LTC_4 and LTD_4 are powerful bronchoconstrictors and are primary components of the slow reacting substance of anaphylaxis (SRS-A; Ch. 25). The release of these mediators *in early phase* leads to broncho-constriction but *in late phase*, inflammation continues, accompanied by pulmonary oedema, mucus secretion, bronchial hyper-reactivity and epithelial damage (see below).

Mast cells also release other leukotrienes (LTB_4) and cytokines (IL-4, IL-5 and IL-13). In the late (delayed) phase, these chemotactic mediators recruit and activate additional inflammatory cells, e.g., eosinophils, basophils and alveolar macrophages which are also rich sources of leukotrienes and cytokines. During this phase, there is also a release of eosinophil cationic protein (ECP; a toxic protein) and eosinophil derived neurotoxin causing damage and loss of epithelium. The epithelial damage means that irritant receptors and C-fibres are more exposed to irritant stimuli—a basis for airway hyper-responsiveness to released chemical mediators. Other putative (famous) mediators of inflammatory process, in delayed phase, are *adenosine* (bronchoconstriction; acting on A_1/A_3 receptors, Ch. 35), *various neuropeptides* (*substance-P* causing mucus secretion and increase in vascular permeability; and *neurokinin-A* causing bronchoconstriction, Ch. 17) and *platelet activating factor* (PAF; producing inflammation, increased vascular permeability, chemotaxis of neutrophils and eosinophils, broncho-constriction and bronchial hyper-reactivity, Ch. 25). (Fig. 48.1)

The normal tone of the bronchial smooth muscle is influenced by a balance between parasympathetic, sympathetic and non–noradrenergic-noncholinergic (NANC) mediators activity. Adenosine also plays an important role in the maintenance of bronchial tone as well. The predominant tone, however, is parasympathetic. Activation of M_3 receptors (on bronchial smooth muscle) by the release of acetylcholine results in an increase in cGMP levels, which leads to bronchoconstriction and an increase in mucus secretions. The sympathetic innervation of the airways is, however, very sparse. Sympathetic nerves innervate only blood vessels (causing vaso-constriction) and glands (inhibiting secretions) *but not bronchial smooth muscle. All sympathetic effects (e.g., bronchodilation and decrease in mucus secretions) are provided by circulating catecholamines.* However, there are β_2 receptors on the bronchial smooth muscle, the epithelium, the glands and on mast cells. β_2-Adrenoceptor stimulation leads to an increase in 3,5-cAMP levels which results in bronchodilation (Fig. 48.1). The neuronal mediators other than ACh and NE also affect airway function. For example, the main NANC inhibitory neurotransmitter is nitric oxide (bronchodilation), while NANC excitatory transmitters are neuropeptides (neurokinin-A and substance-P) released from unmyelinated sensory C-fibres when stimulated by inflammatory mediators and irritant chemicals (e.g., SO_2 and cigarette smoke).

CLASSIFICATION OF DRUGS USED IN THE TREATMENT OF ASTHMA

Bronchodilators

1. ***Selective β_2-Agonist Drugs***
   - ***Short Acting β_2-Agonists (SABAs)***
     Salbutamol (albuterol), Terbutaline, Remiterol, Fenoterol, Pirbuterol, Bitoterol, Levalbuterol
   - ***Long Acting β_2-Agonists (LABAs)***
     Salmeterol, Formoterol, Eformoterol, Bambuterol, Indacaterol, Olodaterol
2. ***Nonselective Sympathomimetics***
   Epinephrine, Ephedrine, Isoprenaline, Orciprenaline (metaproterenol)
3. ***Anti-cholinergic/Anti-muscarinic Drugs***
   - ***Short Acting Muscarinic (Receptor) Antogonists (SAMAs)***
     Ipratropium, Oxitropium
   - ***Long Acting Muscarinic (Receptor) Antagonists (LAMAs)***
     Tiotropium, Glycopyrronium, Aclidinium, Umeclidinium
4. ***Methylxanthines***
   Theophylline, Aminophylline, Diprophylline, Choline-theophyllinate, Doxophylline

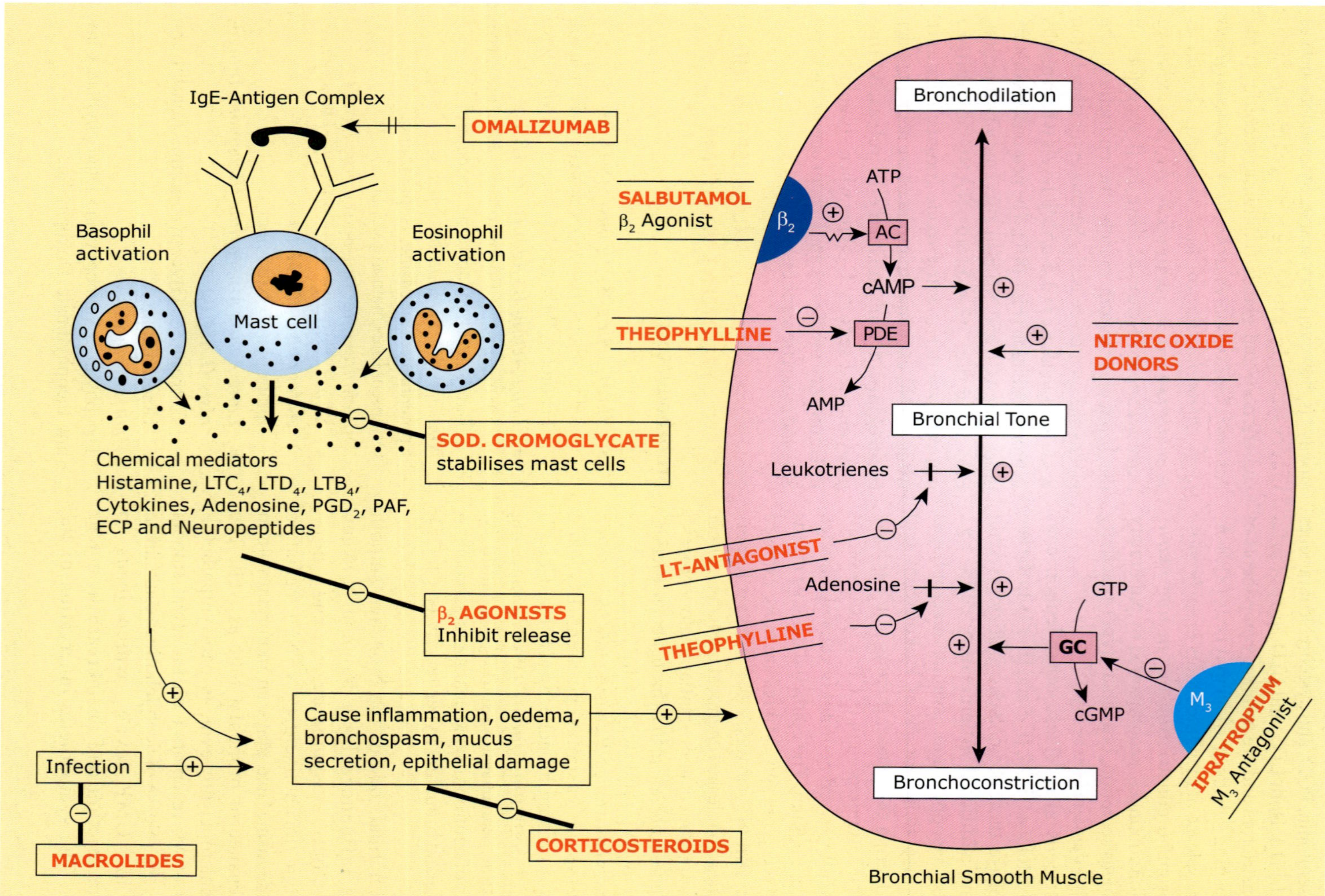

Key: AC—Adenylyl Cyclase; GC—Guanylate Cyclase; PDE—Phosphodiesterase

Fig 48.1 Pathophysiology, Neurohumoral Control and Treatment Strategy for Asthma.

Corticosteroids

1. ***Oral:*** Prednisone, Prednisolone and Methylprednisolone, Dexamethasone, Betamethasone
2. ***Parenteral:*** Hydrocortisone, Methylprednisolone
3. ***Inhalational:*** Beclomethasone dipropionate, Fluticasone propionate/furoate, Budesonide, Flunisolide, Ciclesonide, Triamcinolone, Mometasone

Mast Cell Stabilisers

Sodium cromoglycate (cromolyn sodium), Nedocromil

Leukotriene Modulators

1. *5-Lipoxygenase Inhibitor:* Zileuton
2. *Cysteinyl Leukotriene–Receptor Antagonists (LTRAs):* Zafirlukast, Montelukast, Iralukast, Pranlukast

Monoclonal Anti-IgE Antibody

Omalizumab

Miscellaneous Anti-asthma Drugs

Benralizumab, Tezepelumab, Mepolizumab, Dupilumab, Reslizumab, Nitric oxide donors

DRUG TREATMENT OF ASTHMA

Bronchodilators

When administered in therapeutic doses and by an appropriate route, bronchodilators relieve asthmatic symptoms and improve pulmonary functions by relaxing the bronchial smooth muscle. Since these agents provide a rapid symptomatic relief but do not control the disease process, these are often termed as *relievers* (or *rescue drugs*). These include nonselective sympathomimetics, selective β_2 agonists, methylxanthines and antimuscarinic drugs like ipratropium, titropium and others.

1. Selective β_2-Agonist Drugs

This group of drugs has become the mainstay of modern bronchodilator therapy. The basic pharmacological features of these drugs have been presented in Chapter 12. Here we review their pharmacology relevant to asthma. These agents are subclassified into two classes:

- ***Short acting β_2-Agonists (SABAs)***
  Salbutamol (albuterol), Terbutaline, Remiterol, Fenoterol, Pirbuterol, Bitoterol
- ***Long acting β_2-Agonists (LABAs)***
  Salmeterol, Formoterol, Eformoterol, Bambuterol, Indacaterol, Olodaterol

Both SABA and LABA group of drugs activate β_2-adrenoceptors present on airway smooth muscle and enhance the release of cAMP by activating adenylyl cyclase enzyme (Fig. 48.1) The mast cells have β_2-adrenergic receptors which also respond to them.

Hence these drugs **(a)** relax airway smooth muscle, **(b)** inhibit the release of broncho-constricting chemical mediators from the mast cells, **(c)** inhibit microvascular leakage, and **(d)** increase the mucociliary transport by increasing the ciliary activity. However, *the best characterized actions of β_2-adrenoceptor agonists are relaxation of airway smooth muscle (bronchodilation) and inhibition of mediator release finally leading to reversal of asthmatic attack.*

Most SABA drugs act rapidly with an onset of action of 5–15 min, a peak effect at 30–60 min, and a duration of action of approximately 4–6 hrs. This time course of drug action makes these drugs good agents for use as asthma relievers (or rescue drugs). However, this profile also makes these drugs poor agents for the relief of nocturnal asthma and for prevention of attack although they can be used prophylactically before exposure to a known trigger such as exercise.

Among SABAs salbutamol and terbutaline are most commonly used drugs. These can be administered either by inhalation or orally. However, selectivity of action is less when the drug is given orally. These can also be given by I.V. or I.M. route but inhalational route is more preferred. When inhaled, these drugs produce effective bronchodilation with minimal cardiac stimulation (resulting from β_1 stimulatory effect). Inhaled SABAs are normally the drugs of choice for managing acute attack of bronchial asthma (bronchospasm) because they are less likely to activate other adrenoceptors. Terbutaline is perhaps the only bronchodilator which can be used safely during pregnancy.

LABAs are highly lipid soluble with a half-life much longer (6–12 hrs) than SABAs (2–4 hrs).

The prolonged action of salmeterol is believed to be due to a long lipophilic part in its structure which binds to an "exosite" in the vicinity to β_2-adrenoceptor on airway smooth muscle. As a result, the local availability of drug functions as a slow-release depot that provides the drug to adjacent β_2-receptors over a longer period. The LABAs are not recommended for acute relief of asthma due to their delayed onset of action (30–60 min). As such these drugs have a long duration of action (12–24 hrs), making them good candidates for prevention of bronchial spasm. Although *salmeterol*, *formoterol* and *eformoterol* due to their comparative short onset of action (15–30 min) and long duration of action (12–24 hrs) make them good candidates as relievers/ controllers of asthma attack, these do not affect the underlying inflammation. In fact regular use of *salmeterol*, *formoterol* has been found to be associated with an increased in asthma deaths. Although the exact mechanism of this serious ADR is not known, there is a posibility that these LABAs can improve the chronic symptoms of asthma without affecting the underlying risk of severe asthma exacerbation. Because patients may feel better on LABA durg therapy, they may use lower doses of inhaled corticosteroids or not use inhaled corticosteroids at all. Since inhaled corticosteroids reduce the risk of exacerbation of asthma (for reason see below), the reduction or withdrawal of inhaled corticosteroids may put the patient at increased risk of suffering a fatal asthma attack leading to hospitalization or even death.

It is for these reasons, it is important to note that none of LABAs have been approved for the treatment of bronchial asthma but only for the treatment of chronic obstructive pulmonary disease (COPD). Besides LABAs are particularly useful for treating nocturnal asthma or for long-term prevention of asthma attacks (as controllers or preventers) but *always to be used not alone but with co-inhalation with a corticosteroid or with a SAMA or LAMA*.

The *adverse effects* of β_2-agonists are minimal when they are inhaled and this is a preferred route of their inhalation. Administration by oral route is associated with *muscle tremors* (due to direct stimulation of β_2-receptors in skeletal muscle) and *tachycardia* (due to stimulation of chronotropic β_2 receptors and in high doses β_1 receptors in the heart) and restlessness. Continued use of these agents, especiallty LABAs usually results in desensitization/down-regulation of β_2 receptors that results in diminished responsiveness. Concomitant use of glucocorticoid can prevent or partly reverse this phenomenon. However, concurrent use of glucocorticoids or methyl-xanthines can produce hypokalaemia that should be watched carefully. Recently, there has been a concern over myocardial toxicity from fluorocarbon propellants contained in commercially available aerosol pereparations of β_2-agonists when they are administered by inhalation. Fluorocarbons sensitise the myocardium to toxic effects of catecholamines (albeit in higher doses).

2. Nonselective sympathomimetics

Epinephrine, Ephedrine, Isoprenaline, and Orciprenaline (metaproterenol)

The non-selective sympathomimetics that can be used for the treatment of asthma include epinephrine, ephedrine, isoproterenol and orciprenaline (metaproterenol). Among these, epinephrine activates both α as well as β-receptors, while isosproterenol and metaproterenol activate selectively β-adrenoceptors but do not discriminate between β_1 and β_2-adrenoceptors. However, they have a higher affinity for β_2 receptors which are predominant in bronchial muscle. Because of their non-selective action, which leads to cardiac stimulation, their use has declined.

Epinephrine is now rarely used, but was a drug of choice for the acute attack of asthma when β_2 agonists were not available. When injected S.C., it causes an effective and rapid bronchodilation. Because it stimulates α, β_1 as well as β_2 receptors, its use is associated with troublesome adverse effects, e.g., tachycardia, hypertension, worsening of angina and even arrhythmias. It can be given as aerosol also. It is sometimes used (S.C.) to treat status asthmaticus because besides bronchodilation it also reduces pulmonary oedema as a consequence of pulmonary vasoconstriction due to α-adrenoceptor activation.

Metaproterenol is a longer acting derivative of isoproterenol with more prominent β_2 action. The incidence and severity of side effects are less than isoproterenol. It can be given orally or by inhalation. It has also been superceded by β_2 agonists.

3. Anti-cholinergic/Anti-muscarinic Drugs

- ***Short Acting Muscarinic (Receptor) Antogonists (SAMAs)***
  Ipratropium, Oxitropium
- ***Long Acting Muscarinic (Receptor) Antagonists (LAMAs)***
  Tiotropium, Glycopyrronium, Aclidinium, Umeclidinium

The muscarinic receptor antagonists used for the treatment of asthma include aerosol preparations of ***SAMAs (ipratropium, oxitropium)*** and ***LAMAs (tiotropium, glycopyrronium, aclidinium, umeclidinium).*** However, all these agents are quarternary ammonium compounds and as a result produce less effective bronchodilation than β_2-agonists. They cause bronchodilation by binding to M_3 receptors on airway smooth muscle and thereby preventing the action of acetylcholine (ACh) released from parasympathetic nerves. They act by reducing the cGMP levels in bronchial muscle by blocking M_3 receptors (Fig. 48.1).

However, these drugs do not differentiate between M_2 (presynaptic autoreceptors) and M_3 (postsynaptic) receptors. Hence, subsequent release of ACh due to M_2 receptor blockade usually reduces their effectiveness. When administered by inhalational route, being quaternary compounds, they do not exhibit unwanted anticholinergic side effects due to their poor absorption from bronchial mucosa into systemic circulation. These also decrease mucus secretion (like atropine) but have less drying effect on mucus and minimize the chances of forming mucus plugs (unlike atropine). They do not cross BBB either, and are devoid of CNS side effects. ***Tiotropium*** *is a longer acting derivative of* ***ipratropium***. Combination of ***ipratropium*** with a short acting ***β_2-agonist (salbutamol)*** works better in severe asthma and has longer duration of action than either drug alone. Still, their efficacy in asthma is usually modest compared to their efficacy in COPD (Ch. 49). Side effects in therapeutic doses are negligible, except for bad taste and dryness of mouth after inhalation.

However, LAMAs may produce urinary retention in elderly and therefore, should be given cautiously in patients with BPH.

4. Methylxanthines

Theophylline, Aminophylline, Diprophylline and Choline-theophyllinate, Doxophylline

These drugs have been covered extensively in Ch. 35. The beneficial effects of methylxanthines in asthma are believed to be mediated through: **(a)** inhibition of phosphodiesterase III (present in airway smooth muscle) and IV (present in eosinophil and mast cells), the two specific isoenzymes responsible for the metabolism of cAMP. The cAMP levels, therefore, get elevated leading to bronchodilation, and also by **(b)** blockade of adenosine receptors on airway muscles (A_1) and those present on mast cells (A_3) (Fig. 48.1). Theophylline exhibits bronchodilatory, anti-inflammatory and immunomodulatory effects. The main use of theophylline group of drugs is in the management of asthma and to treat COPD. Theophylline is also used to relieve dyspnoea associated with pulmonary oedema that develops from congestive heart failure. However, theophyllines are generally used as combination therapy with β_2 agonists. Its narrow therapeutic window and the propensity for interactions with many drugs make theophylline a drug of second choice in asthma. Its therapeutic plasma levels should be between 10–20 μg/ml.

At plasma levels above 20 μg/ml there is nausea and vomiting (a CNS stimulant effect). Above 40 μg/ml, there are tremors followed by seizures, agitation, diuresis, arrhythmias and fever. For drug interactions see Ch. 35. Enzyme inducers such as phenytoin, carbamazepine, phenobarbitone and rifampicin decrease theophylline levels. While alcohol, zileuton, cimetidine, erythromycin and ciprofloxacin increase the plasma levels and prolong the half-life of theophylline (leading to adverse effects).

Corticosteroids

These have been dealt extensively in Ch.42 and 69. Only salient features related to asthma are discussed here. Corticosteroids have been the main-stay for decades in the management of asthma. These are also called "controllers/preventers" because they provide long-term control by causing the stabilization of the symptoms due to their anti-inflammatory effects. A major breakthrough in asthma therapy occurred with the success of *inhalation corticosteroids administered by aerosol* dispenser which controlled asthma, avoiding major side effects associated with their systemic use. Currently, inhaled corticosteroids, along with SABA or LABA are the first choice drugs for chronic asthma. Several hours are required for DNA transcription and RNA translation to occur after administering corticosteroids. *Hence, in acute asthma, rapid therapeutic effects can only be obtained when these are used in combination with selective short acting β_2-agonists.*

Many other actions of corticosteroids also help in reversing the pathologic process of bronchial asthma: **(1)** they enhance β_2-adrenergic receptor response by up-regulating the β_2-receptors in lung cells and leukocytes, **(2)** they inhibit the release of prostaglandins and leukotrienes (LTC_4, LTD_4 and LTE_4) and thus prevent smooth muscle contraction, vascular permeability and airway mucus secretion, **(3)** they produce eosinopenia which prevents cytotoxic effects of the mediators released from eosinophils, and **(4)** they inhibit the formation and release of cytokines and chemical mediators (from mast cells and eosinophils) and thus prevent recruitment, proliferation and activation of leukocytes. Hence, corticosteroids are not prophylactic (cannot inhibit an early asthmatic response) but are effective in preventing the late asthmatic responses and in decreasing bronchial hyper-responsiveness.

Aerosolised inhalational corticosteroids**:* Compared to hydrocortisone, prednisone and dexamethasone (which are used systemically), inhalational corticosteroids such as ***beclomethasone, fluticasone, budesonide and ***flunisolide*** are least absorbed into systemic circulation (on inhalation) and produce minimal systemic side effects; these drugs are therefore most suitable for long-term treatment of asthma (along with an inhalational β_2-agonist). In therapeutic doses, side effects such as dryness of mouth, voice changes and oral candidiasis (preventable by oral rinsing) are much less. ***Ciclesonide*** is an inhalational corticosteroids which has a better topical:systemic activity ratio. After inhalation it is degraded by esterases enzymes present in the bronchial epithelium to release active form of ciclesonide which provides the local effects. After absorption also, it gets bound to plasma proteins which further minimises its exposure to glucocorticoid receptors in skin, eye and bone etc and hence carries minimum risk of systemic toxicity.

Oral corticosteroids**:* After the successful use of bronchodilator in acute asthmatic attack, many patients are treated with oral corticosteroids for a period of 7–10 days to suppress symptoms and to prevent relapse. Commonly used drugs include, ***prednisone, prednisolone, and ***methylprednisolone***. Prednisone is a prodrug and is converted to prednisolone in liver. These drugs have a shorter half-life compared to betamethasone or dexamethasone. These are preferred because using a shorter acting drug for a brief period (7–10 days) is generally not associated with adrenocortical suppression and other systemic toxicity. An alternate-day regimen for oral corticosteroids has also been suggested and used (Ch. 42 and 69). There are lesser side effects with this regimen.

***Parenteral corticosteroids**:* These may be used in severe acute asthma as dose can be adjusted as per clinical need. Generally used drugs are hydrocortisone and methylprednisolone.

Mast Cell Stabilisers

The best established of the mast cell stabilizers are ***sodium cromoglycate (cromolyn sodium)*** and ***nedocromil sodium***. Both drugs are chemically related and belong to a chemical group called chromones. These are nonbronchodilating, nonsteroidal drugs used for prophylactic treatment of asthma. Both are available as metered-dose aerosol. Cromolyn sodium powder can also be inhaled through a nebuliser. Both drugs prevent degranulation and subsequent release of chemical mediators from the mast cells. They stabilize mast cells by preventing transmembrane influx of Ca^{2+} ions provoked by antigen-IgE antibody reaction on the mast cell membrane. In addition, they also inhibit leukocyte activation and chemotaxis. The stabilizing effects on mast cells appear to be specific for lung-cell type because they inhibit mast cell degranulation in human lung but not in skin.

There are reports that when taken regularly (2–3 puffs, 3–4 times daily) for prophylaxis, both agents reduce the need for bronchodilator (β_2-agonist) or anti-inflammatory (corticosteroid) treatment (reduction in the dose and frequency). Both drugs are highly ionized and have least systemic absorption (on inhalation) and are well tolerated, making them useful particularly in children. However, throat irritation, dryness of mouth, wheezing or mild headache may occur. These are reserved for prophylactic use in the management of chronic and seasonal asthma and are ineffective in the treatment of acute attacks including status asthmaticus.

Leukotriene Modulators

A newer approach to the treatment of asthma is to prevent the effects of leukotrienes on the airway.

Leukotrienes are powerful mediators of inflammation, cause leukocyte recruitment, stimulate bronchoconstriction and increase capillary permeability leading to pulmonary oedema. In addition, they stimulate mucus secretion and decrease mucociliary clearance (refer Ch. 25). Metabolism of arachidonic acid *via* 5-lipoxygenase pathway yields the cysteinyl leukotrienes—LTC_4, LTD_4 and LTE_4—which activate cysteinyl leukotriene receptor (cys-LT receptor) to cause broncho-constriction (Fig. 48.1). The effects of leukotrienes can be prevented either by inhibiting the leukotriene synthesis or by blocking their stimulatory effect on cys-LT receptors. The synthesis of leukotrienes can be blocked by inhibiting the 5-lipoxygenase enzyme by the drug ***zileuton***, whereas the effects of leukotrienes on cys-LT receptors can be blocked by drugs such as ***zafirlukast, montelukast, pranlukast*** and ***iralukast***. These are mainly used as the adjuvants with inhaled corticosteroids in poorly responding patients. They reduce the dosage of β_2 adrenergic agonists as well of inhaled corticosteroids for maintenance.

Zileuton is given orally at 6 hrly intervals and is well absorbed from GIT. *The notable side effect is hepatotoxicity* (hence withdrawn from several countries). Headache, nausea and GIT distress may also occur. Liver disease is its absolute contraindication.

Zafirlukast is rapidly absorbed after oral administration, but its bioavailability decreases after food. Hence it is administered 2 hrs before meals, at 12 hrly intervals (half-life 10 hrs). It is metabolized by liver by CYP2C9 and hence can inhibit the metabolism of warfarin. Adverse effects include GIT distress and headache.

Montelukast (10 mg OD orally) has the advantage of being administered once daily (usually in the evening) and its bioavailability is not affected by meals. It can be used in children above 5 yrs of age. ***Iralukast*** is similar to montelukast. ***Pranlukast*** is considered to be safest.

In rare cases, treatment of patients with cys-LT receptor antagonists have been reported to be associated with Churg-Strauss syndrome (vasculitis, eosinophilia, and worsening of asthma).

Monoclonal Anti-IgE Antibody

An entirely new approach towards treatment of asthma has involved the development of a mono-clonal antibody targeted to IgE so that the latter cannot bind to its receptors present on mast cells and basophils. ***Omalizumab*** is a recombinant humanized monoclonal anti-IgE antibody which, **(1)** inhibits the binding of IgE to mast cells and basophils, **(2)** inhibits the activation of IgE already bound to mast cells and thus prevents their degranulation and **(3)** down-regulates FcεR-1 (Fc epsilon R-1) receptor present on mast cells and basophils (for meaning of Fc region in antibody, see Ch. 69).

In short, *omalizumab* neutralizes the free IgE in circulation by forming a high affinity IgE-omalizumab (anti-IgE) complex. Thus it is a sort of antibody that is anti- to IgE antibody (anti-antibody to antibody).

Omalizumab is indicated for asthmatic patients who are not adequately controlled by inhaled corticosteroids and who demonstrate sensitivity to aero-allergens. It is not suitable for acute attacks including status asthmaticus (as it is not a bronchodilator). It is well tolerated. However, injection site (I.V., S.C.) reactions (redness, stinging sensation) may occur. Currently, its high cost discourages its use as a first line antiasthmatic drug.

Miscellaneous Anti-asthma Drugs

Nitric Oxide Donors: It is now established that nitric oxide (inhalation) is also useful in bronchial asthma as it relaxes airway smooth muscles. In upper airways it is considered to be a non–noradrenergic non-cholinergic (NANC) neurotransmitter. In place of NO, some NO-donors are being investigated for the treatment of acute severe asthma as well as for the management of pulmonary hypertension.

Chlamydia pneumoniae and *Mycoplasma pneumoniae* infections have also been reported to be causative factors for asthma and hence several patients are benefitted on being treated with an appropriate macrolide, e.g., ***clarithromycin*** (Fig. 48.1).

Benralizumab

It is a humanised IgG1 monoclonal antibody. It is approved as an add-on therapy for severe eosinophilic asthma in more than 12 years of age, given subcutaneously. It binds to the interleukin-5 receptor which is expressed on eosinophils and basophils. It leads to apoptosis of these cells through antibody-dependent cell-mediated cytotoxicity (ADCC). Adverse effects: Headache, pharyngitis, fever and hypersensitivity reactions.

Tezepelumab

Tezepelumab is approved drug by US-FDA for the treatment of bronchial asthma. Mechanism of action: Thymic stromal lymphopoietin (TSLP), a IL-2 cytokine is responsible for chronic inflammation in bronchial asthma. Tezepelumab is a human monoclonal IgG antibody directed against and inhibits TSLP and reduces chronic inflammation. It is used to treat severe asthma as an add-on maintenance therapy. Adverse effects: Injection site pain, redness, swelling, sore throat, joint pain and back pain.

Mepolizumab

It is a humanized IgG1 monoclonal antibody against IL-5. It binds IL-5 and inhibits IL-5 from binding to its receptors on the surface of eosinophils. It is used for add-on maintenance treatment of severe asthma in patients with an eosinophilic phenotype. It can be given in Hypereosinophilic syndrome. Adverse effects: Upper abdominal pain, headache, injection site reactions, fatigue and urinary tract infection.

Dupilumab

It is a monoclonal antibody that inhibits IL-4 and IL-13 signalling by specifically binding to the IL-4 receptor. Given s.c. in eosinophilic phenotype or cortiocosteroid dependent asthma.

TREATMENT OF STATUS ASTHMATICUS

It is a potentially life-threatening acute attack of severe asthma needing immediate treatment. Most often hospitalization is necessary. Usually, a high concentration (40–60%) of O_2 is administered with high flow rate along with high doses of inhaled short acting β_2-agonist. Simultaneously, high dose of systemic corticosteroids are also needed, for example 30–60 mg of prednisolone by mouth or of hydrocortisone sodium succinate, 100–200 mg intravenously. If situation is life-threatening 0.5 mg of ipratropium can also be added through inhalation. Dehydration and acidosis should also be corrected.

Global Initiative for Asthma (GINA) 2022 Treatment Guideline

Stepped Care Approach

Steps 1-2: As-needed low dose ICS-formoterol
Step 3: Low dose maintenance ICS-formoterol
Step 4: Medium dose maintenance ICS-formoterol
Step 5: Add-on Long-acting muscarinic antagonists, ICS-formoterol ± anti-IgE, anti-IL4R, anti-TSLP
Reliever: Administration of ICS-formoterol as reliever reduces the risk of exacerbations compared with using a SABA reliever.

Other controller options having limited indications, or less efficacy in each steps.
Step 1-2: Low dose ICS whenever SABA taken, or daily LTRA, **Step 3**: Medium dose ICS, or add LTRA. **Step 4**: Add LAMA or LTRA, or switch to high dose ICS. **Step 5**: Add azithromycin (adults) or LTRA. As last resort consider adding low dose OCS but consider side-effects.

SABA have limited role in asthma. Whenever SABA is taken alone for acute attack, low dose ICS is combined. LABA and ICS can reduce severe exacerbation of asthma.

ICS—Inhaled corticosteroids; SABA—Short acting β_2-agonist; LABA—Long acting β_2-agonist OCS—Oral corticosteroids, LTRA— Leukotriene receptor antagonist (LTRA); Anti-IL4R —Dupilumab; LAMA—Long-acting muscarinic antagonists; TSLP—Thymic stromal lymphopoietin.

CHAPTER 49 Drug Therapy of Cough and Chronic Obstructive Pulmonary Disease

COMPETENCY PH1.32, PH1.33

Cough is a physiologically useful protective reflex that clears the respiratory tract of the accumulated mucus and foreign substances. Hence, a total abolition of coughing process is not desirable. However, many times it occurs as a symptom of an underlying disorder. In such situations, a long-term cough is quite distressing and exhausting and needs treatment. The cough may be *non-productive (i.e., dry)* or *productive (i.e., tenacious)*. The ***non-productive cough*** is considered as serving no purpose, rather increases discomfort to the patient. For its treatment, antitussive agents are used. An ideal antitussive agent should suppress the *frequency* as well as the *intensity of coughing* without affecting the normal elimination of excessive secretions from the respiratory tract. The ***productive cough*** is characterized by the presence of excessive sputum and may be associated with conditions such as chronic bronchitis and bronchiectasis. In this case, cough suppressants (antitussives) are not effective and are inappropriate but expectorants are used. Expectorants increase the volume and decrease the viscosity of secretions to enhance the propulsion of these secretions upward and outward by ciliary movement and coughing.

ANTITUSSIVES

Three kinds of antitussive are generally used:

Centrally Acting Antitussives

These include opioids like *codeine* and *pholcodeine* and non-opioids such as *dextromethorphan*, *noscapine* and *pipazethate*. All of these, except pipazethate, have been discussed in Chapter 37. Salient characteristics are discussed below. They possess central antitussive actions by virtue of suppressing cough center that mediates the cough reflex.

Codeine: It is a semisynthetic opioid analgesic with potent cough suppressant action and can be administered orally (10 mg BD or TDS). With these therapeutic doses it exhibits lesser addiction liability and lesser constipation. Overdosage can result in respiratory depression, convulsions, postural hypotension and tachycardia.

Pholcodeine: It is structurally related to codeine but is slightly more potent, longer acting and better tolerated than codeine. It causes lesser constipation and drowsiness than codeine and is more suited for long-term use. It is also given orally (10–15 mg BD).

Dextromethorphan: As the name suggests, it is the methylester of the *dextroisomer* of levorphanol. It has least addiction liability, no analgesic action (unlike levorphanol), least constipating effects and minimal drowsiness (unlike codeine). As an antitussive it is as potent as codeine and is given orally (10 mg TDS). It appears to be the most popular cough suppressant and is often used in combination with other agents such as antihistamines and bronchodilators in cough mixtures.

Noscapine: It is a naturally occurring opium alkaloid belonging to benzylisoquinoline group (Ch. 37). It is devoid of analgesic activity, drowsiness, and addiction liability. It has minimal constipating effects and is also a popular cough suppressant. It is given orally (15 mg TDS). High doses may produce nausea, headache and tremors.

Pipazethate: It is a phenothiazine group of antitussive occasionally used in cough mixtures. It has negligible CNS depressants effects. It is also given orally (40 mg TDS).

Though *morphine* is also a powerful cough suppressant, it is seldom used except for the relief of *intractable cough in terminal illness*. For such long-term use constipation is a big problem which can be minimized with the use of lactulose. However, the use of morphine, otherwise, is never considered appropriate for cough.

Central As Well As Peripherally Acting Antitussives

Benzonatate is an antitussive structurally related to the local anaesthetic tetracaine. It not only inhibits the afferent cough impulses to suppress the central cough center, but also inhibits the pulmonary stretch receptors and, therefore, has both central as well as peripheral mode of action. It possesses mild local anaesthetic action as well. It is administered orally (100–200 mg TDS). Side effects include drowsiness, nausea, headache and in high doses, vertigo.

Peripherally Acting Antitussives

Prenoxdiazine acts by inhibiting pulmonary stretch receptors to relieve bronchospasm. It has a moderate antitussive action and is administered orally (100–200 mg TDS). Side effects are mild and infrequent.

Demulcents can also be classified as indirect peripherally acting cough suppressants. They provide a protective coating over sensory receptors on pharynx. These include honey, liquorice, syrup tolu and syrup vasaka.

Local Anaesthetics such as xylocaine and bupivacaine can be applied on pharynx and larynx to reduce the sensitivity of sensory receptors for cough in this area. These are typically used to treat the cough associated with bronchoscopy and can also be tried in patients who are refractory to other cough therapies.

Antitussives, in general, should not be used in cough associated with asthma, or chronic bronchitis or bronchiectasis as they can cause harmful retention and thickening of sputum.

EXPECTORANTS

These drugs either increase the volume or decrease the viscosity (or both) of the respiratory secretions and facilitate their removal by ciliary action and coughing. These act either by *mucokinetic* or by *mucolytic action*.

Mucokinetic Expectorants

These expectorants stimulate the flow of respiratory tract secretions by stimulating the bronchial secretory cells (to increase the volume) and the ciliary movement (to facilitate their removal). They also have a reflex irritant effect on gastric mucosa, which is believed to initiate the reflex secretions of respiratory tract fluid. Commonly used mucokinetic expectorants include essential volatile oils, ammonium chloride, sodium citrate, guaiacol and guaifenesin.

Essential oils (e.g., oil anise, oil eucalyptus) provide only mild expectoration by directly stimulating the bronchial secretory cells. ***Ammonium chloride*** is also traditionally used as cough expectorant in various cough mixtures. It is a gastric irritant which reflexly enhances bronchial secretions. However, in large doses it can produce metabolic acidosis. ***Sodium citrate*** is also used conventionally as expectorant in several cough mixtures. After absorption, citrates get converted to bicarbonates *in vivo* and mucus becomes less viscous in alkaline pH. ***Guaiacol*** and ***Guaifenesin*** are obtained from creosote wood but nowadays are prepared synthetically. These are safe expectorants with proven efficacy. Guaifenesin is less irritating derivative of guaiacol. After absorption, guaifenesin is secreted through bronchial glands to increase airway secretions and mucosal ciliary activity. It is administered orally (100–200 mg BD or TDS).

Mucolytic Expectorants

Mucolytics alter the chemical characteristics of mucus to decrease its viscosity and to facilitate its removal by ciliary action or coughing. Commonly used mucolytics include ***acetylcysteine, carbocysteine, bromhexine, ambroxol*** and ***dornase-alfa.***

Acetylcysteine is a mucolytic that decreases the viscosity of mucus by splitting the disulfide (-S-S-) bonds of mucoproteins. This action is further facilitated by alkaline pH (7–9). Administration is done by nebulisation (3–5 ml of 20% solution) through a face mask in patients of cystic fibrosis and chronic bronchitis. Mechanical suction of liquefied secretions may be necessary because it produces large amounts of secretions, that must be removed. *Side effects* include nausea, vomiting, stomatitis and bronchospasm. Acetylcysteine is also used for the treatment of paracetamol toxicity (Ch. 26). Unlabeled use includes the treatment of dry eyes (keratoconjunctivitis sicca) as 5% acetylcysteine with hyperomellose. Although related to acetylcysteine, ***carbocysteine*** has some other mode of action which is still not clear. The drug has protected -SH group and therefore cannot work through -SH and -S-S- interchange, i.e., it cannot split the disulfide bonds of mucus. It is given orally (250–500 mg TDS). Side effects are similar to acetylcysteine.

Bromhexine is an alkaloid from vasaka plant. It depolymerises mucopolysaccharides of mucus directly and also increases lysosomal enzyme activity that breaks fibre-network of tenacious sputum. Usual oral dose is 8–16 mg TDS. Side effects are mild such as GIT upset and rhinorrhoea. ***Ambroxol*** is a metabolite of bromhexine and has a similar mode of action. It is more useful if mucus plugs are present. Usual oral dose is 30 mg BD or TDS.

Dornase-alfa is a higly purified solution of recombinant human deoxyribonuclease (DNase), an enzyme that selectively cleaves DNA. Purulent pulmonary secretions in cystic fibrosis contain very high amounts of extracellular DNA which is released by degeneration of neutrophils (in response to infection). Dornase-alfa inhalation (2.5 mg once daily) hydrolyses this accumulated DNA in the sputum of the patients of cystic fibrosis and reduces the viscosity of sputum.

CHRONIC OBSTRUCTIVE PULMONARY DISEASE (COPD)

COPD is a disease state characterized by the progressive obstruction of airflow. Unlike asthma, the obstruction of airflow, indicated by an abnormal decline in the forced expiratory volume in one second (FEV_1), is more or less progressive and largely irreversible. COPD is a common disorder, frequently associated with cigarette smoking, respiratory infections, environmental pollution and occupational exposures, e.g., in persons working in cement or cotton industries. COPD is usually associated with *chronic bronchitis* and in later stages *emphysema*.

In chronic bronchitis, there is enlargement of mucous glands, increase in mucus production and thickening of bronchial wall. There is chronic productive cough with excessive sputum production. Patients experience dyspnoea, bronchospasm and frequent respiratory tract infections. In severe cases, irreversible narrowing of the airways occurs which leads to cyanosis, hypoxia and hypercapnia. Severe COPD patient can suffer from right-sided heart failure (*cor pulmonale*), a heart disease characterized by pulmonary hypertension, right ventricular hypertrophy and right heart failure. *Cor pulmonale* is more often associated with chronic bronchitis than with emphysema.

Emphysema is characterized by enlargement of air spaces, destruction of lung parenchyma, loss of lung elasticity and closure of small airways.

Dyspnoea is a prominent symptom along with productive cough, wheezing and recurrent respiratory infection. Patients hyperventilate to maintain oxygen levels in the blood. Some reports also suggest that emphysema may result due to hereditary deficiency of $alpha_1$-antitrypsin.

The inflammatory component of COPD, that leads to airway pathology, differs from asthma, by the fact that COPD patients show increased neutrophil activation as opposed to eosinophil and mast cell activity. In COPD, macrophage activation releases chemotactic factors (LTB_4 and IL-8) from neutrophils. In addition, proteases are also released which destroy lung parenchyma. It is now believed that tumour necrosis factor-α stimulates production of IL-8 and proteases that destroy tissue of alveolar wall.

Management of COPD

The clinical progress of COPD depends on whether bronchitis predominates or emphysema. Most patients with COPD usually have irreversible airway obstruction (unlike asthma). Drugs, therefore, relieve only symptoms without treating underlying pathophysiology. Treatment aims for patients of COPD are **(1)** to lessen airflow obstruction, **(2)** to reduce respiratory symptoms and improve quality of life and **(3)** to prevent and treat secondary complications like hypoxaemia, infections and *cor pulmonale*. Treatment options are given below:

1. The most important therapeutic intervention is to ask the patient to stop smoking. Pharma-cological intervention may also help stop smoking (see Ch. 12, 13, 34 and 38).
2. Influenza vaccine may be given to COPD patients every year and a proper antibiotic therapy should be provided if patient develops purulent sputum.
3. The first-line drug therapy for the treatment of COPD consists of bronchodilators to reduce bronchospasm and wheezing. SABA and LABA drugs should be tried initially since they provide rapid relief and low incidence of side effects on inhalation (Ch. 12 and 48). There are reports that antimuscarinic agents like SAMAs (ipratropium, oxitropium) and LAMAs (tiotropium, glycopyrronium, aclidinium, umeclidinium) are more effective than β_2 receptor acting LABAs and SABAs in COPD patients because the predominant airway muscle tone in COPD patients is parasympathetic. However, they have a slower onset of bronchodilatory effects. Hence, various guidelines suggest that COPD patients are benefitted more from a combined therapy using a SAMA + LABA or LAMA + LABA. Use of alone LABA has no defined place in COPD treatment.
4. A xanthine such as theophylline (Ch. 35 and 48), may also be administered orally in addition to inhaled bronchodilators. Theophylline may improve respiratory muscle function in patients with COPD and because of its positive cardiac inotropic effects could be of value in *cor pulmonale* also. If lung functions show improvement, theophylline is usually continued as maintenance therapy. Persistent nocturnal symptoms such as cough or wheezing may be helped by night-time use of long-acting theophylline.
5. ***Revefenacin***: Revefenacin is a novel biphenyl carbamate tertiary amine agent that belongs to the family of the long-acting muscarinic antagonists (LAMA), anticholinergic drug. It blocks M3 receptors in the smooth muscle, leading to bronchodilation. Revefenacin has been reported to produce a sustained, long-acting bronchodilation with lower anti-muscarinic-related side effects. In clinical trials, revefenacin demonstrated to be of a long duration of action. After reaching maximum concentration, revefenacin concentrations decline in a biphasic manner. This elimination kinetics is observed by a rapid declining plasma concentration followed by a slow apparent bi-exponential elimination. It can be used via nebulizer for maintenance treatment of chronic obstructive pulmonary disease (COPD). *Adverse effects* are cough, nasopharyngitis, upper respiratory tract infection, headache and allergy.
6. Some patients of COPD, who are receiving optimal bronchodilator therapy, exhibit a substantial better response further by administering corticosteroids orally (e.g., prednisolone 30–40 mg per day orally for 15 days). If objective responses are achieved, the recommended guidelines suggest a continued use of *inhalational corticosteroids* (Ch. 48) as these are associated with lesser adverse effects. For the transition from oral to inhaled therapy, the oral glucocorticoids are gradually tapered off and inhaled treatment is started. However, whether glucocorticoids improve the long-term outcome of COPD remains to be confirmed.
7. In the patients with severe COPD and persistent hypoxaemia, the use of domiciliary O_2 therapy for 15 hrs a day reduces the associated mortality and the risk of complications such as cor pulmonale and neuropsychological impairment.
8. The use of mucolytics or expectorants is controversial though they definitely provide modest benefits in reducing exacerbations.

CHAPTER 50

SECTION 10—DRUGS ACTING ON BLOOD & BLOOD FORMING ORGANS

Haematopoietic Agents, Vitamins and Antioxidants

COMPETENCY PH1.35

The haematopoietic machinery, which works in the bone marrow, is primarily involved in the formation of cellular components of blood—erythrocytes, leukocytes and thrombocytes. For its organised functioning, it needs some essential exogenous nutrients such as iron, vitamin B_{12} and folic acid—called haematinics—and certain endogenously derived growth factors such as granulocyte colony stimulating factor (G-CSF), granulocyte- macrophage colony stimulating factor (GM-CSF), erythropoietin, thrombopoietin, interleukin-1 (IL-1) and IL-11, etc. In addition to the above exogenous and endogenous essential nutrients, there are other substances which indirectly help bone marrow function and are labelled as accessory haematinics. These include certain vitamins and minerals like copper, cobalt and manganese. In this chapter, we first summarise different kinds of anaemia due to deficiency of iron, B_{12} and folic acid as well as their treatment and then turn to the clinical use of above haematopoietic growth factors in the management of certain types of anaemia, thrombocytopenia and neutropenia.

TYPES OF ANAEMIA

Anaemia means a decrease in the oxygen carrying capacity of blood due to reduced concentration of haemoglobin or RBCs. On the basis of RBC size and haemoglobin content, the anaemia may be characterised as:

- ***Microcytic hypochromic anaemia***: characterised by small RBC size with low haemoglobin contents; usually caused by iron deficiency.
- ***Macrocytic hyperchromic anaemia* or *Megaloblastic anaemia,*** characterised by larger nucleated primitive RBCs with increasingly pigmented blood smear ; usually caused due to deficiency of vitamin B_{12} and/or folic acid.
- ***Pernicious anaemia*** is a megaloblastic anaemia due to failure of secretion of intrinsic factor by the stomach.
- ***Haemolytic anaemia*** results due to bone marrow depression leading to premature destruction of RBCs. It may result due to adverse reactions of many drugs or due to immune disorder.
- ***Alpastic anaemia*** results due to hypoplasia of bone marrow. Hence, there is a decreased formation of blood cells which may result either due to toxic effects of cytotoxic drugs or due to bone marrow disease. This is usually associated with thrombocytopenia and neutropenia.
- ***Sickle cell anaemia*** is a type of haemolytic anaemia which is characterised by the presence of haemoglobin-S (having altered amino acid structure of polypeptide) in the red cells. On deoxygenation, these molecules of haemoglobin polymerise to form pseudo-crystalline structures (tactoids), which distort the red cell membrane to produce sickle-shaped cells. These cells increase blood viscosity, traverse capillaries poorly and tend to obstruct blood flow to cause thrombosis and infarcts.
- ***Sideroblastic anaemia*** is a refractory anaemia exhibiting sideroblasts in the bone marrow due to inadequate utilisation of iron.

MICROCYTIC HYPOCHROMIC (IRON DEFICIENCY) ANAEMIA

Haemoglobin is the oxygen-carrying component of RBCs. It is made up of haeme + globin. ***Haem*** consists of ferrous (Fe^{2+}) iron chelated between porphyrin rings and the ***globin*** chains conjugated to this complex comprise the haemoglobin. When iron is inadequate, small erythrocytes with insufficient haemoglobin are formed giving rise to microcytic hypochromic anaemia. The clinical features include pallor, fatigue, dizziness, exertional dyspnoea and general symptoms of tissue ischaemia. Iron deficiency could result due to (a) dietary deficiency, (b) faulty absorption, transport and storage, (c) excessive blood loss due to haemorrhage or heavy worm infestation, (d) excessive demand during growth, pregnancy and lactation and (e) during severe infection.

Total body content of iron: The total body iron is about 3.5–4 g in adult male and about 2.5 g in adult female, 70% of which circulates in the blood as haemoglobin. About 15–18% is stored in liver, spleen and bone marrow chiefly as ***ferritin*** and ***haemosiderin***. Ferritin is also present in intestinal mucosa. It is composed of a nucleus of ferric hydroxide with a protein envelope of ***apoferritin*** (which has no iron). Haemosiderin consists of aggregated ferric hydroxide crystals with a partial envelope of apoferritin. Storage iron is always available for haemoglobin synthesis on demand, e.g., in iron deficiency, the body draws iron from these stores for haemopoiesis; but if stores are depleted anaemia develops. The rest of the body iron which is not available for haemoglobin synthesis is present in muscle myoglobin (10–15%), cytochromes (0.3%) and enzymes (0.2%).

Body requirement of iron: Each molecule of haemoglobin has 33% of iron. That means, for a loss of 100 ml of blood (which contains 15 g haemoglobin), there would be a loss of 15 x 0.33 = 50 mg of elemental iron. Average daily requirement of iron for an adult male is 0.5–1 mg, but a menstruating female would need more, i.e., 1–2 mg/day. There is a loss of about 17–18 mg of iron during menstruation which increases the iron demand by 0.6 mg/day more than that required. Iron demand also increases during last 2 trimesters of pregnancy (3–5 mg/day), soon after delivery and also during lactation. Children also need higher amounts (25 mg/kg/day) of iron during their growth.

Liver, egg yolk, meat, chicken, fish are good sources of iron. Pulses, dry fruits, spinach, banana, apple and wheat grains are moderate sources of iron. Humans absorb ferrous iron in the form of haeme which is generally present in meat. In vegetarian food, the iron is in non-haeme form and exists in ferric (Fe^{3+}) state. This needs to be converted to Fe^{2+} state.

Pharmacokinetics of Iron

Maximum iron absorption occurs in the duodenum and proximal jejunum. Haeme iron is absorbed efficiently as such, while non-haeme iron is absorbed primarily in ferrous (Fe^{2+}) form. Ascorbic acid, succinic acid and -SH- group containing amino acids (cysteine; present in gastric juice) facilitate conversion of Fe^{3+} to Fe^{2+} (and thus promote absorption). Iron absorption is hindered by coffee, tea, antacids (of Ca^{2+}, Al^{3+} and Mg^{2+} group) and phosphates. Absorption, storage and excretion of iron within the body is shown in Fig. 50.1.

Iron is absorbed by active transport across the intestinal mucosa where it is converted intracellularly from Fe^{2+} to ferric (Fe^{3+}) iron. If the body does not need iron, then the ingested iron gets bound to *apoferritin* (a protein) to make a apoferritin-iron complex called ***ferritin***, which is then

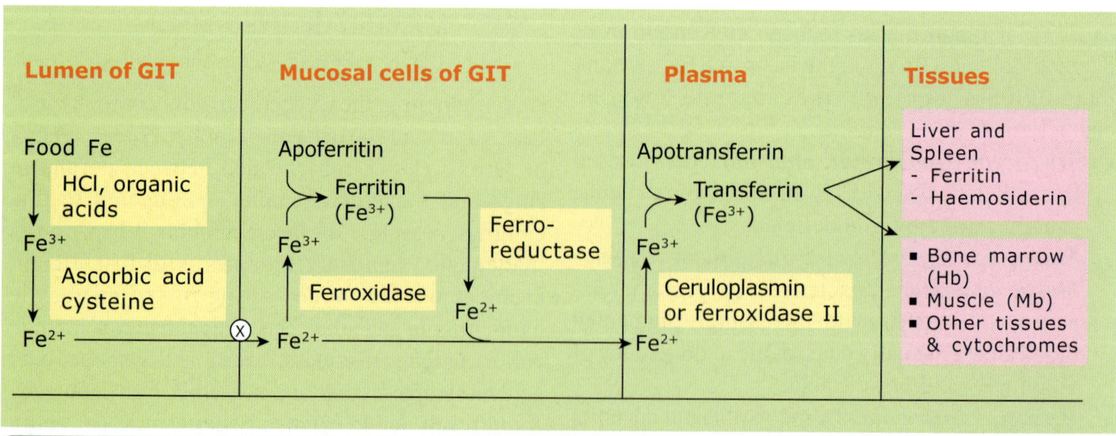

Fig 50.1 Pharmacokinetics of Iron. Hb = Haemoglobin; Mb = Myoglobin

stored virtually in all cells of the body and provides an efficient mechanism for iron storage and release on demand. The rate of iron absorption depends on apoferritin to ferritin ratio. If apoferritin is more than ferritin, the absorption of iron will increase (in iron deficiency anaemia, this ratio is more). If ferritin is more (i.e., saturation of ferritin), absorption of iron would be less (i.e., decrease in absorption due to "mucosal block").

On body's demand for iron, *transferrin* (a transport glycoprotein) enters the plasma and binds with free Fe^{3+} (or Fe^{2+} from ferritin) and carries it to the bone marrow for being used in haemoglobin synthesis. Some Fe^{3+} is stored as ferritin or as haemosiderin-Fe^{3+} in reticuloendothelial cells and some in muscle myoglobin, cytochromes and enzymes of parenchymal cells. Iron stored as haemosiderin, is also found in the monocyte-macrophage system of bone marrow and in the reticuloendothelial cells of the liver.

Iron is remarkably well conserved in the body—only about 0.5–1 mg is excreted on a daily basis. Negligible amounts only are excreted in urine and the major elimination pathway is through the faeces by exfoliation of GIT cells with their intracellular stores of ferritin.

Treatment of Iron Deficiency Anaemia

Iron therapy is indicated in iron deficiency anaemia only. It is rather contraindicated in anaemia of any other cause. Iron preparations can be given orally or parenterally. Oral iron therapy is as good and efficacious as parenteral, provided the iron absorption from GIT is normal.

Oral Iron Therapy: Most of the iron preparations are available as ferrous (Fe^{2+}) salts (sulfate, fumarate, gluconate, lactate, succinate and glycine sulfate etc.). Besides these, some ferric (Fe^{3+}) salts are also available (such as ferric ammonium citrate, iron polysaccharide and ferric hydroxide polymaltose complex). Ferrous salts are better absorbed than ferric salts.

The most commonly used Fe^{2+} preparation is ferrous sulfate. Each 100 mg of ***ferrous sulfate*** provides 20% of elemental iron. Similarly, 100 mg of ***ferrous fumarate, ferrous lactate, ferrous succinate*** and ***ferrous gluconate*** provide 33%, 19%, 12% and 12% of elemental iron, respectively. For full haemopoietic effects in adult, a total of 200 mg of elemental iron should be administered daily in 2 or 3 divided doses after the meals or in between the meals. For children the dose is 3–5 mg/kg to be given in 3 divided doses. Thus, a 325 mg tablet of ferrous sulfate has to be administered orally thrice a day to get optimum benefits (i.e., approximately 200 mg of elemental iron). For prophylactic use, 30 mg of elemental iron per day is sufficient. *Sustained release preparations of ferrous salts are also available but their use has no rationale as most of the iron is absorbed from stomach, duodenum and proximal jejunum and the sustained release drug granules would not stay there for long.*

Lately, ***iron-polysaccharide complex, carbonyl-iron complex*** and ***ferric hydroxide – polymaltose complex*** have also been marketed. All have 100% iron content, carry the least risk of overdose toxicity and have much better GIT tolerance. Albeit, these preparations are much costlier. ***Ferric maltol*** is an oral iron preparation. It dissociates upon uptake from gastrointestinal tract, allowing iron and maltol to be absorbed separately. Food decreases bioavailability of iron after administration of ferric maltol. It is taken orally 1 hr before or 2 hrs after a meal. It is used in iron deficiency anaemia.

Adverse effects depend upon the dose and thus on the elemental iron content. Common complaints include constipation which is more common than diarrhoea, epigastric pain, heart burn, nausea, vomiting, metallic taste and staining of teeth (mainly with oral liquid or chewable preparations).

Parenteral Iron Therapy: Parenteral therapy is reserved for those who are unable to tolerate oral iron or to absorb oral iron preparations or for those who cannot be maintained with oral iron therapy because of acute/chronic blood loss or GIT disorders like sprue or inflammatory bowel disease.

The classical parenteral iron preparation is ***iron dextran*** (I.V. or I.M.), which is a sterile colloidal solution of ferric hydroxide and low molecular weight dextran containing 50 mg of elemental iron per ml of the solution. Other parenteral preparations are ***iron-sucrose complex*** (I.V. or I.M.), ***iron–sodium gluconate complex*** (I.V. or I.M.) and ***iron–sorbitol–citric acid complex*** (only I.M.).

To avoid any risk of hypersensitivity reaction it is always safe to perform a sensitivity test with a small test dose before administering full I.M. or I.V. doses of parenteral iron preparation. These injections are usually supplied with package insert from which the recommended doses can be obtained for patients of different weights and different haemoglobin (Hb) status. However, if the table is not available, the following formula for an equivalent of 50 mg/ml of elemental iron (as in iron dextran) can be used to calculate the dose.

Dose in ml = (0.0476 x Body wt in kg) x (14.8 – Hb g/100 ml) + 1 ml/5 kg body wt (to a max. of 14 ml to replenish the tissue stores).

Using this formula, a 70 kg patient with reported Hb values of 6 g/100 ml would need about a total of 40 ml of iron dextran injection (equivalent to 2 g of elemental iron).

A simplest way to calculate the dose (in mg) for parenteral iron therapy is as follows:

[(14.8 – Hb g/100 ml)x150]+600 mg to replenish the stores = DOSE in mg.

If the dose (mg) is to be converted to the dose in ml, the value obtained is to be divided by 50 (for iron-dextran, as it contains 50 mg/ml of elemental iron). Depending upon the iron contents, this value would differ from one parenteral preparation to another.

Using this formula, a patient with a haemoglobin value of 6 g/100 ml would need about 38.4 ml of iron-dextran injection equivalent to 1.92 g of elemental iron which is very much similar to the values obtained above. In general, most adults who need iron replacement therapy require 1–2 g of elemental iron as replacement or 20–40 ml of iron- dextran. The usual trend is to give the entire dose in a single I.V. infusion, in normal saline, slowly over 6–8 hrs. This avoids local pain and tissue staining, which are the disadvantages of I.M. iron therapy. Iron- sorbitol complex is given only intramuscularly, not I.V., because it binds transferrin and saturates its binding sites. This leads to very high levels of free iron circulating in the blood resulting in iron overdose and toxicity. Use of iron-sucrose complex is preferred in patients undergoing renal dialysis and who are receiving erythropoietin therapy mainly because it is not allergenic and secondly because it efficiently meets the rate of iron demand induced by rapid erythropoiesis.

Intramuscular injection of iron preparations are given deeply in the gluteal region using "Z" track technique to avoid scar formation (due to iron leak) at the injection site. For this the subcutaneous tissue is stretched to one side prior to insertion of needle and then released after the injection has been done. By using this method, the site of injection and the site of drug placement (inside the muscle) do not coincide and thus the scar is not visible. ***Adverse effects—Local***: pain at the site of injection, skin pigmentation and sterile abscess. ***Systemic***: Fever, headache, joint pain, urticaria, lymphadenopathy. Anaphylactoid reaction (palpitation, chest pain, dyspnoea and cardiovascular collapse) may occur with iron-sorbitol preparation but rarely with other preparations. Similarly, metallic taste in mouth occurs commonly with iron-sorbitol compared to other preparations. ***Ferric derisomaltose***: It is a newer parenteral iron given by slow i.v. injection. It is a complex of iron hydroxide and derisomaltose. It is used for iron deficiency anaemia in adults intolerant to oral iron or unsatisfactory response to oral iron. Adverse effects: Hypophosphataemia, tachycardia, anaphylactic reaction, muscle spasms, arthralgia and myalgia.

Iron Toxicity and Treatment

Acute toxicity occurs mostly in young children who have ingested a number of iron tablets (15–20 tabs of ferrous salts are usually fatal). Its manifestations include abdominal pain, vomiting, diarrhoea, haematemesis, cyanosis, dehydration, acidosis, convulsions, shock and death due to cardiovascular collapse. Unfortunately, activated charcoal, a most common and highly effective adsorbent, does not work here as it does not bind iron. ***Desferoxamine***, an iron chelator, is a specific antidote that is given slow I.V. to chelate and remove iron that has already been absorbed. It is then excreted in urine and faeces as a chelated complex. It is capable of removing iron from both ferritin and transferrin but not from haemoglobin, where iron lies in the chelated form already. Alternatively, ***deferiprone*** (oral) can also be used but its main use is to treat iron overload in patients of thalassaemia major. For all these details, refer Chapter 68.

Chronic iron toxicity **(iron overload),** known as haemochromatosis, results when excess iron gets deposited in different organs (heart, liver, kidney and pancreas etc.) that can end up in organ failure and death. Haemochromatosis, without anaemia can be managed by intermittent phlebotomy, wherein one unit of blood is removed every week or fortnight till all excess iron is dislodged and removed. Use of iron chelator desferoxamine is not effective. A new and a selective iron chelator ***deferasirox*** has been approved to treat iron overload associated with thalassaemia. It can be given orally (Ch. 68).

MACROCYTIC HYPERCHROMIC ANAEMIA (MEGALOBLASTIC ANAEMIA)

The pathophysiology of megaloblastic anaemia involves impairment of DNA synthesis and cell proliferation (mitosis) in the precursor cells of RBCs due to vit. B_{12} and folic acid deficiency. The nucleus is present only in the primitive RBCs, not in the mature RBCs. Hence mitosis occurs only in precursor cells, not in mature RBCs (these have only a fixed life span). Deficiency of vitamin B_{12} and folic acid (in the normoblasts) impairs mitosis but not their cytosolic growth; hence the bulk of cytosole increases. As a result, primitive RBCs become very big (*megalobast*) but do not divide, i.e., the number of mature RBCs diminish (*anaemia*) and since their life span is shorter, they are prone to haemolysis (progression to haemolytic anaemia).

Vitamin B_{12}

Mammals cannot synthesise vit. B_{12} for their own requirements. Human needs are satisfied from microbially derived vit. B_{12} in fish, meat, liver, eggs, yeast and milk (but not from vegetables). Commercial source is microbial, from *Streptomyces griseus*.

Deficiency of vit. B_{12} rarely occurs due to insufficient dietary intake as daily requirements are barely 2 μg. Other causes may include: **(a)** decreased absorption or utilisation, **(b)** prolonged chemotherapy (which interferes with purine metabolism) and **(c)** fish tape worm infestation which utilises vit. B_{12} of the host. However, an important cause of vit. B_{12} deficiency is ***pernicious anaemia***. It is a hereditary autoimmune disease in which antibodies develop against ***intrinsic factor*** **(IF)**. These antibodies may either bind to intrinsic factor (IF) and prevent vit B_{12} binding or these may bind to IF-B_{12}-complex to prevent the binding of this 'complex' to IF-receptors present on ileum. The availability of IF decreases in post-gastrectomy patients, diseases of ileum or after surgical removal of ileum (because receptor-bearing area of IF gets reduced).

Chemistry: Vitamin B_{12} is a generic term for cyanocobalamin and hydroxocobalamin. These are the two stable forms of cobalamin and are the only cobalt (Co) containing amino compounds known to occur in nature. This cobalt atom has 6 coordinate bonds that link it with other groups in the molecule of vit. B_{12}. If the cyano (CN) group is attached to Co through the sixth coordination bond, it is called ***cyanocobalamin*** and if the 6th coordination position is occupied by hydroxyl (OH), methyl (CH_3) or 5'-deoxyadenosyl group, these derivatives are called ***hydroxocobalamin, methylcobalamin*** and ***5'-deoxyadenosyl cobalamin***, respectively. Out of these, hydroxocobalamin and cyanocobalamin are stable and are used therapeutically. Methylcobalamin and 5'-deoxyadenosyl cobalamin act as coenzymes and are the active forms of vit. B_{12}, though unstable.

Pharmacokinetics of vit. B_{12} is also unique. It is not lipid soluble and hence for absorption from GIT, it depends heavily on various transfer mechanisms. After ingestion and liberation from the food, it interacts with "*R-proteins*" in the stomach. These proteins protect it from acidic degradation, but still cannot transport it across the enteric mucosa. As the complex reaches duodenum, the pancreatic proteases degrade it to free cobalamin (at alkaline pH). The vit B_{12} is now absorbed onto the ***intrinsic factor*** (IF)—a glycoprotein (apoerythroin) secreted by gastric parietal cells with specific cobalamin-binding properties. The IF-cobalamin complex is then transported across the ileum cell membrane through IF-specific receptors. In the enterocytes, IF liberates cobalamin which is converted to methylcobalamin. A plasma β_2-globulin, ***transcobalamin II***, then binds to methylcobalamin and transports it into portal circulation. If the vitamin is needed, it is taken up by respective cells by endocytosis. If vitamin is in surplus, the cobalamin is moved to the hepatocytes for storage as 5'-deoxyadenosylcobalamin. If it is taken up by cells, the lysosomal enzymes liberate vit. B_{12} from transcobalamin II which is then recycled for further use. Liver can store up to 4–6 mg of vit. B_{12} as 5'-deoxyadenosylcobalamin. If for any reason dietary intake of vit. B_{12} is stopped, the normal hepatic stores can still last for 5 years.

Metabolic functions: The cobalamins are essential cofactors for two main human enzymatic processes:

1) In one enzymatic pathway, methylcobalamin serves as a cofactor for methionine synthase (a cytoplasmic methyl-transferase) and converts homocysteine to methionine and simultaneously 5-methyl tetrahydrofolate to tetrahydrofolic acid (Fig. 50.2). In this reaction, vit. B_{12} serves as a catalyst accepting as well as donating the $-CH_3$ group. Methyl tetrahydrofolic acid donates a $-CH_3$ group to vit. B_{12} (the cofactor). This methyl group is then transferred to homocysteine to form methionine. This methionine then serves as a formate donor and converts tetrahydrofolic acid to formyl tetrahydrofolic acid which serves as a precursor of folic acid polyglutamate. The latter is a cofactor (or a carrier of one-carbon units) in the synthesis of purines and pyrimidines, i.e., DNA synthesis. In vitamin B_{12} deficiency *5-methyl-tetrahydrofolic acid gets trapped* (not converted to THFA). This leads to defective DNA synthesis and ultimately to megaloblastic bone marrow. It is through this mechanism that the metabolic activities of vitamin B_{12} and folic acid are linked together and implicated in DNA synthesis.

2) Deoxyadenosyl cobalamin activates methylmalonyl-CoA mutase, which converts potentially toxic methylmalonyl-CoA to easily metabolised succinyl CoA (Fig. 50.3). In vitamin B_{12} deficiency, an accumulation of methylmalonyl CoA results in faulty (non-physiological) fatty acid synthesis and their incorporation into cell membranes of CNS leading to neurological symptoms related to inadequate myelin synthesis (peripheral neuropathy, dementia, loss of motor and sensory reflexes). There is no role of folic acid in this kind of vit. B_{12} deficiency.

Therapeutic Uses: Neither form of cobalamin is to be given intravenously. Most commonly used preparations are cyanocobalamin, hydroxocobalamin and methylcobalamin. These can be given orally or deep intramuscularly. Hydroxocobalamin is longer acting (highly protein bound) but is associated with the development of antibodies to the transcobalamin II–vit. B_{12} complex (hence lesser in use). Oral therapy needs higher doses. Methylcobalamin is preferred to treat neurological deficits associated with vit. B_{12} deficiency (peripheral neuropathy associated with diabetes, alcohol or drug intake). Intramuscular therapy brings out a rapid change in the bone marrow (from megalobastic to normoblastic erythropoiesis in 2–3 months) with improvement in neurological symptoms.

Daily requirement (adults): 2–3 μg/day
Therapeutic dose (adults): *cyanocobalamin* or *hydroxocobalamin,* 100–1000 μg/day I.M. on alternate days for 2 weeks followed by once a month. *Methylcobalamin* 1000–1500 μg/day orally to correct neurological deficits. ***Adverse effects***: rare.

Folic Acid

Folic acid (pteroylglutamic acid) is also named as “polyglutamate” because each folic acid molecule may have 2–8 molecules of glutamic acid. Humans do not synthesise folic acid and meet their requirements from diet such as green leafy vegetables, fruits, mushrooms, liver, meat, kidney, eggs, milk and yeast. It is one of the B-group of vitamins.

Pharmacokinetics: Absorption occurs primarily in the proximal jejunum. Various carboxypeptidases present in the mucosal membrane

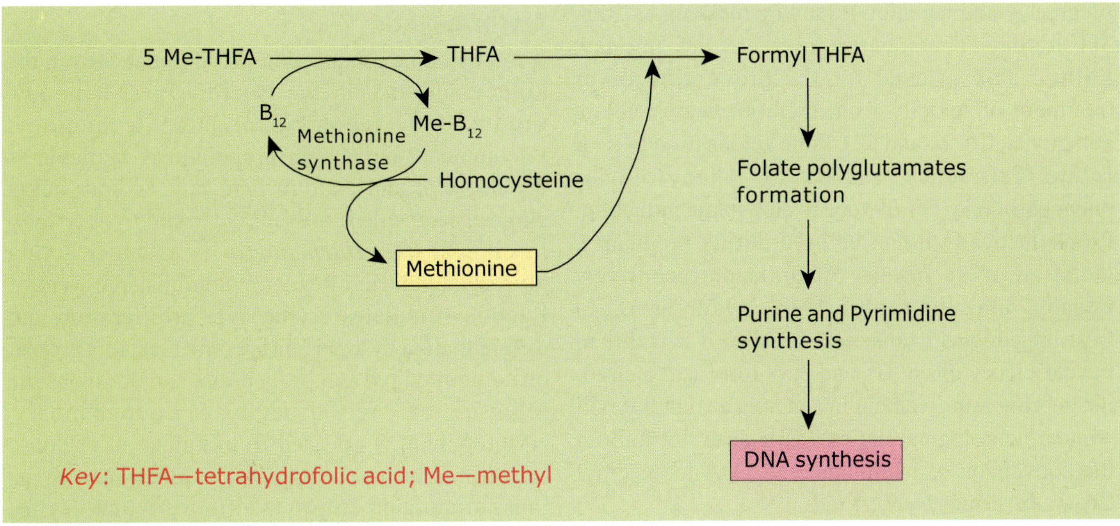

Fig 50.2 Interdependence of Vitamin B_{12} and Folic Acid in DNA Synthesis.

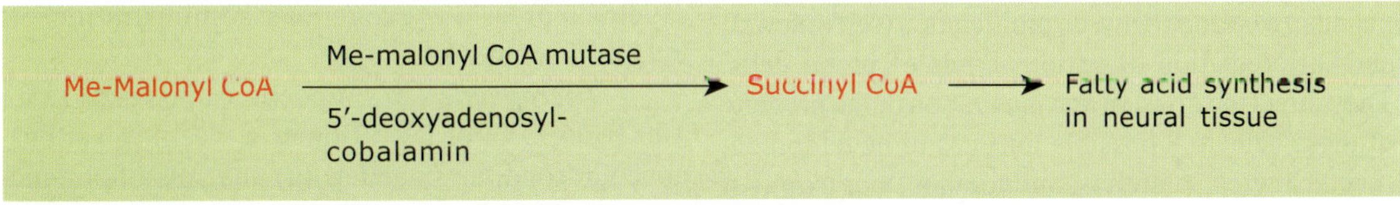

Fig 50.3 Isomerisation of Methylmalonyl CoA to Succinyl CoA by Vitamin B_{12}.

of jejunum, hydrolyse the dietary polyglutamates to folic acid. In the mucosa, before entering the blood stream, this folic acid is reduced by dihydrofolate reductase to tetrahydrofolic acid (THFA), and also methylated to 5-methyltetrahydrofolic acid (5-MeTHFA). Once in the tissues, 5-MeTHFA also gets converted to THFA by vit. B_{12}-dependent methionine synthase (see earlier text). THFA is utilised in the tissues and the rest about 5–20 mg is stored in liver and undergoes enterohepatic circulation similar to vit. B_{12}. Trace amounts of folic acid are excreted in urine and faeces. However, the reabsorption of folic acid is not that smooth as with vit. B_{12} and hence poor dietary intake for about 3 months can result in megaloblastic anaemia.

Metabolic functions: THFA can subsequently be transformed to folate cofactors such as folinic acid (5-formyl-THFA), 10-formyl-THFA and 5,10-methylene-THFA etc. These folate cofactors are interconvertible and serve to donate one-carbon units at various levels of oxidation. Tetrahydrofolic acid keeps on regenerating during such processes and gets recycled. Thus THFA, through 1-C transfer reactions, is involved in the synthesis of purines and pyrimidines which are essential for DNA synthesis (Fig. 50.2).

Deficiency of folic acid results due to: **(a)** dietary lack, **(b)** malabsorption syndrome (coeliac disease or Crohn's disease), **(c)** excessive demand as in pregnancy and anaemia, **(d)** liver disease and renal dialysis (as every time plasma folic acid also gets removed), and **(e)** drug-induced, e.g., after prolonged use of methotrexate (Ch. 26 and 67), phenytoin and phenobarbitone (Ch. 39). Deficiency leads to megaloblastic anaemia and teratogenic effects.

Therapeutic Use and Doses: Daily requirement of folic acid is 50 μg but during pregnancy and lactation it may increase up to 200–300 μg/day. Therapeutic doses are 1–5 mg/day. Folinic acid is used for the prevention of or treatment of toxicity from methotrexate (a folate antagonist, Ch. 26 and 67). Folic acid is used to treat folate deficiency caused by phenytoin or phenobarbitone (Ch. 39) due to enzymatic induction. Prophylactically it can be used during pregnancy, lactation or during use of oral contraceptives. Usually, folic acid is always given with vit. B_{12} to treat megaloblastic anaemia; because if it is due to the deficiency of vit. B_{12} and only folic acid is used, it can bring improvement in anaemia alright but will worsen neurological deficit (as it does not help in the conversion of methylmalonyl CoA to succinyl CoA). ***Adverse effects*** are rare.

HAEMATOPOIETIC GROWTH FACTORS

Haematopoietic growth factors are responsible to maintain a balance between proliferation (self renewal) and differentation of various types of blood cells. They direct the division and maturation of the progeny of these cells to 8 possible lineages of development (erythrocytes, platelets, monocytes, neutrophils, eosinophils, basophils, B-lymphocytes and T-lymphocytes). These endogenous growth factors (**also called cytokine growth factors**) are glycoproteins, which under basal conditions are present in very low concentration. But, in response to any stimulation (anaemia), their concentration can increase by 1000 fold within hours. Cytokines are glycosylated proteins or large peptide mediators released from cells of immune system (macrophages, T- and B-lymphocytes and stromal cells) that regulate host defence system to inflammation. However, the term is gaining more elasticity. There are more than 100 cytokines at present but important among them are: erythropoietin, colony stimulating factors (CSFs), interleukins, chemokines, interferons, growth factors and tumour necrosis factor. They bind to and activate their specific receptors. Here we are concerned with: ***erythropoietin, colony stimulating factors*** (such as ***granulocyte colony stimulating factors*** and ***granulocyte-macrophages colony stimulating factors***) and ***interleukin-11***.

Erythropoietin

It is a cytokine produced in juxtatubular cells in the kidney and also in the macrophages. It is now produced by recombinant DNA technology. Recombinant human erythropoietin is available as *epoetin alfa* and *epoetin beta* but, as both being clinically equivalent, are referred to simply as ***epoetin*** in clinical use. ***Darbepoetin*** is a longer acting glycosylated form of epoetin, administered weekly. Epoetin stimulates erythrocyte proliferation and differentiation by acting on specific receptors present on committed red cell progenitors and promotes the release of reticulocytes. Endogenously, erythropoietin is released from kidney in response to anaemia or myelosuppression. Bone marrow is, thus, stimulated to produce more reticulocytes. However, in renal disease where serum erythropoietin levels do not increase proportionately in response to anaemia/myelosuppression, exogenous administration of epoetin becomes essential.

Therapeutic Uses: Epoetin can be used (25–100 IU/kg S.C. or I.V., 3 times a week) in various anaemic conditions such as **(a)** anaemia of chronic renal failure, **(b)** anaemia resulting from cancer chemotherapy, **(c)** anaemia of AIDS which has been exacerbated by zidovudine treatment, **(d)** anaemia that occurs in premature infants and **(e)** to increase benefits of autologous blood transfusion (collection and reinfusion of patient's own blood). Enhanced erythropoiesis with epoetin increases demands of iron and folic acid. Hence supplementation with iron and folic acid provides better results.

Adverse effects include flu-like symptoms, mild hypertension, encephalopathy with headache, disorientation and occasionally convulsions. Blood viscosity increases as the haematocrit rises, hence there is risk of thrombosis.

Myeloid Growth Factors or Colony Stimulating Factors (CSFs)

CSFs are cytokines. They accelerate the formation of matured colonies of various bone marrow progenitor cells *in vitro*. The CSFs or myeloid growth factors are broadly of two types: ***Granulocyte Colony Stimulating Factors (G-CSFs)*** and

Granulocyte - Macrophages - Colony Stimulating Factors (GM-CSFs).

The recombinant human G-CSF is ***filgrastim*** which is produced in a *E. coli* bacterial expression system using recombinant DNA technology. ***Pegfilgrastim*** is a longer acting analogue of filgrastim which can be given I.V. once per chemotherapy cycle rather than daily till chemotherapy lasts (as with filgrastim).

G-CSF stimulates proliferation and differentiation of neutrophil progenitor cells, activates the phagocytic activity of mature neutrophils and prolongs their survival in circulation. G-CSF in addition, has a remarkable ability to mobilise haematopoietic stem cells and thus to increase their concentration in peripheral blood. This observation has resulted in the use of peripheral blood stem cells (instead of bone marrow cells) in autologous haematopoietic stem cell transplant.

GM-CSF stimulates development of many progenitor cells (granulocytes, erythroids and megakaryocytes). It is virtually a multipotential haematopoietic growth factor. In addition, it also prolongs longevity of matured neutrophils and acts in concert with interleukin-2 and -3 to stimulate proliferation and differentiation of T-cells. It also plays some role in inflammation. Like G CSF, it also mobilises peripheral blood stem cells but to a lesser extent. It is available as ***sargramostim*** which is a recombinant human GM-CSF that is produced in yeast cell expression system. Two other forms—***molgramostim*** (which is bacterially derived) and ***regramostim*** (which is mammalian derived) recombinant GM-CSF—have been developed but are in clinical trials.

Therapeutic Uses of CSFs (G-CSF and GM-CSF) are as follows: **(1)** to reduce the severity and duration of neutropenia induced by cytotoxic drugs during chemotherapy or following bone marrow transplant, **(2)** to stimulate the release of progenitor stem cells in peripheral blood which can be harvested and infused, with or without bone marrow cells, after intensive courses of cancer chemotherapy, **(3)** to prevent persistent neutropenia in advanced HIV infection and **(4)** to treat congenital neutropenia, cyclic neutropenia and neutropenia associated with aplastic anaemia. For all these indications G-CSF is more preferred and commonly used. For the treatment of febrile neutropenia, ***pegfilgrastim*** is considered as a suitable choice for two reasons: **(1)** it can be administered I.V. or S.C. less frequently (only once during the course of chemotherapy) and it shortens the period of neutropenia more than G-CSF, and **(2)** GM-CSF itself induces fever as a side effect and hence not suitable.

Adverse effects: G-CSF is better tolerated than GM-CSF and is, therefore, used more frequently. G-CSF can cause bone tenderness and pain (10–15% of cases) which subsides when the drug is withdrawn. Rarely, it can cause dysuria and vasculitis. GM-CSF frequently produces fever, skin rash, muscle pain and lethargy. Pain and redness at the injection site is also common. If given by infusion it can cause flushing, fall in BP, tachycardia, breathlessness, nausea and vomiting which can be prevented by giving O_2 and adequate I.V. fluids.

Megakaryocyte Growth Factors

These include ***interleukin-11***, a cytokine produced by fibroblasts and bone marrow stromal cells, and ***thrombopoietin***, a protein produced mainly by liver and kidney. ***Oprelvekin*** is a recombinant form of interleukin-11 (IL-11), which is produced by expression in *E.coli.*

IL-11 stimulates the growth of multiple lymphoid and myeloid cells—most notably it increases the number of peripheral platelets and neutrophils. Endogenous ***thrombopoietin (TPO)*** also, independently stimulates the growth of megakaryocytic (platelet) progenitors, and thereby increases the platelet production and increases platelet response to aggregating stimulus. Mice lacking in thrombopoietin or its receptor show marked thrombocytopenia without anaemia or leukopenia. However, trials with human recombinant TPO were abandoned because auto-antibodies against thrombopoietin were found in healthy human subjects.

Therapeutic Uses: ***IL-11*** or ***oprelvekin*** (administered by S.C route) as well as ***thrombopoietin*** are used to treat thrombocytopenia and also for secondary prevention of thrombocytopenia following cancer chemotherapy. IL-11 therapy significantly reduces the need for platelet transfusion in patients receiving chemotherapy for non-myeloid cancers.

Adverse effects of IL-11/oprelvekin are dizziness, headache, and fatigue. There may be anaemia (due to haemodilution) and dyspnoea (due to fluid accumulation in lungs). Occasionally hypokalaemia may result but rarely atrial arrhythmia (usually transient).

Romiplostim and ***eltrombopag*** have been approved for treating idiopathic thrombocytopenic purpura. Eltrombopag is a small molecule TPO receptor agonist administered by oral route, whereas ***romiplostim*** is a recombinant IgG1 Fc-peptide fusion protein (administered by S.C. route) that binds and activates TPO receptor. By activating the TPO receptor both molecules induce a transient increase in the platelet count. However, worsening of thrombocytopenia may develop after termination of treatment with these agents, and bone marrow toxicity (manifesting as bone marrow fibrosis) has also been reported.

VITAMINS

Vitamins are a group of unrelated chemical substances that are needed in smaller quantities for nutrition and metabolic demands of the body. Some are needed for haematopoiesis also. They generally serve as cofactors for enzymes involved in intermediary metabolism. These are mostly obtained from food except for vitamin-D which is synthesised endogenously by the body under the influence of sunlight (Ch. 46). Nicotinic acid is also synthesised from tryptophan endogenously, but the amount produced is inadequate for the maintenance of health. For some vitamins there are *precursors* (e.g., β-carotene for vitamin A) while some vitamins exist in more than one chemical form, called *vitamers* (e.g., pyridoxine, pyridoxal and pyridoxamine are *vitamers* of Vit. B_6).

Classification

1. **Fat-Soluble Vitamins**
   Vitamin A, D, E and K
2. **Water-Soluble Vitamins**
   a) ***Vitamin B-complex Group***: Thiamine (B_1), Riboflavin (B_2), Niacin (B_3), Pantothenic acid (B_5), Pyridoxine (B_6) and Biotin (B_7). These are known as ***energy-releasing B-complex vitamins***. Folic acid and Cyanocobalamin (B_{12}) are known as ***haematopoietic B-complex vitamins.***
   b) ***Non B-complex Group***: Ascorbic acid (vitamin C).

The *fat-soluble vitamins* are generally metabolised slowly and are stored in the liver. Excessive amounts of these vitamins, however, are stored in the body which usually leads to toxicity (hypervitaminosis). In contrast, the *water-soluble vitamins* are less toxic as these are rapidly metabolised and readily excreted in the urine.

Fat-Soluble Vitamins

Vitamin A (Retinol)

- ***Dietary Source***: Carrots, red cabbage, milk, mango, cheese, butter, eggs, fish and liver.
- ***Physiological Role***: **(1)** required for proper vision in dim light (dark adaptation). Vit. A is reduced to an aldehyde (11-*cis*-retinal) which combines with opsins to produce a visual pigment—rhodopsin in retinal rods and cones. This pigment in retina is responsible for the process of dark adaptation, **(2)** maintenance of structural intergrity of epithelial cells all over the body. It inhibits keratinisation and makes epithelium resistant to infection, **(3)** reduces risk of lung and skin cancer being an antioxidant (β-carotene), **(4)** required for proper bone development and bone growth in children, **(5)** activates immune defense mechanisms (lymphocyte proliferation and killer cell functions), and **(6)** involved in spermatogenesis and foetal development.
- ***Deficiency Symptoms***: EYE: night blindness (nyctalopia) with xerosis (dryness) of cornea, Bitot's spots (white patch on conjunctiva) and keratomalacia (ulceration and necrosis of cornea) collectively called xerophthalmia. SKIN: hyperkeratosis. Drying and keratinisation of epidermis. LUNGS: decreased elasticity and increased incidence of infections. RENAL: rough genitourinary epithelium, hence chances of urinary calculi. BONES: faulty modelling of bones. MISCELLANEOUS: risk of lung/skin malignancy; sterility in males; foetal deformities and adverse effects on erythropoiesis.

Any disease that results in fat malabsorption and impaired liver storage can lead to vit. A deficiency. These include sprue, pancreatic disease, biliary tract disease and hepatic disease. Children from low income families, who cannot afford fresh vegetables and milk products are at a great risk of vit. A deficiency.

- ***Therapeutic Doses and Daily Requirements***: For prophylaxis/daily requirements: Adult dose 1000 µg (4000 IU)/day. Therapeutic doses for vit. A deficiency in adults are 50,000 IU–100,000 IU orally for 3 days and then supplementation occasionally.
- ***Drug Interactions***: **(1)** Vitamin E improves its storage and utilisation. Hence used generally in combination, **(2)** Liquid paraffin emulsifies vit. A and leads to its deficiency and **(3)** Use of oral contraceptives increases the levels of vit. A.
- ***Toxicity (Hypervitaminosis-A)*** occurs after regular ingestion of 100,000 IU of vit. A per day for more than 3 weeks. *Chronic toxicity* is manifested as dry and pruritic skin, hair loss, fissures of lips, tenderness of bones, brittle nails, hepatosplenomegaly, oedema, decrease in HDL and increase in triglycerides, headache and fatigue. *Acute toxicity* is manifested as drowsiness, headache, vomiting, papilloedema (due to raised intracranial pressure), abdominal pain, anorexia, diplopia and peeling of skin after 24 hrs.
- ***Vitamin A Analogues***
  1) ***β-Carotene* (precursor of vit. A)** obtained from carrots and red cabbage. Prior to absorption it is converted to vit. A in the wall of intestine and then oxidised to retinoic acid and retinol. Mainly used as an antioxidant. Adult dose 30–300 µg/day (1 mg of retinol = 6 µg of β-carotene).
  2) ***Tretinoin (trans-retinoic acid)***: It is a carboxyacid form (vitamer) of Vit. A and has vit. A activity only in epithelial cells (not in eye or in reproductive system). Used topically for acne vulgaris and to reverse the signs of photoageing.
  3) ***Isotretinoin*** can be used orally for treatment of nodulocystic acne vulgaris and for prevention of skin cancer. Pregnancy is its absolute contraindication. Recently, some idiosyncratic episodes of severe depression with suicidal ideation and suicidal attempts in patients taking isotretinoin, have also been reported. Adult dose 500 mcg/kg daily in 2 divided doses for 3–4 months.
  4) ***Etretinate*** is used orally for refractory psoriasis. Pregnancy is its absolute contraindication.
  5) ***Acitretin*** is a metabolite of etretinate but obtained by a synthetic process using retinoid as a base. It is used by oral route in the doses of 25–50 mg OD in pustular psoriasis, lichen planus and ichthyosis. Pregnancy is its absolute contraindication.
  6) ***Tazarotene*** and ***Bexarotene*** are second generation retinoids, used as gel formulation by topical application in patients of psoriasis and acne. These are significantly abosrbed from skin and should be avoided during pregnancy. Contraception in ladies of child bearing age is necessary during their use.

Vitamin D

It has been covered extensively in Ch. 46.

Vitamin E (Tocoferols)

The most important tocoferol with highest vit. E activity is α-tocoferol.

- ***Dietary Source***: Wheat germ oil, vegetable seed oil, nuts, peas and egg yolk.
- ***Physiological Role***: **(1)** functions as an antioxidant protecting cellular structures from attack by free radicals. Prevents oxidation of coenzyme Q and protects polyunsaturated fatty acids from oxidative breakdown, **(2)** it is an antisterility factor, **(3)** plays an important role in protection against cancer, coronary artery disease, Alzheimer's disease and cataracts (through its antioxidant effects) and **(4)** enhances the use of vit. A by the body.
- ***Deficiency Symptoms***: **(1)** peripheral neuropathy with spinocerebellar degeneration, **(2)** sterility in males and recurrent abortions in females, **(3)** muscular dystrophy and cardiomyopathy, **(4)** haemolytic anaemia in premature infants and **(5)** altered gait and depressed tendon reflexes. The deficiency is believed to occur in patients with biliary, pancreatic or intestinal disease causing steatorrhoea.

- ***Therapeutic Use and Dose Requirements***: Daily requirements are 10–20 mg. Usual adult dose in deficiency is 400 mg/day, children 200 mg/day. It is useful in treating: **(1)** nocturnal muscle cramps (400 mg/day for 6–12 weeks), **(2)** fibrocystic breast disease (600 mg/day for 3–6 months), **(3)** intermittent claudication (400 mg/day for 12–15 weeks), **(4)** acanthocytosis (low levels of circulating vit. E due to genetic absence of β-lipoprotein; 100 mg/week intramuscularly to proctect oxidative fragility of erythrocytes, **(5)** to reduce the risk of retrolental fibroplasia in premature infants exposed to higher oxygen concentrations (100 mg/kg/day, oral), **(6)** to increase the survival time of erythrocytes in patients of G6PD deficiency (100 mg/day) and **(7)** as antioxidant to delay cataract formation, coronary artery disease and neurodegenerative disorders (100–200 mg/day for at least 2–3 years). Vit. E is never given by I.V. route.
- ***Drug Interactions***: **(1)** Liquid paraffin emulsifies vit. E and can cause its deficiency, **(2)** Effects of oral anticogulants are potentiated by vit. E, **(3)** Vit. E can interfere with iron absorption and **(4)** Vit. A, Vit C, selenium and methionine potentiate antioxidant effects of vit. E.
- ***Toxicity***: Rare. However, loose motions, abdominal cramps, lethargy and creatinuria may occur.

Vitamin K

It has been covered extensively in Ch. 51.

Water-Soluble Vitamins

Vitamin B Complex

The vitamins belonging to this group tend to occur together in the food and hence the collective term "Vitamin B Complex". The B-vitamins are obtained from both meat and vegetable products except for vit. B_{12} which occurs only in meat, liver, fish, egg, milk and yeast (but not from vegetables).

Thiamine (Vit B_1)

- ***Dietary Source***: Cereals, pulses, peanuts, yeast, green vegetables, egg and meat. Thiamine is heat labile.
- ***Physiological Role***: **(1)** Its active form (in the body), thiamine pyrophosphate, acts as a coenzyme in carbohydrate metabolism and **(2)** It also plays some role in neuromuscular transmission.
- ***Deficiency Symptoms***: Its dietary deficiency leads to failure of glucose metabolism (aerobic) causing accumulation of pyruvic and lactic acid (BERI-BERI). ***Dry Beri-Beri*** affects CNS and peripheral nervous system causing peripheral neuropathy, numbness, cramps and muscle weakness. ***Wet Beri-Beri*** affects CVS causing palpitation, breathlessness, ECG changes and high-output cardiac failure. In alcoholics, poor diet or neglect of food also leads to thiamine deficiency characterised by Wernicke-Korsakoff syndrome (ophthalmoplegia, memory deficits and ataxia).
- ***Therapeutic Uses*** and ***Doses***: Daily requirements are 1.5–2 mg. For beri-beri, 100 mg/day I.M. or I.V., then 5–10 mg/day orally as maintenance. For Wernicke-Korsakoff syndrome—same as for beri-beri.
- ***Toxicity***: rare, except for sensitivity reactions when given parenterally (occasionally).

Riboflavin (Vit. B_2)

- ***Dietary Source***: Meat, liver, eggs, milk, cheese, sprouted cereals and pulses.
- ***Physiological Role***: It carries its physiological function in its active forms, flavin mononucleotide (FMN) and flavin adenine dinucleotide (FAD), which are coenzymes for flavoproteins involved in several oxidation-reduction reactions. These coenzymes are also involved in carbohydrate metabolism.
- ***Deficiency Symptoms***: Glossitis, angular stomatitis, cheilosis (fissure on lips), vascularisation of cornea, cataract formation, local seborrheic dermatitis of trunk and extremities.
- ***Therapeutic Uses*** and ***Doses***: Daily requirement 1.5–2 mg. In ariboflavinosis 5–20 mg/day. Generally used in combination of other B-complex vitamins. Can be used as an adjunct in the treatment of hypertension, arteriosclerosis, diabetes and obesity.
- ***Toxicity***: Rare

Niacin (Vit. B_3)

Also called as ***pellagra preventing factor.*** Niacin is a mixture of nicotinic acid and nicotinamide.

- ***Dietary Source***: Fish, egg, liver, cereal, pulses and dry nuts.
- ***Physiological Role***: It is converted to active forms, nicotinamide adenine dinucleotide (NAD), or nicotinamide adenine dinucleotide phosphate (NADP), which act as coenzymes in various oxidation-reduction reactions involved in cellular respiration, glycolysis and fat synthesis.
- ***Deficiency Symptoms***: **(1)** Produces symptoms of pellagra (dermatitis, enteritis, stomatitis, headache, dizziness, dementia, insomnia, depression and in severe cases delusion and hallucinations) and **(2)** chronic alcoholics are at more risk of developing pellagra because besides dietary deficiency, absorption of niacin is also impaired in them.
- ***Therapeutic Uses and Doses***: Prophylaxis 15–20 mg/day. For treatment 200–500 mg/day oral. The amino acid *tryptophan* (mainly from animal protein) is a provitamin for niacin, though it is only partly converted to niacin. Maize, Jowar and Bajara eaters are prone to suffer from pellagra because these are almost lacking in tryptophan. Conversion of niacin to its active forms requires the presence of vit. B_1, B_2 and B_6 also. Hence, treatment of pellagra needs, besides niacin, a supplementation of these B-complex vitamins and dietary proteins containing tryptophan. Niacin is also used in treating hyperlipoproteinaemia (Ch. 23).
- ***Toxicity***: As nicotinic acid (Ch. 23)—Flushing of face, pruritus and vomiting. As nicotinamide—rare.

Pantothenic Acid (Vit. B_5)

- ***Dietary Source***: Meat, liver, egg yolk, milk, cereals, legumes, vegetables and fruits
- ***Physiological Role***: It is an essential component of coenzyme-A involved in the metabolism of carbohydrates, fats, proteins and porphyrin to catalyse acetate transfer reactions.
- ***Deficiency Symptoms***: not apparent but believed to cause flatulence, intermittent diarrhoea, leg cramps, paraesthesias and insomnia.
- ***Therapeutic Use*** and ***Doses***: Daily requirements 4–7 mg. For treatment (rarely) 50–100 mg/day. It is generally used as a nutritional supplement in the form of calcium pantothenate along with other B-complex vitamins. Its I.M. injection is sometimes used to treat postoperative paralytic ileus.
- ***Toxicity***: Rare

Pyridoxine (Vit. B_6)

Pyridoxine, pyridoxal and pyridoxamine—all are vitamers and have vitamin B_6 activity.

- ***Dietary Source***: Soyabean, vegetables, cereals, egg, liver and meat.
- ***Physiological Role***: It is involved as coenzyme (pyridoxal phosphate or pyridoxamine phosphate) which are involved in the metabolism of proteins, carbohydrates and fats. Pyridoxal phosphate also plays an important role in the synthesis of GABA (in CNS), haeme (in haemoglobin) and amino acids (tryptophan).
- ***Deficiency Symptoms***: Peripheral neuropathy, glossitis, stomatitis, anaemia, precipitation of epilepsy and growth retardation.
- ***Drug Interactions***: **(1)** Pyridoxine activates the conversion of levodopa to dopamine peripherally and therefore reduces bioavailability of dopamine centrally (Ch. 40). **(2)** Use of isoniazid, in slow acetylators, leads to deficiency of pyridoxine (Ch. 7 and 59). **(3)** Use of hydralazine, cycloserine and penicillamine also lead to vit. B_6 deficiency.
- ***Therapeutic Use*** and ***Doses***: Prophylaxis 2–5 mg/day. Pyridoxine responsive anaemia (50–200 mg/day). Isoniazid induced vit. B_6 deficiency (10–50 mg/day). Mental symptoms in women on oral contraceptives (50 mg/day) and in morning sickness (50–100 mg/day).
- ***Toxicity***: Rare.

Biotin (Vit. B_7)

- ***Dietary Source***: Organ meats including liver, egg yolk (not white), fish, legumes, berries, avacado, cauliflower, mushrooms and dry fruits.
- ***Physiological Role***: It is an important coenzyme involved in carbohydrate and fat metabolism and in the synthesis of fatty acids from glucose.
- ***Deficiency Symptoms***: Anorexia, nausea and vomiting, glossitis, dry and scaly hairs (brittle

hairs and hair loss), nails (brittle and fragile nails) and skin (dry irritated skin, dermatitis) and muscle aches and pains. Biotin is given a nick name of vitamin 'H' which stands from the German words '*Haar*' for hair and '*Haut*' for nail. Biotin is commonly added to hair and skin beauty products, although it is belived that it is not absorbed very well from skin and hair and actually must be ingested to be fully beneficial. Deficiency of biotin is rare. However, spontaneous deficiency can result in persons consuming raw eggs (with whites). Raw egg white contains a heat labile, biotin binding protein called *avidin* which prevents the absorption of biotin from the intestine. Besides, intestinal digestive bacteria are belived to synthesize from biotin on their own. As a result long term use of certain antiepileptic drugs (phenytoil, carbamazepine, valproate, topiramate etc), prolonged use of broad spectrum antibiotics (including fluoroquinolones) which disturb intestinal microbiota, and intestinal malabsorption (Crohn's disease, coeliac disease or leaky guts syndrome) may increase the risk of vit. B_7 deficiency.

- ***Therapeutic Use*** and ***Doses***: Daily requirements are 0.03 mg (30 microgram) for adults, 30 mg for pregnant women and 35 mg for women who are breast feeding. Therapeutic doses are 10–20 mg per day. Generally used in multivitamin preparations.
- ***Toxicity***: Rare

For ***Vitamin B_{12}*** and ***Folic Acid*** refer earlier section of this Chapter.

Vitamin B-Complex Supplements

Together all vitamins in general and vitamins of B-complex group, in particular, support metabolic activity (see above physiological role of each one of them), brain functions, nerve signaling and many other daily functions of a number of organs and tissues. Each one of them also work with one another synergistically. Therefore taking vitamins along with B-vitamins is always the best way to ensure their whole benefit. It should be kept in mind that not all supplements are created in equal quality. High quality multivitamin supplements/products are those that are made from food sources and do not contain fillers and preservatives, some of which may be toxins. An ideal energy supplement is one which is made by assembling together different collaborative nutrients so that the body can recognize the vitamins and minerals and use them in a synergistic manner, similar to how they appear in food sources.

The following example will explain it better. *There are actually eight different chemical forms of Vit B_7 (biotin)*, but only one is naturally occurring, the kind found in food sources; this is called ***D-biotin*** and is thought to be the only type that has complete *Vit. B_7* capabilities. Nutrition scientists in 2004 examined 51 different foods to identify how much *D-biotin* levels was available. They found a wide range of varying *D-biotin* levels within each food. For this reason, many regulators, including US-FDA do not list the amount of biotin in common foods. However, all dietary sources of *Vit B_7 (biotin)* mentioned above contain more than daily requirement, e.g., liver (cooked 100 g: 27–35 mg), egg yellow (one whole: 13–25 mg) salmon fish (cooked 100 g: 4–5 mg), goat cheese (30 g: 0.4–2 mg), avacado (1 whole 2–6 mg), raspberries (1 cup: 2–6 mg), cauliflower (1 cup: 0.2–2 mg) and whole grain bread (1 slice: 0.2–6 mg). This amount of *biotin* in all foods constitute all the eight chemical forums and not the *D-biotin* alone. Therefore food components with high concentrations of varied biotin forms are the best sources of *Vit B_7*, rather than synthetic *biotin,* which may not be *D-biotin*.

Non B-complex vitamin

Vitamin C (Ascorbic Acid)

- ***Dietary Source***: Citrus fruits (lemon, orange, Aamla), black currants, tomatos, potatos, green chilies and cabbage.
- ***Physiological Role***: Serves as a cofactor in a number of oxidation, amidation and hydroxylation reactions. Hence, it plays crucial role in collagen synthesis, adrenal steroidogenesis, biosynthesis of ADH, oxytocin and norepinephrine, conversion of folic acid to folinic acid and to maintain iron in ferrous state for its absorption.
- ***Deficiency Symptoms***: Scurvy (defect in collagen synthesis) characterised by gingival bleed-

ing, gingivitis, lossening of tooth and defects in tooth formation, failure of wound healing, capillaries rupture, haematomas and anaemia.

- ***Therapeutic Uses*** and ***Dose***: Prophylaxis (adult) 50–500 mg daily. For scurvy 1–1.5 g daily. As antioxidant 100 mg/day. In haematinic formulations 150 mg/day (with iron and folic acid). In megadoses (1–2 g/day), it is recommended in common cold, viral infections, cancer prophylaxis and for acidification of urine in UTIs but the outcome is doubtful.
- ***Toxicity***: in therapeutic doses—rare; but if mega doses are taken for longer period, precipitation of renal oxalates stones is possible. Stoppage of megadoses has been reported to cause "rebound scurvy".

ANTIOXIDANTS

Normally for the stability of any atomic orbital, a presence of at least 2 electrons, spinning in opposite directions, is necessary as is seen with most biological molecules which are termed as non-radicals (meaning non-free radicals). A free radical is a molecular species having an unpaired electron and thus is a highly reactive entity (being unstable). Free radicals are formed constantly in human system either as accidental products during metabolism or deliberately during the process of phagocytosis. Apart from these, free radicals can also be generated from toxic environmental polluants, ionizing radiations, ozone, heavy metal poisoning, cigarette smoking and chronic alcohol intake. Free radicals thus formed, being highly reactive, can oxidise biomolecules leading to tissue injury and cell death.

To stabilise itself, a free radical may donate its unpaired electron or may accept one from other biomolecule transforming a non-radical to another free radical to set up a disastrous chain reaction. These free radicals are normally scavenged (removed) by several enzymatic and non-enzymatic antioxidant defense mechanisms (see below). If these defense mechanisms are inadequate, a situation called "oxidative stress" occurs which leads to lipid peroxidation, protein and DNA damage causing tissue injury and cell death. However, if two free radicals combine, the 2 unpaired electrons are shared by each other to form a covalent bond. Their reactivity is thus terminated.

$$x^{\bullet} + x^{\bullet} \rightarrow x\text{–}x$$

Reactive Oxygen Species

Free radicals can be negatively charged, positively charged or electrically neutral. The latter includes inorganic species like hydrogen peroxide (H_2O_2), hypochlorous acid (HOCl) and nascent (singlet) oxygen (O). H_2O_2 and HOCl are not free radicals but are very powerful oxidising agents. Nascent oxygen (O) is a transient atomic state of oxygen which is highly reactive than O_2 and is implicated in the causation of several oxidative processes and photosensitisation reactions. Such highly reactive species, which are not free radicals in true sense are called **R**eactive **O**xygen **S**pecies (ROS).

Promoters of Free Radicals

Several transition metals (e.g., iron and copper) have variable oxidation numbers (i.e., valency) which accordingly can accept a single electron from or donate it to non-radicals.

$$Fe^{3+} + e^- = Fe^{2+} \text{ (or) } Cu^{2+} + e^- = Cu^+$$

As a result, these metals serve as excellent promoters of free radicals. For example, iron and copper ions can convert H_2O_2 into highly reactive free hydroxyl radical ($OH^{\bullet}$) which can accelerate lipid peroxidation and lead to an accumulation of highly cytotoxic end products (see below).

Types of Free Radicals and Damage Produced by Them

Superoxide Radicals ($O_2^{\bullet}$)

It is an oxygen molecule deficient of one electron (also called superoxide ion). These are derived from inevitable leakage from the mitochondrial electron transport chain reactions. These are also generated during metabolism of various drugs by cytochrome P-450 microsomal oxidative system (e.g., of paracetamol or alcohol). Some enzymes also catalyse the formation of these free radicals, e.g., superoxide ($O_2^{\bullet}$) ions and hydrogen peroxide are formed during oxidation of hypoxanthine to xanthine and to uric acid.

Other Free Radicals

Other important free radicals are hydroxyl ($OH^{\bullet}$), peroxyl ($ROO^{\bullet}$) and nitric oxide free radical ($NO^{\bullet}$).

All these free radicals induce oxidative destruction of polyunsaturated fatty acids (PUFAs) of cell membranes (lipid peroxidation). This directly disrupts the integrity and function of biological cell membranes and even destabilises membrane receptors. The cellular components also suffer damage due to reactive aldehyde production. Attack on proteins inactivates enzymes while damage to nucleic acids causes breaks in DNA strands. Free radicals are regarded as carcinogenic because of the damage they inflict on DNA. The cytotoxicity of nitric oxide (NO) results by a bit different mechanism. NO has a very high affinity to even low concentrations of superoxide ion ($O_2^{\bullet}$). In situations of oxidative stress, where superoxide free radicals are in plenty, NO reacts very rapidly to form an unstable peroxynitrite ion ($ONOO^{\bullet}$). The latter instantly gets degraded to hydroxyl ($OH^{\bullet}$) and nitrite ($NO_2^{\bullet}$) free radicals which are responsible for the cytotoxicity of NO.

$$NO + O_2^{\bullet} \rightarrow ONOO^{\bullet} \xrightarrow{H} NO_2^{\bullet} + OH^{\bullet}$$

Free Radicals and Diseases

Free radicals play an important role in the pathogenesis of ***diseases with multiorgan involvement*** such as autoimmune diseases, rheumatoid arthritis, paracetamol and alcohol toxicity, radiation injury, carcinogenesis, amyloidosis and aging; as well as in diseases having specific system/organ involvement such as **(1)** in CNS: Parkinsonism, Alzheimer's disease, Huntington's disease and multiple sclerosis; **(2)** in CVS: myocardial infarction, ischaemic reperfusion injury and atherosclerosis; **(3)** in ENDOCRINES: diabetes mellitus; **(4)** in GIT: peptic ulcer, cirrhosis and pancreatitis; **(5)** in RENAL: nephrotoxicity due to aminoglycosides and heavy metal poisoning; **(6)** in RESPIRATORY SYSTEM: toxicity due to cigarette smoking and **(7)** in EYES: cataract, retinopathy.

Antioxidants and Their Clinical Use

Antioxidants, therefore, can intervene at any of the following levels between the process of free radical generation to the causation of tissue injury: **(1)** blockade of the generation of toxic free radical, **(2)** blockade of the chain reaction set by free radical, **(3)** scavenging of free radical, **(4)** blocking the secondary generation of toxic metabolite or mediator and **(5)** enhancing antioxidant capability. Thus, antioxidants are free radical scavengers which at low concentration can prevent or delay the oxidation of lipids, carbohydrates, proteins and nucleic acids to improve the quality of life by retarding the ageing process. To prevent free radical formation and eventual tissue damage, our body has an array of antioxidant defense system, which allows us to cope with the "oxidative stress" inflicted by them. These are classified as:

Endogenous Antioxidants

Superoxide Dismutase (SOD)

This enzyme found in all cells, scavenges superoxide ion and prevents its accumulation so that cells are protected from oxidative stress. SOD catalyses a dismutation reaction in which one $O_2^{\bullet}$ is oxidised to O_2 while the other is reduced to H_2O_2.

$$O_2^{\bullet} + O_2^{\bullet} + 2H \xrightarrow{\text{SOD}} H_2O_2 + O_2$$

$$2H_2O_2 \xrightarrow{\text{Catalase}} 2H_2O + O_2$$

H_2O_2 which can still oxidise and damage many cellular components is instantly removed by enzymes like ***catalase*** and ***glutathione peroxidase***. SOD can afford protection against ischaemic reperfusion injury, pancreatitis, gastrointestinal ischaemia, myocardial infarction, endotoxic shock and organ transplant.

Glutathione Reduced Form (G-SH)

G-SH is an excellent antioxidant and cytoprotective. It prevents free radical induced oxidation of SH groups of various proteins to disulfide (-S-S-) derivatives. It also protects haemoglobin from getting oxidised by H_2O_2. Glutathione peroxidase (a selenium containing enzyme) scavenges toxic amounts of peroxides, H_2O_2 and free radicals.

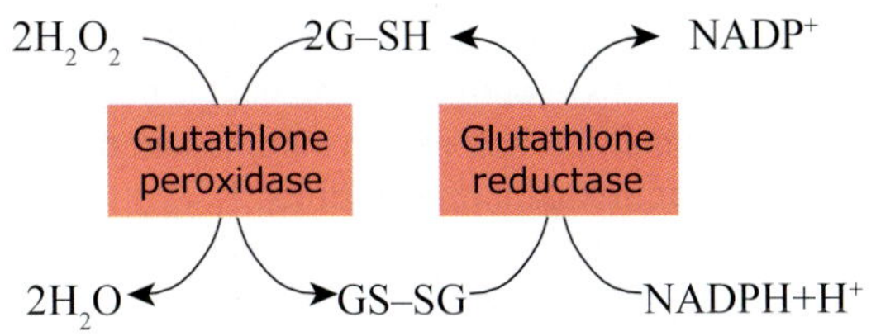

Subsequently, NADPH regenerates G-SH (reduced form) from G-S-S-G (oxidised form) with the help of glutathione reductase. G-SH improves the outcome of organ transplant, cystic fibrosis, reperfusion injury and diseases in AIDS patients.

Carotenoids (β-Carotene)

It is a vitamin-A precursor (see earlier text) which also serves as an antioxidant and reduces the risk of cancers due to free radical damage. It has also been shown to provide protection from heart attack and photo-sensitisation because of its antioxidant properties.

Melatonin

This hormone from pineal gland is also a potent scavenger of free radicals, mainly of $OH^{\bullet}$ radicals. It neutralises nascent oxygen, removes H_2O_2 as well as NO and inactivates peroxynitrite ($ONOO^{\bullet}$) free radical. It catalyses the action of various enzymes involved in the activity of endogenous antioxidants.

Alfa-Tocopherol (Vit. E)

Being antioxidant, supplements of vit. E provides protection against neurological damage, atherosclerosis, thrombotic vascular disease and retrolental fibroplasia (see earlier text).

Ascorbic Acid (Vit. C)

Ascorbic acid reacts with H_2O_2, peroxide and superoxide free radicals and itself gets oxidised to dehydroascorbate in this process. The latter is then reduced back to ascorbic acid by gluthathione reductase. Deficiency of vit C predisposes to atherosclerosis and carcinogenicity. Tobacco (chewing and smoking) is rich in free radicals which damage the DNA, causing throat and lung cancer through the formation of nitrosamine. Both vit C and E inhibit nitrosamine formation.

Miscellaneous

Adenosine inhibits superoxide generation by NADPH oxidase in neutrophils and macrophages. It is an endogenous anti-inflammatory-antioxidant that affords protection against reperfusion injury.

Lactoferrin and ***transferrin*** are circulating iron binding proteins that reduce iron-dependent free radical toxicity and afford natural protection against lung cancer. ***Nicotinamide*** is also used to protect against tissue injury due to oxidative stress.

Agents Augmenting Endogenous Antioxidants

N-acetylcysteine is glutathione precursor while ***ebselen*** is a congener of glutathione peroxidase. Both augment endogenous glutathione peroxidase activity. They serve to promote endogenous antioxidant activity. The former is used as antioxidant in treating paracetamol toxicity and in AIDS patients. ***Desferoxamine*** and ***ceruloplasmin*** bind free Fe^{2+} and also detoxify superoxide anion and thus inhibit iron-dependent lipid peroxidation.

Exogenous (Pharmacological) Antioxidants

Xanthine oxidase promotes superoxidation during reperfusion injury, myocardial infarction, cerebral and gastrointestinal reoxygenation injury. ***Allopurinol*** and ***oxypurinol*** (antigout drugs) are xanthine oxidase inhibitors which also act as antioxidant by inhibiting the process of superoxidation. ***Selegiline*** has also been demonstrated to have free radical scavenging action.

Trace Elements and Minerals

Selenium is a trace element which enhances the antioxidant activity of vitamin E. It also promotes synthesis of glutathione peroxidase as well as stimulates the immune system of the body and therefore, is a most favoured ingredient in various antioxidant formulations. ***Manganese, zinc, copper*** and ***chromium*** are good sources for generating superoxide dismutase, glutathione peroxidase and catalase enzyme.

Antioxidants From Plant Sources

Garlic, grape fruit juice, soyabean (isoflavones), turmeric (curcuminoids), tomato (lycopene, a red carotenoid pigment) and herbal preparations containing bioflavinoids (the phenolic chain breaking antioxidants) also possess good antioxidant properties. These are considered much safer in day-to-day use. These are claimed to reduce the risk of atherosclerosis, myocardial infarction and various cancers. ***Spirulina*** is a blue–green algae from shallow pond water having excellent antioxidant properties. It is a good source for superoxide dismutase (SOD), β-carotene and B-complex vitamins. It is used singly or in combination with other vitamins and minerals in various antioxidant preparations.

CHAPTER 51

Drugs Affecting Coagulation, Fibrinolysis and Platelet Functions

COMPETENCY PH1.25

Haemostasis means limiting the blood loss consequent to bleeding. It should not be confused with a similar term *homeostasis* which means maintenance of body's internal environment within physiological limits. Three basic mechanisms which prevent the blood loss from smaller vessels are: **(1)** ***vascular spasm*** caused by damage (trauma) to smooth muscle which reduces blood loss for several minutes, **(2)** ***platelet plug formation.*** It starts with platelet adhesion (to the exposed collagen of the damaged endothelium) followed by platelet aggregation (by losing their individual membrane and forming a gelatinous mass called *platelet plug*. The platelet plug is loose initially but tightens when reinforced by fibrin threads (see below), and **(3)** ***blood coagulation.*** Thus, blood coagulation is only a part of these important mechanisms of haemostasis.

BLOOD COAGULATION

In the blood vessels, the blood normally circulates in a fluid state. But if it is drawn from the body, and kept for few minutes, it thickens and forms a gel called clot. The process is called ***clotting*** or ***coagulation.*** If clotting takes place abnormally early in an intact blood vessel, the result is ***thrombosis*** but if it takes too long to clot, the result is ***haemorrhage***. The thrombus (or a part of it) which is swept away in blood from its site of formation is called an ***embolus.*** The clotting involves several enzymes and chemical factors known as ***coagulating*** (clotting) ***factors,*** which are noted below:

Factor I (Fibrinogen), **II** (Prothombin), **III** (Tissue Thromboplastin or Tissue Factor; TF), **IV** (Ca^{2+}), **V** (Proaccelerin), **VII** (Proconvertin), **VIII** (Antihaemophilic Factor-A), **IX** (Christmas Factor or Plasma Thromboplastin Component [PTC] or Antihaemophilic Factor-B), **X** (Stuart Factor or Thrombokinase), **XI** (Plasma Thromboplastin Antecedent [PTA], or Antihaemophilic Factor-C), **XII** (Hageman Factor), **XIII** (Fibrin Stabilising Factor or Fibrinase).

The Factor VI is not yet known. Factors II, VII, IX and X are dependent on vitamin K for their synthesis in liver. The factor III (TF) is, rather released from damaged endothelium. Activated platelets release negatively charged phospholipids (PL) which also play important role in coagulation mechanisms.

Clotting is a complex cascade of enzymatic reactions in which each clotting factor activates another factor in a fixed sequence till a fibrin clot is formed (Fig. 51.1). Coagulation process can be divided into 3 stages.

Stage 1: It can proceed either through ***extrinsic pathway*** or via ***intrinsic pathway.***

Extrinsic Pathway: It occurs rapidly, within few seconds after the tissue trauma. It is so named because as a consequence of trauma, a tissue protein called tissue factor (TF) leaks into the blood from cells outside to (*extrinsic to*) blood vessels. TF activates coagulation factor VII to VIIa which in turn activates factor X to Xa. The activated factor Xa then combines with factor V in presence of Ca^{2+} and phospholipids (PL from platelets) to form an active enzyme *prothrombinase* or ***thromboplastin*** (Fig. 51.1).

Intrinsic Pathway: It occurs more slowly and requires several minutes. It is so named because all its factors and activators are contained within (i.e., *intrinsic*) the blood. Unlike extrinsic pathway, outside tissue damage is not needed. However, if endothelial cells get damaged, the blood can come in contact with collagen in the damaged basal lamina. Damaged endothelial cells activate platelets resulting in a release of phospholipids (PL). Contact with collagen of the damaged endothelial cells (or with glass tube of blood collection tube) activates factor XII to XIIa. In turn, XIIa activates XI to XIa, which activates IX to IXa. The activated factor VIIa (from extrinsic pathway) can also activate factor IX to IXa. The activated factor IX joins with VIIIa, phospholipids (PL) from platelets and Ca^{2+} to activate factor X to Xa. The latter then combines with Va, in presence of PL and Ca^{2+} to form the active enzyme *prothrombinase* or ***thromboplastin***. *Thus, the end result of both the pathways is the generation of **Xa** and finally **thromboplastin*** (Fig. 51.1).

Stage 2 and 3: These are called "*common pathways*", because after the formation of Xa, further steps are common in both 2 and 3 stages. ***In stage 2***, thromboplastin and Ca^{2+} catalyse the conversion of prothrombin to thrombin. The latter has three positive feedback effects. The first is through factor Va wherein it accelerates the formation of thromboplastin which in turn produces more thrombin. The second is through platelet activation which promotes their aggregation and release of phospholipids (PL) needed in cascade. The third includes the activation of factor VIII to VIIIa (final step of intrinsic pathway)which along with VIIa (final step of extrinsic pathway) is needed to convert factor X to Xa. ***In stage 3***,

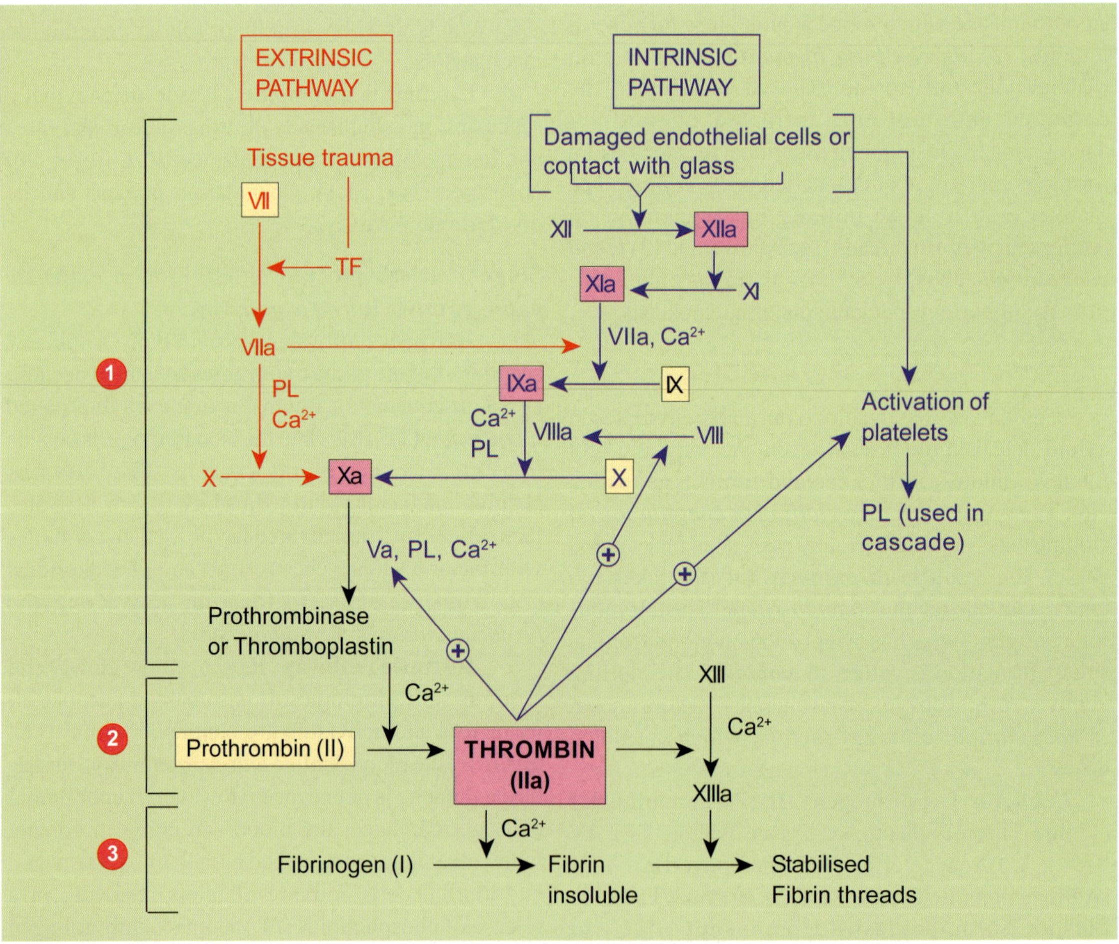

Fig 51.1 The Blood Clotting Cascade. The letter 'a' after any factor denotes its activation, ▭ Synthesis inhibited by warfarin, ▭ Factors inactivated by heparin (mainly IIa and Xa), PL-phospholipid, TF-Tissue Factor

thrombin in presence of Ca^{2+}, converts fibrinogen to loose fibrin threads. These fibrin threads are insoluble, but the strength and stability to these threads is provided by factor XIII which is activated by thrombin. The net result is the formation of sturdy clot.

To prevent the clot becoming larger and larger (because of thrombin activity), the nature has empowered the fibrin with an ability to absorb and inactivate up to 90% of thrombin formed from prothrombin. This prevents the spread of thrombin in the blood and limits the extension of the clot beyond the site of damage.

FIBRINOLYTIC SYSTEM

This system provides checks and balances so that clotting process does not get out of hand for minor reasons in day-to-day life. It also dissolves clots at the site of damage once the damage is repaired. The process of dissolution of a clot is called ***fibrinolysis*** (Fig. 51.2).

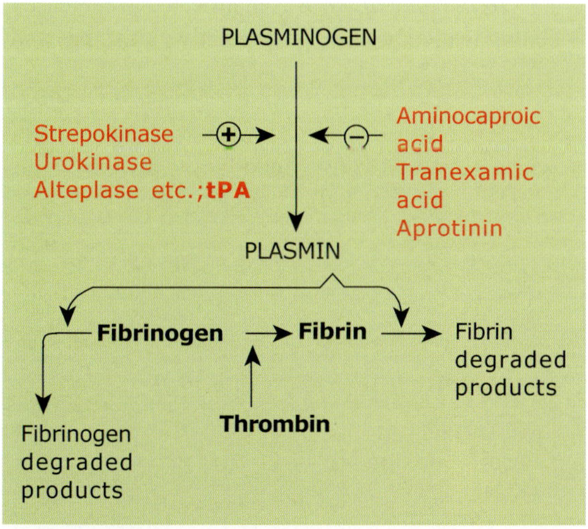

Fig 51.2 Drugs Affecting Fibrinolytic System

When a clot is formed, an inactive plasma enzyme called ***plasminogen*** gets incorporated into the clot. Endothelial cells of most tissues then secrete **t**issue **p**lasminogen **a**ctivator (t-PA) which is released into blood and reaches the site of damage (clot). t-PA in turn activates plasminogen to ***plasmin***—an active enzyme that digests fibrin. The activity of a t-PA is checked by *plasminogen activator inhibitor-1 and 2* (PAI-1 and PAI-2). PAI-1 and PAI-2 inhibit t-PA activity so that circulating plasminogen may not get activated (it is needed for incorporation into clot). Another enzyme *α_2-antiplasmin* also plays an important role in fibrinolytic system. Some of this is bound to fibrin, and thereby protects fibrin from premature lysis by plasmin. Secondly, it inhibits plasmin which escapes into circulation.

NATURAL ANTICOAGULANT MECHANISMS

As discussed above, the clot does not extend beyond a wound site, into the general circulation, partly because fibrin absorbs the thrombin into the clot and inactivates it. Several other mechanisms that control blood clotting also operate:

1) ***Prostacyclin* (PGI_2)**, a metabolite of arachidonic acid, is produced by endothelial cells which opposes the actions of thromboxane-A_2 (TXA_2) and thus inhibits platelet aggregation and release (Ch. 25 and 26).
2) ***Antithrombin III* (AT-III),** a plasma protein which blocks the action of factors XII, XI, IX, X and II (thrombin).
3) ***Protein C*,** is another plasma protein which inactivates factors V and VIII, the two major clotting factors not blocked by AT-III. Protein-C also enhances the activity of t-PA. Protein-C is a vitamin-K dependent endogenous anticoagulant which is activated by thrombin through binding to its receptor *thrombomodulin.*
4) ***Heparan sulfate*,** a proteoglycan related to heparin, is synthesised by endothelial cells. It serves as a cofactor and thus enhances the activity of antithrombin III.

COAGULANTS

Genetically determined deficiencies of clotting factors are of rare occurrence. Examples include: ***classical haemophilia*** (***haemophilia-A*** due to lack of factor VIII) and ***haemophilia-B*** (due to lack of Christmas factor IX). Pure forms of several missing factors are now available, from recombinant technology, but these are too costly and enjoy the status of orphan drugs. On the other hand, acquired clotting defects are more common. These include vitamin K deficiency and excessive oral anticoagulant therapy which require treatment with vitamin K.

Vitamin K (Endogenous Sytemic Coagulant)

Normal clotting depends on adequate amount of vitamin K in the body. Although it is not involved in actual clotting process, it is required for the synthesis of four clotting factors from liver cells: Factors II (prothrombin), VII (proconvertin), IX (Christmas factor) and X (Stuart factor).

Vit. K (K for koagulation in German) is a fat-soluble vitamin found in liver, leafy vegetables and pulses. It is normally produced by the colonic bacteria of the host. γ-Carboxylation of these clotting factors is essential for their activation by Ca^{2+} and phospholipid (PL), and the carboxylase enzyme requires vit. K in its reduced form (KH) as a cofactor. In this process KH is oxidised to K-epoxide (KO). The latter, in turn, is reduced to KH by vit. K reductase, for recycling (Fig. 51.3).

Vitamin K Analogues and Pharmacokinetics

- Natural vit. K or ***Phytonadione*** is obtained from leafy vegetables. It can be given orally or by I.V. injection. It has a rapid onset and prolonged effect. When given orally it requires bile salts for absorption. Hence, deficiency can occur in obstructive jaundice and in any disease involving malabsorption of fats.
- Vitamin K_2 or ***Menaquinone*** is synthesised by intestinal bacterial flora. Hence, inhibition of the growth of intestinal bacteria, from prolonged antibiotic therapy also, leads to vit. K deficiency.
- Vitamin K_3 or ***Menadione*** is a synthetic (water soluble) analogue. Bile salts are not needed for its absorption; can be given orally in case of obstructive jaundice. However, it has slow onset of action.

There is no proper storage of vit. K in the body. It is metabolised in liver and the conjugated glucuronides are excreted in bile and urine.

Deficiency of vit. K is manifested as increased bleeding tendency (e.g., postoperative bleeding) and

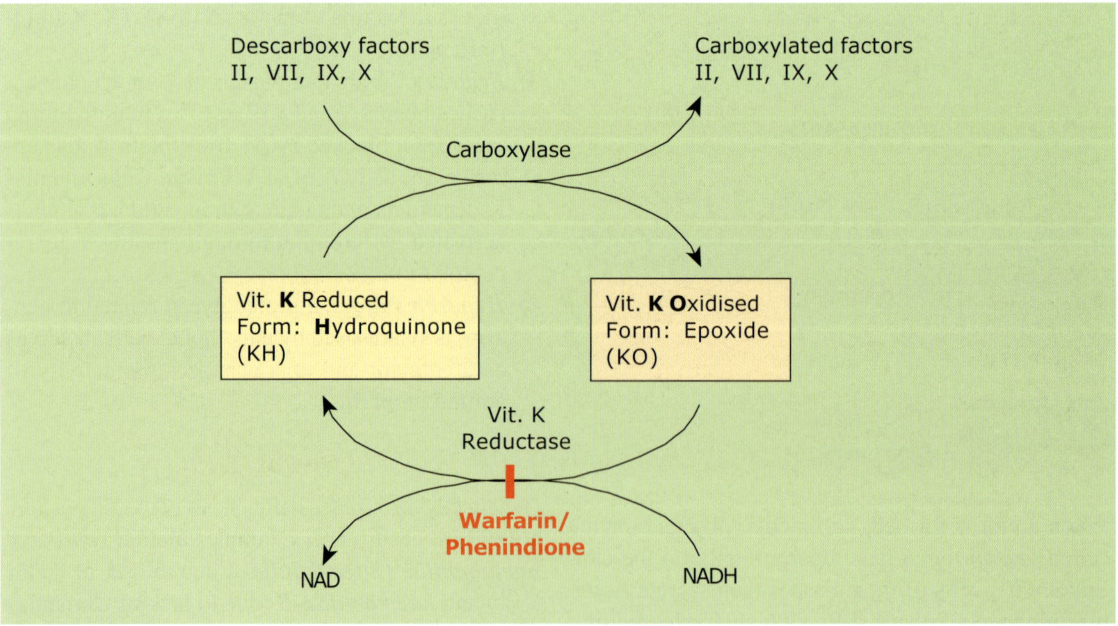

Fig 51.3 Mechanism of Action of Vitamin K and Warfarin

hypoprothrombinaemia. Two groups have greater risk of vit. K deficiency: newborns and patients receiving anticoagulants. Both have low levels of prothrombin and other clotting factors.

Therapeutic Use

(1) ***Prolonged antibiotic use***: Any of the vit. K preparations can be given orally. **(2)** ***Overdose of oral anticoagulants*:** Vit. K is a specific antidote. Vit K_1 may be given I.M. It has a fast onset of action. Vit. K_3 should be avoided because of its delayed onset of action (24 hr), **(3)** ***Newborn or Premature infants***: For reasons, see above. Vit. K_3 (menadione) should be avoided. Firstly because it causes haemolysis in a dose-dependent manner and secondly because it can precipitate kernicterus (it competitively inhibits glucuronidation of bilirubin. Glucuronyl transferase enzymes, as such, are low in neonates. This factor coupled with haemolysis it produces, increases bilirubin load). Vitamin K_1 (1 mg I.M). is usually administered routinely, **(4)** ***Malabsorption Syndrome/ Obstructive Jaundice***: Vit. K_3 orally or K_1 parenterally.

Daily requirements: 50–100 µg/day. But even 5–10 µg/day from exogenous source is sufficient if colonic bacteria is producing it adequately. ***Toxicity***: Not well defined except of vit. K_3 in neonates, as described above. I.V. injection of vit. K should be slow. Dyspnoea, hypersensitivity may result but rarely.

Other Systemic Procoagulants

Plasma Fractions

Treatment of either type of haemophilia (see above) or von Willebrand's disease (vWD)* requires the restoration of the appropriate factors so that IXa/ VIIIa is sufficient. There are variety of factor VIII/IX replacement products available, which are:

a) ***Factor VIII products for treatment of Haemophilia-A***: Antihaemophilic factor, obtained from procine or plasma derived. Ultrapure antihaemophilic factor, obtained from recombinant technology has also been introduced. It does not carry any risk of hepatitis or HIV transmission.

b) ***Factor IX products for treatment of Haemophilia-B***: Two preparations are available—factor IX complex (which contains significant amounts of factors II, VII and X also) and purified factor IX recombinant.

c) ***Mixed factor products for Haemophilia-A, vWD and hypofibrinogenaemia***: These are prepared from single donors. Two preparations are available—**Cryoprecipitated antihaemophilic factor** (primarily contains factor VIII, fibrinogen and vWF but also other factors) and **anti-inhibitor coagulant complex** (a mixed clotting factors preparation).

Desmopressin

Another approach to treat mild haemophilia-A and vWD is to use desmopressin, a synthetic analogue of vasopressin (Ch. 17). The advantages of desmopressin over vasopressin are that: (a) it retains the factor VIII and vWF increasing activity but lacks the vasoconstrictor action of vasopressin and (b) there is no risk of hepatitis or HIV transmission which is inherent with blood derived products. Desmopressin can also be given to the donor before donation of blood to double or triple the amount of factor VIII and vWD recovered. However, it is administered parenterally or insufflated intranasally, not given orally (bioavailability 1%). For preparations see Ch.17.

Antifibrinolytics

These drugs decrease the fibrinolytic activity and are useful in haemophilic patients who may be prone to breakthrough bleeding, after surgery, as the wound is healing.

Aminocaproic acid and Tranexamic Acid

Aminocaproic acid competitively inhibits activation of plasminogen to plasmin. It also has some antiplasmin effects and hence inhibits fibrinolysis. However, the doses used are very high leading to noncompliance (about 5 g to be taken orally every 4 to 6 hrs). ***Tranexamic acid***, an aminocaproic acid analogue, is more potent and hence compliance is better (500 mg orally at 6–8

*Von Willebrand's Disease (VWD) is an autosomal dominant bleeding disorder due to deficiency of von Willebrand factor (vWF). It is synthesised in vascular endothelial cells and is also present in platelets. It has three main functions: (a) stabilisation of factor VIII, (b) to promote platelet adhesion and (c) to stabilise platelet aggregation.

hrly interval). *Side effects* include unwanted deep vein thrombosis and GIT distress.

Aprotinin

In inhibits plasmin, kallikrein and platelet activation and is used for hyperplasminaemia caused by fibrinolytic drug overdose and to prevent blood loss during cardiac bypass surgery (see. Ch. 24).

Miscellaneous

Rutin is a plant glycoside which is being used to prevent capillary bleeding with vit. C, which is claimed to increase its efficacy. Usual dose is 60 mg TDS but the results are doubtful.

Ethamsylate is also claimed to increase capillary wall stability probably by exerting anti-hyaluronidase activity. It inhibits PGI_2 synthesis and hence promotes platelet aggregation. But is has no antifibrinolytic action. It is used to prevent bleeding in postpartum haemorrhage, menorrhagia and also after tooth extraction. Oral dose is 250–500 mg TDS.

Local Haemostatics (Styptics)

Many haemostatics are available for local use to stop bleeding from oozing locations, e.g., tooth sockets, open wounds etc. These are meant only for local applications. Most of them provide a network of fibrin which promotes coagulation.

1) ***Thrombin***, obtained from bovine plasma; when applied topically, particularly in conjunction with a compatible gelatin sponge, operates as a good haemostatic for obvious reasons.
2) ***Fibrin Sealant***, obtained from human plasma, is an even more promising haemostatic. It is used to stop microbleeding and oozing that often accompany dental procedures.
3) ***Gelatin Foams*** can be soaked with saline, fibrin or thrombin to cover or pack bleeding surface.
4) ***Vasoconstrictors***: Temporary haemostasis (e.g., to stop epistaxis) may be obtained by packing a cotton gauze with 1% epinephrine or 0.5% oxymetazoline.
5) ***Astringents***: Tannic acid (1%) is an effective haemostatic. It precipitates proteins, including thrombin.
6) ***Russel's viper venom*** acts like a thromboplastin and applied locally to stop bleeding, but is rarely used.

ANTICOAGULANTS

Anticogulants may be classified as under:

Parenteral Anticoagulants

a) **Heparin**
b) **Low Molecular Weight Heparins**
   Enoxaparin, Dalteparin, Ardeparin, Nadroparin, Parnaparin, Reviparin, Tinzaparin
c) **Synthetic Heparin Derivatives**
   Fondaparinux sodium, Idraparinux sodium
d) **Direct Thrombin Inhibitors**
   - **Hirudin-based Thrombin Inhibitors:** Lepirudin, Bivalirudin, Desirudin,
   - **Synthetic Thrombin Inhibitor**: Argatroban,
e) **Drotrecogin-alfa**

Oral Anticoagulants

a) **Direct Thrombin Inhibitor (DTI)**
   Dabigatran etexilate (Prodrug of debigatran)
b) **Direct Factor Xa Inhibitors (DFXaIs)**
   Rivaroxaban, Apixaban, Betrixaban, Edoxaban
c) **Vitamin K Antagonists**
   - **Coumarin Derivatives**
     Warfarin, Acenocumarol (Ethyl biscoumacetate), Dicumarol (rarely used).
   - **Indanedione Derivatives**
     Phenindione, Anisindione (rarely used).

Parenteral Anticoagulants

Heparin

Heparin (so named as it was first extracted from liver) is a mixture of sulfated mucopolysaccharides with a molecular weight ranging from 10,000–40,000. It is a strong electronegatively charged acidic polymer. It is present together with histamine in all tissues containing mast cells but richest sources are lung, liver and intestinal mucosa. Commercial preparations are obtained from beef lung and pig intestinal mucosa and standardised after biological assay.

Mechanism of Heparin and Low Molecular Weight Heparins

We may recall that antithrombin III (AT-III) plays a crucial role in natural endogenous anticoagulant mechanisms in the body by blocking the activity of activated clotting factors XII, XI, X, IX and II (thrombin). Under physiological settings, these interactions are slow and work on demand and supply basis. *But, heparin accelerates AT-III activity by 1000 folds especially against IIa and Xa.* However, factors like XII, XI and IX are also affected.

Both thrombin (IIa) and factor Xa are sensitive to the inhibitory effects of *high molecular weight heparin–AT-III complex*, but IIa inhibition is much more than Xa. To inhibit thrombin, the long chain heparin molecule serves as a template to which both positively charged AT-III as well as thrombin (IIa) bind (Fig. 51.4A). After binding, heparin induces a conformational change in AT III to expose and make its reactive site more accessible for IIa/Xa binding. The difference between IIa and Xa binding is that Xa needs only to interact with AT-III portion of long chain heparin–AT-III complex (Fig. 51.4B). Once the heparin–AT-III–clotting factor ternary complex is formed, heparin is released for renewed interaction with another AT-III molecule.

On the contrary, only factor Xa is sensitive to the inhibitory effects of low molecular weight heparin (LMWH)–AT III complex, thrombin is not. Reason—LMWH is too small a molecule (compared to heparin) to bind AT-III as well as thrombin simultaneously (Fig. 51.4C).

Although heparin–AT-III complex is a very efficient inhibitor of free thrombin, clot bound thrombin is resistant to inhibition. Heparin in higher doses also *inhibits platelet aggregation* but this action is secondary to its inhibitory effects on thrombin, which itself is a powerful platelet aggregating agent.

Pharmacokinetics

Being a large and highly ionised molecule, heparin is not absorbed from GIT; nor does it cross BBB or placental barrier. Its Ca^{2+} or Na^{+} salts are given by constant I.V. infusion or intermittent I.V. injection or by deep S.C. injection. It is not administered I.M., to avoid haematoma formation at injection site. Low dose S.C. injection is usually preferred for prophylaxis (1–2 hrs before operation and continued till patient is discharged). However, bioavailability by this route is inconsistent and anticoagulant effects appear after an hour. It is metabolised in liver by heparinase and exhibits dose-dependent metabolism. The half-life increases with increasing the dose.

The duration of action of heparin being short (1–5 hrs), its dose is so adjusted that the whole blood clotting time is raised to 2–3 times more than normal or activated partial thromboplastin time (APTT) is raised to 1½–2 times of normal values.

Low Molecular Weight Heparins (LMWH)

Ardeparin, Dalteparin, Enoxaparin, Nadroparin, Parnaparin, Reviparin, and Tinzaparin

Unfractionated heparin (UFH) has a molecular weight (MW) ranging from 5000–30000. On fractionation, it provides high MW heparin and low MW (ranging from 2000-9000) heparins (LMWH). The latter have a shorter polymer length and inhibit activated factor X predominantly but have lesser effect on thrombin (see above and Fig. 51.4C), platelet function and on coagulation in general. Thrombocytopenia is less frequent and chances of haemorrhage are less. The more important advantages of LMWH are their pharmacokinetic features:

1. These can be given S.C. Because of better bioavailability (70–90%) by this route, variability in response is minimised.
2. These have a longer elimination half-life and are eliminated by first order kinetics, so the effects are more consistent and dosing less frequent (once daily, S.C.).
3. These do not prolong aPTT and whole blood clotting time. Hence, response is predictable and monitoring is not required as a routine as with UFH.
4. Dose is given in mg (not in units) can be easily and calculated on body weight basis.

Specific dose regimen for these LMWH may be obtained from the manufacturer's literature.

- Therapeutic uses and adverse effects of heparin and LMWH are discussed in the end as of anticoagulants in general.

Heparin Antagonist

Protamine Sulfate: The need to use a heparin antagonist is rare because the duration of action of heparin being short, the discontinuation of heparin in most cases solves the problem. Even otherwise,

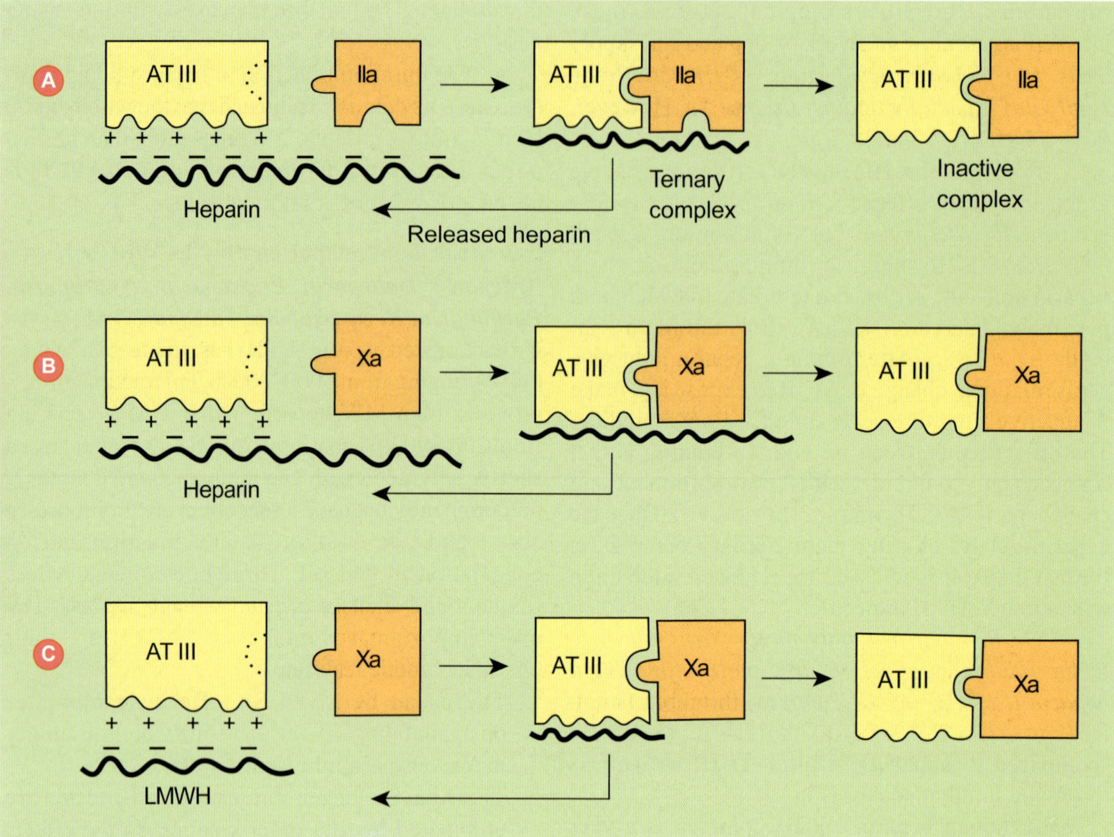

Fig 51.4 Mechanism of Action of Heparin and Low Molecular Weight Heparins (LMWH)

blood transfusion is necessary if bleeding occurs (to compensate the loss). However, in certain situations, e.g., in cardiac/vascular surgery, there becomes a need to terminate heparin action rapidly. *Protamine sulfate* is a specific antagonist for heparin overdose. It is a strongly basic low molecular weight protein which when given I.V. promptly neutralises strongly acidic heparin weight by weight (1 mg of protamine sulfate for 100 U of heparin). Neutralisation of LMWH by protamine is incomplete. Protamine cannot antagonise the actions of fondaparinux. However, the use of excess protamine sulfate should be avoided, as it itself has an anticoagulant effect. Being a basic drug it releases histamine, if given by rapid I.V. injection. Hypersensitivity reaction, flushing and broncho-constriction can occur.

Synthetic Heparin Derivative

Fondaparinux sodium, Idraparinux sodium

Fondaparinux soldium is a synthetic pentasaccharide that causes an antithrombin III–mediated selective inhibition of factor Xa. Neutralisation of factor Xa interrupts the blood coagulation cascade leading ultimately to inhibition of thrombin formation. But, it does not cause inhibition of thrombin by itself because of its shorter polymer length (see above). It is administered S.C. once daily (usual adult dose 2.5 mg). Bioavailability is almost 100% by this route. Half- life is 17–21 hrs which gets prolonged in cases of renal impairment (dosage adjustment becomes necessary). It is excreted unchanged in urine. It has lesser antiplatelet action and hence chances of thrombocytopenia are less frequent. It is generally preferred for thromboprophylaxis of patients undergoing hip or knee surgery and for therapy of pulmonary embolism.

Idraparinux sodium is a long acting congener of fondaparinux, acts similar to this drug by binding with factor Xa and is administered S.C. in once weekly doses.

Direct Thrombin Inhibitors (DTIs)

- **Hirudin-based Thrombin Inhibitors:** Lepirudin, Bivalirudin, Desirudin,
- **Synthetic Thrombin Inhibitor**: Argatroban,

Thrombin is a protease that perform a number of functions in the haemostasis process, e.g., it (1) proteolytically cleave fibrinogen to fibrin, (2) activates factor XIII whioch cross-link fibrin polymer to form a stable clot, (3) activates platelets, (4) induces endothelial release of PGI2, t-PA and PAI-1. In view of these thrombin actions, DTIs would be expected to have profound effects on coagulation. The currently approved DTIs include: lepirudin, bivalirudin, desirudin , argatroban (all given by I.V. route) and dabigatran (given orally). Majority of these agents act by binding to thrombin directly and thereby inhibit its effects in the downstream of blood coagulation cascade. These drugs neither bind to AT III nor to other plasma proteins such as platelet factors.

Herindun is a specific irreversible inhibitor of thrombin obtained from the salivary glands of leech (*Hirudo medicinalis*). There are reports that surgeons had used leeches to prevent thrombosis in fine vessels in reconstructions surgery to attach parts of limbs, digits, toes, etc.

Lepirudin is the recombinant form of hirudin derived from yeast cells. The binding of lepirudin to thrombin prevents, the thrombin-mediated activation of fibrinogen (to form fibrin) and factor XIII (to inhibit fibrin stabilization). The drug has a short half life, administered by I.V. route, and is renally excreted. It is used as anticoagulant in thrombotic events associated with heparin-induced thrombocytopenia in patients of thromboembolic diseases. Its unlabeled use is for prevention of ischaemic complications associated with unstable angina and accute MI including those undergoing coronary stenting and per cutenious angiography and angioplasty. It is monitored by aPTT. *Adverse effects* include haemorrhage, haematuria, and increased transaminases. Patients may develop antibodies directed against thrombin-lepirudin complex. These antigen-antibody complexes are not cleared by kidney and may result in enhanced anticoagulant effect and may limit the long term effectiveness of the agent as anticoagulatnt. There is no antidote to lepirudin. It is a better choice for patients having hepatic insufficiency.

Bivalirudin is another synthetic hidurin-like peptide which acts as thrombin inhibitor. The drug is administered by I.V. route. It has a rapid onset of action with short duration (1 hr, t½ 25 min). It is used in percutaneous coronary angiography and angioplasty (as an alternative to heparin).

Desirudin, like lepirudin, blocks catalytic activity of thrombin and is used to treat deep vein thrombosis and for prophylaxis against deep vein thrombosis during hip replacement.

Argatroban is a synthetic non-peptide molecule that inhibits thrombin and used for the prophylaxis and treatment of thrombisis in patients with heparin-induced thrombocytopenia (as an alternative to lepirudin) including persons undergoing percuteneous coronary intervention (PCI). It has a short duration of action and given by continued I.V. infusion with monitoring of aPTT. Its clearance is not affected by renal disease. Hence, it is a better choice for patients having renal insufficiency.

Drotrecogin-alfa

It is a human recombinant activated Protein-C. It inhibits factor Va and VIIIa and thereby limit pathological thrombosis. It has a shorter plasma half-life (1.5 hrs). Besides its use as anticoagulant, it is given by continuous I.V. infusion to decrease the mortality risk from severe sepsis (associated with organ dysfunction) in adults. Factors contributing to such effect are not clearly understood.

Oral Anticoagulants

a) Direct Thrombin Inhibitor (DTI)

Dabigatran etexilate (Prodrug of debigatran)

b) Direct Factor Xa Inhibitors (DFXaI)

Rivaroxaban, Apixaban, Betrixaban, Edoxaban

A major progress in the area of anticoagulant therapy has been to develop novel orally active thrombin inhibitors like ***dabigatran*** *and novel orally active factor Xa inhibitors like* ***rivaroxaban, apixaban, betrixaban*** **and** ***edoxaban*** (the latter agents decrease thrombin levels indirectly) for primary prevention of venous thrombo-embolic events in adult patients who have undergone elective total hip replacement or total knee replacement surgery and for prevention of stroke and systemic embolism in adult patient with non-valvular atrial fibrillation with one or more risk factors.The anticoagulant therapy with these agents appears to be cost effective since no routine coagulation monitoring is necessary. These have been found equivalent to LMWH in safety and efficacy. In future, they may replace warfarin which has a narrow therapeutic window, requires dosage adjustments and exhibits potential drug interactions. Both group of drugs have been approved for treatment of deep vein thrombosis and prevention of stroke in atrial fibrillation.

Dabigatran and Direct Factor Xa Inhibitor Antidote:

The **n**ovel **o**ral **a**nti**c**oagulants (NOACs) like Rivaroxaban and DTI like dabigatran although exhibit predictible anticoagulant action and improved side effect profile, they lack broad-spectrum reversal agent (s). Pharmacological anticoagulation becomes a clinical problem when anticoagulated patient experience major bleeding, has a traumatic injury, or requires emergency surgery. Such a situation demands a specific antidote to reverse the anticoagulant effect of the concerned drug.

Until recently no treatment was available for dabigatran associated bleeding. ***Idarucizumab***, the Fab fragment of a chimeric human-murine (humanized) monoclonal antibody targeting the DTI, *dabigatran (having an affinity 350 times as high to dabigatran than the thrombin)* has been developed. This drug is a chimeric monoclonal antibody generated from mouse against dabigatran which has been humanized and reduced to a Fab. The drug is available as solution for injection filled aseptically into sterile glass vials containing 50 mL of 50 mg/mL solution (total 2,500 mg/vial). The agent is used by slow infusion in the doses of 1000–4000 mg in 30 min.

Another two drugs which have been developed as antidote for DFXaI are ***Andexanet alfa*** and the other ***Ciraparantag***, a broad spectrum DTI and DFXaI anticoagulant reversal agent. Both antidotes are administered by I.V. infusion.

c) Vitamin K Antagonists

- **Coumarin Derivatives**
  Warfarin,Acenocumarol (Ethyl biscoumacetate), Dicumarol (rarely used).
- **Indanedione Derivatives**
  Phenindione, Anisindione (rarely used).

Introduction of dicumarol (a bis-hydroxycoumarin derivative) in 1940s, provided a new era of relatively inexpensive, self-administered oral anticoagulant therapy. Since then several other coumarin derivatives have been introduced along with other related group called indanediones (these are however more toxic than coumarins and are rarely used these days).

Mechanism of Action: Both coumarin (warfarin and its analogues) and indanedione (phenindione) derivatives act by competitively inhibiting vitamin-K reductase and therefore inhibit the synthesis of clotting factors II, VII, IX and X by the liver. Vitamin K reductase converts the epoxide KO to KH which is a cofactor in γ-carboxylation (activation) of these factors (Fig. 51.3).

Their anticoagulant effects take 1–3 days to develop, because though the concentration of factor VII is decreased earlier, the most important factor prothrombin (factor II) is the last one to be decreased. As the plasma half-life of prothrombin is 2–3 days, the decline in the levels of prothrombin, already in plasma, takes time. Monitoring of coumarin and phenindione drugs therapy is done by estimation of prothrombin time (PT) in blood. Vitamin-K antagonists do not alter bleeding time.

Coumarin Derivatives: Warfarin

Pharmacokinetics: The oral bioavailability of war farin is 100%. Over 99% of warfarin is bound to plasma proteins which results in its low aVd (7.7 L), longer plasma half-life (36 hrs) and several drug displacement reactions. It is metabolised by enzyme CYP2C9 and partly conjugated with glucuronic acid in liver, undergoes enterohepatic circulation, and then finally excreted in urine. Coumarins cross placental barrier; but the active form of the drug is insignificantly excreted through milk.

Warfarin Drug Interactions: Large number of drugs may interact with warfarin. They may either increase warfarin activity resulting in unexpected haemorrhage or may decrease its activity leading to therapeutic failure. Such examples are scattered throughout the text of this book. However, important ones are summarised below:

Warfarin activity is potentiated with concomitant use of:

- *Enzyme inhibitors such as* metronidazole, chloramphenicol, disulfiram, erythromycin, cimetidine, allopurinol, and amiodarone.
- *Drugs which displace warfarin from protein binding sites such as* cotrimoxazole, indomethacin, phenytoin, probenecid and ethacrynic acid
- *Liquid paraffin (habitual use)*: due to emulsification and excretion of vit. K which leads to vit. K deficiency.
- *Inhibitors of platelet aggregation,* e.g., aspirin
- *Drugs which inhibit gut flora and reduce vit. K synthesis*: e.g., broad spectrum antibiotics.
- *Drugs causing hypoprothrombinaemia such as* III generation cephalosporins like cefoperazone, cefamandole and moxalactam
- *Miscellaneous factors*: hepatic disease (decreases the synthesis of clotting factors), hyperthyroidism (enhances catabolism of clotting factors).

Warfarin activity is reduced by the concomitant use of:

- *Enzyme inducers* such as barbituarates, rifampicin, griseofulvin and carbamazepine
- *Drugs that bind to warfarin and inhibit its absorption,* e.g., cholestyramine and sucralfate.
- *Drugs that increase the synthesis of clotting factors,* e.g., estrogen-containing oral contraceptives.
- *Miscellaneous factors*: hypothyroidism (reduced catabolism of clotting factors), hereditary resistance (mutational changes in Vit. K reductase enzyme).

Contraindications: Warfarin should not be used during pregnancy because it may cause abortion as well as birth defects.

Other Coumarin Drugs

Dicumarol: A coumarin derivative. *Side effects:* Very poor GIT tolerance, spontaneous bleeding. Rarely used.

Acenocoumarol is a coumarin derivative. t½ is 18–24 hrs. Biological lag 2–3 days. Dose 8–10 mg orally first day (loading), then 2–8 mg/day as maintenance. *Side effects:* spontaneous haemorrhage, GIT disturbances, stomatitis, dermatitis, urticaria and alopecia.

Ethylbiscoumacetate (Tromexan) is also a coumarin derivative. Shorter t½ 2 hrs. Biological lag 1–3 days. Dose 900 mg first day, then 300–600 mg/day as maintenance. *Side effects:* spontaneous haemorrhage, alopecia, altered taste.

Indanedione Derivatives

Phenindione is a indanedione derivative. *Side effects*: leukopenia, agranulocytosis, haemorrhage, hepatitis, neuropathy, skin rash, fever, dark orange coloured urine. Seldom used.

Anisindione is also a indanedione derivative. *Side effects*: vasculitis, oedema, haepatitis, haematuria, haemorrhage, leukopenia, skin rash, alopecia, diarrhoea and paralysis of accommodation. Rarely used.

Treatment of Warfarin /Phenindione Overdosage/ Poisoning : As a corollary, vit. K [vit.K_1 (phytonadione)] can be used to treat the overdosage toxicity of coumarin/indanedione group of oral anticoagulants. However, in milder episodes, only stopping of warfarin administration usually suffices. Fresh frozen plasma or factor IX concentrate which contains large amounts of prothrombin complex can also be infused.

All such measures, merely restore the normal activity of clotting factors.

Therapeutic Uses of Anticoagulants

Anticoagulants do not dissolve the clot that has already been formed but prevent the thrombous extension, recurrence and embolic complications by reducing the rate of thrombin formation. Heparin is used initially, for its rapid onset of action, while an oral anticoagulant is usually started concurrently. Heparin is then discontinued after 6–7 days, when warfarin has taken its full therapeutic effects.

Prevention and Treatment of Deep Vein Thrombosis and Pulmonary Embolism: Venous thrombi are generally fibrin thrombi and hence anticoagulants are very effective in such situations. Prophylaxis is usually needed for bedridden patients, old, postoperative cases and for patients with hip/leg fracture. For prophylaxis, intermittent low dose ***heparin*** administration (5000 IU, S.C., 8–12 hrly) is generally preferred. ***LMW heparin*** (e.g., ***enoxaparin*** 30 mg S.C., 12 hrly or ***dalteparin*** 5000 U, S.C. per day) may also be used. The main advantage of LMWH over standard heparin is its S.C. administration without laboratory monitoring with minimal risk for thrombocytopenia, osteopenia and spontaneous bleeding. For an established venous thrombosis, a bolus I.V. injection of 5000–10000 U of heparin is given followed by I.V. infusion of 1000 U/hr. Heparin is used for 6–7 days followed by warfarin with a 3 days overlap period. Treatment with warfarin is usually started with 10–15 mg orally per day with a check on prothrombin time. The aim is to reduce plasma thrombin activity to 25% of the normal value. Once the objective has been achieved, a maintenance dose of 5–7 mg/day can be given. Warfarin may soon be replaced by oral thrombin inhibitor ***dabigatran*** and oral Xa inhibitor ***rivaroxaban*** (see above).

Myocardial Infarction: Arterial thrombi are primarily platelet thrombi, hence the antiplatelet drugs are more effective than anticoagulants. However, these can be used to reduce secondary thromboembolic complications. LMWH can be given for shorter period till patient becomes ambulatory. These may also be used during coronary angioplasty and stent placement.

Unstable Angina: To reduce the chances of MI in unstable angina, aspirin + heparin followed by warfarin can be used.

Rheumatic Heart Disease: If there are chances of thrombosis or embolism from atrial fibrillation, warfarin/low-dose heparin/low-dose aspirin can be used to prevent the chances of stroke. However, warfarin is more effective in atrial fibrillation patients with high risk of stroke, while aspirin is reserved for low-risk patients or those who cannot take warfarin.

Cerebrovascular Diseases: Use of antiplatelet drugs is more safe, simpler and efficacious than the use of oral anticoagulants.

Miscellaneous: **(1)** Treatment of disseminated intravascular coagulation, **(2)** Treatment of peripheral (e.g., retinal vessel) embolism, **(3)** During cardiac bypass surgery and in placing artificial heart valves to prevent formation of any thrombous/emboli, **(4)** To prevent clotting in extracorporeal circulation, e.g., during haemodialysis and **(5)** For anticoagulation during pregnancy. In contrast to warfarin, heparin does not cross placenta and is not associated with foetal malformation. Hence, heparin is preferred for such indication.

Adverse Effects of Anticoagulants

Haemorrhage is the commonest adverse effect of parenteral/oral anticoagulant therapy. Chances of haemorrhage are more in presence of renal or hepatic impairment due to reduced rate of elimination.

Adverse effects characteristic of heparin: **(1)** Heparin-induced thrombocytopenia, **(2)** Osteoporosis and spontaneous fractures on prolonged use, **(3)** Transient alopecia and **(4)** Hypersensitivity.

Adverse effects characteristic of warfarin: **(1)** Teratogenic effects. It crosses placenta and can lead to haemorrhagic disorders in foetus and foetal bone deformities, **(2)** Transient alopecia, **(3)** Dermatitis and **(4)** Diarrhoea.

Contraindications

For Heparin Therapy: Bleeding disorders; thrombocytopenia; severe hypertension (risk of cerebral haemorrhage); threatened abortion; bleeding piles; subacute bacterial endocarditis (chances of embolism); tuberculosis (chances of haemoptysis); and concurrent use of aspirin or other antiplatelet drug during therapy.

For Warfarin Therapy: Same as for heparin. In addition: (1) *Pregnancy*: It increases chances of birth defects, specially skeletal abnormalities. (2) *Necrosis of soft tissues* (buttocks and breast), shortly after the start of warfarin therapy (though rarely).

FIBRINOLYTIC DRUGS

These drugs are used to lyse (dissolve) the thrombi (clots) in blood vessels (mainly coronary artery) by activating fibrinolytic system. This system involves an enzymatic activation of plasminogen to plasmin, which in turn dissolves fibrin network (Fig. 51.2). As compared to arterial thrombi, venous thrombi are lysed more easily, and the recent thrombi are lysed better than the older ones.

Six fibrinolytic drugs (plasminogen activators) are available to achieve reperfusion of infarcted area (see also Ch. 20). These are *streptokinase, urokinase, anistreplase, alteplase, reteplase* and *tenecteplase*. These are usually administered intravenously (infusion/bolus) and are increasingly used to treat acute MI, peripheral arterial thrombosis/embolism and for unclotting catheters and shunts. Thrombolytic agents do not distinguish between pathological thrombi and fibrin deposits (at the sites of vascular injury). Hence, haemorrhage is the major side effect of these drugs. As a result, an unsuspected peptic ulcer may bleed following their use. Unfortunately, increased availability of local thrombin at the site of fibrin clot, may enhance rethrombosis after the lysis of the initial clot.

Characteristic Features of Individual Drugs

Streptokinase: It is a protease enzyme obtained from β-haemolytic streptococci. It forms 1:1 complex with proactivator plasminogen which catalyses the conversion of inactive plasminogen to active plasmin. In addition to the lysis of fibrin plug, the complex also catalyses the breakdown of fibrinogen. Compared to the other related drugs its fibrin specificity is less. Half-life is 60–80 min. Being a foreign protein, hypersensitivity reactions (rashes, fever, hypotension, but rarely anaphylaxis) are frequent (3% incidence). Prior presence of antistreptococcal antibodies may reduce its efficacy and due to the formation of antistreptokinase-antibodies it cannot be repeated before one year. However, it is least expensive.

Antistreplase: It is anisolyated plasminogen streptokinase activator complex, and was synthesised to improve the pharmacokinetics of the streptokinase-plasminogen complex. This complex consists of purified human plasminogen with bacterial streptokinase in which the active site of plasminogen has been protected by anisoylation (a process of acetylation). When administered, the acyl group hydrolyses spontaneously releasing the activated streptokinase-proactivator complex to perform fibrinolysis. This modification confers more fibrin specificity compared to streptokinase. The half-life is also more than streptokinase (>90 min). Other features (haemorrhage, hypersensitivity and hypotension) are akin to streptokinase.

Alteplase: It was earlier called "tissue type plasminogen activator (tPA)". It is now prepared by recombinant DNA technology using human tissue culture. It has a low affinity for circulating free plasminogen but rapidly activates plasminogen bound to fibrin in a thrombus. Hence it is highly fibrin specific and has an advantage of hydrolysing only fibrin (not fibrinogen). It seems to be superior to streptokinase and urokinase in dissolving old clots. However, it has a shorter half-life (5–10 min) and shows higher incidence of reocclusion, thus necessitating concomitant use of I.V. heparin also. Side effects are same as of streptokinase except that it has least or no allergenicity. However, it is quite expensive.

Reteplase: It is also a recombinant tissue plasminogen activator which, like alteplase, also initiates local fibrinolysis by binding to fibrin in the clot and converting entrapped plasminogen to plasmin. However, it has a longer half-life (15–20 min). It is administered as two bolus injections of 10 U each at 30 min apart. Side effects are like that of alteplase.

Tenecteplase: It is a genetically engineered mutant form of alteplase, with mode of action similar to reteplase and alteplase. However, it has a longer

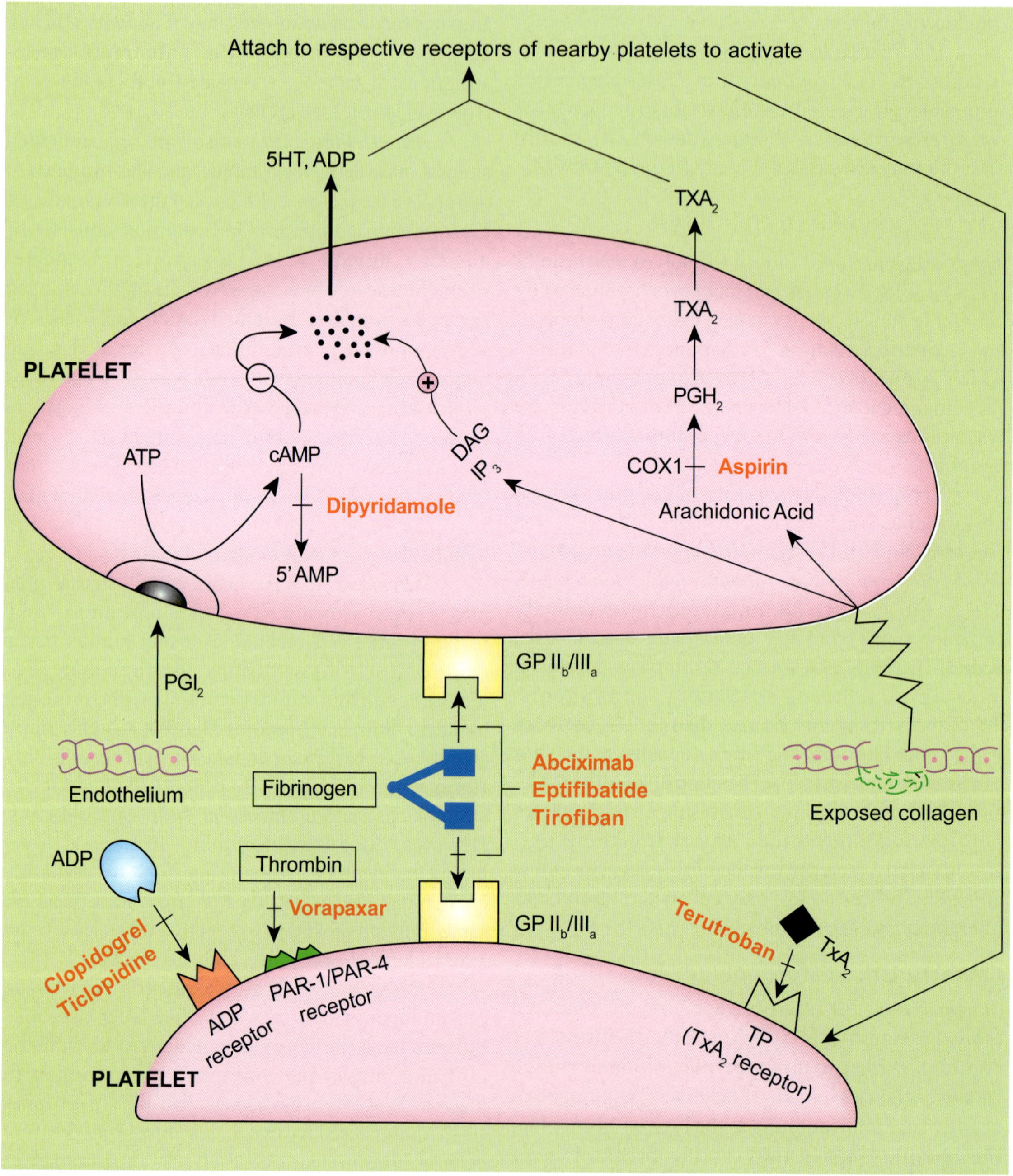

Fig 51.5 Mechanisms Involving Platelet Aggregation and Inhibition

half-life (2 hrs), increased fibrin specificity and increased resistance to plasminogen activated inhibitor-1. It is given as a single bolus injection of 50 mg over 5 sec. Side effects are same as of alteplase. It is very expensive.

Urokinase: It is a protease enzyme, earlier isolated from human urine but now produced from cultured human kidney cells. It is a direct plasminogen activator and can degrade both fibrin and fibrinogen. It is nonallergenic, nonpyrogenic and does not produce hypotension (unlike streptokinase). It also has more fibrin specificity than streptokinase. It has a half-life of 20 min and is used in place of streptokinase or in whom streptokinase cannot be repeated. It is cheaper too and therefore routinely used (slow I.V. injection) in developing countries. A *recombinant pro-urokinase* is also available. It gets converted to urokinase (on binding to fibrin clot), thus making it still more fibrin specific (almost equal to alteplase).

ANTIPLATELET DRUGS

Mechanisms for Platelet Aggregation and Inhibition

Activation and subsequent aggregation of platelets, i.e., high degree of platelet reactivity is a major component of arterial thrombosis and may be involved in initiation of venous thrombosis. The outer membrane of the platelet contains a variety of receptors that respond to signals which promote platelet aggregation or inhibition (i.e., oppose aggregation). These signals, although are many, some of them which have led to the development of clinically useful antiplatelet drugs are discussed below (Fig.51.5):

1) **Platelet Phosphodiesterase (PDE) Inhibitors**: Although ***dipyridamol***, a prototype of this category had existed for many years, ***cilostazol***, an oral PDE-III inhibitor has now been approved for intermittent claudication, PCI and for the prevention and treatment of myocardial and cerebral infarction. In a normal, undamaged blood vessel, platelets are not activated and circulate freely. Prostacyclin (PGI_2), which is synthesised by the normal undamaged endothelium and released into plasma, activates PGI_2 receptor on the platelets that are linked to cAMP (an intra-cellular messenger). PGI_2 receptor activation elevates cAMP levels which inhibit platelet aggregation (by inhibiting the release of ADP and 5-HT from dense granules of platelets—see below). On the other hand, damaged endothelial cells cannot synthesise enough PGI_2. Consequently, intracellular cAMP levels decline which would rather permit platelet aggregation. *cAMP is metabolised to 5'-AMP by phosphodiesterase enzyme and hence any drug which inhibits this enzyme (e.g., **dipyridamole** and **cilostazole**) would increase cAMP levels and inhibit platelet aggregation.* ***Cilostazole*** and ***dipyridamole*** have already been discussed in the text of Ch. 20.

2) **Platelets ADP Receptor Inhibitors**: Within seconds of vascular injury, the exposed collagen of the underlying connective tissue activates the dormantly lying glycoprotein (GP) integrin receptors on the platelets (GPVI) which triggers the release of ADP and 5-HT along with Ca^{2+} and fibrin stabilising factors. This is also known as "*platelet release reaction*". 5-HT, being vasoconstrictor, decreases blood flow to the injured vessel. ADP activates ADP receptors (both $P2Y_1$ and $P2Y_{12}$) on platelets to induce shape change and aggregation ($P2Y_1$ effect) and to increase their adhesiveness ($P2Y_{12}$ effect). *Hence, any drug which inhibits ADP binding to its receptors would also inhibit platelet aggregation (e.g., **ticlopidine, clopidogrel** and **prasugrel**).*

   All these three drugs are thienopyridine derivatives irreversibly block ADP $P2Y_{12}$ receptors and prevent ADP-induced platelet aggregation by inhibiting the conformational change in the platelet membrane and expression of functional GPIIb/IIIa integrin receptors. All three are prodrugs and converted to active metabolite by CYP3A4/5, CYP2C19 and CYP2B6) enzymes in the liver: ***ticlopidine*** to active thiol metabolite (by CYP3 A4/5 > CYP2C19), ***clopidogrel*** to oxidized active metabolite (CYP2C19 >CYP3A4/5 and CYP2B6) and ***prasugrel*** to oxidized metabolite (CYP3A4/5 >>>CYP2C19). CYP2C19 enzyme show polymorphism and depending on **s**ingle **n**ucleotide **p**olymorphism (SNP) inheritance pattern in CYP2C19 (homo- and heterozygous) individuals may be poor metabolizers of clopidogrel. Thus such persons are at increased risk of cardiovascular events due to inadequate formation of clopidogrel active metabolite. The FDA has recommended CYP2C19 genotyping to identify such individuals to alter the prescreption to include alternative antiplatelet drugs. Besides drugs which inhibit CYP2C19 enzyme (omeprazole, fluconazole, ticlopidine) may adversely interact with clopidogrel by not allowing formation of its active metabolite.

Ticlopidine has been approved for prevention of stroke in patient of **t**ransient **i**schaemic **a**ttack (TIA). Because this drug can cause severe neutropenia, patients who are treated with ticlopidine should be tested for **c**omplete **b**lood **c**ount (CBC) every two weeks from a second week to the third month of tretment, and any time they develop an infection. Clopidogrel and prassugrel rarely cause neutropenia and therefore do not require CBC testing and are preferred in patients who cannot tolerate or show neutropenic toxicity to ticlopidine.

Clopidogrel and ***prasugrel*** are approved for patients with unstable angina, STEMI/non-STEMI, thrombotic stroke and intermittent claudication in peripheral arterial disease. Besides, they are also used with aspirin to treat thrombotic cardiovascular events in patients of **a**ccute **c**oronary **s**yndrome (ACS).

For their approved indications ticlodipine is administered in the dose of 250 mg BD, Clopidogrel is given initially in the loading dose of 300–600 mg followed by 75 mg OD and prasugrel is administered initially in the loading dose of 60 mg followed by 5–10 mg OD (see Ch.20 for the use of these drugs in angina pectoris).

Ticagrelor and ***cangrelor*** are other addition in this class of agents. Unlike ***clopidogrel*** and ***prasugrel*** these are not prodrugs and act as a direct reversible inhibitors of $P2Y_{12}$ ADP receptor. Therefore, both drugs have a rapid onset of action and are more potent than prasugrel or clopidogrel. Almost 90% of platelet aggregation is blocked within 2–4 hrs of 180 mg oral loading dose of *ticagrelor*. Maintenance dose is 90 mg once or twice daily.

Cangrelor is a fast acting, potent I.V. $P2Y_{12}$ receptor inhibitor and is approved as an adjunct to PCI for reducing the risk of peri-procedural MI, repeat coronary revascularization, and stent thrombosis in patients not treated with an oral $P2Y_{12}$ receptor inhibitor and/or not being given a GPIIb/IIIa receptor inhibitor.

3. **Platelet Thromboxane A2 (TxA2) Synthesis Inhibitors**: Stimulation of platelet by collagen/ADP also activates platelet membrane phospholipase to synthesise arachidonic acid from membrane phospholipids. It is then converted to TxA_2 by COX-1 in the platelets. TxA_2 is then released into plasma to activate TxA_2 receptors present on other nearby platelets and activate them as well. Release of arachidonic acid also triggers the release of ADP and 5-HT from the platelet granules. All the events further cause platelet activation and aggregation. *Hence, any drug which irreversibly inhibits platelet COX-1, to prevent TxA_2 production (e.g., **aspirin**), would also prevent platelet aggregation.*

Aspirin in low doses have been found to selectively inhibit the synthesis of TxA_2 without having as much effect on PGI_2 , whereas higher doses inhibit the senthesis of both prostaglandins. Therefore the dosage of aspirin used to inhibit platelet aggregation is usually lower than that used for other pharmacologic effects. Unlike other NSAIDs aspirin inhibits thromboxane-A_2 synthesis in platelets by irreversible acetylation of the active serine site of COX-1, the enzyme that catalyzes an early step in TxA_2 synthesis. For this reason, aspirin inhibits platelet aggregation for their total life span (7–10 days). NSAIDs like ***ibuprofen*** also inhibit COX-1 but transiently and reversibly, by competing at the serine catalytic site of COX-1. *Hence concomitant use of ibuprofen (as analgesic-anti-inflammatory drug) and aspirin (as antiplatelet) should be* *avoided because ibuprofen will prevent the access of aspirin to the serine site and would rather antagonise the platelet inhibitory effects of aspirin. If ibuprofen has to be used, asprin should be taken 1 hr before or at least 8 hr after ibuprofen.* For an antiplatelet drug to be effective, it should inhibit platelet aggregation by 80%.

Because aspirin exhibits a longer antiplatelet effect, it is administered once a day (dose 87.5–175 mg) or every other day (dose 350 mg) alone or co-administered with clopidogrel/prasugrel.

4) **Platelet thromboxane A2 Prostaglandin (TP) Receptor Inhibitors/Antagonists**: Receptors for TxA_2 (TP receptors) have also been identified on platelets, vascular smooth muscle cells and endothelial cells. Activation of TP receptors on platelets stimulates platelet aggregation, on vascular smooth muscle cells causes vasoconstriction, while on endothelial cells promotes atherosclerosis. ***Terutroban*** is a selective antagonist of TP receptors located at all the 3 sites. Hence, its triple activity (antiplatelet, vasodilating and anti-atherosclerotic) makes it an innovative antiplatelet drug of unique potential in this series. However, clinical development of terutroban was stopped becasue it was not found to be superior/ or noninferior then compared with aspirin for prevention of ischaemic stroke or cardiovascular event.

5) **Platelet Glycoprotein IIb/IIIa (GPIIb/IIIa) Receptor Inhibitors/Antagonists**:
The last step in the platelet aggregation response to vascular trauma depends on a family of GP IIb/IIIa receptors or fibrinogen binding receptors that are present on the surface of platelet. Normally they remain in an inactive conformation which does not support fibrinogen binding. But on activation of platelets (by ADP/TxA_2/thrombin), the GP IIb/IIIa receptors assume an active conformation which is capable of binding fibrinogen. This leads to the formation of platelet clumps or aggregates (Fig. 51.5). *Any drug which blocks GP IIb/IIIa receptors (e.g.,* ***Abciximab, Eptifibatide*** *and* ***Tirofiban****) and prevents fibrinogen from cross-linking activated platelets would also inhibit thombus growth.*
Abciximab: It is the Fab fragment (antigen-binding fragment) of a chimaric monoclonal antibody that binds to GP IIb/IIIa and inhibits fibrinogen cross-linking of platelets which is the final common pathway of platelet aggregation.

It also binds to αIIb/b3 receptors for vWF present on platelets. vWF also anchor platelets to each other (like fibrinogen). The plasma half-life of abciximab is 30 min. It is initially administered as bolus injection followed by slow I.V. infusion. Though half-life is short yet platelet aggregation remains inhibited for 24 hrs because drug remains bound to αIIb/b3 receptor for a prolonged period. Given with aspirin and heparin during percutaneous angioplasty, it effectively prevents reocclusion, recurrent MI and mortality. ***Major side effect*** is bleeding. However, thrombocytopenia and constipation may occur in 2% of patients but are reversible. It is non-antigenic.
Eptifibatide: It is a cyclic peptide inhibitor of the fibrinogen binding site on GP IIb/IIIa receptor on platelets. It is also given by bolus injection initially followed by slow I.V. infusion. It is similar to abciximab except that it does not bind to αIIb/b3 receptors for vWF. ***Side effect***: bleeding.
Tirofiban: Almost similar to eptifibatide as it does not act on receptors for vWF. Side effects, use and route of administration are similar to eptifibatide/abciximab.

6) **Platelet Thrombin Protease-Activated Receptor-1 (PAR-1) Antagonist**: Thrombin is a protease that fecilitates pathological thrombosis by three well understood actions, e.g., it a) converts fibrinogen to fibring, b) stimulates factor XIII (fibrin-stabilizing factor) to stabilize the fibrin, and c) activates two thrombin receptor PAR-1/PAR-4 expressed on the platelet membrene. Thrombin binding to these receptors results in an enhancement of platelet aggregation.
Vorapaxar is a reversible antagonist of PAR-1, one of the two major PARs on platelets. It

neither inhibits platelet aggregation induced by ADP, TxA_2 or collagen nor affects coagulation parameters *ex vivo*. The drug has been approved for the secondary prevention of MI, stroke in post-MI patients and those with peripheral arterial disease. It is administered orally in a dose of 2.5 mg (of vorapaxar sulphate, containing active drug 2.08 mg) per day. Given orally the drug is absorbed completely, highly protein bound (99%), metabolized by CYP3A4 enzyme and has a long half life (5-13 days). Thus, the drug should be avoided with CYP3A4 inhibitors (increased risk of bleeding, especially when it is given with other antiplatelet drugs) or inducers (reduced drug effect due to increased metabolism) and in patients with hepatic impairment (reduced metabolism, more risk of bleeding). The drug should not be prescribed to patient with prior history of stroke, TIA or intracranial haemorrhage.

Ridogrel

Ridogrel has dual action, a combined thromboxane synthase inhibitor and thromboxane A2 receptor antagonist. It can be used with streptokinase as an adjunctive therapy to reduce the formation of blood clots. While aspirin inhibits cyclooxygenase, the enzyme responsible for producing thromboxane, ridogrel inhibits thromboxane synthesis directly and blocks receptors also. Ridogrel is in different stages of drug development.

Therapeutic Uses of Antiplatelet Drugs

1. **Acute coronary syndrome (ACS)**: Aspirin (75–150 mg/day) or clopidogrel is given for treatment as well as prophylaxis of coronary diseases. It is given for prophylaxis in post-MI patients to prevent reinfarction. Risk of bleeding should be watched. Aspirin and LMWH are given in treatment of ACS.
   - *Unstable angina*: Aspirin and clopidogrel reduces risk of MI and death.
   - *Non- ST elevation MI (NSTEMI)*: Aspirin and clopidogrel combination is given for about 12 months. Ticagrelor can also be combined.
   - *ST-elevation MI (STEMI)*: Aspirin (300 mg/day) and prasugrel are given in patients who undergo percutaneous coronary intervention (PCI). Aspirin + abciximab/tirofiban/eptifibatide can be given to decrease restenosis after coronary angioplasty. Heparin should also be given.
   - For coronary artery bypass graft, aspirin + prasugrel/abciximab/eptifibatide should be given.
2. **Prosthetic heart valves**: Formation of microthrombi on the artificial heart valves may lead to generation of emboli. Aspirin reduces formation of microthrombi on artificial heart valves. Dipyridamole can be combined with aspirin.
3. **Arteriovenous shunt**: Aspirin or Prasugrel can be used for patency of arteriovenous shunt during venous grafting and dialysis.
4. **Stroke and Transient Ischemic Attack (TIA)**: Aspirin and dipyridamole are used to prevent stroke and transient ischemic attack. Clopidogrel can be given. Oral anticoagulants are not effective.
5. **Venous thromboembolism**: Anticoagulants are more effective. Antiplatelets can be used as a prophylaxis.
6. **Intermittent claudication**: Aspirin and clopidogrel can be used in peripheral vascular disease.

CHAPTER 52

SECTION 11—CHEMOTHERAPY OF MICROBIAL DISEASES

Introduction to Chemotherapy

COMPETENCY PH1.42, PH1.43

While doing research on microbes and the diseases caused by them, Paul Ehrlich (1913) realised that if a particular dye could stain a particular species of microbe, these could be killed selectively by certain drugs as well. ***Chemotherapy***, therefore, means the treatment of systemic/topical infection with drugs that have selective toxicity for an invading pathogen (living or multiplying) without harming the host cells. In most instances, this selective toxicity is relative, rather than absolute, requiring a proper dose of a drug that is toxic to the microorganism but being tolerated by the host. Chemotherapy usually takes advantage of the biochemical and physiological differences that exist between microorganisms (prokaryotes) and the human beings (eukaryotes).

The term ***antimicrobial agents*** is broader in meaning because it includes drugs synthesised in the laboratory (precisely called ***antibacterial agents***) as well as those obtained from fermentation of microorganisms (***antibiotics***). There are many antimicrobial agents wherein the key portion of the chemical structure is derived from the microbial source but its chemical structure is then modified by attaching different chemical moieties (called ***semisynthetic antibiotics***). Hence, the distinction between the terms "antibacterials", "antibiotics" and "semisynthetic antibiotics" is somewhat blurred and has lost the original precise meaning in today's context. We shall be using these terms for which they stand for, but virtually many texts and many physicians use these terms interchangeably.

Again, these days, the term chemotherapy has been extended to cover "cancer chemotherapy" as well, because the same definition can cover this aspect also. However, in this introductory chapter we stick to the original meaning, i.e., treatment of infectious diseases caused by the microbes (i.e., bacteria, fungi and viruses) and the parasites (i.e., protozoa and helminths). That leaves the mysterious proteinaceous agents, lacking nucleic acids, called ***prions*** (Ch. 66) which cause certain fatal diseases, and defy proper classification.

In today's context, the older term "***commensals***" has also lost its meaning. It is now difficult to distinguish between commensals—microorganisms that are parasites without causing disease—and the disease-causing microorganisms, since it is now clear that many so-called "commensals" can also cause disease if the immune system of the host is compromised.

Antimicrobial agents may act as either *bacteriostatic* or *bactericidal*. ***Bacteriostatic*** drugs arrest the growth and replication of the bacteria and thus limit the spread of infection. In case of antifungal drugs the term used is ***fungistatic***. Examples of bacteriostatic drugs include: macrolide group of antibiotics, oxazolidinones, chloramphenicol, tetracyclines, sulfonamides, trimethoprim, clindamycin, nitrofurantoin and ethambutol (see following chapters). A bacteriostatic agent often is adequate in uncomplicated infections because the host defenses usually help eradicate the microorganism. However, for a neutropenic individual, such a bacteriostatic agent is usually ineffective. ***Bactericidal agents***, on the other hand, kill or irreversibly damage the multiplying bacteria, so that the total number of viable organisms decreases. Examples include: beta-lactam antibiotics, cotrimoxazole, aminoglycosides, fluoroquinolones, vancomycin, polymixins, bacitracin, isoniazid, pyrazinamide and rifampicin (see related chapters). For antifungal drugs, the equivalent term is ***fungicidal***. Such a classification of antimicrobial drugs as bacteriostatic or bactericidal has its own limitations. A given agent may show the bactericidal actions under some conditions but bacteriostatic actions under others, depending on the concentration of the drug and the target bacteria. For example, chloramphenicol is 'static' against gram-negative rods but 'cidal' against pneumococci; and many antibacterial agents are 'static' when used alone (sulfonamides or trimethoprim) but become bactericidal when used in combination (e.g., cotrimoxazole, Ch. 53). Bactericidal drugs are preferred over static drugs under circumstances in which host defenses are impaired or for management of complicated infections, e.g., tuberculosis, endocarditis and meningitis. Thus the susceptibility of the pathogen is not the only criterion for the efficacy of an antibiotic.

DIFFERENCE BETWEEN PROKARYOTIC AND EUKARYOTIC CELLS

Living organisms are classified as either ***prokaryotes*** (as of bacteria) or as ***eukaryotes*** (as of mammals, protozoa, fungi and helminths). In a separate category are viruses which need to utilise the metabolic machinery of the host cells as they lack their own biochemical machinery for generating energy or for any sort of protein synthesis. Treatment of viral diseases therefore poses a peculiar problem in target oriented drug attack, while antiprotozoal, antifungal and anthelmintic drugs are not only toxic to these parasites but are toxic to the host cells also. The major differences between the prokaryotes and eukaryotes are as under:

- Prokaryotic cells are smaller in size (0.1–5 μm) while eukaryotic cells are large (10–100 μm).
- Prokaryotic cells are enveloped by a rigid cell wall which is made up of peptidoglycan (except in mycoplasma). Eukaryotic cells are enveloped by a flexible plasma membrane.

  In Gram-positive bacteria, there is a plasma membrane beneath this cell wall. This consists of phospholipid bilayer and proteins but no sterols (as in fungi). It functions as a selectively permeable membrane with specific transport mechanisms for various nutrients (Fig. 55.4A). The function of the cell wall is to provide support to this membrane which is subject to an internal osmotic pressure due to hypertonic fluid inside the bacterial cell cytoplasmic membrane. In Gram-negative bacteria, on the contrary, there is also an outer membrane, outside the cell wall, and the peptidoglycan cell wall is thus sandwiched between this outer membrane and the inner cytoplasmic membrane (Fig. 55.4 B). This outer membrane consists of lipopolysaccharides with narrow porin channels which serves as barrier to the permeability of various antibiotics.
- In prokaryotic cells, distinct subcellular organs like mitochondria, nucleus and lysosomes are absent, while in eukaryotic cells these are distinctly present.
- Prokaryotic cells have ill-defined nucleus, while in eukaryotic cells, nucleus is well defined and is surrounded by a membrane.
- In prokaryotic cells, the enzymes related to energy metabolism are bound to cell membrane, while in eukaryotic cells these are located in mitochondria.
- In prokaryotes, cell division takes place by fission, while in eukaryotes it takes place by mitosis. Further, in prokaryotes a network of tubules and filaments are absent in the cytoplasm, while in eukaryotes these essential constituents of cytoskeleton are present.
- Ribosomes, the centres of protein synthesis, are also different in prokaryotes and the eukaryotes. The difference in the nature of these cytoplasmic nucleoproteins provides the basis for the selective toxicity of an antibiotic to the invading pathogen only (and not to the host cells). The bacteria possess 70S ribosomal units in their cytoplasm which, when fractionated chromatographically, separate into 30S and 50S ribosomal subunits. The mammalian ribosomes are 80S which can be fractionated into 60S and 40S subunits. The unit "S" denotes the *Svedberg unit,* which measures the sedimentation rate and not the mass; and hence 60S + 40S does not mean that it should be equal to 100S (instead of 80S).

  One Svedberg unit = 10^{-13} sec and hence the sedimentation rate of 60S ribosomal unit shall be 60 x 10^{-13} sec. Most antibiotics inhibit 30S (aminoglycosides and tetracyclines) or 50S (erythromycin and chloramphenicol) subunits of bacterial ribosomes and hence exhibit selective toxicity towards bacteria than host cells. However, some antibiotics (chloramphenicol) also inhibit mammalian mitochondrial 30S and 50S ribosomes and therefore are toxic to the host cells as well. Having outlined the essential structures of the bacterial cell, we need now to consider how different antibacterial drugs act upon the invading organisms.

SITE AND MECHANISM OF ACTION OF ANTIBIOTICS

Antimicrobials affect the viability of micro-organisms by four different mechanisms (Fig. 52.1):

1) Inhibition of cell wall synthesis
2) Alteration of cell membrane integrity
3) Inhibition of ribosomal protein synthesis
4) Suppression of DNA synthesis

Microbial cell wall synthesis inhibition and alteration of membrane integrity are extra-cytoplasmic sites of action while inhibition of DNA and ribosomal protein synthesis are intra-cytoplasmic sites of action. Drugs that affect bacterial cell wall or membrane integrity and DNA synthesis are usually bactericidal (but not always) while those affecting protein and folic acid synthesis (see below) are usually bacteriostatic (though not always true, see above).

1. Inhibition of Bacterial Cell Wall Synthesis

All penicillins, cephalosporins, monobactams and carbapenems inhibit bacterial cell wall synthesis (Fig. 55.3) by binding to one or more of penicillin binding proteins (PBPs), which in turn inhibits the final transpeptidation step (cross bridging) of peptidoglycan (the building blocks) synthesis in bacterial cell wall. The formation of an imperfect cell wall leads to an osmotic drive of the fluid from outside of the environment to inside of the hypertonic fluid of the bacteria. As a result the bacteria swells and bursts to die. The lysis of the bacteria is also facilitated by an ongoing activity of cell wall autolysing enzymes (murein hydrolases and autolysins). The details can be found in Ch. 55.

2. Alteration of Cell Membrane Integrity

Polymixins function as cationic detergents and disrupt the bacterial cell membrane osmotic integrity by displacing Ca^{2+} and Mg^{2+} from membrane lipid phosphates (Ch. 57). This ends up in the leakage of intracellular constituents and the death of bacteria. Some antifungal antibiotics such as amphotericin-B bind to ergosterol present in fungal cell membrane and alter its permeability by forming pores through which K^+, Na^+, H^+, Mg^{2+} and other macromolecules leak out, leading to cell death (Ch. 60). The azole group of antifungal drugs also *inhibit ergosterol biosynthesis* which results in damaged leaky fungal cell membrane (Ch. 60).

3. Inhibition of Ribosomal Protein Synthesis

Ribosomes are involved in the protein synthesis by the bacteria. Ribosomes are different in eukaryotes and prokaryotes. The bacterial ribosome consists of a 50S and 30S subunit which when combine, form 70S subunit while in the mammalian ribosomes the 60S and 40S subunits combine to form 80S subunit. This difference provides the basis for the selective antimicrobial action of some antibiotics. The protein synthesis in bacteria takes place in the following steps (Fig 52.2 A-D):

a) Messenger RNA (m-RNA), which is transcribed from DNA, becomes attached to the 30S subunit of the ribosome. The 50S subunit then binds to 30S subunit to constitute 70S subunit. This unit moves along the m-RNA so that the successive codons of the m-RNA pass along the ribosome from the acceptor site (A-site) to the peptidyl site (P-site). A stage is now set for protein synthesis. This stage is called formation of ***initiation complex***. Codon means a triplet of 3 nucleotides carrying the codes for a specific amino acid needed for protein synthesis.

   A transfer RNA (t-RNA) with its existing amino acid chain (A_1–A_3) is already attached at the P-site of the complex by complementary codon: anticodon pairing. The incoming t-RNA carries another amino acid residue (A_4) to be added to the growing peptide chain.

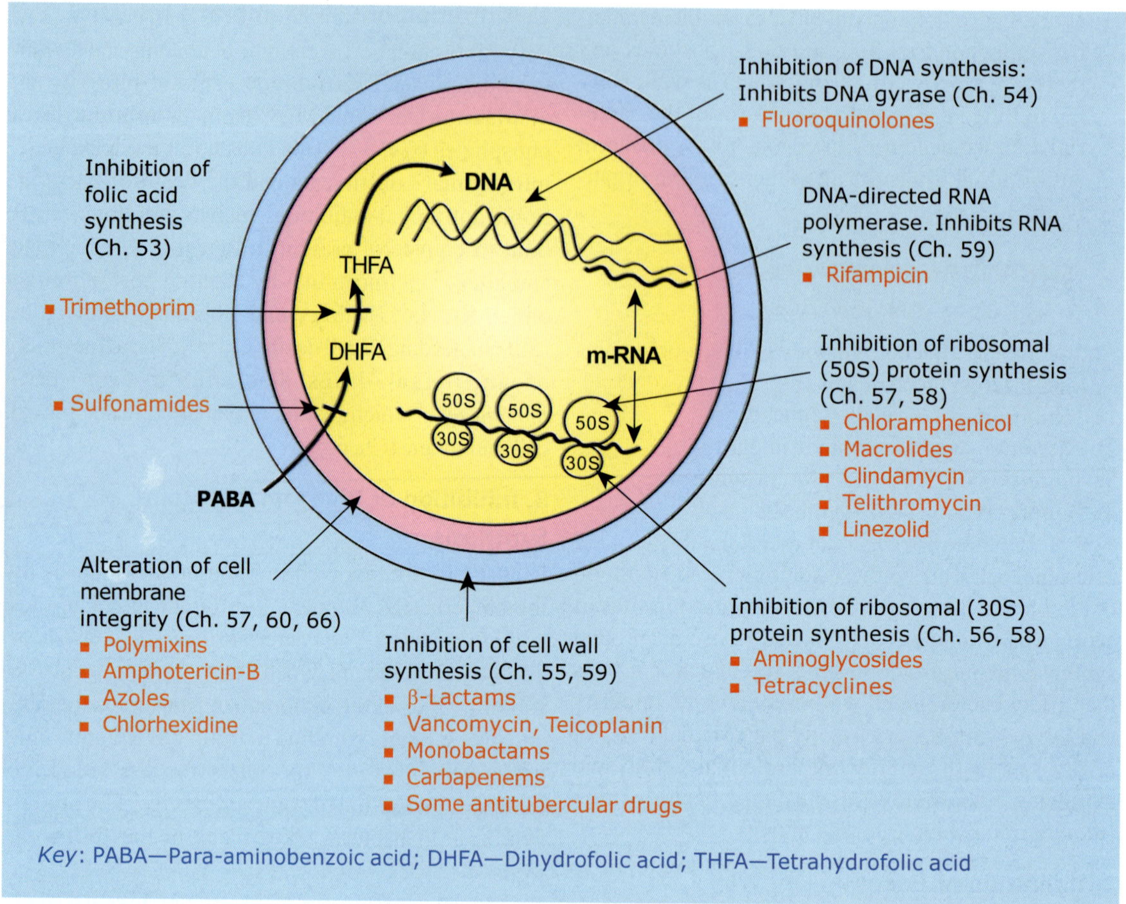

Fig 52.1 Classification of Some Antimicrobial Agents by Their Mechanism & Site of Action

b) The incoming aminoacyl t-RNA with a new amino acid (A_4) binds to the acceptor site (A-site) by complementary base pairing.

c) The peptide chain (A_1–A_3) on the t-RNA attached to the P-site is then transferred to the t-RNA linked to A-site. This process is called ***transpeptidation***. The t-RNA at the P-site has lost its peptide and transferred it to aminoacyl t-RNA of the A-site which now consists of 4 amino acid (A_1–A_4) peptide chain.

d) This t-RNA which has lost its peptide chain is then ejected out from the P-site, while the t-RNA at the A-site (with 4 amino acid chain) is ***translocated*** to the P-site. The freed A-site is now ready to receive a new t-RNA, with new amino acid (A_5) and relevant anticodon attached to it. The whole process is then repeated. During the process of translocation the ribosome moves on one codon relative to the messenger. Usually several ribosomes, i.e., ***polysomes***, simultaneously translate on a single m-RNA template.

Aminoglycosides group of antibiotics (refer Ch. 56 for details) bind to 30S ribosomal units of the bacteria and prevent the formation of the "initiation complex" which is the prerequisite for peptide synthesis. They also interfere with the assembly of polysomes which results in the accumulation of nonfunctional ribosomes (monosomes). Macrolide group of antibiotics (erythromycin group) inhibit bacterial

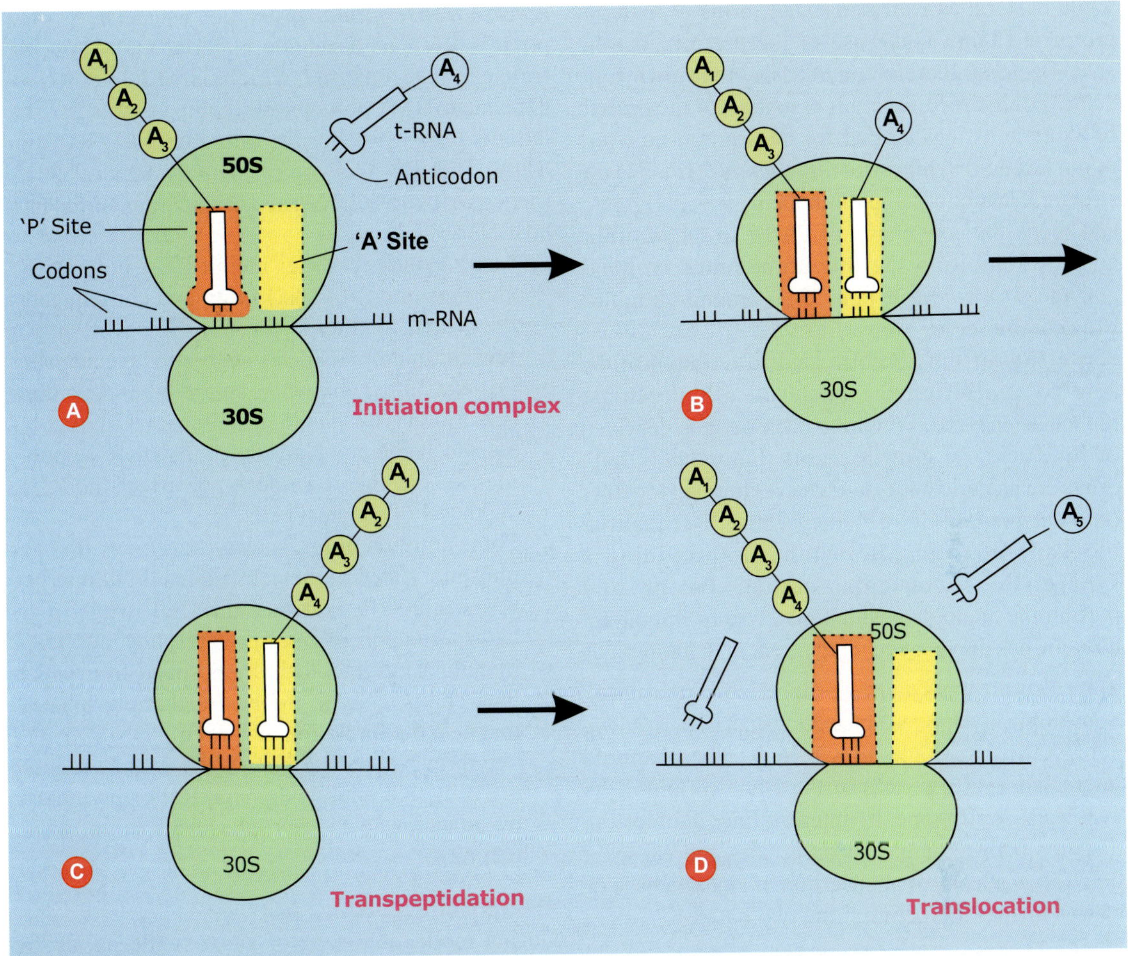

Fig 52.2 Steps in Bacterial Protein Synthesis

protein synthesis by binding reversibly to the P-site in the 50S ribosomal unit (Ch. 57). As a result the translocation of the growing peptide chain from the A-site to the P-site is hindered. The same holds true for clindamycin and telithromycin (Ch. 57). Linezolid (Ch. 57) binds to 50S ribosomal unit near the interface with 30S subunit and thus inhibits the formation of "initiation complex". Streptogramins (Ch. 57) also bind to 50S ribosomal unit but prevent the extrusion of the newly synthesised peptide chain from the ribosome leading to bacterial death. Chloramphenicol (Ch. 58) also inhibits bacterial 50S ribosomal subunits but prevents the binding of aminoacyl t-RNA to A-site of 50S ribosomal unit. Tetracyclines (Ch. 58) inhibit 30S ribosomal unit to prevent attachment of aminoacyl t-RNA to the A-site of 50S ribosomal subunit. All these antibiotics, therefore, act by prematurely terminating the protein synthesis of bacteria.

4. Suppression of DNA Synthesis

The nucleic acid synthesis can be inhibited by five different mechanisms:

1) By inhibiting the synthesis of folates, purines and pyrimidines

One of the prime examples of difference that has proved to be useful in chemotherapy is that humans cannot synthesise folic acid but acquire it from diet, while bacteria as well as asexual forms of malarial protozoa cannot make use of the preformed folic acid. Bacteria, therefore, synthesise their own folic acid. Tetrahydrofolic acid is essential for the growth of bacteria as it is crucial for one-carbon transfers in nucleic acid synthesis. *Sulfonamides* (Ch. 53) are structural analogues of p-aminobenzoic acid (PABA) and block the conversion of PABA to dihydrofolic acid by inhibiting the dihydropteroate synthase enzyme. *Trimethoprim* (Ch. 53) is another drug that blocks the next step (Fig. 52.1, 53.2), i.e., conversion of dihydrofolic acid to tetrahydrofolic acid by inhibiting the bacterial dihydrofolate reductase enzyme. When the bacteria gets deprived of folic acid, its growth ceases. Individually both drugs are bacteriostatic, but when combined together (*cotrimoxazole*, Ch. 53) they cause a sequential blockade of folic acid synthesis, providing a synergistic bactericidal action. Purine and pyrimidine analogues which give rise to fraudulent nucleotides have been discussed in Chapter 67.

2) By altering base pairing properties of template

Some topically applied antiseptics such as *acriflavine* act by this mechanism (Ch. 66). These agents intercalate (get inserted) in the DNA to inhibit its synthesis. Acriflavine, by intercalating, doubles the distance between adjacent base pairs and causes a deletion of a base, or an insertion of an extra base or causes mispairing between the two bases.

3) By inhibiting either DNA or RNA polymerase

DNA polymerase has a catalysing as well as proof reading functions during the synthesis of new DNA strand. RNA polymerase (or DNA dependent-RNA polymerase) synthesises all RNAs in prokaryotes from their DNA; and ***transcription*** is a process in which RNA is synthesised from DNA. There are three types of RNAs: m-RNA, t-RNA and r-RNA (ribosomal RNA). The r-RNA is actually an integral part of ribosome (in both prokaryotes and eukaryotes) which is necessary for (a) assembly of ribosomes, (b) binding of m-RNA to the functional ribosomal units and (c) for peptidyl chain transfer process in the ribosomes. All these are essential steps in protein synthesis by bacteria (Fig. 52.2). Some of the oncogenic viruses, called ***retroviruses***, show a unique nucleic acid synthesis by way of ***reverse transcription***. Instead of usual DNA, they possess RNA as a genetic material and a reverse transcriptase enzyme which is rather a RNA-dependent-DNA polymerase (compare above). The latter is responsible for the formation of DNA from RNA. This DNA is complementary to viral RNA (hence written as cDNA) and can be transmitted into host-DNA as *provirus*.

- Many anticancer drugs inhibit RNA polymerase and thus prevent transcription and consequently the protein synthesis (Ch. 67). However, only a few antimicrobial agents act by this mechanism. For example, *rifampicin,* an antitubercular drug (Ch. 59), acts by inhibiting the bacterial RNA polymerase. It does not bind to mammalian RNA polymerase and therefore does not affect the RNA synthesis of the host cells.
- Some antiviral drugs, such as *acyclovir*, first get phosphorylated in the cells infected with herpes virus (Ch. 61). Various antiviral drugs, e.g., *zidovudine* and *didanosine,* are phosphorylated by cellular enzymes to the triphosphate form which then competes with the host cell triphosphates, that help the formation of "proviral DNA" by the "viral reverse transcriptase" (Ch. 62). *Foscarnet* is a drug that inhibits the viral RNA polymerase by attaching to the pyrophosphate binding site (Ch. 62).

4) By inhibiting DNA gyrase

During replication stage of DNA synthesis, as the double helical strands of DNA separate from one end, the positive supercoils (overbinding) are formed at the other end. The phenomenon of positive supercoiling can be easily understood by comparing DNA helix with two twisted ropes which are tied at one end. If one person holds the ropes at the tied end (in a fixed position) while another person tries to pull them apart from the other side, there would obviously be a tangling (overbinding or supercoiling) in front of the point of their separation. This problem of supercoiling that comes in the way of bacterial DNA replication is overcome by a group of enzymes called DNA topoisomerases (DNA gyrase).

In Gram-negative bacteria, DNA gyrase (topoisomerase II) is responsible for continuously introducing negative supercoils into DNA. Its function is to cut both the strands of bacterial DNA and then reseal them to overcome the process of supercoiling. In Gram-positive bacteria, this problem is overcome by topoisomerase IV but in a slightly different manner. It separates the catenated (interlinked) daughter DNA molecules (that are the products of DNA replication) and then reseals the strands. Fluoroquinolone group of antibiotics (Ch. 54) block the cutting and resealing activity of DNA gyrase and also block the decatenating (delinking) action of topoisomerase IV. Eukaryotic cells do not contain DNA gyrase but have an almost similar type of DNA topoisomerase II that removes overwinding of eukaryotic DNA strands during their replication. Therapeutic doses of fluoroquinolones do not inhibit mammalian topoisomerase.

5) By directly damaging DNA and its functioning

Many anticancer drugs do make a covalent bonding with the bases of DNA and prevent their replication. Hardly any antibacterial drug works by this mechanism. However, an antiprotozoal drug, metronidazole, partly acts by this mechanism. The 5'-nitro group of metronidazole (Ch. 65) is first reduced in sensitive obligate anaerobes to cell toxic free radicals (nitro, nitroso and hydroxylamine) that damage the protozoal DNA or inhibit its synthesis.

BACTERIAL RESISTANCE TO ANTIBIOTICS

Unfortunately with the advancement of chemotherapy, bacteria have also matched their inventive power in developing their self defences against these therapeutic agents. Since the population of most of the bacteria gets doubled in just 30 min, there may be several generations of the same bacteria in couple of hours and this provides ample opportunity for them for genetic adaptations. Resistance to chemotherapeutic agents can also develop in protozoa and in malignant cells. The term ***drug resistance*** refers to unresponsiveness of microorganisms to an antimicrobial agent after its repeated use. A similar term, ***tolerance***, is used in relation to human beings when there is a need to increase the dose in order to produce the pharmacological response of equal magnitude and duration. However, a term ***"antibiotic tolerance"*** is sometimes used when the antibiotic no longer kills the micro-organism but merely inhibits its growth or multiplication. Tolerant microorganisms start to grow after the antibiotic is stopped, whereas resistant microorganisms multiply even in the presence of antibiotics.

Resistance in bacterial populations can be spread from person to person by bacteria; from bacterium to bacterium by plasmids and from plasmid to plasmid by transposons and integrons (Fig. 52.3). Antibiotic resistance could be ***intrinsic*** (natural) or ***acquired***. For example, *Mycobacterium tuberculosis* have always been resistant to common antibiotics and *Pseudomonas aeruginosa* is intrinsically resistant to many antibiotics because of the inability of antibiotics to cross its outer membrane or bind to target sites. This type of resistance poses no significant clinical problem as only the proper drugs are to be selected. The ***acquired resistance*** develops subsequently at a later stage due to widespread and irrational use of antibiotics. This type of resistance develops either by gene transfer or by mutation or by modification in biochemical mechanisms.

1. Genetic Methods of Antibiotic Resistance (Fig. 52.3)

A) Chromosomal Methods: Mutations

Mutation refers to a change in the DNA structure of a gene. The spontaneous mutation in bacterial cells occurs at a frequency of approximately one per million cells. The mutation rate of bacteria is therefore quite low. However, during the course of therapy, the 'sensitive' bacteria may die but the resistant ones continue to grow and multiply resulting in "***selection of mutants***". Such mutants therefore, confer resistance to the antibiotic. Although mutants resulting from chromosomal mutations have reduced pathogenicity, it is a big clinical problem in infections caused by mycobacteria (tuberculosis and leprosy) and by methicillin resistant *Staphylococcus aureus* (MRSA; an imprecise name because MRSA is resistant to most of the antibiotics and because methicillin is no longer used clinically).

B) Extrachromosomal Mechanisms: Plasmids

Plasmids are actually vectors serving as a carriers of DNA molecule. Most bacteria contain such extrachromosomal genetic elements, that can replicate independently and freely in cytoplasm. Plasmids which carry genes resistant to antibiotics (*r-genes*) are called *R-plasmids*. These *r-genes* can get readily transferred from one *R-plasmid* to another plasmid or to chromosome. Much of the drug resistance encountered in clinical practice is plasmid mediated.

i) Methods of Transfer of r-Genes From One Bacterium to Another

The transfer of resistant genes can occur between bacteria of the same species or of different species. There are three mechanisms for gene transfer.

Conjugation: It is the main mechanism for the spread of resistance or even multidrug resistance (if r-genes are transferred between different species). The conjugative plasmids, that contain the transfer r-genes, make a connecting tube (sex pili) between the two bacteria through which the plasmid itself can pass. This is commonly observed with bacterial population at high density, as in the gut, because the resident microflora can serve as a reservoir for the resistant genes which can be transferred to other organisms that later invade the host.

Transduction: A less common method of transfer of resistance is by transduction by which the plasmid DNA enclosed in a bacterial virus (bacteriophage) is transferred to another bacterium of the same species. It is usually observed in the transmission of resistant genes between strains of staphylococci and between strains of streptococci.

Transformation: This method for developing resistance poses the least clinical problems. It involves the ability of certain bacteria to pick up free DNA from the environment (i.e., from a cell belonging to closely related or the same strain). The new DNA is then incorporated into the genome of the bacteria which then becomes resistant (Fig. 52.3).

ii) Transfer of r-Genes Between Plasmids Within The Bacterium

By Transposons: Transposons are DNA segments that cannot self-replicate but can self-transfer between plasmids or from plasmid to chromosomes. In such a process of transfer of resistance, the donor plasmid, containing a transposon, cointegrates with the acceptor (or target) plasmid. During the process of cointegration the transposon can now replicate. Both the plasmids then separate and each contains the r-gene carrying the transposon (Fig. 52.3). Some strains of staphylococci and enterococci acquire resistance transferred by transposons. As a result these organisms can cause virtually untreatable nosocomial (those acquired in hospital) infections.

By Integrons: Resistance, mainly the multidrug resistance, can also be spread by a larger mobile DNA unit called "*integron*", which can be located on a transposon. Each integron is packed with multiple *gene cassettes*, each consisting of a resistant gene attached to a small recognition site. These gene cassettes are encoded with several bacterial functions including resistance and virulence. Currently the gene cassettes have been identified for all antibiotics except for fluoroquinolones. Integrons cannot promote self transfer (as they lack transporter genes) but they are commonly associated with and work with transposons and conjugative plasmids.

2. Biochemical Mechanisms of Resistance to Antibiotics

A) By Producing an Enzyme That Inactivates The Antibiotic (Fig 52.4A)

Inactivation of β-Lactam Antibiotics

Staphylococcus aureus, Neisseria gonorrhoea, Haemophilus influenzae and some enteric Gram-negative rods are the principal bacteria which produce *beta-lactamase enzyme* that cleaves the β-lactam ring and inactivates many β-lactam antibiotics. However, some β-lactamases have a preference for penicillins while some for cephalosporins and hence cross resistance is not complete. Similarly, newer β-lactam antibiotics (monobactams and carbapenems) and third/fourth generation cephalosporins are resistant to degradation by β-lactamase enzymes (Ch. 55).

Inactivation of Chloramphenicol

Chloramphenicol is inactivated by *chloramphenicol acetyltransferase* produced by resistant strains of gram-negative and gram-positive bacteria. The r-genes are borne on plasmids (Ch. 58). The Gram-

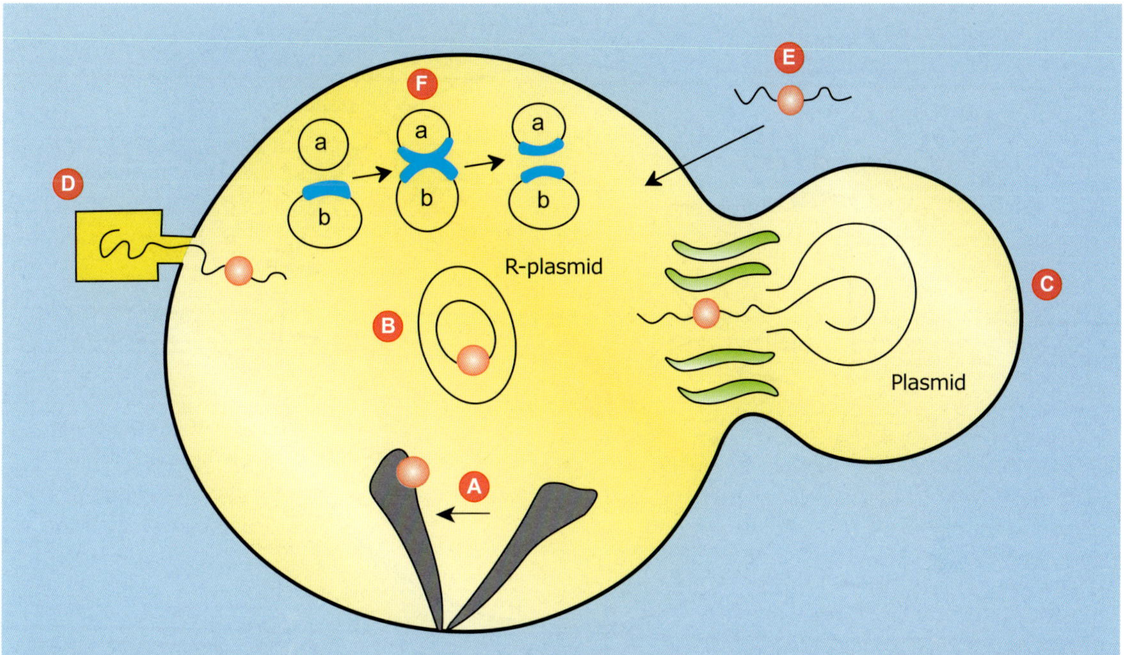

(A) Chromosomal mutation. **(B)** R-plasmid containing r gene. **(C)** Conjugation between two bacteria having exchange of plasmid DNA containing r-gene. **(D)** Transduction with a bacterial virus (bacteriophage) carrying r-gene to target bacteria. **(E)** Transformation by picking up free DNA from the environment. **(F)** Transfer and replication of a transposon carrying r-genes. Plasmid-b contains a transposon encoded with resistant gene. After the process of cointegration, both plasmids, a and b, now contain the transposon.

Fig 52.3 Genetic Methods of Antibiotic Resistance

negative bacteria exhibit five-fold higher resistance compared to Gram-positive bacteria, because in the Gram-negative bacteria the enzyme is present constitutively (available even when the substrate drug is absent) while in Gram-positive bacteria this enzyme is inducible (synthesised only when drug is present even in sub-therapeutic concentrations).

Inactivation of Aminoglycosides

Aminoglycosides are inactivated by *acetyl transferases, phosphotransferases* and *adenylyltransferases* present in both Gram-negative and Gram-positive organisms. The resistant genes are carried on plasmids and also on transposons (Ch. 56).

B) Prevention of Drug Accumulation in The Bacterium (Fig 52.4B and C)

The bacterial envelope may undergo biochemical alteration, either not allowing influx or promoting efflux of the drug. Efflux pumps are cytoplasmic membrane transport proteins (similar to P-glycoprotein in human beings; Ch. 5 & 6) which commonly operate in *E. coli, P. aeruginosa, S. typhi, Staph. aureus, Strepto. pyogenes, Strepto. pneumoniae* and *N. gonorrhoeae* as well as in myobacteria and enterococci. These chromosomal or plasmid-mediated efflux transporter proteins protect the bacterial cell from foreign chemical invasion and are regulated by a number of genes. For tetracyclines, these efflux pumps are the major

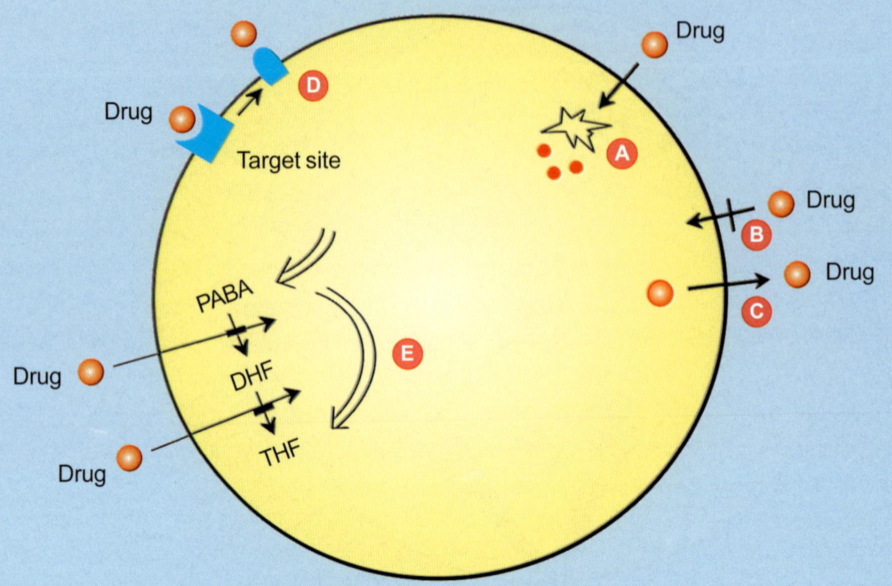

(A) Enzymatic inactivation of drug. **(B)** Preventing influx of the drug. **(C)** Promoting efflux of the drug. **(D)** Modification of the target site. **(E)** Using alternative pathways for metabolic requirements.

Fig 52.4 Biochemical Mechanism For Development of Bacterial Resistance

mechanism for the resistance (Ch. 58) and are becoming increasingly so for fluoroquinolones (Ch. 54) and erythromycin (Ch. 57). Some Gram-negative bacteria inhibit the plasmid-mediated synthesis of porin channels, which obstructs the "influx" of hydrophilic penicillins, e.g., of ampicillin, to confer resistance (Ch. 55). Mutations in the components of bacterial envelope have been reported to reduce the accumulation of tetracyclines, chloramphenicol, aminoglycosides and β-lactam antibiotics.

C) By Modification/Protection of the Target Site (Fig 52.4D)

Resistance resulting from the altered target sites include ribosomal point mutations for the tetracyclines (Ch. 58), macrolides and clindamycin (Ch. 57); altered DNA gyrase and topoisomerase for fluoroquinolones (Ch. 54) and modified penicillin binding proteins (PBPs) in *Strepto. pneumoniae* leading to penicillin resistance (Ch. 55). Point mutation means the replacement of only one base pair in the DNA structure. Another example includes the resistance of *Mycobacterium tuberculosis* to rifampicin that results by a change of only one amino acid in the β-subunit of the DNA-directed RNA-polymerase.

D) Use of Alternative Pathways for Metabolic/ Growth Requirements (Fig 52.4E)

Resistance can also occur by developing an alternative pathway that bypasses the reaction inhibited by the antibiotic. Thus sulfonamide resistance may occur from overproduction of PABA and some enteric organisms evade β-lactam antibiotics by overproducing β-lactamase.

E) By Quorum Sensing (QS)

In the past few years (2005–2010) it has been identified that the microbes communicate with each other and exchange signaling chemicals **(autoinducers)** which allows the bacterial population to co-ordinate gene expression for virulence, conjugation, mobility, apoptosis and antibiotic resistance etc. This process has been termed **"Quorum Sensing (QS)"**. A single autoinducer from a single microbe is incapable of inducing any such change but when its colony reaches a critical density (*quorum*), a threshold of autoinduction is reached and gene expression starts. Several chemically distinct classes of QS-signal molecules have been identified in Gram-negative bacteria viz., AHLs, AIP, AI-2 and AI-3. Among these, autoinducer-2 (AI-2) QS-system appears to be shared by both Gram-negative and Gram-positive bacteria. Any drug that can inhibit these signals for virulence or adhesiveness may minimise the risk of microbial growth as well as development of resistance to antibiotics. To-date, a number of compounds have been synthesised which inhibit QS-system in different bacteria and include AHL, AIP and AI-2 analogues and some that are structurally unrelated to QS-signals. These are under investigation and, in the coming years, it is likely that the problem of drug resistant infections can be solved.

PRINCIPLES OF ANTIBIOTIC DOSING

Four important characteristics that have a significant influence on the frequency of dosing of any antibiotic are: **M**inimum **I**nhibitory **C**oncentration (MIC)**,** **C**oncentration **D**ependent **K**illing **E**ffect (CDKE), **T**ime **D**ependent **K**illing **E**ffect (TDKE) and **P**ost-**A**ntibiotic **E**ffect (PAE). A clear understanding of these concepts is therefore essential for achieving optimal efficacy and for reducing microbial resistance.

Minimum Inhibitory Concentration: The goal of the antibiotic therapy is to aid body's defences to clear the tissues of the microbial pathogens by achieving antibiotic levels in the infected area equal to or greater than the **M**inimum **I**nhibitory **C**oncentration (MIC). The MIC is the lowest antibiotic concentration that prevents the growth of microorganism after a 24-hr incubation period with a standard organism inoculation (of 10^4 to 10^5 cfu/ml). There is also another term called **M**inimum **B**actericidal **C**oncentration (MBC), which means the lowest concentration of an antibiotic that causes complete destruction of the organism or permits survival of less than 0.1% of the inoculum. Because the concentration of the antibiotic cannot be measured at the site of infection, the serum antibiotic concentration and the MIC serve as surrogate (alternative) markers to assess or quantify the antibiotic activity. Although useful, the MIC also has certain inherent limitations as it is an *in vitro* measure and tells nothing about the true antibiotic activity at the locus of infection.

Antibiotics Exhibiting Concentration-Dependent Killing (CDK) and Time-Dependent Killing (TDK): Bactericidal effects of the antimicrobial drugs can be classified as either concentration-dependent or as time-dependent. Some antibiotics are much more effective if higher blood concentrations are reached periodically. These exhibit **concentration-dependent killing** (CDK). Others are more effective if blood levels are maintained above the MIC for as long a duration as possible. These exhibit **time-dependent killing** (TDK). The length of time above MIC is most important for the efficacy of antibiotics having TDK effect. To sum up, for drugs whose killing action is concentration dependent, the rate and extent of killing action increases with increasing drug concentration; while for drugs whose killing action is time-dependent, the bactericidal activity continues as long as their serum concentrations are maintained above the MIC for the entire interval between the doses (increasing the dose does not enhance their bactericidal activity). The antibacterial activity of aminoglycosides, fluoroquinolones and metro-nidazole is concentration dependent while that of β-lactams and vancomycin is time-dependent.

Post-antibiotic Effect (PAE): A persistent suppression of bacterial growth after a brief exposure of an antimicrobial agent is known as post-antibiotic effect (PAE). In PAE, the inhibition of bacterial growth is seen even when the antibacterial agent is no longer present in the bacterial medium or even when its concentration is well below MIC. The

PAE, therefore, reflects the time required for the bacteria to return to normal growth. The longer the time the bacteria needs for return to logarithmic growth (after an exposure to antimicrobial agent), the greater is the PAE of that antibiotic. Virtually many antibiotics may exhibit PAE but the duration is most significant with those which act by inhibiting bacterial protein/DNA synthesis (e.g., aminoglycosides, fluoroquinolones, tetra-cyclines, chloramphenicol and rifampicin, i.e., with those having CDKE) and least with those which act by inhibiting bacterial cell wall synthesis, i.e., with those having TDKE (e.g., β-lactams and vancomycin). β-Lactams have a shorter PAE (1–2 hrs) in gram-positive organisms but no PAE in Gram-negative species; while aminoglycosides, fluoroquinolones, rifampicin, tetracyclines and chloramphenicol ***show significant PAE*** mainly against Gram-negative and also against some Gram positive organisms.

For aminoglycosides and fluoroquinolones, it was noted that an initial high antibiotic concentration and increased time of exposure prolongs the PAE. Therefore, with a high single daily gentamicin dose, the PAE can be as long as 5–10 hr. The antitubercular drug, rifampicin, not only has a prolonged PAE but also prolongs the PAE of other antitubercular drugs synergistically (hence antitubercular drugs can be administered twice or thrice weekly with rifampicin). The PAE is usually a result of disruption in bacterial ribosomal or DNA gyrase functions whose resumption requires time, once these are inhibited by drugs like aminoglycosides and fluoroquinolones. The antibacterial agents can also be classified on the basis of their CDK/TDK activity and their PAE as follows:

Group I: ***Agents that show concentration-dependent killing (CDK) with prolonged PAE.***
These include aminoglycosides (Ch. 56), fluoroquinolones (Ch. 54), metronidazole analogues (Ch. 65) and rifampicin (Ch. 59). These agents kill bacteria more rapidly if their serum concentrations are kept appreciably above MIC. Hence, a higher dose with wider dosage intervals can be chosen with this group of drugs, e.g., gentamicin can be administered in a single dose (7 mg/kg I.M., once daily) rather than in a dose of 1.5 mg/kg I.M. 8 hrly.

Group II: ***Agents that show time-dependent killing (TDK) with shorter PAE.***
Examples include β-lactam antibiotics (Ch. 55), clindamycin (Ch. 57), macrolides (except azithromycin and clarithromycin, Ch. 57). The aim of therapy with these agents is to maintain the serum concentrations above MIC/MBC for as long as possible during the dose intervals (i.e., to maximise the exposure time to the drug). Hence, β-lactams with shorter half lives are given at 6 hrly or 8 hrly intervals. Recent trials have even suggested that continuous infusion of cephalosporins (such as cefazolin) is more useful in the treatment of serious infections.

Group III: ***Agents that show time-dependent killing (TDK) with prolonged PAE.***
These include newer macrolides such as azithromycin, clarithromycin (Ch. 57) and longer-acting tetracyclines (Ch. 58). For these agents, although the duration of antibacterial exposure is important, the clinical effectiveness is not compromised if their concentration falls below the MIC/MBC as they possess longer and persistent PAE (besides longer t½).

ANTIMICROBIAL SPECTRUM

Antimicrobial agents that are active against a single or limited group of pathogens are said to have a ***narrow spectrum,*** e.g., antitubercular drugs which act mainly on *Mycobacterium tuberculosis* and procaine penicillin-G or cloxacillin which act primarily on Gram-positive bacteria. Agents which act against a wide range of pathogens (i.e., Gram-positive, Gram-negative, Spirochetes, Chlamydia and Rickettsia etc) are called ***broad-spectrum*** drugs. Antibiotics that are effective against Gram-positive organisms and also against some Gram-negative pathogens (e.g., amoxycillin and ampicillin) are referred to as ***extended-spectrum*** drugs. A broad-spectrum antibiotic is more likely to cause *superinfection* or *pseudomembranous colitis* (PMC) by destroying the normal flora of the gut which prevents the growth of other pathogenic flora (see below).

SUPERINFECTION AND PSEUDO-MEMBRANOUS COLITIS (PMC)

The native indigenous bacterial flora present in GIT and oral cavity provides resistance to colonization, and limits the growth of other pathogenic flora. Antibiotic therapy markedly reduces this flora allowing invasion by opportunistic organisms such as *Proteus*, resistant *Staphylococci* and *Pseudomonas* etc. This is termed as ***superinfection***, which is manifested as antibiotic-induced diarrhoea and colitis. Superinfection due to *Clostridium difficile* or *Candida* (a fungus) is more serious and leads to ***pseudomembranous colitis*** (PMC), which is characterised by bloody diarrhoea, abdominal distension with pain, dehydration and blood leukocytosis. This is often seen with amoxycillin, third generation cephalosporins and clindamycin. Treatment of PMC is done with metronidazole (500 mg orally, TDS for 10 days) or with vancomycin (125 mg orally QID for 10 days). Other therapies have also been tried and these include: vancomycin + rifampicin, teicoplanin, bacitracin and reestablishment of colonic flora with probiotics (*Lactobacilli* and *Saccharomyces boulardii*).

CLASSIFICATION OF PATHOGENIC MICROBES

As a handy reference, important pathogenic microbes, their morphological characteristics and the diseases they are associated with, are classified as under:

I. Bacteria

- HIGHER FORMS: These are gram-positive branching filamentous organisms resembling fungi in morphology.
  - ***Actinomycetes***
    - *Actinomyces israelii*: cervicofacial, abdominal lesions.
    - *Nocardia asteroides*: pulmonary, brain abscess.
  - ***Streptomycetes***
    - Non-pathogenic. Useful sources for obtaining several antibiotics.
- LOWER FORMS: Average diameter 1 μm. Can be stained as gram positive or gram negative.
  - ***Cocci*** (Spherical)
    Staphylococci (variable sized clusters)
    Streptococci (in chains);
    Diplococci (in pairs)
    Gaffkyae (spherical flat form of 4)
    Sarcinae (two adhering flat groups of 4)
  - ***Bacilli*** (straight rod shaped)
  - ***Vibrios*** (curved cylinder rods)
  - ***Spirilla*** (rigid elongated spiral shaped; causative agent for rat-bite fever).

For further classification of bacilli and cocci, see below:

- SPECIAL GROUP: No Gram stain. Koch stain is positive.
  - ***Acid-Fast Bacilli***
    - *Mycobacterium avium intracellulare*: Atypical mycobacteria; causes disseminated tuberculosis type disease in AIDS patients.
    - *Mycobacterium kansasii:* Atypical mycobacterium; causes tuberculosis type lung diseases.
    - *Mycobacterium tuberculosis*: various types of tuberculosis.
    - *Mycobacterium leprae*: Leprosy.

II. Spirochetes

Organisms with no rigid cell wall, slender and spiral in shape. Cells are contractile (unlike spirilla). Stained by silver impregnation method.

- *Treponema pallidum*: aerobic pathogen; causes syphilis.
- *Treponema oralis*: aerobic, causes orofacial infections.
- *Borrelia burgdorferi*: aerobic pathogen, causes Lyme disease (tick bites).
- *Borrelia recurrentis*: aerobic pathogen, causes relapsing fever (body lice).
- *Leptospira interrogans*: anaerobic pathogen, causes Weil's disease (from rodents—hepatocellular involvement with atypical pneumonia), also meningitis.

III. Rickettsiae

Rigid cell wall, spherical, rod-shaped, Gram-negative organism.

- *Rickettsia Sp.*: causes Rocky Mountain spotted fever, Typhus fever (conveyed through the skin from lice, fleas, ticks and mites).
- *Coxiella burnetii*: causes Q fever (vector-ticks; world-wide occurrence).

IV. Chlamydiae

Rigid cell wall, spherical rod-shaped Gram-negative organism, 0.3 μm in diameter, 2 μm in length. Possesses RNA, DNA in the cytoplasm (like bacteria) but can grow only inside other cells, like virus. Hence intermediate between virus and bacteria.

- *Chlamydia psittaci*: causes psittacosis (from exposure to birds; malaise, high fever, cough with muscle pain).
- *Chlamydia trachomatis*: causes trachoma, inclusion conjunctivitis, urethritis, cervicitis and lymphogranuloma venereum (sexually transmitted disease).
- *Chlamydia pneumoniae*: causes pneumonia.

V. Miscellaneous (Atypical) Microbes

- *Mycoplasma pneumoniae*: Smallest cellular organism (dia. 100–250 nm), no rigid cell wall, can acquire variety of structures depending upon osmolality of medium. Plasma membrane contains cholesterol (unlike bacteria); cytoplasm contains RNA-DNA (like bacteria). Causes atypical pneumonia.
- *Ureaplasma urealyticum*: belongs to mycoplasma group. Cause nonspecific urethritis.
- *Pneumocystis carinii*: Traditionally considered as a protozoan (because of its morphology) but closely related to fungus (by molecular analysis). Causes pneumonia in AIDS patients and opportunistic lung infections in immunocompromised hosts.

FURTHER CLASSIFICATION OF COCCI AND BACILLI

Gram-Positive Cocci

- *Staphylococcus aureus*: aerobic, usually β-lactamase producing. Causes abscesses, septicaemia, bacteraemia, osteomyelitis and endocarditis.
- *Streptococcus pyogenes* (β-haemolytic): aerobic, causes pharyngitis, sinusitis, otitis media, rheumatic fever, glomerulonephritis and septicaemia.
- *Viridans group of Streptococcus* (VGS), e.g., *S.milleri* and *S.mutans*: (α-haemolytic), aerobic; cause bacterial endocarditis, bacteraemia and orofacial infections. *S.mutans* causes dental caries.
- *Strepto.viridans*: aerobic, causes bacterial endocarditis, bacteraemia.
- *Strepto.faecalis* (Non-haemolytic, Enterococcus sp.): aerobic, causes endocarditis, bacteraemia, urinary tract infections.
- *Strepto.pneumoniae* (α-haemolytic; Pneumococcus): aerobic diplococci. Causes pneumonia, meningitis, sinusitis.
- *Peptostreptococcus*: anaerobic; causes brain, lung, puerperal and dental abscess.

Gram-Negative Cocci

- *Neisseria gonorrhoeae*: aerobic diplococci; also called gonococci; causes gonorrhoea (urethritis/cervicitis).
- *Neisseria meningitidis* (meningococcus): aerobic diplococci; causes meningitis.
- *Moraxella (Branhamella) catarrhalis*: aerobic; causes pneumonia, sinusitis, otitis media.

Gram-Positive Bacilli

- *Clostridium tetani*: anaerobic rods, causes tetanus.
- *Clostridium perfringens*: anaerobic rods; causes gas gangrene.
- *Clostridium difficile*: anaerobic rods; causes pseudomembranous colitis.
- *Clostridium botulinum:* anaerobic rods; causes botulism (food poisoning).
- *Corynebacterium diphtheriae*: aerobic/anaerobic rods; causes diphtheria.
- *Listeria monocytogenes*: aerobic rods; causes meningitis, bacteraemia.
- *Bacillus anthracis*: aerobic rods; causes pneumonia and anthrax.

Gram-Negative Bacilli

a) Enterobacteriaceae

- *Escherichia coli*: aerobic rods; causes UTI, dysentery, other infections.
- *Salmonella typhi*: aerobic rods; causes typhoid, paratyphoid fever, food poisoning.
- *Shigella*: aerobic rods; causes gastroenteritis and bacillary dysentery.
- *Klebsiella*: aerobic rods; causes hospital associated UTI and pneumonia.
- *Proteus mirabilis* and *P. vulgaris*: aerobic rods; cause UTI, other infections.
- *Enterobacter aerogenes*: aerobic rods; causes UTI.
- *Helicobacter pylori*: aerobic rods; causes peptic ulcer.
- Coliform bacteria are commensals present in colon. In situations like liver failure these invade and become pathogenic. Some (*Klebsiella* and *Proteus*) produce ammonia which aggravates encephalopathy.

b) Others

- *Haemophilus influenzae*: aerobic rods; causes sinusitis, bronchitis, pneumonia and meningitis.
- *Haemophilus ducreyi*: aerobic rods; causes chancroid (sexually transmitted disease, ulcers on genitals).
- *Pseudomonas aeruginosa*: UTI, pneumonia and hospital acquired infection in burn cases.
- *Yersinia pestis*: aerobic rods, causes plague.
- *Brucella abortus*: aerobic rods, causes brucellosis (from ingestion of raw milk of infected cattle).
- *Francisella tularensis*: aerobic rods, causes tularemia (from skinning infected wild rabbits).
- *Legionella pneumophila*: aerobic rods; causes Legionnaire's disease (pneumonia type multisystem disorder).
- *Campylobacter sp.*: aerobic rods; causes gastroenteritis.
- *Vibrio cholerae*: aerobic (Vibrio sp.), causes cholera.
- *Serratia sp.*: aerobic rods; causes nosocomial opportunistic infections.
- *Acinetobacter sp.*: aerobic; causes nosocomial opportunistic infections.
- *Bordetella pertussis*: aerobic rods; causes whooping cough.
- *Fusobacterium sp.*: anaerobic rods; causes alveolar abscess, lung abscess and gingivitis.
- *Bacteroides fragilis*: anaerobic rods; causes oral, pharyngeal, lung, brain abscess.
- *Porphyromonas sp.:* anaerobic; causes acute orofacial infections.
- *Prevotella sp.:* anaerobic; causes acute orofacial infections.
- *Burkholderia pseudomallei:* aerobic Gram-negative bacilli; causes melioidosis (generalised infection with pneumonia, septicaemia and abscess formation. Diabetics are more prone to this infection; an emerging disease in India).

CHAPTER 53 Sulfonamides

COMPETENCY PH1.42

Sulfonamides are structural analogues of p-amino benzoic acid (PABA). The structural similarity of both is shown in Figure 53.1. Since sulfonamides are synthetic derivatives, these are labeled as "*antibacterial agents or synthetic antimicrobials*" rather than as antibiotics as latter are those antimicrobials that are obtained from microorganisms.

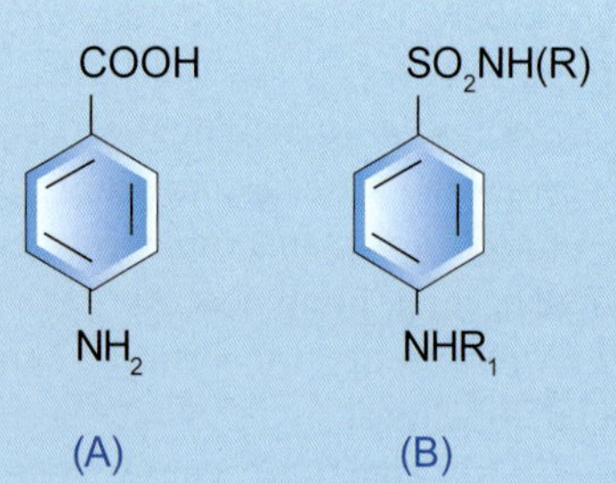

Fig 53.1 Structures of p-Amino Benzoic Acid (A), and Sulfonamide Derivatives (B)

MECHANISM OF ACTION

Human cells are freely permeable to exogenously given folic acid but bacterial cells are not. Hence, the bacteria has to synthesise its own folic acid (from PABA) for its growth and multiplication, while humans acquire it from the diet. The active form of folic acid is tetrahydrofolic acid or folinic acid, which is an important coenzyme responsible for the synthesis of bacterial proteins (from amino acids) and of bacterial RNA and DNA (from nucleic bases). Structurally, folic acid consists of three components: a pteridine moiety + PABA + glutamate. Bacterial folic acid synthesis takes place according to synthetic steps shown in Fig. 53.2.

SULFONAMIDES, being structural analogues of PABA, enter the synthetic sequence in place of PABA by competing for the enzyme dihydropteroic acid synthetase (also called folic acid synthetase) and thus form a non-functional analogue of folic acid which is of no use to bacteria. Hence, its growth ceases (bacteriostatic action). Human cells can directly absorb folic acid and therefore bypass the sulfonamide-induced block of PABA inclusion. Hence sulfonamides are selectively toxic to the bacteria and not to the host cells.

TRIMETHOPRIM (see below) is another drug which is a structural analogue of the pteridine portion of dihydrofolic acid but, unlike sulfonamides, it blocks the conversion of dihydrofolic acid to tetrahydrofolic acid (active form) by competitively inhibiting the enzyme dihydrofolate reductase. Trimethoprim has a much higher affinity for bacterial dihydrofolate reductase compared to protozoal and a least affinity for mammalian dihydrofolate reductase.

ICLAPRIM is a trimeth-roprim analogue with improved activity (see below).

PYRIMETHAMINE (see below), like trimethoprim, also blocks dihydrofolate reductase but has a greater activity against protozoal dihydrofolate reductase. Though it has negligible activity against bacterial, it unfortunately has some activity against mammalian dihydrofolate reductase. Hence, during its therapy it is advisable to administer folinic acid (citrovorum factor). Protozoa are impermeable to folinic acid and hence antiprotozoal effect is not lost but the depletion of tetrahydrofolic acid and the consequent side effects are prevented.

Looking to the mechanism of action of sulfonamides it is implied that their antibacterial effects can be overcome by excess of PABA. That is why some local anaesthetics such as *procaine*, which is a PABA ester, can antagonize the effects of sulfonamides. Their action is also antagonized by the presence of pus (as it contains PABA) and by

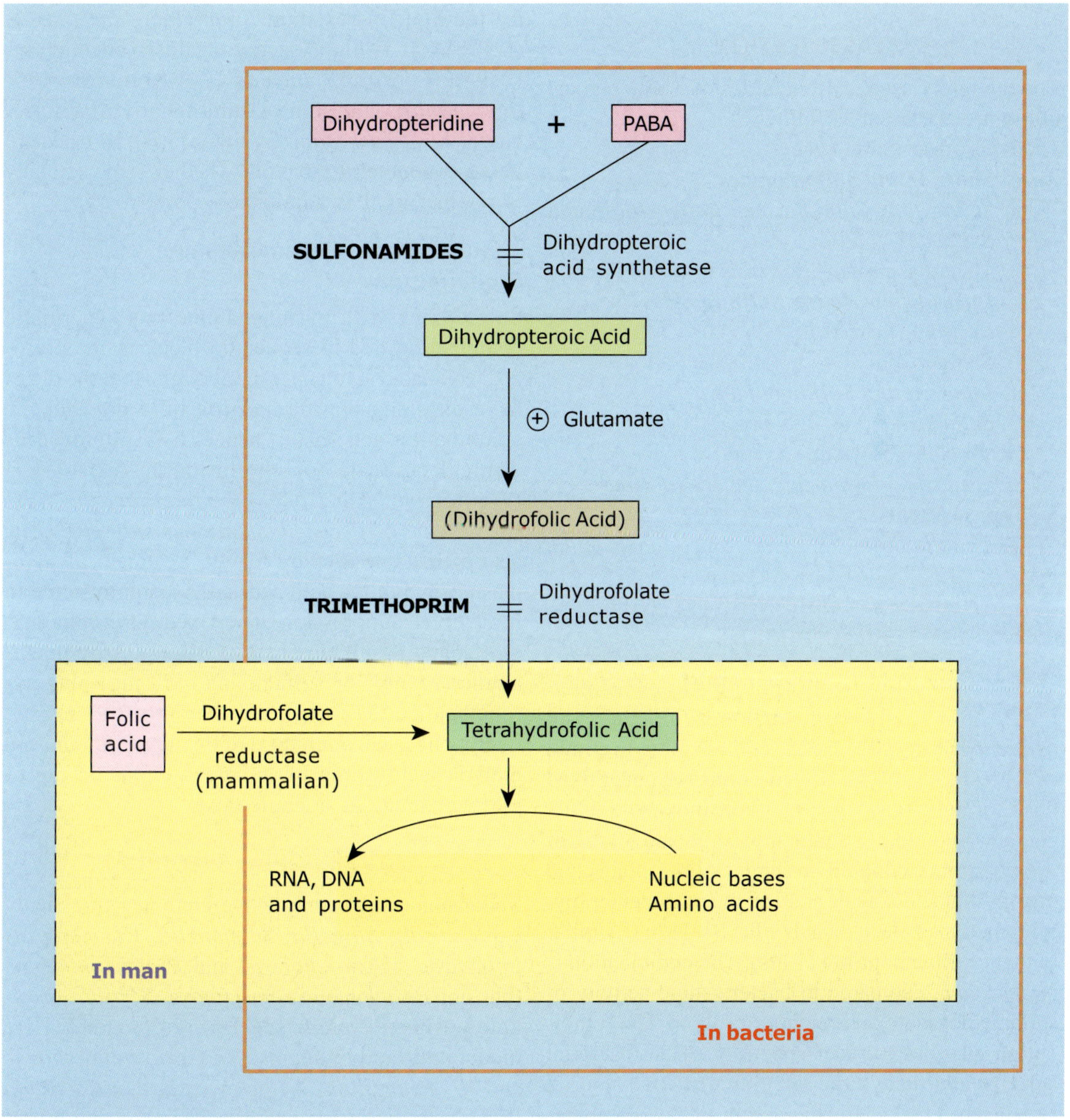

Fig 53.2 Bacterial Folate Synthesis and Sites of Action of Sulfonamides and Trimethoprim. Pyrimethamine also inhibits dihydrofolate reductase but preferentially of protozoa.

the products of tissue breakdown since these contain thymidine and purines, which bacteria can use to bypass the need of folic acid.

CLASSIFICATION

Though rarely used, sulfonamides of some clinical utility are classified as follows:

1. **Orally absorbable Agents**
   - ***Short Acting Sulfonamides***
     Sulfacytine, Sulfadiazine, Sulfisoxazole and *Sulfamethizole*
     Their plasma half-life varies from 6–9 hours.
   - ***Intermediate Acting Sulfonamides***
     Sulfamethoxazole (t½ 10–12 hrs) and *Sulfamoxole*
   - ***Long Acting Sulfonamides***
     Sulfadoxine (t ½ 7–8 days).
2. **Orally Non-absorbable Agents**
   Sulfasalazine, Olsalazine and *Balsalazine*
3. **Topical Agents**
   Silver Sulfadiazine, Mafenide and *Sulfacetamide*

SYNERGISTIC COMBINATIONS WITH SULFONAMIDES

1. Cotrimoxazole (Generic name)

It is a combination of ***sulfamethoxazole*** and ***trimethoprim*** as a fixed dose combination, in a ratio of 5:1 respectively (for why this ratio, see under fixed dose formulations, Ch. 6). A cotrimoxazole tablet contains 400 mg of sulfamethoxazole and 80 mg of trimethoprim. A double strength tablet contains 800 mg of sulfamethoxazole and 160 mg of trimethoprim. Sulfamethoxazole has a half-life (10–11 hrs) similar to that of trimethoprim (11 hrs). The combination is *bactericidal*, compared to bacteriostatic activity of sulfamethoxazole or trimethoprim alone. The combination also has a wider spectrum of antibacterial activity and delays the development of bacterial resistance. The synergistic action of this combination results due to the blockade of folic acid synthesis at two sites in a sequence. The usual oral dose of double strength (DS) cotrimoxazole tablet is one tablet at 12 hrly interval (800 mg of sulfamethoxazole + 160 mg of trimethoprim).

Iclaprim is a new trimethoprim analogue. Intravenously administered iclaprim is more effective and better tolerated than trimethoprim and equally effective as linezolid (Ch. 57) in persons suffering from skin and soft tissue infections caused by methicillin-resistant *Staphylococcus aureus* (MRSA). It is highly active against vancomycin-resistant *Staph. aureus* (VRSA), *Strepto. pneumoniae* and some Gram-negative bacteria. Under *Fast-track status* by FDA, phase III trials are being conducted to explore whether same efficacy is retained if it is administered orally.

2. Sulfadoxine + Pyrimethamine Combination

Sulfadoxine with pyrimethamine is a synergistic combination due to sequential block in the protozoal folic acid synthesis (see above). Both the drugs have ultralong plasma half-life (>95 hrs) but the combination acts faster, hence, it is employed as clinical curative for choloroquine-resistant *P. falciparum* (Ch. 64). *Pyrimethamine* plus *sulfadoxine* or *pyrimethamine* plus *sulfadiazine* is also a first line therapy for the treatment of toxoplasmosis. Folinic acid is usually coadministered to limit myelosuppression. The fixed-dose combination contains sulfadoxine (500 mg) plus pyrimethamine (25 mg) or sulfadoxine (750 mg) plus pyrimethamine (37.5 mg), i.e., in a ratio 20:1 respectively. The usual adult dose of treating *P. falciparum* malaria is 1500 mg of sulfadoxine plus 75 mg of pyrimethamine as a single dose.

ANTIMICROBIAL SPECTRUM

Sulfonamides are mainly active Gram-negative bacilli, e.g., *E. coli*, *Shigella*, *Salmonella*, *Haemophilus influenzae*, *Vibrio cholerae* and *Proteus mirabilis* (but not *Pseudomonas aeruginosa*, *Serratia* or indole-positive *Proteus* species). Sulfonamides are moderately active against *Neisseria gonorrhoeae* and *N. meningitidis*. Actinomycetes like *Nocardia*, Rickettsiae like *Chlamydia trachomatis* and a protozoan parasite *Toxoplasma gondii* are also quite sensitive.

The antibacterial spectrum of cotrimoxazole is similar to sulfonamides except that it is more potent with low incidence of bacterial resistance. Sulfadoxine + pyrimethamine combination is also used as a second line agent in the treatment of malaria (Ch. 64), and also for the treatment of toxoplasmosis (see below).

RESISTANCE

Gonococci, Staphylococci, Meningococci, Streptococci, *E. coli* and *Shigella* usually develop resistance to sulfonamides soon. Cotrimoxazole has a very low order of resistance even for *E. coli* (1.5% of incidence) and Staphylococci (0.55% incidence). Sulfonamide resistance may occur as a result of *mutations* that may cause either **(a)** overproduction of PABA to overpower the inhibition due to sulfonamides or, **(b)** alteration in the nature of dihydropteroic acid synthetase enzyme that has a low affinity for sulfonamides or, **(c)** loss of permeability of sulfonamides through bacterial membrane or, **(d)** an appearance of alternative pathway for PABA synthesis.

PHARMACOKINETICS

Sulfonamides are well absorbed when given orally, except for the agents designed for local gut effects. These are never administered subcutaneously or intramuscularly as their solutions are alkaline and injections are painful. Sodium salts of sulfonamides in 5% dextrose can be given I.V. but except for cotrimoxazole, these are rarely used intravenously. Topical sulfonamides can be absorbed through skin but the amount absorbed is usually low. However, a burn area larger than 20% of total body surface can absorb enough drug to result in toxicity, especially if accompanied by renal dysfunction. These are widely distributed and pass through BBB as well as placental barrier. Sulfonamides show good accumulation in prostatic fluid. Longer acting sulfonamides such as sulfamethoxazole and sulfadoxine are highly protein bound (85–93%). These are metabolized as acetylated conjugates in the liver. Acetylated metabolites are inactive and have low solubility in acidic urine. This leads to precipitation of crystalluria and renal toxicity.

CLINICAL USES

Sulfonamides are rarely used as single agents these days. These have been largely replaced by the fixed-dose combination of trimethoprim-sulfamethoxazole (cotrimoxazole). In addition, topical sulfonamides and those for ulcerative colitis are also being used (see below). Nevertheless, singly they can be used in some clinical situations discussed below:

Orally Absorbable Sulfonamides

1. Acute uncomplicated urinary tract infections (UTI) caused by *E. coli* and other pathogens usually respond to a short acting sulfonamide—*sulfisoxazole*.
2. These can also be used alone as third choice drugs in the following conditions. However such uses are outmoded these days.

   (a) Nocardiosis, (b) Chancroid due to *Haemophilus ducreyi* and (c) Lymphogranuloma due to *Chlamydia*.

Cotrimoxazole

Present indications for cotrimoxazole include the following:

Urinary Tract Infections (UTIs): Coliform bacteria including *E. coli* and *Proteus mirabilis*, the commonest cause of UTI, generally are susceptible to cotrimoxazole, through resistance of *E. coli* has emerged. Acute but uncomplicated cases respond rapidly. Courses of 5–10 days of cotrimoxazole-DS tablets given twice daily is an effective therapy for most UTIs. A single dose therapy with four tablets of cotrimoxazole-DS formulation has been recommended for acute cystitis.

Prostatitis: Since cotrimoxazole gets concentrated in prostatic fluid, one DS tablet twice daily for 3 weeks is effective in acute prostatitis. For chronic prostatitis, the treatment may continue for 6–12 weeks. If the patient is allergic to sulfonamide, trimethoprim alone can be effectively used, because being a basic drug it is trapped in the acidic prostate tissue and prostatic fluid.

Respiratory Tract Infections: Cotrimoxazole is a frequent choice for the treatment of acute sinusitis, bronchitis and otitis media due to *Pneumococcus* and *Haemophilus* species. One DS tablet twice a day is generally used.

Typhoid: Though the first choice drug is ciprofloxacin, cotrimoxazole may be used an alternative drug, in a dose of one DS tablet twice a day for 2 weeks. A 10–12 weeks course eradicates carrier state of *Salmonella typhi* also.

Bacterial Diarrhoeas and Dysentery: Acute gastroenteritis due to *Shigella* and *Yersinia enterocolitica*, traveler's diarrhoea due to *E. coli* and cholera due to *Vibrio cholerae* respond well with cotrimoxazole, although ciprofloxacin or norfloxacin are the drugs of choice. The usual dose for adults is one cotrimoxazole-DS tablet twice daily for 7 days.

Nocardiosis: Cotrimoxazole is the drug of choice for pulmonary lesions or brain abscess due to *Nocardia*.

Sexually Transmitted Diseases: Cotrimoxazole-DS Tablet twice a day for 7–10 days is one of the drugs of choice for chancroid due to *Haemophilus ducreyi*. Nonspecific urethritis, lymphogranuloma due to *Chlamydia* and gonorrhoea due to *Neisseria gonorrheae* may also be treated with cotrimoxazole with cure rates comparable to standard therapy.

Pneumonia: Cotrimoxazole is a drug of choice for treating pneumonia due to *Pneymocystis carinii* in neutropenic and AIDS patients. Cotrimoxazole DS one tablet four times a day for 2–3 weeks is used as curative, while one DS tablet once a day may be used prophylactically.

Melioidosis: Cotrimoxazole (or a combination of sulfadiazine, sulfamerazine and sulfamethazine) can also be used as an alternative drug for treating melioidosis caused by *Burkholderia pseudomallei*. However, prolonged treatment for several months is needed.

Intravenous Cotrimoxazole: Intravenous cotrimoxazole, in 5% dextrose solution, is preferred to treat moderate to severe *Pneumocystis carinii* pneumonia, shigellosis, typhoid fever, nocardiosis and Gram-negative bacterial sepsis. An I.V. solution usually contains 80 mg of trimethoprim plus 400 mg of sulfamethoxazole per 5 ml which is then diluted in125 ml of 5% dextrose solution. It is then administered by I.V. infusion over a period of 60–90 minutes.

Oral Sulfonamide Plus Pyrimethamine

Sulfadiazine plus ***pyrimethamine*** has been used to treat and prevent recurrences of toxoplasmosis while ***sulfadoxine*** plus ***pyrimethamine*** is used to treat chloroquine-resistant falciparum malaria. For details see Ch. 64.

Oral Non-absorbable Sulfonamides

Sulfasalazine is widely used in the treatment of ulcerative colitis (Ch. 29) and in rheumatoid arthritis (Ch. 26). It is poorly absorbed through GIT and is degraded by the bacterial flora of the colon to 5-aminosalicylic acid (5-ASA, mesalazine) and sulfapyridine. 5-ASA acts as anti-inflammatory agent in ulcerative colitis while sulfapyridine serves as a carrier moiety for 5-ASA, which otherwise cannot reach large bowel unless combined with sulfapyridine. Unlike ulcerative colitis where 5-ASA is an active component, sulfapyridine appears to be an active component in rheumatoid arthritis. Olsalazine and balsalazine are some newer agents.

Topical Agents

Sodium sulfacetamide (10% , 20% or 30%) ophthalmic solution or ointment is an effective treatment for trachoma due to *Chlamydia trachomatis* and for bacterial conjunctivitis.

Silver sulfadiazine is a least toxic topical sulfonamide ointment and is preferred over mafenide for prevention of infection in burn cases. It is active against large number of Gram-negative bacteria including *Pseudomonas*. It slowly releases Ag^+ which also provides an additional antimicrobial action. It is well tolerated. However, sulfadiazine can be absorbed from the abraded skin to produce systemic side effects.

Mafenide is a sulfonamide analogue. It is used topically and has good activity against Gram-positive and Gram-negative bacteria. The advantage is that it is active even in the presence of pus and is effective also against *Pseudomonas* and *Clostridia* which are not inhibited by commonly used sulfonamides. It is also used in burn cases; but irritation at the site of application and metabolic acidosis that it produces (being carbonic anhydrase enzyme inhibitor) reduces its usefulness.

ADVERSE EFFECTS

1. ***Crystalluria and Renal toxicity***: Acetylated metabolites of sulfonamides are less soluble in acidic urine and get precipitated in kidney and renal tubules causing crystalluria and renal obstruction. The risk can be minimized by (a) taking adequate intake of water, (b) increasing the urinary excretion of sulfonamides by making urine alkaline or (c) using triple sulfa combination such as of *sulfadiazine* + *sulfamerazine* + *sulfamethazine*. The antibacterial action of three sulfonamides is additive while their solubilities are independent of their total concentration. Besides this, the latter drugs are relatively more soluble in acidic urine than other sulfonamides.
2. ***Hypersensitivity reactions***: These are manifested in the form of (a) rashes particularly at mucocutaneous junctions, (b) Stevens-Johnson syndrome characterized by erythema multiforme, ulcerations of mucous membranes of mouth and genitalia, and malaise, (c) eosinophilia and (d) drug fever, which usually appears after the 7th or 10th day of drug treatment.
3. ***Kernicterus in neonates***: In neonates the blood-brain-barrier is not fully developed. Sulfonamides displace bilirubin from the protein binding sites. The free bilirubin then passes through BBB and gets deposited in basal ganglia and subthalamic nuclei, causing kernicterus—a toxic encephalopathy. Sulfonamides therefore, should be avoided in neonates or in women during the last trimester of pregnancy.
4. ***Haemolytic anaemia***: It is a rare complication, but can develop in persons with a genetic deficiency of glucose-6-phosphate dehydrogenase (G6PD). Routinely, agranulocytosis and thrombocytopenia are of rare occurrence with sulfonamides.

Adverse Effects of Cotrimoxazole

All adverse effects of sulfonamides are also shared by cotrimoxazole. However, a higher incidence (approximately 50%) of drug fever, hypersensitivity reactions and agranulocytosis, has been reported when cotrimoxazole is used in AIDS patients. Trimethoprim probably increases the haematological toxicity of sulfamethoxazole. Long-term use of cotrimoxazole in susceptible persons with folate deficiency (malnourished cases or alcoholics) may end up with megaloblastic anaemia. Toxicity can be prevented by giving folinic acid.

DRUG INTERACTIONS

Sulfonamides and cotrimoxazole increase the activity of oral anticoagulants, sulfonylureas and methotrexate by displacing them from their protein binding sites. On the contrary, sulfonamides are displaced from plasma binding sites by aspirin and several NSAIDs.

CHAPTER 54 Quinolones

COMPETENCY PH1.42

Fluoroquinolones (FQs) like sulfonamides, are the synthetic antimicrobial agents. Prior to fluoroquinolones *nalidixic acid,* which is a simple quinolone derivative, was being commonly used to treat urinary tract infections caused by Gram-negative aerobic microorganisms. However, it is not used to treat systemic infections because, being 98.5% protein bound, its systemic antibacterial levels can only be achieved at the cost of toxicity (see below). However, a major breakthrough was achieved in late 1980s with the introduction of 6-fluorinated-4-quinolones such as ***ciprofloxacin*** and analogues, because this group of antibacterial agents has a broader antimicrobial activity with fewer side effects and comparatively slower rate for microbial resistance.

CHEMISTRY

The FQs have a basic structure of 6-Fluoro-4-quinolone-3-carboxylic acid (Fig. 54.1).

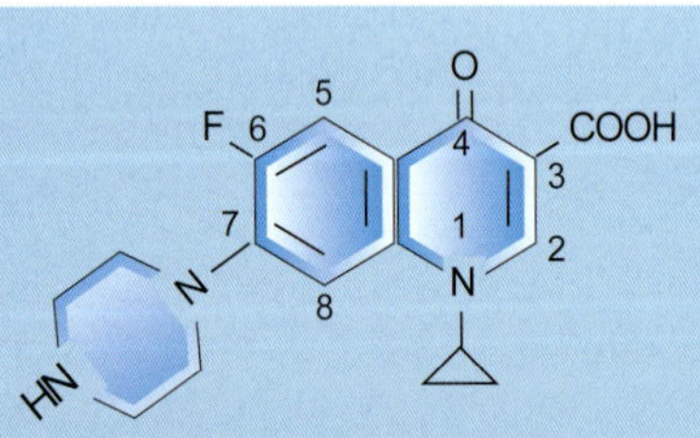

Fig 54.1 Chemical Structure of Ciprofloxacin

The common feature of all FQs is that they have a -COOH group at position-3, a -CO group at position-4 and a fluorine at position-6. The -COOH group at position-3 and a -CO group at position-4 increases hydrophobicity and therefore facilitates drug entry into Gram-negative bacteria by passive diffusion while fluorine at position-6 increases activity against Gram-negative organisms. Further alterations in the basic structure have yielded drugs having longer half-life with activity against Gram-positive organisms and anaerobes.

MECHANISM OF ACTION

FQs enter the bacterial cells by passive diffusion through porin channels. Intracellularly, in Gram-negative bacteria, these drugs inhibit the enzyme DNA gyrase (also called topoisomerase II) and thus prevent replication of bacterial DNA during bacterial growth and reproduction. They also inhibit topoisomerase IV, mainly in Gram-positive bacteria, and thus interfere with the separation of replicated chromosomal DNA into the respective daughter cells during cell division (see also Ch. 52 about DNA gyrase).

In addition, inhibition of bacterial DNA gyrase also leads to extensive filamentation, vacuole formation and degradation of chromosomal DNA by exonucleases whose production is signalled by damaged DNA. All these actions confer bactericidal activity onto FQs.

In place of DNA gyrase or topoisomerase IV, the mammalian cells possess a conceptually similar but structurally different type of enzyme called mammalian topoisomerase II. The latter, like bacterial DNA gyrase, also relaxes (removes) the positive supercoiling of eukaryotic DNA to prevent its tangling during replication. FQs, however, inhibit eukaryotic topoisomerase II only at a very high concentration and hence these are least toxic to the host but selectively toxic to the bacteria.

CLASSIFICATION

The FQs were earlier classified according to generations, much like cephalosporins (Ch. 55), depending on the time of their introduction into clinical practice but now these are grouped according to their antibacterial spectrum.

- **First Generation***
  Norfloxacin, Ciprofloxacin, Ofloxacin, Pefloxacin and *Lomefloxacin*
- **Second Generation**
  Levofloxacin and *Prulifloxacin*
- **Third Generation**
  Gatifloxacin, Sparfloxacin and *Gemifloxacin*
- **Fourth Generation**
  Moxifloxacin, Trovafloxacin, Alatrofloxacin and *Finafloxacin*
  *Some text classify *nalidixic acid* as first generation drug; but it is a quinolone not fluoroquinolone.

ANTIMICROBIAL SPECTRUM

First generation drugs (i.e., ciprofloxacin group) These are most effect against:

- **Gram-negative aerobes** which include Enterobacteriaceae *(E. coli, Klebsiella, Salmonella, Shigella* and *Proteus mirabilis);* other Gram-negative bacteria such as *Haemophilus influenzae, H. ducreyi, Legionella pneumophila, Pseudomonas aeruginosa,* and to some extent *Vibrio cholerae.*
- **Some Gram-negative cocci** such as *Neisseria gonorrhoeae* and *N. meningitidis.*
- Recently ciprofloxacin has gained popular attention in providing **protection against *Bacillus anthracis*** (Gram-positive bacilli), a major bioterrorism agent. Otherwise, these drugs are least effective against other Gram-positive bacilli. These have moderate activity against Gram-positive cocci such as *Staphylococcus aureus.*
- Among other microorganisms, these are **effective against *Mycobacterium tuberculosis*,** and Rickettsiae such as *Chlamydia trachomatis* and *Chlamydia pneumoniae.*
- These drugs show no activity against methicillin-resistant *Staph. aureus* (MRSA), *Streptococcus pneumoniae* and anaerobes such as *Bacteroides fragilis* and *Fusobacterium* species. These are not reliably active against *Mycoplasma pneumoniae* either.

Second generation drugs have similar spectrum as of first generation **plus better activity against Gram-positive cocci** such as *Streptococcus pneumoniae* and **for other microorganisms** like *Mycoplasma, Legionella* and *Chlamydia.*

Third generation drugs have **enhanced activity against Gram-positive cocci** such as *Streptococcus, Staphylococcus* and *Enterococcus* **as well as for** *Mycobacterium tuberculosis, Mycoplasma pneumoniae* and *M. avium complex* in AIDS. These are active against anaerobes also.

Fourth generation drugs, not only show **enhanced activity against Gram-positive organisms, but exhibit significantly greater activity against anaerobes** (for details see individual agents).

Fluoroquinolones, like aminoglycosides (Ch. 56), exhibit ***concentration dependent killing*** and a ***post-antibiotic effect*** (Ch. 52) which usually persists for 3 to 6 hrs. Only ***moxifloxacin, trovafloxacin*** and ***finafloxacin*** have reliable activity against anaerobes.

RESISTANCE

Resistance is related to mutations in the DNA gyrase (in Gram-negative bacteria) and mutation of topoisomerase IV (in Gram-positive bacteria).

Enterococcus, Streptococcus, some *Enterobacteriaceae, Pseudomonas aeruginosa* and *Bacteroides fragilis* display resistance through modification of porin channel and by development of efflux mechanism. All these modes of resistance are chromosomally mediated. Incidence of cross resistance does occur, but with *moxifloxacin,* the chances are the least.

FIRST GENERATION FLUOROQUINOLONES

Examples: Norfloxacin, Ciprofloxacin, Ofloxacin, Pefloxacin and Lomefloxacin

Pharmacokinetics

In this group, *norfloxacin* has a poor bioavailability (30–35%). Its plasma levels are therefore not sufficient to treat systemic infections. For others, oral bioavailability ranges from 80–100%. An average plasma protein binding is only 20–40% and therefore tissue penetration of these drugs is high. These drugs get concentrated in mucosal tissues of GIT, genitourinary and respiratory tract; in prostate, lungs, heart and macrophages. These drugs penetrate placental barrier and concentrate in amniotic fluid. These are metabolised in liver and eliminated through kidney.

Despite their short half-life, which ranges from 3–5 hrs *(norfloxacin)* to 8–10 hrs *(pefloxacin),* these agents can be administered twice daily because of their post-antibiotic effect which varies from 3–6 hrs.

Therapeutic Uses

Norfloxacin is less potent than ***ciprofloxacin*** and is not used to treat systemic infections because of its poor bioavailability. It has restricted use in urinary, genital and GIT infections only**.** *Pseudomonas* and Gram-positive cocci are not inhibited by norfloxacin. ***Ofloxacin*** is intermediate between norfloxacin and ciprofloxacin in activity against Gram-negative bacteria; but it has slightly *better action against Gram-positive organisms and still better action against Chlamydia and Mycoplasma compared to ciprofloxacin.* ***Pefloxacin*** is similar to ciprofloxacin but penetrates tissues better and accumulates in CSF in high concentration than other drugs in this group. It also attains higher plasma concentration as it is completely absorbed and exhibits cumulation on repeated dosing. ***Lomefloxacin*** is also similar to ciprofloxacin but *has a longer plasma half-life* and needs single daily dose administration. It is more active against some Gram-negative bacteria and *Chlamydia.*

Urinary Tract Infections

Commonly used drugs are *norfloxacin* (400 mg BD), *ciprofloxacin* (500 mg BD), *ofloxacin* (400 mg BD), *pefloxacin* (400 mg BD) and *lomefloxacin* (400 mg OD) orally for 4–6 weeks to treat lower urinary tract infections.

Acute Bacterial Diarrhoea

These drugs do not disturb the normal anaerobic bacterial flora of colon and provide a high faecal concentration. Hence these are favourable drugs for treating acute enteric bacterial infections. *Norfloxacin* (400 mg BD) or *ciprofloxacin* (500 mg BD) or *ofloxacin* (200 mg BD) orally, for 5 days, are as effective as cotrimoxazole for treating traveller's diarrhoea.

Salmonella typhi Infection

The high efficacy of FQs, with low incidence of complications and least chances of relapse, has made them as one of the most preferred drugs in the management of typhoid fever. The FQs in this group, *viz, ciprofloxacin* (500 mg BD x 10 days), *ofloxacin* (400 mg BD x 10 days) and *pefloxacin* (400 mg BD x 14 days) have been reported to produce a cure rate of 100% while *norfloxacin* (400 mg BD x 14 days) produces cure rate of 90–92%. The patient unable to take ciprofloxacin orally may be treated with 200 mg I.V., 12 hrly, in the beginning and then switched over to oral route after defervescence. Being bactericidal and due to good intracellular accumulation and adequate levels in bile and faeces, these drugs prevent carrier state also.

Despite these claims, some nonresponders to ciprofloxacin are being increasingly reported. After a widespread nonprudent use, these drugs may also suffer from the same drawback of the development of resistance.

Sexually Transmitted Diseases

Norfloxacin (800 mg), *ciprofloxacin* (250–500 mg), *ofloxacin* (400 mg), *pefloxacin* (800 mg) and *lomefloxacin* (400 mg) as a single oral dose provide a cure rate of 95% in cases of gonorrhoea due to *Neisseria gonorrhoeae.* Gonococcal urethritis, cervicitis and proctitis can be treated with a single oral dose of ciprofloxacin (500 mg). For chancroid (due to *Haemophilus ducreyi),* ciprofloxacin (500 mg BD x 3 days, orally), provides 98% cure rate. The only FQ in this group that is effective against both *Chlamydia trachomatis* and *N. gonorrhoeae* is ***ofloxacin*** (400 mg daily orally for 7 days).

Soft Tissue and Wound Infections

Ciprofloxacin (500 mg BD x 7 days), *ofloxacin* (400 mg BD x 10 days), *pefloxacin* (400 mg BD x 7 days) and *lomefloxacin* (400 mg OD x 7 days) are used to treat skin and soft tissue infections caused by Gram-negative organisms. If used along with clindamycin or metronidazole (to cover anaerobes), *ciprofloxacin* is quite effective to treat diabetic foot. Ciprofloxacin (500–750 mg BD orally for 6 weeks) has been proved as an effective therapy for malignant otitis externa.

Respiratory Infections

Although these are not the drugs of choice, yet *ciprofloxacin* (500 mg BD x 7 days), *ofloxacin* (400 mg BD x 10 days), *pefloxacin* (400 mg BD x 7 days) and *lomefloxacin* (400 mg OD x 10 days) can provide clinical cure rate up to 90% in cases of bronchitis and sinusitis if the infection is due to Gram-negative pathogens.

Anthrax

Ciprofloxacin in a dose of 500 mg BD orally x 60 days has been used effectively for post-exposure treatment of inhalational/cutaneous anthrax (that may occur due to bioterrorism). If there is gastrointestinal or oropharyngeal involvement, ciprofloxacin 400 mg every 12 hrly should be given intravenously in conjunction with any two of the following drugs: rifampicin, ampicillin, imepenem, clindamycin or clarithromycin. A combined three-drug therapy should continue for 60 days. Whenever clinically appropriate this combination therapy may be switched over to ciprofloxacin oral therapy later.

Miscellaneous Uses

- Among these FQs, only *ciprofloxacin* and *ofloxacin* are used, in combination with other antitubercular drugs, to treat multidrug resistant tuberculosis and *Mycobacterium avium complex* infection in AIDS.
- Accumulation of *pefloxacin* in CSF is higher than any other FQs in this group. Hence, it is preferred to treat meningitis due to Gram-negative organisms.
- For chronic bacterial prostatitis *ciprofloxacin* (500 mg BD x 28 days), *ofloxacin* (300 mg BD x 42 days) or *pefloxacin* (400 mg BD x 28 days) provides excellent results. The group as a whole exhibits good accumulation in prostatic fluid.
- *Lomefloxacin* is a preferred drug for use in surgical prophylaxis (transurethral procedures or transrectal prostate biopsy).
- *Ciprofloxacin,* in particular, is used as prophylaxis in neutropenic patients to minimise the chances of Gram-negative bacteraemia. In neutropenic cancer patients with fever, it is given along with gentamicin.
- *Ciprofloxacin* is indicated in the treatment of cystic fibrosis (a lower respiratory tract infection) where *Pseudomonas aeruginosa* is the predominant pathogen.
- Almost all FQs of this group are used in ophthalmology as eye drops/ointments for superficial ocular infections due to susceptible strain.

SECOND GENERATION FLUOROQUINOLONES

Examples: Levofloxacin and Prulifloxacin

Pharmacokinetics

After oral absorption the bioavailability of these drugs is 95–100%. Hence, their oral and I.V. doses are similar. Their protein binding is poor (30–45%) and hence have a wider distribution in body fluids and tissues but penetration into CSF is relatively poor. These have relatively longer half-lives *(levofloxacin* 8 hrs; *prulifloxacin* 10 hrs), which permits once daily dosing. The primary route of elimination of these drugs is renal. *Prulifloxacin* is a prodrug of *ulifloxacin* (active metabolite).

Therapeutic Uses

Levofloxacin has an extended spectrum against Gram-positive bacteria (especially *Streptococcus pneumoniae*), atypical pathogens *(Chlamydia, Mycoplasma)* and also against anaerobes. These are equally effective against Gram-negative organisms including *Pseudomonas, Legionella, Proteus* and *Moraxella catarrhalis.*

Its main use is in: **(1)** acute bacterial exacerbation of chronic bronchitis, **(2)** community acquired pneumonia, **(3)** nosocomial pneumonia, **(4)** acute sinusitis, **(5)** uncomplicated skin and soft tissue infections, **(6)** uncomplicated UTI, **(7)** complicated UTI and **(8)** ophthalmic practice as eye drops or ointment for bacterial conjunctivitis and corneal ulcer. Its usual dose is 500 mg orally, once daily.

Prulifloxacin also has an extended spectrum of activity against Gram-negative organisms (especially *E. coli, Pseudomonas, Proteus, Haemophilus, Klebsiella* and *Moraxella catarrhalis*) as well as against Gram-positive organisms (especially *Streptococcus pneumoniae, Enterococcus* and *Staphylococcus aureus*). *Prulifoxacin* is mainly used to treat **(1)** acute uncomplicated urinary tract infection, **(2)** complicated lower urinary tract infection and for **(3)** acute exacerbation of chronic bronchitis. Its usual dose is 600 mg orally once daily.

THIRD GENERATION FLUOROQUINOLONES

Examples: Sparfloxacin, Gatifloxacin and Gemifloxacin

Pharmacokinetics

Gatifloxacin, Sparfloxacin and *Gemifloxacin* are readily absorbed from the GIT after oral administration with an almost absolute bioavailability. All are widely distributed into body tissues and fluids and are poorly bound to plasma proteins. All of them have a longer half-life (*Gatifloxacin* 8–10 hr, *Gemifloxacin* 8–10 hr, *Sparfloxacin* 18 hr).

Therapeutic Uses

These drugs exhibit enhanced activity against Gram-positive cocci (*Streptococcus pneumoniae, Staphylococcus aureus* and *Enterococcus*), *Mycobacteria* and anaerobes such as *Bacteroides fragilis*. These are primarily used to treat pneumonia, acute sinusitis, exacerbations of chronic bronchitis, UTIs, as an adjuvant drug in the treatment of tuberculosis, to treat infection due to *Mycobacterium avium complex* in AIDS patients and in Chlamydial genital infections (e.g., gonococcal urethritis in males).The usual dose schedule for *Sparfloxacin* is a loading dose of 400 mg on the first day followed by a maintenance dose of 200 mg daily. The standard dose *of Gemifloxacin* is 320 mg orally once a day. The usual dose *of Gatifloxacin* is 400 mg orally, once daily. It has been withdrawn from Indian market (see under adverse effects).

FOURTH GENERATION FLUOROQUINOLONES

Examples: Moxifloxacin, Trovafloxacin, Alatro-floxacin and Finafloxacin

Pharmacokinetics

These are orally well absorbed. Bioavailability is 90–92% for *moxifloxacin* and 88–90% for *trovafloxacin, alatrofloxacin.* These are primarily metabolised by liver *via* phase II conjugation. Their elimination half- life is longer (12–15 hrs for *moxifloxacin* and 10–12 hrs for *trovafloxacin),* allowing once daily dosing. *Trovafloxacin* also appears in breast milk. *Alatrofloxacin* is a prodrug for *trovafloxacin.* Alatrofloxacin is usually given intravenously while trovafloxacin can be given orally or intravenously.

Therapeutic Uses

Some fluoroquinolone like *moxifloxacin* exhibits enhanced activity against *Streptococcus pneumoniae* and against penicillin or erythromycin resistant Gram-positive bacteria and against many anaerobes, while retaining the favourable activity of FQs against Gram-negative organisms. It is mainly used to treat **(1)** community acquired pneumonia, **(2)** acute bacterial exacerbations of chronic bronchitis, **(3)** acute bacterial sinusitis and **(4)** complicated skin or soft tissue infections. Its usual dose is 400 mg orally once daily.

Trovafloxacin/Alatrofloxacin are highly active against *Streptococcus pneumoniae*, other Gram-positive bacteria and have an extended spectrum against anaerobes. It has good activity against penicillin-resistant strains. Due to its hepatotoxicity (see below) its use is reserved only for life-threatening infections and that too for a maximum duration of 15 days. It has been withdrawn from many European countries (not from USA) for this reason. Its use is restricted to treat (1) nosocomial pneumonia, (2) community acquired pneumonia, (3) complicated intra-abdominal infections or gynaecological infections and (4) skin/soft tissue infections including diabetic foot infection. Because of its good accumulation in CSF it is being tried in cerebral meningitis. Its usual dose is 200 mg I.V./orally, once daily.

Finafloxacin is a novel fluoroquinolone. The unique features of finafloxacin, which set it aside from other fluoroquinolones, are that **(1)** its antibacterial activity markedly increases at acidic pH, i.e., it become more efficacious in tissues and body compartments acidified due to infection or inflammation; **(2)** it has a very high safety profile, i.e., no hepatotoxicity, renal toxicity, cardiotoxicity or phototoxicity; **(3)** it has widest spectrum, i.e., against Gram-positive, Gram-negative, anaerobic and atypical pathogens; **(4)** it has a longer t ½ supportive of once daily dosing (oral or I.V.). Clinical options for its trial include *H. pylori* eradication, urinary tract infection, community acquired pneumonia, severe exacerbations associated with bronchitis and COPD, cystic fibrosis infections, complicated intra-abdominal infection, acute otitis externa and skin infections.

ADVERSE EFFECTS OF FQs

Compared to other antimicrobial agents, the FQs are relatively safe. The adverse reactions commonly seen with FQs are confined to GIT, CNS and cardiovascular system, but these are dose-dependent. Normally, these are mild and do not need discontinuation of the therapy. The most common side effects are ***nausea, vomiting, diarrhoea,*** headache, dizziness and ***skin rash***. FQs have been associated with ***tendonitis*** and ***tendon rupture*** on prolonged use. Joint erosions (arthropathy) and reversible arthralgia has been observed in younger and growing animals administered with FQs. However, when FQs were used to treat cystic fibrosis in children no such adverse effects were seen. Nevertheless, caution seems necessary while using them in children. Adverse effects associated with individual FQs are as under:

- ***Ciprofloxacin:*** Recently its use for prophylaxis or treatment of anthrax infection has been associated with damage to muscle ligaments; ***Lomefloxacin:*** Photosensitivity (2%); ***Pefloxacin:*** Photosensitivity (1%). Dose adjustment is needed in patients having liver disease; ***Sparfloxacin:*** Higher incidence of photosensitivity (5%) than with other FQs. Cardiotoxicity: QTc prolongation (3%); ***Levofloxacin:*** QTc prolongation – lesser incidence; ***Gatifloxacin:*** QTc prolongation and photosensitivity. Gatifloxacin causes episodes of hypo-, as well as hyperglycaema (hence, risky in diabetics). It has recently been withdrawn from the market. ***Moxifloxacin:*** QTc prolongation (3%). Post marketing case reports are suggestive of phototoxicity and lowering of seizure threshold but incidences are rare (0.1–1%); and ***Trovafloxacin/Alatrofloxacin***: Hepatotoxicity; use has been restricted only to life-threatening infections.

DRUG INTERACTIONS

- Oral absorption of FQs is decreased with Al^{3+}, Mg^{2+} and Ca^{2+} containing antacids and also with Zn^{2+}, Fe^{2+} salts and sucralfate. These form chelation complexes with FQs resulting in their decreased absorption.
- Plasma concentration of theophylline is increased by majority of FQs due to inhibition of its metabolism. *Ofloxacin* has little effect while *lomefloxacin, levofloxacin* and *sparfloxacin* have no effect on theophylline metabolism.
- All FQs interact with warfarin resulting in its decreased metabolism and enhanced effects. However, *levofloxacin* and *sparfloxacin* have no effect on warfarin metabolism.
- FQs which prolong QTc interval should be used with caution in those receiving Class IA (quinidine or procainamide) or Class III antiarrhythmics (amiodarone, sotalol or ibutilide) and in patients receiving other drugs known to increase QTc interval (erythromycin, cisapride, antidepressants, astemizole and terfenadine).
- Morphine decreases oral absorption of *trovafloxacin.*

CONTRAINDICATIONS

- Pregnancy and children (see adverse effects)
- Drugs which prolong QTc interval are contraindicated in patients of cardiac arrhythmias and in those having hypokalaemia.

URINARY ANTISEPTICS

Urinary antiseptics are those antimicrobial agents which are concentrated primarily in renal pelvis and the bladder, and therefore used to treat UTI. These cannot be used to treat systemic infections because effective plasma concentrations are not achieved with their therapeutic doses (see below). Their usefulness is limited to cure chronic lower UTI where eradication of bacteria by short-term systemic therapy has not been possible.

Nalidixic Acid

It is a non-fluorinated quinolone which is rapidly excreted in urine and is 98% protein bound. These two pharmacokinetic properties do not allow an attainment of reasonable plasma concentration of free drug, for therapeutic use in systemic infections. It is rarely used nowadays because of the availability of more efficacious and less toxic FQs. It is active against Gram-negative coliform bacteria (except *Pseudomonas*) but resistance develops soon.

Nitrofurantoin

It is a nitrofuran derivative. It blocks bacterial carbohydrate metabolism by inhibiting its acetyl-CoA synthesis. Susceptible bacteria also enzymatically reduces nitrofurantoin to generate nitroanion superoxide and other toxic reactive intermediates which damage bacterial DNA also. It is primarily bacteriostatic but acts as bactericidal in higher concentration and in acidic urine. It loses its antimicrobial action at pH 8. Hence, sufficient plasma concentration of active drug is not attained at plasma pH of 7.4. Consequently it is not useful to treat systemic infections.

Nitrofurantoin is primarily active against Gram-negative bacteria (*E. coli* and *Proteus mirabilis*) and to some extent Gram-positive organisms such as *Staphylococcus aureus* and *Enterococcus faecalis*. Most indole-positive *Proteus, Klebsiella, Serratia* and *Pseudomonas* are resistant. Cross resistance with other antimicrobials has not been reported. The singular indication of nitrofuran toin is the treatment as well as long-term prophylaxis of lower UTIs caused by susceptible bacteria (mainly *E. coli*). Acidifying agents such as vitamin-C and cranberry juice increase its effectiveness. Usual dose is 100 mg TDS orally for 10 days.

Nausea and vomiting are the most commonly observed adverse effects which can be lessened if the drug is given with milk or food and taken in between the meal. Nausea is less with macrocrystalline formulation and with sustained release preparation. Peripheral neuritis, intrahepatic cholestatis and hepatitis and a pulmonary reaction with fibrosis are some complications on long-term use. Haemolytic anaemia can occur in G6PD deficient cases. Urine of patients taking nitrofurantoin becomes dark brown due to its metabolites. It antagonises the action of nalidixic acid. Probenecid inhibits its tubular secretion. This reduces its concentration in urine and can decrease its efficacy in UTI therapy.

Urinary Analgesics: Phenazopyridine

It is a dye which exerts analgesic effects in UTIs and provides symptomatic relief from burning sensation, dysuria and urgency due to cystitis. It is devoid of antibacterial activity. *Adverse effects* include nausea and epigastric distress. Urine colour turns orange red due to its metabolites. It is used as urinary tract analgesic. Usual dose is 200 mg TDS orally. When used concomitantly with an antimicrobial agent, its use should not exceed 2 days.

CHAPTER 55 Inhibitors of Bacterial Cell Wall Synthesis

COMPETENCY PH1.42

β-Lactam antibiotics are widely prescribed drugs that share a common structure and mechanism of action, i.e., inhibition of bacterial cell wall synthesis. The β-lactams are comprised of four different groups of antibiotics, *viz,* penicillins, cephalosporins, monobactams and carbapenems. All of them have a β-lactam ring, as a common feature, in their chemical structure (Fig. 55.1).

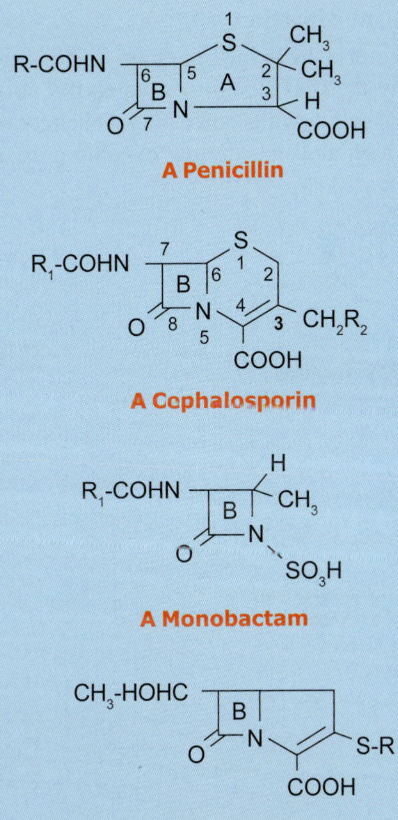

Fig 55.1 Comparison of Basic Nuclei of Four β-Lactam Antibiotics. The ring marked B in each structure is the β-lactam ring.

PENICILLINS

Penicillin was originally obtained from the fungus *Penicillium notatum*, but at present the high-yielding source is another fungus *Penicillium chrysogenum* (see below).

- All penicillins consist of a sulfur containing thiazolidine ring (A), fused with a β-lactam ring (B) to which a side chain is attached at position-6 (-NHCOR; Fig. 55.1).
- The active moiety of the penicillin structure is 6-amino penicillanic acid (6-APA) which consists of an *intact* β-lactam ring (B), having a NH_2 group at position-6, joined to thiazolidine ring (A) (Fig. 55.2). Obviously, therefore, penicillins are classified as β-lactam antibiotics.
- Large quantities of 6-APA are nowadays produced from the cultures of *P. chrysogenum*. This mold contains large amounts of fungal amidases which hydrolyses penicillin side chain at position-6. A variety of semisynthetic penicillins are then obtained from this basic material by attaching appropriate side chain at position-6. The nature of the side chain governs mainly the pharmacokinetics but also the antimicrobial spectrum. In natural penicillin (***penicillin-G***), the R in the side chain is benzyl ($CH_2C_6H_5$); but in semisynthetic penicillins, this R is anything other than benzyl moiety.
- Most of the penicillins are available as their Na^+ or K^+ salts formed at the COOH group at position-3 of thiazolidine ring. However, some amine salts, such as ***procaine penicillin-G*** and ***benzathine penicillin-G*** are also available as depot injections. These are used as sustained release preparations of penicillins.

- The β-lactam ring of penicillins can be degraded by β-lactamase enzyme produced by the invading bacteria. β-Lactam ring can also be hydrolysed by gastric acid. The resultant product *penicilloic acid* (Fig. 55.2) is devoid of any antibacterial activity. However, it combines with the host proteins and acts as an antigenic determinant of penicillin-induced hypersensitivity.

Mechanism of Action

Since bacteria have no mechanism to regulate osmolarity, they have to utilise a supportive structure around the cell to withstand osmotic changes due to inherent high and outside low osmotic pressure of the environment. Hence, majority of bacteria are surrounded by a thick cell wall that confers stability and rigidity to their cell structure. Their cell wall is composed of peptidoglycan. The latter is composed of parallel "glycan" (polysaccharide) chain crosslinked by "peptide chains" (Fig. 55.3), hence the term "peptidoglycan". This peptidoglycan layer, which envelops the cell, does not allow bacteria to swell and prevents its death due to lysis.

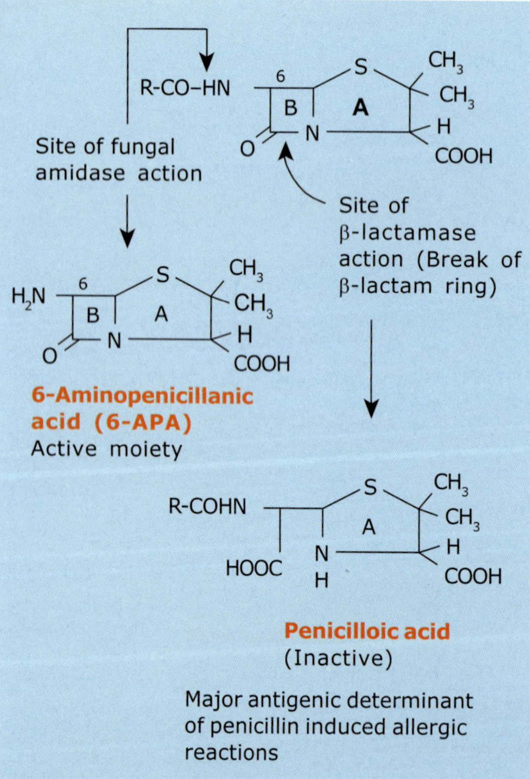

Fig 55.2 Biosynthesis of 6-Amino-penicillanic Acid From Fungal Amidase of *Penicillium chrysogenum* and Degradation of Penicillin by β-Lactamase Enzyme

The glycan chain consists of the repeating units of two aminosugars: N-acetylmuramic acid (NAcM) and N-acetylglucosamine (NAcG). The pentapeptide side chain (L-alanyl-D-glutamyl-L-lysyl-D-alanyl-D-alanine) is linked to the N-acetyl muramic acid sugar (NAcM). These peptide chains are cross linked to other peptide chains by a pentaglycine bridge which extends from the L-lysine residue of one peptide chain to the D-alanine residue of another peptide chain (Fig. 55.3). This cross bridging between the peptidoglycan strands provides necessary strength to the bacterial cell wall. The process of cross-bridging is called as the *transpeptidation* reaction and is catalysed by penicillin binding proteins (PBPs) which are the transmembrane surface enzymes present in the bacteria.

Penicillins compete for and inhibit this PBPs catalysed process of transpeptidation. The formation of an imperfect cell wall leads to an osmotic drive of the fluid from outside of the environment to the inside of the bacteria which then swells and bursts to die. The death of the bacteria, however, is not solely due to osmotic drive but also results from the activation of autolysing enzymes called murein hydrolase or autolysins. Penicillins, therefore, are bactericidal drugs acting through the inhibition of cell wall synthesis and lysis of the bacteria. Since rapid cell wall synthesis takes place when bacteria are multiplying, penicillins are lethal in the multiplying phase rather than the dormant phase of the bacteria.

Three types of PBPs are found in cytoplasmic membrane of all bacterial species. PBP-1 is the major transpeptidase involved in peptidoglycan synthesis during elongation. It cleaves the terminal D-ala and connects the remaining D-ala to L-lys of

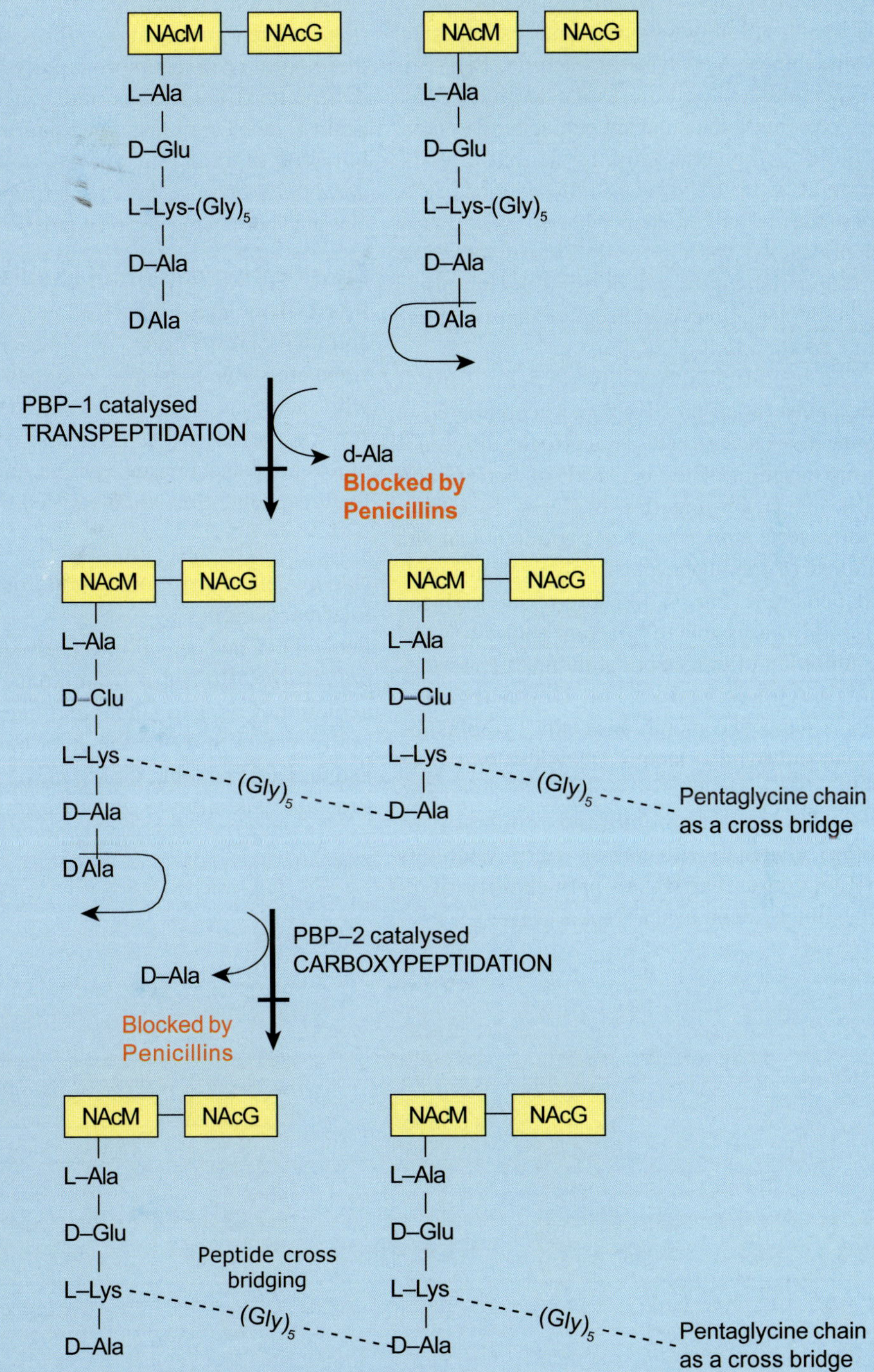

Fig 55.3 Biosynthesis of Peptidoglycan Cell Wall by the Bacteria and its Inhibition by Penicillins

adjacent peptidoglycan strand by pentaglycine bridge. Its inhibition by penicillin causes imperfect cell wall synthesis and lysis of bacteria. PBP-2 is carboxypeptidase. It hydrolyses the terminal D-ala residue, present on the adjacent pentapeptide chain, to promote further cross-linking at that site. Its inhibition leads to the formation of spherical cells, instead of the normal rod-shaped bacilli. PBP-3 is an endopeptidase. It splits cross-linking involved in septum formation during cell division. Its inhibition results in filamentation wherein cells cannot separate from one another during cell division.

The bactericidal activity of penicillins is greater against Gram-positive bacteria compared to Gram-negative bacteria. This relates to the difference in the organisation of the cell wall of both Gram-positive and Gram-negative bacteria. In Gram-positive bacteria a *thick layer* of peptidoglycan and teichoic acid (a polyol phosphate polymer) surrounds the cell membrane (Fig. 55.4A). Their peptidoglycan layer is easily accessible to β-lactam antibiotics and hence inhibition of transpeptidation reaction (cross-linking) becomes easier. The Gram-negative organisms have two membranes, the cytoplasmic membrane and an outer membrane, with a *thin layer* of peptidoglycan sandwiched between the two (Fig. 55.4B). The outer membrane consists of lipopolysaccharides with narrow porin channels which function as barriers to permeability of β-lactam antibiotics and hence weaker activity. However, some penicillins with hydrophilic character (e.g., ampicillin and amoxycillin) can diffuse through these porin channels more rapidly and significantly than natural penicillins and hence show activity against some Gram-negative bacteria also (see below) but still remain inactive against *Pseudomonas aeruginosa* because these bacteria are lacking in such classical permeable porin channels (Fig. 55.4).

Classification and Antimicrobial Spectrum

Penicillins are classified according to their antimicrobial spectrum. Within each of these groups some are stable to gastric acid (can be given orally) while some are labile (given parenterally). Similarly some are resistant to β-lactamase degradation while others are β-lactamase sensitive. Including all these features, penicillins are classified as follows (Table 55.1 A and B).

Narrow Spectrum Penicillins (Table 55.1A)

Pharmacokinetics

Penicillin-V and penicillin-G are referred to as *natural penicillins*. Both are β-lactamase sensitive, but penicillin-V is acid stable and hence can be given orally. Penicillin-G, on the other hand, is acid labile and therefore suitable for I.M. or I.V. administration. Procaine penicillin-G and benzathine penicillin-G are the depot intramuscular formulations of penicillin-G. They have a delayed but a sustained

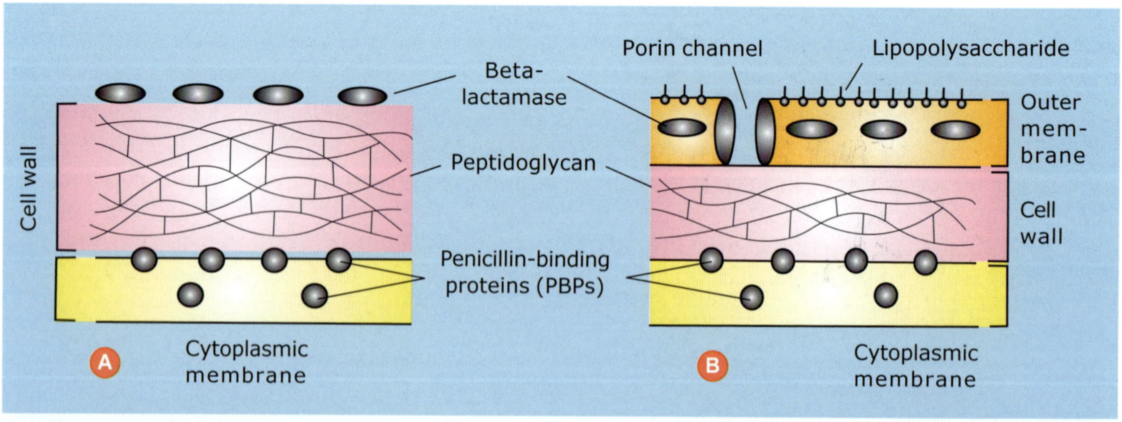

Fig 55.4 Structure and Comparison of (A) Gram-positive and (B) Gram-negative Bacterial Cell Envelops.

Table 55.1A Narrow Spectrum Penicillins

β-Lactamase Sensitive (NATURAL PENICILLINS)		β-Lactamase Resistant (ANTISTAPHYLOCOCCAL PENICILLINS)	
Acid Stable	**Acid Labile**	**Acid Stable**	**Acid Labile**
Penicillin-V (Phenoxymethyl penicillin) (oral)	Penicillin-G (Benzyl penicillin) (I.M., I.V.)	Cloxacillin (oral, I.M.)	Methicillin (I.M., I.V.)
	Procaine penicillin-G (I.M. depot inj.)	Dicloxacillin (oral, I.M.)	Nafcillin (I.M., I.V.)
	Benzathine penicillin-G (I.M. depot inj.)	Flucloxacillin (oral, I.M.)	

Table 55.1B Extended Spectrum Penicillins

All are sensitive to β-lactamase degradation	
Acid Stable (AMINOPENICILLINS)	**Acid Labile** (ANTIPSEUDOMONAL PENICILLINS)
Ampicillin (oral/parenteral)	Carbenicillin (parenteral)
Bacampicillin (oral/parenteral)	Ticarcillin (parenteral)
Talampicillin (oral/parenteral)	Piperacillin (parenteral)
Amoxycillin (oral/parenteral)	Mezlocillin (parenteral)
	Azlocillin (parenteral)

absorption and consequently have a prolonged half-life. A single 600,000 unit I.M. dose of procaine penicillin-G yields clinically effective concentration for 12–24 hrs. Similarly a single I.M. dose of 1.2 million units of benzathine penicillin-G can provide plasma levels which are sufficient to protect against β-haemolytic streptococcal infection for 3 weeks. Penicillin-G concentration in most tissues are equal to those in serum except in eye, prostate and CNS where its penetration is poor. However, if meninges are inflammed, as in bacterial meningitis, the permeability of penicillin increases so as to provide CSF concentration sufficient to kill susceptible strains of pneumococci and meningococci.

Penicillin-G is excreted by the kidneys. Its 90% elimination occurs *via* tubular secretion while only 10% is excreted *via* glomerular filtration. *Probenecid* blocks tubular secretion of penicillin and has been used to increase the plasma concentration and to prolong the half-life of penicillins. Renal failure prolongs the half-life of penicillins also. Hence, their dose must be reduced accordingly. *Methicillin* and *nafcillin* are acid-labile, hence these are not suitable for oral administration. *Cloxacillin* and *dicloxacillin* are acid stable, well absorbed and can be given orally; but their absorption is impaired by food. Hence these should be administered 1–2 hrs before or after food. Methicillin use has declined. Nafcillin is cleared primarily by biliary excretion while cloxacillin and dicloxacillin are eliminated by both renal and biliary route. Thus no dosage adjustment is required for these drugs in renal failure. Flucloxacillin is similar to dicloxacillin.

Antimicrobial Spectrum and Uses

Narrow spectrum, β-lactamase sensitive group (penicillin-V and penicilin-G etc) – are highly effective against Gram-positive cocci and bacilli; equally effective against spirochetes; moderately active against Gram-negative cocci and actinomycetes but have negligible activity against Gram-negative bacilli and bacteroides.

- **Gram-positive cocci**: Natural penicillins are highly active against: *Streptococcus pyogenes* (pharyngitis, otitis media); *Streptococcus pneumoniae* (pneumonia); *Streptococcus viridans* and *S. faecalis,* i.e., *enterococcus* (subacute bacterial endocarditis, SABE). Though 18–25 million units of penicillin-G can inhibit enterococci, simultaneous administration of gentamicin (an aminoglycoside, Ch. 56) is needed to treat enterococcal endocarditis. This combination, being synergistic, acts as bactericidal to enterococci.

  A single injection of benzathine penicillin-G (1.2 million units I.M.), is satisfactory for treating *rheumatic fever* as it prevents colonisation of *β-haemolytic Streptococci*. The same dose given intramuscularly once every 3–4 weeks, for 5 years after the attack, provides satisfactory prophylaxis against reinfection with β-haemolytic streptococcal pharyngitis (rheumatic fever).
- **Gram-positive bacilli**: Penicillin-G is the drug of choice for infections caused by the following Gram-positive bacilli: *Clostridium tetani* (cause tetanus); *Clostridium perfringens* (cause gas gangrene); *Corynebacterium diphtheriae* (cause diphtheria); *Bacillus anthraecis* (cause anthrax) and *Listeria monocytogenes* (cause *Listeria* meningitis, listeriosis). For diphtheria, tetanus and gas gangrene, antitoxin and other measures are more important, penicillin-G has adjuvant role.

Spirochetes like *Treponema pallidum* (cause syphilis) are also highly sensitive to penicillins. Benzathine penicillin-G (2.4 MU I.M. once a week for 2–3 weeks), is effective in the treatment of syphilis. Alternatively, 1.2 MU of procaine penicillin-G can be given I.M. every day for 10 days.

Penicillin-G is only moderately active against: Gram-negative cocci such as *Neisseria meningitidis* (cause meningitis) and *Neisseria gonorrhoeae* (cause gonorrhoea). However, *N. gonorrhoeae* has developed partial resistance and alternative regimens such as flouroquinolones (Ch. 56) and some cephalosporins (see following text) are more beneficial. Similarly, for meningitis, higher doses of I.V. penicillin-G are needed. These are also effective against Actinomycetes like *Actinomyces israelii* (cranio-facial/thoracic/abdominal abscess).

Penicillin-G has insignificant activity against *Bacteroides* and Gram -negative bacilli.

Narrow Spectrum, β-lactamase resistant group (cloxacillin, dicloxacillin, methicillin and ***nafcillin***) have the antimicrobial spectrum similar to penicillin-G as described above, but these are additionally effective against β-lactamase producing *Staphylococci* and hence called ***antistaphylococcal penicillins***. Methicillin is no longer used because of nephrotoxicity, yet for historical reasons *Staphylococcus aureus* resistant to cloxacillin or nafcillin are labeled as methicillin resistant *Staphylococcus aureus* (MRSA). Nafcillin is preferred for parenteral use while cloxacillin and dicloxacillin can be given orally. These are used to treat infections such as osteomyelitis, septicaemia, endocarditis and cellulitis caused by susceptible strains of staphylococci. Cloxacillin, in addition, can also be used to treat mild staphylococcal skin infection such as impetigo.

Extended Spectrum Penicillins

All these penicillins are β-lactamase sensitive, but aminopenicillins (***ampicillin*** and ***amoxycillin*** group) are acid stable (can be given orally) while carboxypenicillins (***carbenicillin*** and ***ticarcillin***) and ureidopenicillins (***piperacillin, mezlocillin*** and ***azlocillin***) are acid labile (given only I.V. or I.M.). (Table 55.1B).

Pharmacokinetics

The pharmacokinetics of ampicillin and amoxycillin are similar. Both have adequate oral bioavailability. Ingestion of food decreases the bioavailability of ampicillin but not of amoxycillin. Therefore, oral doses of ampicillin must be administered 1 hour before or after meals. Ampicillin achieves therapeutic concentrations in CSF during inflammatory conditions but amoxycillin does not; hence amoxycillin is not suitable for meningitis therapy. Their primary route of excretion is through kidney. Bacampicillin and talampicillin are prodrugs of ampicillin. Bacampicillin, talampicillin and amoxycillin disturb the intestinal flora to a much lesser extent, hence incidence of diarrhoea is less.

Carbenicillin, ticarcillin, piperacillin, mezlocillin and azlocillin are parenteral penicillins available as sodium salts and hence these must be administered with caution to the patients of congestive heart failure. They achieve only low concentration in CSF. All undergo renal elimination, and require dose adjustment in renal failure. Carbenicillin is also available as indanyl sodium salt. This formulation is acid stable and can be given orally. Among them, mezlocillin has significant hepatic metabolism and requires dose adjustment in patients with hepatic insufficiency.

Antimicrobial Spectrum and Uses

This group retains the antimicrobial spectrum of penicillin-G. However, ***ampicillin group of antibiotics,*** because of their hydrophilic character, have enhanced ability to penetrate through porin channels of the Gram-negative bacteria. ***Hence, these have an extended spectrum against some Gram-negative bacteria also,*** but not against *Pseudomonas aeruginosa* as these bacteria are lacking in porin channels.

Gram-negative bacilli covered by ***ampicillin*** group of antibiotics include: *Bordetella pertusis* (whooping cough), *Haemophilus influenzae* (pneumonia, otitis media, sinusitis), *E. coli* (UTI), *Salmonella typhi, Proteus mirabilis* (UTI) and *Shigella*. This group of antibiotics is not active against *Pseudomonas, Klebsiella, Serratia, Citrobacter*, indole-positive *Proteus* and other Gram-negative aerobes. Presently, fluoroquinolones have replaced ampicillin for treating UTI, for treating typhoid fever (as amoxycillin prolongs the carrier state) and for treating bacillary dysentery due to *Shigella*. ***Amoxycillin*** is also used in multidrug regimens for eradication of *Helicobacter pylori* in duodenal and gastric ulcers (Ch. 27).

Ampicillin and amoxycillin are also very effective against *Streptococcus viridans* and enterococci (SABE) and pneumococci, but not against other Gram-positive cocci such as *Staphylococcus*. For SABE, ampicillin 2 g I.V., every 6 hrs, may be used in place of penicillin-G. Concurrent use of gentamicin provides synergistic effects. These drugs have moderate activity against Gram-negative cocci such as gonococci and meningococci. A single dose of 3.5 g of ampicillin +1 g of probenecid is adequate for gonococcal urethritis. Ampicillin (not amoxycillin) is also effective in meningitis caused by *Listeria monocytogenes*. An usual dosage of 250–500 mg TDS of amoxycillin is equivalent to the same amount of ampicillin QID daily.

Piperacillin group of penicillins have comparable spectra of activity against many Gram-positive and Gram-negative organisms as described above. But the special feature of these penicillins is their activity against *Pseudomonas aeruginosa* and indole-positive *Proteus* which are not inhibited by penicillin-G or aminopenicillins. Hence, these are called ***antipseudomonal penicillins*** also. Among carboxypenicillins, *carbenicillin* has become obsolete and has been replaced by more potent and better tolerated drug ***ticarcillin***. However, ***carbenicillin-indanyl sodium***, which is an acid stable formulation, is being used orally for less serious or chronic UTI due to *Pseudomonas* or *Proteus*. The ureidopenicillins such as ***piperacillin, mezlocillin*** and ***azlocillin*** have similar clinical outcome in *Pseudomonas* infection as with *ticarcillin* except that these are also active against *Klebseilla pneumoniae* and *Enterobacter*. These drugs are used for serious infections due to *Pseudomonas, Proteus* or *Klebseilla* as in burns, septicaemia, UTI and in immuno-compromised patients. Usually a combination of piperacillin with gentamicin is preferred.

Penicillin Units

The activity of natural penicillins (e.g., penicillin G) is defined in terms of units. Crystalline sodium penicillin-G contains 1600 units per mg. In other words 1 unit of penicillin-G = 0.625 μg; or 625 mg of penicillin-G = one million units. Semisynthetic penicillins are prescribed by weight basis rather than units, e.g., amoxycillin 500 mg 8 hrly orally.

Resistance to Penicillins

Bacterial resistance to penicillins may arise from one or more than one of the following mechanisms:

1) ***Inactivation of β-lactam ring by β-lactamase***: Over 300 β-lactamases have been identified. Some bacteria such as *Staphylococcus aureus, Haemophilus influenzae* and *E. coli* produce β-lactamase with a narrow substrate specificity which can hydrolyse penicillins but not cephalosporins. Other β-lactamases such as those produced by *Pseudomonas*, *Enterobacter*, *Neisseria gonorrhoeae* and *Moraxella catarrhalis* have a broader degradative activity and can hydrolyse both penicillins and cephalosporins. Some bacteria have chromosomal (penicillin inducible) genes for producing β-lactamases. Other bacteria acquire β-lactamase genes *via* plasmids or transposons. Transfer of such β-lactamase genes contributes to the proliferation of resistant organism and therapeutic failure. Efforts to overcome this problem have led to the development of β-lactamase inhibitors (see below).
2) ***Modifications of penicillin binding proteins (PBPs)***: Resistant bacteria like methicillin resistant *Staphylococcus aureus* (MRSA), *Streptococcus pneumoniae* and *Enterococcus* produce mutant PBPs which have low affinity to penicillins and other β-lactam antibiotics.
3) ***Reduction of penicillin permeability to reach PBPs***: Some bacteria reduce the antibiotic access to PBPs through porin channels. For example, in resistant bacteria such as *Pseudomonas aeruginosa*, the porin mutants block the penicillin transfer across the outer membrane.
4) ***Activation of antibiotic efflux mechanisms***: Some Gram-negative bacteria may produce an efflux pump that efficiently ejects antibiotic from the periplasm back across the outer membrane before it can bind to PBPs, e.g., efflux of nafcillin by *Salmonella typhi* and efflux of imipenem by *Pseudomonas aeruginosa*.

β-Lactamase Inhibitors

These agents resemble β-lactam antibiotics only structurally but do not possess any significant antimicrobial action. They bind irreversibly to the catalytic site of susceptible β-lactamases (produced by bacteria) to prevent hydrolysis of penicillins (suicide inhibitors). These can inhibit plasmid-mediated β-lactamases which are responsible for transferred drug resistance, such as those produced by methicillin-sensitive *Staphylococcus aureus, H. influenzae, H. ducreyi, E. coli, Klebsiella pneumoniae, Proteus mirabilis, Neisseria gonorrhoeae, Salmonella* and *Shigella*. These are unable to inhibit chromosomally mediated β-lactamases found in *Enterobacter, Pseudomonas aeruginosa*, *Citrobacter* and *Serratia* and organisms producing inducible forms of (extended spectrum) β-lactamases.

Currently seven β-lactamase inhibitors are available: ***clavulanic acid*** (derived from *Streptomyces clavligerus*), ***sulbactam*** (semisynthetic), ***tazobactam*** (structural analogue of sulbactam), ***avibactam***, ***vaborbactam, relebactam, zidebactam***. Only clavulanic acid is orally absorbed; others are used parenterally (I.V. or I.M.). According to their common pharmacokinetic features, clavulanic acid is combined with amoxycillin; sulbactam with ampicillin; and tazobactam with piperacillin, and are available as fixed dose combinations.

Addition of clavulanic acid with amoxycillin extends the antimicrobial spectrum of amoxycillin against β-lactamase producing bacteria, e.g., *Streptococcus pneumoniae, H. influenzae* and *Moraxella* (otitis media, sinusitis and respiratory tract infections), methicillin sensitive *Staphylococcus aureus* (MSSA), *Klebsiella pneumoniae* (nosocomial pneumonia), penicillinase producing *Neisseria gonorrhoeae* (gonorrhoea), β-lactamase producing anaerobes (intra-abdominal abscess), *E. coli*, *Proteus* and *Klebsiella* (urinary tract infections). All β-lactamase inhibitor combinations require dose adjustment in patients with renal insufficiency because these are excreted by kidney. Available fixed dose combinations are:

- Amoxycillin 250/500 mg + Clavulanic acid 125 mg; Tablets/Caps
- Ampicillin 1 g + Sulbactam 0.5 g; I.V. or I.M. Injection
- Piperacillin 2 g + Tazobactam 0.25 g; I.V. or I.M. Injection
- Ceftazidime+Avibactam
- Meropenem+Vaborbactam
- Imepenem/Cilastatin+ Relebactam

Adverse effects are rare except GI intolerance, stomatitis and rashes. For preparations see under amoxycillin group.

Adverse Effects to Penicillins

One of the remarkable features of penicillins is their relative freedom from direct toxic effects except the hypersensitivity reactions which at times may become life-threatening.

1. **HYPERSENSITIVITY REACTIONS**: The incidence varies from 5–8% of the patients receiving penicillins. The major antigenic determinant is penicilloic acid (Fig. 55.2), but minor determinants like benzyl penicillin itself or sodium benzylpenicilloate can also combine with host proteins and become antigenic. Allergic reactions of penicillins can be classified as *immediate, accelerated* or *late hypersensitivity* reactions.

   Immediate hypersensitivity reactions are most common and occur within 20 min of parenteral administration of penicillins. These appear to be mediated by IgE antibodies against the minor determinants. Manifestations include urticaria, pruritus, wheezing, sneezing and rhinitis which in 0.05% cases may pass-over to ***anaphylaxis***, which is the extreme form of immediate hypersensitivity characterised by diffused pruritus, hypotensive shock, angioneurotic oedema, choking and finally loss of consciousness and death. Management includes administration of adrenaline (S.C./I.M.), corticosteroids (I.V./I.M.), antihistamine (I.M.) with supportive measures such as O_2 inhalation, I.V. fluids or plasma expanders.

   Accelerated hypersensitivity reactions usually occur within 72 hrs of penicillin administration, and are mediated by IgE antibodies against major antigenic determinant. Manifestations include rash, fever and urticaria but rarely angioneurotic oedema. Fatality is extremely rare.

   Late hypersensitivity reactions occur after 72 hrs of penicillin administration, and are mediated by IgE and IgM antibodies against the major antigenic determinant of penicillin. Manifestations include morbiliform, urticarial or erythematous eruptions, local inflammatory reactions, lymphadenopathy, splenomegaly, serum sickness and Coombs positive haemolytic anaemia.

   Ampicillin or amoxycillin, at times, also produce non-urticarial maculopapular rash after 3–4 days of the start of oral therapy. This type of non-allergic reaction is more frequent if ampicillin/amoxycillin are taken during viral fever or when these are used along with allopurinol.

2. GIT SIDE EFFECTS: Diarrhoea is more common with ampicillin but less with amoxycillin, bacampicillin or talampicillin. Glossitis, stomatitis and abnormal taste sensation may result after oral use.
3. MISCELLANEOUS EFFECTS: Oxacillin can cause reversible elevations in SGOT and SGPT values. Methicillin can cause interstitial nephritis. High doses of carbenicillin (also ticarcillin) may produce reversible increase in prothombin time leading to bleeding problem. High dose of carbenicillin are neurotoxic also. ***Penicillin injected in a syphilitic patient may produce Jarisch-Herxheimer reaction*** characterised by shivering, fever, myalgia and even collapse due to sudden release of spirochaetal breakdown products. The reaction may last up to 72 hrs.

Drug Interactions

ANTAGONISTIC COMBINATIONS: **(1)** Oral penicillins (penicillin-V, ampicillin etc.) may be antagonised by bacteriostatic antibiotics (tetracyclines, chloramphenicol, erythromycin etc.) as they will diminish the bactericidal effect of penicillins by inhibiting the bacterial growth (see earlier text). **(2)** Penicillins and aminoglycosides (e.g., gentamicin) should not be mixed, in the same syringe, as they inactivate each other. These should be injected separately. **(3)** Ampicillin with allopurinol may cause non-urticarial maculopapular rash. **(4)** Hydrocortisone inactivates ampicillin if mixed in the I.V. fluid.

SYNERGISTIC COMBINATIONS: **(1)** Probenecid prolongs the action of penicillins by decreasing its tubular secretion (see above). **(2)** β-lactamase inhibitors extend the spectrum of penicillins against β-lactamase producing cocci and bacilli (see above). **(3)** Procaine penicillin-G with gentamicin is a synergistic bactericidal combination against *Streptococcus viridans* and *Strepto. faecalis* in SABE. **(4)** Piperacillin and gentamicin is a very effective synergistic combination against *Pseudomonas* and *Proteus*. **(5)** A fixed dose combination of ampicillin or amoxycillin 250 mg with cloxacillin 250 mg has been promoted as a synergistic combination useful in postoperative and respiratory infections. In this formulation ampicillin (or amoxycillin) is active against Gram-negative bacteria but its dose is inadequate while cloxacillin acts against staphylococci but its dose also has been halved. This increases the chances of developing resistance. Hence the use of such formulation is not only irrational but harmful.

CEPHALOSPORINS

All cephalosporins, or their chemical analogues cefamycins, consist of a dihydrothiazine ring fused to a β-lactam ring (B) containing an appropriate side chain at position-7 (Fig. 55.1). The active nucleus of cephalosporins and cefamycins is isolated from the fungus *Cephalosporinium acremonium* and from *Streptomyces lactamdurans*, respectively; but most of the drugs in use today are semisynthetic or synthetic and are obtained by chemical modification at position-3 or 7.

Cephalosporins are similar to penicillins chemically, in mechanism of their action, and in adverse effects. Except for first generation drugs, rest are more resistant to β-lactamase (cephalosporinase) degradation and therefore have a broader spectrum of activity against Gram-negative bacteria and anaerobes compared to penicillins. *However, no cephalosporin is active against Enterococcus faecalis, MRSA and Gram-positive bacilli.*

Mechanism of Action

Cephalosporins possess a mechanism of action identical to penicillins, i.e., inhibition of transpeptidation process leading to the formation of imperfect cell wall; osmotic drive from the outside isotonic environment of the host cell to the inside of the hypertonic bacterial cytoplasm; and finally activation of the autolysin enzyme leading to the lysis of bacteria. Hence cephalosporins are also bactericidal drugs.

Classification and Antimicrobial Spectrum

Cephalosporins have been classified according to their "generation" which is based on their antibacterial spectrum, stability to β-lactamases and the year of introduction. First generation drugs were introduced in 1960s, second generation in 1970s, third generation in 1980s and fourth generation somewhere in 1997–98. Cephalosporins discovered later have been tentatively placed in fifth generation.

First Generation Cephalosporins

Examples: ***Cephalexin*** (oral), ***Cefadroxil*** (oral), ***Cephradine*** (oral/parenteral), ***Cefazolin*** (parenteral).

Pharmacokinetics

Oral cephalosporins are generally well absorbed. ***These do not cross BBB*** (not suitable for treating brain abscess or meningitis). Metabolism is not a major elimination path for these cephalosporins. ***These are primarily excreted through kidney.*** As usual probenecid increases their plasma concentration and prolongs their half-life by inhibiting their renal tubular secretion. Except for cefadroxil which is given 12 hrly, others are administered on 6–8 hrly basis. ***All are sensitive to β-lactamase enzyme degradation.***

Antimicrobial Spectrum and Uses

⊕ Cocci > ⊖ Bacilli > ⊕ Bacilli > ⊖ Cocci > Anaerobes

These drugs have appreciable activity against Gram-positive cocci such as streptococci, pneumococci and methicillin sensitive staphylococci, but do not inhibit MRSA and *Enterococcus faecalis*. They show moderate activity against Gram-negative bacteria like *E. coli*, *Klebseilla pneumoniae*, and indole-negative *Proteus mirabilis* EXCEPT *Pseudomonas*, *Salmonella*, *Enterobacter*, indole-positive *Proteus*, *Serratia* and *Acinetobacter*. These have insignificant activity against Gram-positive bacilli. Interestingly anaerobic Gram-positive cocci are sensitive (e.g., peptococci) but anaerobic Gram-negative bacteria (e.g., *Bacteroides fragilis*) are not.

Except for *cefazolin*, other cephalosporins of this group should not be relied upon in serious systemic infections. However, these can be used for the treatment of UTIs, for minor staphylococcal infections or for infection like cellulitis or soft tissue abscess. These are ineffective in meningitis (do not cross BBB). Compared to other cephalosporins, ***cefazolin*** has better penetration to tissues. Hence, it is the drug of choice in surgical prophylaxis before cardiac surgery and orthopaedic prosthesis procedures (See appendix III).

Second Generation Cephalosporins

Examples: ***Cefaclor*** (oral), ***Cefuroxime*** (oral or parenteral), ***Cefprozil*** (oral), ***Cefotetan*** (parenteral), ***Cefamandole*** (parenteral), ***Cefoxitin*** (parenteral). Chemically *cefotetan* and *cefoxitin* are cephamycins, but for all purposes these are considered as cephalosporins.

Pharmacokinetics

Cefaclor, cefuroxime axetil and cefprozil can be given orally and have good bioavailability. Cefuroxime axetil is an ester prodrug formulation in which the ester is hydrolysed during drug passage through the intestinal mucosa. The free cefuroxime then enters the systemic circulation. Among these drugs ***only cefuroxime crosses BBB and achieves therapeutic concentrations in CSF***. Except for cefaclor, ***these drugs are more stable to β-lactamase degradation.*** Their intramuscular injections are painful and hence are preferably administered by I.V. route. ***These are excreted unchanged through kidney.*** Probenecid competes with their tubular secretion and increases their half-life and plasma concentration.

Antimicrobial Spectrum and Uses

As we proceed from first generation to second generation cephalosporins, the antimicrobial spectrum shifts as follows:

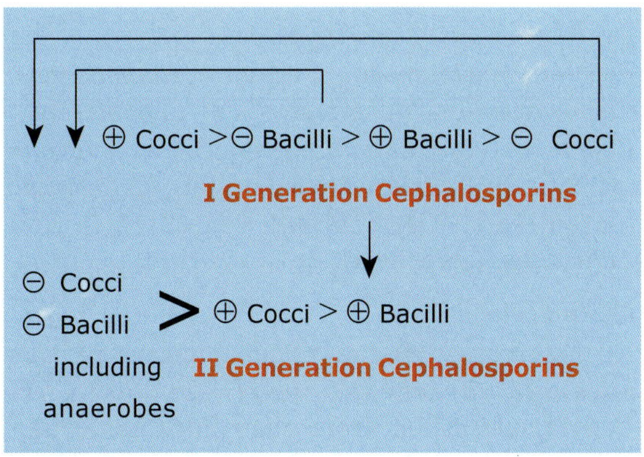

Thus, all second generation drugs are less active against Gram-positive cocci and bacilli compared

to first generation drugs, rather they have an extended Gram-negative coverage including some anaerobes. For example, ***cefoxitin*** and ***cefotetan*** have good anaerobic activity and are useful in such anaerobic infections as lower abdominal (peritonitis, diverticulitis) and some gynaecological infections.

Cefaclor and ***Cefprozil*** are more active than first generation drugs against *H. influenzae, M. catarrhalis, E. coli* and *Proteus mirabilis* and are primarily used to treat upper respiratory infections. ***Cefuroxime*** is resistant to degradation by β-lactamase producing Gram-negative bacteria, e.g., penicillinase-producing *Neisseria gonorrhoeae, H. influenzae* and *Klebsiella pneumoniae*; hence it is used to treat community-acquired pneumonia and for single dose I.M. therapy of gonorrhoea due to PPNG. Since it attains relatively higher CSF levels it is also used to treat meningitis, though third generation drugs are more preferred. It is also active against Gram-positive cocci like *S. pneumoniae* and *S. pyogenes* (equal to first generation drugs) but not against *Staph. aureus*. ***Cefamandole*** is very similar to cefuroxime in structure and antibacterial activity and is preferred for treating sexually transmitted diseases. The use of second generation cephalosporins has lately declined because of two reasons: firstly because penicillin + β-lactamase inhibitor combination is a better alternative against *B. fragilis,* and secondly for infections due to Gram-negative organisms, third and fourth generation cephalosporins are more preferred.

Third Generation Cephalosporins

The third generation drugs include: ***Cefixime*** (oral), ***Cefpodoxime*** (oral), ***Ceftibuten*** (oral), ***Cefdinir*** (oral), ***Cefditoren*** (oral), ***Ceftolozane*** (oral), ***Cefoperazone*** (parenteral), ***Ceftriaxone*** (parenteral), ***Cefotaxime*** (parenteral), ***Ceftazidime*** (parenteral) and ***Ceftizoxime*** (parenteral).

Pharmacokinetics

All these drugs, regardless of inflammation, ***provide adequate therapeutic levels in the CSF. Ceftriaxone*** differs from other third generation drugs by its long plasma half-life (7–8 hrs) and high protein binding (90%), so the drug is administered once daily. ***Cefotaxime*** is the one cephalosporin in this group which is metabolised to an active metabolite, desacetyl cefotaxime. ***Cefoperazone*** and ***ceftriaxone*** are the two drugs which ***are excreted through bile*** and no dosage adjustment is required in renal insufficiency. ***Urinary excretion is the major elimination route for other cephalosporins*** and therefore require dosage adjustment in renal insufficiency. An increase in cephalosporin plasma concentration occurs with probenecid which blocks the renal tubular secretion of these cephalosporins. ***All are highly resistant to degradation by β-lactamases produced by Gram-negative bacteria.***

Antimicrobial Spectrum and Uses

As we proceed from second generation to third generation cephalosporins, the antimicrobial spectrum changes as follows:

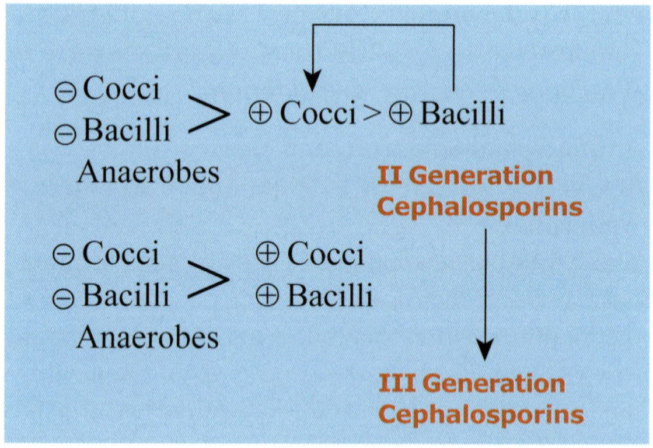

These drugs are highly active against Gram-negative cocci, Gram-negative bacilli and anaerobes. Thus they have an excellent activity against *N. gonorrhoeae, N. meningitidis, E. coli, Enterobacter, H. influenzae, Klebsiella pneumoniae,* and *Proteus mirabilis*. ***Cefoperazone*** and ***ceftazidime*** are very active against *Pseudomonas aeruginosa.* In general, these drugs are considered to be the drugs of choice for serious infections caused by *Klebsiella, Enterobacter, Proteus, Serratia* and *Haemophilus* species. These are generally less active than first generation drugs against Gram-positive cocci.

Ceftriaxone is very effective in treating meningitis (*except due to Listeria monocytogenes).* A single I.M. dose of 250 mg is effective in treatment of gonorrhoea and chancroid. It is excellent for treatment of community acquired pneumonia caused by pneumococci, *H. influenzae* and *Staph aureus*. It is also efficacious in treating complicated UTIs, abdominal sepsis and septicaemias. It can be used to treat multidrug resistant typhoid fever, though doses are relatively high (4 g I.V. daily for 2 days followed by 2 g I.V. per day till 2 days after fever subsides).

Cefotaxime, like ceftriaxone, has been utilised effectively for treating meningitis and community acquired pneumonia (see above). A single 0.5–1 g I.M. dose is effective in treating gonorrhoea. It has been used in respiratory, genitourinary and abdominal infections, septicaemia, anaerobic and hospital acquired infections.

Cefoperazone is more active than cefotaxime against *Pseudomonas* (but less active than ceftazidime). It is good for *Salmonella typhi* and *B. fragilis* also. It is used for pseudomonal UTIs, bacteraemia and infections in immunocompromised patients. Other uses like meningitis, gonorrhoea and septicaemia are common to other drugs of this series.

Ceftazidime has an excellent activity against *Pseudomonas* (better than cefoperazone) and other Gram-negative bacilli. Ceftazidime + aminoglycosides is a treatment of choice for pseudomonal meningitis. It is useful for nosocomical infections also.

Ceftizoxime is more active against *B. fragilis* than cefotaxime, otherwise similar.

Cefixime and ***Cefpodoxime*** are orally administered. In a dose of 200–400 mg BD, *cefixime* is used to treat respiratory, urinary, biliary infections. In a single 400 mg oral dose it provides effective treatment of uncomplicated gonorrhoea. It is not active against *Staph.aureus* and *Pseudomonas*. *Cefpodoxime* is similar to cefixime but it is active against *Staph.aureus* also. Usual dose is 200 mg BD.

Ceftibuten, Cefdinir and ***Cefditoren pivoxil*** are also orally active. These are active against both Gram-positive and Gram-negative bacteria. These are used to treat community acquired pneumonia, chronic bronchitis, otitis media, sinusitis, pharyngitis, tonsilitis and skin infections. *Cefdinir* is given as 300 mg BD while *ceftibuten* as 400 mg once daily. Usual dose of *cefditoren pivoxil* is 400 mg orally BD.

In neutropenic, febrile immunocompromised patients, third generation cephalosporins are often used with aminoglycosides. However, their use with aminoglycosides is controversial as these are nephrotoxic while cephalosporins, though themselves not nephrotoxic, may considerably increase the nephrotoxicity of aminoglycosides.

Ceftolozane + tazobactum (TOL-TAZ) is a novel third generation cephalosporin currently available in combination with β-lactamase inhibitor. When administered in 1 hr I.V. infusion (in the doses of 2000+1000 mg / 1000+500 mg / 500+250 mg, respectively) I.V. infusion, the co-formulated solution is found to be useful for *Pseudomonas aeriginosa* (PA) and other Gram-negative bacilli as this cephalosporin is not a substrate for several PA efflux system.

Like penicillins, other types of β-lactamase inhibitors like clavulenic acids are available with 3rd generation Cephalosporins. They are well known in Indian market.

Fourth Generation Cephalosporins

The fourth generation cephalosporins include ***Cefepime***, ***Cefpirome*** and ***Cefozopran*** (all parenteral).

Pharmacokinetics

Cefepime is given by I.M./I.V. injection (1–2 g 8 hrly). Its plasma half-life is 2 hrs. It is widely distributed in body tissues and fluids and accumulates well in CSF. It is eliminated 85–90% through kidney. *Cefpirome* and *cefozopran* are less commonly used.

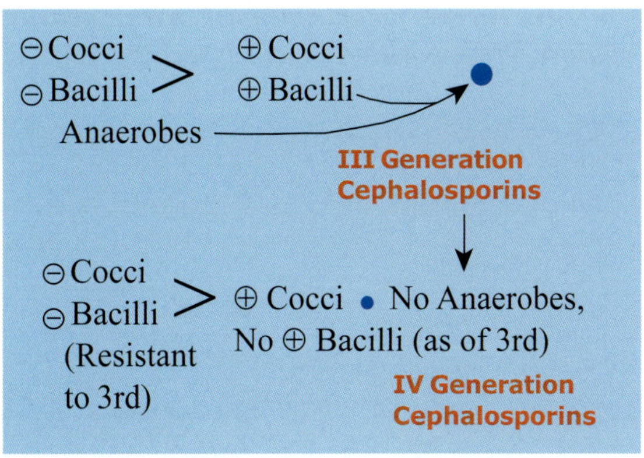

Antimicrobial Spectrum and Uses

As we proceed from 3rd generation to 4th generation, the antimicrobial spectrum shifts as follows (flow chart):

Both drugs are ***resistant to degradation by several forms of β-lactamases***. Against Gram-positive cocci (methicillin sensitive *Staph. aureus, S. pneumoniae*), their activity is similar to 3rd generation drugs but these are ***highly active against Gram-negative organisms,*** e.g., *P. aeruginosa*, *Enterobacteriaceae*, *Haemophilus*, *Proteus* and *Neisseria*; and *against bacteria that were resistant to earlier group of cephalosporins*. These are used against hospital acquired pneumonia, bacteraemia and septicaemia. These are also useful in UTIs, respiratory tract infections and as empiric therapy for febrile neutropenic patients.

Fifth Generation Cephalosporins

Examples: ***Ceftaroline, Ceftobiprole*** and (both parenteral).

Although they also inhibit cell wall synthesis, these have a bit different mode of action and a unique antimicrobial spectrum. They effectively bind to and inhibit an altered penicillin binding protein-2a (PBP-2a) produced by MRSA and penicillin resistant *Streptococcus pneumoniae,* which is not inhibited by majority of cephalosporins in clinical use.

Antimicrobial Spectrum and Uses

As we proceed from IV generation to V, the antimicrobial spectrum changes as follows (see flow chart):

(1) *There is notable increase in their activity against Gram-positive cocci (especially MRSA, penicillin resistant Strepto. pneumoniae, Strepto.pyogens and Enterococcus).* (2) *These retain the activity of Fourth generation against Gram-negative bacilli (especially E. coli, Haemophilus influenzae, Klebsiella pneumonae and Pseudomonas)*. These have limited activity against anaerobes.

Ceftaroline fosamil has been approved by for the treatment of community acquired bacterial pneumonia and acute bacterial skin infections including MRSA.

Ceftobiprole has been approved for the treatment of community acquired pneumonia and skin and skin structure infections inlcuding non-limb threatening diabetic foot infections without bone involvement. It is a broad spectrum cephalosporin with activity against Gram-positive cocci, including MRSA and MRSE, penicilline-resistance Strepto. pneumoniae, Enterococcus, faecalis as well as many Gram-negative bacilli including AmpC producing *E.coli* and *P.aeruginosa.* The drug demonstrates post- antibiotics effect against MRSA and *Strecpto. pneumoniae*. Ceftobiprole shows limited activity against and anaerobes such as *Bacteroides fragilis*. The drug is administered I.V. and after a single 30 min infusion of a 500 mg dose reaches blood concentration of 35 mcg/mL. It has a half life of 3.5 hrs.

Both Fifth generation cephalosporins are excreted primarily by kidney. Hence, dose adjustment is essential in renally compromised patients. None of them inhibits major CYP-450 isoenzymes. Hence, such drug interactions are not

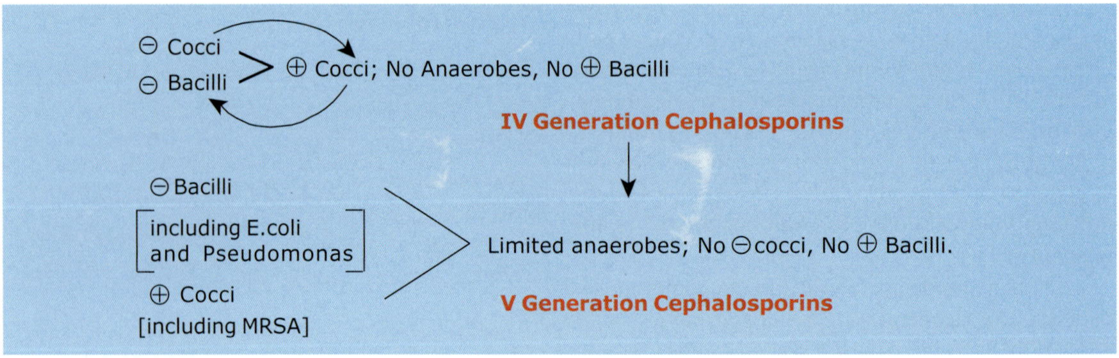

relevant either. Both have high safety profile except nausea, diarrhoea and rash.

Adverse Effects to Cephalosporins

- The cephalosporins have a good safety profile. Though the incidence of ***hypersensitivity reactions*** is very less compared to penicillins, yet fever (1%), skin rash (1–4%) eosinophilia (3–8%) and haematological abnormalities (1–2%) can occur. The anaphylactic reactions to cephalosporins are rare (less than 0.02%). The issue of cross-sensitivity between cephalosporins and penicillins has never been resolved satisfactorily. However, if a patient had anaphylaxis or angioedema following penicillin use, cephalosporins as a rule should be avoided, because the frequency of allergic reactions to cephalosporins is 1.7–2% in patients with a history of type-I penicillin reaction.
- ***Superinfection, pseudomembranous colitis*** **(PMC)** and ***diarrhoea*** could result from the use of 3rd, 4th and 5th generation cephalosporins (see Ch. 52).
- ***Coagulation abnormalities*** (bleeding) may be an uncommon but a serious side effect of some cephalosporins like *cefamandole*, *cefoperazone* & *cefotetan*. They cause hypo-prothrombinaemia and bleeding disorders by destruction of vitamin-K producing colonic bacteria and by reducing the synthesis of vit. K-dependent clotting factors. Administration of vitamin K can prevent this problem.
- High doses of ***ceftriaxone*** can result into ***pseudolithiasis*** (gall bladder sludge) which disappears after discontinuation of the therapy. Ignorance of this effect usually leads to uncalled for laparotomy.
- Local irritation can produce severe pain after I.M. injection of many cephalosporins.

Drug Interactions

1. Antacids decrease the absorption of cefaclor, cefdinir and cefpodoxime.
2. Food decreases the oral absorption of cefuroxime and cefpodoxime.
3. Cefoperazone, cefotetan and cefamandole, may induce disulfiram (antabuse) type reaction after consuming alcohol due to inhibition of aldehyde dehydrogenase.
4. Probenecid enhances plasma levels and duration of action of those cephalosporins which are secreted through renal tubule.
5. Aminoglycosides should not be mixed, in the same syringe, with cephalosporins.
6. Like penicillins, combination of cephalosporins with *sulbactam* and *clavulanic acid* are also available which have an extended spectrum against β-lactamase producing bacteria.

OTHER BETA-LACTAM ANTIBIOTICS

The newer classes of β-lactam antibiotics are the ***monobactams*** and ***carbapenems***. Their mechanism of action is same as that of penicillins, i.e., inhibition of cell wall synthesis.

1. Monobactams

Examples: ***Aztreonam, Tigemonam & Carumonam***.

Aztreonam is the only monobactam currently in clinical use. Others are in the process of approval. It is a monocyclic β-lactam (i.e., monobactam) lacking the thiazolidine ring (A) of penicillins (Fig. 55.1). Aztreonam has low affinity for PBPs in streptococci, staphylococci and anaerobes and ***therefore its spectrum and utility is limited to aerobic Gram-negative microorganisms only. It is stable to most β-lactamases.*** In its spectrum of activity it resembles aminoglycosides (Ch. 56), *hence it is preferred for all sorts of Gram-negative infections in patients with renal impairment where aminoglycosides are to be avoided.* It is active primarily against *Entero-bacteriaceae, Pseudomonas, Klebsiella, Proteus, Citrobacter, Yersinia enterocolitica, Pasturella, Salmonella, Shigella, Haemophilus, Serratia and Neisseria* etc.

Its oral bioavailability is poor and hence given I.M. or I.V. (1 g, 8 hrly). The drug achieves therapeutic concentration in CSF in the presence of inflammed meninges and serves as an alternative to cephalosporins for the therapy of meningitis caused by Gram-negative bacilli. An inhalational formulation of aztreonam has been approved by FDA for treatment of cystic fibrosis due to *P. aeruginosa*.

It rarely causes allergic reactions in the patients with a history of type-I hypersensitivity to penicillins. Side effects are not serious except diarrhoea, skin rash or pain at the site of injection.

2. Carbapenems

Examples: ***Imipenem, Meropenem, Ertapenem, Doripenem, Faropenem*** and ***Razupenem.***

The carbapenems are also structurally related to β-lactam antibiotics (Fig. 55.1). Four carbapenems, viz, *imipenem*, *meropenem*, *ertapenem* and *doripenem* (approved in October 2007) are in clinical use at present. *Razupenem* is still in phase III clinical trials. ***These have a wider spectrum of antimicrobial activity, i.e., Gram-negative rods including Pseudomonas aeruginosa, Gram-positive organisms and anaerobes. These are resistant to many β-lactamases also.*** Carbapenems are, therefore, drugs of choice for the management of infections caused by *E. coli*, *K. pneumoniae*, *Proteus mirabilis*, indole- positive *Proteus*, *H. influenzae*, *P. aeruginosa*, *Enterobacter*, *Acinetobacter*, *Citrobacter*, *Clostridium perfringens*, *Serratia*, *Bacteroides*, MSSA and *Streptococcus pneumoniae*. Strains of *P. aeruginosa* may develop resistance with carbapenems, so simultaneous use of an aminoglycoside is recommended for such purpose. ***Meropenem*** has slightly greater activity than ***imepenem*** against Gram-negative aerobes, while ***ertapenem*** is slightly less active than both against *P. aeruginosa,* otherwise there is hardly any difference in their activity except for their pharmacokinetics. Carbapenems with or without aminoglycosides is considered as effective treatment for febrile neutropenic patients. *Clostridium difficile*, *Corynebacterium*, MRSA and *Enterococcus faecium* are resistant to carbapenems. ***Razupenem*** is a novel carbapenem which has high activity against multidrug-resistant Gram-positive and Gram-negative (i.e., extended spectrum β-lactamase producing) bacteria.

Carbapenems are given by I.M./I.V. injection because their oral bioavailability is poor. The more preferred route of their administration is I.V. as their I.M. injection is painful. Among these, ***imipenem*** is hydrolysed by renal dehydropeptidase present in renal brush border, resulting in lower urinary concentration. It is therefore administered with ***cilastatin*** which inhibits this enzyme and prevents its degradation. ***Ertapenem, doripenem*** and ***meropenem*** are not degraded by renal dehydropeptidase. *Imipenem* may cause nausea, vomiting, diarrhoea, skin rash and even seizures (in high doses). *Meropenem, ertapenem* and *doripenem* do not cause seizures and are safer than imipenem.

Patients allergic to penicillins may be allergic to carbapenems. ***Faropenem*** can be given orally. It is well tolerated except for diarrhoea and at times rash.

The usual dose of ***imipenem*** is 0.25–0.5 g I.V., 6–8 hrly; of ***meropemem*** 0.5–1 g I.V., 8 hrly; of ***doripenem*** 0.5 g I.V. infusion, 8 hrly. ***Ertapenem,*** because of its longer t½, can be given 1 g I.V./I.M. once daily. Its I.M. injection, being painful, is available with 1% xylocaine. ***Faropenem*** can be administered orally, 150–200 mg, 6–8 hrly.

OTHER ANTIBIOTICS THAT INHIBIT CELL WALL SYNTHESIS

The drugs included in this group are ***vancomycin*** (a glycopeptide), ***teicoplanin*** (a newer glycopeptide), ***daptomycin*** (a lipopeptide), ***bacitracin*** (a polypeptide), ***fosfomycin*** (a phosphonic acid derivative) and ***cycloserine*** (an analogue of D-alanine). All inhibit cell wall synthesis of bacteria but by different mechanisms.

Glycopeptides

1. Vancomycin

Vancomycin is obtained from *Streptococcus orientalis*. It inhibits Gram-positive bacterial cell wall synthesis by complexing with D-alanyl-D-alanine portion of the terminal end of peptidoglycan pentapeptide (Fig. 55.3). Further elongation and cross-linking of peptidoglycan is thus prevented. The cell wall becomes weak and susceptible for lysis. It also damages the cell membrane and alters cytoplasmic membrane permeability. The drug is, therefore, bactericidal. However, because of its larger molecular size, it cannot traverse the outer cell membrane of Gram-negative bacteria. ***Vancomycin is exclusively active against aerobic as well as anaerobic Gram-positive species*** such as Streptococci as well as Staphylococci ***(including***

MRSA), enterococci, peptostreptococci, *Corynebacterium diphtheriae, Listeria, Clostridium tetani, C. perfringens* and *Bacillus anthracis*. It is not effective against Gram-negative rods.

Parenteral vancomycin is primarily used for infections caused by methicillin-resistant *Staph aureus* (MRSA) or for *Staph. epidermidis* infections associated with the use of intravascular catheters or with continuous peritoneal dialysis. It is also effective for the treatment of *Staph. enterocolitis* and endocarditis. A combination of vancomycin + gentamicin is synergistic against enterococci and is useful in enterococcal endocarditis. Vancomycin orally is effective in controlling pseudomembranous colitis (PMC) when *C. difficile* colitis is not responding to metronidazole. High grade resistance of pneumococci to penicillin is also an indication for its use. To avoid development of resistance, it has been suggested that the use of vancomycin should be limited to the treatment of serious infections caused by MRSA, or for PMC not controlled by metronidazole or to treat infections where the use of other antibiotics should be avoided.

It is poorly absorbed from GIT, if given orally. Its oral use is restricted to treat antibiotic-associated PMC. Its preferred route of administration is intravenous (500 mg I.V., QID or 1 g I.V., BD). 90% of the unchanged drug is excreted through kidney. Doses have to be adjusted in renal failure. ***Adverse effects*** include "red neck syndrome" (due to histamine release) which can be prevented by giving slow infusion or by increasing dose interval. Minor incidences include ototoxicity, nephrotoxicity, skin rash, reversible neutropenia, eosinophilia, chills and fever.

2. Teicoplanin and Ramoplanin

Teicoplanin is very similar to vancomycin in its mechanism of action, antibacterial spectrum and clinical use. ***It is more active than vancomycin against enterococci but equally effective against MRSA***. It is used as prophylaxis against endocarditis, peritonitis (associated with continued peritoneal dialysis) and to treat PMC or infections in immunocompromised patients. Cross-sensitivity with vancomycin is rare and it can be used in patients intolerant to vancomycin.

Unlike vancomycin (which may cause tissue necrosis) it can be given I.M. as well as I.V. Its plasma half-life is 50 hrs. It is given as a loading dose of 400 mg I.V. on 1st day followed by maintenance dose of 200 mg from the 2nd day. Unlike vancomycin, it rarely causes "red neck syndrome" or nephrotoxicity. However, occasional bronchospasm has been reported.

Ramoplanin is an analogue of teicoplanin. It is administered orally, and not absorbed systemically. It is under fast-track approval by FDA for treating *Clostridium difficile* induced pesudomembranous colitis (PMC) and to eliminate vancomycin-resistant *Enterococcus* (VRE) colonization in GIT.

3. Telavancin, Dalbavancin and Oritavancin

These are second generation glycopeptides similar to vancomycin and teicoplanin (see below) in mode of action, spectrum of activity and clinical uses.

Telavancin

It is a semisynthetic lipoglycopeptide derivative of vancomycin. Its half-life is 8 hrs allowing once daily I.V. dosing (8 mg/kg). Like vancomycin, it inhibits bacterial cell wall synthesis but exhibits a rapid bactericidal effect unlike vancomycin which is a slow acting bactericidal agent. Besides telavancin also acts through an additional mechanism similar to deptomycin which disrupts bacterial cell membrane due to its lipophilic side chain. As a result it is more potent than vancomycin against MRSA and is used as an alternative to vancomycin, linezolid and daptomycin for treating skin and soft tissue infections. It is a last choice antibiotic for ventilator-associated and hospital acquired pneumonia as well as catheter-induced urinary and systemic infections. Its use, however, is limited due to its adverse effects-renal toxicity, teratogenicity and prolongation of QTc interval.

Dalbavancin

It is a semisynthetic lipoglycopeptide derivative of teicoplanin and exhibits the same mechanism of action as vancomycin and teicoplanin. The drug shows enhanced bactericidal activity against MRSA, coagulase- negative staphylococci and enterococci but does not act on the vancomycin resistant enterococci. It has a extremely long half-life (6–11 days) allowing once weekly I.V. dosing by infusion. It has been approved for treatment of skin and soft tissue infections caused by MRSA and catheter-related bloodstream infections where it seems to be superior to vancomycin. *Dalbavancin* does not cause infusion-related reaction and nephrotoxicity. GIT upset has been reported in some cases after administration of the drug.

Oritavancin

It is a synthetic glycopeptide. Like dalbavancin, it possesses long half-life permitting once weekly I.V. dosing by infusion and display increased activity against MRSA, vancomycin resistant staphylococci and enterococci (against latter neither telavancin nor dalbavancin show antibacterial activity). It has been approved for use in treating serious skin and soft tissue infections caused by staphylococci (including MRSA), streptococci; both drugs can also be used for treatment of enterococcal infections. Oritavancin, like vancomycin has similar toxic effects except the much lower risk of nephrotoxicity. Both telavancin and oritavancin have been reported to interfere with the commercially available anticoagulant assays, and may give falsely prolonged prothrombin time, activated partial thromboplastin and activated clotting time (PT, aPTT, aCT). This may also result in a falsely elevated INR. Therefore it is advised that blood should be drawn for these assays at the time of trough plasma concentration of these drugs.

Miscellaneous Group

1. *Daptomycin*

It is a new lipoglycopeptide antibacterial drug similar to vancomycin. However, vancomycin acts in a time-dependent manner, whereas deptomycin shows a concentration-dependent antibacterial activity. It is used for I.V. treatment of complicated resistent Gram-positive infections of the skin and soft tissues caused by organisms like MRSA and vancomycin-resistance enterococci as an alternative to linezolid and quinupristin/dalfopristin. With gentamicin it shows greater antimicrobial synergy against enterococci and MRSA, than vancomycin. It is a useful alternative to vancomycin but cannot be used to treat pneumonia as it is inactivated by pulmonary surfactant.

2. *Bacitracin*

Bacitracin is a mixture of polypeptide-antibiotics produced by *Bacillus subtilis*. Unlike penicillins, it does not contain a β-lactam ring. Bacitracin is primarily a ***topical antibiotic***. It is not absorbed from GIT following oral administration. It is highly active against *Staphylococcus aureus*, *Streptococcus pyogenes* and *Clostridium difficile*. Gram-negative organisms except *Neisseria* and *H. influenzae* are resistant. It can be given by mouth to treat PMC associated with *Clostridium difficile*. As ointment or as eye drops it is used in conjunction with other agents such as neomycin, polymyxin-B and sometimes with corticosteroid. Systemic absorption may lead to nephrotoxicity.

3. *Fosfomycin*

It is a phosphonic acid derivative. It is bactericidal against a range of Gram-positive and Gram-negative bacteria including *Staph. aureus*, some streptococci and most of enterobacteriaceae, *H. influenzae*, *P. aeruginosa* and *Neisseria* species. *Bacteroides* are resistant. There is no cross resistance with other antimicrobials. It demonstrates synergistic effects when combined with penicillins, cephalosporins, aminoglycosides or fluoroquinolones. A single 3 g oral dose is used to treat uncomplicated lower UTIs in women.

It is poorly absorbed from GIT but *fosfomycin trometamol* salt can be used both orally as well as parenterally. It is excreted 90–95% unchanged through kidney. *Adverse effects* include GIT distress, skin rash, visual disturbances, exacerbation of asthma and cholestatic jaundice (on prolonged use). The drug is safe in pregnancy.

4. *Cycloserine*

The drug is D-alanine analogue. It acts by disrupting bacterial cell wall synthesis via inhibiting two enzymes that convert L-alanine to D-alanine (racemase) and its subsequent interlinking to D-alanyl-D-alanine (ligase) during the formation peptidoglycan.

It is an orally effective drug which acts against many Gram-positive and Gram-negative bacteria.

However, it is exclusively used as a second line drug to treat tuberculosis due to *Mycobacterium tuberculosis* (Ch. 59) where it serves as a part of multidrug regimen. It is completely absorbed from GIT; widely distributed and crosses BBB and placental barrier. It is largely excreted unchanged by glomerular filtration. Plasma half-life is 10 hrs which is prolonged in renal impairment. *Adverse effects* include dose related CNS toxicity such as headache, vertigo, tremors, psychotic manifestations and seizures. These reactions subside after dose reduction or on discontinuation of the drug. Serum aminotransferase values may be raised. Folate or vitamin B_{12} deficiency can occur when used with other antitubercular drugs.

Levocycloserine is under trials for the treatment of Gaucher's disease (hereditary disorder involving reticuloendothelial hyperplasia).

CHAPTER 56 Aminoglycosides

COMPETENCY PH1.42

Aminoglycosides are bactericidal antibiotics which interfere with the ribosomal functions and inhibit the protein synthesis of bacteria (see Ch. 52 and mechanism of action discussed below). *Streptomycin,* and all other aminoglycosides whose name end with the suffix *"mycin",* are obtained from the genus of fungus *Streptomyces;* while *gentamicin,* and others whose names end with the suffix *"micin"* are obtained from the genus of bacterium *Micromonospora.* The names of the semisynthetic derivatives, e.g., *netilmicin* and *plazomicin* also end with the suffix "micin".

CHEMISTRY

The term aminoglycosides stems from their structure characterised by two aminosugars joined to a aminocyclitol (a nonsugar) moiety by a glycosidic (-O-) bond (see Ch. 2 also). In majority of aminoglycosides, the aminocyclitol moiety is 2-deoxystreptamine which is placed centrally in between two aminosugars as shown below:

aminosugar -O- 2-deoxystreptamine -O- aminosugar

However, in streptomycin, the aminocyclitol is streptidine which is not placed centrally as in other aminoglycosides. Rather, it is placed laterally to the aminosugar (streptose), which in turn is joined to another aminosugar (*N*-methyl-L-glucosamine). These two aminosugars are jointly called streptobiosamine (see below).

Streptidine -O- Streptose aminosugar -O- N-methyl-L-glucosamine aminosugar

(Streptose aminosugar + N-methyl-L-glucosamine aminosugar = **Streptobiosamine**)

The group includes Streptomycin, Gentamicin, Sisomicin, Netilmicin, Kanamycin, Tobramycin, Amikacin, Neomycin, Paromomycin, Soframycin and Spectinomycin. The latter, however, is not a true aminoglycoside because, though it is obtained from the genus *Streptomyces* its aminocyclitol is not connected to any aminosugar.

MECHANISM OF ACTION

Initially, the aminoglycosides penetrate through the bacterial cell wall, to periplasmic space, through porin channels by passive diffusion. *That is why, β-lactam antibiotics which weaken or inhibit the bacterial cell wall synthesis, facilitate the passive diffusion of aminoglycosides if given together* (synergistic action, Ch. 55). Subsequently, further transport of aminoglycosides across the cytoplasmic membrane takes place by energy and O_2 dependent active transport. *Since such transport cannot take place under anaerobic conditions, aminoglycosides are inactive against anaerobic bacteria* (see below).

These drugs then bind to 30S ribosomal subunits of the bacteria and prevent the formation of "initiation complex" which is the prerequisite for peptide synthesis (Fig. 52.2). Lack of the formation of "initiation complex" causes the 30S subunit to misread the genetic code on mRNA. Incorrect amino acids are thus incorporated into the growing peptide chain, which are of no use for bacterial growth.

The formation of improper ''initiation complex" also blocks the movement of ribosomes, resulting in a mRNA chain attached with single ribosomes (monosomes). Thus aminoglycosides also interfere in the assembly of polysomes, which results in the accumulation of nonfunctional ribosomes.

POST-ANTIBIOTIC EFFECT (PAE)

Aminoglycosides exhibit ***concentration-dependent killing***, i.e., their increased concentration kills an increasing proportion of bacteria at a rapid rate. They also possess significant ***post-antibiotic effect (PAE)***, which means that they continue to suppress the bacterial growth for several hours even when their serum concentration falls below their MIC. It is likely that the disruption in 30S ribosomal function accounts for this post-antibiotic effect (residual bactericidal efficacy) because resumption of bacterial ribosomal functions requires time for the synthesis of new ribosomes after their inhibition with aminoglycosides. The PAE of aminoglycoside can explain why these drugs can be given in a single daily dose despite their short half-life (1–3 hrs).

Clinical trials of single daily dosing of aminoglycosides have been conducted on adults, pregnant women and children for a variety of indications, including serious infections, and it has been confirmed that single daily dosing of aminoglycosides are at least as effective and no more toxic (even less toxic) than multiple dosing as has been the usual practice. Uptake of aminoglycosides across the brush border of proximal renal cortical tubular cells is a capacity-limited saturable process. Therefore, giving a single large dose results in an enhanced bactericidal activity with lesser renal accumulation to cause nephrotoxicity (or even ototoxicity). Giving aminoglycoside as a single daily dose results in a higher peak tissue concentration than if the total daily dose were divided and administered at 8 or 12 hrly interval.

While single daily dosing of aminoglycosides for 4 to 5 days is justified in most patients having serious infections, it may not be suitable in the following situations: **(a)** In the cases of renal insufficiency where selection of appropriate dose is particularly critical and repeating the same dose could be disastrous, and **(b)** when aminoglycosides are given to provide synergism with β-lactam antibiotics in enterococcal endocarditis.

ANTIBACTERIAL RESISTANCE

Three principal mechanisms for the development of resistance have been identified: **(1)** Synthesis of plasmid-mediated bacterial transferase enzymes that can inactivate aminoglycosides. These enzymes are 6'-acetyltransferase, 2'-phosphotransferase, 3'-phosphotransferase and 4'-adenylyltransferase, which inactivate aminoglycosides by acetylation, phosphorylation and adenylylation, respectively. **(2)** Due to decreased transport of aminoglycoside into the bacterial cytosol. This may result from mutation or deletion of porin channel or proteins involved in transport or by making the oxygen + energy-dependent transport system nonfunctional. **(3)** By deletion or alteration of the target receptor protein on 30S ribosomal subunit because of mutations to prevent attachment of the drug with the 30S ribosomal subunit.

PHARMACOKINETICS

Aminoglycosides are highly polar, basic drugs which do not permit their membrane permeability. As a result, these have very poor oral bioavailability; virtually the entire oral dose is excreted in faeces. These are, therefore, given parenterally (I.V. or I.M.) or applied locally (as ointments or eye drops). These are poorly distributed and poorly protein bound. When given parenterally they fail to reach intraocular fluid or CSF. As they do not penetrate most cellular compartments, they do not undergo any significant metabolism. Nearly all of an I.V. dose (90–95%) is cleared by kidney through glomerular filtration resulting in fairly high urinary concentration which makes them useful in most UTIs. Use of urinary alkaliser increases their effectiveness in the treatment of UTI, because these drugs are more active at alkaline pH rather than acidic.

Their excretion is directly proportional to creatinine clearance of the patient. Though normal half-life varies from 1.5–3 hrs, it may increase to 24–48 hrs in patients with renal insufficiency. These are only partly removed by peritoneal or haemodialysis. Hence dose adjustment is needed to avoid toxicity in patients with renal insufficiency. Normally, the dose interval is kept constant but the dose is scaled down as desired. However, in view of their post-antibiotic effect some clinicians prefer to keep the dose as constant but increase the interval between the two doses.

The simplest formula uses the serum creatinine levels to adjust the doses in renal insufficiency as shown below:

$$\text{Dose for a case of renal insufficiency} = \frac{\text{Normal therapeutic dose}}{\text{Serum creatinine value (mg/dL)}}$$

Thus, if a 70 kg normal patient (serum creatinine value 1 mg/dL) receives 350 mg/day (I.M.) of gentamicin (5 mg/kg/day), then the same person with a serum creatinine value of 3.5 mg/dL would receive 350/3.5, i.e.. 100 mg/day (I.M.) which may be administered in two equally divided doses (i.e., 50 mg BD, I.M.). However, the most precise method for calculating the dose for such patient must use creatinine clearance values of an individual because aminoglycoside clearance is directly proportional to his creatinine clearance value. The calculation of dose by this method is discussed in Chapter 6.

ANTIBACTERIAL SPECTRUM

The activity of aminoglycosides is primarily directed against Gram-negative aerobic bacilli *(E. coli, Klebsiella, Shigella, Proteus,* including *Enterobacter* and *Pseudomonas aeruginosa,* **except *Salmonella*)**. Most enterobacteriaceae are sensitive to aminoglycosides. **Only a few Gram-positive cocci** (*Staphylococcus aureus, Streptococcus viridans* and *faecalis,* not others) **are inhibited by these drugs**. However, there are some differences among the aminoglycosides in their efficacy towards specific microorganisms. These differences are highlighted under individual drugs. **Aminoglycosides are not effective against Gram-positive bacilli, Gram-negative cocci and anaerobes.**

INDIVIDUAL DRUGS AND CLINICAL USES

Streptomycin

Ribosomal resistance to streptomycin develops fast, which has limited its usefulness as a single agent except for few indications cited below. In plague, tularemia and brucellosis, streptomycin (1 g/day I.M.) is used effectively but in combination with an oral tetracycline. Streptomycin and penicillin combination therapy, for 2 weeks, is effective for subacute bacterial endocarditis (SABE) due to *Strepto. viridans* and *Strepto. faecalis* as well as for bacteraemia, but gentamicin is more preferred. Earlier, it was the first line drug for the treatment of tuberculosis (TB). Presently, it has been kept as a reserve drug among the Anti-TB first line drugs. However, it should be used only in combination with other anti-TB drugs to prevent emergence of resistance (for other details see Ch. 59).

Gentamicin

It is the most commonly used aminoglycoside, often acting synergistically with ampicillin, benzathine penicillin-G, ticarcillin, ceftriaxone and vancomycin. For septicaemia, sepsis and fever in immuno-compromised patients, it is used in combination with penicillins. For pelvic infections it is combined with metronidazole (to enlarge spectrum against *B. fragilis).* For SABE, it is used along with benzathine penicillin-G. For coliform infection (as in UTIs) it is combined with ampicillin or ceftriaxone, while for pseudomonal infections it is usually combined with ticarcillin. A combination of vancomycin with gentamicin is synergistic against enterococci and is useful against enterococcal endocarditis in patients with a history of penicillin allergy. It is administered in a dose of 3–5 mg/kg/day, I.M. in divided doses at 8 hrly interval for 7–10 days. Once daily dose of 5–7 mg/kg is equally effective, and even less toxic, than 8 hrly dosing. Topically (0.1–0.3%) it is used as cream, ointment or eye drops for the treatment of infected burns, wound and bacterial conjunctivitis. However, it is inactivated by purulent exudates of wounds. Hence it is not useful in presence of pus.

Sisomicin

It is similar to gentamicin but exhibits greater efficacy against *Pseudomonas* and beta-haemolytic *Streptococci*. It is generally used interchangeably with gentamicin in the same doses and for similar therapeutic uses. Neither it is resistant to degradation by aminoglycoside inactivating enzymes nor does it offer any advantage over gentamicin in terms of toxicity.

Tobramycin

It is also clinically interchangeable with gentamicin

and the difference in their toxicities is also inconsequential (though a few reports suggest that tobramycin is less nephrotoxic). Its current status is its usefulness against infections due to *Pseudomonas, Proteus* and *Acinetobacter* resistant to gentamicin.

Netilmicin

It is a semisynthetic derivative of sisomicin. It is relatively resistant to aminoglycoside-inactivating enzymes and thus serves as a better alternative to gentamicin or tobramycin resistant infections caused by indole-positive *Proteus, Pseudomonas, Klebsiella. E. coli* and *Staph. aureus.* The doses and routes of administration are same as for gentamicin. It is therapeutically interchangeable with gentamicin or tobramycin and has similar toxicities, though there are a few reports to support that it has lesser ototoxicity.

Arbekacin

Arbekacin shows potent broad spectrum concentration-dependant antimicrobial activity against MDR bacteria including methicellin-reistent *Staphylococcus aureus* (MRSA) and Gram-negative pathogens (such as *Pseudomonas* spp., *Acinobacter* spp., *Enterobater* spp., *K.pneumoniae, E.coli*). Arbekacin remains stable and resist inactivation in presence of aminoglycoside-modifying enzymes (AMEs) produced by MRSA and other sensitive Gram-negative bacteria for which gentamicin, tobramycin, amikacin fail to work due to their inactivation.

This antibiotic was approved in Japan in 1990 under the trade name Habekacin for the treatment of sepsis and pneumonia by MRSA but because of its novelty that it is not destroyed by AMEs, it has been approved in India in 2017 (still not approved in USA and Europe) for use in bacterial infections resistant to β-lactams and aminoglycosides (vide supra). It is marketed as an I.V. injectable formulation of 200 mg/4 mL to be given in the doses of 1–3 mg/kg or 200 mg/24 hr to reach the target concentration of (C_{peak}) of 10–15 mcg/mL and C_{trough} < 2 mcg/mL.

It produces ototoxicity and nephrotoxicity and neuromuscular blockade. The nephrotoxicity, as such is less in patients with normal renal function (crCL ≥80ml/min) but TDM is required if crCL is low. It shows a t½ of 3.5 hrs and a PAE of an equal duration (2.3–3.5 hrs) enabling it to be given by once daily I.M. or slow I.V. dosing.

Plazomicin

It shows potent concentration-dependent antibacatieral activity against both the **E**xtended **S**pectrum **β-L**actamase (**E**SBL)-**p**roducing **E**nterobacteriaceae (EPE) and Carbapenemase (-producing) **C**arbapenem-**r**esistant **E**nterobacteriaceae (CRE) which are currently resistant to all currently available aminoglycosides (Plazomicin MIC 1 mcg/mL vs. 4–8 mcg/mL of amikacin and gentamicin). The drug has been approved for the treatment of complicated **U**rinary **T**ract **I**nfection (cUTI) including Pyelonephritis and **B**lood **S**tream **I**nfections (BSI) caused by EPE and CRE pathogens who have limited or no alternative treatment.

Plazomcin is available as 500 mg/10mL single dose vial. The dose is I.V. 15 mg/kg per 24 hr for 4–7 days for cUTI. It can produce ototoxicity, nephrotoxicity and neuromuscular blockade. TDM is required and dose adjustements are needed if renal function is compromised. Hypersensitivity reaction and *C.difficile* diarrhea may occur during the course of therapy.

Kanamycin and Amikacin

Kanamycin produces higher ototoxicity and nephrotoxicity, it is reserved as second line injectable anti-TB drug (Ch. 59).

Amikacin is a less toxic, semi-synthetic derivative of kanamycin and is next commonly used aminoglycoside than gentamicin. It is resistant to the enzymes that inactivate gentamicin and tobramycin and hence used against gentamicin/tobramycin-resistant Gram-negative bacilli such as *Pseudomonas, Proteus* and *Serratia.* It is also effective in multidrug resistant *Mycobacterium tuberculosis* (including streptomycin-resistant strains) but is used in combination with other anti-TB drugs. Usual dose is 7.5–15 mg/kg/day I.M. or I.V. in two equally divided doses at 12 hrly interval.

Neomycin and Framycetin

Neomycin and Framycetin (Soframycin) are too toxic for parenteral use. Neomycin and framycetin are now limited to topical use. Neomycin, however, has some restricted oral use also. Leaving aside *Pseudomonas* and streptococci which are resistant, these drugs are active against some Gram-positive and Gram-negative bacteria.

(1) Neomycin with polymyxin-B solution is used as an irrigant in the urinary bladder to prevent bacteriuria associated with the use of indwelling catheter. **(2)** Neomycin is often combined with bacitracin (to extend spectrum for Gram-positive organisms) and polymyxin-B (to extend spectrum against *Pseudomonas)* to prevent infection in minor cuts, wounds and burns as well as to treat superficial external ear and eye infections. Such combinations are available as ointment or eye/ear drops. **(3)** Neomycin is also used orally as preoperative intestinal antiseptic (1 g TDS or QID) a day before surgery along with erythromycin (250 mg QID) to reduce aerobic bowel flora. **(4)** Neomycin (1 g TDS or QID with reduced protein intake) is useful in hepatic coma, as it suppresses ammonia-producing coliform bacterial flora. Blood ammonia levels therefore get decreased and encephalopathy (widespread degeneration of brain tissue) is thus prevented. Blood urea levels also get decreased because lesser ammonia is now available for conversion to urea. However, lactulose (Ch. 29) is more preferred as it is much less toxic.

Framycetin ointment is used for skin infections, otitis externa, furunculosis, burns and scalds. Eye drops are used for ophthalmic infections.

Paromomycin

Paromomycin (1 g QID orally for 2 weeks) can be used to treat intestinal amoebiasis. It is also used orally to treat cryptosporidiosis in immunocom-promised patients. It is an infection with *Cryptosporidium parvum*, a coccidian protozoa found in intestinal tract of humans and domestic animals. It is presented with chronic watery diarrhoea with abdominal cramps which becomes severe in AIDS patients.

Spectinomycin

Spectinomycin is used in a single dose of 40 mg/kg I.M. (up to a maximum of 2 g) as an alternative treatment for gonorrhoea in patients who are allergic to penicillin. *Adverse effects* include pain at the site of injection; occasional fever and nausea; but nephrotoxicity or ototoxicity are very rare.

ADVERSE EFFECTS

All aminoglycosides are nephrotoxic, ototoxic and produce curare type neuromuscular blockade.

Nephrotoxicity

Among aminoglycosides, *neomycin, gentamicin, amikacin* and *tobramycin* are more nephrotoxic than streptomycin. This toxicity is encountered when therapy is continued for several days and in settings of renal insufficiency, biliary obstruction or hepatitis. Nephrotoxicity results in the rise in serum creatinine levels (> 1.5 mg/dL). A concurrent use of loop diuretics (furosemide and ethacrynic acid) or of other nephrotoxic agents such as vancomycin, amphotericin-B, polymyxin-B, cisplatin and cyclosporine potentiate the nephrotoxicity. The aminoglycoside-induced nephrotoxicity is nearly always reversible.

Ototoxicity

Aminoglycosides cause impairment of 8th cranial nerve function. They accumulate in the endolymph and the perilymph of the inner ear leading to vestibular and cochlear damage which may be irreversible. Vestibular damage is characterised by vertigo, ataxia and loss of balance while cochlear damage leads to hearing loss and tinnitus. Vestibular toxicity is more with *streptomycin* and *gentamicin* while cochlear toxicity is more with *neomycin* and *amikacin. Tobramycin* has both types of ototoxicity. *Netilmicin* has been claimed to have low ototoxicity but reports are inconclusive. The aminoglycoside-induced ototoxicity is worsened by coadministration of vancomycin, furosemide, ethacrynic acid while lessened by Ca^{2+}.

Neuromuscular Blockade

Among aminoglycosides *streptomycin* can cause neuromuscular junction blockade (see Ch. 14). This is usually relevant in patients of myasthenia gravis only or in situations where some other skeletal muscle relaxant is to be coadministered (as the blockade may be aggravated). The neuromuscular blockade can be reversed by an administration of I.V. calcium gluconate or I.M. neostigmine.

CHAPTER 57 Macrolides, Ketolides, Lincosamides, Oxazolidinones & Other Antibacterial Drugs

COMPETENCY PH1.42

The antimicrobial agents covered in this chapter are: **(a)** Protein synthesis inhibitors which act mainly by binding to 50S ribosomal subunits. These include macrolides, ketolides, lincosamides, streptogramins and oxazolidinones. Chloramphenicol also acts by the same mechanism but has an entirely different spectrum of activity and hence discussed separately under broad-spectrum antibiotics (Ch. 58); **(b)** A miscellaenous group of drugs that have only limited use and act by diverse mechanisms. These include polymyxin-B, colistin (polymyxin-E), mupirocin and fusidic acid.

MACROLIDES

The term "macrolides" means a multimembered lactone ring structure to which one or more deoxysugar molecules are attached. The prototype macrolide is ***erythromycin*** which has a 14 member lactone ring attached with two deoxysugar moieties and is derived from *Streptomyces erythreus*. ***Roxithromycin***, ***clarithromycin*** and ***azithromycin*** are semisynthetic derivatives of erythromycin. ***Spiramycin*** is also related to erythromycin but is obtained from *Streptomyces ambafaciens*.

Mechanism of Action

Macrolides inhibit protein synthesis by binding reversibly to the 'P' site of the 50S ribosomal subunit of the bacteria. Precisely, these drugs inhibit the translocation step (Fig. 52.2) wherein t-RNA with its growing peptide chain is translocated (shifted) from the 'A' site to the 'P' site. As a result, the ribosome cannot move on one codon further towards right, relative to m-RNA. In other words the 'A' (acceptor) site (due to inhibition of translocation) does not become free to accept the next incoming t-RNA charged with desired amino acid. The protein synthesis thus stops (for details refer Ch. 52 & Fig. 52.2). Macrolides do not inhibit the 60S or 40S ribosomal units of mammalian cells, nor do these drugs permeate through mitochondrial membrane of the host cells; this accounts for their selective toxicity.

Antimicrobial activity of macrolides is enhanced by alkaline pH, because these are weakly basic drugs and increased pH results in more of the unionised form of the drug for penetration into the bacterial cells.

Resistance

Resistance to macrolides results primarily from modification of the receptor sites on the 50S ribosomes, through a methylation reaction (ribosomal protection) which results in a decreased binding of the drug. Efflux systems represent another predominant mechanism of macrolide resistance (but not of lincosamides or streptogramin-B). Another form of resistance to macrolides is their failure to permeate through bacterial cell membrane. Some resistant enterobacteriaceae produce esterases enzymes that hydrolyse macrolides. Active efflux mechanism and methylase production account for the vast majority of resistant strains in Gram-positive organisms.

Antibacterial Spectrum

Antimicrobial spectrum of macrolides, in general, overlaps considerably with that of ampicillin. Erythromycin, therefore, is used in patients allergic to the penicillins. However, individual drugs have differing activity against different microorganisms. The macrolides are effective against a number of organisms cited below:

1. **Gram-positive cocci**: ***Streptococcus pneumoniae***, ***Strepto. pyogenes*** and *Staphylococci* (most of penicillin-resistant staphylococci are now macrolide resistant also).
2. Gram-negative cocci: *Neisseria gonorrhoeae* and *Moraxella catarrhalis*.

3. **Gram-positive bacilli**: ***Corynebacterium diphtheriae***, *Bacillus anthracis*, *Listeria monocytogenes* and *Clostridium tetani*.
4. **Gram-negative bacilli**: ***Legionella pneumophila***, ***Bordetella pertussis***, ***Bartonella henselae***, *Haemophilus influenzae*, *H. ducreyi*, ***Campylobacter jejuni***, and *Helicobacter pylori*.
5. Acid-Fast Bacilli: *Mycobacterium kansasii*, *Mycobacterium avium intracellulare*, *Mycobacterium avium complex* and *Mycobacterium leprae*.
6. Spirochaetes: *Treponema pallidum*
7. **Miscellaneous Organisms**: ***Mycoplasma pneumoniae***, ***Ureaplasma urealyticum***, ***Chlamydia trachomatis***, *Chlamydia pneumoniae* and *Chlamydia psittaci*.

- The microorganisms listed in **bold face** are highly sensitive to ***erythromycin***.
- Strains resistant to macrolides include *Peptostreptococcus, Actinobacillus, Pasteurella, Fusobacterium*, *B. fragilis*, MRSA, enterobacteriaceae (including *Salmonella*) and *Mycobacterium tuberculosis*. *H. influenzae* has lately become resistant.
- ***Roxithromycin*** has the same spectrum as of erythromycin but it is more potent against *Moraxella catarrhalis* and *Legionella*; and less potent against *Bordetella pertussis*.
- ***Clarithromycin*** has increased activity against *Moraxella catarrhalis*, *Legionella pneumophila*, *H. influenzae* and *Chlamydia trachomatis*, compared to erythromycin. In addition it is highly active against *Mycobacterium avium complex*, *Mycobacterium leprae*, *Helicobacter pylori* and *Toxoplasma gondii* (see uses).
- ***Azithromycin*** has an extended spectrum compared to erythromycin. It has a higher activity against *H. influenzae*, *Moraxella catarrhalis*, *Chlamydia trachomatis*, *Mycoplasma pneumoniae*, *Mycobacterium avium complex*, *Campylobacter jejuni*, *H. ducreyi* and *N. gonorrhoeae*. It is also effective against *Toxoplasma gondii*.
- ***Spiramycin*** also resembles erythromycin in its spectrum, though it has weaker activity. However, it is highly efficacious against *Toxoplasma gondii* and *Cryptosporidium* (causes watery diarrhoea with abdominal cramps).

Pharmacokinetics

- ***Erythromycin*** free base is destroyed by gastric acid and therefore administered orally with an enteric coating that dissolves in duodenum. Food interferes with its absorption. Ester forms (stearate or ethylsuccinate) or ester salts (estolate) are available to overcome this problem and to protect it from acid degradation. Lactobionate, the water soluble salt of the drug, is available for I.V. administration. I.M. injections are painful and usually not preferred. Erythromycin estolate is the best absorbed oral preparation that can be taken without any regard to meals.

  Erythromycin is well distributed and produces therapeutic concentrations in tonsillar tissue, middle ear fluid, lungs and prostatic fluid. It achieves high concentration in alveolar macrophages and neutrophils. CSF levels are only 15–20% of plasma levels. It is metabolised by liver and primarily excreted through bile and lost in faeces. Only 5% is excreted through urine, hence doses need not be adjusted in renal failure. Plasma half-life is about 1.5 hrs.
- ***Roxithromycin*** is a semisynthetic derivative of erythromycin. It is a long acting (t½ 12 hrs), acid stable macrolide. Food does not interfere with its oral absorption. Longer half-life makes it suitable for twice daily dosing.
- ***Clarithromycin***, an O-methyl derivative of erythromycin, is also an acid stable macrolide. Food does not interfere with its oral absorption. Its longer half-life (t½ 6–7 hrs) permits twice daily dosing. It is metabolised in liver to 14-hydroxyclarithromycin which also has good antimicrobial activity. The drug and its metabolite are excreted through kidney. Dose adjustments are needed in patients with compromised renal functions.
- ***Azithromycin*** is more acid stable with wider tissue distribution (except CSF). Therapeutic concentrations are achieved in lung, genital tissue, liver, prostate and also in phagocytes, macrophages and fibrolasts from where it is slowly released. Elimination half-life is about 68 hrs, which permits once daily dosing, and shortening the duration of treatment (3 days). Food interferes with its

absorption; hence it is administered either 1 hr before or 2 hrs after meals. It does not inhibit cytochrome P-450 enzymes in liver (see under adverse effects). It is largely excreted unchanged in the bile; renal excretion is only 5–10%. It also exhibits significant ***post-antibiotic effect***.

- ***Spiramycin*** is incompletely absorbed from GIT but is given orally as well as intravenously. It has high tissue distribution except in CSF. It is metabolised in liver and excreted (90%) in the bile and only 10% in urine. It is also secreted through breast milk. Plasma half-life is 8 hrs.

Therapeutic Uses

- At present there are relatively few indications for ***erythromycin*** use. It is a first choice drug for:

  (1) atypical pneumonia caused by *Mycoplasma pneumoniae*, **(2)** Legionnaire's pneumonia, **(3)** whooping cough due to *B. pertussis*, **(4)** eradication of *Corynebacterium diphtheriae* from pharyngeal carriers, though antitoxin is the primary treatment.

  It is a second choice drug for treating: **(1)** Campylobacter gastroenteritis (but fluoroquinolones are more preferred), **(2)** chancroid due to *H. ducreyi*, though doses are higher (2 g/day for 7 days) where it is as effective as cotrimoxazole and **(3)** chlamydial conjunctivitis and urethritis. Erythromycin can also be used as prophylaxis against endocarditis during dental procedures in individuals with valvular heart disease though clindamycin, which is better tolerated, has largely replaced it. Erythromycin is effectively being used to treat acute orofacial infections in dentistry, as an alternative to β-lactam antibiotics. Usual oral dose of erythromycin is 250 mg 6 hrly but higher doses are required to treat Legionnaire's pneumonia and chancroid.

  Non-Chemotherapeutic Use: **(1)** *Erythromycin* possesses anti-inflammatory effects distinct from its antimicrobial actions by decreasing proinflammatory cytokines release from the phagocytes, which may prove useful in the management of rheumatoid arthritis, cystic fibrosis, chronic sinusitis and asthma. **(2)** *Erythromycin,* being a motilin receptor agonist, can be used to improve gastric emptying in cases of diabetic gastroparesis (Ch. 28). Motilin is a regulatory peptide of GIT that stimulates phasic contractions of the stomach leading to enhanced gastric emptying.

- Therapeutic uses of ***roxithromycin*** are similar to erythromycin but it is more preferred for treating otitis media, sinusitis and pneumonia caused by *Moraxella catarrhalis* and pneumonia caused by *Legionella*. However, it is less potent against *B. pertussis* (whooping cough). Usual oral doses are 150 mg at 12 hrly intervals.

- ***Clarithromycin*** and erythromycin are virtually similar with respect to their use except that clarithromycin has some additional indications of potential value. Clarithromycin is very effective against *Mycobacterium avium complex*, *H. influenzae, Toxoplasma gondii*, *Mycoplasma leprae* and *H. pylori*. *Mycobacterium avium complex* (MAC), which includes both *M. avium* and *M. intracellulare* is a common cause of disseminated disease in the later stages of AIDS and is difficult to treat. Combination of clarithromycin 500 mg BD+ ethambutol 15 mg/kg once daily is an effective therapy to suppress the disease. Clarithromycin + minocycline is used for the treatment of lepromatous leprosy caused by *M. leprae*. Clarithromycin 500 mg + omeprazole 20 mg + amoxycillin 1 g each, administered twice daily for 14 days is very effective for the treatment of peptic ulcer caused by *H. pylori* (Ch. 27). It is also used to treat toxoplasmosis encephalitis caused by *Toxoplasma gondii* and to treat exacerbations of chronic bronchitis due to *H. influenzae*. The recommended doses of clarithromycin are 200–500 mg BD.

- ***Azithromycin*** is almost similar to clarithromycin with respect to its clinical use except that it is more active against *H. influenzae, Moraxella catarrhalis* and *Legionella*. It is highly active against *Chlamydia*. Thus a single 1 g dose of azithromycin is extremely efficacious in the treatment of chlamydial cervicitis and urethritis (as an alternative to doxycycline). Azithromycin 500 mg once daily is used for suppression or treatment of disseminated infections caused by *M. avium complex* in AIDS patients. However, clarithromycin + ethambutol combination is considered superior to azithromycin alone. Community acquired pneumonia is also treated with azithromycin given as 500 mg loading dose followed by 250 mg once daily for next 4 days. Other uses of azithromycin are similar to clarithromycin. A 500 mg once daily dose for 3 days is usually sufficient for most infections. Azithromycin 500 mg/day x 3 days is quite effective in treating periapical abscess.

Indications and uses of ***spiramycin*** are similar to erythromycin but it has only restricted use, e.g., treatment of *Toxoplasma gondii* to prevent transmission of infections from mother to fetus. Usual adult dose for most infections is 6–9 MU by mouth daily in 3 divided doses for 5 days. For toxoplasmosis it is 2–3 MU three times a day for 3 weeks, to be repeated after a gap of 2 weeks till parturition.

Adverse Effects

Serious toxicity with macrolides is rare but can be occasionally significant.

1. Among allergic reactions, rashes, fever, eosinophilia and skin eruptions may occur with the use of erythromycin estolate. Hypersensitivity reactions are less common with other salts of erythromycin or with other macrolides.
2. Cholestatic hepatitis is much more common with erythromycin estolate than with other macrolides. It is characterised by jaundice, fever, leukopenia and eosinophilia which disappear after its discontinuation. It is considered to be a result of the hypersensitivity reaction to estolate ester salt. Incidence of cholestatic hepatitis is less with clarithromycin and rare with azithromycin.
3. Erythromycin use is also associated with severe epigastric pain which results from stimulation of gastric smooth muscle motilin receptors (see above and Ch. 28). Azithromycin and clarithromycin are lesser stimulants of motilin receptor (lesser GI side effects).
4. Erythromycin in a dose exceeding 4 g/day is associated with reversible ototoxicity (hearing loss). Tinnitus has been observed even with the therapeutic doses of azithromycin when used for more than 5 days.
5. I.V. administration of erythromycin is associated with thrombophlebitis, which can be minimised by slow rates of infusion.

Drug Interactions

1. ***Erythromycin*** and ***clarithromycin*** inhibit CYP3A4 isoenzyme which can lead to significant drug-drug interactions. Thus, they can inhibit the metabolism and increase the serum levels of theophylline, carbamazepine, statins, warfarin, pimozide, terfenadine and cisapride leading to respective drug toxicities. ***Azithromycin*** does not inactivate CYP3A4 and therefore is free of these drug interactions.
2. Macrolides may seriously decrease digoxin metabolism, and increase its bioavailability, by inhibiting the microbial flora responsible for degrading digoxin.

MACROCYCLIC ANTIBIOTIC

Fidaxomicin

It is a narrow spectrum orally effective antibiotic with bactericidal activity against *C.difficile*, *staphylococci* and *enterococci*, but not Gram negative bacilli. It acts by inhibiting protein synthesis through blockade of RNA polymerase. This drug is a safe alternative to vancomycin for *C.difficile* diarrhoea in the doses of 200 mg BD. Most common adverse effects are nausea, vomiting, headache, abdominal pain, diarrhoea and constipation.

LINCOSAMIDES

The lincosamide family of antibiotics includes ***lincomycin*** and ***clindamycin***. Lincomycin is now obsolete and is no longer in use.

Mechanism of Action and Antibacterial Spectrum

The receptor site for lincosamides is same as that of macrolides. They bind to 50S ribosomal subunits resulting in bacteriostatic inhibition of bacterial protein synthesis.

Clindamycin is highly active against streptococci, pneumococci (except enterococci) and staphylococci (except MRSA). *Bacteroides fragilis*, *Clostridium* (except *Clostridium difficile*) and other anaerobes are usually susceptible. It also shows excellent activity against *Corynebacterium acnes*. In combination with other drugs (see below) it is very effective against *Toxoplasma gondii* and *Pneumocystis carinii.*

Pharmacokinetics

Clindamycin is well absorbed orally. Food does not interfere with its absorption. It penetrates well in most tissues, including bones and phagocytes, excepting CSF. It is metabolised in liver and is primarily excreted in urine and also through bile. Its plasma half-life is 2.5 hrs.

Resistance

Resistance to clindamycin occurs by three mechanisms: **(1)** alterations of the 50S ribosomal subunit by adenine methylation (ribosomal protection like macrolides), **(2)** chromosomal mutation of 50S ribosomal protein (receptor alteration) or **(3)** drug inactivation by a plasmid mediated adenyl transferase.

Clinical Uses

Clindamycin is chiefly used in treating serious anaerobic infections notably due to *Bacteroides fragilis* and susceptible staphylococcal and streptococcal infections such as liver abscess, lung abscess, staphylococcal bone and joint infections, septicaemia and pelvic inflammatory disease (for which it is given with aminoglycoside). It is also used in the prophylaxis of endocarditis in penicillin allergic patients. It can also be applied topically in the treatment of acne. The usual adult dose by mouth is 150–300 mg every 6 hrs.

Clindamycin (300–450 mg QID orally) + primaquine (30 mg/day) for 21 days is an alternative to cotrimoxazole for the treatment of *Penumocystis carinii* pneumonia in AIDS patients. Oral clindamycin (600 mg QID) + pyrimethamine (75 mg/day orally) for 6 weeks are used to treat AIDS patients with toxoplasmic encephalitis (as an alternative for patients who cannot tolerate sulfonamide + pyrimethamine).

Adverse Effects

1. In some patients, clindamycin-associated diarrhoea and pseudomembranous colitis may develop which may prove fatal. This appears to be due to toxins produced by *C. difficile*. The drug should be withdrawn, if this occurs; and metronidazole or vancomycin be used to treat pseudomembranous colitis. Other GIT side effects include nausea, vomiting, abdominal cramps and metallic taste.
2. Higher I.V. doses of clindamycin may result in neuromuscular blockade similar to that of aminoglycosides.
3. Hypersensitivity reactions including rashes, urticaria and stomatitis can occur.

KETOLIDES

Examples: ***Telithromycin*** and ***Cethromycin***

In this group, only ***telithromycin*** is in clinical use (introduced in 2004). Ketolides are 14-membered ring macrolides specifically designed for activity against microorganisms responsible for community acquired respiratory tract infections. Telithromycin is a semisynthetic derivative of erythromycin having a 3-keto group which is crucial in conferring sensitivity to macrolide resistant strains. The mechanism of action of telithromycin is exactly similar to erythromycin. However, an overall enhanced activity of telithromycin, compared to erythromycin, results due to: **(1)** a tighter binding of the drug to the ribosomes of the bacteria and **(2)** a decreased incidence of the development of resistance. The structural modification, as in telithromycin, makes it a poor substrate for the efflux-pump mediated drug resistance. Ketolides exhibit longer ***post-antibiotic effects*** also.

Though telithromycin undergoes first-pass metabolism (30%), its oral bioavailability is good. It achieves high tissue concentration in respiratory fluid, saliva, alveolar macrophages and bronchial mucosa. It is metabolised in the liver and eliminated by a combined biliary (77%) and urinary (18%) routes of excretion. Its plasma half-life is 13.5 hrs. The **antibacterial spectrum** of telithromycin demonstrates enhanced activity against erythromycin resistant Gram-positive cocci, e.g., *Strepto. pyogenes, Strepto. pneumoniae* and *Staph. aureus*; Gram-negative cocci, e.g., *Moraxella catarrhalis*, *N. gonorrhoeae* and *N. meningitidis*; Gram-negative bacilli, e.g., *H. influenzae* and *Legionella pneumophila* and to some anaerobes like *Peptostreptococcus* and *Bacteroides fragilis*.

Telithromycin is **mainly indicated for** macrolide-resistant community acquired pneumonia, acute exacerbations of chronic bronchitis, sinusitis and streptococcal pharyngitis. The usual dosage of telithromycin is 800 mg once daily orally for 10 days. ***Adverse effects*** are mild. Diarrhoea and nausea may occur but no pseudomembranous colitis (modestly active against *Clostridium difficile* also). Like erythromycin, telithromycin also inhibits CYP3A4 and may **(1)** increase blood levels of theophylline, midazolam and simvastatin, **(2)** prolong the QT interval if administered with cisapride, terfenadine and pimozide and **(3)** CYP3A4 inhibitors (like itraconazole) increase its serum concentration.

Cethromycin is more potent than telithromycin, not only against macrolide-susceptible strains but also against macrolide-resistant *Streptococci* and *Enterococci* (except macrolide-resistant *Staph. aureus*). Resistance mechanisms involved are similar to telithromycin (i.e., ribosomal protein mutations and tRNA dimethylation). It has cleared phase III clinical trials.

OXAZOLIDINONES

Examples: ***Linezolid, Radezolid, Torezolid and Tedizolid***

Linezolid is the first totally synthetic new antibiotic of oxazolidinone group.

Mechanism of Action: It inhibits bacterial protein synthesis by binding to the A-site of 50S ribosomal subunit near the interface with 30S subunit, where the amino acid moiety of aminoacyl tRNA normally binds. Oxazolidinones block productive interations of aminoacyl tRNA with the A-site in peptidyl transfarase centre.

Thus the formation of the "*initiation complex*", required for bacterial protein translation (Fig. 52.2), is prevented. This unique mechanism of inhibiting the very first step of the bacterial protein synthesis, minimises the possibility of cross resistance with other antibiotics.

Antimicrobial Spectrum and Uses: Linezolid is effluxed out by Gram-negative bacteria and hence its antimicrobial spectrum is restricted to Gram- positive pathogens only, that lack these specific efflux pumps. Hence, the drug is reserved for the treatment of infections caused by multidrug resistant Gram-positive bacteria. Therefore, it is very useful against infections caused by vancomycin-resistant *Enterococcus faecium* and MRSA (endocarditis, bacteraemia); nosocomial and community acquired pneumonia caused by *Staphylococcus aureus* (including MRSA) and penicillin-sensitive *Strepto. pneumoniae*; complicated skin infections from MRSA and penicillin-resistant *Strepto. pyogenes*. It is also active against some Gram-positive bacilli, e.g., *Corynebacterium diphtheriae*, *Bacillus anthracis*, *Bacteroides fragilis*, *Clostridia* and *Listeria monocytogenes*. It has also been approved for paediatric use and diabetic foot infections. The recommended dose is 500 mg BD (oral/I.V.).

Pharmacokinetics: The oral bioavailability of linezolid is 100% and hence dose adjustment is not required when switching from I.V. to oral and vice versa. Food does not interfere with its absorption. It is metabolised in liver and excreted in urine as free drug and its inactive metabolite (a part is excreted through faeces also). It has a plasma half-life of 4–6 hrs. Post-antibiotic effect lasts for 1.5 hrs. It is not a substrate for any of the cytochrome P-450 isoenzymes.

Adverse Effects: are reversible thrombocytopenia (if used for more than 15 days), reversible neutropenia (if the patient is predisposed to bone marrow suppression) and reversible optic neuropathy (on prolonged use). This results because linezolid binds to mitochondrial 70S ribosomes. Hence, weekly monitoring of platelet counts are required if the drug is to be used for more than a week. Minor adverse effects include diarrhoea (but rarely pseudomembranous colitis as it is active against *C. difficile*), headache, taste alteration and oral candidiasis.

Drug Interactions: Linezolid is a reversible inhibitor of MAO enzyme and may lead to "cheese reaction" with food containing tyramine (Ch. 34). It can also precipitate "serotonin syndrome" (confusion, hypertension, seizures, tachycardia, and muscle rigidity, even death) if used concomitantly with selective serotonin reuptake inhibitors such as fluoxetine (Ch. 34).

Radezolid, Torezolid and Tedizolid are second generation oxazolidinones (structural analogues of linezolid). These oral drugs are more effective members of this chemical class, e.g., these drugs are 4–6-fold more active than linezolid against *staphylococci* and *enterococci* and up to 4-fold higher activity against anaerobes. All three agents appear to have lower rates of myelosuppression and neuropathic toxicity and are relatively safer than linezolid. All these new oxazolidinones are expected to be used in the treatment of serious multidrug resistant infections like uncomplicated skin and skin structures infections and community aquired pneumonia including infections due to Gram-positive bacteria which were sensitive to linezolid but have become resistant to it now.

STREPTOGRAMINS (PRISTINAMYCIN)

It is a synergistic combination of streptogramin-B (***quinupristin***) and streptogramin-A (***dalfopristin***) in a 30:70 ratio, respectively. Both streptogramins bind to different sites of 50S subunit of 70S ribosome and prevent the extrusion of the newly synthesised peptide chain from the ribosome, leading to cell death. Its spectrum closely resembles vancomycin and linezolid. It is used to treat bacteraemia caused by vancomycin-resistant *Enterococcus faecium* (*E. faecalis* is somehow resistant) and skin infections from *Staphylococcus aureus* (including MRSA) and *Strepto. pyogenes*. It is also effective in treating nosocomial pneumonia caused by MRSA, vancomycin resistant *Enterococcus faecium* and *Strepto. pneumoniae*. The usual dose is 7.5 mg/kg every 8–12 hrs, intravenously.

The combination is rapidly metabolised via nonenzymatic reactions to active metabolites. Elimination is mainly by faecal route. Elimination half-life for quinupristin is 0.85 hrs while for dalfopristin is 0.7 hrs. However, the combination has a prolonged post-antibiotic effect and hence can be administered at 12 hrly interval.

Adverse effects include pain at the site of infusion and moderate infusion-related arthralgia-myalgia syndrome. Streptogramins decrease the liver metabolism of Ca^{2+} channel blockers, cyclosporine, statins, diazepam, warfarin, terfenadine, opioids and cisapride (inhibits CYP3A4). Among these, the dose reduction of only cyclosporine may be necessary.

POLYMYXIN-B AND COLISTIN

Both are peptide antibiotics, which being very toxic are rarely used now except topically. Colistin is polymyxin-E, and has a structural similarity to polymyxin-B. It is available as colistin sulfate for oral use and as colistimethate sodium for parenteral use. Both polymyxin-B and colistin (polymyxin-E) function as cationic detergents and disrupt the bacterial cell membrane osmotic integrity by displacing Ca^{2+} and Mg^{2+} from membrane lipid phosphates. This ends up in the leakage of intracellular constituents and the death of bacteria. Polymyxins have a bactericidal action on most Gram-negative bacilli except *Proteus*, *Serratia*, *Providencia* and *Bacteroides fragilis*. But these are remarkably effective against *Pseudomonas aeruginosa*. Polymyxins demonstrate antimicrobial synergy with other antibiotics like bacitracin and neomycin.

Polymyxin-B is not absorbed from GIT (except in newborn). It is not absorbed from the intact skin either. Polymyxin-B sulfate is used primarily topically, often in combination with other drugs, in the treatment of skin, ear and eye infections. It can be given orally for oropharyngeal decontamination or the suppression of intestinal flora in patients with high risk of endogenous infections. Colistin sulfate can be given orally for treating GIT infections. Colistimethate sodium has been used by inhalation in the management of respiratory infections, especially cystic fibrosis. It has also been used as subconjunctival injection for eye infection and for bladder irrigation. Both colistin preparations are also used topically for skin, ear and eye infections.

Adverse effects include neurotoxicity (paraesthesia, ataxia and slurred speech) and nephrotoxicity (haematuria, proteinuria, electrolyte disturbances and tubular necrosis). They cause histamine release which may lead to flushing and bronchoconstriction. They also possess potent neuromuscular blocking properties and may cause respiratory paralysis in patients of myasthenia gravis.

MUPIROCIN

Mupirocin is obtained from *Pseudomonas fluorescens*. It is rapidly inactivated after absorption and hence not suitable to treat systemic infections. It is used as ointment topically.

It inhibits bacterial RNA and protein synthesis by binding to isoleucyl-t-RNA synthetase. This prevents incorporation of isoleucine into the bacterial proteins. The antimicrobial spectrum for mupirocin includes Staphylococci (including MRSA) and Streptococci. Gram-negative aerobes are usually not sensitive. Anaerobes and enterococci are usually resistant. Mupirocin is used for topical treatment of impetigo, folliculitis, burns and leg ulcers. It is also used intranasally for eradication of nasal colonization with MRSA in adult patients and health care workers. Adverse effects are rare.

PLEUROMUTILINS

Retapamulin

It is a first drug of this chemical group. This compound is used for minor bacterial skin infections like inpetigo as topical treatment. It's mechanism of action is similar to linezolid and steptogramins, i.e., the drug binds to a pocket in the A-site (like linezolid) of the peptidyl transferase centre where aminoacyl tRNA also binds but its binding also extends to P-site (like steptogramins). Adverse reaction to retapamulin are mild and manifest as local irritation and itching at the site of application.

FUSIDIC ACID

It also inhibits bacterial protein synthesis, but by interfering with elongation of peptide chain (it inhibits elongation factor-G). It is particularly active against penicillinase-producing *Staphylococcus aureus*, *Corynebacterium* and *Clostridium*. It is highly lipid soluble agent which readily penetrates the skin. Hence when applied locally, it is useful in deeper skin infections such as boils, impetigo and pyoderma. Adverse effects are rare except local irritation.

BEZLOTOXUMAB

It is a human monoclonal antibody which binds to *Clostridium difficile* toxin B and neutralizes its effects. It is given intravenously to reduce recurrence of *Clostridium difficile* bacterial infection in adults. Adverse effects are nausea, headache, fever, infusion related reactions and increased risk of heart failure.

CHAPTER 58 Broad-Spectrum Antibiotics: Tetracyclines and Chloramphenicol

COMPETENCY PH1.42

The tetracyclines and chloramphenicol are a group of broad-spectrum bacteriostatic antibiotics, whose widespread use (or say misuse) has resulted in many resistant strains of bacteria which has ultimately minimised their clinical usefulness. Paradoxically, the clinical use of tetracyclines (and possibly of chloramphenicol also) has had a recent surge in the interest that has resulted due to an almost complete lack of the use of these drugs by the clinicians during last 2 decades, with a concomitant loss of tetracycline or chloramphenicol resistant bacteria from our environment.

TETRACYCLINES

As is implied by the name, tetracyclines possess a four cyclic anthracycline ring structure. Different substitution on these rings affects individual pharmacokinetics which leads to certain variations in clinical usefulness.

Mechanism of Action

Initially, these drugs enter the cytoplasm of Gram-positive bacteria by an "energy-dependent active transport system". In Gram-negative bacteria these drugs pass through the outer membrane by passive diffusion through the porin channels. Once inside the bacterial cell, tetracyclines inhibit the bacterial protein synthesis by binding to their 30S ribosomal subunit and by subsequently blocking the attachment of aminoacyl t-RNA to the "A" site (of the mRNA-ribosome complex). As a result the peptide chain fails to grow (Fig. 52.2). Tetracyclines are bacteriostatic. The carrier involved in the active transport of tetracyclines is absent in the host mammalian cells. Moreover these drugs do not bind to mammalian 60S or 40S ribosomal units. This explains their selective toxicity to the bacteria only, and not to the host cells.

Antibacterial Spectrum

Currently **tetracyclines are highly active against** *Rickettsiae*, *Chlamydia psittaci, C. trachomatis* and *C. pneumoniae*. These drugs are also **highly efficacious against** spirochaetes such as *Borrelia burgdorferi* and *B. recurrentis*. **Some other atypical pathogens** like *Mycoplasma pneumoniae* and *Ureaplasma urealyticum* **are also very sensitive**.

Some **selective Gram-negative bacilli** such as *Vibrio cholerae, Brucella abortus, Actinomyces israelii, Francisella tularensis, Yersinia pestis, Helicobacter pylori* and *Propionibacterium acnes* **are also quite sensitive**. Some Gram-positive bacilli such as *Bacillus anthracis, Clostridium perfringens* and *C. tetani* are also modestly inhibited (but of no clinical usefulness).

Almost all Gram-positive and Gram-negative cocci and notable Gram-negative bacilli (e.g., *E. coli, Enterobacter, Proteus, Pseudomonas aeruginosa, Klebsiella, Salmonella, Shigella* and *B. fragilis*) have now become resistant. *Entamoeba* and *Plasmodia* are inhibited at higher concentrations (hence used as adjuvant drugs).

Resistance

There are four main mechanisms by which a bacteria develops resistance to tetracyclines. These are: **(a)** decreased cell permeability of the drug, **(b)** increased drug efflux from bacterial cell by an energy-dependent process, **(c)** ribosomal protection and **(d)** enzymatic inactivation of the drug. Among these, the drug efflux is the most important mechanism, as there are at least 300 different active efflux proteins capable of extruding tetracyclines from the bacterial cell.

Classification

- **Group I: Shorter Acting (t½ 6–10 hrs)**
  TETRACYCLINE, CHLORTETRACYCLINE and OXYTETRACYCLINE.

- **Group II**: **Intermediate Acting (t½ 12–13 hrs)** DEMECLOCYCLINE and METHACYCLINE
- **Group III**: **Long Acting (t½ 18–20 hrs)** DOXYCYCLINE and MINOCYCLINE

Pharmacokinetics

Tetracyclines are variably absorbed from GIT with significant differences in their bioavailability: Chlortetracycline (30%); demeclocycline, oxytetracycline and tetracycline (60–80%); minocycline and doxycycline (95–100%). *Food retards absorption of all tetracyclines except doxycycline and minocycline.*

Dairy products like milk or curd, Ca^{2+}, Mg^{2+} and Al^{3+} (present in antacids), Fe^{2+} (present in iron preparations) and $NaHCO_3$ (in antacids) significantly impair tetracycline absorption either by chelation or by altering gastric pH. The chelated complex of these divalent or trivalent metal ions with tetracyclines are not absorbed.

Tetracyclines are widely distributed throughout the body tissues and fluids excepting CSF. They get deposited in teeth, bones and in tumours which have high Ca^{2+} contents (e.g., gastric carcinoma). The serum protein binding for tetracycline, chlortetracycline and oxytetracycline is low (20–60%); for demeclocycline and methacycline is moderate (40–80%) but for doxycycline and minocycline is high (80–95%). All of them cross placental barrier.

These are metabolised in the liver and are concentrated in the bile or excreted in urine. Urinary excretion ranges from 70–75% for tetracycline, oxytetracycline and chlortetracycline. *Doxycycline and minocycline are primarily excreted through bile. With renal impairement, only doxycycline and minocycline can be administered with safety without dose adjustment.* Other tetracyclines may accumulate in conditions of renal failure and if doses are not adjusted a possible hepatotoxicity may ensue. Minocycline is also excreted through saliva and tears. All tetracyclines are secreted through breast milk.

Clinical Uses

The tetracyclines are the drugs of first choice for the treatment of Rocky Mountain spotted fever, Typhus fever (caused by *Rickettsia*); psittacosis, granuloma inguinale, pneumonia (caused by *Chlamydia*); nonspecific urethritis (*Ureaplasma urealyticum*); atypical pneumonia (*Mycoplasma pneumoniae*); Lyme disease (*Borrelia burgdorferi*) and relapsing fever (*B. recurrentis*).

These are also effective in the treatment of brucellosis (*Brucella abortus*), tularaemia (*F. tularensis*) and plague (*Y. pestis*) (where these are used along with gentamicin); bacteraemia and abscesses (*Pasteurella*); trachoma, inclusion conjunctivitis, nonspecific urethritis/cervicitis (*C. trachomatis*) and for abdominal/thoracic lesions (*Actinomyces israelii*).

Other conditions where tetracyclines may be used are: **(a)** Amoebiasis—along with metronidazole (Ch. 65), **(b)** Malaria—along with quinine or with sulfadoxine + pyrimethamine combination for chloroquine-resistant *P. falciparum* malaria (Ch. 64), and **(c)** Acne–because of their antioxidant effect on the degranulated neutrophils in the acidic contents of sebaceous material, **(d)** Peptic ulcer due to *H.pylori* – where these are used as adjuvant drugs (Ch.27).

The recommended oral doses are: Tetracycline 250 mg 6 hrly; Oxytetracycline 250 mg 6 hrly; Demeclocycline 300 mg 12 hrly; Doxycycline 100 mg 12 hrly 1st day, then 100 mg daily; Minocycline 100 mg 12 hrly. Except for demeclocycline and methacycline, which are administered by oral route, others can be given orally as well as intravenously.

Doxycycline with its longer half-life and lack of nephrotoxicity (biliary excretion) is a popular choice for patients with pre-existing renal disease. It can also be given I.V. It is the treatment of choice for early stage Lyme disease and in the prophylaxis of anthrax. ***Demeclocycline*** inhibits the actions of ADH in the renal tubules and has been used in the treatment of inappropriate (excess) secretion of ADH (see below and Ch.17).

Minocycline 100 mg orally BD for 5 days is used to eradicate the meningococcal carrier state from the nasopharynx. Despite some conflicting pharmacokinetic data, patients with impaired renal functions do not usually require adjustment in dosage. Minocycline is effectively used for the treatment of swimming pool granuloma caused by *Mycobacterium marinum*. It is also used to treat chronic facial dermatoses.

Adverse Effects

1. Oral administration can cause nausea, vomiting, epigastric burning and stomatitis. Chronic use can cause fungal esophagitis which can be recognised by dysphagia. Withdrawal of the drug is usually curative in initial stage, otherwise antifungal therapy may be required. Superinfection may result in intestinal *Candida albicans* infection, whereas *Staph. aureus* or *Clostridium difficile* overgrowth can lead to enterocolitis.
2. Staining of both the deciduous and permanent teeth and retardation of bone growth usually occurs if tetracyclines are administered after the first trimester of pregnancy or when given to children below 10 years of age.
3. Hepatotoxicity may occur particularly during pregnancy. On prolonged use these drugs may also lead to elevated blood urea levels. Hence a combination of uraemia and jaundice may at times be fatal.
4. Except doxycycline and minocycline (see text, above) other tetracyclines are occasionally nephrotoxic on prolonged use, and may accumulate to toxic levels in patients with impaired renal functions. The renal toxicity (***Fanconi's syndrome***) has also been observed with the use of tetracycline preparations after expiry date. It is characterised by azotaemia (blood urea) and kindney damage due to formation of toxic metabolites, viz., epitetracycline and epianhydro-tetracycline.
5. Intravenous injection can cause phlebitis. Intramuscular injection is painful and causes local irritation and should be avoided.
6. Pulmonary eosinophilic syndrome (eosinophilia and hilar lymphadenopathy) can occur with even 10 days of therapy with tetracyclines. The symptoms disappear following discontinuation of the drug.
7. Pseudotumor cerebri (in adults) and bulging fontanelles is another complication of chronic use of tetracyclines but usually resolves with cessation of the therapy.
8. MINOCYCLINE induces vestibular toxicity (vertigo, ataxia) because of its accumulation in lipid rich cells of inner ear. Increased usage of minocycline can induce skin pigmentation that is unrelated to the photosensitivity seen with other tetracyclines. In light-skinned patients, thyroid staining becomes visible through the overlying skin of the neck, but the endocrine functions of the gland are not affected. Symptoms resolve in few months after drug discontinuation.
9. DEMECLOCYCLINE and DOXYCYCLINE can induce photosensitivity to sunlight or u.v. light. It is manifested as sun-burn type reaction.
10. DEMECLOCYCLINE antagonises renal actions of ADH and can induce nephrogenic diabetes insipidus.

Drug Interactions

1. Al^{3+}, Ca^{2+}, Zn^{2+}, Mg^{2+} and iron preparations decrease tetracycline absorption by chelation. $NaHCO_3$ alters gastric pH and reduces absorption of tetracyclines.
2. Enzyme inducers such as barbiturates, phenytoin and carbamazepine reduce serum levels of tetracyclines.
3. Tetracyclines inhibit intestinal flora that produces vitamin K, and therefore may potentiate the anticoagulant effects of warfarin.

Contraindications

Renal impairment, hepatic insufficiency, pregnancy, lactation and in children below 10 yrs of age. Tetracyclines after expiry date should never be used (see above). Intrathecal injections should be avoided.

GLYCYLCYCLINES

Tigelcycline is a glycylcycline antibiotic. It is a minocycline analogue. It binds with a higher affinity to 30S ribosomal subunits and is 20-fold more potent than tetracycline in inhibiting bacterial protein synthesis.

It has a broad-spectrum bacteriostatic action against tetracycline as well as multidrug-resistant pathogens. Tigecycline is active against Gram-positive cocci including MRSA; vancomycin-resistant enterococci (VRE) and multidrug-resistant *Strepto. pneumoniae*; Gram-negative cocci, e.g.,

N. gonorrhoeae and *M. catarrhalis;* Gram-positive anaerobes like *Clostridium* and *Bacteriodes;* and β-lactamase producing Gram-negative bacilli like *H. influenzae,* and *E. coli,* and is equally potent against *Mycobacterium pneumoniae.* Pseudomonas, Proteus and Providencia are resistant. It is approved for the treatment of complicated skin and soft tissue infections and also for intra-abdominal infection. It is administered I.V. as a 100 mg loading dose followed by 50 mg I.V. every 12 hrs.

It is eliminated through bile (dose adjustment not needed in renal impairment). Nausea-vomiting is the major side effect. It is not metabolised by cytochrome-P450, hence usual drug interactions are rare.

CHLORAMPHENICOL

Chloramphenicol (chloromycetin) is a broad-spectrum antibiotic isolated from *Streptomyces venezuelae.* It is unique among naturally occuring antibiotics in that it contains a nitro group as nitrobenzene moiety.

Mechanism of Action and Resistance

Its mode of action is similar to macrolides (Ch. 57). It inhibits bacterial protein synthesis by binding to the 50S ribosomal subunit. It is bacteriostatic to most pathogens but is bactericidal to *H. influenzae.* Chloramphenicol-induced inhibition of mitochondrial protein synthesis, by inhibiting eukaryotic mitochondrial 70S ribosomes, probably is responsible for the associated host toxicity.

Resistance to chloramphenicol develops due to: **(1)** ribosomal protection which results in decreased affinity for the drug to the ribosomal binding site, **(2)** decreased permeability to the drug, and **(3)** production of plasmid as well as chromosomal mediated chloramphenicol acetyltransferase that metabolises chloramphenicol to an inactive form.

Antimicrobial Spectrum and Clinical Use

Chloramphenicol is active against a wide range of Gram-negative organisms, e.g., *Salmonella typhi, Haemophilus influenzae* and *Neisseria meningitidis*; Gram-positive organisms, e.g., *Streptococcus pneumoniae*; and against most anaerobic bacteria including penicillin-resistant *Bacteroides fragilis.*Other common pathogens sensitive to chloramphenicol are spirochaetes, rickettsiae, *Mycoplasma* and *Chlamydia* (like tetracyclines).

Because of the propensity to induce bone marrow depression and aplasia, the use of chloramphenicol is no longer justified in treating minor infections. However, it can be used as an alternative drug for some and a choice of drug for a few infections discussed below:

1. Since effective CSF levels are obtained, it is a preferred treatment for meningitis caused by *H. influenzae, N. meningitidis* and *Strepto. pneumoniae,* particularly if the patient is hypersensitive to β-lactams. However, with the advent of III generation cephalosporins such as ceftriaxone and cefotaxime, its use has declined. Dose of 50–75 mg/kg/day in equally divided doses 6 hrly for 2 weeks is quite effective for this condition.
2. Earlier, chloramphenicol had been the drug of choice for typhoid fever. Later, its use declined due to its toxicity and development of resistant strains of *S. typhi.* Moreover, being bacteriostatic, it does not cure carrier state and relapse occurred in 10% of the cases. However, it is cheaper and defervescence takes place earlier than with drugs used currently. With a dose of 500 mg QID the fever subsides within 3–4 days. Thereafter, a dose of 250 mg QID should be continued for another 7 days to cure intestinal lesions. Shorter therapy can lead to relapse but the bacilli remain sensitive and relapse can be treated again as described above. However, as chloramphenicol has not been used for this purpose for the last two decades, there has been a loss of chloramphenicol-resistant genes from *S. typhi.* Other antimicrobials of choice for treating typhoid fever are: ciprofloxacin (Ch. 54), ceftriaxone, cefoperazone and cefotaxime (Ch. 55).
3. Another indication for chloramphenicol is for the treatment of serious anaerobic infections (pelvic and brain abscess) caused by penicillin-resistant *B. fragilis.* However, clindamycin and metronidazole are more preferred for this purpose.

4. Chloramphenicol is also widely used topically for treating conjunctivitis and external ear infections. When given systemically, it attains high concentration in ocular fluid and hence is preferred to treat endophthalmitis caused by sensitive strains.

Pharmacokinetics

Chloramphenicol is rapidly and completely absorbed after oral administration. Chloramphenicol palmitate is used for oral suspension. It is degraded into chloramphenicol by pancreatic lipase in duodenum. It can be administered either orally or I.V. It is widely distributed in different body compartments including CSF. It is metabolised in liver by glucuronyl conjugation and excreted through urine. Plasma half-life is 3–5 hrs.

Adverse Effects

The most documented adverse effects are on haematopoietic system.

1. ***Dose-related bone marrow depression*** is characterised by anaemia, leukopenia and thrombocytopenia, which is reversible on discontinuation of chloramphenicol. It is seen most frequently when daily dose exceeds 3–4 g/day for 1–2 weeks. It is a direct toxic effect of the drug resulting from inhibition of host mitochondrial enzyme synthesis (inhibition of mitochondrial 70S ribosomes). Hepatic and renal insufficiency predisposes to this type of toxicity. Periodic blood counts should be advised.
2. ***Non-Dose related or Idiosyncratic aplastic anaemia***, though rare (1:40,000), is a serious adverse effect. It is irreversible, even fatal and probably has a genetic cause. It is quite unpredictable and may occur even after ocular administration or after a single dose oral administration.
3. ***Gray Baby Syndrome***: Neonates cannot adequately conjugate chloramphenicol to form the glucuronide. They also have slow rates of glomerular filtration and tubular secretion. Consequently, high levels of free chloramphenicol may accumulate to cause potentially fatal neonatal toxicity, characterised by abdominal distension, progressive cyanosis (gray body), hypothermia, vomiting, loss of hunger and ultimately cardiovascular collapse and death.
4. ***Superinfection,*** as seen with tetracyclines.

Drug Interactions

Chloramphenicol is a potent enzyme inhibitor and inhibits the metabolism of morphine (severe respiratory depression), of chlorpropamide (aggravate hypoglycaemia) and of warfarin (causing bleeding).

CHAPTER 59

Chemotherapy of Tuberculosis and Leprosy

COMPETENCY PH1.44, PH1.45, PH1.46, PH1.55

Tuberculosis (TB) is an infectious disease caused predominantly by *Mycobacterium tuberculosis* and among the leading causes of mortality in the world. India accounts for 25% of the global TB burden. Pulmonary TB is the most common site for pathological lesions but it also affects other sites, which is called extrapulmonary TB. The infection is usually due to inhalation of infected droplet nuclei and the lung is generally the first organ to be affected. Pulmonary TB usually occurs after a period of dormancy in a previously infected individual. The onset is gradual but deceptive. Symptoms include low grade fever (99^0F) in the evening, night sweats, malaise, fatigue, weight loss and a blood streaked productive cough. Spread of pulmonary TB to the pleura results in pleural effusion as a part of inflammatory reaction (pleurisy). Later, the tubercular bacilli may disseminate and the hypersensitivity reaction to mycobacterial proteins may cause extensive tissue damage and virtually any organ of the body may be involved. *Miliary tuberculosis* is a massive dissemination of tubercle bacilli throughout the body including liver and spleen that do not have a high O_2 tension.

Mycobacteria other than *M. tuberculosis* are called non-tuberculous or *atypical mycobacteria*. These are present in the environment and can cause disease similar to tuberculosis. Some of them are: *M. kansasii,* which produces milder but chronic pulmonary disease resembling tuberculosis; *M. marinum* causes swimming pool granuloma; *M. scrofulaceum,* causes cervical lymphadenitis and *M. leprae,* which causes leprosy. *M. avium complex* (MAC) includes both *M. avium* and *M. intracellulare*. MAC is an important and common cause of disseminated TB type of pulmonary disease seen most commonly in immunocompromised patients, e.g., those with AIDS. This chapter describes the drug treatment of TB, leprosy and diseases caused by MAC.

Since a major portion of the tubercle bacilli becomes intracellular and resides in the macrophages, it is inaccessible to the majority of antibiotics as these cannot penetrate easily. Moreover, the mycobacteria are well known for developing resistance to any single drug. Combination of drugs are therefore needed to overcome resistance during the course of therapy. The answer as to why a multiple drug combination lowers the chances of development of resistance is simple. Suppose, the frequency of drug 'A' resistant mutants, in an active tuberculosis pocket, is about one bacillus in 10^6. This resistant bacillus will be readily selected out if the drug 'A' is administered alone. But if a second drug 'B', having a similar incidence of drug resistance (i.e., 1 in 10^6) is combined with the drug 'A', the probability of this bacillus to get resistant to both the drugs is reduced to 1 in 10^{12}. Therefore, it is advisable to combine at least two or more anti-TB drugs to which the *Mycobacterium* is susceptible. Since the response of the therapy is also slow, the treatment must continue for months depending on the drug that has been used. The risk of adverse reactions is therefore a major concern in proper drug selection. Key points in the treatment of tuberculosis are: **(1)** The therapy must contain two or more drugs to avoid development of resistance, **(2)** the drugs must be taken regularly (strict drug compliance) and **(3)** the drug therapy must continue for a sufficient duration to achieve adequate therapeutic results.

Traditionally, the drugs used in the treatment of TB are classified into:

First Line Drugs (FLDs): These drugs display a high anti-TB efficacy and acceptable toxicity. This class of drugs are the first to be selected for the treatment any type of clinical TB manifestation. A three or four drugs' combination of FLDs is used for a specified period as per **National Tuberculosis Elimination Programme** (NTEP-2021) prescribed regimens to avoid development of resistance.

Second Line Drugs (SLDs): These drugs exhibit low anti-TB efficacy and higher toxicity or both. This class of drugs are only used if there is resistance to FLDs or these are contraindicated for some reason.

CLASSIFICATION OF ANTI-TB DRUGS

First Line Drugs (FLDs)

First Line Oral (FLO) Drugs

1. Isoniazid (INH/H)
2. Rifampicin (R)
3. Pyrazinamide (Z)
4. Ethambutol (E)

Second Line Drugs (SLDs)

Second Line Oral (SLO) Drugs

1. Fluoroquinolones
   - Levofloxacin (Lfx)
   - Moxifloxacin (Mfx)
   - Gatifloxacin (Gfx)
2. Ethionamide (Eto)
3. Prothionamide (Pto)
4. Cycloserine (Cs)
5. Terizidone (Trz)
6. Para-aminosalicylic Acid (PAS)
7. Thiacetazone (Taz)
8. Rifabutin/ Rifapentine

Second Line Injectable (SLI) Drugs

9. Kanamycin (Km)/Amikacin (Am)
10. Capreomycin (Cm); 11. Streptomycin (S)

Newer Anti-TB Drugs

1. Bedaquiline
2. Delamanid

Repurposed Anti-TB Drugs

1. Linezolid (Lzd)
2. Clofazimine (Cfz)
3. Amoxicillin+Clavulanic acid (Amoxi-clav)
4. Imipenem+ Cilastatin
5. Meropenem

First Line Anti-TB Drugs

TB therapy normally begins with four FLDs: ***INH + rifampicin + pyrazinamide + ethambutol*** for 2 months followed by a course of two drugs ***INH + rifampicin*** (in regimens before 2017) but now (after 2017) with three drugs: +ethambutol also for the next 4 months. The treatment would consist of 2-month (8 weeks) of IP with H,R,Z,E administered in daily dosage as fixed dose combination (FDC) tablets as per patient weight-wise 4 bands. Z is stoped after 2 months and only FDC tablets of H,R,E are given in CP of 4-month (16 weeks) as per weight band. (see Table 59.1).

First Line Oral (FLO) Drugs

1. Isoniazid (INH/H)

Isonicotinic acid hydrazide or INH is a very potent synthetic anti-TB agent which has structural resemblance to pyridoxine.

Mechanism of Action and Resistance: Isoniazid inhibits the synthesis of α-mycolic acids (the waxy lipids), which are essential components of mycobacterial cell wall (along with peptidoglycan). Interestingly, INH is a prodrug and the mycobacterial enzyme catalase peroxidase converts it to its biologically active form to block mycolic acid synthesis. The drug is bactericidal to actively growing tubercle bacilli but not to dormant organisms which are only inhibited. It is primarily an antitubercular drug having activity only against *M. tuberculosis* and also to one atypical mycobacteria, *M. kansasii*. It acts on extracellular as well as on intracellular tubercle bacilli (present within macrophages) and is equally active in acidic and alkaline medium.

The most common mechanism of INH resistance is the mutation in catalase-peroxidase gene responsible for activation of INH. Another mechanism is through mutation in the promoter gene *inh*A involved in mycolic acid biosynthesis.

Pharmacokinetics: INH is well absorbed orally and readily distributed in pleural, peritoneal and synovial fluids. CSF concentrations can reach up to 100% if the meninges are inflammed. It is metabolised in liver, by N-acetyltransferase, to acetylisoniazid. Genetic variation has been observed in its rate of N-acetylation (Ch. 7) which is inherited as autosomal recessive trait. Most of Eskimos, Japanese and about 30–40% of Indians are usually ***rapid acetylators***. Plasma half-life of INH in such population is 1 hr. While Egyptians, Mediterranean Jews, Swedes and about 60–70% of Indians are ***slow acetylators*** ($t^{1/2}$ 3 hrs). The acetylator status of an individual may influence the nature of INH toxicity but not the antitubercular response (if INH is administered once daily) because its plasma concentration normally remains above its inhibitory concentration.

Adverse Effects: Peripheral neuritis and hepatotoxicity are the two major, but acetylator status-dependent, adverse effects. ***Peripheral neuritis***

(paresthesias, numbness) is more common with ***slow acetylators*** because of two reasons: **(a)** INH-induced increase in the excretion of pyridoxine in urine and **(b)** because the accumulated INH inhibits pyridoxine kinase which converts pyridoxine to its active form pyridoxyl phosphate. This neurotoxicity can be prevented by prophylactic use of vitamin B_6 (10–40 mg/day). Though incidence is low (0.2–0.5%), ***hepatotoxicity*** is another potentially serious side effect of INH. The risk of hepatitis is higher (2%) in people aged 50–65 yrs, or in persons with underlying liver disease or in alcohol drinkers or ***in fast acetylators*** (fast metabolism of INH provides high concentrations of hepatotoxic metabolites acetylisoniazid and acetylhydrazine). The drug should be discontinued at the onset of symptoms such as nausea, loss of appetite, abdominal pain and on rise in aminotransferases enzymes by three-fold. ***Other adverse effects*** include allergic reactions (fever, rashes), xerostomia, haematological changes and convulsions in seizure prone patients. Drug induced systemic lupus erythematosus has also been reported. **Drug interactions** are not alarming except: **(1)** Aluminium hydroxide (as in antacids) inhibits the absorption of INH, **(2)** Alcohol increases the risk of hepatitis and **(3)** INH inhibits the metabolism of phenytoin and carbamazepine.

Dose: Typical adult dose is 300 mg once daily orally or 5 mg/kg/day. If given thrice weekly, then 600 mg thrice a week, i.e., 10 mg/kg/day. For serious infections or meningitis 600 mg once daily orally. Duration of treatment is related to drug combination used.

2. Rifampicin (rifampin; R)

Rifampicin is a semisynthetic derivative of a macrocyclic antibiotic rifamycin.

Mechanism of Action and Resistance: Rifampicin, binds to and inhibits bacterial DNA-dependent RNA polymerase so that it cannot synthesise new RNA. Mammalian RNA polymerase does not bind to the drug. The RNA synthesis of the host cells is therefore unaffected. The drug is bactericidal for both intracellular and extracellular *M. tuberculosis*. The bactericidal action is exerted on all forms of TB bacilli, but show a robust killing effect on slowly dividing organism called spurters. In addition to *M. tuberculosis*, rifampicin is also active against *M. leprae, Staph. aureus, N. meningitidis, H. influenzae, Brucella* and *Legionella*. It has good sterilizing and resistance preventing action, when used in combination with other drugs. Rifampicin resistance results from a point mutation in ***rpo***B gene (the gene present on β-subunit of **R**NA **po**lymerase), thereby preventing the binding of the drug to RNA polymerase. Hence, if used alone, resistance develops rapidly.

Pharmacokinetics: Rifampin is well absorbed after oral administration. It penetrates in all tissues, tubercular cavities, placenta and is significantly protein bound. Adequate CSF levels are achieved if meninges are inflammed. It is excreted mainly through liver into bile and undergoes enterohepatic circulation. It is a potent enzyme inducer.

Doses and Clinical Use: As antitubercular drug its usual daily dose is 600 mg (10 mg/kg/day) as a single dose before breakfast. It can also be administered as 600 mg in a single dose, before breakfast, *thrice a week*. Other indications for rifampicin include: **(1)** treatment of leprosy in combination with dapsone (see following text), **(2)** for prophylaxis of meningococcal (oral dose of 600 mg BD for 2 days) and *H. influenzae*-caused meningitis (oral dose of 600 mg/day for 4 days) and carrier state, **(3)** for prosthetic valve endocarditis, and **(4)** for treating brucellosis, in combination with doxycycline (first choice combination).

Adverse Effects: ***Hepatitis*** is the major adverse effect and the risk may be increased if used with INH or in patients with underlying liver disease. However, it is dose-dependent and reversible. Occasional adverse effects include rashes, GI disturbances, dizziness, fatigue and ***flu-like syndrome*** (more seen when the drug is given intermittenlty ratherthan when given on daily basis) characterised by fever, chills, myalgias and thrombocytopenia. Rifampin imparts a harmless ***red orange colour to urine.***

Drug interactions result because of its enzyme inducting properties (induction of cytochrome P-450 isoforms). Hence, it accelerates the metabolism of several other drugs such as oral contraceptives, anticoagulants and protease inhibitors used in HIV patients, which may result in therapeutic failure.

3. Ethambutol (E)

Ethambutol is a synthetic tuberculostatic drug, active against *M. tuberculosis, M. kansasii* and *M. avium-intracellulare*.

Mechanism of Action: It has been found to inhibit arabinosyl transferase enzyme to prevent polymerisation of arabinoglycans, which are essential constituents of the mycobacterial cell wall. Drug resistance occurs due to point mutations in the *emb B* gene that encodes the arabinosyl transferase enzyme involved in mycobacterial cell wall synthesis.

Oral bioavailability of ethambutol is about 80%. It is widely distributed in all body fluids including CSF.

Doses and Clinical Use: It is commonly included as a fourth drug along with INH, rifampin and pyrazinamide in the treatment regimen of tuberculosis. If used alone, resistance develops rapidly. Usual daily dose is 800–1000 mg orally (15 mg/kg/day). It can also be given in a dose of 1600 mg/day (30 mg/kg/day) thrice a week orally. It is also used in combination with clarithromycin and rifabutin, in the treatment of *M. avium-intracellulare* infection in AIDS patients (see following text). Higher doses are needed to treat tuberculous meningitis.

Adverse Effects: Ethambutol if used in a dose of 25 mg/kg/day for more than 9 months can cause ***retrobulbar neuritis impairing visual acuity and red-green colour discrimination.*** Though this adverse effect is dose related, it reverses slowly after drug discontinuation. Periodic visual acuity and field of vision testing is desirable during treatment period. ***It should also be avoided in children below 5 yrs*** where it is difficult to assess visual acuity and red-green colour blindness. Ethambutol decreases renal excretion of urates and may ***precipitate gouty arthritis.*** Mild GIT intolerance, rashes, fever and dizziness are also possible.

4. Pyrazinamide (Z)

Pyrazinamide is the pyrazine derivative of nicotinamide. Because of its hepatotoxicity, its use had declined earlier. But pyrazinamide, in reduced doses and in combination, has reemerged as the third most important antituberculosis agent.

Mechanism of Action: The drug is thought to enter *M. tuberculosis* by passive diffusion and is converted to pyrazinoic acid (its active metabolite) by bacterial pyrazinamidase enzyme. The active metabolite then inhibits mycobacterial fatty acid synthase-I enzyme and disrupts mycolic acid synthesis needed for cell wall synthesis. It is bactericidal to *M. tuberculosis* and is active at low (acidic) pH. It is highly effective on intracellular mycobacteria (can work in acidic environment of phagocytes). A mutation in the gene (*pcnA*) that encodes pyrazinamidase enzyme is responsible for drug resistance which can be minimised by using drug combination therapy.

The drug is well absorbed after oral administration, and is widely distributed in all tissues, macrophages, tubercular cavities and in meninges. Plasma half-life is 9–10 hrs.

Adverse Effects: ***Hepatotoxicity*** is seen in about 15% of recipients of this agent but is less evident with the lower doses currently being used. It may may cause ***hyperuricaemia*** and possibly acute gouty arthritis. Other adverse effects include nausea, vomiting, anorexia, drug fever and malaise. PZA should be avoided during pregnancy.

Dose: 1500 mg (25 mg/kg/day) orally, once a day. It can also be given in two equally divided doses. If given thrice a week it should be administered in a dose of 2000 mg/day (35 mg/kg/day).

Second Line Oral Anti-TB Drugs

Second Line Oral (SLO) Drugs

These are the alternative for SLDs that are useful in cases of resistance to FLDs.

1. Fluoroquinolones (FQs): FQs are important recent additions to the therapeutic regimen used against *M. tuberculosis* as bactericidal agents especially in multidrug-resistant strains. These are also very effective when used as a part of combined regimen in HIV-infected patients (see following text and Ch. 54). ***Levofloxacin (Lfx), moxifloxacin (Mfx)*** and ***gatifloxacin (Gfx)*** inhibit 90–95% of the strains of susceptible tubercular bacilli including *M. avium complex* (MAC) and *M. fortuitum*. Due to good penetration into the cells, these are capable of killing intracellular pathogens, and because of their convenient dosage schedule and good tolerability, these are being increasingly included in combination regimens against multidrug-resistant tuberculosis and MAC infection in AIDS patients. These can be substituted in drug combinations if any first-line drug is contraindicated. All drugs are given orally and the recommended doses for Cfx are 750 mg BD or 500 mg TDS and for Ofx are 400 mg BD. Lfx is the levo isomer of Ofx and is preferred over Ofx because of its potency and once daily dose schedule (500 mg once daily). Mfx is given as 400 mg once daily. Recent studies have suggested that the use of Mfx (with other drugs) reduces the duration of therapy for drug-susceptible TB.

2. Ethionamide (Eto): Structurally, it is a sulphur containing isoniazid-like drug but exerts a tuberculostatic effect. It acts by blocking the synthesis of mycolic acid. The drug is rarely used, as in recommended dose of 1 g/day it is seldom tolerated because of intense gastric irritation and neurological toxicity (dizziness, encephalopathy, peripheral and even rarely optic neuritis). It is also hepatotoxic. Hence, one has to settle for a daily dose of 500–750 mg which leads to a faster development of resistance.

3. Prothionamide (Pto): The drug is an interchangeable congener of ethioamide and exibits similar pharmacokinetic and pharmacodynamic properties but safety-wise it is better tolerated than ethionamide. It is given orally in once daily dosing (15–20 mg/kg, both in children and adult (max.1g). Twice daily dosing may be considered if patients are unable to tolerate once daily regimen. Prothionamide is a WHO Group 4 drug for the treatment of drug resistant TB.

4. Cycloserine (Cs): It is a broad-spectrum d-alanine containing antibiotic which acts by inhibiting bacterial cell wall synthesis. It is tuberculostatic to *M. tuberculosis* and is also effective against *E. coli, Staph. aureus, Enterococcus, Nocardia* and *Chlamydia* (Ch. 55). It is readily absorbed after oral administration and mainly excreted unchanged by the kidney. Hence, the drug is very useful in treating renal tuberculosis and also for the treatment of multidrug-resistant tuberculosis. Usual dosage is 500 mg BD orally. Peripheral neuropathy, dizziness, tremors convulsions and, psychotic behavioural changes are some major side effects. Vitamin B_6 100 mg/day can reduce the neurological toxicity.

5. Terizidone (Trz): Terizidone is combination of two molecules of cycloserine and one molecule of terephthalaldehyde and is a broad spectrum antibiotic. It exerts a potent and extended anti-TB activity, and possesses remarkable effects against not only strains causing pulmonary TB or urinary tract infections but also strains which have become resistant to existing anti-TB drugs. Terizidone is a WHO Group 4 drug for the treatment of drug resistant TB.

Its mode of action is similar to cycloserine, i.e., it acts by inhibiting cell wall synthesis by impairing peptidoglycan formation. Given orally in the dose of 250 –750 mg OD, the drug is completely absorbed, maximum concentration in blood achieved in 2–4 hrs. The drug is excreted unchanged in urine where its concentration is much higher than the blood even after 30 hrs of administration exceeding its antitubercular MIC. This makes it an ideal drug for the treatment of renovesicular TB.

Terizidone is recommonded for both pulmonary and extra-pulmonary TB caused by strains of *M. tuberculosis* or *avium.* It is not recommonded for use as monotherapy. Toxic reactions are rarely observed with this drug even on prlonged therapy.

6. Para-Aminosalicylic Acid (PAS): PAS is a structural analogue of PABA. It exhibits bacteriostatic action against *M. tuberculosis* by inhibiting the folate synthesis of the bacteria. Lately its use even as a second-line drug has declined as better and safer drugs are available as alternatives. With PAS there is always a poor compliance due to GIT intolerance. Common side effects are: hypersensitivity reactions that include include skin rashes, lupus-like reactions, drug fever, joint pain and hepatitis. Doses: 8–12 g/day orally in 2 or 3 divided doses.

7. Thiacetazone (Thz): Because of its low cost and efficacy in combination with isoniazid, it was once used as a first-line drug for tuberculosis. It is no longer used now because of its ototoxicity and life-threatening hypersensitivity reactions (hepatitis, neutropenia and thrombo-cytopenia).

8. Rifabutin/Rifapentine: ***Rifabutin (Mycobutin)*** is a structural analogue of rifampicin. It shares with rifampicin its **(a)** common mechanism of action, **(b)** common spectrum of activity against Gram-positive and Gram-negative organisms, and **(c)** common molecular basis for the development of resistance. Hence, there is a complete cross-resistance between these two drugs.

Rifabutin, however, differs from rifampicin in the following features: **(a)** it is a less potent inducer of cytochrome P-450 enzymes and causes lesser drug interactions with protease inhibitors and nonnucleoside reverse transcriptase inhibitors which are commonly used drugs in HIV-coinfected patients, **(b)** it has better activity than rifampicin, against *M. avium complex* (MAC), **(c)** It is not only active against *M. tuberculosis* but also active against some rifampicin-resistant strains such as *M. leprae* and *M. fortuitum*. and **(d)** it has a longer plasma half-life (45 hrs).

Rifabutin is used either alone or in combination with pyrazinamide in the treatment of latent TB. It can be used in place of rifampicin for the treatment of TB in HIV-infected patients. The most important use of rifabutin, in the HIV- infected population, is the prevention and treatment of disseminated MAC. Recommended dosage is 300 mg/day (5 mg/kg/day, orally).

Adverse effects include skin rash, GI intolerance, neutropenia, hepatitis and red-orange discolouration of urine (like rifampicin). Rifabutin is also an enzyme inducer and may decrease plasma concentrations of theophylline, oral anticoagulants, protease inhibitors and non-nucleoside reverse transcriptase inhibitors, etc (but less than rifampicin). On the other hand fluconazole increases rifabutin plasma concentration resulting in pseudo-jaundice and polymyalgia syndrome.

Rifapentine is a longer acting (t½ 13–15 hr) analogue of rifampicin. Its mechanism of action, cross resistance, enzyme induction, toxic profile and clinical use is identical to rifampicin. It is not used alone but in a 3–4 drug combination regimen. Recommended dose is 600 mg once or twice weekly. Though it also induces CYP3A4 isoenzyme, its potential for drug-drug interaction is lower than that of rifampicin but greater than that of rifabutin.

Second Line Injectable (SLI) Drugs

9. Kanamycin (Km), Amikacin (Am): Both drugs, being aminoglycoside antibiotics (Ch. 56), have significant ototoxicity and nephrotoxicity. Hence for the treatment of multidrug-resistant TB one of these is considered as a second choice after streptomycin and even capreomycin. The standard regimen for MDR-TB in RNTCP includes Km (not Am) because it costs less but in some contries Am is preferred because of its being less toxic. An additional use of Am is in the treatment of disseminated *M. avium complex* in AIDS patients. Most *M. tuberculosis* strains that are resistant to streptomycin are sensitive to amikacin. The recommended dosage for amikacin are 15 mg/kg/day I.M. or I.V. for 5 days a week for 2 months and then 1 g/day thrice weekly for another 4 months. As per WHO guidelines of 2016, both of these drugs along with Capreomycin are now classified as Group B SLIs.

10. Capreomycin (Cm): It is a tuberculocidal polypeptide antibiotic. It is effective against *M. tuberculosis, M. kansasii* and *M. avium*. It is poorly absorbed from GIT and hence must be given parenterally (1 g/day I.M.). *Adverse effects* of Cm are similar to those of aminoglycosides and include ototoxicity and nephrotoxicity. Though rarely used, Cm is an important drug for the treatment of multidrug-resistant TB.

Newer Anti-TB Drugs

Several new drugs for the treatment of tuberculosis are undergoing clinical trials these days. Two of them: **Bedaquiline** and **Delamanid** have been approved for use individually in combination with other anti-TB drugs to treat pulmonary tuberculosis.

1. **Bedaquiline (Bdq)**: Bdq is a diaryl-quinoline derivative that exerts a bactericidal action through its unique ATP Synthase enzyme inhibitory effect in the mycobacterial mitochondria. It depletes the bacteria of its energy source of ATP and as a result has a potential to remain active against MDR strains of *M.*

tuberculosis. Bdq shows cross resistance with clofazimine as both drugs are substrate for the cell wall efflux transporter of mycobateria.

Given orally the drug is rapidly absorbed (fatty meal facilitates its absorption). In circulation the drug remains highly protein bound (>99%) and slowly gets metabolized by CYP3A4 enzyme to several metabolites, one of which (M2) shows 4–6 times less anti-TB potency. Due to their high circular and cellular protein binding, both Bdq and its active M2 metabolite exhibit a long terminal half-life of about 5 months. Because of the involvement of CYP3A4 enzyme in its metabolism, Bdq may show interaction with drugs which inhibit or induce this enzyme.

Currently Bdq is approved and is available with conditional access under the RNTCP for the treatment of MDR-TB in combination therapy with atleast 3 other anti-TB drugs for which sensitivity testing has shown that the patient is susceptible to. If drug susceptibility testing is not available than Bdq should be used with at least 4 other drugs to which the patient is likely to be susceptible.

The recommended dose of Bdq is 400 mg a day for two weeks and then 200 mg taken three times a week (with at least 48 hours between doses) for the next 22 weeks. The drug is available as 100 mg tablet, which should be swallowed whole with water and preferably taken with food to maximise its absorption. Hepatotoxicity and cardiac conduction toxicity (prolongation of the QTc interval) are some adverse reactions observed with Bdq.

2. **Delamanid (Dlm)**: A bicyclic nitro-dihydro-imidazo-oxazole derivative, Dlm is a new potent tuberculocidal drug that also demonstrates post-antibiotic effect. It does not show any cross resistance or antagonistic activity to any of the anti-TB FLDs. It inhibits biosynthesis of methoxy-mycolic acid and keto-mycolic acid, the two key components of mycobacterial cell wall. Dlm is a prodrug that is bioactivated to des-nitro-metabolite by the mycobaterial-**d**eazaflavin (F420)-**d**ependent **n**itro-reductase (ddn) coenzymes. Among anti-TB drugs, Dlm has the lowest MIC (0.006–0.05 mcg/mL) against the drug susceptible- and DR-TB isolates, and is active against both the replicating and dormant extra- and intra-cellular bacilli. Its bioavailability is estimated to be between 25–47%. It is extremely (> 97%) protein bound, with high aVd (2100 L), and a half life 30–38 hrs. Very little (< 5%) Dlm is excreted in urine. It is primarily (95%) metabolized in blood by albumin with secondary (5%) contribution by liver CYP450 enzymes, mainly CYP3A4, CYP2D6 and CYP2E1.

The drug is available as 50 mg film-coated tablets and the adult dose is 100 mg twice daily for 24 weeks. Its oral absorption is increased when administered with meal. Despite its long t½ Dlm is given in twice daily doses to achieve higher concentrations of its active metabolite faster and maintain the same on long-term basis. Common side effects associated with Dlm are nausea (38%), vomiting and dizziness (30%). However, like Bdq, Dlm can cause QT prolongation and therefore is not recommended to be given with Bdq and other QT-prolonging drugs like moxifloxacin and clofazimine, and even alone when QTcF interval is more than 500 ms on repeated ECG. One of the strongest points for Dlm is its inability to be metabolized by CYP450 enzymes, making it a favourable drug for the treatment of TB in HIV patients.

Dlm has been recommended by WHO for children with MDR-TB above 6 years of age on compassionate basis; the dose is 50 mg BD for age 6–11 years (or 20–30 kg body weight) and 100 mg BD for age >12 years (or >35 kg body weight) for six months.

Repurposed Anti-TB Drugs

1. Linezolid (Lzd): Linezolid (discussed in Ch. 57) has been found to be very effective against both drug-susceptible as well as drug-resistant *M. tuberculosis,* and has been successfully used as a component of multidrug regimen in patients with drug-resistant TB. However, its adverse effects on prolonged use (which becomes necessary for the treatment of TB) may limit its usefulness. Adverse effects which should be watched carefully and seriously include dose-dependent and reversible bone marrow suppression and peripheral neuropathy which may be irreversible. Incidentally, the oral dose used is 600 mg once a day (i.e., half of the usual dose; as it is given 600 mg BD in normal course) which may reduce the incidence of these adverse effects. As per WHO guidelines of 2016, it is now classified as Group C core SLO drug along with Clofazimine.

2. Clofazimine (Cfz): As described below (p 778), Cfz, besides leprostatic has also been found to have tuberculostatic and good sterilizing activity. As a result, it is now classified by WHO as Group C drug along with Lzd. It is administered as per patient weight-wise bands in the dose of 50–200 mg/day as anti-TB drug.

TREATMENT OF TUBERCULOSIS

The goal of treatment of tuberculosis is to ensure high cure rates, prevent emergence of drug resistance, minimize relapses and cut the chain of transmission through early diagnosis and treatment. Treatment of tuberculosis is not only a matter of individual health; it is also a matter of public health. All practitioners who undertake to treat a patient with tuberculosis must not only prescribe a standard regimen, but also have the means to assess compliance to regimen and address poor compliance in order to ensure that treatment is completed.

Revised National Tuberculosis Control Program (RNTCP) is launched in 1997. RNTCP is renamed as ***National Tuberculosis Elimination Program (NTEP)*** in 2020. The goal is to achieve a rapid decline in burden of TB, morbidity and mortality while strategies towards elimination of TB by 2025.

Principle of Treatment for Tuberculosis

Short course chemotherapy regimen is administered to treat and cure TB patients as short as period of 6 months. Reduction in the duration of treatment regimens is possible because of the combination therapy. The first line antituberculosis drugs are initiated as a daily Fixed Dose Combination (FDC) according to the body weight of patient.

Objectives of Multi-Drug Therapy (MDT)

Objectives of MDT are to prevent the development of drug resistant bacilli, to prevent relapse of TB, to decrease morbidity and mortality, combination therapy reduces duration of treatment, to decrease transmission of TB and faster sputum conversion.

Bacterial Subpopulation in Tuberculosis

- ***Rapidly growing bacteria***: Inside wall of lung cavity, bacteria will divide. Isoniazid acts rapidly and kills bacteria inside cavity
- ***Slow multiplying bacteria***: Inside macrophage and inflamed sites at acidic pH. Pyrazinamide acts on slow growing bacteria.
- ***Spurters***: Bacteria resides within caseous material. Rifampicin acts on spurters and intermittently dividing bacteria.
- ***Dormant***: Bacteria remans inactive for prolonged time. Bedaquiline is effective on the dormant phase of bacteria.
- ***Pyrazinamide*** and ***rifampicin*** have good sterilizing activity. Ethambutol helps in faster sputum conversion and slows development of resistance.

Classification by History of Previous TB Treatment

- *New case*: TB patient who has never taken anti-TB drugs or has taken them for < 1 month.
- *Previously treated* patients have received anti-TB drugs for 1 month or more from any source in the past.

DRUG-SENSITIVE TB (DS-TB)

In patient with drug sensitive TB, the bacilli are susceptible to all first-line drugs for TB. It can be newly diagnosed TB case or previously treated case.

Treatment is given in two phases:

- *Intensive phase (IP)* consists of 8 weeks (56 doses) of isoniazid (H), rifampicin (R), pyrazinamide (Z) and ethambutol (E) daily.
- *Continuation phase (CP)*, consists of 16 weeks (112 doses) of isoniazid, rifampicin and ethambutol daily.

The CP can be extended upto 24 weeks in various conditions like tuberculosis of CNS, skeletal muscles, disseminated TB, etc.

Role of intensive phase: The objective of combining four drugs in the intensive phase (IP) is to achieve rapid killing of actively multiplying bacillary population.

Role of continuation phase: Continuation phase (CP) for longer time will ensure elimination of persisters which are responsible for relapses.

Regimen for Drug-Sensitive (DS) Tuberculosis

The H and R sensitive cases of TB and cases with unknown sensitivity pattern, the treatment regimen is given in Table 59.1.

Table 59.1 Regimen for drug sensitive TB for adults and children

Type of TB case	Intensive phase	Continuation phase
New and previously treated cases (H and R Sensitive/ unknown)	2HRZE	4HRE

The daily dosage of commonly used first line drugs are given in Table 59.2.

If a patient does not take drugs as recommended in IP or CP, the regular schedule should be started, continued and completed (56 doses of IP and 112 doses of CP). *Patient should adhere* to the number of doses to be administered.

Recording of Adverse Events

Adverse events must be recorded with details like date, symptoms, duration, management of adverse event and outcome. *Common adverse effects*: Isoniazid – Peripheral neuropathy, skin rash, hepatitis, sleepiness; Rifampicin – Abdominal pain, nausea, vomiting, hepatitis, generalised cutaneous reactions; Pyrazinamide – Arthralgia, hepatitis, gastrointestinal; Ethambutol – Retrobulbar neuritis.

The daily dose of drugs for tuberculosis is according to the body weight of patient (Table 59.3).

Treatment of Paediatric TB

For children having tuberculosis, daily dosages are as per 6 weight categories (Table 59.4). If age of patient is up to 18 years and weight <39 kg, should be treated using paediatric weight category. But, if weight of children is >39 kg, should be treated as per adult weight category (Table 59.4).

Chemoprophylaxis; TB Preventive Therapy (TPT)

TPT is recommended to prevent progression of TB infection to TB disease in contacts of drug-sensitive TB patients. Children are more susceptible to TB infection, more likely to develop active TB disease. They are more likely to develop severe forms of disseminated TB. Children < 6 years of age, who are close contacts of a TB patient, should be evaluated for active TB.

Isoniazid Preventive Therapy (IPT)

INH should be used for TPT to prevent TB infection to TB disease. It is recommended that, first rule out the active TB disease and then start TPT.

The dose of INH for preventive therapy is 10 mg/kg body weight, administered daily for a minimum period of 6 months.

Management of TB in Patients with Liver Disorders

Many anti-TB drugs are hepatotoxic. Liver functions should be monitored. If the serum alanine aminotransferase level is >3 times normal before the initiation of treatment, the following regimens should be considered:

- **Containing two hepatotoxic drugs (options)**:
  a) 9 months: Isoniazid, Rifampicin, plus Ethambutol – 9HRE
  b) 2 months: Isoniazid, Rifampicin, Streptomycin and Ethambutol, followed by 7 months of Isoniazid and Rifampicin – 2SHR + 7HR
  c) 6–9 months, Rifampicin, pyrazinamide and ethambutol – 6–9 RZE
- **Containing one hepatotoxic drug**: 2 months of Isoniazid, Ethambutol and Streptomycin, followed by 10 months of Isoniazid and Ethambutol – 2SHE + 10HE.

Table 59.2 Drug dosages for first-line anti-TB drugs

Drug	Adult	Children	Maximum in children
Isoniazid (H)	5 mg/kg daily (4–6 mg/kg)	10 mg/kg daily (7–15 mg/kg)	300 mg
Rifampicin (R)	10 mg/kg daily (8–12 mg/kg)	15 mg/kg daily (10–20 mg/kg)	600 mg
Pyrazinamide (Z)	25 mg/kg daily (20–30 mg/kg)	35 mg/kg daily (30–40 mg/kg)	2000 mg
Ethambutol (E)	15 mg/kg daily (12–18 mg/kg)	20 mg/kg daily (15–25 mg/kg)	1500 mg

Table 59.3 Daily dose schedule for adults (as per weight category)

Weight category* (kg)	Number of tablets (FDCs)	
	Intenstive phase (HRZE)	Continuation phase (HRE)
	75/150/400/275	75/150/275
25–34	2	2
35–49	3	3
50–64	4	4
65–77	5	5
>75	6	6

**During treatment, if the weight of the patient increases by more than 5 kg and crosses the next weight category then patient should be given the next higher weight category FDC drugs*

- **Containing no hepatotoxic drugs**: 18–24 months of Streptomycin, Ethambutol and Levofloxacin – 18–24 SLE.

TB in Pregnant and Lactating Women

A recommended dose and duration of anti-TB drugs are essential for successful outcome of pregnancy. The first-line drugs for TB are safe for use in pregnancy. Injectable drug, Streptomycin should not be used during pregnancy, as it is ototoxic to the foetus. Lactating mother should receive a full course of first line drugs for TB. Vitamin B_6 should be given to mother (10 mg/kg) and infant (5 mg/day).

Latent Tuberculosis Infection (LTBI)

LTBI is termed as the presence of *M. tuberculosis* bacteria in the body without signs and symptoms, or radiographic evidence of TB. Isoniazid should be used for at least 6 months in LTBI to reduce subsequent progression of TB.

TB and HIV

The primary impact of HIV on TB is that the risk of developing TB becomes higher in patients with HIV. Similarly, Tuberculosis is the most common opportunistic infection amongst HIV-infected individuals. Implementation of Isoniazid preventive treatment (IPT) for all HIV patients is recommended.

Table 59.4 Drug dosage for paediatric TB

Weight category (kg)	Number of tablets (dispersible FDC)			
	Intenstive phase		Continuation phase	
	HRZ	E	HR	E
	50/75/150	100	50/75	100
4–7	1	1	1	1
8–11	2	2	2	2
12–15	3	3	3	3
16–24	4	4	4	4
25–29	3 + 1A	3	3 + 1A	3
30–39	2 + 2A	2	3 + 1A	2

A—Adult; FDC—(HRZE = 75/150/400/275; HRE = 75/150/275).

For drug details and regimens used in patients having HIV and TB, refer Ch. 62.

Co-trimoxazole is given routinely for the prevention of opportunistic infections in HIV-infected persons; this strategy is called **Cotrimoxazole Prophylaxis Therapy**. *Dose*: 960 mg (800 mg sulfamethoxazole + 160 mg trimethoprim) daily.

DRUG-RESISTANT TB (DR-TB)

The management of DR-TB is very complex. It is important to prevent development of DR-TB. The implementation of the DOTS strategies must be strengthened at community level.

Definition of Drug Resistant Tuberculosis (DR-TB)

- **Mono-resistant (MR)**: A TB patient, whose biological specimen is resistant to one first line anti-TB drug only.
- **Poly-Drug Resistant (PDR)**: The bacilli are resistant to more than one first-line anti-TB drug, but not both INH and Rifampicin.
- **Multi Drug Resistant (MDR)**: A TB patient, resistant to both isoniazid and rifampicin with or without resistance to other first-line anti-TB drugs.
- **Rifampicin Resistant (RR)**: Resistance to rifampicin detected with or without resistance to other anti-TB drugs excluding INH. Patients, who have any Rifampicin resistance, should also be managed, as if they are an MDR TB case.
- **Extensively Drug Resistant (XDR)**: MDR-TB case whose biological specimen is additionally resistant to a fluoroquinolone (ofloxacin, levofloxacin or moxifloxacin) and a second-line injectable anti-TB drug (kanamycin, amikacin or capreomycin).

Classes of Anti-TB Drugs Recommended for Treatment of DR TB patients (WHO)

The anti-TB drugs are grouped based on efficacy, experience of use and drug class and aligned with revised classification as per WHO consolidated guidelines for treatment of drug resistant TB. They were classified into three groups: (1) Oral H mono/poly DR TB regimen; (2) Shorter MDR-TB regimen; (3) Oral longer M/XDR-TB regimen.

Regimen for DR TB Treatment

For M/DR-RR TB patients: Select 3 drugs from Group A (Lfx/Mfx, Bdq and Lzd) and 1 drug from Group B (Cfz and Cs). Ensure that the treatment starts with atleast four anti-TB agents. If the regimen cannot be composed with drugs from Groups A and B alone, Group C drugs are added to complete regimen (Table 59.5).

Table 59.5 Grouping of anti-TB drugs for longer MDR regimen

Groups & Steps	Drug	Abbreviation
Group A	Levofloxacin OR Moxifloxacin Bedaquiline Linezolid	Lfx Mfx Bdq Lzd
Group B	Clofazimine Cycloserine OR Terizidone	Cfz Cs Trd
Group C	Ethambutol Delamanid Pyrazinamide Imipenem-cilastatin Meropenem Amikacin (OR Streptomycin) Ethionamide OR Prothionamide p-aminosalicylic acid	E Dlm Z Ipm-Cln Mpm Am S Eto Pto PAS

Other drugs that are not included in Groups A-C are:

- Kanamycin and Capreomycin, which were associated with poorer outcomes when used and are therefore no longer recommended for use in MDR TB regimens.
- Gatifloxacin and high-dose Isoniazid were used in very few patients and thioacetazone was not used at all. Gatifloxacin is not currently available following its withdrawal from the market due to concerns about dysglycaemias.
- Thioacetazone is unlikely to have a role in longer regimens and is not currently available in a quality-assured formulation.
- Clavulanic acid should be included in MDR/RR TB regimens only as a companion agent to the carbapenems (Imp-Cln and Mpm). It should be given with every dose of carbapenem and should not be counted as an additional effective TB agent.

The standard regimens are given in Table 59.6.

- **All oral H mono-poly DR TB regimen**: Patients with Isoniazid (H) resistance or poly DR TB, regimen is given for 6 months with no separate IP and CP. Duration can be extended to 9 months in certain conditions. In CNS, skeletal and milliary TB, treatment may be given up to one year.
- **Shorter MDR TB regimen**: Total duration of shorter MDR TB regimen is for 9–11 months, depending on IP duration. IP should be given for at least 4 months. After fourth month, if sputum microscopy is negative then CP should be initiated. IP should be extended to 5th or 6th month at the end of 4th and 5th month of treatment if sputum microscopy and culture remains positive. This will be done for a maximum of 2 months (i.e., total duration of IP is not >6 months). Duration of CP is fixed for 5 months.
- **All oral longer MDR TB regimen**: Total duration of all oral longer MDR TB regimen is 18–20 months. At the end of 6th month of treatment, the patient must be reviewed based on the 5th month culture result.

Tapper the dose of Lzd to half (300/150 mg) will be based on 4th month culture result. If culture result remains positive, the regimen is extended by 1 more month. However, the duration of new drugs (Bdq or Dlm) is limited to 24 weeks only.

Table 59.6 Standard regimen for initiating treatment of MDR/RR TB or H mono-poly DR TB

Regimen class	Intensive phase	Continuation phase
All oral H mono-poly DR TB regimen	(6) Lfx,R,E,Z	
MDR/RR TB		
Short MDR TB regimen	(4–6) Mfx,Km/Am,Eto,Cfz,Z,H,E	(5) Mfx,Cfz,Z,E
Bedaquiline-containing regimen	(4–6) Bdq (6 m) Lfx,Cfz,Z,E,H,Eto	(5) Lfx,Cfz,Z,E
Oral longer M/XDR-TB regimen	(18–20) Bdq (6 m or longer) Lfx,Lzd,Cfz,Cs	

- If Lfx resistance: Replace Lfx with Mfx for 9 months.
- If Mfx or Z can't be used: Replace with Lzd. If Lzd also cannot be given, replace with Cfz + Cs for 9 months.
- If Mfx and Z can't be used, add 2 drugs of 3: Lzd,Cfz,Cs for 9 months.

Table 59.7 Sequence of using replacement drugs to modify the regimen

Regimen	Replacement situations	Proposed drugs after replacement
All oral longer regimen (Lfx,Bdq, Lzd,Cfz,Cs)	In initial 6 months of treatment	
	If Lfx cannot be used, replace with Mfx	Mfx,Bdq,Lzd,Cfz,Cs
	If Mfx cannot be used, replace with 1 drug	Bdq,Lzd,Cfz,Cs + 1 drug from replacement sequence*
	If Bdq cannot be used, replace with Dlm	Lfx,Dlm,Lzd,Cfz,Cs
	If Dlm cannot be used, replace with 1 drug	Lfx,Lzd,Cfz,Cs + 1 drug from replacement sequence*

***Replacement sequence**: Z,Am,Eto,PAS,E,Imp/Cln or Mpm + Amx/Clv in given order.

Extension of IP beyond 8th month is not recommended and patient should be switched to CP.

- Sequence of using replacement drugs to modify the regimen is given in Table 59.7.

Patients who Miss Doses

In shorter MDR-TB regimen, all missed doses during IP must be completed prior to switching the patient to CP. Similarly, all missed doses during CP must be administered prior to ending treatment.

Patients who are "Lost to Follow-up"

Patients who are "lost to follow-up" (interrupt treatment continuously for 1 month or more): First evaluate the patient. If there are signs of impending treatment failure for any MDR RR TB patient with or without additional resistant to second line drugs, the patient should be switched to an oral longer DR-TB regimen. If patient is on Bdq regimen, Bdq course will be reloaded (started afresh). Patients who initiated on Bdq/Dlm containing regimen and return after treatment interruption of 1 month or more will be declared as "loss to follow up." Such patients would not be considered eligible for administration of same drug (Bdq/Dlm) anymore.

Treatment for Mycobacterium Avium Complex (MAC)

MAC infection is very common in HIV-infected patients. As a rule, the disease caused by nontuberculous or so-called "atypical" mycobacteria is often less severe than tuberculosis and is not communicable from person to person. MAC includes two atypical mycobacteria—*M. avium* and *M. intracellulare*. Infections due to MAC are common cause of pulmonary and disseminated disease in late stages of AIDS. Such infections usually do not respond to conventional antitubercular drugs. The most common drug regimens are as under:

- Rifampicin 450–600 mg OD;
- Ethambutol 800 - 1200 mg OD;
- Clarithromycin 1 gm OD
- Add injection Amikacin 750 mg to 1 g thrice weekly for the first 2–3 months.

Intensive phase is for 3 months and can be extended to a maximum of 6 months with all four drugs. Continuation phase of treatment will be with the same drugs except amikacin.

Role of Corticosteroids in Tuberculosis

Corticosteroids should be avoided in patients of TB. However, they can be given under certain conditions as follows:

1. In pleural, pericardial and meningeal TB: To prevent pleural adhesions, pericarditis and neurological deficits.
2. To control hypersensitivity reactions due to anti-TB drugs.
3. AIDS with severe complications of tuberculosis.

Prednisolone or dexamethasone can be given. The drug should be gradually tapered to prevent HPA axis suppression. Steroids are contraindicated in intestinal TB due to risk of perforation.

TREATMENT OF LEPROSY

Leprosy is a chronic granulomatous infection caused by an acid-fast bacilli *Mycobacterium lepare* which is related to tubercle bacilli. *M. leprae* cannot be grown on culture media, so drug sensitivity testing *in vitro* is not possible. The *M. leprae* lie within the macrophages and remain dormant but alive. Hence, though a large number of persons may be infected by *M. leprae*, only a few suffer clinically. Clinical leprosy, therefore, is a consequence of deficient cell mediated immunity in susceptible individuals. Infection is usually transmitted from person to person when bacilli are shed from the nose and skin lesions of the infected patients. It then affects the peripheral nervous system, the skin and various tissues.

For the purpose of categorising patients for chemotherapy, leprosy may be classified as:

1. ***Paucibacillary leprosy*** is a noninfectious leprosy with few bacilli. Also called *tuberculoid leprosy*. Important features are: **(a)** < 5 hypoaesthetic skin lesions; **(b)** normal or only partially deficient cell mediated immunity; **(c)** bacilli are rarely found in biopsies; **(d)** lepromin test is positive. Lepromin is an extract of tissue infected with *M. leprae*, used in skin test to determine tissue resistance to leprosy; **(e)** there are prolonged remissions with periodic exacerbations.
2. ***Multibacillary leprosy*** is an infectious leprosy with numerous bacilli. It is mainly a *lepromatous leprosy*. The important features of this type of leprosy are: **(a)** more than 5 hypoaesthetic but diffused skin lesions with mucous membrane infiltrations; **(b)** cellular immunity is largely deficient; **(c)** skin and mucous membrane have numerous bacilli; **(d)** lepromin test is negative; **(e)** the disease later progresses to anaesthesia of distal parts and wounds.

Classification of Antileprosy Drugs

Sulfones: Dapsone
Phenazine derivatives: Clofazimine

Antitubercular drugs: Rifampicin

Antibiotics:

a) *Fluoroquinolones*: Ofloxacin, Sparfloxacin, Pefloxacin
b) *Macrolides*: Clarithromycin
c) *Tetracyclines*: Minocycline

Dapsone

Dapsone is closely related to sulfonamides and shares a common mechanism of action, i.e., inhibition of bacterial folic acid synthesis. It is thus leprostatic. Dapsone is the most widely used sulfone for the long-term therapy of both types of leprosy. However, resistance usually emerges in some population of *M. leprae,* especially in lepromatous leprosy patients if it is used as a monotherapy. Therefore, the combination of dapsone with rifampicin and/or clofazimine is recommended for treatment of leprosy. The usual adult dose is 100 mg/day orally for 3–5 years (for children 1–2 mg/kg/day to a maximum of 100 mg/day). Dapsone is also useful in the treatment and prevention of *Pneumocystis carinii* pneumonia in AIDS patients (*prophylaixs*: 100 mg/day; *treatment*: dapsone 100 mg/day plus trimethoprim 15–20 mg/kg/day for 21 days).

Dapsone is well absorbed after oral administration and is widely distributed throughout the body fluids and tissues. It tends to remain in skin, muscle, kidney and liver up to 3 weeks after the therapy is stopped. Skin heavily infected with *M. leprae* may contain 10–15 times as much dapsone as normal skin. It is acetylated in liver, excreted in bile and undergoes enterohepatic circulation. About 70% is excreted in urine. Plasma half-life is 1–2 days.

Adverse Effects: Dapsone is usually well tolerated. However, it may produce nonhaemolytic anaemia and methaemoglobinaemia in persons having G6PD deficiency. Anaemia may be watched; dapsone may be avoided if Hb is less than 7 g %. Some other mild side effects include nausea, loss of appetite, pruritus, drug fever, reversible neuropathy and hepatotoxicity.

During dapsone therapy for lepromatous leprosy some reactive episodes may occur. These are known as *lepra reactions*. These are of two types. ***Type 1 lepra reactions*** are delayed hypersensitivity reactions to *M. leprae* antigens (Type IV hypersensitivity). It is characterised by cutaneous ulceration, and multiple nerve involvement. It can also be seen during dapsone therapy for tuberculoid leprosy. Prompt treatment with corticosteroids is necessary to prevent nerve damage. ***Type 2 lepra reactions***, also known as ***erythema nodosum leprosum,*** represent a humoral antibody response (Type III hypersensitivity) to dead bacteria. It is of abrupt onset, existing lesions enlarge, become red, inflammed and painful. This reaction can be treated with clofazimine or corticosteroid or thalidomide. Clofazimine does not act as rapidly as corticosteroids or thalidomide. It might suit for mild type-2 lepra reaction only.

Clofazimine

It is a phenazine dye which binds preferentially to mycobacterial DNA to inhibit mycobacterial growth. It is leprostatic and tuberculostatic drug with anti-inflammatory properties. This is a major advantage of clofazimine over other antileprosy drugs and, therefore, it has a valuable place in the management of lepra reaction ***(erythema nodosum leprosum)***.

Clofazimine is used for dapsone-resistant leprosy or in patients intolerant to dapsone. Recommended doses are 100 mg/day orally (but 50 mg/day is preferred in combination therapy). The antileprotic effect of clofazimine has a biological lag of 6–7 weeks, and hence it is preferred as a component of multidrug therapy of leprosy.

Its oral absorption is quite variable. Major elimination is through faeces. Plasma half-life is 60–70 hrs. It is widely distributed in tissues including phagocytes.

The most disturbing ***side effects*** of clofazimine are two: (1) red-brown discolouration of skin, especially in fair complexioned people and (2) abdominal pain with loose stools due to deposition of clofazimine crystals in the intestinal mucosa. It is to be avoided in pregnancy. Mild side effects include conjunctival pigmentation and phototoxicity.

Rifampicin

Rifampicin has been discussed earlier in this chapter. It is bactericidal to *M. leprae* also. Though it rapidly renders leprosy patients noncontagious (kills 99.9% *M. leprae* in 5–6 days), resistance develops after prolonged treatment. Hence it is not used alone but as a component in multidrug therapy of leprosy so as to shorten the duration of treatment. Usual dose in lepromatous leprosy is 600 mg/day but single 600 mg/month is preferred in combination therapy to minimise its hepatotoxicity and the chance of enzymatic induction.

Fluoroquinolones

Ofloxacin (400 mg/day orally) if used as monotherapy, has been reported to kill 99.9% of *M. leprae* in 3 weeks period. However, it is used as an alternative drug, and not as a main drug, in the treatment of leprosy (see below) for the patients who have rifampicin intolerance or resistance. Ciprofloxacin, incidentally, is inactive but ***ofloxacin, pefloxacin*** (400 mg, BD) and ***sparfloxacin*** (400 mg once on first day, followed by 200 mg/day) are highly active.

Clarithromycin

It has a weaker activity than rifampicin, against *M. leprae* but is the only macrolide antibiotic which also has antileprotic activity. Clarithromycin (500 mg/day) can kill 99.9% of bacteria but in 8 weeks. It is also one of the alternative drugs for the treatment of leprosy. For other details refer Ch. 57.

Minocycline

It is an only tetracycline which is active against *M. leprae*. However, it is less active than rifampicin but more active than clarithromycin. If clofazimine cannot be used because of unacceptable skin pigmentation, minocycline 100 mg/day may be substituted in standard regimen. For other details refer Ch. 58.

Antileprotic Drugs under Investigation

Under recent preliminary trials the antileprotic activity of bedaquline (see earlier text) was found to be equal to rifampicin or moxifloxacin but significantly greater than minocycline. These data suggest that bedaquline may prove to be an important drug in the management of leprosy.

Mycobacterium Indicus Pranii (MIP) Vaccine

Mycobacterium indicus pranii (MIP) is a rapidly growing, non-pathogenic mycobacterium, shares several antigens with *M. leprae*. The MIP vaccine is developed by the National Institute of Immunology, India. It is safe and well accepted. It accelerates bacterial clearance and hastens recovery of leprosy patient. It has both immunotherapeutic, as well as immunoprophylactic properties against leprosy.

WHO REGIMEN FOR LEPROSY TREATMENT

- **For Multibacillary (Lepromatous) Leprosy**:
  Rifampicin 600 mg once monthly (supervised) +
  Dapsone 100 mg daily (self-administered) +
  Clofazimine 300 mg once monthly (supervised) +
  Clofazimine 50 mg daily (self-administered)
  Duration of treatment is for 12 months.
- **For Paucibacillary (Tuberculoid) Leprosy**:
  Dapsone 100 mg daily (self-administered) +
  Rifampicin 600 mg once monthly (supervised)
  Duration of treatment is for 6 months.
- **Alternative Regimens**:
  Clofazimine + Any two other drugs (ofloxacin, clarithromycin, minocycline, etc.) daily for 6 months followed by clofazimine + minocycline or ofloxacin daily for further 18 months.
- **Post-exposure Prophylaxis for Leprosy**: Single dose of rifampicin is recommended for contact of multibacillary leprosy.

CHAPTER 60 Antifungal Drugs

COMPETENCY PH1.57

Fungal infections are called "mycoses". Unlike bacteria, fungi are eukaryotic. They have a rigid cell wall composed mainly of chitin (instead of peptidoglycan), followed by a cell membrane which contains ergosterol (rather than cholesterol found in mammalian membrane). Fungi can be divided into four classes: **(1)** ***Yeasts*** (which reproduce by budding). The only pathogenic yeast is *Cryptococcus neoformans* which causes meningitis. **(2)** ***Yeast-like fungi*** (which partly grows like yeast and partly as filaments called hyphae). The only pathogenic fungus in this group is *Candida albicans* which causes oral/ vaginal thrush and systemic candidiasis. Another yeast-like fungus causing superficial mycoses is *Pityrosporom orbiculare* (which causes pityriasis versicolor or tinea versicolor presented as distinct hyperpigmented macules with fine scaling over the face, trunk and proximal extremities). **(3)** ***Moulds*** (filamentous fungi which reproduce by forming spores). Pathogenic moulds are called *dermatophytes* (e.g., *Trichophyton* sp., *Microsporum* sp and *Epidermophyton* sp., all causing skin or nail infections called tinea or 'ringworm'). Dermatophytoses (or tinea infection) is further classified according to body site affected: *Tinea barbae* (beard), *T. capitis* (scalp), *T. corporis* (body), *T. cruris* (groin),*T. manuum* (hand), *T. pedis* (athlete foot) and *T. unguium* (nails). Another pathogenic mould causing systemic fungal infection is *Aspergillus fumigatus* causing pulmonary aspergillosis and **(4)** ***Dimorphic fungi*** (which can grow as filaments or as yeast). Most fungi causing systemic infections are dimorphic fungi, e.g., *Histoplasma capsulatum* (causing histoplasmosis characterised by cough, fever, multiple pneumonic infiltrates in lungs followed by dissemination), *Coccidioides immitis* (causing coccidiomycosis characterised by pulmonary tuberculosis with dissemination), *Blastomyces dermatides* (causing blastomycosis presented as pneumonitis followed by dissemination). Another dimorphic fungus which causes subcutaneous mycoses is *Sporothrix* sp. (causing sporotrichosis presented as granulomatous lesions with lymphatic spread).

CLASSIFICATION OF ANTIFUNGAL AGENTS

- ***Inhibition of fungal cell wall synthesis (Echinocandins)***
  Caspofungin, Micafungin and Anidulafungin
- ***Bind to fungal cell membrane ergosterol and increase membrane permeability (Polyene Group)***
  Amphotericin-B, Nystatin
- ***Inhibition of ergosterol + lanosterol synthesis (Allylamine Group)***
  Terbinafine (see also topical agents)
- ***Inhibition of ergosterol synthesis (Azole Group)***
  Ketoconazole, Fluconazole, Itraconazole, Voriconazole and Posaconazole (see also topical Azoles), Isavuconazole
- ***Inhibition of nucleic acid synthesis***
  5-Flucytosine
- ***Disruption of mitotic spindle and inhibition of fungal mitosis***: Griseofulvin
- ***Newer Drug***: *Ibrexafungerp*
- ***Topical Agents***
  Ciclopi+rox, Tolnaftate, Clioquinol, Naftifine, Butenafine and Topical Azoles (Miconazole, Clotrimazole, Butaconazole, Econazole, Oxiconazole, Sulconazole, Terconazole and Tioconazole)

Antifungal drugs described in this chapter have been categorised into three major headings: (1) Drugs used for systemic fungal infections, (2) Drugs given systemically to treat superficial fungal infections and (3) Drugs used topically to treat superficial fungal infections. Precisely speaking, such distinction is arbitrary because as discussed below, azole group of antifungal drugs and even amphotericin-B can be used systemically as well as topically.

DRUGS USED TO TREAT SYSTEMIC FUNGAL INFECTIONS

Echinocandins

Three echinocandins are in current use: ***caspofungin, micafungin*** and ***anidulafungin***

Mechanism of Action: They cause fungal cell wall lysis by inhibiting the synthesis of 1,3-β-glucan, an essential component of the cell wall of susceptible fungi (Fig. 60.1). Mammalian cell wall does not require 1,3-β-glucan. Hence, selective toxicity to the fungi and not to the host.

Therapeutic Use: They are used for the treatment of invasive *Aspergillus* infection and *candidiasis* (oesophageal, intra-abdominal peritonitis etc.). Caspofungin is orally not absorbed and hence infused slowly (initially 70 mg is infused slowly and then 50 mg/day infusion). It is well tolerated.

Adverse Effects: Common adverse effects are minor and include thrombophlebitis, abnormal liver functions, sensation of warmth, flushing, headache and rashes. A combination of caspofungin with cyclosporine should be avoided because of the risk of hepatotoxicity.

Drug Interactions: Enzyme inducers increase the clearance of caspofungin while caspofungin increases the clearance of tacrolimus.

Micafungin and ***anidulafungin*** are more potent analogues of caspofungin.

Amphotericin-B (Polyene Group)

It is a polyene group of antifungal-antibiotic whose chemical structure is composed of a large lactone ring (as in macrolides) with several conjugated double bonds.

Mechanism of Action: Amphotericin-B binds to the ergosterol, a fungal cell membrane sterol (see above), and alters the permeability of the fungal cell membrane by forming pores (channels) through which K^+, Na^+, Mg^{2+}, H^+ and other macromolecules leak out, leading to cell death (Fig. 60.1). The principal sterol of the mammalian cell membrane is cholesterol for which amphotericin-B has much less affinity. Therefore, the drug shows selective toxicity against fungal cells than mammalian cells. Nevertheless, some binding to human membrane sterols does occur which accounts for the drug toxicity. *Resistance to amphotericin-B* is associated with a replacement of ergosterol by other sterols in fungal plasma membrane. When this happens, a parallel fall in virulence also occurs, so resistance has not been a problem clinically with amphotericin-B except for rare instances involving *Candida* other than *C. albicans*. Fungi that lack ergosterol are not susceptible to the drug.

Pharmacokinetics: It is poorly absorbed from GIT. Oral administration is thus effective only against fungal infections of instestine, and not for treatment of systemic fungal infections. It is, therefore, administered by slow I.V. infusion. However, it is insoluble in water and is therefore prepared as a colloidal suspension with sodium desoxycholate for I.V. infusion. Several new formulations as liposomal amphotericin-B and lipid complex of amphotericin-B are now available. Liposomal amphotericin-B incorporates the drug into small unilamellar lipid vesicles; while amphotericin-B lipid complex is a non-liposomal formulation that complexes the drug with two phospholipids. An active drug from these lipid moieties, can be selectively transferred to ergosterol containing fungal membrane, without interfering with cholesterol-containing human cell membrane, thereby reducing the risk for nephrotoxicity.

Peak antifungal activity of the drug occurs at pH 6.0 to 7.5. The drug is widely distributed in most tissues (except in CSF unless administered intrathecally). It is 90% bound to plasma proteins and in tissues to cholesterol-containing membranes to some extent. Most of the drug is metabolised in liver and then slowly excreted by the kidney over a period of several days. Plasma half-life is about 15 days. Since plasma concentrations are not affected much, so dose adjustments are not needed in renal and hepatic impairments.

Antifungal Spectrum and Therapeutic Uses: Amphotericin-B is most commonly used to treat serious disseminated yeast group and some mould group of fungal infections in immuno-compromised hospitalised patients. It is also administered systemically to treat superficial candidiasis (see below). After the advent of azole

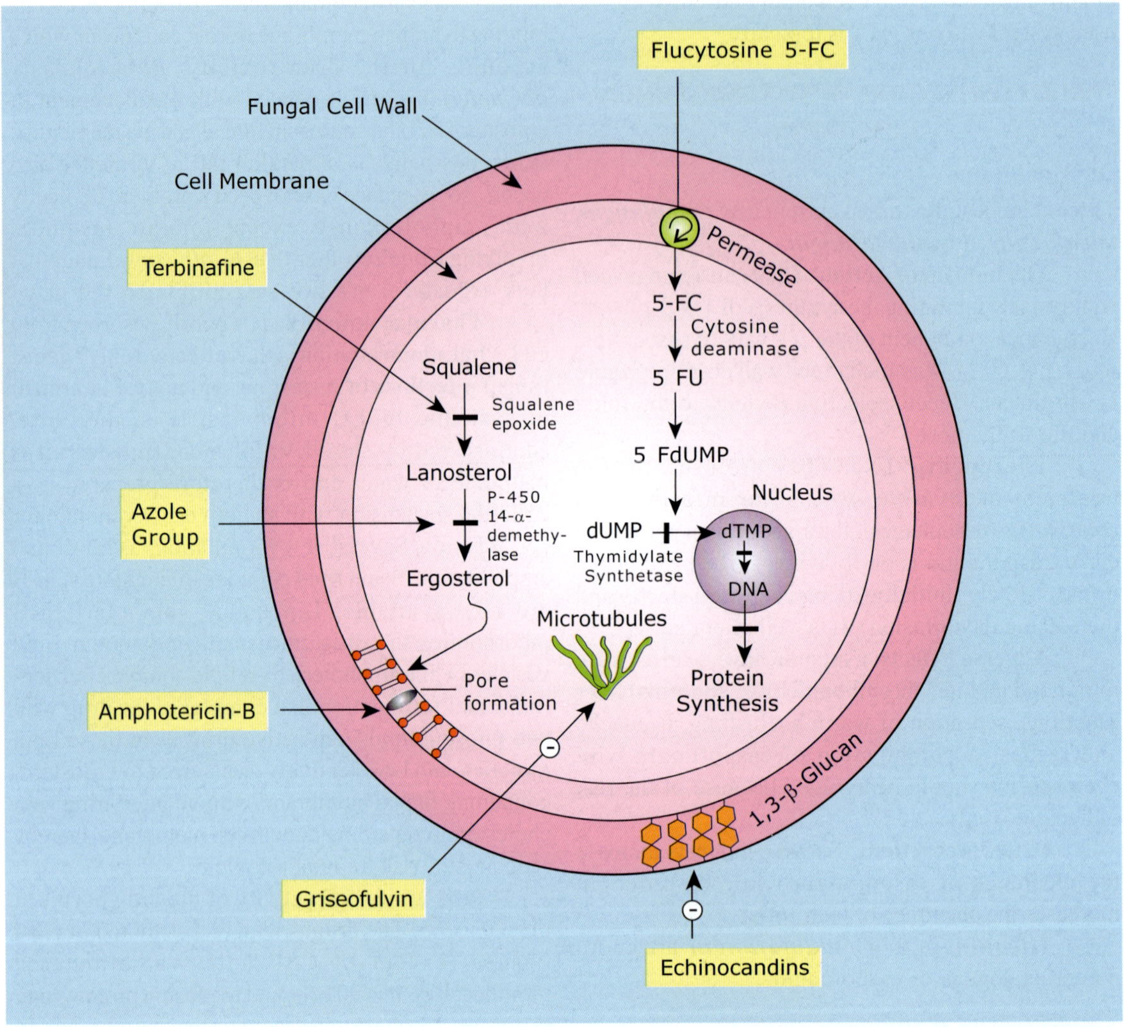

Fig 60.1 Mechanism of Action of Various Antifungal Drugs. Representative Antifungal Drugs are Shown in Yellow Boxes; refer text for details

group of antifungal drugs (e.g., fluconazole), which have an advantage of ease of administration and reduced toxicity profile, the use of amphotericin-B has lately declined. However, it still remains a drug of choice in the following order of fungal infections:

1) Treatment of invasive aspergillosis in immunocompromised and non-immunocompromised patients.
2) Mucormycosis (an opportunistic fungal infection in lungs).
3) Disseminated rapidly progressing histoplasmosis.
4) Rapidly progressive coccidioidomycosis, meningeal coccidioidomycosis and for paracoccidioidomycosis in immunosuppressed host.
5) Rapidly progressive blastomycosis. Blastomycosis in normal hosts no longer requires amphotericin-B treatment.
6) Non-AIDS cryptococcal meningitis (used with fluconazole or with flucytosine).

7) ***Topical Use***: It is also used topically (3% cream, lotion, ointment) to treat oropharyngeal candidiasis and cutaneous candidiasis. Mycotic corneal ulcers and keratitis can be cured with topical eye drops or by direct subconjunctival injection.
8) ***Other Use***: It is a reserve drug for resistant cases of Kala azar and mucocutaneous leishmaniasis.

The drug has no antibacterial activity. The usual therapeutic dose of amphotericin-B deoxycholate complex is 0.5–0.6 mg/kg/day as slow I.V. infusion in 5% glucose for 4 hrs. Treatment lasts till a total dose of 1–2 g is administered. Amphotericin-B and flucytosine have synergistic action on systemic candidiasis and cryptococcosis. Once the progression of fungal disease is arrested, after administering amphotericin-B, maintenance therapy can be continued with an azole group of antifungal agent.

Adverse Effects: **(1)** *The commonest, most serious, long-term toxicity of amphotericin-B administration is* ***nephrotoxicity*** (renal tubular necrosis, hypokalaemia and hypomagnesaemia secondary to renal tubular acidosis, azotaemia and even irreversible damage if the total dose exceeds 5 g). Keeping patient well hydrated by prior infusion of 1 L of normal saline reduces the risk of renal toxicity. Concomitant diuretic therapy should be avoided. Liposomal amphotericin-B carries a lesser risk for nephrotoxicity. **(2)** Hypochromic normocytic anaemia is common, but thrombocytopenia and leukopenia are less common. **(3)** Intrathecal administration may lead to arachnoiditis and seizures. **(4)** Hepatic impairment with jaundice can occur but rarely. **(5)** *Infusion related toxicity* is manifested as chills, tachypnoea, fever, vomiting and modest hypotension, but anaphylaxis is extremely rare. These reactions can be managed by administering paracetamol, diphenhydramine (antihistamine), K-supplements and hydrocortisone (a corticosteroid).

Being most toxic antifungal-antibiotic in use today, it is labelled as "amphoterrible" drug.

Drug Interactions: Flucytosine has synergistic actions with amphotericin-B because amphotericin-B facilitates permeation of flucytosine through the fungal cell membrane. Aminoglycosides and other nephrotoxic drugs enhance the renal toxicity of amphotericin-B. Concomitant use of diuretics should be avoided (see above).

Azole Group of Antifungal Drugs

These are synthetic antifungal drugs with broad-spectrum fungistatic or fungicidal properties depending upon drug concentration. Azoles can be divided into two groups: *the imidazole group* (2 nitrogens in the azole ring) and *triazole group* (3 nitrogens in the azole ring). Antifungal imidazole for systemic infections is only ketoconazole. Others are used topically to treat superficial fungal infections (see below). The representative drugs belonging to triazole group are fluconazole, itraconazole, voriconazole and posaconazole. Some are used only topically to treat superficial fungal infections (see below).

Mechanism of Action: Azole group of antifungal drugs bind to the fungal cytochrome P-450-dependent 14-α-demethylase enzyme, that is responsible for the demethylation of lanosterol to ergosterol. The ergosterol synthesis is therefore hindered, which results in damaged leaky fungal cell membrane (Fig. 60.1). However, an addition of ergosterol in culture media fails to reverse their antifungal effect *in vitro*, hence other antifungal mechanisms have also been ascribed to these agents. Azoles inhibit fungal respiration under aerobic conditions, hence blockade of respiratory-chain electron transport seems to be a more plausible alternative mechanism for their antifungal effects.

Antifungal Spectrum and Therapeutic Uses: Compared to imidazoles, triazoles tend to have fewer side effects, better absorption, better drug distribution in body tissues and fewer drug interactions. Itraconazole, fluconazole, voriconazole, and posaconazole are therefore preferred antifungal drugs compared to ketoconazole. Individual drugs have their own useful antifungal spectrum and clinical use and hence would be discussed individually.

Ketoconazole

Pharmacokinetics: Ketoconazole is well absorbed from the GIT provided the gastric contents are acidic. Therefore, the drugs that increase gastric pH, such as antacids and H_2 receptor blockers markedly reduce its absorption. Likewise its bioavailability is reduced in achlorhydria. Such patients should be given acidifying agents (like orange juice) before ketoconazole administration.

It is readily distributed to most body compartments but penetration into CSF is negligible; hence it is ineffective in the treatment of fungal meningitis. The drug is metabolised in the liver and excreted in the bile. Plasma half-life is 8–10 hrs but saturation of metabolism occurs shortly, which prolongs its half life and permits once-a-day dosing. Since only small amounts of active drug appear in urine, it is not effective in the treatment of fungal cystitis.

Therapeutic Uses: Ketoconazole has only restricted use (see adverse effects), and has been replaced by newer triazoles in the treatment of histoplasmosis and coccidioidomycosis. Ketoconazole is useful in silent non-CNS blastomycosis and in silent coccidioidomycosis. It is also effective against oropharyngeal candidiasis even in patients of AIDS. For this indication it is given orally. Ketoconazole is ineffective in the treatment of cryptococcosis, mucormycosis, aspergillosis and sporotrichosis.

Adverse Effects: Nausea, vomiting and anorexia occur commonly but these adverse effects can be minimised by taking ketoconazole with food. Pruritus, allergic dermatitis and reversible elevations in liver enzymes are also common, but hepatitis is rare. It markedly inhibits the synthesis of testosterone and estradiol which may lead to gynaecomastia and irregular menstrual cycles respectively. These hormonal effects have led to the use of ketoconazole as a potential adjunct in the drug therapy of prostatic carcinoma.

Drug Interactions: Ketoconazole inhibits mammalian cytochrome P450 (CYP3A4) more than fungal cytochrome P450. This leads to several drug interactions noted below:

1) Ketoconazole increases the serum concentrations of cisapride, terfenadine, astemizole and quinidine leading to fatal ventricular fibrillation and arrhythmias. It also raises the plasma concentrations of warfarin, cyclosporine, tacrolimus and HMG-CoA reductase inhibitors (except pravastatin and fluvastatin)
2) Rifampicin and phenytoin accelerate ketoconazole metabolism and reduce its efficacy.

Other drug interactions include:

1) H_2 receptor blockers, proton pump inhibitors and antacids decrease ketoconazole absorption by decreasing gastric acidity.
2) Ketoconazole (and azoles in general), since they inhibit the synthesis of ergosterol, should not be used along with amphotericin-B, because the depletion of membrane ergosterol reduces the binding sites for amphotericin-B.

Fluconazole

Pharmacokinetics: Fluconazole does not need acidic pH for its absorption from GIT, as does ketoconazole. The half-life is 27–37 hrs, permitting once daily dosing in patients with normal renal functions. About 80% of the drug is excreted unchanged in the urine, while about 10% is excreted unchanged in the faeces. Dosage reductions are required in the presence of renal insufficiency. Fluconazole has the least effect, of all the azoles, on hepatic microsomal enzymes. It can be administered orally as well as parenterally (I.V.).

Therapeutic Uses: Fluconazole, given orally, is very effective in the treatment of vulvovaginal, oropharyngeal, mucocutaneous and systemic candidiasis. A 3-day course of oral fluconazole is effective treatment for candida urinary tract infections. Candida endophthalmitis can be successfully treated with fluconazole. It is an acceptable alternative therapy for meningeal cryptococcosis, meningeal coccidioidomycosis and silent coccidioidomycosis. Its use obviates the need for intrathecal amphotericin-B. However, fluconazole displays no activity against aspergillus and other filamentous fungi. The usual oral dose is 150–400 mg once daily.

Adverse Effects: Fluconazole is well tolerated. Nausea, vomiting, diarrhoea, headache and rashes have been reported in 2–3% of patients. Increase in serum transaminase and alopecia have been observed as a common adverse effect in patients receiving prolonged therapy. Fluconazole has least effect on mammalian cytochrome P450. Therefore, drug interactions are mild and are of no clinical significance.

Itraconazole

Pharmacokinetics: Chemically, fluconazole and itraconazole are triazole derivatives but pharmacologically these are distinct. Itraconazole requires low gastric pH for its absorption (fluconazole does not). Oral bioavailability of itraconazole is variable, only 50–60% when taken with food (fluconazole bioavailability is 90%). Itraconazole is highly protein bound (99%), while fluconazole is 10–12% protein bound. Itraconazole has wider tissue distribution excepting CSF (fluconazole levels in CSF are 80% of serum levels). Itraconazole is metabolised in liver and excreted in bile (80% of fluconazole is excreted unchanged in urine). It has a longer half-life of 30–35 hrs. It is more specific for fungal cytochrome P450 dependent 14-α-demethylase as compared to ketoconazole, but is less specific than fluconazole.

Therapeutic Uses: Itraconazole is most useful in long-term suppressive treatment of disseminated or chronic pulmonary histoplasmosis in AIDS patients. It is also very useful in oral treatment of non-meningeal blastomycosis. It appears to be the drug of choice for cutaneous and extracutaneous sporotrichosis except meningitis and has a lower relapse rate in the treatment of disseminated coccidioidomycosis and indolent paracoccidioidomycosis than does fluconazole. Itraconazole and voriconazole are the two triazole antifungal agents which are most useful in the treatment of invasive aspergillosis in non-immunocompromised patients. Additional, but important, uses of itraconazole include treatment of oropharyngeal and cutaneous candidiasis, ringworm (e.g., Tinea capitis or T. corporis), fungal nail infections (Tinea unguium) and extensive Tinea versicolor. Although an unlabeled use, itraconazole is a drug of choice for treatment of pseudallescheriasis not responding to amphotericin-B. Usual recommended doses are 200–400 mg once daily.

Adverse Effects: Although well tolerated, itraconazole may be associated with headache, nausea and epigastric distress. Higher doses may cause hypokalaemia, hypertension and oedema. Serum transaminase enzyme levels may rise transiently. Itraconazole, unlike ketoconazole, does not suppress steroidogenesis. In recent years some cases of congestive heart failure in patients taking itraconazole have been reported through pharmacovigilance.

Drug Interactions: Although itraconazole inhibits mammalian cytochrome P450 to a lesser extent than ketoconazole, yet the following drug interactions are of concern with itraconazole:

1) Absorption of itraconazole is impaired by antacids, H_2 blockers, proton pump inhibitors and drugs that contain buffers, e.g., antiretroviral drug didanosine.
2) Itraconazole inhibits the metabolism of cisapride, astemizole and terfenadine. The resultant increase in their plasma concentration results in severe cardiac arrhythmias and death.
3) Similarly, itraconazole inhibits the metabolism of triazolam and midazolam and potentiates as well as prolongs the hypnotic effects of these drugs.
4) Rifampicin, phenytoin and carbamazepine accelerate the metabolism of itraconazole and reduce its efficacy.

Voriconazole

Pharmacokinetics: Voriconazole is a second generation triazole that has some distinguishing features compared to itraconazole and fluconazole. Like fluconazole, it has high oral bioavailability (96%), low protein binding (55%) and good CSF penetration but unlike fluconazole it undergoes extensive hepatic metabolism (through CYP2C19) and only 2% of free drug is excreted in urine. Unlike itraconazole and ketoconazole, gastric acid is not necessary for its absorption. Unlike fluconazole and itraconazole its plasma half-life is only 6 hrs. Dosage reduction is necessary in severe hepatic insufficiency but not with renal insufficiency.

Therapeutic Uses: It appears to be the best choice drug for primary therapy of invasive aspergillosis. Voriconazole is most useful in esophageal candidiasis. It is more active than amphotericin-B against certain moulds like *Fusarium* and *Pseudallescheria boydii* and can be used as first line therapy for these infections. Majority of candida isolates, resistant to fluconazole, are sensitive to voriconazole. Recommended doses are 200 mg 12 hourly.

Adverse Effects: Although voriconazole is generally well tolerated, about 30% of patients may experience transient visual changes such as blurred vision, altered colour perception and photophobia. These are usually reversible and normalise within one hour. Occasionally, rashes (5–6% of cases), nausea and elevated hepatic enzymes have been noted. Voriconazole, on prolonged use, has been reported to cause prolongation of the QTc interval.

Drug Interactions: Inhibitors or inducers of CYP2C19 may increase or decrease voriconazole plasma concentration. Rifampicin, rifabutin, phenytoin and ritonavir accelerate voriconazole metabolism and reduce its efficacy. On the other hand, the metabolism of sirolimus, tacrolimus, cyclosporine and warfarin is retarded by voriconazole leading to their significant accumulation. Grape fruit products may increase serum voriconazole levels.

Posaconazole

It is a triazole licensed in 2006.

Therapeutic Uses: Broader spectrum against candida, aspergillus infections in severely immuno-compromised patients. It is equally effective in mucormycosis and zygomycosis (for which till date only amphotericin-B was available). It is valuable alternative for fluconazole-resistant oropharyngeal candidiasis.

Adverse Effects: Well tolerated except headache, GIT distress and occasional elevation of liver enzymes.

Drug Interactions: Inhibits CYP3A4 isozymes and hence may increase the plasma levels of tacrolimus and cyclosporine resulting into toxicity.

Isavuconazole

It is a newly approved azole. It is used in fungal infections like mucormycosis. It is approved for rare fungal infection like invasive aspergillosis. It is an inhibitor of CYP3A4 metabolizing enzyme. Adverse effects: Nausea, vomiting, diarrhoea, hypokalaemia, dyspnoea, peripheral edema and insomnia. It does not prolong QT interval.

Flucytosine (5-Fluorocytosine; 5-FC)

5-FC is a fluorinated analogue of cytosine and is structurally related to the antineoplastic agent 5-fluorouracil. While devoid of anticancer activity, it is a potent antifungal agent.

Mechanism of Action: Flucytosine is transported into the fungal cells with the help of cytosine permease enzyme where it is converted to 5-fluorouracil by the fungal cytosine deaminase enzyme. 5-Fluorouracil is then further metabolised to 5-fluorodeoxyuridine monophosphate. The latter being the competitive inhibitor of thymidylate synthetase, blocks the formation of thymidine monophosphate from deoxyuridine monophosphate and inhibits the fungal DNA synthesis (Fig. 60.1). Mammalian cells are virtually devoid of cytosine deaminase which prevents the conversion of 5-FC to 5-Fluorouracil. Hence the drug is selectively toxic to the fungi and not to the host.

Pharmacokinetics: 5-FC is orally well absorbed (90–95%). It has a plasma half-life of 3–6 hrs and is excreted unchanged in the urine. Levels rise rapidly in renal impairment leading to toxicity.

Therapeutic Uses: 5-FC has a limited antifungal spectrum and is generally used as a part of combination therapy for candidiasis and cryptococcal meningitis (with amphotericin-B) or for chromoblastomycosis (with itraconazole). When it is used as monotherapy, resistance and therapeutic failure are common. When used with amphotericin-B, there is an increase in fungal uptake of 5-FC and hence the synergistic effects against candidiasis and cryptococcosis. Coadministration also permits reduction in the dose of amphotericin-B. Recommended doses are 50–150 mg/kg/day in divided doses every 6 hrs.

Adverse Effects: The major toxicity of 5-FC is bone marrow depression leading to leukopenia and thrombocytopenia. Because of baseline leukopenia, 5-FC is often not tolerated by end-stage HIV infected patients with disseminated candida/cryptococcal infection. Because it is normally given with highly nephrotoxic amphotericin-B, 5-FC serum levels should be closely monitored in patients with renal insufficiency. An elevation of hepatic enzymes and reversible hepatomegaly occurs in about 5% of the patients receiving 5-FC. Lastly it may cause nausea, vomiting, epigastric distress and skin rash that may result from the formation of 5-fluorouracil by the fungi and other intestinal microbes. There seems to be a narrow therapeutic window, with an increased risk of toxicity at higher drug levels. As a result it is nicknamed as 'fluotoxin'.

Ibrexafungerp

Ibrexafungerp is a newer antifungal that acts by inhibiting the synthesis of β-1,3-glucan synthase. Echinocandins bind to the FKS1 domain of β-1,3-glucan synthase, while Ibrexafungerp binds at an alternate site which allows them to maintain their activity against fungal infections that are resistant to echinocandins. It is given orally 300 mg twice daily. Half-life is approximately 20 hrs. It is approved by US-FDA for the treatment of vulvovaginal candidiasis. Adverse effects: Diarrhoea, nausea, abdominal pain, skin rash, elevated transaminases and vaginal bleeding.

DRUGS GIVEN SYSTEMICALLY FOR TREATING SUPERFICIAL FUNGAL INFECTIONS

The drugs discussed below are used systemically not to treat systemic fungal infections but to treat superficial mycoses, e.g., candidiasis and dermatophytoses (ringworm, tinea infection).

Griseofulvin

Griseofulvin is a fungistatic drug derived from *Penicillium griseofulvum*.

Pharmacokinetics: Ineffective topically, griseofulvin is administered orally but is variably absorbed from GIT. Micronisation of the drug particles and ingestion with a fatty meal improves its bioavailability. Although most of the administered drug is inactivated in the liver by dealkylation, its plasma half-life is approximately 24 hrs. The drug binds to keratin precursor cells and newly synthesised keratin in the stratum corneum of the skin, hair and nails making them resistant to fungal invasion.

Mechanism of Action: Griseofulvin causes disruption of the mitotic spindle and eventually arrests fungal mitosis at metaphase (Fig. 60.1). It also binds to newly synthesised keratin making it resistant to fungal invasion.

Therapeutic Uses: Its only use is in the systemic treatment of dermatophytosis caused by *Microsporum, Trichophyton* and *Epidermophyton* (broadly speaking tinea infections of skin, hair and nails). Duration of therapy depends on the site of infection and is usually longer. Such long duration of treatment is needed to allow the replacement of the fungal infected keratin by the fungal resistant new keratin. Nail infections require longer time because the growth of new fungal-resistant nail is slow. Recommended dose for the microfined griseofulvin is 500–1000 mg/day in 2 divided doses orally.

Adverse Effects: Headache, nausea, vomiting, photosensitivity and peripheral neuritis. Hepatotoxicity can occur in patients with acute intermittent porphyria. As an inducer of cytochrome P-450 it can decrease the effectiveness of warfarin and oral contraceptives. Paradoxically, it causes disulfiram-like reaction with ethanol (vomiting, headache, flushing and tachycardia). Itraconazole and terbinafine are more safe and more efficacious than griseofulvin and therefore more preferred nowadays.

Terbinafine

Terbinafine is a synthetic allylamine group of antifungal agent.

Pharmacokinetics: Its oral bioavailability is 50–70%. It is highly lipophilic and keratophilic resulting in high concentrations in stratum corneum, sebum, hair and nails. It has a prolonged terminal half-life of about 15 days because of the very slow release of the drug from skin, nails and adipose tissue. It has negligible effect on cytochrome P-450 enzyme system. Dosage adjustments are required in renal and hepatic insufficiency.

Mechanism of Action: Terbinafine inhibits fungal enzyme squalene epoxidase which converts squalene to lanosterol (Fig. 60.1). Reduced lanosterol production decreases ergosterol production which affects fungal cell membrane integrity and function. Thus, like azoles it also decreases ergosterol biosynthesis but unlike azoles it inhibits squalene epoxidase rather than cytochrome P-450 dependent 14-α-demethylase enzyme system (see earlier text). Like griseofulvin it is also keratophilic but unlike griseofulvin it is fungicidal.

Therapeutic Uses: It can be used systemically (250 mg/day in two divided doses) as well as topically. Orally it is specifically used to treat onychomycosis of toenail/fingernail while topically to treat tinea infections (ringworm, athlete foot etc.). Unlabeled use includes topical treatment of cutaneous candidiasis and pityriasis versicolor.

Adverse Effects: Terbinafine is generally well tolerated. However, it causes headache, GIT upset and liver enzymes elevation. It may cause symptomatic hepatobiliary dysfunction (but rarely). There are no clinically relevant drug interactions either.

TOPICALLY USED ANTIFUNGAL AGENTS

Nystatin

Nystatin is a polyene antifungal drug having a chemical structure similar to amphotericin-B and a mechanism of action also identical to amphotericin-B. Being too toxic for systemic use, nystatin is used primarily to treat candidal infections of the mucosa, skin, GIT and vagina. Nystatin is not absorbed to a significant degree from skin, mucous membranes or the GIT. Hence, chances of toxicity are rare. The major complaint on oral use is its bitter and foul taste. The topical use of amphotericin-B has already been discussed.

Topical Azoles

CLOTRIMAZOLE, MICONAZOLE, KETOCONAZOLE, BUTACONAZOLE, ECONAZOLE, OXICONAZOLE, SULCONAZOLE, TERCONAZOLE, TIOCONAZOLE and SERTACONAZOLE.

A plethora of topical azoles is available for the treatment of superficial mycoses. These are effective for tinea corposis, tinea pedis, tinea cruris, tinea versicolor, cutaneous, oropharyngeal and vulvovaginal candidiasis. Absorption is negligible, and adverse effects are rare. These are available as skin ointment, cream, lotion, vaginal cream and as vaginal tablets. Shampoo form of ketoconazole is also available for treating seborrheic dermatitis. Topical azoles + corticosteroid fixed-dose combinations are also available. *Oteseconazole* is recently approved azole used to reduce the incidence of recurrent vulvovaginal candidiasis (RVVC) in females.

Topical Allylamines

TERBINAFINE, BUTENAFINE and NAFTIFINE

Naftifine is available as 1% cream for topical use primarily for cutaneous dermatophytosis and candida infections. It is as effective as topical azoles for these conditions. *Butenafine* is structurally related to naftifine and is available as 1% cream to be applied once daily for superficial dermatophytosis (tinea infections). *Terbinafine* (see above) is also used as 1% cream for treatment to tinea pedis, tinea cruris, tinea corporis and tinea versicolor.

Ciclopirox

It is available as 1% cream and lotion for the topical treatment of dermatomycosis, cutaneous candidiasis and tinea versicolor. Higher concentration (8%) can also be used for the treatment of mild to moderate onychomycosis of fingernails and toenails. It acts by inhibiting the membrane uptake of amino acids and ions needed for the fungal growth.

Tolnaftate

It is a synthetic antifungal drug. It distorts hyphae and mycelial growth of yeast-like fungi and moulds. It is effective in the topical treatment of dermatomycosis and tinea, but relapses are common. Infections of the palms, soles, and nails are usually unresponsive to tolnaftate alone.

Clioquinol

Topically it can be used to treat dermatophytosis, tinea barbae, seborrhoeic dermatitis and pityriasis versicolor. It is also useful as vaginal cream for monilial and trichomonas vaginitis. It is available as 3–8% cream.

Benzoic Acid and Sodium Thiosulfate

Sodium thiosulfate is a weak fungistatic. Its 20% solution, if applied twice daily for a month, is effective in pityriasis versicolor. It is not useful in other superficial mycosis. *Benzoic acid* is also a weak fungistatic which is sometimes used in combination with salicylic acid (Whitfield ointment: Benzoic acid 6% + Salicylic acid 3%). When applied on hyperkeratotic lesion, salicylic acid due to its keratolytic action, helps to remove the infected tissue and promotes the penetration of benzoic acid into the fungal infected lesion.

CHAPTER 61

Antiviral Drugs for Non-retroviral Infections

COMPETENCY PH1.48

Virus is an ultramicroscopic infectious parasite responsible for significant morbidity and mortality in populations worldwide. These microorganisms consist of a core genome of nucleic acid (either RNA or DNA; not both) contained in a protein shell (capsid) which in many viruses is also surrounded by a lipoprotein membrane called envelope (Fig. 61.1). The whole structure (genome + capsid + envelope) constitutes a virion (the intact virus particle).

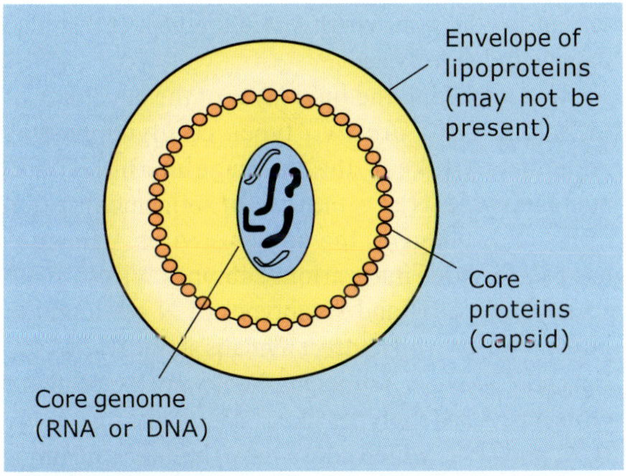

Fig 61.1 Basic Components of Virus Particle (Virion)

A virus is active only when it is within the host cells. Hence viruses are called obligate parasites (obligate = entirely dependent on). These host cells may be mammalian (mammalian virus) or insect (arbovirus) or plant (plant virus) or bacteria (bacteriophage). Virus outside the host cells is inert as it cannot replicate independently. They have to use energy generating, RNA or DNA replicating, and protein synthesising machinery of the host cells for their growth. They not only replicate in host cells but direct them to make new viral particles. Therefore, it is very difficult to find an antiviral drug that would selectively inhibit or kill the virus without being toxic to the infected host cells.

CLASSIFICATION OF VIRUSES

Viruses are basically classified as ***DNA viruses*** or ***RNA viruses***, depending upon the genomic material in their core. Their classification and the diseases they produce is noted below:

DNA Viruses

(1) ***Adenoviruses*** (upper respiratory tract and eye infection). **(2)** ***Hepadnaviruses*** (hepatitis-B). **(3)** ***Herpesviruses*** which is subclassified as **(a)** *Herpes simplex Virus Type-1* (HSV-1; causes oral herpes, ocular herpes, viral encephalitis, and herpes keratitis); **(b)** *Herpes simplex Virus Type-2* (HSV-2; genital herpes); **(c)** *Varicella zoster Virus* (VZV; chicken pox, herpes zoster or shingles); **(d)** *Cytomegalovirus* (*CMV*; infectious mono-nucleosis); **(e)** *Epstein-Barr Virus* (*EBV*; infectious mononucleosis, B-cell lymphoma). **(4)** ***Papillomaviruses*** (warts). **(5)** ***Poxviruses*** (small pox). **(6)** ***Parvoviruses*** (erythema infectiosum, aplastic anaemia).

RNA Viruses

(1) ***Picornaviruses*** (includes *Poliovirus* causing polio and *Hepatovirus* causing hepatitis-A); **(2)** ***Orthomyxoviruses*** (includes *Influenza virus* type A,B,C causing various types of influenza; H_1N_1 *Virus*, which causes swine flu, is a subtype of *Influenza virus-A*); **(3)** ***Paramyxoviruses*** (includes *Rubulavirus* causing mumps; *Morbillivirus* causing measles and *Respiratory syncytial virus* causing lower respiratory tract infections); **(4)** ***Rhabdoviruses*** (causing rabies); **(5)** ***Arboviruses*** (these are arthropod-borne viruses and includue *Toga (alfa) virus* causing chikungunya and encephalitis; *Flavivirus* causing Dengue and yellow fever and *Bunyavirus* causing encephalitis); **(6)** ***Rotavirus*** (causing gastroenteritis in children); **(7)** ***Retrovirus*** (includes *Human immunodeficiency virus* causing AIDS and *Human T-cell leukaemia virus* causing

T-cell leukaemia); **(8)** ***Arenavirus*** (causing viral meningitis) and **(9)** ***Coronavirus*** (causing upper respiratory tract infections).

VIRAL REPLICATION

Fig. 61.2 A and B depict the replication cycle of a DNA virus and a RNA virus, respectively. Specific receptor sites on the DNA virus recognise the corresponding surface proteins on the host cells and get attached (step 1; Fig. 61.2A). The virus then penetrates the host cell membrane by endocytosis (step 2). During penetration, if the virus has an envelope, the envelope merges with the host cell membrane, i.e., only the capsid along with the genome enters the interior of the cell. Within the cell the capsid is removed (step 3) to free the genome containing DNA. Once the viral genome enters the cell nucleus, its DNA is transcribed into viral m-RNA by the host cell's RNA polymerase (step 4). Host cell's ribosomes then utilise the viral m-RNA for the synthesis of viral proteins and enzymes (step 5). During this process the regulatory proteins are synthesised first, which in turn initiate the transcription of the early genes responsible for replication of viral DNA by viral DNA polymerase (step 6). After the DNA is replicated the late genes are transcribed and translated to produce structural proteins required for an assembly of new virions (genome+capsid with or without envelope). Following their production, the viral components are assembled to form a mature virus particle (step 7). The release of progeny virus takes place through budding of the host cell (step 8). After this, usually the host cell is not lysed, but with certain viruses, the host cells are lysed and damaged.

Most RNA viruses (unlike DNA viruses) complete their replication in the cytoplasm without involving host cell nucleus. However, some, e.g., influenza virus, are transcribed in the host cell nucleus (Fig. 61.2B). In the replication cycle of influenza (RNA) virus, the step 1 (attachment) and 2 (endocytosis) are same as for DNA virus. The M_2 proteins (ion channels) of the virus then allow an influx of H^+ into the interior of virion which promotes dissociation of ribonucleoprotein (RNA+nucleoproteins) segments (step 3). The latter, for most RNA viruses, is then released in the cytoplasm, except for influenza virus where this viral genome gets entry into the host cell nucleus (step 4). Viral RNA polymerase now synthesises viral m-RNA from genomic viral RNA (step 5), which is then translated by host cell ribosomes to synthesise (a) **n**on**s**tructural proteins (NS proteins which direct the synthesis of more viral RNA) and (b) structural proteins (which are needed for the assembly of new virions) (step 6). Replication of viral RNA can also take place via replicative form of c-RNA (complementary RNA) using viral RNA polymerase (step 7). Rest of the steps such as assembly of virus particles (step 8) followed by budding and release of progeny virus (step 9) take place similar to DNA virus. Neuraminidase enzyme, present in virions, plays an important role for the release of progeny virus. The release of progeny RNA virus usually takes place through budding and protrusion of the host cell except for the poliovirus where the host cell is also damaged due to lysis.

Attached to the lipid layer of the envelope of influenza virus are two types of glycoproteins peplomers (spikes): the haemagglutinin (H) and neuraminidase (N). On the basis of antigenic variation of H and N antigens, the influenza virus A,B and C has been divided into various subtypes. Viruses with 15 subtypes of H and 9 subtypes of N are found in birds. Viruses which infect humans show 3H (H_1, H_2, H_3) and 2 N (N_1, N_2) subtypes. For example, influenza virus type A has subtypes like H_1N_1 (swine flu), H_1N_2, H_2N_2 and H_3N_2 which cause most human epidemics of influenza.

ANTIVIRAL THERAPY FOR NON-RETROVIRAL INFECTIONS

Viral diseases can be controlled by vaccination or by antiviral drug therapy or by stimulating host defence mechanisms. Vaccines are available to prevent measles, smallpox, chickenpox, rubella, mumps, poliomyelitis, yellow fever and hepatitis-B. However, the vaccines cannot prevent the spread of active infection within the host, hence they are of no use once the infection has occurred. Nevertheless, passive immunity can be provided with human immune globulins to assist the body's own defence mechanisms. Intravenously administered immune globulins can provide immediate passive

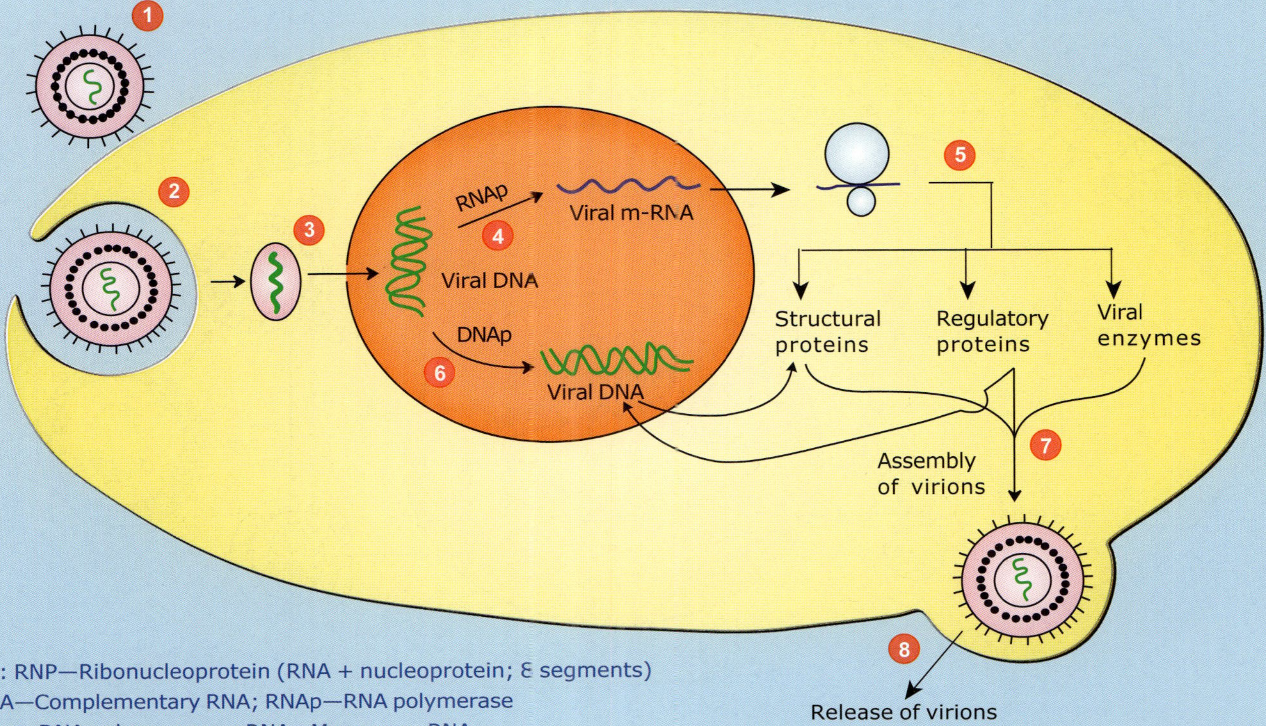

Key: RNP—Ribonucleoprotein (RNA + nucleoprotein; Ɛ segments)
cRNA—Complementary RNA; RNAp—RNA polymerase
DNAp—DNA polymerase; mRNA—Messenger RNA

Fig 61.2A Replicative Cycle of DNA Virus

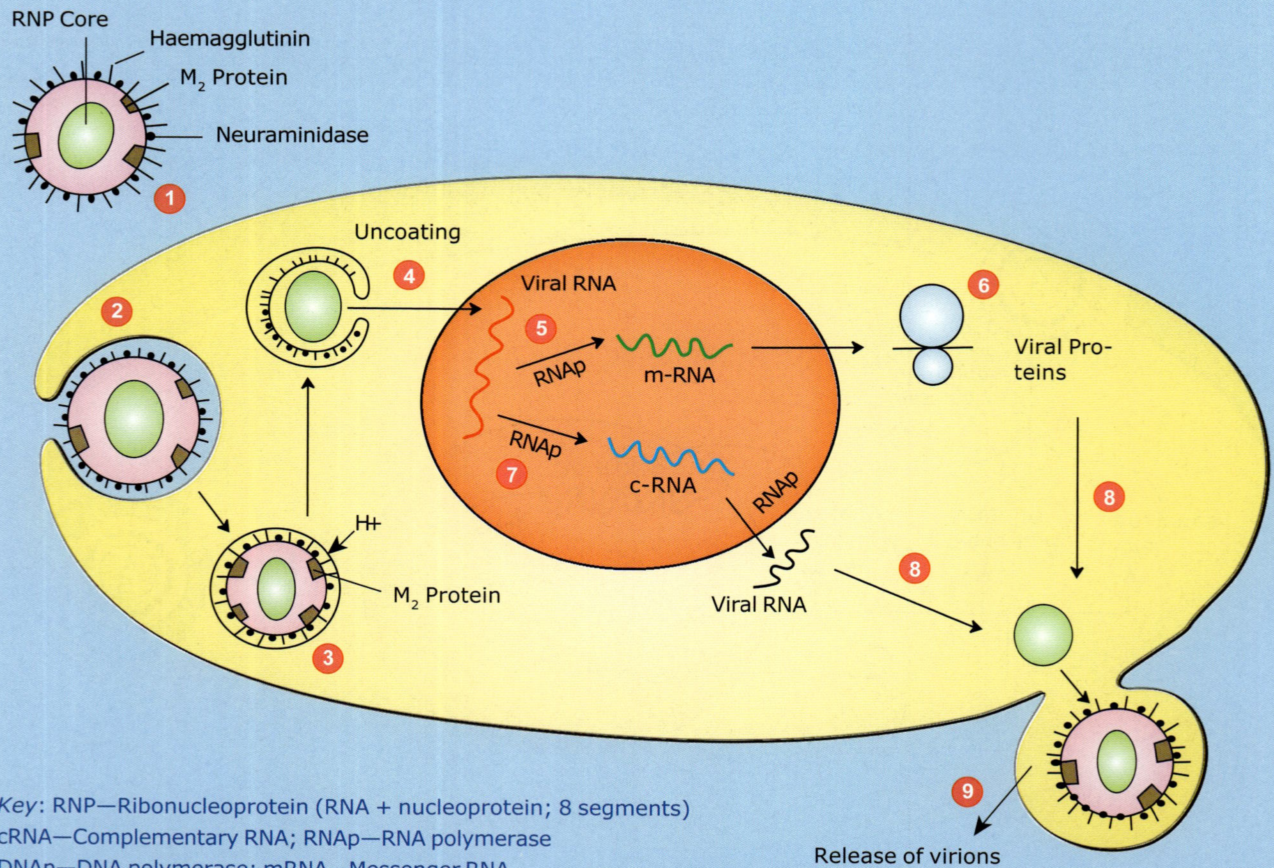

Key: RNP—Ribonucleoprotein (RNA + nucleoprotein; 8 segments)
cRNA—Complementary RNA; RNAp—RNA polymerase
DNAp—DNA polymerase; mRNA—Messenger RNA

Fig 61.2B Replicative Cycle of RNA (Influenza) Virus

immunity, while with I.M. immune globulins the occurrence of peak plasma concentration may take 2–3 days.

For an antiviral agent to be optimally active, the patient must have a competent host immune system that can eliminate or effectively halt virus replication. Immunocompromised patients are more prone to frequent viral infections that may recur when antiviral drugs are stopped. The chemotherapy of viral infections may involve inhibition of any of the steps in viral attachment, uncoating, penetration, replication, growth and release of progeny virions as shown in Figure 61.2 A and B.

MECHANISM BASED CLASSIFICATION OF ANTIVIRAL DRUGS (ANTI-RETRO VIRAL DRUGS EXCLUDED)

- **DNA Polymerase Inhibitors**
  Purine Analogues
  Acyclovir, Valacyclovir, Ganciclovir, Valganciclovir, Famciclovir, Penciclovir, Cidofovir, Adefovir, Entecavir, Vidarabine, Valomaciclovir
  Pyrimidine Analogues
  Idoxuridine, Trifluridine, Telbivudine
  Non-Nucleosides
  Foscarnet
- **m-RNA Synthesis Inhibitors**
  Ribavirin, Fomivirsen
- **Inhibitors of Viral Penetration and Uncoating**
  Amantadine, Rimantadine, Docosanol
- **Neuraminidase Inhibitors**
  Zanamivir, Oseltamivir, Peramivir, Laninamivir
- **Immunomodulators**
  Interferons, Palivizumab, Imiquimod

Since anti-viral therapy is available for most of the vital infections, in the following text the anti-viral drugs will be discussed as per their therapeutic application in diseases cause by different viruses.

THERAPEUTIC CLASSIFICATION OF ANTI-VIRAL DRUGS (anti-retroviral drugs excluded)

- **Drug for Herpes Virus and Cytomegalo Virus Infections**
  Acyclovir, Valacyclovir, Ganciclovir, Valganciclovir, Penciclovir, Famciclovir, Vidarabine, Cidofovir, Idoxuridine, Trifluridine, Foscarnet, Docosanol, Fomivirsen, Valomaciclovir.
- **Drugs for Influenza Virus Infection**
  Ribavirin, Amantadine, Rimantadine, Oseltamivir, Zanamivir, Peramivir, Laninamivir
- **Drugs for Hepatitis B Virus Infection**
  Entecavir, Telbivudine, Interferons, Adefovir dipivoxil, Tenofovir
- **Drugs for Hepatitis C Virus Infection**
  Ribavirin, Interferons, Boceprevir, Sofosbuvir
- **Drugs for Respiratory Syncytial Virus (RSV) Infection**
  Ribavirin, Palivizumab
- **Drugs of papilloma Viruses Infection**
  Imiquimod

Drug for Herpes Virus and Cytomegalo Virus Infections

Acyclovir and Valacyclovir

Mechanism of Action: ***Acyclovir*** is a guanosine analogue which is converted to its active metabolite via three phosphorylation steps. First, viral thymidine kinase converts it to acyclovir monophosphate. Then, host cell enzymes (guanidylate kinase) convert this monophosphate to acyclovir diphosphate and finally to an active form, acyclovir triphosphate. This active metabolite inhibits viral DNA polymerase and prevents its replication by terminating the elongation of the viral DNA chain (blocks step 6; Fig. 61.2A). Two reasons account for its selective toxicity: **(a)** In the non-infected host cell, the phosphorylation of acyclovir occurs to a limited extent only and **(b)** acyclovir triphosphate inhibits viral DNA polymerase 10–30 times more effectively than the host cell DNA polymerase.

The specific mechanisms of viral resistance against acyclovir include: **(1)** mutations that lead to a decreased thymidine kinase activity, **(2)** elaboration of the viral thymidine kinase with altered substrate specificity and **(3)** DNA polymerase resistance to acyclovir binding.

Pharmacokinetics: Orally administered acyclovir has only 20–30% bioavailability. Hence, peak plasma concentrations are sufficient only for prophylaxis or treatment of highly susceptible infections such as genital herpes. About 90% of the dose is excreted unchanged in the urine. In normal healthy persons, the plasma half-life is 3–4 hrs but is actients with renal failure.

Antiviral Spectrum and Clinical Use: Acyclovir is highly effective against *Herpes Simplex Virus-1 (HSV-1),* which causes herpes labialis (cold sores), herpes esophagitis, herpes keratitis, herpes encephalitis and ocular herpes; *Herpes Simplex Virus-2* (HSV-2), which causes genital herpes; and *Varicella Zoster Virus* (VZV), which produces chickenpox and shingles. It has comparatively weaker activity against *Epstein-Barr Virus* (EBV) and *cytomegalovirus* (CMV).

Oral acyclovir is used in the treatment of HSV-1 and HSV-2 infections and for VZV infections. Parenteral acyclovir is effectively used in the treatment of chronic and recurrent mucocutaneous HSV infections in immunocompromised patients, VZV infections and in herpes encephalitis. Acyclovir ointment is used in the treatment of early genital herpes but not for recurrent disease. Ophthalmic acyclovir ointment is used in the treatment of herpes keratoconjunctivitis. Usual oral dose of acyclovir is 400 mg TDS or 200 mg 4–5 times a day.

Adverse Effects and Drug Interactions: No serious toxicity occurs with oral and topical use of acyclovir. Intravenous therapy can cause phlebitis, rash and mild hypotension but nephrotoxicity is rare although dosage must be reduced in patients with renal insufficiency. Cyclosporine and other nephrotoxic agents may increase the risk of renal toxicity of acyclovir. Probenecid inhibits the renal excretion of acyclovir.

Valacyclovir is the L-valine ester (a prodrug) of acyclovir. Valacyclovir after oral administration gets rapidly converted to acyclovir during its first-pass through intestine and liver. Its mechanism of action, pharmacological effects and clinical uses are same as of acyclovir except **(1)** the bioavailability of the resultant acyclovir after oral valacyclovir dosing is 4–5 times more of orally administered acyclovir, **(2)** its efficacy is similar to acyclovir but requires less frequent oral dosing. It is currently used in the treatment of VZV infections and recurrent genital herpes (oral bioavailability of resultant acyclovir is comparable to that of I.V. acyclovir), **(3)** It is more effective than acyclovir in treating herpes zoster, and **(4)** there is no I.V. formulation available. Usual oral dose is 1 g BD or TDS for 7–10 days.

Ganciclovir and Valganciclovir

Ganciclovir is hydroxymethylated analogue of acyclovir, and has a similar mechanism of action. After conversion to ganciclovir triphosphate by herpes virus specific thymidine kinase, it is incorporated into viral DNA, which inhibits viral DNA polymerase, thereby terminating its replication. The principal mechanisms of resistance to ganciclovir are also similar to acyclovir and involve: (a) mutation of protein kinase gene and (b) mutation of DNA polymerase.

Pharmacokinetics: Because of the poor oral bioavailability (8–10%), ganciclovir is usually administered intravenously for the treatment of active viral infections. Oral administration is usually reserved to prevent relapse once the infection has been suppressed. Following I.V. administration it shows high accumulation in vitreous humour. It is hardly metabolised and excreted unchanged in urine. The plasma half-life is about 3–4 hrs.

Antiviral Spectrum and Clinical Use: Parenteral ganciclovir is used for the treatment of serious and vision-threatening retinitis due to cytomegalovirus (CMV) in immunocompromised cases. It is also effective for the treatment of acyclovir-resistant HSV infections. Its approved indication is prevention of CMV infection in organ transplant patients and in immunocompromised individuals. Recently, its intravitreal implants are being used for the treatment of CMV retinitis in AIDS patients. Ganciclovir triphosphate exhibits 100-fold more accumulation in CMV infected cells (compared to normal cells) and is preferentially incorporated into viral DNA by viral polymerase; hence the selective efficacy of the drug against CMV infections. Usual dose for induction is 5 mg/kg BD, I.V.; maintenance dose: 5 mg/kg/day.

Adverse Effects and Drug Interactions: The most common serious side effect of ganciclovir is myelosuppression, which may or may not be reversible after stopping the drug. This is because the mammalian bone marrow cells are sensitive to growth inhibition by ganciclovir. It has an increased potential for dose-related neutropenia, anaemia and thrombocytopenia. In animal studies, ganciclovir is teratogenic, carcinogenic and causes a decrease in sperm production. Other adverse effects include fever, phlebitis and pain. Adjustment of doses is necessary in renal impairment.

Zidovudine (Ch. 62) with ganciclovir may potentiate myelosuppression. Cyclosporine with ganciclovir may potentiate nephrotoxicity. Ganciclovir increases didanosine (Ch. 62) levels, whereas probenecid increases ganciclovir serum levels.

Valganciclovir is a L-valine ester (prodrug) of the antiviral drug ganciclovir. It is well absorbed from the GIT and is rapidly metabolised to ganciclovir. The bioavailability of the resultant ganciclovir is about 60%. Its bioavailability is increased when given with food. Formulation for intravenous use is not available. Its mode of action, clinical uses, adverse effects and drug interactions are same as for ganciclovir. Oral valganciclovir is comparable to I.V. ganciclovir for the treatment and suppression of CMV retinitis in AIDS patients. Usual oral dose for induction is 900 mg BD, maintenance dose is 900 mg once a day.

Penciclovir and Famciclovir

Penciclovir is a guanine nucleoside analogue and is structurally related to acyclovir. It is less potent than acyclovir as an inhibitor of viral DNA polymerase. Acyclovir-resistant HSV strains (that have mutants of thymidine kinase) are also resistant to famciclovir and penciclovir. Bioavailability of oral penciclovir is uncertain. It is available as 1% topical cream. The active triphosphate form of penciclovir persists intracellulary in infected cells for a longer time (half-life 8–20 hrs).

Famciclovir is the diacetyl ester (prodrug), that is converted to penciclovir during its first pass from the gut to the systemic circulation. The bioavailability of the resultant penciclovir following famciclovir administration is about 75–80%. Its plasma half-life is 2–3 hrs. It is excreted unchanged in the urine. Dose adjustments are necessary in renal insufficiency.

Topical penciclovir is used for the treatment of herpes labialis. Famciclovir is currently approved for the treatment of acute localised VZV infections (shingles). It is as effective as acyclovir in the treatment of HSV-1 and HSV-2 infections. *Adverse effects* include fatigue, GIT distress, anorexia and headache. Drug interactions are similar to acyclovir. Usual oral is 500 mg TDS for 7 days.

Vidarabine

It is an adenine nucleoside analogue obtained from *Streptomyces antibioticus*. Like acyclovir it also inhibits viral DNA synthesis by blocking DNA polymerase. It also acts as DNA chain terminator. Viral DNA polymerase is more susceptible to inhibition by vidarabine compared to host DNA polymerase. Resistance occurs as a result of DNA polymerase mutation.

Because of its poor GIT absorption, poor lipid solubility and its deamination to weakly active metabolite, vidarabine is used only topically as an ophthalmic ointment. It is mainly used for the treatment of HSV keratoconjunctivitis, and superficial keratitis in patients not responsive to or hypersensitive to idoxuridine. Because of its topical use in eye, side effects are also limited to lacrimation, irritation and photophobia. Concomitant use of ophthalmic corticosteroids should be avoided as it may spread HSV infection, may increase intraocular pressure and may promote cataract.

Cidofovir

Cidofovir is an analogue of cytidine that gets converted to cidofovir diphosphate which inhibits viral DNA polymerase. It also acts as an alternative substrate for viral DNA polymerase. It has very poor oral bioavailability and is applied topically or given intravenously. Although plasma half-life is 2–3 hrs, its disphosphate form persists within host cells for longer periods which permits once a week I.V. dosing. It is not metabolised significantly and is excreted unchanged in urine. Intravenous cidofovir is usually administered with probenecid (which blocks its tubular secretion and also reduces its nephrotoxicity). Cidofovir (I.V.) is used for the treatment and prophylaxis of CMV retinits and HSV mucocutaneous lesions. It has also been used in the treatment of acyclovir-resistant infections and for post-exposure prophylaxis against smallpox and for anogenital warts. Usual I.V. dose for induction is 5 mg/kg once in a week and for maintenance 5 mg/kg every 15 days. The most common *adverse effect* is nephrotoxicity (proteinuria, azotaemia and elevated serum creatinine levels). Nephrotoxic agents (e.g., aminoglycosides, amphotericin-B) should not be administered during the therapy. Foscarnet also potentiates its nephrotoxicity. Other effects include decrease in intraocular pressure, uveitis and neutropenia.

Cedofovir 3% gel has been reported to arrest hair growth (beard) and thus can be used to treat hirsutism.

Idoxuridine

Idoxuridine is an iodinated derivative of deoxyuridine. As with acyclovir, the triphosphate derivative of idoxuridine, inhibits viral DNA synthesis by blocking viral DNA polymerase. In addition, incorporation of idoxuridine into viral DNA leads to chromosomal breakage and altered synthesis of viral proteins. However, similar incorporation of idoxuridine into DNA of normal host cell accounts for its toxicity. Viral resistance commonly develops because idoxuridine is inactivated by viral deaminase and nucleotidase enzymes. It has only topical ophthalmic use for the treatment of HSV infections of eyelid, cornea and conjunctiva. *Side effects* include local irritation, corneal clouding, photophobia and lacrimation. Teratogenic effects have been reported in animals.

Trifluridine

Trifluridine is a trifluoromethyl derivative of idoxuridine. Trifluridine triphosphate is preferentially incorporated into viral DNA and inhibits viral DNA polymerase. Although more potent than idoxuridine it also inhibits cellular DNA synthesis and therefore is cytotoxic.

Trifluridine is used as a topical ophthalmic solution for the treatment of keratoconjunctivitis and recurrent keratitis due to HSV-1 and HSV-2. It is also effective in treating patients unresponsive to topical idoxuridine or vidarabine. *Adverse effects* include transient burning, palpebral oedema, hyperaemia and increased intraocular pressure.

Foscarnet

Foscarnet is an inorganic pyrophosphate derivative. It does not require phosphorylation for inhibiting viral DNA polymerase, but inhibits herpetic DNA polymerase activity by blocking the pyrophosphate binding site on the enzyme. The cleavage of the pyrophosphate moiety from the newly attached nucleotide is thus prevented which in turn inhibits viral chain elongation. It is 100 times more selective for herpes DNA polymerase than for mammalian DNA polymerase. Foscarnet has a very poor oral bioavailability, hence administered intravenously. It accumulates in aqueous humour and bones and eliminated unchanged in urine.

It is given by a slow I.V. infusion for the treatment of acyclovir-resistant mucocutaneous HSV infections in AIDS patients and CMV retinitis in immunocompromised patients. It is a good alternative for treating acyclovir-resistant infections because it does not require viral thymidine kinase and is not phosphorylated like acyclovir. Hence the thymidine kinase mutant cannot pose any resistance to foscarnet action. Dose 90 mg/kg I.V. 12 hrly for induction; 90 mg/kg/day for maintenance.

Its major *adverse effects* are renal toxicity and electrolyte disturbances. Renal toxicity is manifested as elevated serum creatinine levels which is often reversible but nephritis and necrosis (if result) may not be reversible. Electrolyte disturbances include hypocalcaemia, hypomagnesaemia and hypokalaemia which may lead to neurological and cardiovascular disturbances. Malaise, nausea and vomiting, headache, anaemia, leukopenia and liver dysfunction are other manifestations of foscarnet toxicity. Acyclovir, aminoglycosides, NSAIDs, amphotericin-B, ritonavir and saquinavir potentiate renal toxicity of foscarnet while pentamidine increases the risk of renal toxicity as well as electrolyte disturbances.

Docosanol

Docosanol is a long chain saturated alcohol, which in some countries is available as over-the-counter ointment of herpes labialis. It is active against lipid enveloped viruses such as some HSV strains, CMV and some RNA virus, e.g., influenza virus and paramyxovirus. It prevents the entry (penetration) of the virion into the host cell by inhibiting the fusion between the viral envelope and the host plasma membrane (step 1& 2; Fig. 61.2A, B). Development of resistance is not a problem with docosanol as it does not affect the actual process of viral replication. It is used only topically as a cream. Adverse effects are rare.

Fomivirsen

Fomivirsen is an oligonucleotide that is primarily an anti-CMV agent. It binds to m-RNA and thus inhibits the synthesis of immediate early proteins needed for viral replication (Step 6; Fig. 61.2B). Resistance to fomivirsen is least common (as its mechanism of action is different from other antiviral drugs). The drug has selective accumulation in retina and vitreous humour. It is injected intravitreally for the treatment of CMV retinitis in patients with AIDS; and in patients who have not responded to other therapies.

Adverse effects include iritis, vitreitis and increased intraocular pressure. Cidofovir increases the risk of ocular inflammation.

Valomaciclovir

This drug inhibits the DNA polymerase of Herpes zoster and Epstein-Barr viruses. Currently this agent is being evaluated for the treatment of shingles and infectious mononucleosis.

Drugs for Influenza Virus Infection

Ribavirin

Ribavirin is a synthetic analogue of guanosine with a broad spectrum antiviral activity (DNA as well as RNA virus). It inhibits the synthesis of viral m-RNA (blocks step 5; Fig. 61.2B) and DNA by depleting intracellular nucleotide reserves. Host cell enzymes successively convert ribavirin to its monophosphate, diphosphate and triphosphate form. The monophosphate inhibits viral GTP synthesis. The triphosphate form inhibits viral RNA polymerase. Resistance to ribavirin is uncommon as it simultaneously delays the mutation rate of RNA viruses.

Its oral absorption is rapid, first-pass is extensive, yet bioavailability is 65%, which is increased to 75% with a fatty meal. It is also administered as aerosol. It is metabolised in liver. The free drug as well as metabolite is excreted in the urine. Plasma half-life is 9–10 hrs but the terminal half-life is 20–36 hrs.

In aerosol it has been used to treat influenza and infections due to respiratory syncytial virus (but recent clinical trials reveal inconsistent benefits). It is used by I.V. to reduce mortality in Lassa fever (a serious arena virus infection). It is highly effective against influenza-A and influenza-B viruses. Oral ribavirin (800–1200 mg per day) + subcutaneous interferon alfa-2b (3 million units 3 times weekly) is synergistically effective in the treatment of chronic hepatitis-C viral (HCV) infections. Monotherapy with either drug alone is not effective.

Adverse effects include worsening of respiration in patients with pre-existing chronic obstructive pulmonary disease. It also carries potential mutagenic, carcinogenic and teratogenic risk. Additional side effects include anaemia, hypotension and deterioration in cardiac functions.

Amantadine and Rimantadine

Amantadine is a synthetic tricyclic amine and ***rimantadine*** is its α-methyl analogue. Both share a similar pharmacological profile. Both drugs are effective against influenza-A virus and have negligible activity against influenza-B virus and mumps virus. They inhibit uncoating of influenza-A viral RNA, within the infected host cells, thus preventing its replication (step 4; Fig. 61.2B). Precisely, they inhibit the viral M_2 protein (Fig. 61.2B), present within the influenza-A viral membrane, and thus prevent H^+ mediated dissociation of ribo-neucleoprotein (RNP) core segment, which is prerequisite for viral replication (step 3). Influenza-B virus contains a different protein (other than M_2) in its membrane. In certain strains of influenza-A virus, the pH changes that result from M_2 inhibition alter the conformation of haemagglutinin and hence block viral assembly also. They have no effect on viral RNA polymerase activity. Point mutations in M_2 proteins is responsible for the development of resistance to amantadine and rimantadine.

Both are rapidly absorbed from the GIT. Plasma half-life varies with age (amantadine: 17 hrs in young adults and 30 hrs in elderly; rimantadine: 25 hrs in young adults and 33 hrs in elderly). Amantadine is mostly excreted unchanged (95%) in the urine. Rimantadine is partly metabolised in liver. Its conjugated metabolites and some free drug (25%) is excreted in urine.

Amantadine and rimantadine are administered orally for prevention and for treatment of influenza-A viral infections (dose for both 100 mg BD or 200 mg OD). They reduce the duration of fever and other complaints by 1 to 2 days. Amantadine prophylaxis reduces infection rates by 50% and illness rate by 60%. Due to high rate of development of resistance, both agents are no longer recommended for the prevention and treatment of influenzae.

An additional use of amantadine, unrelated to its antiviral activity, is in the therapy of Parkinson's disease (Ch. 40).

The *side effects* are dose related and are more common with amantadine than with rimantadinewhich appears to be safer since display fewer side effects. For adverse effects refer to Ch. 40.

Oseltamivir and Zanamivir

Both the drugs are neuraminidase inhibitors and, therefore, are effective against a variety of influenza strains. Orally administered ***oseltamivir*** is converted by hepatic esterases to an active form—oseltamivir carboxylate. The latter has 80% bioavailability. Its plasma half-life is 8 hrs and is eliminated mainly in urine. Oral bioavailability of ***zanamivir*** is only 5%. It is administered by a disk inhaler. Its plasma half-life is about 3.5 hrs and is excreted in urine.

Both the drugs can be used for the treatment of acute uncomplicated influenza A (including H_1N_1 virus; swine flu) or influenza B infections. Dose: Oseltamivir 75 mg BD orally for treatment; 75 mg OD orally for prevention. For zanamivir 10 mg BD inhalation for treatment; 10 mg per day for prevention. For best results, treatment should begin within 2 days of the symptom onset because replication of influenza virus peaks at 30–72 hrs after the onset of illness.

The common side effects include nausea, vomiting, vertigo, seizures and aggravation of diabetes for *oseltamivir*; while bronchospasm, bronchosecretions and nasal discomfort for *zanamivir*.

Peramivir

This is a new neuraminidase inhibitor which has been approved by FDA for the emergency treatment of hospitalised patients with H_1N_1 influenza infection. Its oral bioavailability is very poor and hence used I.V. for patients showing resistance to oseltamivir or zanmivir inhalation. It is currently the only I.V. option for treating swine flu.

Laninamivir

Laninamivir is a new long acting inhaled neuraminidase inhibitor which has retained activity against oseltamivir resistant influenza virus and is being evaluated for resistant cases of H_1N_1 infections.

Drugs for Hepatitis B Virus (HBV) Infection

Entecavir

Entecavir is an orally effective (0.5 mg–1 mg OD) guanosine nucleoside analogue that competitively inhibits viral DNA polymerase and hence its replication. It is used for the treatment of patients with chronic hepatitis-B in adults with or without AIDS (including lamivudine-resistant cases). Oral bioavailability is 100% but decreases with food (to be taken on empty stomach). Half-life is 15 hrs. *Adverse effects* are mild such as headache, fatigue, nausea and dizziness.

Telbivudine

It is a thymidine nucleoside analogue which is phosphorylated to an active triphosphate form that inhibits hepatitis-B viral DNA polymerase and prevents viral replication. It is used to treat chronic hepatitis-B. Common adverse effects include elevations in creatine phosphokinase, headache, nausea and vomiting. Patients resistant to lamivudine (Ch. 62) are resistant to telbivudine also.

Adefovir dipivoxil

Adefovir is an analogue of adenosine monophosphate. It is phosphorylated by cellular kinases to an active diphosphate derivative that competitively inhibits hepatitis-B virus (HBV) DNA polymerase. Adefovir also gets incorporated in viral

DNA and causes chain termination. Oral bioavailability is 40–60%. It is excreted unchanged in urine. Plasma half-life is 6–8 hrs. It is mainly used for the treatment of chronic HBV infection and is effective even in lamivudine (Ch. 62) resistant strains of HBV. Its usual oral dose is 10 mg OD. Major *adverse effect* is nephrotoxicity but the risk is low if treatment duration lasts for less than one year. Other effects include lactic acidosis and hepatomegaly. Ibuprofen increases its oral bioavailability by 23–25%.

Interferons

The enhanced production of cytokines called *interferons* is one of the body's important defences against viral infection. In addition to their antiviral activity, interferons exert cellular antiproliferative and immunoregulatory effects. Interferons (IFNs) can be classified according to 3 major groups: α, β and γ. IFN-α is synthesised primarily by human leucocytes; IFN-β from human fibroblasts while IFN-γ, which is a lymphokine, produced by T-lymphocytes as a part of the immune response to viral and nonviral antigens. Commercial synthesis of IFNs is done by recombinant DNA technology in bacterial cultures. IFN-α and IFN-β exert potent antiviral effects while IFN-γ has antiviral as well as immunomodulatory effects.

IFNs bind to specific cell surface receptors and affect viral replication at multiple steps: inhibition of viral penetration, uncoating, m-RNA synthesis leading to suppression of protein synthesis, assembly of virions and their release. In the ribosomes of the host's cells, IFNs induce the production of enzymes that inhibit the translation of viral m-RNA into viral proteins and thus stop the replication of the virus. Additional antiviral effects may result from activation of macrophages and natural killer (NK) cells along with modulation of cell surface proteins to facilitate immune recognition. All DNA or RNA viruses are sensitive to IFNs to a greater or lesser degree. Endogenous IFNs are just responsible for making most viral infections self-limiting.

Various IFN preparations can be administered subcutaneously, intramuscularly, intravenously or intra-lesionally (as in genital warts). These do not cross BBB and are eliminated through phagocytosis or by catabolism in the kidney and liver.

Clinical Uses of IFNs are as under:

IFN-α-2a: Chronic HBV infection; chronic hepatitis-C infection; AIDS related Kaposi's sarcoma; hairy cell leukaemia and chronic myelogenous leukaemia. Dose: 3 mU, three times weekly, S.C. or I.M.

IFN-α-2b: is indicated for the treatment of chronic HBV; chronic hepatitis-C (in combination with ribavirin); malignant melanoma; condylomata acuminata (anogenital warts caused by human papilloma virus); and non-Hodgkin's lymphoma. Dose: 3 mU, three times weekly; S.C. or I.M.

IFNs are now used as an adjunct in the treatment of viral infections including AIDS (Ch. 62). A complex of polyethylene glycol with IFNs (Pegylated interferon-α-2b) has improved outcomes in chronic hepatitis-B and -C, presumably from more sustained blood levels of IFNs (longer t½). Pegylated interferon alfa-2a and -2b are given once weekly S.C.

Adverse effects include fever, weakness, nausea, vomiting, headache, myalgia and flu-like symptoms. Long-term toxicity includes dose-related bone marrow depression, rashes, alopecia, cardiovascular, hepatic and thyroid dysfunction, insomnia, depression. IFNs in higher doses may cause miscarriage. Immunosuppressed transplant recipients should not receive IFNs. Interferons inhibit cytochrome-P450 enzymes and therefore decrease the clearance of theophylline.

Tenofovir

Tenofovir, a nucleotide analogue of adenosine is primarily a anti-retroviral drug but also shows a potent activity against HBV. This drug shows good activity against lamivudine- and entecavir- resistant HBV isolates but has reduced activity against adefovir- resistant strains.

The common adverse effects of the drug in patients with HBV infection on nausea, abdominal pain, diarrhoea, fatigue, dizziness and rash.

Drugs for Hepatitis C Virus (HCV) Infection

Boceprevir

Boceprevir is an oral HCV protease NS3/4A inhibitor and is used along with pegylated-interferon alfa 2a/2b and ribavirin. Used alone it shows fast resistance and as a result is approved for combined therapy with other anti-HCV agents. The drug is metabolised by CYP3A4/5 pathways and is inhibitor of P-glycoprotein transporter. Therefore, co-administration of this drug with many other agents (phenytoin, rifampicin, lovastatin, simvastatin, sildenafil, midazolam, etc) may show adverse interactions.

Sofosbuvir

This drug is a nucleotide analogue that inhibits HCV RNA-dependent RNA polymerase in patients with HCV infection having viral genotype 1,2,3 or 4. It is an orally effective agent, administered in once daily doses (400 mg) in combination with ribavirin and pegylated interferon alfa-2a/2b or inteferon alfa-2b for a period of 12 weeks or longer (24 weeks when infection is due to HCV genotype 3). Like boceprevir, this drug is also a P-gp transporter inhibitor and may show adverse interaction with other co-medicated drugs which are also substrate for P-gp. Common side effects observed with the drug are nausea, headache and fatigue. It should be given cautiously in patients with severe renal impairment as its safety in such patients has not been estabilished.

Glecaprevir and Pibrentasvir

Glecaprevir and pibrentasvir are used in combination for hepatitis C infection. This contains two new antiviral drugs: Glecaprevir (NS3/4A protease inhibitor) and pibrentasvir (inhibits NS5A protein) involved in viral replication. Both drugs inhibit P-glycoprotein and BCRP (Breast cancer resistance protein). Adverse effects: Headache, fatigue nausea, diarrhoea and pruritus.

Elbasvir and Grazoprevir

Elbasvir and grazoprevir are used in combination. Elbasvir is an inhibitor of HCV NS5A, which is essential for viral RNA replication and virion assembly. Grazoprevir is an inhibitor of HCV NS3/4A protease which is necessary for the proteolytic cleavage of the HCV-encoded polyproteins. This combination is used orally for chronic hepatitis C virus (HCV) genotype 1 or 4 infection in adults or for use with ribavirin in certain patient populations. Adverse effects: Nausea, vomiting, fatigue, headache, diarrhoea, irritability, depression, anaemia and dyspnoea.

Voxilaprevir

Voxilaprevir is an inhibitor of NS3/4A protease enzyme. It is used in combination with sofosbuvir (NS5B nucleotide polymerase inhibitor) and velpatasvir (NS5A inhibitor). It is used in chronic Hepatitis C virus infection who had previously failed treatment with other drugs. Voxilaprevi and velpatasvir combination is used for sustained virological suppression. Adverse effects: Headache, fatigue, diarrhoea and nausea.

Drugs for Respiratory Syncytial Virus (RSV) Infection

Palivizumab

Palivizumab is a humanised monoclonal antibody directed against the highly specific antigenic site (F-glycoprotein) present on the cell surface of respiratory syncytial virus (RSV). It neutralises RSV and inhibits its fusion with host cell membrane (step 2; Fig. 61.2B). It is used to prevent lower respiratory tract infection due to RSV in high-risk infants and children and in those with bronchopulmonary dysplasia. Dose: 15 mg/kg I.M. once a month for 5 months. *Adverse effects* are rare except pain at the I.M. injection site, and a transient elevation in serum aminotransferase levels. It has negligible immuno-genicity in humans.

Drugs of Papilloma Viruses Infection

Imiquimod

It is a topical antiviral agent (5% cream) used in the treatment of external genital and perianal warts/condyloma acuminata due to human HPV. It acts as an immune response modifier and induces cytokines including IFN-α. Side effects are rare except local erythema and itching. Pigmentary skin changes may occur.

CHAPTER 62 HIV and Antiretroviral Drugs

COMPETENCY PH1.48, PH1.55

Acquired immunodeficiency syndrome (AIDS) was first characterized in 1980s and attributed to Human Immunodeficiency Virus (HIV), which is a single stranded RNA retrovirus. In other viruses (Ch. 61), RNA is transcripted from DNA, but in retrovirus, DNA is transcripted from RNA (reverse transcription; *retro = reverse*) by an enzyme called reverse transcriptase (viral RNA-dependent-DNA polymerase). In fact, there are two viruses associated with AIDS: HIV-1 and HIV-2. Most HIV infections worldwide are caused by HIV-1, while HIV-2 infections occur in Western Africa and India, but not showing significant spread from these places (being less virulent). In this text we refer to both as HIV. In other viral infections the host defences try to gain the upper hand. Hence the majority of viral infections (except in immunocompromised hosts) are self-limiting; but in HIV infection the cell mediated immunity collapses due to continued decline in $CD4^+$-T lymphocyte cells. As a result, massive opportunistic infections and malignancies appear (AIDS-related complex) leading to death. Thus occurrence of AIDS is the end stage of chronic HIV infection.

REPLICATIVE CYCLE OF HIV

The structure of HIV is basically the same as of other viruses except that its envelope contains surface proteins composed of knob-like glycoproteins (gp120) linked to a transmembrane stalk (gp41). These glycoproteins are antigenic and facilitate viral attachment to $CD4^+$ cells of T lymphocytes. Secondly, their core genome contains RNA along with three genes: ***gag, pol*** and ***env.*** The ***gag*** and ***pol*** genes code for the formation of reverse transcriptase, integrase and protease enzymes while ***env*** genes code for the formation of envelope proteins gp120 and gp 41 (Fig. 62.1A).

HIV can infect T lymphocytes, macrophages, Langerhans cells and even dendritic cells of CNS. But the prime target of viral attachment is the helper T-lymphocytes which have $CD4^+$ epitopes expressed on their surface. The surface glycoproteins, gp120, on the HIV envelope bind to $CD4^+$ and also to chemokine coreceptor (CXCR4) present on these T cells. Another viral glycoprotein, gp41, causes fusion of the viral envelope with the plasma membrane of the T-cells (step 1; Fig. 62.1B). For binding to macrophages, the chemokine coreceptor is CCR5. As the disease advances and immune surveillance fails there is shift from CCR5 binding to CXCR4 binding. After fusion of the virus with host cell membrane, the virus enters the target cells (step 2).

After entering the host cell and uncoating (step 3), the viral reverse transcriptase (RT) synthesises DNA from viral RNA (step 4). This viral DNA then enters the host cell nucleus and is integrated into the host genome, by the viral enzyme integrase, producing provirus (step 5). The provirus DNA is then transcribed into both new genomic RNA (step 6) and m-RNA (step 7). The latter is translated into viral proteins by host ribosomes (step 8 and 9). The new virions then assemble the genomic RNA and polypeptides and undergo a process of maturation in which the viral protease enzyme cleaves the polypeptide into functional structural proteins and viral enzymes (step 10). The resultant mature virion then buds out from the cell membrane to infect other susceptible cells until eventually the immune response fails (step 11).

DRUG THERAPY OF HIV INFECTION

The replicative cycle of HIV presents many opportunities for the targeting of antiviral drugs against HIV. But majority of drugs available today have serious adverse effects, unwelcome drug interactions and have to be taken life long, because HIV cannot be eradicated completely. The virus may be lying latent in the memory T cells, integrated into host genome, forming a source of potential

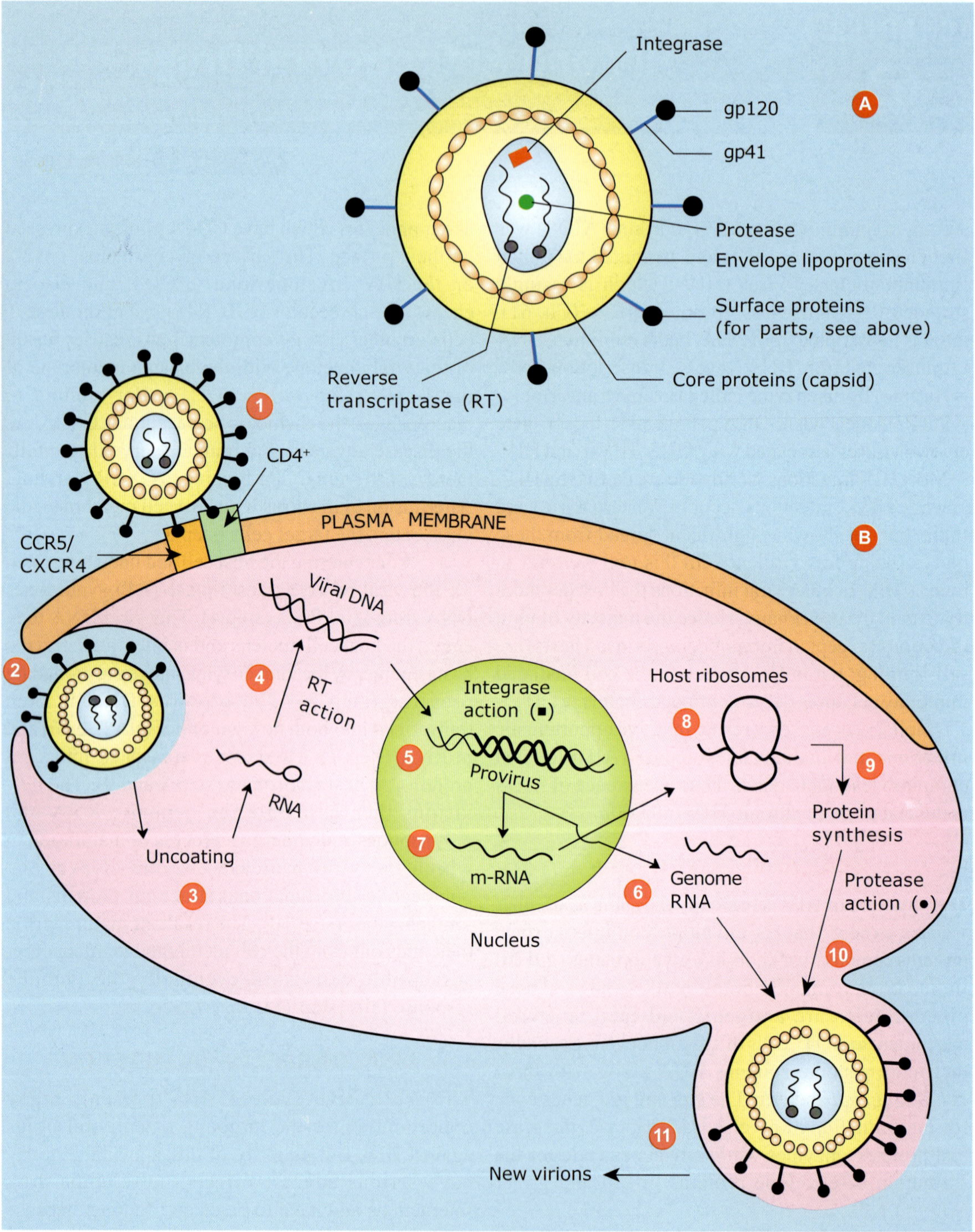

Fig 62.1 (A) Basic Components of Human Immunodeficiency Virus (HIV) and (B) Its Replicative Cycle (for details refer text).

reactivation any time after stopping the drug. Since the HIV virus has a high mutation rate, cross resistance between the drugs may also become the problem in the near future. To sum up the situation, it can be said that HIV virus has not yet been out-smarted.

MECHANISM BASED CLASSIFICATION OF ANTI-RETROVIRAL DRUGS

I. ***Nucleoside Reverse Transcriptase Inhibitors (NRTIs)***
Zidovudine, Stavudine, Lamivudine, Abacavir, Emtricitabine, Didanosine

II. ***Non-Nucleoside Reverse Transcriptase Inhibitors (NNRTIs)***
Efavirenz, Nevirapine, Delavirdine, Etravirine, Rilpivirine.

III. ***Nucleotide Reverse Transcriptase Inhibitors (NtRTIs)***
Tenofovir

IV. ***Protease Inhibitors (PIs)***
Saquinavir, Indinavir, Nelfinavir, Amprenavir, Fosamprenavir, Ritonavir, Lopinavir, Atazanavir Tipranavir, Darunavir

V. ***Entry/Fusion Inhibitors***
Enfuvirtide,

VI. ***CCR5 Inhibitors***
Maraviroc

VII. ***Integrase Inhibitors (also called Integrase Strand Transfer Inhibitors: (INSTIs)***
Raltegravir, Elvitegravir, Dolutegravir, Bictegravir

VIII. ***Newer Antiretroviral Drugs in Pipe-line***
Bevirimat, Elvucitabine, Vicriviroc

NUCLEOSIDES AND NUCLEOTIDES: GENERAL COMMENTS

There are two types of nucleic acids, namely DNA (deoxyribonucleic acid) and RNA (ribonucleic acid). Nucleic acids are the polymers of nucleotides (as proteins are polymers of amino acids). A *nucleotide* unit of RNA/DNA consists of: a heterocyclic nitrogenous base, a pentose sugar and a phosphate. The nucleotide without a phosphate is called a *nucleoside*. In other words, a *nucleotide* = *base+sugar* + *phosphate* while a *nucleoside* = *base* + *sugar* only.

The nitrogenous bases found in nucleotide/nucleoside belong to two groups: Purines and Pyrimidines. The purines are of two types: Adenine and Guanine; while the pyrimidines are of three types:
Cytosine, Thymine and Uracil. RNA consists of two purines (adenine and guanine) and two pyrimidine bases (cytosine and uracil). Though, DNA also carries two purines (adenine and guanine) and two pyrimidine bases (cytosine and thymine), the difference lies only in the type of pyrimidine base which is uracil in RNA but thymine in DNA.

The pentose sugar in RNA is ribose while in DNA is deoxyribose. The latter has a H in place of OH at 2-C atom (i.e., one oxygen less) of ribose structure (Fig. 62.2). A nucleoside containing a base linked to ribose is called as ribonucleoside and those which have the base joined to deoxyribose are called deoxyribonucleosides. Therefore, if adenine (purine base) is linked to ribose it is called *adenosine ribonucleoside*; cytosine + ribose is *cytidine ribonucleoside*; uracil + ribose is *uridine ribonucleoside*; guanine + ribose is *guanosine ribonucleoside*; while thymine + deoxyribose is *thymidine deoxyribonucleoside*.

The basic chemical skeleton of two types of nucleosides are given below (Fig. 62.2A, B).

NUCLEOSIDE REVERSE TRANSCRIPTASE INHIBITORS (NRTIs)

Examples: ***Zidovudine, Stavudine, Lamivudine, Abacavir, Emtricitabine*** and ***Didanosine.***

Mechanism of Action

1) These drugs are first converted to their active triphosphate metabolites by host cell kinase enzymes. The triphosphate form of these drugs then competes with viral nucleoside triphosphates for their access to viral reverse transcriptase (RT) enzyme and hinders its action to produce complementary DNA from RNA (blocks step 4: Fig. 62.1B).
2) NRTIs either lack 3'-OH group, present in nucleoside (see stavudine structure, Fig. 62.3A) or have an azido group ($-N_3$) in place of 3'-OH

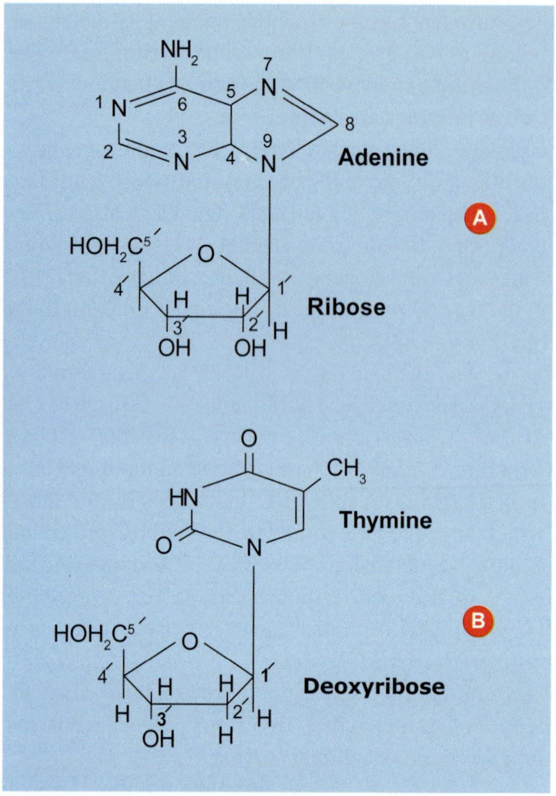

Fig 62.2 Chemical Structures of (A) Adenosine Ribonucleoside and (B) Thymidine Deoxyribonucleoside.

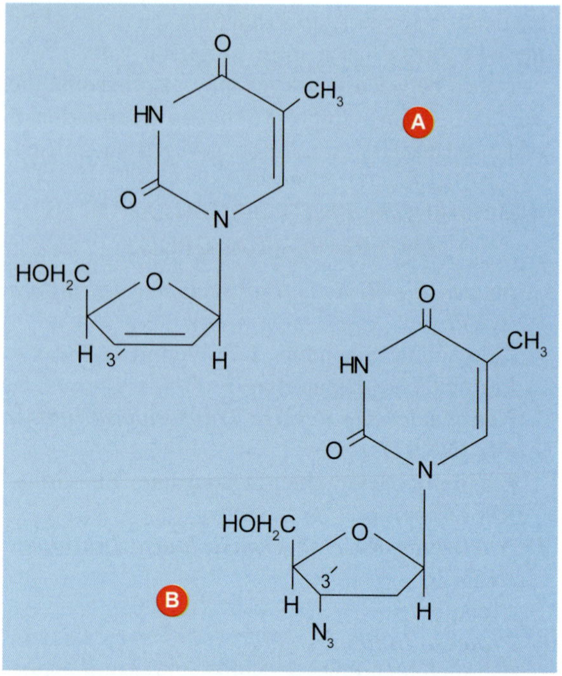

Fig 62.3 Chemical Structures of (A) Stavudine and (B) Zidovudine

(as in zidovudine, Fig. 62.3B). Hence these are also falsely incorporated into a growing viral DNA chain by viral RT. This results into the termination of the DNA chain elongation.

These drugs therefore block the HIV replication and consequently the infection of the new cells rather than treating the already infected cells.

Therapeutic Uses

These drugs are generally used in combination with other drugs to avoid development of resistance. A multidrug therapy is needed to counteract the rapid mutation rate of HIV and also to minimize drug toxicity. The multidrug **H**ighly **A**ctive **A**nti-**R**etroviral **T**herapy (HAART) needs synergistic combination of NRTIs and protease inhibitors; because, working with different mechanisms, the combined drugs produce a sequential blockade of viral reproduction at two different steps. HIV cannot develop mutants simultaneously to different drugs working by two different mechanisms. Popular combination choices include: two NRTIs + one NNRTI or one/two protease inhibitors (PIs), i.e., NRTIs (2) + PI (1) **or** NRTIs (2) + NNRTI (1) **or** NRTIs (2) + PI (1) + Ritonavir (PI). The preferred drug regimens are: Zidovudine + Lamivudine + Efavirenz OR Zidovudine + Lamivudine + Lopinavir/Ritonavir.

Following are some other alternatives: NRTI (1) + NNRTI (1) + PI (1) **or** NRTI (1) + NNRTI (1) + PI (2). Resistance, which results due to mutation in reverse transcriptase, is usually a problem with NRTIs if used as monotherapy.

Toxicity

NRTIs inhibit cellular as well as mitochondrial DNA polymerase along with various cellular kinases resulting in toxicity. Initially, the immune system is not much disturbed, hence the drug toxicity is less. At the later stage of infection when the cell mediated immunity starts declining, the drug toxicity is more. All NRTIs cause fatal lactic acidosis, severe hepatomegaly and hepatic steatosis. Women, obese persons and alcoholics are more prone to such toxicity. Prolonged use of NRTIs also leads to such toxicity, and if this occurs the drug should be withdrawn.

Salient Features of Individual Drugs

Zidovudine (AZT)

It is a thymidine analogue in which 3'-OH group is replaced by azido (N_3) group (Fig. 62.3B). It provides an effective but palliative treatment of HIV-1, HIV-2 and human T-cell lymphotrophic virus (HTLV-I and II). It is also used for postexposure prophylaxis for health care workers. Its oral bioavailability is 60–65% and t½ is 1–3 hrs. As a preventive measure zidovudine significantly reduces the incidence of neonatal HIV infection when the HIV-infected mother is given zidovudine (100 mg, 5 times a day) after 14 weeks of gestation until birth. The newborn then receives zidovudine syrup (2 mg/kg 6 hrly) from birth till six weeks of age. The success rate of preventing such vertical transmission of HIV is only 25%. The usual recommended dose is 200 mg TDS or 300 mg BD orally. It is mostly used in combination with lamivudine or with lamivudine + abacavir.

Adverse effects (besides above) include headache, nausea, vomiting, anorexia, fatigue, insomnia, myopathy and myositis. Prolonged use may lead to bone marrow toxicity, anaemia and neutropenia, which may necessitate dose reduction or drug discontinuation (erythropoietin may be added if the therapy has to be continued).

Concurrent use of myelosuppressant drugs (e.g., interferon-α, cotrimoxazole, dapsone, foscarnet, ganciclovir and valganciclovir) should be avoided. Ribavirin inhibits the phosphorylation of zidovudine, while zidovudine inhibits the phosphorylation of stavudine. Hence zidovudine should not be combined with ribavirin or stavudine. Nelfinavir decreases the plasma levels while probenecid, fluconazole and lamivudine increase plasma levels of zidovudine.

Stavudine (d4T)

Stavudine is a thymidine nucleoside analogue that is devoid of a 3'-OH group (Fig. 62.3A) and is used for the therapy of HIV infections as a part of multidrug regimen (stavudine + lamivudine) as well as for postexposure prophylaxis. Its oral bioavailability is high (85–90%); t½ 1–2 hrs. The recommended adult oral dose of stavudine is 30–40 mg BD.

The main *adverse effect* is peripheral neuropathy, that is dose-dependent. Doses adjustment is necessary for patients with renal insufficiency and peripheral neuropathy. Other adverse effects include pancreatitis and joint pain. Headache, diarrhoea, skin rash, vomiting, stomatitis, insomnia and anorexia are also common. Lactic acidosis is more frequent with stavudine than with any other NRTIs. Concurrent administration of other neuropathic drugs (didanosine, zalcitabine and isoniazid) should be avoided. It should not be administered with zidovudine (see above).

Lamivudine (3TC)

Lamivudine is a cytosine nucleoside analogue that is devoid of a 3'- OH group and is active against HIV-1, HIV-2 and hepatitis-B virus. As with other antiretroviral drugs, it is used as a part of multidrug regimen (see above) and also for postexposure prophylaxis. The combination of zidovudine + lamivudine strongly enhances $CD4^+$ counts. It is the best tolerated NRTI. Its oral bioavailability is high (85–90%); t½ 5–7 hrs.

The usual adult dose for treating HIV infection is 150 mg BD; but for treating hepatitis-B infection is 100 mg/day. The mode of action against HBV is, however, different. The monophosphate form of lamivudine is incorporated into the viral DNA by HBV-DNA polymerase resulting into termination of DNA chain elongation.

Most common *adverse effects* are: nausea, headache, fatigue and insomnia. There is an increased risk of pancreatitis in children (but rarely in adults). Dose adjustment is necessary in patients with renal insufficiency. Lamivudine and zalcitabine inactivate each other by inhibiting each other's phosphorylation. Cotrimoxazole inhibits renal elimination of lamivudine.

Abacavir (ABC)

It is a guanosine nucleoside analogue devoid of a 3'-OH group and is indicated for the therapy of HIV-1 infection in adults and children as well as for postexposure prophylaxis. It is mostly used in combination with zidovudine + lamivudine. The usual adult dose is 300 mg BD. Its oral bioavailability is high (80–85%); t½ 1.5 hr.

The *adverse effects* include generalised hypersensitivity reactions occurring within 6 weeks of the initiation of the therapy. These may be rare but are fatal. If hypersensitivity occurs, rechallange must be avoided. Other side effects could be headache, nausea, vomiting, fatigue, skin rash and possible increase in episodes of myocardial infarction. It is partly metabolised by alcohol dehydrogenase, hence concomitant intake of alcohol may increase the plasma levels of abacavir.

Emtricitabine (FTC)

It is a cytosine nucleoside analogue, structurally related to lamivudine. It is used in combination with a protease inhibitor and/or a NNRTI for treatment of HIV infection in adults. A usual combination includes emtricitabine + tenofovir + efavirenz OR emtricitabine + tenofovir. It has a longer half-life which provides a rationale for once-daily dosing. The usual adult dose is 200 mg orally once daily. Oral bioavailability to excellent (93%); t½ is 10 hr.

It is best tolerated, least toxic drug of this series. Prolonged use leads to hyperpigmentation of skin. Hepatotoxicity and pancreatitis may result if used along with other drugs that are by themselves hepatotoxic. No significant drug interaction has yet been reported. Doses are to be adjusted in patients of renal insufficiency.

Didanosine (ddI)

Didanosine is an adenosine nucleoside analogue devoid of a 3'-OH group and having activity against HIV-1, HIV-2 and HTLV-I. As a part of multidrug regimen it is used to treat HIV infection and for postexposure HIV prophylaxis. The usual adult dose is 250 mg BD, 30 min before or 2 hrs after meal. Oral bioavailability is 42% (decrease with food, tetracyclins and fluoroquinolones); t½ 1.5 hr.

Major *adverse effects* include diarrhoea, peripheral neuropathy, hyperuricaemia, pancreatitis and optical neuritis. Except for diarrhoea, other toxicities are dose related. Hence it is contraindicated in patients of gout, pancreatitis, peripheral neuropathy and in those having visual problems. Zalcitabine with didanosine increases the risk of peripheral neuropathy while stavudine with didanosine increases the risk of pancreatitis as well as of peripheral neuropathy. Ganciclovir and valganciclovir, increase blood levels of didanosine.

NON-NUCLEOSIDE REVERSE TRANSCRIPTASE INHIBITORS (NNRTIs)

Examples: ***Nevirapine, Efavirenz, Delavirdine, Etravirine, Rilpivirine***

Mechanism of Action

NNRTIs do not require activation through phosphorylation. They bind directly to the catalytic site of viral reverse transcriptase causing enzyme inactivation and inhibition of viral DNA synthesis (blocks Step 4; Fig. 62.1B). If used alone, resistance develops due to mutations in reverse transcriptase. Monotherapy with these agents, therefore, is not recommended. Cross resistance has been noticed in between NNRTIs but not between NNRTIs and NRTIs or between NNRTIs and protease inhibitors.

Therapeutic Uses

All NNRTIs are active against HIV-1 reverse transcriptase only. Their use with NRTIs or protease inhibitors provide synergistic effects against HIV due to sequential blockade at two different steps required for viral reproduction.

Adverse Effects

NNRTIs share certain adverse effects such as skin rashes including Stevens-Johnson syndrome, and elevation in the levels of liver enzymes. Individual drug toxicity is discussed below.

Drug Interactions and Contraindications

Certain drug interactions due to induction or inhibition of cytochrome P450 enzymes are also common to all. Since protease inhibitors are also metabolised by cytochrome P450 enzymes, NNRTIs may either increase or decrease their plasma levels (see below). NNRTIs, therefore, should be used with caution in patients with hepatic disease.

Individual Drugs

Nevirapine (NVP)

Nevirapine is used for the treatment of HIV infection in adults and children as a component of multidrug antiretroviral therapy. The recommended oral dose for adult is 200 mg BD. A single 200 mg oral dose of nevirapine has been found to be effective in preventing vertical (mother-to-newborn) transmission of HIV, if administered at the onset of labour. Thereafter, a single 2 mg/kg oral dose is to be given to the neonate within 3 days after birth. Oral bioavailability is high (95%); t½ 25–30 hrs and penetrate well into the CSF.

Characteristic *side effects* include life-threatening skin rashes including Stevens-Johnson syndrome and fulminant hepatitis with fever, within the first 6 weeks of the initiation of therapy. Intermittent monitoring of liver function tests is therefore essential. Other side effects include: headache, nausea, diarrhoea and dizziness. The dose may be escalated slowly to decrease frequency of side effects.

Nevirapine is a moderate inducer of CYP3A4 and may increase its own clearance. It decreases the plasma levels of some protease inhibitors (such as amprenavir, indinavir, lopinavir and saquinavir), azole group of antifungal agents and ethinyl estradiol based oral contraceptives. Nevirapine levels may decrease in presence of enzyme inducers such as rifampicin.

Efavirenz (EFV)

Efavirenz is used to treat HIV-1 infections in adults and children. It is also used as postoperative prophylaxis. The recommended adult dose is 600 mg orally OD. It is not to be taken with fatty meals. Oral bioavailability is 50%; t½ 50 hrs.

The principal *adverse effects* involve CNS: dizziness, nightmares, insomnia, headache and euphoria, which get resolved during continuation of the therapy. Other adverse effects include skin rash, nausea, vomiting, diarrhoea, elevated liver enzymes and serum cholesterol levels. Teratogenic effects have been reported in monkeys exposed to efavirenz (caution! pregnancy).

Several drug interactions are possible with efavirenz as it is an inducer for CYP3A4 and inhibitor for CYP2C9 and CYP2C19. It is also a self inducer. Concurrent use of cisapride, midazolam, triazolam and ergot alkaloids may result in life-threatening toxicities. It increases the plasma levels of protease inhibitors like nelfinavir and ritonavir. On the contrary, it decreases the plasma concentration of other protease inhibitors, specially of saquinavir. Phenobarbital, rifampicin and herbal preparations like St. John's wort may decrease the plasma levels of efavirenz.

Delavirdine (DLV)

Delavirdine is used for the treatment of HIV-1 infection in adults only as a part of combination therapy. The usual adult dose is 400 mg TDS. Oral bioavailability is high (85%); t½ 5–6 hrs. It use has declined because of three times daily dosing schedule.

Main *adverse effects* include skin rash and pruritus which resolve on continuation of therapy. Other side effects include diarrhoea, headache, nausea, vomiting and elevated hepatic enzymes.

If didanosine or antacids are to be used, the dosing of delavirdine is to be withheld by 1 hr as they decrease its oral bioavailability. It is metabolised by and inhibits CYP3A4 and thus it increases the plasma concentration of several protease inhibitors such as amprenavir, indinavir, lopinavir, ritonavir and saquinavir. Hence, dose reduction of these drugs should be considered if these are administered concurrently. Plasma levels of delavirdine are reduced by phenytoin, phenobarbitone, carbamazepine and rifampicin. Being teratogenic in rats, pregnancy should be avoided during delavirdine therapy.

Etravirine (ETV)

Etravirine (200 mg B.D. orally) is indicated for use, in combination with at least two additional antiretroviral drugs, in the treatment-experienced (not is treatment-naive patients) adults who demonstrate documented resistance to other NNRTIs. As food increases its bioavailability, it should be administered following the meal. Adverse effects include nausea and rash. It is an inducer of CYP3A4 and an inhibitor of CYP2C9 and CYP2C19. Hence, it should not be used concomitantly with carbamazepine, phenytoin, unboosted protease inhibitors, other NNRTIs, ketoconazole, St. John wort and rifampicin.

Rilpivirine (RPV)

Rilpivirine is reserved for use in only treatment-naive

patients with HIV-1 RNA load of 100,000 copies for per mL and that too in combination with atleast two other ARV drugs. (emtricitabine and tenofovir, with which it is available in FDC formulation. The drug should be administered with meal (preferably of high fat content to increase its absorption). The drug's absorption is facilitated by acid environment and therefore it should not be co-medicated with antacid, H_2 blockers and PPIs. It is highly bound to plasm proteins and is metabolise by CYP 3A4. It is a long acting drug with a terminal halflife is 50 hrs. Drug-drug interaction may occur with agents effecting CYP3A4 enzyme induction or inhibition.

The common side effect seen with rilpivirine a treatment are headache, insomia, depression and increase in serum aminotransferases. In some patients an elevated blood cholesterol and abnormal body fat redistribution syndrome have been observed. A QTc prolongation has been reported with higher doses of the drug.

NUCLEOTIDE REVERSE TRANSCRIPTASE INHIBITORS (NtRTIs)

Tenofovir (TFV)

Tenofovir available as two prodrug ester forms: tenofovir **d**isoproxil **f**umarate (TFV-DF) and tenofovir **a**la**f**enamide (TFV-AF) is an analogue of adenosine-5'-monophosphate (i.e., it is a nucleotide analogue; see above; some texts, however, classify it under NRTIs). These prodrugs are first hydrolysed in liver to TFV which is subsequently phosphorylated to an active tenofovir **di**phosphate (TFV-DP). The latter molecule like NRTIs discussed above, competitively inhibits HIV reverse transcriptase enzyme and causes termination of chain elongation after getting incorporated into viral DNA (blocks step 4, Fig. 62.1B). *Note that NtRTIs are active as diphosphates, unlike NRTIs which require conversion to triphosphate.*

Tenofovir is used along with other anti-HIV drugs in the treatment of HIV infection in adults in a dose of 300 mg once daily after meals. Its oral bioavailability is 25% which is increased to 40% after meals. Plasma half-life is 17 hrs.

Tenofovir is usually well tolerated. However, nausea, vomiting, diarrhoea and osteomalacia (in animal studies) have been observed. As with NRTIs, hepatomegaly, pancreatitis and lactic acidosis may be carefully watched. Tenofovir increases the plasma levels of didanosine leading to toxicity (pancreatitis, hepatotoxicity, lactic acidosis). It decreases serum concentration of atazanavir.

PROTEASE INHIBITORS (PIs)

Examples: ***Saquinavir, Indinavir, Nelfinavir, Fosamprenavir, Ritonavir, Lopinavir, Atazanavir, Tipranavir, Darunavir***

Mechanism of Action

The protease inhibitors (PIs) competitively inhibit the viral protease enzyme and prevent the cleavage of gag-pol poly proteins necessary for virion production. This results in the production of immature, noninfectious virions (block step-10; Fig. 62.1B). This isoform of protease is not present in the host; *hence PIs are better option for therapeutic intervention.*

Therapeutic Uses

Combination therapy with PIs and other antiretroviral drugs significantly improves the clinical efficacy by blocking HIV replication at different stages in the intracellular life cycle. These agents are active against HIV-1 and HIV-2 infection. Cross resistance between *indinavir* and *ritonavir* can occur but has not been noted with other PIs. *Amprenavir* (>4 years), *lopinavir* (6 months), *nelfinavir* and *ritonavir* (>2 years) are the only PIs approved for paediatric use.

Adverse Effects

These include diarrhoea, nausea and abdominal discomfort. In addition, PIs are liable to produce hyperglycaemia, fat redistribution and hyperlipidaemia. These also have a risk potential for increased bleeding episodes particularly in haemophilics. Individual drug toxicity is discussed in the following text.

Drug Interactions

All PIs are competitive inhibitors of drugs metabolised by CYP3A4 family. Hence, life-thereatening toxicities (due to increased plasma levels) may result with concurrent use of the following drugs: cisapride (arrhythmias), ergot alkaloids (vasospasm); statins (rhabdomyolysis); midazolam and triazolam (respiratory depression). Benzodiazepines as a rule are contraindicated with PIs. Enzyme inducers like phenytoin, pheno-barbitone, carbamazepine, dexamethasone and rifampicin may decrease the plasma levels of PIs. Drugs such as clarithromycin, itraconazole and ketoconazole may increase the plasma levels of PIs. St. John's wort antagonises antiviral actions of PIs.

Popular Drug Combinations

Indinavir + Zidovudine + Lamivudine
Nelfinavir + Zidovudine + Didanosine
Ritonavir + Lopinavir + Stavudine + Lamivudine
Ritonavir + Indinavir + Stavudine + Didanosine

Individual Drugs

Saquinavir (SQV)

Saquinavir hard gel capsule (Saquinavir-H) or tablets have a very poor bioavailability (4%) but saquinavir-S (soft gel capsule) has a better bioavailability (13%). Fatty meal enhances the bioavailability of both but not to therapeutically useful levels. Maximum bioavailability is obtained when saquinavir-H is combined with low doses of ritonavir (boosted therapy). t½ of saquinavir is 8 hrs. Saquinavir-H alone is usually administered as 600 mg TDS orally, 2 hrs after full meal. The drug combination of saquinavir-H (1000 mg BD) with ritonavir (100 mg BD) exhibits an improved antiviral efficacy as well as a reduction in GIT side effects. Ritonavir increases the plasma levels of saquinavir by inhibiting its first-pass metabolism. Soft gel capsule formulation has been withdrawn. Remaining features are similar to other PIs (see above).

Fosamprenavir (FPV)

Fosamprenavir is a prodrug of amprenavir (which was available as a drug in its own right but was withdrawn from the market as a result of development of serious toxicity like lactic acidosis, seizures and depression produced due to presence of propylene glycol in which the drug was formulated) that has an advantage of better bioavailability (80%) due to its high hydrophilicity. Moreover, it is better tolerated than amprenavir. It is recommended to be given in combination with other ARV drugs like ritonavir (usual dose: 700 mg BD with ritonavir 100 mg BD). This drug should be avoided in severe hepatic insufficiency. Antacids decrease its absorption.

Indinavir (IDV)

It shares pharmacological features common to other PIs. The recommended adult dose is 800 mg orally TDS or 800 mg BD + ritonavir 100 mg BD. Oral bioavailability is 65%. Food decreases its bioavailability. t½ is 1–2 hr. Its characteristic side effects are nephrolithiasis, urolithiasis and possibly renal insufficiency (high incidences of nephrolithiasis have been reported with combination therapy with ritonavir). Hence, large intake of water is usually recommended. Additionally, it causes reversible hyperbilirubinaemia, alopecia, paronychia (nail infection) and anaemia.

Nelfinavir (NFV)

It is probably the most commonly used PI as it has a relatively low toxicity profile. Its usual adult dose is 750 mg orally BD (t½ 5 hr). Food increases its bioavailability. Common side effects (besides discussed above) are diarrhoea and flatulence, which resolve after continued use. It is the only PI that cannot be boosted by ritonavir, because it is not extensively metabolised by CYP3A4.

Ritonavir (RTV)

Though a potent protease inhibitor, it is not well tolerated and hence usually given in combination with *lopinavir* (see below). It is also used in low doses to increase the effectiveness of other PIs (e.g., saquinavir, fosamprenavir and indinavir). Usual adult dose is 600 mg orally BD. Oral bioavailability is 75%. Food increases its bioavailability. Its t½ is 3–5 hr.Ritonavir is rarely used as a sole PI owing to its poor tolerability in therapeutic doses. It is primarily used in low doses (100 mg BD) as a pharma-cokinetic booster for concomitantly used other PIs. Being a potent CYP3A4 enzyme inhibitor, it markedly increases the plasma concentration of other PIs leading to improved viral suppression.

Additional side effects include altered taste, anorexia, peripheral paraesthesias, elevated triglycerides and hepatic transaminases. Ritonavir has the highest incidence for potential drug interactions. Besides those discussed above, it should not be used in conjunction with amiodarone, bepridil, propafenone, quinidine or pimozide. Being a potent inhibitor of CYP3A4, it increases the plasma levels of these drugs to cause toxicity.

Lopinavir + Ritonavir (LPV+RTV)

This is the only PI fixed dose combination used for the treatment of HIV-1 and HIV-2 infections. Ritonavir markedly reduces the metabolism of lopinavir resulting in its increased plasma levels. This property has an added advantage as it increases the half-life of lopinavir. This combination is not only synergistic but exhibits milder side effects than either drug alone.

Atazanavir (ATV)

It is a azapeptide PI active against HIV-1 and HIV-2. It has a good oral bioavailability (75%) which is further enhanced by intake of food. Its absorption is acid-dependent. Hence H_2 blocker/proton pump inhibitors decrease its absorption. A combination of atazanavir + low dose ritonavir is as efficacious as lopinavir + ritonavir combination. Its side effects are like that of indinavir and include nausea, diarrhoea, reversible hyperbilirubinaemia, hyperglycaemia and hyper-cholesterolaemia. It is the only PI that has no effect on lipid profile. Drug interactions are as described for other PIs. Efavirenz decreases atazanavir plasma levels.

Darunavir (DRV)

It is approved by FDA for the treatment of patients with HIV resistant mutants. It is to be coadministered with ritonavir. Lopinavir and saquinavir decrease, while indinavir increases its plasma levels.

Tipranavir (TPV)

It is approved for treating patients not responsive to other PIs (treatment-experienced patients). It is also coadministered with ritonavir to increase its bioavailability.

FUSION/ENTRY INHIBITORS

Enfuvirtide (EVT)

It is a polypeptide and the only drug available in this category. It binds to gp41 subunit of viral envelope glycoproteins and thus prevents the entry of HIV-1 into $CD4^+$ cells by interfering with the *fusion* of viral and host cell membrane (blocks step 1 & 2; Fig. 62.1B). Its usual adult dose is 90 mg orally BD given *subcutaneously*. Its metabolism does not involve cytochrome-P450 enzyme system. Its elimination half-life is 3–4 hrs. It is used along with other antiretroviral drugs for the treatment of advanced HIV-1 infections (in patients with extensive viral resistance).

Adverse effects include local reaction (nodule) at the injection site, skin rash, eosinophilia and pneumonia like manifestations. Till date no drug-drug interaction or cross resistance with other antiretroviral drugs has been reported.

Fostemsavir

Fostemsavir is a prodrug of temsavir, a HIV-1 attachment inhibitor that works by binding directly to the glycoprotein 120 (gp120) subunit on the surface of the virus. Fostemsavir blocks HIV from attaching to CD4+ T cells, which prevents virus to enter and multiply in host cells. It is used for the treatment of multidrug-resistant HIV-1 infection in adults. Adverse effects: Nausea, headache, diarrhoea, abdominal pain, fatigue, allergy and sleep disturbances.

Ibalizumab

It is a CD4-directed post-attachment HIV-1 inhibitor. Recombinant humanized monoclonal antibody; blocks HIV-1 from infecting CD4+ T cells and blocks the entry of HIV-1 virus particles into the host cells. It is used i.v. for HIV-1 infection in adults with multidrug-resistant infection, used in combination with other ART drugs.

CHEMOKINE RECEPTOR-5 (CCR-5) ANTAGONIST

Maraviroc (MRV)

It is the only member at present for this novel class of anti-HIV agents. It binds to CCR-5 receptor (one of the two coreceptors) present on host CD4 cell membrane and prevents the entry of the virus into the host cell.

Precisely, maraviroc prevents interaction of viral gp120 with CCR-5, a chemokine coreceptor (step 1; Fig. 62.1B). It is used along with other ARVs, only in highly treatment-experienced (resistant) adult patients infected with HIV that binds to CCR-5 receptor only (called R5 HIV or CCR-5 tropic HIV infections). These viruses use only CCR-5 receptor exclusively present on macrophages (and not CXCR4 coreceptor present on T-cells) for their entry into the host CD4 cell.

Main adverse effect is hepatotoxicity; others include cough, rash, fever, muscular/joint pain and GIT distress. Dosage depends on concomitant drug used: **(1)** when used with enzyme inducers (like phenytoin, carbamazepine, rifampicin, St. John wort, efavirenz and etravirine), it is used in a dose of 600 mg BD; **(2)** when used with enzyme inhibitors (like delavirdine, ketoconazole, itraconazole and clarithromycin), it is administered in a dose of 150 mg BD orally.

INTEGRASE INHIBITORS/INTEGRASE STRAND TRANSFER INHIBITORS (INSTIS)

Raltegravir (RTG), Elvitegravir (ETG), Dolutegravir (DTG), Bictegravir

These are new class of agents that work by inhibiting the viral enzyme integrase, thereby, preventing the insertion of HIV pro-viral genetic (DNA) material into the host cell genome (step 5; Fig. 62.1B) and halting the viral replication process. These drugs bind not only to aminoacid residues of integrase protein but also megnesium ions chelated by acid active site residues which are complexed with DNA. This complex make the DNA to angle its position in such a manner that prevents the strand transfer.

These drugs are used, along with other ARVs, only in treatment-experienced adult patients demonstrating resistance to the therapy. These drugs since not metabolised by cytochrome P-450 system, drug interactions are not clinically significant. However, rifampicin decreases raltegravir levels. Antacids and iron bind to integrase, hence their dosing should be separated by 2 hrs. All these agents have been approved for the treatment of patients with HIV in combination with other anti-retroviral drugs.

Dolutegravir shows a higher resistance-resisting activity than raltegravir and elvitegravir do, and therefore dolutegravir remains active against many HIVs that are resistant to the other two INSTIs. Dolutegravir is available as single tablet regimen (STR) with abacavir and lamivudine. *Adverse effects* include nausea, diarrhoea, headache, fever, and myopathy.

NATIONAL GUIDELINES FOR HIV CARE AND TREATMENT 2021

Anti-Retroviral Therapy (ART) consists of the use of a combination of at least three Anti-Retroviral (ARV) drugs from different classes to inhibit the replication of HIV and reduce viraemia to undetectable levels. ART was earlier known as Highly Active Antiretroviral Therapy (HAART).

Principles of Antiretroviral therapy

Use combination of at least three antiretroviral drugs from different classes to inhibit the replication of HIV and reduce viremia to undetectable level.

Goals of therapy

To inhibit viral replication (viral load <50 copies/ml), to restore CD4 count to normal level, to prevent drug resistance by starting combination anti-retroviral treatment (ART), to reduce morbidity, mortality and improve quality of life and immune status.

Initiating antiretroviral therapy (ART)

Start ART to all symptomatic patients. The introduction of the 'Treat All' recommendation supports the rapid initiation of ART, including the same-day initiation where there is no clinical contraindication. Rapid ART initiation is defined as ART initiation within seven days from the day of HIV diagnosis. Taking ART is a lifelong commitment, and the first 6 months of therapy are especially important which predicts drug response. Clinical and immunological improvement and viral suppression are expected when individuals adhere to ART. In most adults and children, CD4 cell counts rise by 40 to 60 cells/year when ART is initiated, and immune recovery starts (CD4 > 200 cells/mm^3).

Which drugs are selected?

Drugs are selected on basis of their efficacy, safety, durability, convenience, drug interactions and cost. The basic principle for first-line ART for treatment-naive adult and adolescent patients is to use a triple drug combination from two different classes of ARVs. (National AIDS Control Organisation [NACO], 2021)

The preferred first-line ART regimen for adults: Tenofovir (TDF 300 mg) + Lamivudine (3TC 300 mg) + Dolutegravir (DTG 50 mg) regimen (TLD) as FDC in a single pill once a day (in morning or at a fixed time every day). This regimen can be used for the treatment of all adults, adolescents, pregnant women including those with HIV-1, HIV-2, women exposed to single dose nevirapine in the past and those co-infected with TB or Hepatitis.

In cases where the preferred first-line ARV regimen cannot be used, the alternative regimens are mentioned in Table 62.1.

Table 62.1 Alternate first-line ART in adults and adolescents

Condition	Alternate First-line Regimen
HIV with body weight <30 kg	Abacavir 600 mg + Lamivudine 300mg, one tablet + Dolutegravir (50 mg) once daily in the morning
HIV on Rifampicin-containing Anti-tuberculoid therapy (ATT) regimen	Tenofovir (300 mg) + Lamivudine (300 mg) + Dolutegravir (50 mg). Additional dose of Dolutegravir 50 mg until 2 weeks after completion of ATT.
Women of childbearing potential who do not wish to take Dolutegravir -based ART	Tenofovir (300 mg)+Lamivudine (300 mg)+Efavirenz (600mg). If Efavirenz is contraindicated, Tenofovir (300 mg) + Lamivudine (300 mg) + [Lopinavir (200 mg) + ritonavir (50 mg) twice daily]

Immune Reconstitution Inflammatory Syndrome (IRIS)

It is the worsening of signs and symptoms of HIV due to inflammatory response by a immune system following the initiation of ART. IRIS occurs within 2–12 weeks of the initiation of ART, although it may present later (usually between 6 weeks to 6 months). Symptoms are lymph nodes enlargement, severe fever, painful lesions, organ dysfunction, reactivation of are TB and Cryptococcosis. Management: If mild, observation with continuing ART. Management of infections by antimicrobial therapy to eliminate the pathogen. Short-term therapy with corticosteroids or non-steroidal anti-inflammatory drugs can be given to reduce the inflammation, Prednisolone 1.5 mg/kg orally. Temporary cessation of ART must be considered, only if potentially life-threatening forms of IRIS develop.

Pregnant or Breastfeeding Women with HIV

Parent to child transmission (PTCT) is a major route for transmission of new HIV infection in children. PTCT contributes to about 4% of HIV infections in India. *The preferred regimen for PTCT*: Tenofovir (TDF) + Lamivudine (3TC) + Dolutegravir (DTG) as FDC to be given once daily.

If Women Presenting Directly in Labour having HIV

Intra-partum: Initiate TDF (300 mg) + 3TC (300 mg) + DTG (50 mg) & continue postpartum also.

Infant ARV Prophylaxis

Viral -load testing of all HIV positive pregnant women should be done during 32 to 36 weeks of pregnancy (regardless of duration of ART). The HIV-exposed infants are categorized as low risk or high risk. Low-risk infants are infants born to mothers with suppressed viral load (<1000 copies/ml): give Syrup Nevirapine (NVP) or Syrup Zidovudine (if NVP will not be effective) from birth till 6 weeks of age. High-risk infants are infants born to HIV-positive mother not on ART: give Syrup NVP + Syrup Zidovudine from birth till 6–12 weeks of age.

Management recommendations for TB diagnosed in patients already receiving ART (Table 62.2).

TREATMENT FAILURE

Treatment failure refers to the loss of antiviral efficacy to the current regimen. Virological failure means incomplete suppression of viral replication. Under the national programme, it is defined as a plasma viral load value of ≥1,000 copies/mL at or after 6 months of ART.

Formulation of second-line ART

For treatment failure of first-line ART, second-line ART should be started. If Zidovudine (AZT) is used in first line, NRTI choice in second line is Tenofovir (TDF). If TDF/ABC is used in first line, NRTI choice could be AZT, unless contraindicated. Continuing Lamivudine reduces viral fitness and must be part of second-line ART. If patient had NNRTI in first line, Integrase Strand Transfer Inhibitor (INSTI); Dolutegravir will be preferred. (Table 62.3).

Initiation of third-line ART

For treatment failure of second-line ART, third-line ART should be started. If treatment adherence is poor or major opportunistic infection is identified, it is upmost importance to improve adherence and/or treat opportunistic infection. Initiation of third-line ART: it should include new drugs with minimal risk of cross-resistance to previously used regimens. As per recent NACO guideline, dolutegravir (50 mg) and darunavir should be started in combination (Table 62.4).

- **Pre-exposure prophylaxis**: It is administration of antiretrovirals prior to HIV infection. It is preferred for homosexual men, women and i.v. drug abusers. Give tenofovir (300 mg) daily + emtricitabine (200 mg) + Lamivudine 300 mg daily.
- **Post-exposure prophylaxis**: It includes accidental needle stick or sharp injury or contact with blood. Preferred regimen for adults: Tenofovir (300 mg) + Lamivudine (300 mg) + Dolutegravir (50 mg) (FDC: One tablet OD) within 2 h of exposure and administered daily for 28 days. For children: Zidovudine + Lamivudine + Dolutegravir (50 mg). Alternative regimen is Tenofovir + Lamivudine + Lopinavir/Ritonavir.

Table 62.2 ART regimens for patients diagnosed with TB

ART regimen when TB is diagnosed	Management
(AZT or TDF or ABC) + 3TC + EFV	Continue with (AZT or TDF or ABC) + 3TC + EFV. Anti-Tubercular Therapy (ATT): 2HREZ + 4HR
(AZT or TDF or ABC) + 3TC + NVP	Substitute NVP with EFV and continue EFV thereafter even after TB treatment is completed. ATT: 2HREZ + 4HRE
Two NRTIs (AZT or TDF or ABC) + ritonavir boosted PI	ATT: 2HRZE + 4HRE daily regimen. modify ATT. Rifampicin must be replaced with Rifabutin.

Table 62.3 Regimen for failure to first line ART

Failing First line ART	Recommended Regimens
TDF + 3TC + EFV/NVP	Hb ≥9 g/dl: AZT + 3TC + DTG Hb <9 g/dl, DTG + ATV/r + existing NRTI
AZT + 3TC+ NVP/EFV	TDF + 3TC + DTG
TDF + 3TC + DTG	Hb ≥9 g/dl: AZT + 3TC + ATV/r Hb <9 g/dl: DTG + ATV/r + existing NRTI
AZT + 3TC + DTG	TDF + 3TC + ATV/r

AZT—Zidovudine; ABC—Abacavir; TDF—Tenofovir 3TC: Lamivudine; EFV—Efavirenz; NVP—Nevirapine; ATV/r—Atazanavir/ritonavir; LPV/r—Lopinavir/ritonavir; DTG—Dolutegravir.

Table 62.4 Third line ART regimens

Previous regimen failed	Preferred third line regimen
2 NRTI + NNRTI as first line, PI-based second line	DRV/r + DTG + existing NRTI
2 NRTI + NNRTI as first line, INSTI-based second line	LPV/r or DRV/r + DTG + 2 NRTIs including 3TC.
2 NRTI + PI as first line, DRV/r BD second line	DTG + DRV/r BD + 2 NRTIs including 3TC

DRV/r—Ritonavir boosted Darunavir; INSTI—Integrase Strand Transfer Inhibitor.

CHAPTER 63

Anthelmintics

COMPETENCY PH1.47

The helminths (worms) are macroscopic, multicellular organisms having their own digestive, excretory, reproductive and nervous system. The helminths could be *nemathelminths* (round bodied worms) or *platyhelminths* (flat bodied worms).

Nemathelminths include **Nematodes** such as roundworms (*Ascaris lumbricoides*), hookworms (*Necator americanus or Ancylostoma duodenale*), whipworms (*Trichuris trichiura*), threadworms (*Strongyloides stercoralis*), pinworms (*Enterobius vermicularis*), filarias (*Wuchereria bancrofti* or *Brugia malayi*), onchocerca (*Onchocerca volvulus*) and guinea worms (*Dracunculus medinensis*).

Platyhelminths are of two types: **Trematodes (flukes)** and **Cestodes (tapeworms).**

Trematodes include, blood flukes (schistosomiasis or bilharziasis), liver flukes (clonorchiasis), intestinal flukes (fasciolopsiasis) and lung flukes (paragonimiasis). **Cestodes** (tapeworms) include beef tapeworm (*Taenia saginata*), pork tapeworm (*Taenia solium*), fish tapeworm (*Diphyllobothrium latum*) and dwarf tapeworm (*Hymenolepis nana*).

The drugs used to get the body rid off the helminths (worms) are called ***anthelmintic drugs,*** which may serve as either ***vermicide*** (kill) or ***vermifuge*** (expel) to the infesting helminth. Antihelminths attack the parasite cells but not the mammalian cells and hence have selective toxicity to the helminths only. Most available anthelmintic drugs exert their antiparasitic effects by interfering with **(a)** neuromuscular functions, **(b)** microtubular functions, **(c)** Ca^{2+} permeability and **(d)** energy metabolism.

Most of the **nematodes** (roundworms, hookworms, whipworms, pinworms and threadworms) are found primarily in intestine where they attach to the mucosa and feed on host blood and tissue fluid. The symptoms may be manifested as vague abdominal pain, diarrhoea, pruritus and if infestation is severe, anaemia. However, threadworm infestation in small intestine may remain asymptomatic for years but in immunocompromised person there may be a widespread tissue invasion (dissemination) which could be serious. In most nematodal infestations, particularly with pinworms, the characteristic symptom is perianal pruritus due to migration of female worm through the anus to the perianal skin. Other nematodes (filarial worms, guinea worms) live in blood, lymphatics and other tissues and are referred to as blood and tissue nematodes. The filarial worms differ from other nematodes in that they are thread-like and are found in blood, tissues and lymphatics. The infective larvae enter following the bite of infected fly or mosquito. Larvae then enter lymphatics and lymph nodes causing fever, eosinophilia, and lymphadenitis. Chronic infestation may cause elephantiasis as a consequence of lymphatic obstruction. If filarial worms migrate to other subcutaneous tissues, these may produce nodules and blindness (onchocerciasis). Guinea worm infestation is acquired by ingesting *Dracunculus medinensis* larvae which inhabit the ponds and step wells. They penetrate intestinal wall and migrate through connective tissue. The fully developed female worm surfaces anywhere under skin to discharge its larvae externally. There is painful vesicle, ulcer, cellulitis usually on leg and secondary infection. Onchocerciasis infestation is caused by nematode of genus *Onchocerca*. Adult worms live in a tangled mass in the subcutaneous tissue of infected humans. Degenerating microfilaria elicit a granulomatous reaction and eosinophilia. Inflammatory reactions may occur in the lungs, liver, spleen and kidney. Damage to the eyes (river blindness) is caused by living or dead microfilaria (see above).

Trematodes (flukes) are hermaphroditic, nonsegmented flattened helminths. The larvae are acquired either through ingestion of food (vegetables or fish) or through skin penetration. After ingestion, those trematodes which mature in the intestinal tract are called *intestinal flukes*; others may migrate and mature in liver and bile ducts (*liver flukes*); some may migrate through the abdominal cavity to the lungs (*lung flukes*). Intestinal flukes cause diarrhoea, abdominal pain and anorexia. Liver flukes produce bile duct obstruction, jaundice, liver enlargement and diarrhoea. Chronic infestation may cause cirrhosis of liver. Lung flukes may cause coughing, haemoptysis and chest pain. *Schistosomes* (blood flukes) are a distinct type of trematodes. Their sexes are separate and these are cylindrical at the anterior but flattened at the posterior end. Three species of Schistosoma (*S. haematobium, S. mansoni* and *S. japonicum*) are the causative agents of schistosomiasis. Cercariae (free swimming state in the development of this fluke) penetrate the skin or mucosa of the final host (humans) where they pass through the lung, reach the liver and mature. After maturation these migrate to veins where the adults mate and release the eggs. In mesenteric veins, the eggs secrete certain enzymes which enable them to pass through the intestinal walls (*S. mansoni and S. japonicum*) or bladder (*S. haematobium* in vesicular veins). Some eggs reach liver or lungs via circulation. Much of the pathology associated with schistosome infection is attributed to immune reactions to the eggs of the parasite. The manifestations are haematuria, frequent and painful micturition, and uraemia (*S. haematobium*); abdominal pain, diarrhoea with blood-stained mucus, ascites, hepatomegaly and haematemesis (*S. mansoni*); and features resembling those with *S. mansoni* plus neurologic manifestations (*S. japonicum*).

Cestodes (tapeworms) are ribbon-shaped parasitic worms of the genus *Taenia*. These are mainly intestinal parasites, though a few invade other tissues in the larval stage. The scolex (or the head) of these worms is the hold-fast segment with suckers to attach with intestinal wall. Anthelmintics detach the scolex and help expulsion of the worm. The fertilised eggs are released from the worm and discharged into the environment. Cestodes require development in a second or intermediate host. Infestation in humans occurs from eating undercooked meat or fish that is infested with cysts containing larvae. Tapeworms have no digestive system and depend on the host for their nutrients; hence vitamin-B deficiency is a common manifestation, but vague complaints such as abdominal discomfort, hunger pangs and at times anorexia may be observed. If the larval stage of the tapeworm develops in extraintestinal tissues it is called cysticercosis (pea-like ovoid bodies under the skin), or hydatid disease (echinococcosis—cysts growing in liver or lungs).

MECHANISM OF ACTION OF DIFFERENT ANTHELMINTICS

Against Nematodes

Unlike humans, the locomotor muscles of nematodes have both cholinergic and GABAergic innervation and their neuromuscular junction has both excitatory cholinergic-nicotinic (N_N) and inhibitory GABAergic receptors.

Pyrantel pamoate and ***Levamisole*** are the N_N receptor agonist and also cause release of ACh by inhibition of acetylcholinesterase. Therefore, they produce depolarising neuromuscular blockade. Affected helminths are thus unable to maintain their attachment to the intestinal lumen and are expelled in the faeces.

GABAergic neurotransmission in humans is predominantly in CNS, not in the periphery as in nematodes. Anthelmintic drugs cannot cross BBB and act peripherally. ***Piperazine*** is a GABA receptor agonist and activates GABA-gated Cl^- channel in nematode muscles. Flaccid paralysis of nematode results due to Cl^- dependent hyperpolarisation and the paralysed worms are expelled alive. ***Ivermectin*** also activates Cl^- channels but it acts primarily on nematode specific glutamate-gated Cl^- channels which are also inhibitory due to subsequent hyperpolarisation. These glutamate-mediated voltage-gated Cl^- channels are found on the pharyngeal muscles of nematodes only and are physiologically related to the vertebrate GABA-gated Cl^- channels. ***Diethylcarbamazine*** is a piperazine derivative, yet its mode of action is entirely different. It alters the microfilarial membrane surface characteristics so that they are subsequently phagocytosed by tissue fixed monocytes (not by circulating phagocytes). It also hyperpolarises the worm's musculature (perhaps due to the piperazine moiety) so that these are expelled. It also blocks the production of prostaglandins, resulting in capillary vasoconstriction and impairment of the passage of microfilariae. However, its exact mode of action is yet not clear.

For ***thiabendazole*** mode of action, see under albendazole (below).

Doxycycline is a recent addition to the armoury of anthelmintics (see under individual drugs). It eradicates *Wolbachia,* an intracellular bacteria which is an endosymbiont of filarial parasite and is responsible for oogenesis and reproductive ability of adult female filarial parasite.

Against Trematodes

Metrifonate is an organophosphorous compound whose mode of action resembles *pyrantel pamoate* (see above). Its active metabolite, dichlorvos, inactivates acetylcholinesterase and potentiates depolarising neuromuscular blockade of *Schistosoma haematobium.*

Oxamniquine intercalates in the parasitic DNA leading to the death of schistosome by blocking its nucleic acid and protein synthesis. The fluke probably first esterifies oxamniquine to produce a reactive metabolite that alkylates parasite DNA.

Bithionol uncouples parasite-specific (fumarate reductase-mediated) oxidative phosphorylation. Thus by blocking the ATP synthesis, it inhibits the energy derived by the helminth from the anaerobic metabolism.

For ***triclabendazole*** mode of action, refer albendazole (see below).

Against Cestodes

Niclosamide appears to uncouple oxidative phosphorylation in adult cestode. The result is an expulsion of dead worm in the faeces. It inhibits the anaerobic incorporation of energy-rich inorganic phosphates into ATP, which is detrimental to the parasite.

Against Trematodes As Well As Cestodes

Praziquantel causes influx of Ca^{2+} from endogenous stores of the cestodes resulting in intense contractions and subsequent expulsion of the worm from the GIT. In Schistosomes (flukes), praziquantel-induced influx of Ca^{2+} damages the tegument, causing vacuolations (holes) which exposes the hidden parasite antigens. The antibodies, in the host, then bind to these antigens and destroy them by phagocytosis.

Broad-Spectrum Anthelmintics

These are ***benzimidazole group*** of anthelmintics and include ***thiabendazole, mebendazole, albendazole*** and ***triclabendazole***. All share a common mechanism of action. However, thiabendazole and triclabendazole have only restricted use (see below).

Benzimidazoles have a different mode of action. Cytoskeletal structures of helminths include microfilaments, microtubules and β-tubulins. Under normal conditions microtubule assembly is dependent on β-tubulin function wherein β-tubulin dimers are continually being polymerised from one end and then depolymerised at the other end of the microtubules. Benzimidazoles bind to β-tubulins and prevent their assembly, i.e., polymerisation, resulting in breakdown of cytoplasmic microtubules. This leads to the selective and irreversible inhibition of glucose uptake by these organisms. The end result is depletion of parasite's glycogen stores, reduced formation of ATP, disruption of metabolic pathways and ultimately parasitic death. Since these drugs bind to parasite β-tubulin with much higher affinity, serum glucose concentration of the human host is not affected and hence the selective toxicity of these drugs to helminths only.

INDIVIDUAL DRUGS

In the following text, all anthelmintic drugs are arranged alphabetically and discussed. Table 63.1 summarises major helminth infections, drugs of choice and the alternative drugs to treat such infections. Their mechanism of action has already been discussed above.

Benzimidazoles

Benzimidazoles constitute an important category of drugs in treating various helminth infections. Four of these, *albendazole, mebendazole, thiabendazole* and *triclabendazole* are described here. Albendazole and mebendazole have a broader range of anthelmintic activity against nematodes and cestodes including cutaneous and visceral larva

Table 63.1 Choice of Drugs For Helminthic Infestations

Worm Infestation	First Choice Drugs	Second Choice Drugs
Nematodes		
Ascaris lumbricoides (Roundworms)	Mebendazole, Albendazole, Pyrantel pamoate	Piperazine, Levamisole
Necator americanus *Ancylostoma duodenale* (Hookworms)	Mebendazole Albendazole Pyrantel pamoate	Levamisole
Trichuris trichiura (Whipworm)	Mebendazole Albendazole	Thiabendazole Oxantel pamoate
Trichinella spiralis (Trichinosis)	Mebendazole Albendazole	Thiabendazole
Enterobius vermicularis (Pinworm)	Mebendazole Pyrantel pamoate	Albendazole Piperazine
Strongyloides stercoralis (Threadworm)	Ivermectin	Albendazole Thiabendazole
Wuchereria bancrofti *Brugia malayi* (Filaria)	Diethylcarbamazine	Ivermectin
Onchocerca volvulus (Onchocerciasis)	Ivermectin	Diethylcarbamazine
Dracunculus medinensis (Guinea worm)	Metronidazole (see Ch. 65)	Thiabendazole
Cutaneous larva migrans (Creeping eruption)	Albendazole Ivermectin	Thiabendazole (Topical/oral)
Visceral larva migrans	Albendazole	Diethylcarbamazine Mebendazole
Intestinal capillariasis	Albendazole	Mebendazole, Thiabendazole
Trematodes (Flukes)		
Schistosoma haematobium (Bilharziasis)	Praziquantel	Metrifonate

contd.

Worm Infestation	First Choice Drugs	Second Choice Drugs
Schistosoma mansoni *Schistosoma japonicum* (All blood flukes)	Praziquantel Praziquantel	Oxamniquine —
Clonorchis sinensis (Liver fluke)	Praziquantel	Albendazole
Fasciola hepatica (Sheep liver fluke)	Bithionol Triclabendazole	—
Paragonimus skrjabini (Lung fluke)	Triclabendazole Praziquantel	Bithionol
Cestodes (Tapeworms)		
Taenia saginata (Beef tapeworm)	Praziquantel Niclosamide	Mebendazole
Diphyllobothrium latum (Fish tapeworm)	Praziquantel Niclosamide	—
Taenia solium (Pork tapeworm)	Praziquantel Niclosamide	—
Hymenolepis nana (Dwarf tapeworm)	Praziquantel	Niclosamide
Cysticercosis Hydatid disease	Albendazole Albendazole	Praziquantel

migrans. Thiabendazole and triclabendazole, however, have only restricted use.

Albendazole

It is a broad spectrum oral anthelmintic.

Pharmacokinetics: Its oral absorption is quite variable but fatty meals increase its absorption by five folds. It is rapidly metabolised in liver to an active sulfoxide metabolite which has a wide distribution into different tissues, bile, CSF and the hydatid cysts. Elimination half-life is 8–12 hrs.

Clinical Uses: Albendazole is a broad-spectrum anthelmintic agent particularly against intestinal nematodes and cestodes as well as against liver fluke (a trematode, *Clonorchis sinensis*). It is considered a drug of choice for various **nematodes** such as *Ascaris lumbricoides* (common roundworm), *Trichuris trichiura* (whipworm), *Ancylostoma duodenale* and *Necator americanus* (hookworms). For such infestations the recommended dose, for adults and children above 2 yrs, is 400 mg orally as a single dose at night. For children of 1–2 yrs of age, the dose is 200 mg OD. No preparation or post-drug purging is required. For heavy infestations the dose may be repeated for 3 days. Albendazole can be considered as an alternative drug for the treatment of *Strongyloides stercoralis* (threadworm; 400 mg OD for 3 days) and *Enterobius vermicularis* (pinworm; 400 mg OD to be repeated after 2 weeks). Albendazole plus diethylcarbamazine or ivermectin is a synergistic combination for treating or controlling lymphatic filariasis.

It is also a preferred drug to treat cutaneous larva migrans (400 mg OD for 5 days) and visceral larva migrans (400 mg BD for 28 days). It is a drug of choice for various cestodes, e.g., cysticercosis (*Taenia solium*—pork tapeworm—larva stage) and hydatid disease (echinococcosis; a cyst in the lung or liver containing larva of *Taenia echinococcus*). For both these conditions, the recommended dose schedule is 400 mg BD for 28 days with fatty meals. However, for cysticercosis corticosteroids are usually given along with albendazole to prevent inflammation caused by the dying organism; while for hydatid disease better therapeutic results are obtained when albendazole is used along with praziquantel.

It is also a second choice drug for a trematode, e.g., *Clonorchis sinensis* (liver fluke; 400 mg BD for 7 days). Albendazole is administered on an empty stomach when used against intraluminal worms but with a fatty meal when used against tissue parasites.

Adverse Effects: Albendazole is well tolerated and side effects are rare if used for a short period (up to one month). However, if used for 3 months (as needed for hydatid disease) the following toxicities were observed: epigastric distress, headache, alopecia, fatigue and lassitude, insomnia and transient aminotransferase enzyme elevation. Albendazole is teratogenic in animals, hence its long-term use in pregnancy should be avoided.

Mebendazole

Mebendazole is a prototype benzimidazole having wide spectrum of anthelmintic activity.

Pharmacokinetics: Absorption of orally administered mebendazole is erratic (10%). Absorption is increased if the drug is ingested with fatty meals. It is extensively metabolised to decarboxylated metabolites in liver that are excreted mainly in urine but a part of the absorbed drug is excreted in the bile also. Half-life is 2–6 hrs.

Clinical Uses: Mebendazole is still considered a drug of choice for the treatment of *Ascaris lumbricoides* (round-worm), *Trichuris trichiura* (whip-worm), *Necator americanus* and *Ancylostoma duodenale* (hook-worm). For these infestations, the recommended dose schedule is 100 mg BD for 3 consecutive days. The drug provides a cure rate of 95–100% in pinworm (*Enterobius vermicularis*, oxyuris) infestation. For control of pinworm infestation a single dose of 100 mg is taken once, which is repeated after 2 weeks (to eradicate ova that have developed later).

Owing to its broad-spectrum anthelmintic effects, mixed infections (ascaris + hookworm OR ascaris + hookworm + whipworm) frequently respond to therapy. It is considered as an alternative drug for the treatment of trichinosis (200 mg TDS initially, increasing over 3 days to 400 mg TDS and then continued for next 10 days), intestinal capillariasis (200 mg BD for 21 days), visceral larva migrans (100 mg TDS for 5 days) and *Taenia saginata* (beef tapeworm; 200 mg BD for 4 days). In dracontiasis (guinea worm) and *Clonorchis sinensis* (liver fluke) its efficacy is doubtful. Mebendazole chewable tablets are also available. No post-drug purging is necessary with its use.

Adverse Effects: As with albendazole, short-term therapy with mebendazole is nearly free of side effects. Abdominal discomfort, nausea, vomiting and diarrhoea have been observed. With higher doses, rash, urticaria and elevation of aminotransferase enzymes have been reported. Mebendazole is contraindicated in patients of liver cirrhosis. It is teratogenic in a few animal species and hence contraindicated in pregnancy.

Thiabendazole

Thiabendazole was the first benzimidazole introduced in 1960. It is rarely used now, except in special conditions.

Pharmacokinetics: It is rapidly absorbed after oral administration. It chelates with iron but not with calcium. Half-life is 1.2 hrs.

Clinical Uses: Though thiabendazole also has a broad spectrum of activity, it has presently been replaced by safer drugs such as albendazole and ivermectin. It is used as an alternative agent to treat *Strongyloides stercoralis* (threadworm), cutaneous larva migrans (creeping eruptions) where it can be applied topically or given orally, and trichinosis. The recommended dose schedule is 25 mg/kg/day (max. 1.5 g) in two divided doses for 2 days.

Adverse Effects: It has more adverse effects compared to other benzimidazoles. Dizziness, nausea, vomiting and anorexia are more common. Pruritus, rash, headache, drowsiness and neuropsychiatric problems are less common. Liver failure and Stevens-Johnson syndrome can occur but rarely. Urine of the patient smells like asparagus because of the excretion of the metabolite asparagine. The drug is contraindicated in pregnancy, hepatic and renal disease.

Triclabendazole

Triclabendazole is a narrow spectrum benzimidazole used primarily in veterinary medicine. Recent studies have shown that triclabendazole when given as a single dose of 10 mg/kg, is the drug of choice for treating human fascioliasis (*Fasciola hepatica*; sheep liver fluke). The cure rate was 90% on repetition of the course after a week. Human beings are, however, only accidentally infected by *F. hepatica,* which primarily affects cattle and sheep. Eating contaminated fresh-water plants initiates the infection. Unlike infestations with other flukes, fascioliasis does not respond to praziquantel and hence the importance of triclabendazole. Triclabendazole, also recently, has been reported to be efficacious in the treatment of *Paragonimus skrjabini* (lung fluke) infestation in a dose of 10 mg/kg orally daily, for 3 days. Human beings become infected by eating undercooked crabs or cray fish. This infection is also refractory to praziquantel but responds to triclabendazole.

The drug is well tolerated. No significant side effects have been reported.

Bithionol

Bithionol is orally well absorbed and is the drug of choice for the treatment of fascioliasis (sheep liver fluke) and parogonimiasis (lung fluke). It is given in a dose of 30–50 mg/kg (in 2 divided doses) orally on alternate days for 10 to 15 days. WHO recommends a regimen of 30 mg/kg daily for 5 days to treat fascioliasis. *Adverse effects* include anorexia, nausea, vomiting, diarrhoea, dizziness, headache and skin rashes (as a reaction to antigens released from dying helminths). It should be avoided in children below 8 yrs of age.

Diethylcarbamazine

Diethylcarbamazine is a synthetic piperazine derivative and is available as citrate salt.

Pharmacokinetics: It is rapidly absorbed from the GIT and is widely distributed in tissues except fat. It is excreted in urine unchanged or as N-oxide metabolite. The plasma half-life of the drug is 2–3 hrs if urine is acidic but 8–10 hrs if urine is alkaline. Dose adjustments are needed in renal impairment and in patients having urinary alkalosis. Complete excretion of the drug from the body takes 48 hrs.

Clinical Uses: It is the drug of choice for treatment of lymphatic filariasis due to *W. bancrofti* (bancroftian filariasis), *B. malayi* (brugian filariasis) and *Loa loa* (loiasis). It is active against both microfilarial and adult worms. Its combination with albendozle provides synergistic response compared to diethylcarbamazine alone. It is no longer used to treat onchocerciasis for which ivermectin is the drug of choice. It is also used to treat visceral larva migrans (toxocariasis). The recommended doses for filariasis, loiasis and toxocariasis are similar, i.e., 50 mg on day one, 50 mg TDS on day 2, 100 mg TDS on day 3 and then 2 mg/kg TDS for 2–3 weeks. Complete cure may require 2–3 repeated courses. Antihistamine and corticosteroid cover is needed to limit the allergic reaction to dying filariae. Diethylcarbamazine may also be used for chemoprophylaxis of loiasis (300 mg weekly) and of filariasis (50 mg monthly orally). Diethylcarbamazine is also preferred to treat tropical eosinophilia (2 mg/kg orally TDS for 7 days).

Adverse Effects: Adverse effects during treatment with diethylcarbamazine are of two types: pharmacological dose dependent effects and allergic reactions to the dying filariae parasite.

Adverse effects to the first type include headache, weakness, malaise, anorexia, nausea, vomiting, dizziness and lethargy. Reactions to dying microfilariae are mild in bancroftian, more intense in brugian filariasis but could be severe in loiasis and specifically in onchocerciasis. These are manifested by fever, lymphadenopathy, cutaneous swelling, leukocytosis, eosinophilia, oedema, rashes, proteinuria and at times renal haemorrhage and encephalopathy. In onchocerciasis, the microfilariae dying in the eye lead to optic neuritis and visual field loss.

Doxycycline

It has been observed that an intracellular bacteria *Wolbachia* (order: Rickettsia) lives inside the filarial (*Wuchereria bancrofti*) and onchocerca nematodes, as an endosymbiont with these parasites. These bacteria are transmitted maternally through the cytoplasm of parasite eggs and are necessary for the oogenesis in the adult female parasites. Later it was found that the eradication of these bacteria by doxycycline made the adult female filarial parasite incapable to reproduce. Clinical trials have revealed that 200 mg/day, 8-week course of doxycycline eliminated 95% of microfilariae. Further trials suggested that a combination of doxycycline + ivermectin can provide complete amicrofilaraemia (approval awaited). It is probably the first report that even the bacteria are necessary for oogenesis in nature (may be for a parasite) and that a disease which has affected over 90 million people world-over can be controlled by using simply doxycycline instead of far more toxic diethylcarbamazine which can precipitate reactions to dying microfilariae.

Ivermectin

Ivermectin is a semisynthetic macrocyclic lactone and is a mixture of avermectin-B1a and -B1b, which are derived from *Streptomyces avermitilis*.

Pharmacokinetics: It is absorbed from GIT following oral administration. It has a plasma half-life of 12 hrs. It is excreted mainly in the faeces. The drug has a wide distribution in the body.

Clinical Uses: Ivermectin has a wide spectrum of activity as it is active not only against filarial nematodes but against other nematodes and some parasites also.

It is the drug of choice in onchocerciasis as it reduces the microfilarial load without the toxicity seen with diethylcarbamazine. A single dose of 150 mcg/kg orally, for patients over 5 yrs of age, is given every 6 months on empty stomach for treatment of onchocerciasis. Corticosteroids may be used to avoid inflammatory eye reactions. Annual treatment can prevent blindness from ocular onchocerciasis. In lymphatic filariasis it reduces microfilarial load to nearly zero level but does not kill the adult worms. In loiasis it does reduce microfilaraemia but its potential to produce neurotoxicity in these patients discourages its use.

Ivermectin is very useful in treating disseminated strongyloidiasis (200 mcg/kg orally daily on two consecutive days). There are some reports of ivermectin being effective in the treatment of cutaneous larva migrans. Ivermectin (200 mcg/kg single oral dose) is also effective in the treatment of pediculosis (lice infestation) and scabies.

Adverse Effects: These include fever, pruritus, arthralgia, postural hypotension, tachycardia, oedema, lymphadenopathy, sore throat, cough and headache. Ivermectin should not be used in pregnancy and should be avoided in children below 5 yrs of age. The side effects, if troublesome, can be minimised by giving antihistamine and analgesics/corticosteroids.

Levamisole

Levamisole is an active levo-isomer of tetramisole and has a restricted use to treat ascariasis and hookworm infestation. For ascariasis a single oral dose of levamisole 50 mg (for children having 10–20 kg body weight), 100 mg (for children having 21–40 kg body weight) and 150 mg for adults are recommended. For hook worm or mixed roundworm–hookworm infection in adults, 300 mg is given orally as a single dose over 2 days. Children are given 6 mg/kg orally once for 2 days.

Levamisole is also used as immunostimulant as it restores depressed T-cell functions. There are reports that patients with slow spreading vitiligo respond to levamisole (150 mg once daily orally for 2 consecutive days in a week) within 3–4 months period. There have been favourable reports that levamisole, in a dose of 150 mg daily in divided doses given for 3 days at the first sign of mouth ulceration provides beneficial results. It is also used as an adjunct drug in malignancy. Reports reveal that recurrences of colorectal cancer are inhibited by adjuvant treatment with levamisole and fluorouracil following resection of tumours.

When given as a single dose for treatment of roundworm or hookworm infestation, levamisole is well tolerated and side effects are limited to nausea, vomiting, abdominal discomfort and headache. Long-term use results in influenza-like syndrome, hypersensitivity, arthralgia, muscle pain, abnormal taste in mouth and rarely thrombocytopenia.

Metrifonate

It is an organophosphorous compound that is effective only against *Schistosoma haematobium* (bilharziasis). It has a good oral absorption. It is still considered as an alternative drug for treating *S. haematobium* infestation because it is not effective against eggs and these continue to pass into urine for several months of the killing of adult worms. It is usually given as a single oral dose of 7.5–10 mg/kg TDS at intervals of 2 weeks.

Metrifonate is generally well tolerated but may cause cholinergic side effects (see mechanism of action above) such as diarrhoea, tremors, nausea, vomiting, bronchospasm and sweating. Atropine antagonises these effects without affecting the drug's efficacy. It is contraindicated in pregnancy, recent insecticide exposure, or with depolarising neuromuscular blocker such as succinylcholine.

Niclosamide

Niclosamide is a chlorinated salicylamide, and is used for the treatment of most cestodes (tapeworm) infection. It is not absorbed from the GIT; hence high concentrations can be achieved in the lumen. The drug affects the scolex and proximal segments of most cestodes (*T. saginata, T. solium, D. latum* and *H. nana*) resulting in their detachment from the intestinal wall and evacuation by the normal peristaltic action. However, the drug is not ovicidal. With the availability of better drugs (praziquantel and benzimidazoles) the use of niclosamide has lately declined. The recommended adult dose of niclosamide is 2 g OD orally in the morning on an empty stomach. The tablet is to be chewed thoroughly, and then swallowed with water. Niclosamide is not effective against cysticercosis and hydatid disease.

No serious side effects are observed with niclosamide use except for abodminal discomfort, nausea and loose stools. Consuming alcohol with niclosamide results in antabuse type reaction.

Oxamniquine

It is a tetrahydroquinoline derivative, that has a restricted range of efficacy, being active only against *Schistosoma mansoni* infestation. It is given orally and is readily absorbed from GIT. Intersubject variations in the serum concentration of the drug have been reported and hence chances of therapeutic failure exist. Interestingly, the fluke esterifies oxamniquine to produce a reactive metabolite that alkylates flukes DNA (see mechanism). Though not active against *S. haematobium* and *S. japonicum*, oxamniquine has been successfully used in combination with metrifonate for the treatment of mixed schistosomal infections.

With oxamniquine, CNS side effects are common: drowsiness, dizziness and dullness with headache. Seizures may occur but rarely and with higher dose. Other effects include nausea, colic, pruritus and urticaria. It is contraindicated in pregnancy and in epileptic patients.

Piperazine

Piperazine, nowadays, is an alternative drug for the treatment of ascariasis and pinworm (*Enterobius vermicularis*) infestation. It is not used for other helminth infestations. It is given orally and is readily absorbed from the GIT. For ascariasis the dosage of piperazine is 4 g once a day for 2 consecutive days (for adults) while for enterobiasis the dosage is 2 g once a day for 7 days. Concomitant use of senna purgative at night helps expulsion of worms, but is not necessary.

Adverse effects include nausea, vomiting, abdominal pain and headache. Neurotoxic and allergic reactions are rare. It is contraindicated in pregnancy because its nitrosamine metabolite has carcinogenic and teratogenic potential. It should be avoided in patients of epilepsy and in those having impaired renal and hepatic functions. Concomitant use of piperazine and pyrantel pamoate should be avoided as they have antagonistic mode of action (see mechanism).

Praziquantel

Praziquantel is a synthetic isoquinoline-pyrazine derivative.

Pharmacokinetics: It is readily absorbed (80%) after oral administration. It undergoes significant first pass in the liver and is converted to inactive hydroxylated metabolites. Plasma half-life 1–3 hrs. Plasma concentration increases when the drug is taken with a high carbohydrate meal. Bioavailability is reduced with concomitant use of phenytoin, carbamazepine and dexamethasone.

Clinical Uses: Praziquantel is a drug of choice for all sorts of schistosomiasis, possessing activity against male and female adults and immature stages. For *S. mansoni* and *S. haematobium* the dose is 20 mg/kg orally BD, while for *S. japonicum* and *S. mekongi* the dose is 20 mg/kg orally TDS; but the dose intervals in both cases are to be kept between 4–6 hrs. In addition, it is very effective against other flukes also (75 mg/kg once or in 2 instalments for 1 or 2 days) except *F. hepatica*.

It is also used effectively in the treatment of tapeworm infestations (*T. solium, T. saginata, D. latum* and *H. nana*). For *T. solium* and *T. saginata* it is administered as a single dose of 10 mg/kg in the morning, while for *D. latum* and *H. nana* it is administered as a single dose of 15–25 mg/kg in the morning. Hence its dose schedules are simpler while efficacy is similar to niclosamide against tapeworm infestations.

Praziquantel and albendazole are considered equivalent in treating neurocysticercosis. 50 mg/kg daily in 3 divided doses for 15 days kills the larvae lodged in brain and other tissues. Corticosteroids reduce the bioavailability of praziquantel and hence their concomitant use is controversial.

Adverse Effects: These include drowsiness, dizziness, headache, nausea, vomiting, abdominal pain, pruritus, urticaria, skin rashes with eosinophilia (due to release of proteins from dying worms). The safety of praziquantel in children below 5 yrs of age is not established. It should also be avoided in pregnancy. Praziquantel is contraindicated in ocular cysticercosis because of the risk of severe eye damage resulting from occlusion due to dead parasites.

Pyrantel Pamoate and Oxantel Pamoate

Pyrantel pamoate is a tetrahydropyrimidine derivative and oxantel pamoate is its analogue.

Pharmacokinetics: Only a small proportion of the dose of pyrantel pamoate is absorbed from the GIT. High levels are therefore achieved in the intestinal tract. It is active against luminal helminths.

Clinical Uses: Pyrantel pamoate is active against several nematodes: *Ascaris lumbricoides* (roundworm), *Ancylostoma duodenale* and *Necator americanus* (hookworm) as well as *Enterobius vermicularis* (pinworm). For these indications the standard dose is 10 mg/kg of the free base (max.1 g) given orally as a single dose. For pinworms, the dose is repeated after 2 weeks. For heavy infestations with *N. americanus* a consecutive 3-day course may be needed. Pyrantel is not effective against whipworms (*Trichuris trichiura*) but oxantel is. Hence a combined formulation of these two drugs is available in many countries to achieve a broad-spectrum nematodal activity.

Adverse Effects: Pyrantel pamoate has no major adverse effects. Yet, headache, dizziness and drowsiness may occur. Its safety in pregnancy and in children below 2 years has not been established.

CHAPTER 64 Antimalarial Drugs

COMPETENCY PH1.47

Until 1880, the occurrence of malaria was considered to be associated with bad air ("mal-aria"). Later it was established that malaria is a tropical disease caused by sporozoites of Plasmodium that are transmitted to humans by the bite of an infected female mosquito of the genus *Anopheles* (Greek word meaning *worthless*) which has previously sucked the blood from a person infected with malaria. Malaria is prevalent in Central and South America, Mexico, Haiti, Dominican Republic, Central and South Africa, Middle East, India, Pakistan, Bangladesh, Thailand, Vietnam and China. By now, all attempts to eradicate malaria have failed due to emergence of both drug-resistant strains of malarial parasites and insecticide-resistant strains of *Anopheles*. As a result, the annual global incidence of malaria is approximately 200 million cases and it ranks as one of the leading causes of mortality in the world today. The symptoms of malaria include chills and rigors followed by fever, headache and sweating. In chronic malaria there is progressive splenomegaly. Symptoms become apparent only 7–10 days after being bitten by an infected mosquito. The incubation period of malaria is 10–30 days.

LIFE CYCLE OF MALARIAL PARASITE

The malarial parasite is a single cell protozoan called *Plasmodium*. The main clinically important species of plasmodium are *Plasmodium falciparum, P. vivax, P. ovale, P. malariae and P. knowleski* but out of these 5 types, only *P. falciparum* and *P. vivax* are the most common forms which cause malaria. These two species are common in India also.

The malarial parasite (*Plasmodium*) has a complex life cycle that consists of a *sexual cycle* which takes place in female anopheline mosquito (definitive host) and an *asexual cycle* which occurs in human beings (intermediate host; Fig. 64.1). Initially, a female mosquito is infected by biting a malarial patient whose blood contains male and female gametes of the parasite. Though the blood is digested, the gametes are resistant to the digestive juice of the mosquito. Fertilisation takes place in the mosquito gut and after differentiation and multiplication, the oocysts (encysted zygotes) liberate matured *sporozoites* (spores) which then migrate and stay in the insect's salivary glands. In the event of next bite by this mosquito, these *sporozoites* are passed into the blood stream of another human to begin the asexual cycle. No available drugs are lethal to sporozoites, hence infection cannot be prevented by the drugs at this stage. The sporozoites can survive hardly for an hour in circulation and hence these seek shelter in liver parenchymal cells where they divide and develop into multinucleated *schizonts*. This is called the ***pre-erythrocytic state*** of the life cycle during which the host remains asymptomatic. The *primary tissue schizonts* present in the liver mature within 8–21 days to form mononucleated *merozoites* which are then liberated by the liver and released into the blood stream (Fig. 64.1).

If the species is *P. falciparum*, all merozoites enter the phase of ***erythrocytic schizogony*** (asexual reproduction or division of the plasmodium in the RBC of human host). In this phase the merozoites bind to and invade the erythrocytes and form *trophozoites* (motile intracellular parasite—a stage during the growth of protozoa). During their maturation within the red cell, the host's haemoglobin is digested and transported to parasite's food vacuole where it provides a source of amino acids; while the free haem which would be toxic to the Plasmodium is rendered harmless by polymerisation to haemozoin by parasitic haem polymerase. Following mitotic replication of its nucleus, the parasite in the red cells which are called blood-schizonts, after schizogony, produce more merozoites. The RBCs, infected with merozoites, eventually rupture causing the release

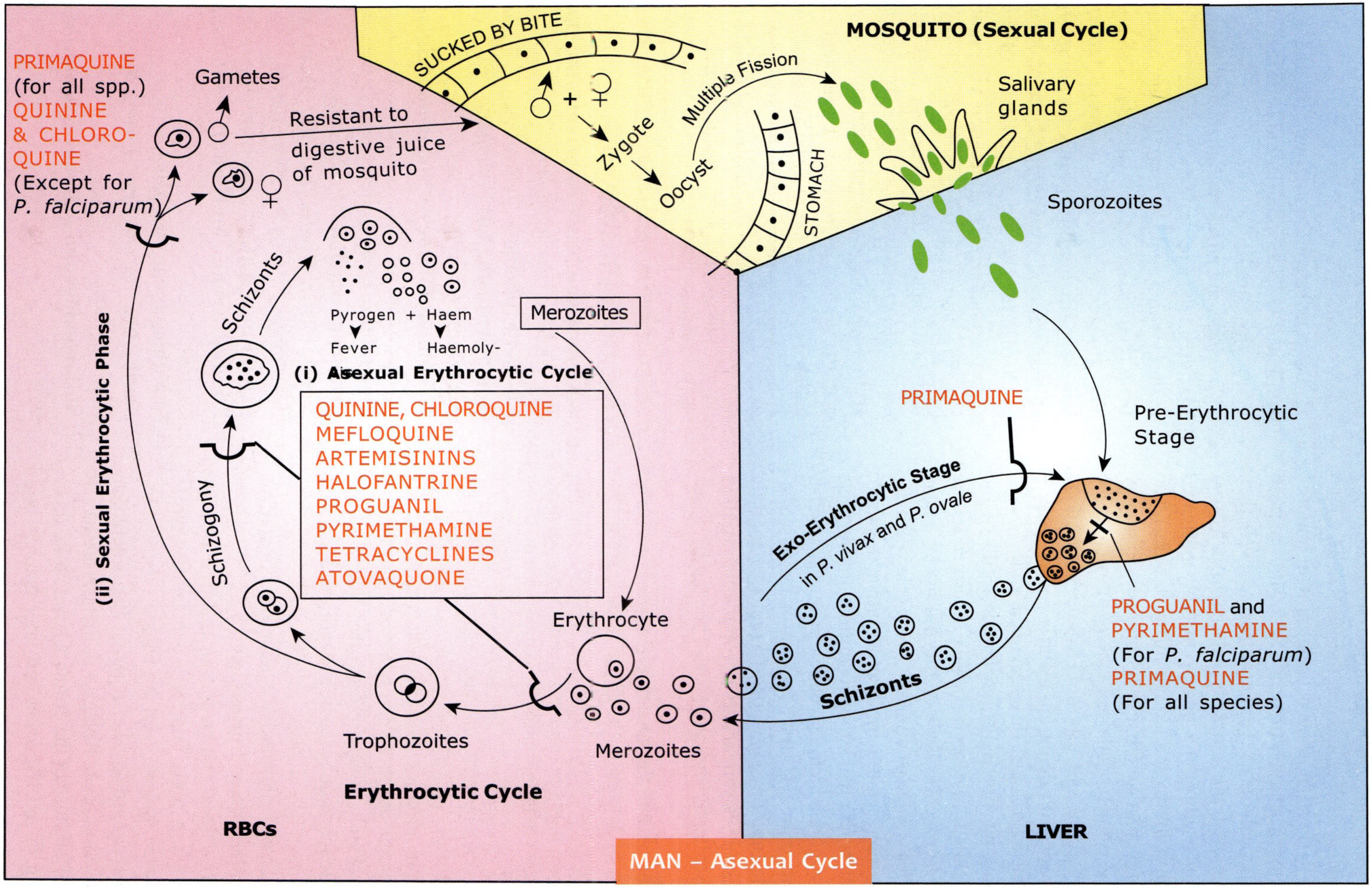

Fig 64.1 Life Cycle of Malarial Parasite and Sites of Antimalarial Drugs Action

of thousands of merozoites in the bloodstream along with pyrogens, TNF-α and polymerised haem, which gives rise to the symptoms associated with malaria. The liberated merozoites then bind to and invade fresh erythrocytes and the ***asexual erythrocytic cycle*** then starts again. If all the schizonts and merozoites, from the asexual erythrocytic phase, are not eradicated completely (due to inadequate drug therapy), the malarial fever may subside temporarily but may reappear again when surviving merozoites enter the erythrocytic phase again. This is termed as ***recrudescence*** of falciparum malaria.

Some merozoites, on entering the erythrocytes, differentiate into the male and female forms of the parasites called *gametocytes*. This is termed as the ***sexual erythrocytic phase*** of the life cycle. These gametocytes can only complete their cycle when the diseased person is bitten by the mosquito at this time. The gametes then reach the mosquito's gut, fertilise to form a zygote which then develops into an oocyst. The rupture of oocysts releases sporozoites (asexual form of plasmodium, i.e., spores) which then migrate to the mosquito's salivary glands and enter another human host after the mosquito's next bite (as discussed above).

If the plasmodial species is *P. vivax* or *P. ovale*, then a part of schizonts (after the release from pre-erythrocytic and erythrocytic schizogony phase), reenter liver parenchymal cells and form dormant hypnozoites (sleeping form of parasite) which are capable of reactivation and good cause relapse of malaria weeks, months, or even years after the first malaria episode. This phase is called ***exoerythrocytic state.*** The hibernation of hypnozoites may last for several months but these can be reactivated later to schizonts which release merozoites that undergo erythrocytic schizogony leading to ***relapse*** of malarial fever.

The main plasmodial species implicated in causing human malaria are as under:

- *P. vivax* causes benign tertian malaria. Benign because it is rarely fatal. It is less severe than *P. falciparum* malaria. Tertian, because there is fever on every 3rd day, i.e., a gap of 48 hrs between two onsets of fever. Relapses of malaria are likely to occur because of the dormant hypnozoite form residing in the liver that can later emerge into merozoites after a few months interval (see above and Fig. 64.1).
- *P. ovale* infection has periodicity and *relapses* similar to *P. vivax* malaria, but is milder and can be readily cured.
- *P. falciparum* causes malignant tertian malaria. Malignant, because it is the most severe form of malaria which could be fatal. Tertian, because the fever recurs after every 3rd day (i.e., 48 hrs gap). The infected RBCs have a special tendency to adhere with healthy RBCs forming clusters called "*rosettes*" (resembling circular ornament). Such rosettes can block capillaries of the vital organs and adversely affect their vital functions, causing renal failure and encephalopathy (cerebral malaria). *P. falciparum* does not have an exoerythrocytic stage. Hence if the erythrocytic stage is eradicated relapses do not occur (Fig. 64.1). However, if treatment is inadequate *recrudescence* may occur (see above).
- *P. malariae* causes quartan malaria as it has 72 hrs cycle. It has no exoerythrocytic state but relapses may occur. Such malarial infection is of rarer occurrence.

CLASSIFICATION OF ANTIMALARIAL DRUGS

• Based on Chemical Structure

1. **4-Aminoquinolines**: *Chloroquine, Amodiaquine, Piperaquine, Pyronaridine*
2. **Chincona Alkaloids**: *Quinine*
3. **Quinoline-methanol**: *Mefloquine*
4. **Acridine**: *Mepacrine, Quinacrine*
5. **8-Aminoquinolines**: *Primaquine, Bulaquine, Tafenoquine*
6. **Biguanides**: *Proguanil*
7. **Diaminopyrimidines**: *Pyrimethamine*
8. **Artemisinin Semisynthetic Derivatives**: *Artesunate, Artemether, Arteether*
9. **Artemisinin Synthetic Derivative**: *Arterolane*
10. **Phenanthrene methanol**: *Halofantrine, Lumefantrine*
11. **Naphthoquinone**: *Atovaquone*
12. **Antibiotics**: *Tetracycline, Doxycycline, Clindamycin*
13. **Sulfonamides and Sulfones**: *Sulfadoxine, Dapsone*

• Based on Affected Plasmodial State

Schizonticides

These drugs kill the schizonts of the malarial parasite.

i) *Tissue (Hepatic) Schizonticides*

These drugs destroy the hepatic schizonts soon after infection (Fig. 64.1). ***Primary tissue schizonticides*** act on pre-erythrocytic state, e.g., ***proguanil* and *pyrimethamine***. But, these drugs are active against the pre-erythrocytic state of *P. falciparum* only (not of *P. vivax* & *P. ovale*). ***Secondary tissue schizonticides*** act on exo-erythrocytic state in liver, e.g., ***primaquine.*** *However, primaquine acts on the pre- as well as exoerythrocytic stages of all plasmodial species*. Hence, primaquine is the only available drug at present as tissue schizonticide and subclassification therefore, becomes immaterial.

ii) *Blood Schizonticides*

These drugs destroy the blood schizonts (merozoites → schizonts → merozoites) and prevent erythrocytic schizogony to terminate the attack of malarial fever (Fig. 64.1). These may be subgrouped as ***(a) fast-acting high-efficacy blood schizonticides*** such as *chloroquine, quinine, mefloquine, lumefantrine, artemisinin* and *atovaquone*. These can be used singly to terminate the attack of malaria promptly; ***(b) slow-acting low-efficacy blood schizonticides*** such as *pyrimethamine + sulfadoxine, proguanil,* and *doxycycline*. These can be used only in combination if the aim is to terminate the clinical attack.

Gametocides

These drugs destroy the gametocytes or make them ineffective in the host's blood so that mosquitoes cannot transmit the disease (Fig. 64.1), such as *primaquine* (for all the 4 species of plasmodium), *chloroquine* and *quinine* (against *P. vivax, P. ovale* and *P. malariae* only; except *P. falciparum*).

Sporontocides

These drugs make the gametocytes ineffective within the body of the mosquito. *Pyrimethamine* and *proguanil*, which are blood schizonticides, are also sporontocides.

However, use of these drugs as gametocide/ sporontocide provides no clinical advantage as their use in one infected person would not prevent widespread transmission of malaria in the population.

• Based on Clinical Use

Causal Prophylactics

No "*true causal prophylactic drug*" is available at present. Such a drug is supposed to destroy the sporozoites prior to their invasion into the liver parenchymal cells of the human host. However, certain drugs can be used for "*causal prophylaxis*". These drugs prevent the maturation of sporozoites to schizonts within the infected hepatic cells. None of the available tissue schizonticidal drugs are entirely satisfactory in this regard. *Proguanil* and *pyrimethamine* are causal prophylactic against *P. falciparum* only (not against *P. vivax* or *P. ovale*); while *primaquine*, though effective against all plasmodial species, lacks favourable toxic profile for its routine use in causal prophylaxis. However, if G6PD levels are normal, it can be used in a dose of 0.5 mg/kg daily for causal prophylaxis as long as the person remains in an endemic malarial region.

Suppressive Prophylaxis (Chemoprophylaxis)

Drugs used for such purpose do not affect the hepatic phase of the malarial parasite but destroy the merozoites released from the liver so that the very development of the erythrocytic stage is prevented. Such drugs are mainly blood schizonticides. Suppressive prophylaxis is employed during the periods of exposure to infected mosquitoes and for some weeks to follow.

Suppressive Cure

If the suppressive prophylaxis is continued for a longer period, the hepatic phase of hypnozoites becomes extinct or exhausted. Thus if *chloroquine* 300 mg weekly is taken for 3 months, after the attack of *P. vivax* malaria or after leaving the endemic area, the hepatic phase of *P. vivax* becomes extinct. Suppressive cure is like a radical cure but by an extended suppressive prophylaxis therapy.

Clinical Cure

The asexual erythrocytic schizogony state of malarial parasite is responsible for clinical symptoms (chills, rigor, fever) of malaria and therefore the blood schizonticides can be used to terminate an acute attack of malaria (clinical cure). The *fast-acting high-*

efficacy blood schizonticides such as *chloroquine, quinine, mefloquine, artemisinin, lumefantrine* and *atovaquone* can be used singly to treat attacks of *P. falciparium* malaria where any delay in the treatment may be fatal. Since *P. falciparum* displays no exoerythrocytic cycle, the clinical cure itself can provide radical cure. However, if the blood is not cleared of the malarial parasite totally, *recrudescence* of falciparum malaria may occur. For chloroquine- resistant falciparum malaria, *quinine* is an effective schizonticide as an alternative. *P. vivax* and *P. ovale* malarial infection also respond well but as their exoerythrocytic phase persists, subsequent relapses may occur which can be treated by repeating the course. The *slow-acting low-efficacy blood schizonticides* such as *proguanil, pyrimethamine* with *sulfadoxine*, and *tetracyclines* can also be used for clinical cure but these are rather used in combination.

Radical Cure

Eradication of both *exoerythrocytic* as well as *erythrocytic state* of malarial parasite leads to radical cure of malaria. As discussed above, an adequate clinical cure of *P. falciparum* (with chloroquine) results in radical cure. However, a proper drug is needed for the radical cure of *P. vivax* or *P. ovale* malaria to prevent relapse due to reactivation of hypnozoites (exoerythrocytic stage) at a later stage. The drug that accomplishes radical cure in *vivax* malaria is *primaquine* administered as 15 mg orally daily for 15 days. Usually primaquine is given immediately after the use of chloroquine to achieve a high radical cure rate (primaquine phosphate as 26 mg = 15 mg base).

INDIVIDUAL ANTIMALARIAL DRUGS

Chloroquine

Chloroquine is a synthetic 4-aminoquinoline derivative available as chloroquine phosphate for oral use.

Pharmacokinetics: Chloroquine can be given orally or by I.M. injection or by slow I.V. infusion. It is almost completely absorbed from GIT. The drug has a large aVd and is extensively bound to liver and other body tissues including cornea and RBCs. It is metabolised by the liver. Initial half-life is 3–4 days but as it is slowly released from the tissues, the terminal half-life may be extended to 1–2 months.

Mechanism of Action: Chloroquine has a preferential accumulation in parasitised erythrocytes. Being a basic drug it diffuses freely into the parasite lysosome. Inside, at the acidic pH of the lysosome it gets ionised (impermeable) and gets trapped inside the parasite. Its accumulation in parasite's food vacuoles, inhibits peptide formation and reduces the synthesis of amino acids necessary for parasite viability. It also inhibits the parasite enzyme haem polymerase and thus protects the host's haem from being converted to haemozoin (see above under life cycle). Free haem is toxic to the malarial parasite.

Antimalarial Action and Clinical Use: Asexual erythrocytic state (+); gametocidal (+) only in *P. vivax* and *P. ovale*, not for *P. falciparum*; pre- and exoerythrocytic state (–). Resistance to chloroquine among the strains of *P. falciparum* is most common and results due to mutations in putative chloroquine transporter (PfCRT). The drug is effective in all types of malaria excepting chloroquine-resistant *P. falciparum* malaria. It is used for chemoprophylaxis in visitors temporarily residing in an area where *P. falciparum* malaria is not resistant to chloroquine. It is also used in providing the suppressive cure of *P. vivax* malaria (after leaving the endemic area) by giving an extended suppressive prophylactic (chemo-prophylaxis) therapy. It is very effective in providing the clinical as well as radical cure of *P. falciparum* malaria not resistant to chloroquine. In *P. vivax* and *P. ovale* malaria it provides clinical cure but relapses usually occur unless chloroquine therapy is followed by *primaquine* (15 mg OD for 15 days). For all these details refer above.

In addition to its antimalarial use, chloroquine has been used in the treatment of rheumatoid arthritis (Ch. 26) and for amoebic abscess not responding to metronidazole (Ch. 65).

Adverse Effects: Chloroquine is usually well tolerated in the doses used for chemoprophylaxis. With doses used to treat the clinical attack of malaria, nausea, vomiting, dizziness, headache, urticaria and blurred vision may occur occasionally. Larger doses sometimes may precipitate retinopathies. Bolus I.V. injection of chloroquine may cause hypotension and T-wave abnormalities in ECG.

Contraindications and Drug Interactions: **(1)** Its use should be avoided in patients with retinal and visual field abnormalities; **(2)** Chloroquine aggravates the attacks of psoriasis or porphyria and therefore contraindicated in such patients; **(3)** In G6PD deficient persons its use may result in haemolytic anaemia; **(4)** Ca^{2+} and Mg^{2+} containing antacids decrease its absorption and **(5)** Concomitant use of metoclopramide with chloroquine sometimes precipitates paradoxical extrapyramidal side effects. Chloroquine is considered safe in pregnancy and in younger children above 2 years of age.

Amodiaquine

Amodiaquine is similar to chloroquine. It was withdrawn several years ago because of the risk of agranulocytosis (1:2000) and hepatotoxicity when the drug is used for chemoprophylaxis. Incidentally, this drug has been reintroduced in several countries not only because it is cheap but the chloroquine-resistant *P. falciparum* malaria generally responds to amodiaquine combination regimens such as: artesunate + amodiaquine or pyrimethamine - sulfadoxine + amodiaquine. Recent trials have shown that with combination regimens the chances of serious toxicity are rare and therefore it can also be used as a replacement for chloroquine in area with high prevalence of resistant falciparum malaria.

Piperaquine and Pyronaridine

Piperaquine a bisquinoline-derived chloroquine analogue is an established antimalarial drug developed in China and available in several southeast-asian countries. It acts like chloroquine by inhibiting heme digestion pathway in host erythrocytes but shows a slower onset of action due to its large aVd and long t½ (35 days). This longer t½ may be beneficial in reducing the rate of relapse following the treatment. It exerts antimalarial activity against both *P.vivax* and *P.falciparum* including the chloroquine-resistant strains, where its schizonticidal activity is equal to chloroquine against sensitive but more robust against resistant *P.falciparum*. The tolerability, efficacy, pharma-cokinetic profile and low cost of piperaquine make it a promising drug against malaria. As the resistantance to well established antimalarial drug is fast developing, especially in southeast-asian countries, piperaquine use has been reserved in fixed dose combination therapy with dihydroartemisinin (8:1/960 mg + 120 mg, respectively) or arterolone, an orally effective trioxolone synthetic derivative of artemisinin, developed in India (7:1/750 mg + 150 mg, respectively). In clinical trials, these combinations were found equally efficacious/non-inferior to artesunate + mefloquine combination.

Pyronaridine is an amodiaquine analogue and has been in use, in China, for almost last 15 yrs. It is being used with artesunate for the treatment of chloroquine- resistant *P. falciparum* malaria and *P. vivax* malaria. It is effective orally and has low toxicity.

Quinine

Quinine is an alkaloid derived from cinchona bark and has been used in the treatment and prevention of malaria since 1820.

Pharmacokinetics: Quinine is usually given orally but can also be given by slow I.V. infusion (see above for how to use). It is well absorbed after oral ingestion. It is widely distributed in body tissues. It is primarily metabolised in liver and excreted in the urine (t½ 10–11 hrs).

Mechanism of Action: Its mechanism of antimalarial action is not clear. Like chloroquine, it inhibits the parasite's haem polymerase but it is not so extensively concentrated in the malarial parasite as chloroquine does. It is believed to act as a protoplasmic poison to the parasite and poisons the parasite's feeding mechanism and hampers the supply of amino acids and peptides.

Antimalarial Action and Clinical Use: Asexual erythrocytic state (+); gametocidal activity (+) only in *P. vivax* and *P. ovale* but not for *P. falciparum*; pre- and exoerythrocytic state (–). Some resistance of *P. falciparum* malaria to quinine has been reported from Southeast Asian countries like Thailand, yet till date quinine is now the main antimalarial drug for treating chloroquine-resistant *P. falciparum* malaria. Resistance is conferred by increased expression of P-glycoprotein, which effectively pumps the drug out of the parasite.

The treatment should begin with a loading dose to achieve effective plasma concentrations rapidly. It can be administered slow I.V. in divided doses or by slow continuous I.V. infusion. The therapy should be changed to oral as soon as the condition of the patient improves to tolerate oral medication. Aside from its use as an antimalarial drug, quinine is also used to treat nocturnal leg cramps observed in the patients of varicose veins, diabetes and arthritis. Quinine + clindamycin is a first-line therapy for the treatment of babesiosis (a tick-borne malaria like disease) also.

Adverse Effects: Being bitter in taste, compliance is poor. Being irritant to gastric mucosa, can cause nausea and vomiting. Bolus I.V. administration can lead to hypotension and cardiac arrhythmias. Higher plasma levels lead to ***cinchonism***—a toxic state characterised by sweating, tinnitus, blurred vision, headache, diarrhoea and cardiac arrhythmias. It is potentially neurotoxic in higher doses. Haematological toxicity includes haemolysis especially in G6PD deficient cases. Quinine stimulates insulin release and may cause hypoglycaemia. Hence, it is usually infused with 5% glucose solution. In severe *P. falciparum* malaria glucose consumption by the parasite is also increased, which also causes hypoglycaemia. All this leads to hypoglycaemic coma which may be erroneously confused with coma due to cerebral malaria. Though pathogenesis is uncertain, *black water fever* is a rare consequence of erratic use of quinine for fever due to other reasons. This type of hypersensitivity is manifested by marked haemolysis with renal failure (it may result even during quinine therapy for malaria).

Contraindications and Drug Interactions: **(1)** Persons having visual and auditory problems; **(2)** Persons with cardiac abnormalities; **(3)** Al^{3+} and Mg^{2+} containing antacids decrease its absorption; **(4)** Quinine raises plasma levels of digoxin and **(5)** Quinine should not be given concurrently with mefloquine, as both drugs adversely affect cardiac conduction.

Mefloquine

Mefloquine is chemically related to quinine. Orally administered mefloquine is well absorbed. It is not given parenterally because of pain and local irritation at the site of injection. It is highly protein bound, extensively distributed in body tissues, undergoes enterohepatic circulation and eliminated slowly ($t\frac{1}{2}$ 20 days) allowing weekly dosing for chemoprophylaxis and single dose regimen for clinical cure.

Its ***mechanism of action*** resembles quinine. As with quinine, resistance of *P. falciparum* to mefloquine is caused by an increased expression of P-glycoproteins. It is potent blood schizonticide against *P. falciparum, P. vivax* and *P. ovale*. It is neither tissue schizonticidal nor gametocidal. It is used for chemoprophylaxis or for clinical cure but not for severe or complicated malaria as it cannot be used intravenously and in such situation a rapid acting drug such as quinine is more preferred.

Adverse effects, when mefloquine is used for chemoprophylaxis, are nausea and vomiting. When mefloquine is used for treatment of an acute attack, the neuropsychiatric side effects may be observed in 0.5% of the patients which include vertigo, confusion, vivid dreams, hallucination enxiety and seizures (though rare). There have been a few reports of abnormal AV conduction also. Mefloquine should be avoided during pregnancy. It should not be coadministered with quinine or halofantrine (aggravates conduction defects). Mefloquine chemoprophylaxis should be discontinued if neuropsychiatric symptoms develop (though incidence is rare).

Quinacrine and Mepacrine

Quinacrine and mepacrine are erythrocytic schizonticides which being more toxic and less effective than chloroquine are no longer used in clinical practice. Yet these are marketed in some countries. Vertigo, abdominal cramps, nausea and vomiting and rarely psychosis are the major adverse effects. Long-term use causes discolouration of skin and eyes.

Primaquine

Primaquine is a synthetic 8-aminoquinoline derivative.

Pharmacokinetics: The drug is well absorbed orally. Though widely distributed, it is not bound extensively to the tissues. It is rapidly metabolised by liver and excreted in urine ($t\frac{1}{2}$ 3–6 hrs). Its metabolites, though active, have a higher potential for toxicity.

Mechanism of Action: Its mechanism of action is not clear. Lately, it has been observed that its quinone metabolite inhibits the coenzyme-Q governed respiratory processes of the parasite in the exoerythrocytic state. However, these oxidising metabolites are also responsible for the haemolytic side effects of the drug.

Antimalarial Action and Clinical Use: Pre-erythrocytic state (+), exoerythrocytic state-hypnozoites (+), gametocidal (+), asexual erythrocytic state (–). Resistance among *P. vivax* is rare and is not a clinical problem. Primaquine finds its greatest use in providing the radical cure and to prevent relapse for *P. vivax* and *P. ovale* malaria (for dosage regimen, see earlier text). Primaquine and tafenoquine are the only two drugs effective against the exoerythrocytic and pre-erythrocytic forms of all malarial parasites. However, the G6PD status of the patient should be evaluated prior to prescribing a 14-day course of primaquine or one-day treatment with tafenoquine.

Non-antimalarial Use: A combination of clindamycin plus primaquine offers improved tolerance over high-dose cotrimoxazole in treating moderate *Pneumocystis jiroveci* pneumonia.

Adverse Effects: It is well tolerated in recommended doses. With higher doses or prolonged use GIT distress, nausea, headache, pruritus and leukopenia (rarely) can occur. In individuals with G6PD deficiency (as observed in black race and Mediterranean people), primaquine can cause fatal haemolytic anaemia (for reasons, see Ch. 7). Primaquine is contraindicated in pregnancy because the foetus is G6PD deficient and thus is at risk of haemolysis.

Other congeners of primaquine are bulaquine, etaquine and tafenoquine. ***Bulaquine,*** developed in India, is a prodrug for primaquine. Its clinical use, adverse effects and contraindications are similar to primaquine. It is given in a dose of 25 mg/day for 5 days starting on 2nd day of chloroquine therapy. Neither primaquine nor bulaquine can be given parenterally as both can produce marked hypotension.

Tafenoquine

Tafenoquine (TQ) is a more potent and longer acting (plasma t½ 15 days) analogue of primaquine (t½ 6–8 hrs) approved by FDA (in 2018) for single dose anti-relapse therapy against *P. vivax*. It shows a strong activity against both pre-erythrocytic (primary schizonts) as well as exo-erythrocytic (secondary schizonts) liver hypnozoites and gametocyte, and a weak activity against erythrocytic stage of *P. vivax* as well as *P. falciparum*.

It is indicated for radical cure (prevention of relapse) in only one 300 mg dose coadministered with standard dose of (erythrocytic schizonticidal/suppressive agent like) chroloquine. The dose of primaquine for the same indication is one daily dose (15 mg base/26 mg tablet) for 14 days but ***TQ*** works like primaquine in one dose only. Therefore, in future single-dose anti-relapse ***TQ*** therapy may replace primaquine 14 dose/day anti-relapse and radical cure therapy as its 14-day long treatment compliance is difficult to maintain and chance of failling treatment is high. ***TQ*** is going to be an alternative medication for radical cure (along with a suppressive treatment), chemoprophylaxis and terminal prophylaxis/ presumptive anti-relapse therapy (PART). Like primaquine, ***TQ*** can produce GIT adverse effects and haemolysis in 6-G-PD deficient patients.

Pyrimethamine–Sulfonamide/Dapsone Combinations

Pyrimethamine is structurally related to trimethoprim. Its mode of action and clinical use have already been discussed in Chapter 53. Malarial parasites, like bacteria, cannot utilise preformed folic acid and therefore have to synthesise their own folic acid required for their growth and development. Pyrimethamine selectively inhibits the plasmodial folate reductase enzyme that converts dihydrofolic acid to tetrahydrofolic acid (active form). The nonavailability of the latter prevents the synthesis of pyrimidines and purines which are essential for plasmodial nucleic acid synthesis. Pyrimethamine is well absorbed after oral administration. Its elimination half-life is 3–4 days and hence it can be administered once a week.

Pyrimethamine is a slow acting erythrocytic schizonticide for all four human malarial species. It exhibits weak activity against pre-erythrocytic state of *P. falciparum*. It has no gametocidal activity. If used alone, resistance develops rather rapidly by mutation in the dihydrofolate reductase enzyme of the malarial parasite. Hence it is not used alone as antimalarial drug but is highly effective when used in combination with sulfonamides (sulfadoxine or sulfamethopyrazine) or with dapsone.

The sulfonamides or the sulfones (dapsone) rather inhibit the plasmodial dihydropteroate synthase enzyme that is the key enzyme involved in the formation of dihydrofolic acid from PABA (Fig. 53.2). The combination causes a sequential blockade of folic acid synthesis, attacking the same pathway at different points. These combinations, therefore, not only have synergistic action but also have least chances of developing resistance.

Sulfadoxine + pyrimethamine or dapsone + pyrimethamine are no longer recommended for chemoprophylaxis of malaria because of resistance and toxicity (exofoliative dermatitis, Stevens-Johnson syndrome). These combinations are, therefore, used for clinical cure of *P. falciparum* malaria. The sulfadoxine + pyrimethamine combination can also be used as an adjunct with quinine to treat chloroquine-resistant *P. falciparum* malaria (for doses, see earlier text).

Other Uses: Pyrimethamine (50–75 mg/day) with sulfadiazine (2–4 g/day) for 1–3 weeks is the first line therapy for toxoplasmosis in immunodeficient patients. Folinic acid is added to the therapy to counteract inevitable megaloblastic anaemia. The doses are then reduced to 50% and continued for another 4–5 weeks. Alternatives include pyrimethamine + clindamycin (or clarithromycin or azithromycin).

Adverse effects are mild if used carefully in therapeutic doses. In high doses pyrimethamine may inhibit mammalian dihydrofolate reductase and may induce megaloblastic anaemia; hence if used during pregnancy, folic acid supplements must be added. Other toxic symptoms include anorexia, vomiting, atrophic glossitis and CNS stimulation including seizures. The pyrimethamine + sulfadoxine combination can cause serious skin reactions, Stevens-Johnson syndrome, allergic alveolitis and blood dyscrasias. Large doses of pyrimethamine + dapsone combination can cause haemolytic anaemia, agranulocytosis and eosinophilic alveolitis.

Proguanil (Chloroguanide)

Like pyrimethamine, it is also a inhibitor of plasmodial dihydrofolate reductase. It is rapidly absorbed after oral administration. Its elimination half-life is 16 hrs (administered once daily).

It has a slow action against the erythrocytic forms of all the four human malarial species. It has an additional schizonticidal effects on pre-erythrocytic state but not on the hypnozoites of *P. vivax*. Proguanil alone is no longer recommended for chemoprophylaxis because of the chances of developing resistance but the combination of chloroquine (300 mg/week) and proguanil (200 mg/day) is often preferred as an alternative to mefloquine because the combination is less toxic than mefloquine. Interestingly, when *proguanil* or *atovaquone* are used as monotherapy, *P. falciparum* becomes resistant readily but the resistance to the combination is rarely observed. Hence, a combination of 250 mg of ***atovaquone*** + ***proguanil*** (100 mg) once daily 2 days prior to and 7 days after the exposure is a preferred regimen for chemoprophylaxis of *P. falciparum* malaria; while ***atovaquone*** (1000 mg) + ***proguanil*** (400 mg) once daily for 3 consecutive days is a preferred regimen for the treatment of chloroquine-resistant *P. vivax* and multidrug-resistant *P. falciparum* malaria. Presently, atovaquone + proguanil is the only recommended drug combination for the self-treatment of malaria. The combined formulation should be taken with food.

The ***adverse effects*** are much less severe than with pyrimethamine. With folic acid supplements, it is considered safe for use during pregnancy. Paradoxically, it is remarkably safe when used in combination with chloroquine/atovaquone/doxycycline.

Atovaquone

Initial use of atovaquone, as an antimalarial drug, led to disappointments because of treatment failures due to rapidly developing resistance. Lately, the interest in atovaquone has been revoked due to the findings that proguanil potentiates its antimalarial action and that the use of the fixed dose oral combination of atovaquone + proguanil not only prevents emergence of resistance but is better tolerated and safer than either drug used alone. For more details refer discussion on proguanil.

The mechanism of action of atovaquone is not clear. It probably disrupts the plasmodial mitochondrial electron transport of the respiratory process. This results in the collapse of plasmodial mitochondrial membrane functions and inhibition of pyrimidine and ATP synthesis.

Atovaquone is administered only orally. Its bioavailability is poor and erratic but increased by fatty meal. It is highly protein bound (99%). It has a long plasma half-life (2–3 days), partly also due to enterohepatic recycling. It is excreted unchanged exclusively in faeces.

Therapeutic uses of atovaquone include: **(a)** Chemoprophylaxis and treatment of *P. falciparum* malaria where it is used in combination with proguanil (for dosage schedule refer proguanil). The combination has a very potent activity against asexual erythrocytic stage of *P. falciparum*. It is also active against pre-erythrocytic state but not against *P. vivax* hypnozoites; **(b)** Acute oral treatment of mild to moderate *Pneumocystis carinii* pneumonia in patients intolerant to cotrimoxazole (750 mg TDS, orally for 21 days); **(c)** Treatment or suppression of *Toxoplasma gondii* encephalitis.

The adverse effects include abdominal pain, nausea, vomiting, headache, rash (rare) and reversible elevation in liver enzyme. Concurrent use of metoclopramide, tetracycline or rifampicin reduces atovaquone plasma levels by 40–50%; hence if an antiemetic has to be used metoclopramide should be avoided (prefer promethazine).

Artemisinin Semisynthetic & Synthetic Derivatives

Artemisinin Semisynthetic Derivatives

Artemisinin (*Qinghaosu* in Chinese), **artesunate**, **artemether** and **arteether** are sesquiterpene lactone endoperoxides that have been obtained from a Chinese herb *Artemisia annua*. Artemisinin, chemically a cyclic endoperoxide sesquiterpine lactose is a prodrug and is rapidly metabolised to an active metabolite *dihydroartemisinin*. Artesunate, artemether and arteether are the semisynthetic derivatives of artemisinin with improved potency and better bioavailability. ***Artesunate*** is the water soluble hemisuccinate ester of dihydroartemisinin. It can be given orally, I.V., I.M. or rectally. ***Artemether*** is a oil soluble methylether of dihydroartemisinin. It can be used orally or I.M. ***Arteether*** is a oil soluble ethylether of dihydroartimisinin. It is administered I.M. only. Newer derivatives of artemisinin include *sodium artelinate* and *arteflene*. The aqueous solutions of these derivatives, compared to artesunate, are more stable.

Mechanism of action of artemisinin derivatives involves two steps. Initially, the intraparasitic heme or ferrous protoporphyrin-IX (a catabolic product of haemoglobin present in the parasitic food vacuole) catalyses breakdown of endoperoxide (-O-O-) bridge of the artemisinin molecule. This is followed by the generation of highly reactive free radicals that damage the parasite membrane by covalently binding to membrane proteins and other cellular proteins, one of which is ***P.falciparum*** **s**arco**e**ndoplasmic **r**eticulam **C**a^{2+} **AT**Pase (Pf SERCA), critical for the parasite survival.

The plasma half-life of artesunate is less than one hour, that of artemether is 4–11 hrs (depending on route of administration), while arteether has a longer elimination half-life (23 hrs).

Compared to other antimalarials, these act rapidly and are many fold active against the asexual erythrocytic state of *P. vivax, P. ovale* and *P. falciparum* malaria. These drugs have little gametocidal action but do not have any effect on pre-erythrocytic or exoerythrocytic (hypnozoites) state of liver.

Artemisinin Synthetic Derivative

Arterolane

Arterolane is a trixolone-derived synthetic analogue of artemisinin that has emerged from a focused research conducted in India to find out peroxide antimalarial agents. It is a rapidly but short acting drug (halflife 1–3 hrs) and more potent than currently available semi-synthetic artemisinin derivatives like, artesunate, etc.

After administration, the drug localizes to parasite cytosol and food vacuoles and exerts a rapid schizonticidal effect by acting on all stages of asexual schizogony of all malarial parasites including chloroquine- and mefloquine- resistant *P.falciparum.* Presently arterolone is available in combination with piperaquine (see above) because both have large aVd, one is short acting (the former) and the other long acting (the latter). Both arterolone and piperaquine are metabolized by oxidation mediated mainly by CYP3A4. The chances of drug interaction should be kept in mind when this combination is used with drugs which are metabolized by this enzyme. The efficacy of arterolone and piperaquine combination is well proven in all clinical trials where it has shown a cure rate of more than 95% with fever and parasitaemia clearance within 24-48 hrs.

Therapeutic uses of Artemisinin Derivatives: The use of these drugs is restricted to the clinical cure of severe falciparum malaria including cerebral malaria and chloroquine- or multidrug-resistant malaria. Their use for chloroquine-sensitive *P. falciparum* malaria or for other uncomplicated malaria is not justified as other effective drugs are available. Similarly, their use for chemoprophylaxis of malaria is also irrational because of their shorter half-lives, which translates into recrudescence of malaria and treatment failure. However, these are not cross resistant with other antimalarial drugs.

Artemisinin-based Combination Therapies (ACTs)

The standard treatment of malaria now employs ACTs and the drugs used in combination with artemisinin derivatives are called ACT partner drugs. Currently 5 ACT regimens have been recommended by WHO for the treatment of *P. falciparum* malaria. These are comparatively safer and well tolerated. These include: **(1)** Artemether + Lumefantrine(ACT-AL); **(2)** Artesunate + Mefloquine (ACT-As/MQ); **(3)** Artesunate + Sulfadoxine Pyrimethamine- (ACT-As/S/P); **(4)** Artesunate + Amodiaquine (FEC-As/AQ); **(5)** Artesunate + Pyronaridine (ACT-As/Py); **(6)** Dihydroartemisinin + Piperaquine (ACT-DHA/PPQ); and **(7)** Arterolane + Piperaquine (ACT-ART/PPQ).

Adverse effects to artemisinin derivatives are rare. These are better tolerated than most antimalarials. Intravenous artesunate is equally effective and much safer than quinine given intravenously. Yet, nausea, vomiting, abdominal pain, itching and temporary QT prolongation may occur.

Halofantrine and Lumefantrine

Halofantrine is a phenanthrene-methanol group of antimalarial drug with potent blood schizonticidal properties against all four human malaria species. It is not active against any hepatic stage of malarial parasite. It has no gametocidal activity either. Its oral bioavailability is erratic but enhanced with food. Its mechanism of action is unknown but may involve possible inhibition of plasmodial proton pump.

Because halofantrine displays erratic bioavailability and manifests potentially lethal cardiotoxicity and cross resistance with mefloquine, its use is highly restricted to treat multidrug-resistant falciparum malaria (500 mg QID for one day, to be repeated after one week). In view of its cardiotoxicity and erratic bioavailability it is not used for malarial chemoprophylaxis.

The most common ***adverse effects*** are abdominal pain, vomiting, cough, rash, pruritus, transient rise in liver enzyme levels. Of greater concern is its cardiotoxicity: prolongation of QT and PR interval and dose-related defects in cardiac conduction. Concurrent use of mefloquine worsens its cardiotoxicity. The drug is contraindicated in cardiac patients with conduction defects. Being embryotoxic in animal studies, it should be avoided in pregnancy.

Lumefantrine is a new drug with structural similarities to mefloquine and halofantrine. However, it is not used alone but used in combination with artemether as both provide a synergistic antimalarial effect against multidrug-resistant *P. falciparum* malaria; The combination does not appear to cause cardiotoxicity (as seen with halofantrine) and hence can be given with fatty meal to maximize bioavailability. The coformulated tablet (with artemether) is to be taken twice daily for 3 days (see preparations above).

Antibiotics

None of the antibiotics can be used as single agent for the treatment of malaria because of their slower mode of action. ***Tetracycline*** and ***doxycycline*** are blood schizonticidal for all human malarial parasites, but these have no activity against any of the liver stages. Doxycycline (100 mg/day orally) or tetracycline (250 mg QID or 500 mg BD) can be used as a second-line therapy for chemoprophylaxis of malaria in chloroquine-resistant *P. falciparum* areas. ***Doxycycline*** (200 mg/day) can be combined with ***quinine*** or ***artesunate*** to treat multidrug-resistant falciparum malaria. For other details refer Chapter 58. Similarly, ***clindamycin*** (20 mg/kg/d orally, divided TDS x 7 days) with ***quinine*** (650 mg TDS orally for 3–7 days) is one of the suggested regimens for chloroquine-resistant falciparum malaria. For other pharmacological details of clindamycin refer Chapter 57. Antimalarial activity of azithromycin and some fluoroquinolones is under evaluation.

REGIMENS FOR TREATMENT OF MALARIA

The National Drug Policy for Malaria (2013) has advocated that all fever cases clinically suspected of malaria should be investigated for confirmation of malaria either by microscopy or Rapid Diagnostic Test (RDT). According to the ***National Vector Borne Control Program (NVBDCP)*** guidelines for diagnosis and treatment of malaria 2014, the rational management of malaria case is as follows. The National Framework of Malaria Elimination (NFME) in India 2016–2030 is currently working with aim to eliminate malaria by 2030 from India.

Treatment of Uncomplicated Malaria

Acute attack of chloroquine sensitive *P. vivax, P. ovale, P. malariae*

Oral chloroquine is the drug of choice. Dose of chloroquine is given in Table 64.1.

Uncomplicated *Plasmodium falciparum* Malaria

ACT regimen + Primaquine single dose (on day 2)

Various options are given below:

a) ACT regimens: Artesunate 4 mg/kg 100 mg BD orally for 3 days
 +
 Sulfadoxine and Pyrimethamine (S/P): S (1500 mg;25 mg/kg) and P (75 mg; 1.25 mg/kg) on day 1
 +
 Primaquine single dose 0.75 mg/kg on day 2

b) Artemether 20 mg + lumefantrine 120 mg combination taken with fatty meal to increase absorption. It is given as twice daily for 3 days.
 +
 Primaquine 0.75 mg/kg single dose on day 2.
 The dose of combination is according to the body weight of patient (Table 64.2).

c) Artesunate 4 mg/kg orally once daily for 3 days
 +
 Mefloquine 25 mg/kg in two divided doses (to minimise nausea, vomiting) on day 1 followed by 15 mg /kg on day 2 and 10 mg/kg on day 3
 +
 Primaquine 0.75 mg/kg single dose on day 2.

d) **Alternative to ACT regimens**:
 Quinine sulphate 8 mg base/kg orally TDS for 7 days
 +
 Doxycycline 100 mg per day for 7 days or Clindamycin 600 mg twice daily for 7 days.
 - As quinine and mefloquine share cross resistance, evidence of easy drug resistance when used as monotherapy, lack of safety profile data with large stat dose in children and neuropsychiatric symptoms as adverse effect–use of mefloquine regimens is better avoided when quinine is also being administered in countries like India.
 - In North Eastern states of India, regimen with sulfadoxine-pyrimethamine (SP) is not advised, (b) or (c) is recommended. The reason is the reported resistant malarial strain to sulfadoxine-pyrimethamine combination; due to mutations leading to treatment failure rates in >10% cases.

Uncomplicated Mixed Infection (*Plasmodium vivax and falciparum*)

Artemisinin-based combination therapy (ACT) regi-

Table 64.1 Dosage regimen for uncomplicated *Plasmodium vivax* malaria

Chloroquine	0 hr	6 hrs	24 hrs	48 hrs	Total dose
Regimen 1	10 mg/kg	5 mg/kg	5 mg/kg	5 mg/kg	25 mg/kg
Regimen 2	5 mg/kg	–	10 mg/kg	5 mg/kg	25 mg/kg
Plus					
Primaquine*	0.25 mg/kg once daily for 14 days to prevent relapse				

*Primaquine eliminate hypnozoites in liver, prevents relapse.
Preferred: Chloroquine 600 mg base (10 mg/kg) followed by 600 mg base 10 mg/kg on second day and 300 mg base (5 mg/kg) on third day.

Table 64.2 Combination of Artemether (20 mg) & lumefrantrin (120 mg) as per wt. category

Body weight	Start dose	8–12 hrs	Day 2	Day 3
5–14 kg	1 tablet	1 tablet	1 tablet twice	1 tablet twice
15–24 kg	2 tablets	2 tablets	2 tablets twice	2 tablets twice
25–34 kg	3 tablets	3 tablets	3 tablets twice	3 tablets twice
35 kg and above	4 tablets	4 tablets	4 tablets twice	4 tablets twice

Table 64.3 Antimalarials for severe or complicated *P. falciparum* malaria

Drug option	Dosage
Artesunate	2.4 mg/kg intravenous (IV) stat then at 12 hrs and 24 hrs and then once a day. Once the patient is able to swallow, complete the course of 7 days by Artesunate + Sulfadoxine-pyrimethamine (Except North-Eastern state) Artemether + Lumefantrine in North-Eastern state
Artemether	3.2 mg/kg (loading dose) followed by 1.6 mg/kg daily once the patient is able to swallow, complete the course by Artesunate + Sulfadoxine-pyrimethamine
Alternative to artesunate Quinine dihydrochloride	Quinine loading dose—20 mg salt/kg diluted in 500 ml of 5% dextrose and every 8 hrs till the patient can take orally. Then oral quinine 600 mg TDS should be substituted to complete 1 - week therapy + Tetracycline or doxycycline or clindamycin is for 7 days

men as above plus primaquine for 14 days as for vivax malaria. Glucose-6-phosphate dehydrogenase (G-6PD) screening is highly recommended. In G6PD deficient children, dose of primaquine is 0.6-0.8 mg/kg once a week for 6 weeks.

For severe or complicated *P. falciparum* malaria (Cerebral malaria)

For severe or complicated malaria, patient should always be hospitalized. Parenteral drugs are administered. Antimalarials given in severe or complicated *P. falciparum* malaria are shown in Table 64.3.

Other Treatment

- ***Supportive care***: Supplemental oxygen, intravenous fluids, proper positioning in unconscious, care of eyes, mucosa, skin, nasogastric feeding and depending on close monitoring of vitals are as important as specific treatment.
- ***Cerebral malaria***: For convulsions, lorazepam or midazolam is administered. Steroids are contraindicated. Mannitol and other anticerebral edema treatment is not required as raised intracranial pressure (ICP) is not a feature of cerebral malaria and it can be harmful.
- ***Hyperpyrexia***: Common in children and at times may lead to convulsions. Tepid sponging and paracetamol 15 mg/kg can be used.
- ***Disseminated intravascular coagulation (DIC)***: For spontaneous gastrointestinal bleeding and subcutaneous bleeding, fresh frozen plasma is administered. Subcutaneous low molecular weight heparin is reserved for cases with clinical and laboratory evidence of DIC.

Table 64.4 Treatment of malaria during pregnancy

Malaria	Pregnancy first trimester	Second & third trimester
Uncomplicated *P. vivax* malaria	Chloroquine (3 days)	Chloroquine (3 days)
Uncomplicated *P. falciparum* malaria	Quinine (7 days) & Clindamycin (7 days). *Alternative*: Oral ACT (3-day regimen)	ACT
Complicated or severe *P. falciparum* malaria	I.V. Quinine or I.V. Artesunate followed by oral ACT	I.V. Artesunate followed by oral ACT

Regimens for Chemoprophylaxis of Malaria

a) ***For travel in Chloroquine sensitive malaria***: Chloroquine phosphate 500 mg (300 mg base) once a week, start 1 week before travel to endemic area and continued till 4 weeks after leaving the area.

b) ***For travel in Chloroquine resistant P. falciparum malaria***: *Short-term chemoprophylaxis*: It is indicated in people who plan to stay up to 6 weeks in high endemic areas of falciparum malaria. Doxycycline 1.5 mg/kg, once daily, maximum dose 100 mg in children above 8 years. To start 2 days before arrival and continue 4 weeks after leaving endemic area. *Long-term chemoprophylaxis*: It is indicated in people who plan to stay for >6 weeks in high-endemic areas of falciparum malaria. Mefloquine 5 mg/kg, maximum dose 250 mg, weekly. Started 2 weeks before and continue 4 weeks after leaving endemic areas.

c) ***To prevent relapse (for terminal prophylaxis)***: Primaquine 30 mg daily taken shortly before or after the person leaves the endemic areas and continued for 2 weeks.

Treatment of malaria during pregnancy is given in Table 64.4.

CHAPTER 65 Antiamoebic and Other Antiprotozoal Drugs

COMPETENCY PH1.47

Protozoal infections are a major cause of diseases in the countries where sanitary conditions are inadequate. However, with increasing world travel, the protozoal diseases are no more confined to these countries only, but have affected the developed countries as well. Unlike prokaryotic bacterial cells, the unicellular protozoan cells are more or less eukaryotic and hence have metabolic functions closer to human host cells. Consequently protozoal diseases (amoebiasis, giardiasis, trichomoniasis, trypanosomiasis, toxoplasmosis and leishmaniasis) are difficult to treat and most of the antiprotozoal drugs have a serious toxicity profile. Different protozoal infections and the drugs used to treat them are discussed below.

CHEMOTHERAPY OF AMOEBIASIS

Amoebiasis is an intestinal infection with *Entamoeba histolytica*. Diagnosis is made by identifying *E. histolytica* from 2 or 3 samples of fresh faeces. The amoebic infection could be asymptomatic or may present as mild to moderate colitis or as dysentery or as liver abscess. Drug therapy is needed not only for the acutely ill patient but also for the asymptomatic carrier because the dormant *E. histolytica* may prove to be a potential source of infection to others.

Life cycle of *E. histolytica* is shown in Figure 65.1. *E.histolytica* exists in two forms: CYSTS that can survive outside the body for several weeks and TROPHOZOITES that are labile, live inside the body and are invasive in nature. Cysts are ingested through food or water that is contaminated with infective cysts. Inside the lumen these are converted to trophozoites which survive on intestinal bacterial flora. These luminal trophozoites can be carried towards the rectum, get converted to cysts in between the pathway and expelled in faeces to cause infection in other persons. Some trophozoites may multiply and invade to ulcerate the mucosa of the large intestine. This leads to dysentery (blood and mucus in the stool) or chronic intestinal amoebiasis (vague colicky pain and amoeboma). At a later stage, the trophozoites may pass into the blood stream and may spread to the liver through the portal vein to produce amoebic liver abscess. On rare occasions (years later) amoebic abscess may be found in lungs or the brain. Tissue phase is only secondary to intestinal amoebiasis. Hence, in tissues, only trophozoites are present not the cysts. Antiamoebic drugs are classified according to the site where they act (Fig. 65.1) as follows:

Classification

- **Tissue amoebicides**
  a) Intestinal and Extraintestinal Amoebicides
    - *Metronidazole, Tinidazole, Ornidazole, Secnidazole, Satranidazole, Nimorazole (All are nitroimidazole derivatives)*
    Emetine, Dehydroemetine (Both are alkaloids).
    - *Nitazoxanide*
  b) Extraintestinal Amoebicides
    - *Chloroquine*
- **Luminal (Intestinal) amoebicides**
  - Amides: *Diloxanide furoate*
  - 8-Hydroxyquinolines: *Diiodohydroxyquin (Iodoquinol)*
  - Antibiotics: *Tetracyclines, Paromomycin*

INTESTINAL AND EXTRAINTESTINAL AMOEBICIDES

Metronidazole and Analogues

Metronidazole is a nitroimidazole derivative which is selectively toxic not only to amoebae, but to certain other protozoa, most anaerobic bacteria and certain helminths as well (see below).

Pharmacokinetics: Orally administered metronidazole is readily absorbed. It distributes well

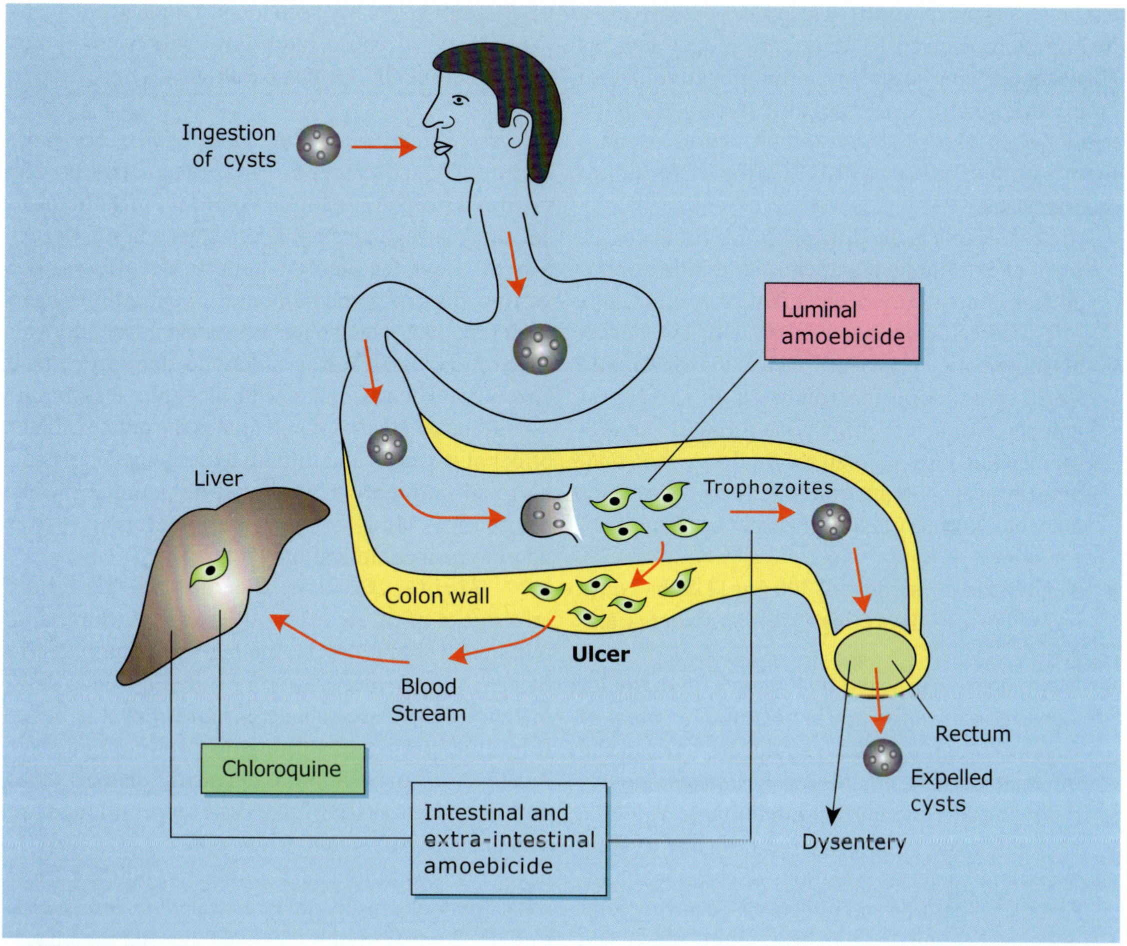

Fig 65.1 Life Cycle of *E. histolytica* and Site of Action of Different Antiamoebic Drugs

throughout the body tissues and fluids. Therapeutic levels can be found in vaginal and seminal fluids, CSF, saliva and breast milk. Its plasma half-life is about 8 hrs, which is increased in patients with impaired renal function. The parent drug and its metabolites are excreted in the urine.

Mechanism of Action: Anaerobic protozoan parasites (including amoebae) possess an enzyme, pyruvate-ferrodoxin oxidoreductase (P-FOR), which is not found in mammalian cells. This enzyme is involved in energy production (carbon recycling) and other metabolic functions through electron transfer reactions. The nitro group in metronidazole serves as an electron acceptor and thus in turn gets reduced. Reduced metronidazole is cytotoxic to anaerobic bacteria/protozoa and disrupts replication, transcription and repair process of DNA that results in cell death. It has no effect on aerobic organisms as their cellular aerobic environment prevents reduction of metronidazole and thereby its activation for cytotoxicity.

Antimicrobial Spectrum and Clinical Uses: Metronidazole is highly active against *E. histolytica, Giardia lamblia, Trichomonas vaginalis* (in both males and females), *Blastocystis hominis, Balantidium coli* and a helminth *Dracunculus* *medinensis* (guinea worm). It also finds extensive use in infections caused by anaerobic cocci such as *Peptococcus* and anaerobic Gram-negative bacilli (e.g., *Bacteroides*). Anaerobic Gram-positive bacilli, such as *Clostridia*, which causes pseudomembranous colitis (PMC), also respond to metronidazole.

- Metronidazole is the drug of choice for the treatment of extraluminal amoebiasis. It kills trophozoites but not the cysts and effectively eradicates intestinal and extraintestinal amoebiasis. For an asymptomatic cyst passer, metronidazole should be used in combination with intraluminal amoebicide such as diloxanide furoate. The recommended dose regimen for moderate intestinal amoebiasis is 400 mg orally TDS for 7 days; for amoebic dysentery and liver abscess, 800 mg TDS for 7 days.
- Metronidazole in a dose of 200 mg TDS for 7 days or 2 g/day for 3 days is highly effective in giardiasis.
- Metronidazole in a dose of 400 mg TDS orally for 7 days is highly effective in treating *Trichomonas vaginitis*. Vaginal tablets should also be used and the male partner should also be treated concurrently to prevent recurrent infection.
- Metronidazole is an effective drug for treating anaerobic bacterial infections such as brain abscess, endocarditis and infections occurring after colorectal surgery or appendicectomy where it is generally used with gentamicin. The recommended dose schedule is 15 mg/kg by I.V. infusion over 1 hr followed by 7.5 mg/kg I.V. infusion every 6 hrs till oral therapy could be started (400 mg TDS for another 7 days).
- Oral metronidazole in a dose of 500 mg TDS is very effective, convenient and safer drug to treat pseudomembranous colitis due to *Clostridium difficile*. It may be used with vancomycin.
- Metronidazole with tetracycline is an effective combination in treating ulcerative gingivitis and stomatitis.
- Metronidazole is effective in treating guinea worm infestation (Ch. 63) and in eradicating *H. pylori* infection (Ch. 27).
- Metronidazole has been found to induce mutagenesis and to cause radiosensitisation but is not used clinically for this purpose.

Adverse Effects and Drug Interactions: The most frequently observed adverse effects of metronidazole are: nausea, vomiting, metallic taste and epigastric distress. The urine becomes dark red-brown. Less frequently, neurotoxic effects like vertigo, dizziness and numbness of extremities have been reported, which may necessitate its withdrawal. Metronidazole inhibits aldehyde dehydrogenase enzyme and hence if taken with alcohol, a disulfiram-type reaction occurs. It potentiates the anticoagulant effect of warfarin and lithium toxicity by decreasing its renal elimination. It should be avoided during pregnancy and in persons suffering from neurological complications.

Tinidazole: It is an equally efficacious analogue of metronidazole except that it is eliminated more slowly, having a plasma half-life of 12–14 hrs, hence it is more suited for once daily or twice daily dose schedule. Moreover, it is better tolerated than metronidazole producing lesser incidence of nausea (1%), epigastric distress (1%) and metallic taste (2%). Recommended dose schedules for *amoebiasis* are 600 mg BD for 5–7 days; *trichomoniasis* and *giardiasis*, 600 mg for 7 days (or 2 g single dose); *anaerobic infections*: initially 2 g followed by 500–600 mg BD for 5 days. For use in *H. pylori* infections see Ch. 27.

Ornidazole: It is also slowly metabolised; plasma half-life is 12–14 hrs. Its clinical use, dose regimen and toxicity profile is almost identical to tinidazole.

Satranidazole: Similar to tinidazole in all aspects except that it is slightly more potent and does not cause neurological toxicity and disulfiram-type reaction with alcohol; otherwise its plasma half-life, clinical use and side effect profile is similar to tinidazole. Recommended dose schedules for *amoebiasis* are 300 mg BD for 5 days and for *giardiasis* as well as *trichomoniasis* are 600 mg orally as single dose.

Secnidazole: Its clinical use, potency and side effect profile is similar to metronidazole except that it has a longer plasma half-life of >20 hrs and has a post-antiprotozoal effects. Recommended dose schedule for *amoebiasis, giardiasis* and *trichomoniasis* are 2 g as single dose orally, while for *hepatic amoebiasis* it is 1.5 g once daily orally for 5 days.

Nimorazole: It is similar to metronidazole in all aspects except for dose schedule. For *amoebiasis* or *giardiasis* 1 g BD orally for 5–7 days; for *trichomoniasis* 2 g orally as single dose, with main meal, to be repeated after one month.

Emetine and Dehydroemetine

Emetine is an alkaloid derived from *Cephaelis ipecacuanha*. Dehydroemetine is its synthetic analogue. Both are effective against tissue trophozoites of *E. histolytica* but have no effect on cysts. Both act by inhibiting protein synthesis in amoeba. Both are administered parenterally, as their oral absorption is erratic and because these themselves being emetic would be vomited out. These are given by S.C. or I.M. injection but never intravenously. Both accumulate in tissues, particularly in liver, and are eliminated slowly (taking 1–2 months) via the kidneys. Hence, these drugs should be given only till patient becomes asymptomatic and in any case for not more than 10 days. Dehydroemetine is, however, less cumulative.

These drugs, because of their toxicity profile (see below), are rarely used these days and have been almost completely replaced by metronidazole and its analogues. Yet, these can be used in severe amoebic dysentery or amoebic liver abscess in situations where metronidazole cannot be used. A luminal amoebicide like diloxanide furoate must always follow their use to eradicate cyst forming trophozoites.

Serious toxicity of major concern is their cardiotoxicity which includes hypotension, tachycardia, cardiac arrhythmias and myocarditis. Hence, these should be administered in hospital settings with complete bed rest. Dehydroemetine is less cardiotoxic. Being tissue irritant, pain and tenderness and even abscess formation at the site of injection is most common. Nausea and vomiting are most frequent due to stimulation of CTZ. Other adverse effects include diarrhoea, abdominal cramps and muscle weakness. These drugs should not be used in patients with cardiac or renal disease, in children or in pregnancy. If these alkaloids have to be used, dehydroemetine is preferred over emetine. Usual recommended dose is 60 mg I.M. once daily for 3–5 days (maximum 10 days).

Nitazoxanide

Nitazoxanide is a nitrothiazolyl-Salicylamide prodrug and like metronidazole is activated in the intestine. It has a broad spectrum of activity against protozoa (*Entamoeba histolytica, G. lamblia, Cryptosporidium parvum,* particularly in children), helminths (round worm, tape worm) and anaerobic bacteria (*Helicobacter sp., Clostridia difficile, Bacteroides fragilis*).

After oral administration (dose: 500 mg BD for 3 days in adult; for ***Cryptosporidium diarrhoea*** the dose is 100–200 mg BD for 3 days (for children). It is rapidly obsorbed and hydrolised in the intestine to an active metabolite tizoxanide. Being a structural analogue of thiamine pyrophosphate, the active metabolite inhibits P-FOR that is involved in the conversion of pyruvate to acetyle CoA in the protozoa and bacteria.

Unlike metronidazole, it is free of mutagenic effects and well tolerated by the patient. Adverse effects include GI upset, occasional nausea, flatulence, enlarged salivary glands, pruritus, dizziness and rarely fever.

EXTRAINTESTINAL AMOEBICIDES

Chloroquine

Chloroquine is highly concentrated in liver and destroys trophozoites of *E. histolytica*. As a result it is very effective in treating hepatic abscess, amoeboma and extraintestinal amoebiasis (500 mg twice daily orally for initial 2 days and then 500 mg once daily for 21 days). Amoeba does not develop resistance to chloroquine. It is not effective against cysts, hence a luminal amoebicide must always be given after chloroquine to abolish luminal cycle. For other pharmacological details refer Chapter 64.

LUMINAL AMOEBICIDES

Diloxanide Furoate

Diloxanide furoate is an effective luminal amoebicide but is not active against tissue trophozoites. However, it is very effective in mild intestinal amoebiasis and in asymptomatic cyst passers as it kills trophozoites that produce cysts. Diloxanide furoate, being ester, is hydrolysed in the gut to diloxanide and furoic acid. About 80–90% of free diloxanide gets absorbed systemically but has no systemic antiamoebic action despite absorption. About 10–20%, which remains unabsorbed, is the real antiamoebic substance; but because of poor tissue amoebicidal action it is primarily a luminal amoebicide and not useful in amoebic dysentery. Recommended dose schedule is 500 mg orally TDS for 10 days. Its combined use with metronidazole or tinidazole is quite popular. Diloxanide furoate does not produce serious adverse effects and is very well tolerated. However, flatulence is a common complaint.

8-Hydroxyquinolines

Iodoquinol (diiodohydroxyquin) is a halogenated 8-hydroxyquinoline. Like diloxanide furoate it is commonly used with metronidazole to treat luminal amoebiasis. It kills the cysts forming trophozoites but not the trophozoites present in intestinal wall or extraintestinal tissues. Its mechanism of action is unknown but may act as contact amoebicide.

Systemic iodoquinol has a plasma half-life of 12 hrs. Other uses are: giardiasis and local treatment of monilial and trichomonal vaginitis. It is also used to treat superficial fungal skin infections (Ch. 60). Recommended doses for treatment of intestinal amoebiasis are: Iodoquinol 600 mg TDS orally. In therapeutic doses, side effects are mild such as nausea, green coloured stools and pruritus (rare). However, its prolonged use may cause goiter and iodism (chills, fever, angioedema and inflammation of mucous membranes) because of iodine overload. Repeated and indiscriminate use of iodoquinol in relatively high doses may cause subacute myelo-optic neuropathy (SMON) leading to visual impairment and blindness (particularly in children).

It is not recommended during pregnancy and for children.

Antibiotics

These are used as alternative drugs in the management of mild to moderate intestinal amoebiasis along with other luminal agent such as diloxanide furoate (also with metronidazole). They reduce the normal gastrointestinal bacterial flora on which the amoebae thrive for their growth. Tetracycline and doxycycline (Ch. 58), do not have a direct effect on the protozoa while paromomycin (Ch. 56) has a direct amoebicidal action also, besides reducing the GIT bacterial flora. These have no effect against extraintestinal amoebic infections.

CHEMOTHERAPY FOR GIARDIASIS

Giardia lamblia resembles *E. histolytica* in that it also exists in two forms: an active trophozoite confined to upper small intestine and a cyst produced in lower bowel and excreted in the faeces. Giardiasis is characterised by episodic watery diarrhoea and malabsorption. Many drugs useful in amoebiasis are also effective in giardiasis. Their dose schedules are: ***Metronidazole*** 200 mg TDS orally for 7 days; ***Tinidazole*** 600 mg daily for 7 days or 2 g as single dose; ***Secnidazole*** 2 g as a single dose orally; and ***Furazolidone*** 100 mg QID or TDS orally for 7 days. Furazolidone is a nitrofuran derivative which is active not only against *Giardia, Trichomonas* but also against some Gram-negative bacilli such as *Salmonella* and *Shigella*. It has been used as an alternative drug for treating giardiasis (inferior to metronidazole or tinidazole), diarrhoea due to food poisoning and bacillary dysentery. Side effects are mild and include nausea and dizziness. Being excreted in urine, the colour of urine becomes orange-red.

CHEMOTHERAPY FOR TRICHOMONIASIS

Trichomoniasis is a genital infection produced by *Trichomonas vaginalis*. In males trichomoniasis is frequently asymptomatic but in females it is characterised by vulvovaginitis with frothy pale yellow discharge. Relapses are common unless both male and female partners are treated simultaneously.

Additionally, intravaginal drugs may also be needed to prevent recurrences. Oral drugs used are: ***Metronidazole*** 400 mg TDS orally for 7 days or 2 g as a single dose; ***Tinidazole*** 600 mg daily for 7 days or 2 g as single dose; ***Secnidazole*** 2 g as a single dose; and ***Nimorazole*** 2 g as single dose with meals. A repeat course may be given after 6 weeks.

Drugs used intravaginally include: natamycin, hamycin, povidone-iodine, clotrimazole (and its combination with metronidazole or tinidazole) and iodoquinol. These are to be inserted intravaginally at bed time for a specified period.

CHEMOTHERAPY OF TRYPANOSOMIASIS

Trypanosomiasis refers to two types of chronic and eventually fatal diseases caused by the species of *Trypanosoma.* This disease is not prevalent in India, except in Africa and America.

The *African trypanosomiasis* (African sleeping sickness) follows the bite of a tsetse fly infected with the protozoan *Trypanosoma brucei.* The ensuing illness passes through two stages: the haemolymphatic stage characterised by lymph node enlargement, fever and headache, and the meningo-encephalopathic stage characterised by mental disturbances and drowsiness (sleeping sickness) as the disease progresses.

The *American trypanosomiasis* (*Chagas' disease*) is caused by *Trypanosoma cruzi.* It is quite different from African type in its clinical and pathological presentation such as cardiomyopathy, mega-colon and mega-esophagus and other gastrointestinal lesions. *T. cruzi* infection is carried by infected triatomine bugs which feed on human blood.

Treatment of African Trypanosomiasis

The main drugs used to treat African sleeping sickness are ***suramin***, with ***pentamidine*** as an alternative, in the haemolymphatic phase of the disease. For the meningo-encephalopathic phase ***melarsoprol*** is a choice. ***Eflornithine*** is an alternative drug which is effective in both the phases.

Suramin

It is a first choice drug for early haemolymphatic African trypanosomiasis. Since it does not cross BBB, it is not effective against advanced CNS stage of the disease. Its mechanism of action is not clearly understood. The drug binds firmly to the host plasma proteins. The drug-protein complex then enters the trypanosome by endocytosis. The drug is then liberated by lysosomal proteases to exert detrimental action on trypanosomal enzymes.

Suramin is not absorbed orally and is administered by slow I.V. injection (as 10% solution). It is tightly bound to plasma proteins and is released slowly with a terminal elimination half-life of 50 days. A drug-sensitivity test is advisable before starting the treatment. Combination with pentamidine usually improves efficacy. Melarsoprol + Suramin combination is usually preferred if there is advanced CNS involvement.

Adverse Effects: The immediate reaction to suramin could be potentially fatal, with nausea, vomiting, shock, loss of consciousness and even death which may follow its injection (and hence the test dose). Abdominal pain, mouth ulcers and urticaria may also result. At a later stage paraesthesia, hyperaestheia of palm and soles, fever, polyuria, polydipsia, lacrimation, proteinuria and haematuria may occur. If renal casts appear, the treatment must cease.

Pentamidine

Pentamidine is quite active against *Trypanosoma brucei-gambiense*, *Pneumocystis Jiroveci* and *Leishmania donovani.* It is not active against *T. cruzi.* It binds to protozoal DNA and inhibits DNA replication and function.

It is administered either intramuscularly or as aerosol. I.V. injection is avoided as it causes sharp fall in blood pressure, and tachycardia. The drug is bound avidly by the tissues and is slowly eliminated, with plasma half-life of about 12 days. Since it does not enter the CSF it is ineffective against the meningoencephalitic stage of trypanosomiasis. It is used as an alternative drug to suramin for treating the haemolymphatic stage of *T. brucei.* It can also be used with suramin. Its sequestration in tissues accounts for its prophylactic use in trypanosomiasis. It is also an alternative drug for the treatment of *P. jiroveci* pneumonia. Although more toxic and less effective than cotrimoxazole it is used as an alternative drug as prophylaxis against pneumocystosis in immunocompromised patients. Pentamidine is also an alternative drug for visceral leishmaniasis (Kala azar) especially when sodium stibogluconate therapy has failed or is contra-indicated.

Adverse reactions: Rapid drug infusion is risky as it may produce rapid fall in blood pressure, headache, vomiting, dyspnoea and tachycardia. Pain at the site of I.M. injection is common and sterile abscess may develop. Pancreatic β-cells toxicity is common. This may induce hypoglycaemia which may be followed by hyperglycaemia. Reversible renal insufficiency is also common which must be carefully watched. Other adverse effects include rash, metallic taste and fever. Inhaled pentamidine is safer but may cause coughing and bronchospasm.

Melarsoprol

Melarsoprol is a trivalent arsenical. Its use is reserved for treating meningo-encephalitic stage of African trypanosomiasis. It acts by binding to -SH- groups in protozoal enzymes and proteins, thereby altering their cellular structure and inhibiting their functions. Trypanosomal enzymes are more sensitive than those of the host. Mammalian cells are less permeable to the drug and thus protected from its toxic effects. Nevertheless, the drug is very toxic. It is administered as 2.2% solution in propylene glycol by slow I.V. infusion. A characteristic pharmacokinetic feature of melarsoprol is that its therapeutically significant concentration is achieved in the CSF that has a lethal effect on trypanosomes infecting the CNS.

The most important toxicity is the reactive encephalopathy characterised by cerebral oedema, seizures, coma and death. It is due to immune reaction resulting from rapidly dying trypanosomal parasites. A concurrent administration of prednisolone reduces the symptoms. Other toxic effects include peripheral neuropathy, hypertension, myocardial damage, albuminuria, fever, abdominal pain, vomiting and hypersensitivity reactions. The use of the drug is contraindicated in leprous patients (precipitation of lepra reaction). Severe haemolytic reactions occur in patients having G6PD deficiency.

Eflornithine

Eflornithine is an irreversible inhibitor of trypanosomal ornithine decarboxylase and thus inhibits the biosynthesis of protozoal polyamines (putrescine and spermidine). The polyamines are required for cell division and differentiation in protozoa. The human as well as protozoan enzymes are equally susceptible by the drug but mammalian enzymes have a rapid turnover while the parasite enzyme pool is fixed. The mammalian cells can replenish their polyamine pool through uptake from extracellular polyamines whereas trypanosomes divide within host blood which has an insignificant level of polyamines. These differences likely play a role in selective toxicity. Eflornithine (I.V.) is currently used to treat West African trypanosomiasis caused by *T. brucei-gambiense*. It has a good accumulation in CSF making it useful in advanced CNS disease state of African trypanosomiasis. It is much less toxic than melarsoprol. *Adverse effects* include vomiting, diarrhoea, anaemia, thrombo-cytopenia and seizures but these effects are reversible.

Treatment of American Trypanosomiasis

Nifurtimox

Nifurtimox is trypanocidal to *T. cruzi*. It is given orally and is effective in the treatment of the acute form of American trypanosomiasis but is less effective once the disease becomes chronic. Thus it often fails to prevent progression of GIT and cardiac manifestations that are most undesirable consequences of chronic *T. cruzi* infection. It has also been successfully used in *T. brucei-gambiense* infection with CNS involvement. A combination of gamma-interferon + nifurtimox appears to be more efficacious.

Being a nitrofuran, nifurtimox undergoes reduction to nitroamine radical and eventually generates hydrogen peroxide, hydroxyl and superoxide free radicals. These highly reactive free radicals are toxic to trypanosome because the parasite is devoid of catalase, an enzyme that protects the damage inflicted by free radicals. Mammalian cells are partly protected from such free radical damage by the presence of enzymes such as catalyse, glutathion peroxidase and superoxide dismutase.

Major toxicities include: immediate hypersensitivity reactions leading to anaphylaxis; delayed hypersensitivity reactions such as dermatitis, icterus (jaundice) and fever; GIT problems and anorexia that may be so severe as to cause weight loss; peripheral neuropathy, psychic problems, headache, nausea and vomiting are common.

Benznidazole

Oral ***benznidazole*** appears to have an efficacy similar to that of nifurtimox for the treatment of American trypanosomiasis (Chagas disease). Its plasma half-life is 12 hrs. Its mechanism of action is same as for other nitroimidazoles. However, it is better tolerated than nifurtimox. Side effects include epigastric distress, nausea, rash and peripheral neuropathy.

CHEMOTHERAPY OF LEISHMANIASIS

Leishmanias are transmitted from animal to humans, and from human to humans by the bite of infected sandflies. Three principal diseases result from leishmania infection. *Leishmania donovani* causes visceral leishmania (Kala azar); *L. tropica* and *L. major* produce cutaneous leishmaniasis while *L. braziliensis* causes mucocutaneous leishmaniasis. In *visceral leishmaniasis* the protozoa infect the reticuloendothelial cells causing enlargement of lymph nodes, liver and spleen. *Cutaneous leishmaniasis* remains localised to the site of inoculation where it forms a raised disfiguring ulcerative lesion. The *mucocutaneous leishmaniasis* is characterised by ulceration of mucous membranes of nose, mouth and pharynx.

Sodium Stibogluconate

Sodium stibogluconate and a related drug *meglumine antimonate* are pentavalent antimonial compounds. Their mechanism of action is not yet clear. Since none of these drugs is active *in vitro*, it has been proposed that their conversion to the trivalent antimony compound is essential for their activity. Recently it has been established that Sb^{3+} induces a rapid efflux of glutathione and trypanothione from the protozoal cell and also inhibits trypanothione reductase resulting in a decrease in trypanothione and glutathione levels as well as in a loss of "thiol reduction potential" necessary for cellular function.

Both sodium stibogluconate and meglumine antimonate are generally considered as first choice drugs for visceral and cutaneous leishmaniasis. These drugs are gastric irritants and therefore are administered by intravenous (preferred) or intramuscular routes. These drugs are eliminated in two phases. The first has a short half-life (2 hrs) while the second has a much longer half-life (>30 hrs) and reflects the conversion of Sb^{5+} to Sb^{3+}. Sequestration of Sb^{3+} in macrophages also contributes to a prolonged antileishmanial effect.

Adverse effects are usually reversible. These include pain at injection site (when given I.M.), pancreatitis, elevation of liver transaminase levels, muscle and joint pain, abdominal pain, nausea and skin rashes. QT prolongation may occur in electrocardiogram but such changes also are reversible.

Miltefosine

It is an alkylphosphocholine analogue recently introduced for the oral treatment of visceral (Kala azar) and also for cutaneous leishmaniasis. A 100 mg daily dose orally for 28 days provides excellent clinical results in adults. It is the first orally effective and safer drug for treating visceral leishmaniasis and compared to other drugs it may become the treatment of choice in near future. It has been approved for this indication in India. It inhibits key enzymes involved in the metabolism of surface glycolipids found in leishmania species. It is orally well absorbed and has a plasma half-life of 8 days.

Adverse effects include nausea and vomiting (in 50–60% of patients) but it is short-lived. Transient elevations in liver transaminases and serum creatinine values have also been observed. The drug being teratogenic is contraindicated in pregnancy. Since it has haemolytic activity, it should not be given intravenously.

Miscellaneous Agents

These include ***pentamidine*** (discussed earlier) and ***amphotericin**-B* (Ch. 60). Amphotericin-B through quite effective in treating visceral and mucocutaneous leishmaniasis but is seldom used because of difficulty

Table 65.1 Drug Treatment of Other Protozoal Infections

Protozoal Infection	Drugs of Choice	Alternative Drugs
Cryptosporidiosis	Paromomycin 500 mg TDS or QID, orally for 10 days (Ch. 56) OR Nitazoxanide 500 mg BD, orally for 3 days (Adult). Children: 100–200 mg BD orally for 3 days	Azithromycin 500 mg daily for 3 weeks orally (Ch. 57)
Pneumocystosis	Cotrimoxazole (Ch. 53)	Pentamidine (see text) Trimethoprim (Ch. 53) Dapsone (Ch. 59) Clindamycin (Ch. 57) Primaquine (Ch. 64) Atovaquone (Ch. 64)
Toxoplasmosis	Pyrimethamine + Clindamycin + Folinic acid (Ch. 64) Spiramycin in pregnancy (Ch. 57)	Pyrimethamine + Sulfadiazine + Folinic acid (Ch. 53) or Azithromycin (Ch. 57) or Clarithromycin (Ch. 57) or Atovaquone (Ch. 64)

in I.V. administration, high cost of lipoid preparations and unacceptable toxic profile.

CHEMOTHERAPY OF OTHER PROTOZOAL INFECTIONS

Other protozoal infections of clinical relevance and with cognizable frequency of occurrence include *cryptosporidiosis* due to *Cryptosporidium* sp. *Pneumocystosis* due to *Pneumocystis jiroveci* (previously *carinii)* and *Toxoplasmosis* due to *Toxoplasma gondii*. *Cryptosporidium* is a coccidian protozoa found in intestinal tract of humans and domestic animals. Cryptosporidiosis is presented with chronic watery diarrhoea and abdominal cramps. *Pneumocystis jiroveci*, tradionally has been considered as a protozoan because of its morphology but molecular analysis has shown it to be closely related to fungi. It causes opportunistic lung infection in an immunocompromised host. Toxoplasmosis due to *Toxoplasma gondii* could be congenital or acquired. Congenital form results by transmission from mother infected during pregnancy to foetus. Manifestations are hydrocephalus or microcephaly associated with convulsions, tremors or paralysis. In acquired form, the *Toxoplasma gondii* invades lymph nodes and spleen. It may present with features of pneumonia or enlarged lymph nodes.

Drug treatment of these protozoal infections are summarised in Table 65.1.

CHAPTER 66

Antiseptics—Disinfectants

COMPETENCY PH1.62

Till now we have discussed those antimicrobials which could be used to treat systemic infections. These had a high margin of safety and could be administered systemically. However, while providing medical care to the patients, numerous instruments, glasswares and environmental surfaces get contaminated with patient's saliva, blood or pus, which are potential source for transmission of infection particularly to hospital staff. Hence, it is necessary to protect health care workers and also other patients from transmission of infection and its consequences.

Such antimicrobials that are used for chemical methods of disinfection or antisepsis are called ***germicides***. These have a low margin of safety and are for non-systemic use. Germicides can be further classified as ***disinfectants*** or as ***antiseptics***. There are some ancillary terms also, like ***sterilisation, pasteurisation, decontamination, sanitation*** and ***preservation,*** which create confusion due to an overlap in their meaning.

Disinfectants are those germicides or chemical substances which are used to destroy or inhibit the growth of pathogenic vegetative bacteria (not their spores) *on inanimate (non-living) surfaces* such as glasswares or surgical instruments. For example, formaldehyde, phenols, ethyl alcohol, soaps, lysol and caustics.

Antiseptics are those germicides or chemical substances which are used to destroy pathogenic bacteria (not the spores) *on animate (living) surfaces* such as skin and mucous membranes. The differences between disinfectants and antiseptics seems to be small and overlapping as some antiseptics in higher concentrations may work as disinfectants while some disinfectants in lower concentrations may serve as antiseptics. Nonetheless, disinfectants fall under the control of Environmental Protection Agency of the Government while antiseptics, because they are used on living tissues, fall under the control of Drug Control Agency of the Government. Antiseptics can be used on skin, eye or mucous membranes (as in mouth washes).

Sterilisation is the ultimate goal of any infection control protocol. It is a process that kills all living microorganisms *including spores*, viruses and fungi. Usually sterilisation is affected by autoclaving at 15 lb pressure of steam at 120^{0}C for at least 1/2 hr, but other methods such as infra-red, ultraviolet or gamma radiation are also used.

Decontamination means marked reduction or destruction of viable pathogenic organisms to a level that will allow a healthy person's natural defences to prevent any infection (for example, decontamination of water). ***Sanitisation*** means reduction in microbial load from an inanimate surface to a level set forth by Public Health Department or Environmental Agency. These levels are considered acceptable for the health of the population. ***Pasteurisation*** is a process of heating milk or other liquids or semisolids for about 30 min at 60–80^{0}C, which kills the non-sporulating microorganisms and prevents the growth of food-borne pathogens for a specified period of time. ***Preservation*** means to preserve the efficacy and to prevent the deterioration of a drug formulation up to its expiry period. A preservative may protect the drug from oxidation (antioxidants) or may kill or inhibit the growth of microorganisms inadvertently introduced during manufacture or its use (antimicrobial/antifungal preservatives).

Antimicrobial preservatives are used in sterile preparations such as eye drops and multidose injections to maintain sterility during use. These are also used in cosmetics, foods and non-sterile pharmaceutical formulations such as oral liquids, ointments and creams to prevent microbial spoilage. Commonly used preservatives are *benzyl alcohol* (2%), *benzoic acid and its salts* (0.2%), the *parabens* (alkyl esters of p-hydroxybenzoic acid, 0.2–0.25%), *phenyl mercuric salts* (0.002% in eye drops and 0.001% in injections) and *thiomersal* (0.001–0.01%). Preparations that should not contain these preservatives include those for injecting into CSF, eye or heart.

The most commonly used *antioxidant preservatives* are *alkyl gallates* (0.001–0.01%), *butylated hydroxyanisole* (0.02%) and *butylated hydroxytoluene* (0.02%). Concomitant use of citric acid or edetic acid along with antioxidant preservatives increases their efficacy.

An ideal antiseptic would be one which has (1) an ability to kill the vegetative form of all pathogenic organisms; (2) an effectiveness even on shorter exposure; (3) an effectiveness at room temperature and (4) selective toxicity (i.e., toxic to microorganisms but not to the host cells). Besides, it should be non-corrosive and less expensive. Truly speaking, these ideal features are unlikely to be achieved. In practice, therefore, an antiseptic reduces the number of viable pathogenic microorganisms on skin surface to levels that will allow a healthy person's natural defences to prevent transmission of infection. Handwashing is rather a most effective method to prevent transmission of infection. Regular hand washing, without any disinfectant minimises the side effects such as drying, irritation and sensitisation of the skin.Even simple cleansing with soap and water is less damaging than antiseptics to wounds, because the use of topical antiseptics has been reported to delay healing to some extent.

The various antiseptics and disinfectants can be classified according to their mechanism of action or according to their chemical characteristics. In the present text both ways to classify have been blended to one. Pirons, as a rule, are resistant to antiseptics and disinfectants (see below).

CLASSIFICATION OF ANTISEPTICS

1. **Which act by precipitating (coagulating) bacterial proteins**
   Aldehydes: Formaldehyde, Glutaraldehyde
   Phenols: Phenol, Cresol, Lysol, Chloroxylenol, Eugenol, Hexachlorophene, Triclosan
   Alcohols: Ethyl alcohol, Isopropyl alcohol
   Heavy metal salts: Silver nitrate, Zinc-calamine lotion
2. **Which act by complexing with sulfhydryl (SH) groups of bacterial enzymes**
   Mercurial antiseptics: Mercurochrome, Nitromersol
3. **Which act by oxidising the sulfhydryl (SH) groups of bacterial enzymes**
   Chlorophores: Chlorinated lime, Chloramine-T, Sodium hypochlorite
   Iodophores: Povidone-iodine, Tincture iodine
   Oxidising Agents: Hydrogen peroxide, Potassium permanganate, Peracetic acid
4. **Which alter the properties of bacterial cell membrane**
   Cationic surface active agents: Chlorhexidine, Cetrimide, Cetylpyridinium chloride, Benzalkonium chloride, Dequalinium chloride
5. **Miscellaneous Agents**
   Dyes: Acriflavine, Aminacrine, Gentian violet
   Others: Nitrofurazone, Boric acid

INDIVIDUAL AGENTS

Which Act by Precipitating (Coagulating) Bacterial Proteins

Aldehydes

Aldehydes are broad-spectrum germicidal agents. Their antimicrobial spectrum includes: Gram-positive bacteria (+), Gram-negative bacteria (+), bacterial spores (+), tubercle bacilli (±), viruses (+) and fungi (+). ***Formaldehyde*** is a pungent gas. Its 37% aqueous solution is called ***formalin.*** Its 4–5% diluted solutions are used for preserving dead tissues. It is now occasionally used to disinfect surgical instruments and glasswares. Though a quite effective disinfectant, its use has declined because of its pungent odour and tendency to cause sensitisation (eczematoid reactions) with repeated contact. ***Glutaraldehyde*** is less pungent, less irritating and a better disinfectant than formaldehyde. A 2% solution is used to disinfect surgical instruments, glasswares and endoscopes etc. (used as immersion disinfectant). Alkalisation activates glutaraldehyde activity but reduces its stability. Activated solutions have a shelf life of only 14 days.

Prions are unique as they are devoid of DNA or RNA yet can self replicate (although their incubating peroid lasts up to 20 yrs). These are not the microorganisms but are the proteinaceous infectious particles, which replicate in the brain cells where they produce vacuoles and deposition of misfolded prion proteins. Prion (native form) is designated as PrP^{C} while the infectious form derived from Prp^{C} is designated as PrP^{SC}. Prions produce transmissible fatal disease like Crutzfeldt-Jakob disease (spongiform encephalopathy), Gerstmann-Straussler-Scheinker Syndrome (cerebellar ataxia with dementia) and fatal familial insomnia. It can be transmitted by surgical procedures or eating beef of a cattle suffering from a mad cow disease etc. Prions are resistant to all disinfectants (except for concentrated sodium hypochlorite solution but that too partially), even to sterilisation, heat or U.V. radiation. For a confirmed case of prion infection, the surgical/medical instruments after use must be incinerated.

Phenols

Phenol is no longer used as disinfectant because of its corrosive nature, toxicity upon absorption and carcinogenic effects. Phenols also are broad-spectrum germicides. Their antimicrobial actions include: Gram-positive bacteria (+), Gram-negative bacteria (+), tubercle bacilli (+), viruses (+) and fungi (+). Phenols are effective in presence of detergents also. Phenol has now been replaced by other phenolic substitutes that have equivalent antimicrobial actions with much lower human toxicity. ***Cresol*** (from coal-tar) is a mixture of 3 isomers of methylphenol. It is more active and less toxic than phenol. It has been used as a surface disinfectant. ***Lysol*** is 50% soapy emulsion of cresol and is widely used as disinfectant in hospital and domestic practice for washing hands. ***Chloroxylenol*** is a non-corrosive, non-irritating phenol substitute having efficacy equal to phenol but less toxic. Dettol is a commercial preparation that contains 4.8% chloroxylenol in 9% terpinol and 13% absolute alcohol. Dettol is used for surgical disinfection. Skin antiseptic creams and antiseptic soaps contain 0.8% chloroxylenol; mouthwashes contain 1% chloroxylenol. Because it can penetrate epithelial surfaces, chloroxylenol is an effective alternative to chlorhexidine in many antiseptic handwash preparations with almost no sensitisation potential. ***Eugenol*** has a weak antimicrobial action but has an analgesic action. It is used in toothpastes and mouthwashes. ***Hexachlorophene*** is quite an effective antiseptic when used with soaps. It has a tendency to accumulate on skin and reduces bacterial load on skin by 90–95% within 3–4 days. It has a good deodorant action also. Soaps and talcum powders containing more than 2% hexachlorophene are banned because of its cutaneous absorption and neural toxicity (cerebral oedema and convulsions). ***Triclosan*** is a chlorinated bisphenol antiseptic used in soaps and handwashes in a concentration of 2%. It has also been used (0.3%) in mouthwashes and toothpastes (as it has an additional anti-inflammatory action). It is also devoid of sensitising effects.

Alcohols

Most frequently used alcohols for antiseptic purposes are ***ethanol*** and ***isopropyl alcohol (isopropanol)***. They are rapidly active against various microbes that includes: Gram-positive bacteria (+), Gram-negative bacteria (+), tubercle bacilli (+), viruses (±) and fungi (±). The optimal bactericidal concentration is 70% for ethanol and 90% for isopropanol. Since these are not sporicidal, have variable action against viruses and fungi and lack residual action due to quick and complete evaporation, these are not used as sterilants. These are damaging if applied onto corneal tissue, mucous membranes, ulcers or to delicate skin (scrotum). These are used as skin antiseptic before I.M. or I.V. injection. These can also be used as disinfectant on inanimate objects *except* those having leather coverings (as on dental chairs or those having plastic coatings).

Heavy Metal Salts

Heavy metal salts of mercury or silver are now rarely used as disinfectants. Use of mercury salts has become obsolete. However, ***thiomersal*** (0.001–0.01%) is still being used, but as preservative only. Its higher concentration causes hypersensitivity reactions. ***Silver nitrate*** eye drops (0.1%) are still useful in the prophylaxis of gonococcal ophthalmitis in the newborn. But antibiotic ointments have now replaced silver nitrate for this indication. ***Silver sulfadiazine ointment*** is still being used. It releases silver and works synergistically with sulfadiazine to suppress bacterial growth in burn cases. It is highly active against *Pseudomonas*. ***Zinc salts*** are only mild antiseptics. These are primarily astringents. ***Zinc sulfate*** (0.1–1.0%) is used in eye drops as antiseptic. ***Zinc oxide+calamine*** (Fe_2O_3) is a mild antiseptic, dermal protective and adsorbent. It is available as zinc-calamine lotion.

Which Act by Complexing With Sulfhydryl (-SH-) Groups of Bacterial Enzymes

Inorganic salts of mercury are outdated but organic mercurial antiseptics are more active and less toxic than their inorganic salts. ***Mercurochrome*** (merbromin or mercurodibromo fluorescein, 2%) is a weak skin antiseptic with poor penetrability. However, it stains skin with brilliant yellow-red colour. ***Nitromersol*** (0.01–0.02%) is also a mercurial antiseptic used for disinfecting skin prior to surgery. Nitromersol occasionally may give rise to hypersensitivity reactions.

Which Act by Oxidising the Sulfhydryl (-SH-) Group of Bacterial Enzymes (Oxidising Agents)

These are either ***iodophores*** **or** ***chlorophores*** or other oxidising agents such as ***hydrogen peroxide*** or ***potassium permanganate solution.***

Iodine and Iodophores

Iodine is a rapidly acting broad-spectrum (bacteria, viruses and fungi) germicide. It has variable action against bacterial spores and tubercle bacilli. Its 1:20,000 solution has the capability to kill most vegetative forms of bacteria within one minute. Thus iodine makes a nearly ideal disinfectant/antiseptic. It was originally used as *tincture iodine* wherein elemental iodine was mixed with KI to increase its solubility in aqueous-alcoholic solution. However, it had the disadvantages of discolouring skin and other material, having an odour and being painful on skin abrasions and open wounds. The development of *iodophores* has led to a wider acceptance of iodine as a disinfectant. ***Iodophores*** are the soluble complexes of iodine with large molecular natural polymers such as polyvinyl pyrrolidone or polyethyl glycols from which free iodine is released slowly. Iodophores have little or no odour, reduce discolouration of surfaces and serve as a reservoir for sustained release of free iodine to react with the susceptible microorganisms. The most popular iodophore is ***povidone-iodine***, which is a polyvinyl pyrrolidone complexed with iodine. In higher concentration (5%) it is used on boils, burns, otitis externa, ulcers, monilial/trichomonal/nonspecific vaginitis, furunculosis and tinea infections. A 10% solution can be used to disinfect endoscopes and surgical instruments. Lower concentrations (1%) can be used in mouthwash. Povidone iodine (5%) when used with spray-wipe-spray technique is an effective surface disinfectant.

Chlorine and Chlorophores

Chlorine is a very effective germicide in a concentration of 0.25 ppm (except for *M. tuberculosis*). It is more active in acidic or neutral medium. It is primarily used to disinfect drinking water supplies. Nowadays, chlorinated compounds that slowly release hypochlorous acid (HOCl) in solution are preferred over gaseous chlorine. These chlorinated compounds are called ***chlorophores***. These are least irritating and easy to handle. Commonly used chlorophores are as under:

- ***Sodium hypochlorite solution*** (NaClO): It is unstable, and hence not used frequently as an antiseptic. However, 5% solution is used as disinfectant on inanimate objects. Its 4% solution is sometimes used in dentistry for root canal treatment.
- ***Dakin's solution (surgical chlorinated soda solution)***: It is a 0.5% sodium hypochlorite solution buffered with boric acid. It is used as antiseptic for wound irrigation.
- ***Chlorinated lime (bleaching powder)***: It contains 30–35% w/w of available chlorine. On exposure to moisture, it decomposes to liberate chlorine. Though onset of action is quick but is short lasting. It is a useful disinfectant for swimming pools, water tanks, drains and toilets. It is also used to disinfect ponds during epidemics of cholera.
- ***Chloramine-T***: It is an organic chlorophore. It is slowly active than sodium hypochlorite solution. It is less irritant and more stable and is

used to treat minor wound infection, as skin antiseptic, as hard surface disinfectant and for the treatment of drinking water.

Oxidising Agents

Hydrogen peroxide has a broad spectrum germicidal action against bacteria, tubercle bacilli, spores, viruses and fungi when used in appropriate concentration. However, it has poor penetrability and loses potency on keeping. It liberates nascent oxygen which oxidises necrotic matter and kills microbes. It is used for cleansing wounds, abscesses, for loosening and removing slough and ear wax. In dentistry it is used to clean septic sockets in root canal and as a mouth freshener in mouth washes. Concentrations of 10–20% of H_2O_2 are sporicidal. Hydrogen peroxide is now used to disinfect respirators, acrylic resin implants and soft contact lenses.

Peracetic acid ($CH_3.COO.OH$), prepared from H_2O_2 and acetic acid (CH_3COOH) is a more potent bactericidal and sporicidal agent than H_2O_2. The food processing industry and breweries extensively use peracetic acid as disinfectant as its breakdown products are not toxic, and have no odour or taste. As a result, subsequent rinsing is not required, which saves time as well as money.

Potassium permanganate also liberates oxygen which oxidises bacterial proteins and enzymes; but it loses activity in contact with organic matter (gets decolourised). A 1:5000 to 1:10,000 solution is bactericidal and is used for gargling, for irrigating cavities and for cleaning weeping eczema. Higher concentrations are used to disinfect wells during cholera epidemics. It is also used for gastric lavage in morphine poisoning (oxidises morphine). However, its use has declined because its higher concentrations are irritant and stains the tissues as well as clothing. It promotes rusting and hence is not suitable to disinfect surgical equipments.

Which Alter the Properties of Bacterial Cell Membrane

a) **Cationic surface-active agents** are large complex molecules containing a quaternary ammonium, or pyridinium or piperidinium group. Having a detergent like action, these lower the surface tension and damage the bacterial cell membrane leading to an alteration in cell membrane permeability and leakage of vital nutrients like K^+, Mg^{2+} and phosphorous (bacteriostatic action). These are highly effective against Gram-positive bacteria, moderately against Gram-negative bacteria and fungi but are ineffective against bacterial spores, tubercle bacilli and viruses. A number of these agents are good cleansing agents and are often formulated with other agents to serve as broad-spectrum disinfectants. Some of them are used as preservatives, others in mouthwashes and in sore throat remedies. These can also be used for disinfecting glasswares and surgical gloves after which they should be thoroughly washed. These are inactivated by anionic detergents (soaps, see below).

- ***Chlorhexidine*** is a cationic biguanide which is highly effective against Gram-positive bacteria, moderately active against Gram-negative bacteria and ineffective against tubercle bacilli, spores, viruses and fungi. It exhibits residual activity after repeated use. Combination of chlorhexidine with cetrimide, called ***Savlon liquid antiseptic*** (chlorhexidine gluconate 1.5% + cetrimide 3%) exhibits enhanced efficacy. Chlorhexidine is formulated as lotions, washes and creams for preoperative cleansing of skin (0.5% solution in 70% alcohol); for cleaning of wounds (0.05% aqueous solution); for mouth infection including candidiasis (0.1–0.2% mouth wash) and for reducing dental plaque accumulation (0.1–0.2% aqueous solutions in mouth wash). A gel containing 0.25% chlorhexidine with xylocaine has been used in catheterisation and cystoscopy. Solutions containing 0.002–0.005% of chlorhexidine are used for disinfection of hydrophilic contact lenses. It is also used extensively in obstetrics (1% cream) and for surgical scrub and in neonatal bath.
- ***Benzalkonium chloride***: Its 1:1000 solution is used for preoperative disinfection of intact skin; 1:2000 solution is used for cleaning wounds while 1:10,000 solution is used for irrigation of bladder. It is also used as preservative/antiseptic in eye drops.

- ***Dequalinium chloride*** is used as an antiseptic in various gum paints and lozenges.
- ***Cetrimide*** is used as 1–3% solution to clean roadside accident wounds because it efficiently removes dirt and congealed blood. In combination with chlorhexidine (***Savlon***, see above) it is one of the commonly used antiseptic & disinfectant for surgical instruments.
- ***Cetylpyridinium chloride*** is similar to cetrimide. It is being used in mouthwashes and lozenges.

b) **Anionic surface-active agents**: These include common soaps and dodecylsulfate/phosphate detergents. These are effective primarily because of their cleaning and emulsifying ability. These have been combined with hexachlorophene/chloroxylenol to enhance their antimicrobial activity.

Miscellaneous Agents

a) **Dyes**

- ***Acriflavine*** is a orange yellow acridine dye, active against mainly Gram-positive bacteria and gonococci. Its efficacy is not reduced by the presence of organic matter and is enhanced in alkaline medium. It is non-irritating and is used for chronic ulcers, wounds and simple burn dressings (0.1–0.5% cream). Staining constitutes its disadvantage. ***Aminacrine*** is similar to acriflavine except that it is non-irritating and non-staining.
- ***Gentian violet*** is a roseaniline dye active against Gram-positive bacteria and fungi. Its 0.5–1% alcoholic solution is used for chronic ulcers, infected eczema and wound. Staining is its disadvantage.

b) **Furan Derivatives**

- ***Nitrofurazone*** (Furacin) is bactericidal to Gram-positive, Gram-negative, aerobic and anaerobic bacteria. It acts by inhibiting enzymes involved in carbohydrate metabolism of bacteria. Its 0.2% cream is used in burn dressings and skin grafting. Local toxicity is minimal except sensitisation (rare).

A number of other antibiotics such as neomycin, bacitracin, polymyxins, sodium fusidate, mupirocin and chloramphenicol are also used as ointments to treat local mucocutaneous infections. These have been discussed in appropriate chapters.

Boric acid is a bacteriostatic, weak antiseptic, used in eye and ear drops, prickly heat powders and in boroglycerine paint (to treat stomatitis and glossitis). Its use for irrigating bladder, cleaning wounds and for burn dressing is not recommended as its systemic absorption causes diarrhoea, vomiting, visual disturbances and renal toxicity.

CHAPTER 67

SECTION 12—CHEMOTHERAPY OF NEOPLASTIC DISEASES

Anticancer Drugs

COMPETENCY PH1.49

The term cancer refers to a disease of cells that show uncontrolled proliferation, dedifferentiation (anaplasia), invasiveness and the ability to metastasise (spread to distant parts of the body). The appearance of such abnormal characteristics reflects their chromosomal abnormality including an expression of abnormal gene sequences (called oncogenes). When such cells proliferate excessively, they form local tumours which can compress or invade nearby normal cellular structures. A small core of cells within this tumour, which retain the ability to undergo repeated proliferation and to metastasise, are called tumour stem cells. These have colony forming capability and can readily survive in the multicellular environment of the host. The extent of metastasis and deterioration in metabolic processes, resulting from cancer, leads to eventual death of the patient, unless the neoplasm is successfully eradicated by the treatment.

There are four main approaches to treat cancer: (1) Surgical resection, (2) Radiotherapy, (3) Chemotherapy and (4) Immunotherapy (use of monoclonal antibodies). Chemotherapy can be used alone or as an adjunct to other forms of therapy. Chemotherapy of cancer, as compared to antibacterial chemotherapy, presents potential problems. Microorganisms (prokaryotic cells) are qualitatively different from human cells (eukaryotic cells). But, cancer cells and normal cells are so similar that normally a drug which is cytotoxic to cancer cells is cytotoxic to normal cells also. Hence, selectivity of an anticancer drug is very limited.

TYPES OF NEOPLASM (TUMOURS)

Neoplasm can be *benign* or *malignant*. Benign tumours are generally slow growing, resemble normal cells, remain localised and are usually not harmful. The terms *cancer* or *malignant neoplasms* are synonymous. They proliferate rapidly, manifest dedifferentiation, invasiveness, and the ability to metastasise. The malignant neoplams inflict damage to the surrounding cells and are harmful if left untreated.

Tumours are categorised according to their tissue of origin:

Benign tumors' names usually end with **"*oma*"**, for example, *Papilloma* (from surface epithelium), *Adenoma* (from glandular epithelium), *Melanoma* (from pigment cells), *Myoma* (from muscle tissue), *Fibroma* (from fibrous tissue), and *Neurofibroma* (from nerve sheath), etc.

Malignant neoplasms are either ***Solid tumours*** or ***Haematological malignancies***.

i) ***Solid tumours*** are of the following types: *Carcinomas* are solid tumours of surface epithelial tissue. These include oral cancers, cancer of head and neck, lung, breast, prostate and colon. *Adenocarcinomas* are malignant tumours of glandular epithelial tissue. *Sarcomas* include tumours of connective tissue such as bone (*osteosarcoma*) or muscle (*leiomyosarcoma*). *Neurofibrosarcoma* is a tumour of nerve sheath, while *Myeloma* is a tumour of haematopoietic tissue of bone marrow (e.g., *multiple myeloma*–a malignant proliferative tumour of plasma cells in bone marrow).

ii) ***Haematological malignancies*** include the following:

- ***Lymphomas*** are malignant neoplams of lymphoid tissue, classified as *Hodgkin's lymphoma* and *non-Hodgkin's lymphoma* (B-cell and T-cell origin).Lymphomas, mainly non-Hodgkin's lymphoma may be nodal or extranodal.

- ***Leukaemia*** is the neoplastic proliferation of haematopoietic and lymphoid tissue. In *acute leukaemia*, the severe anaemia and bleeding problems are commonly seen and result from overproduction of immature cells (blasts) which consequently prevent the normal production of RBCs and platelets. In *acute lymphoid/lymphoblastic leukaemia* (ALL), the neoplasmic proliferation affects lymphoid cell lines (usually B-cells) with lymphocytosis; while in *acute myeloid/ myelogenous/non-lymphoblastic leukaemia* (AML) the neoplastic proliferation affects myeloid cell lines (mainly haematopoietic tissue involving granulocyte precursors from myeloblasts). If untreated, ALL and AML are usually fatal (mostly within months).

  Chronic leukaemia, [chronic myeloid leukaemia (CML) and chronic lymphocytic leukaemia (CLL)] have easily recognisable late precursors series of leukocytes circulating in large number as the predominant leukaemic cell type and the patients tend to have more indolent behaviour. Cytogenetic abnormality called philadelphia (Ph) chromosome is seen in 90–95% of CML. Ph chromosome is formed by reciprocal balanced translocation between part of long arm of chromosome (9;22). CML may also undergo transformation to AML or ALL (rerely).

  Myelodysplastic syndrome are low-grade neoplasms of haematopoietic stem cells in bone marrow, characterised by cytopenia of one or more cell lines in peripheral blood and dyshaematopoietic changes in bone marrow. These are also known as "smouldering leukaemia" or "pre-leukaemia" as some of the patients undergo trans-formation to acute myeloid leukaemia.

AETIOLOGY OF CANCER

The following factors have been implicated in the aetiology of cancer:

1. **Viruses:** Both DNA and RNA viruses have been implicated in the aetiology of cancer. **DNA viruses** that are associated with the cause of various neoplasms are Human Papilloma virus, Epstein-Barr virus, Human Herpes virus-8. Hepatitis B virus. **RNA viruses** implicated in the aetiology of cancer are: Human T-cell lymphotropic virus (HTLV-I and HTLV-II). HTLV-I causes Adult T-cell leukaemia /lymphoma and HTLV-II causes T-cell variant of hairy cell leukaemia.
   Hepatitis C.virus (RNA virus) is involved in the causation of 70–80% cases of hepatocellular carcinoma.
2. *Environmental and occupational hazards* such as exposure to ionising and UV radiation and exposure to various chemical carcinogens like azodyes, asbestos, benzene and polyvinyl chloride.
3. *Diet and habits* such as high-fat and low-fiber diet; tobacco smoking and alcohol consumption.
4. *Use of drugs* like immunosuppressants and some alkylating agents (see below).
5. *Genetic factors* such as inherited genetic mutations, expression of oncogenes and repression of tumour suppressor genes.

The point mutations in genes, which often result due to action of certain viruses and chemical carcinogens, predominantly contribute to causation of cancer. Two types of genetic changes usually lead to cancer:

a) *Activation* of *proto-oncogenes* to *oncogenes*. Proto-oncogenes are normal genes which control normal cell division, apoptosis and differentiation. These get transformed to oncogenes by carcinogens. About 100 types of oncogenes have been identified.

b) *Repression or inactivation of tumour suppressor genes (antioncogenes)*. These genes protect normal cells from malignant changes; but in different cancers, mutations of these genes occur which lead to their inactivation. About 35 types of tumour suppressor genes have been found.

CHARACTERISTICS OF CANCER CELLS

1. Uncontrolled Proliferation

The genetic changes, discussed above, confer autonomy of growth to cancer cells so that their proliferation is now not subject to normal physiological processes. The factors that lead to an uncontrolled proliferation of cancer cells include:

a) ***Growth factors*** (such as Epidermal Growth Factor, EGF; Insulin-like Growth Factor, IGF; Platelet Derived Growth Factor, PDGF; Transforming Growth Factor-β, TGF-β; and Vascular Endothelial Growth Factor, VEGF) and ***their receptors*** (e.g., EGFR, IGFR, PDGFR *and* VEGFR). Growth factor action stimulates a quiescent cell (lying in G_0 phase) to divide, i.e., to start with G_1 phase. Growth factors act through receptor tyrosine kinases or receptor-coupled other kinases to stimulate the production of cell cycle transducers (see below)

b) ***Cell cycle transducers***: These are of 2 types: **(i)** ***Positive regulators of cell cycle*** which facilitate the progress of cell cycle through different phases ($G_0 \rightarrow$ M phase). These include 2 families of protein called ***cyclins*** (so named because these proteins undergo a process of synthesis and breakdown during each cell division) and ***cyclin-dependent kinases*** **(cdk's)**. Each cdk is inactive until it binds to its respective cyclin. The binding enables the cdk to phosphorylate the desired protein or enzyme. After carrying out the phosphorylation, the cyclin is degraded. The activity of these cyclin-cdk complex is modulated by various negative regulatory forces which act at the check point -1 or -2 of the cell cycle (mainly at the check point -1; Fig., 67.1); **(ii)** ***Negative regulators of the cell cycle***: These include Rb proteins (so named because mutations of Rb genes are associated with **R**etino**b**lastoma tumours), protein p21 (which is under the control of p53 gene), other **c**dk **i**nhibitory **p**roteins (CIP family) and **in**hibitors of **k**inases (Ink family). Interplay of all these inhibitors (see text below, under cell cycle) arrest the cell cycle in check state (mainly at check point 1) if any unphysiological event occurs (e.g., DNA damage or aberrant DNA synthesis). If at this point, the DNA repair is done the cell cycle proceeds as usual from G_1 to S phase. If not, the p53 genes would trigger the process of apoptosis by initiating the cascade of proteases (mainly of caspases).

c) ***Disposal of abnormal cells by apoptosis***: It is a programmed cell death. Development of resistance to apoptosis/inactivation of proapoptotic factors/activation of anti-apoptotic factors is the main cause of development of cancer. Apoptosis prevents cancer by monitoring the cancerous changes as it acts as a first line defence against mutations—disposing cells with abnormal DNA that could become malignant. Physiologically apoptosis is involved in the shedding of the intestinal lining, regression of mammary gland cells after lactation and the death of term-expired neutrophils. The apoptosis can take place by 2 pathways which ultimately activate the effector caspases (proteases family); **(i)** *Death receptor pathway* which stimulates tumour necrosis factor (TNF) receptor family that finally activates caspase-8 and **(ii)** *Mitochondrial pathway* which promotes transcription of p53 genes that finally activates caspase-9.

d) ***Tumour-directed angiogenesis of blood vessels***: This factor influences the total tumour mass because the growth of solid tumour depends on the development of its own blood supply (angiogen esis) in response to VEGF produced by growing tumour.

e) ***Telomerase expression***: *Telomeres* are the protective caps over the distal extremity of a chromosomal arm. As a small metal cap over the laces of an office file protects them from damage during daily use, telomeres protect the chromosomes from degradation and entanglement with other chromosomes. Telomeres are *long* in immortalised (cancer) cells and markedly *short* in normal cells, because with each round of cell division a portion of telomere gets eroded and ultimately becomes nonfunctional. At this stage the DNA replication ceases and the cell becomes senescent (old). In malignant cells, telomeres are long and prevent the loss of "end oncogenes". Many malignant tumours express an enzyme *telomerase* that maintains and provides stability to telomeres as well as confers "immortality" on cancer cells (i.e., allows them to proliferate indefinitely). The search for newer anticancer drugs now attempts to capitalise on inhibition of telomerase enzyme.

2. Dedifferentiation

Normally when daughter cells get matured, they eventually differentiate and behave like their parent cell of origin to carry out the predetermined programmed functions (e.g., the muscle cells would start contracting). However, cancer cells do not differentiate, e.g., the cells of pancreatic tumour do not behave as normal pancreatic cells either in function or morphology.

3. Invasiveness

Normal cells are not found outside their tissue of origin, e.g., cardiac cells are not found in liver. If any cell accidentally escapes, it would undergo apoptosis and die. The cancer cells, because of mutations in their genes, have no such constraint over them and can slip inside nearby organs.

4. Metastasis

Cancer cells can disseminate to distal organs through blood and lymphatics and grow, e.g., bony malignancy occurring in femur can metastasise in lungs. The tumour-induced growth of new blood vessels locally (see above) makes the metastasis even easier. A series of genetic modification confers resistance on them towards normal regulatory factors and enables them to establish "extraterritorially".

THE CELL CYCLE

A proper understanding of cell cycle is essential for rational use of anticancer drugs. The cells reproduce themselves through cell division. The first kind of cell division—*the somatic cell division*—involves nuclear division (by *mitosis*) and cytoplasmic division (by *cytokinesis*). The whole process ensures that each daughter cell gets the same number and kind of chromosomes as the original parent cell. The second type of cell division is called *reproductive cell division*, by which sperm and egg cells are produced. This division involves a nuclear division (with cells containing haploid (n) number of chromosomes) called *meiosis* followed by a cytoplasmic division called *cytokinesis*.

When we discuss cell cycle, particularly in relation to cancer, we restrict our discussion to somatic cell (body cell) division because in majority of cancers, the cell division takes place by mitosis (leaving aside few germ cell tumours where cell division is by meiosis). Human cells, except for gametes, contain 23 pairs of chromosomes. When a cell reproduces, it must produce duplicates of all its chromosomes so that its hereditary traits may be passed on to its successive generations.

Cell Cycle Phases

G_0 Phase: Most cells do not divide constantly and spend a varying amount of time in quiescent (calm) state outside the cell cycle. This phase is termed as **G_0 (G_{zero})**. Neurons, skeletal muscle and cardiac muscle cells increase in bulk through hypertrophy and spend their life time in G_0 state. On the contrary, bone marrow cells, GIT cells and skin cells divide constantly. The growth factor action (or other stimulus such as wound) provides momentum for the start of cell cycle (Fig. 67.1). Growth factors stimulate the production of positive as well as negative regulators of cell cycle through signal transduction (see above). The cell cycle, in itself, consists of two major activities: the *interphase* **(G_1 → S → G_2** phase**)** and *the cell division* (mitosis, i.e., **M**-phase and cytokinesis).

Interphase: When the cell is in-between one mitosis and the next, it is said to be in interphase. It is during interphase that the replication of chromosomes, occurs. Also the DNA, the RNAs and the proteins, needed to produce structures that are required for doubling all cellular components (before mitosis), are manufactured. Interphase consists of three distinct phases: **G_1, S** and **G_2** phase.

G_1 phase is a growth (or gap) phase during which cells are engaged in metabolism and production of substances required for forthcoming cell division and growth. In **S** (synthesis) **phase**, DNA and chromosomes are replicated. S-phase is followed by another growth phase, **G_2 phase** (or a gap period between S phase and mitosis) where the cell prepares itself for mitotic division into two daughter cells. In G_1 and G_2 phase there are no events related to chromosomal or DNA replication. These phases simply serve as preparatory ground or gaps in DNA synthesis.

Cells that are destined to never divide again (e.g., nerve cells, skeletal muscle cells) are permanently arrested in G_1 phase; but once a cell enters in the S-phase, it is bound to go through the mitosis (M-phase). An entry of the cell into the S-phase or M-phase is controlled at ***two check points*** in the cell cycle (Fig. 67.1): one at the start of S- and the other at the start of M-phase. In the quiescent G_0 cells the Rb protein is not phosphorylated. The unphosphorylated Rb protein serves as a brake, keeping the cells in G_1 by inhibiting the genes essential for passing into S-phase. In mid G_1, the cyclin-cdk complex phosphorylates the Rb protein to release this brake (check point 1). If there is DNA damage, the tumour suppressor gene p53 stops the cycle at check point 1, allowing the physiological repair. If repair fails apoptosis is initiated. Once check point 1 is cleared the process cannot be reversed and the cell is committed to enter into S-phase. Any abnormal DNA synthesis or DNA damage in S-phase or G_2-phase can further stop the cell cycle at check point-2 by inhibiting the formation of cyclin B–cdk 1 complex.

Mitosis (M-Phase) or Nuclear Division: Though a continuous phase, it can precisely be divided further into four stages.

i) ***Prophase (Pro = before)***
Till now, the chromosomes (though duplicated) are still in a form of tangled mass filled inside the nucleus. In prophase they condense into visible chromosomes (i.e., two sister chromatids joined at centromere). Nuclear membrane now disintegrates and condensed chromosomes are released into cytoplasm.

ii) ***Metaphase (Meta = after)***
In this second stage of mitosis, the centromeres of the chromatid pair (collectively a chromosome and its copy) line up at the exact centre of the mitotic spindle in an equatorial plane (Fig. 67.1).

iii) ***Anaphase (Ana = upward)***
In this third stage of mitosis, centromeres divide and identical sets of chromosomes move to the opposite poles of the cell. The separated sister chromatids are referred to as daughter chromosomes.

iv) ***Telophase (Telo = end)***
This end stage of mitosis is essentially the opposite of prophase. During telophase, the identical sets of chromosomes at opposite poles of the cell uncoil and revert to their thread-like chromatin form. A new nuclear envelope is re-formed around chromatin mass. Nucleoli reappear and spindle disappears.

Cytokinesis or Cytoplasmic Division

In this stage (after mitosis), a division of parental cytoplasm and organelles takes place. A cleavage furrow is formed around the center of the cell, which gradually deepens and separates the cytoplasm and the organelles into two equal and different portions. The separated two daughter cells now have equal and separate portion of cytoplasm, organelles and its own set of identical chromosomes. The daughter cells may now undergo differentiation or remain in G_0 phase, or if stimulated, may enter into interphase (G_1-S-G_2), mitosis (M-phase) and cytokinesis.

Length of Cell Cycle

The length of G_1 phase of cell cycle is highly variable. Typically it takes about 8–10 hrs but it may be even nonexistent (in rapidly dividing cells), to days, weeks or years (in other types of cells). The S-phase takes about 6–8 hrs; G_2 phase about 4–6 hrs and mitosis and cytokinesis about 1–2 hrs. Together, the various phases of cell cycle require about 18–24 hrs in mammalian cells.

Cell Cycle Sites of Anticancer Drugs

Anticancer drugs may also be classified broadly (see Table 67.1), according to their cell cycle cytotoxic effects. Combination of chemotherapeutic agents that are active in different phases of cycle (see below) can result in a greater cell kill. Anticancer drugs falling into cell cycle specific and cell cycle–nonspecific category are shown in Fig. 67.1 and discussed in Table 67.1. Drugs that are cytotoxic to the cells nonselectively at any point in the cycle are called ***"cell cycle-nonspecific drugs"***, while ***the cell cycle-specific drugs*** exhibit phase selectivity (either at G_1 or S or G_2 or M-phase).

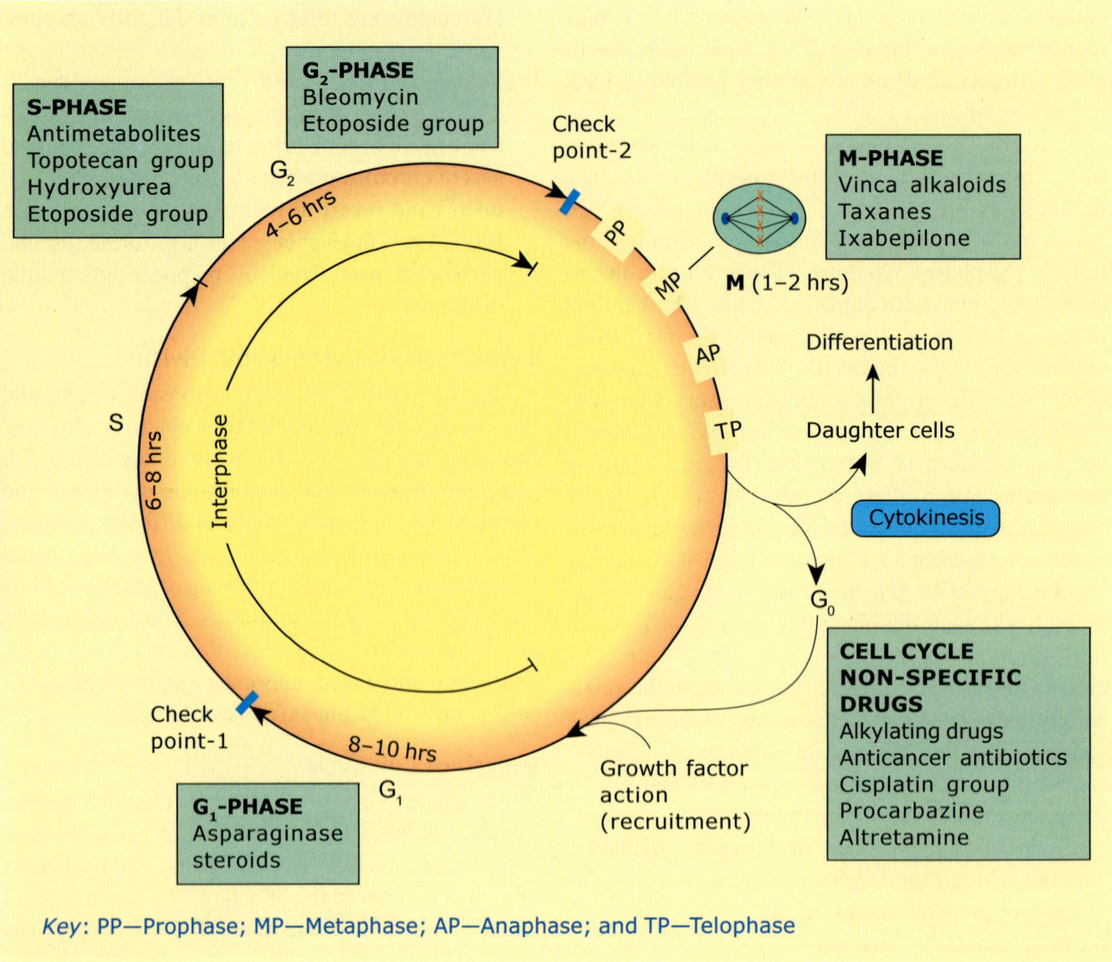

Fig 67.1 Main Phases of Cell Cycle and Cell Cycle Specificity of Anticancer Drugs

DRUGS USED IN CANCER CHEMOTHERAPY

The classification, mechanism of action, major clinical use in cancer treatment and adverse effects of more than 100 anticancer drugs has been summarised in Table 67.1 and in Figure 67.2. In this table, the differences in the mechanism of action of individual drugs have been covered mainly in those group of anticancer drugs which have only a smaller number of drugs. However, in groups having a large number of drugs, like antimetabolites and monoclonal antibodies, some details pertaining to each drug's mode of action are required. These are furnished below:

Antimetabolites

Folic Acid Analogues

Methotrexate,Pemetrexed, Pralatrexate

By competitively inhibiting the dihydrofolate reductase enzyme, methotrexate and other two d rugs deprive the cancer cells of various folate coenzymes and essential components of DNA such as purines, methionine and thymidine monophosphate (dTMP), leading to cell death (Fig. 67.3). The cells in S-phase

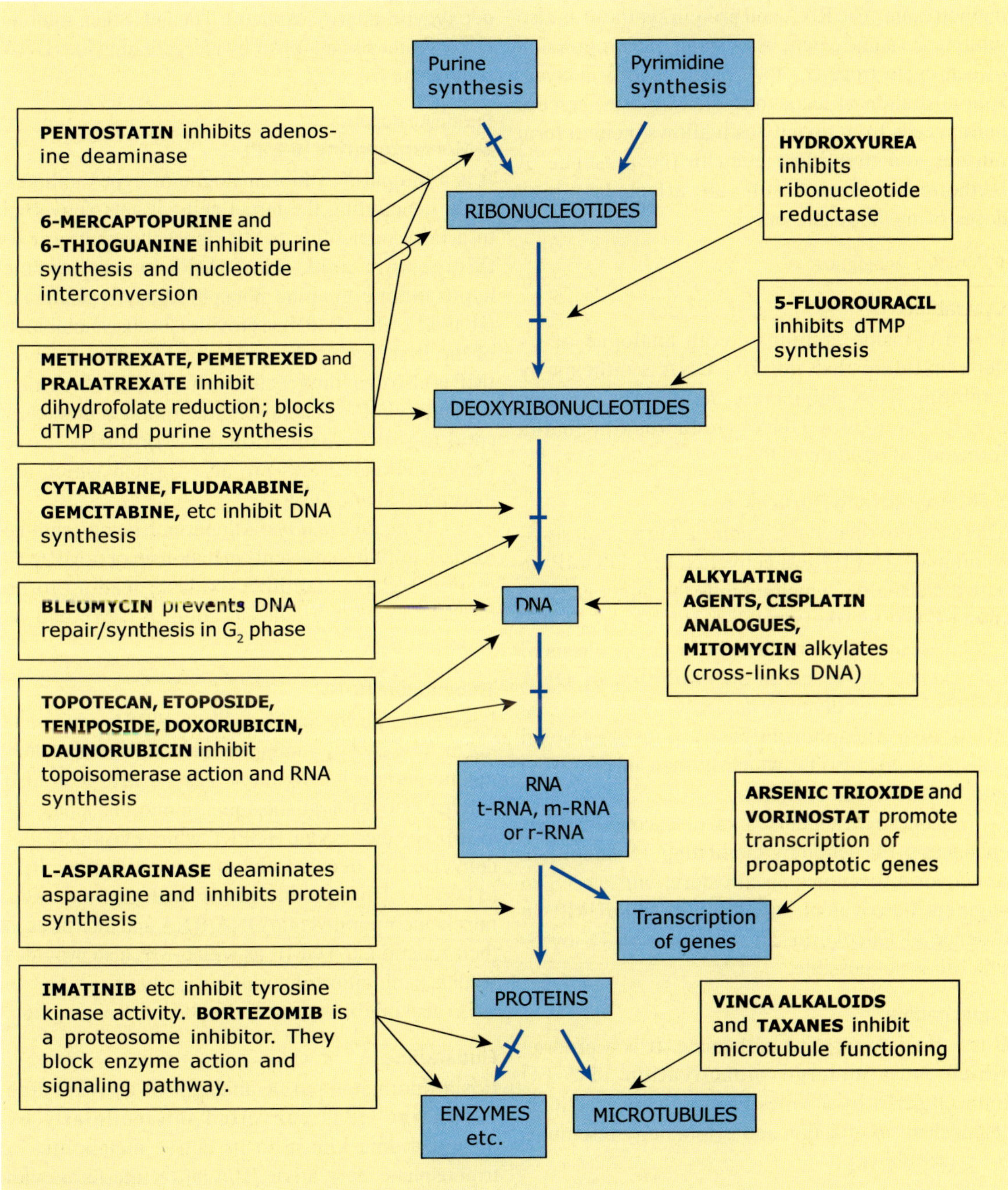

Fig 67.2 Sites of Action of Important Anticancer Drugs. Monoclonal antibodies provide either antibody-dependent celluar cytotoxicity (ADCC) or complement-dependent cytotoxicity (CDC) or direct induction of apoptosis.

are more sensitive to the cytotoxic effects of methotrexate. The RNA and protein synthesis is also inhibited to some extent. As a result, the progression of cell cycle from G_1- to S-phase is also delayed. Administration of leucovorin (folinic acid) rescues normal cells from toxicity as it allows them to form purines and thymidine even in the presence of methotrexate (normal cells are affected by high doses of methotrexate only).

Pyrimidine Analogues

Cytarabine

It is a cytosine arabinoside–an analogue of 2'-deoxycytidine that inhibits DNA synthesis by inhibiting DNA polymerase activity. It also gets incorporated into DNA which results in the formation of fraudulent DNA.

5-Fluorouracil and Floxuridine

These are fluorinated pyrimidines. Intracellularly 5-fluorouracil (5-FU) gets converted to 5-FdUMP, an active metabolite, which inhibits the target enzyme thymidylate synthetase (TS). Inhibition of this enzyme leads to a derangement in the synthesis of dTMP. The net result is an inhibition of DNA synthesis due to thymine depletion (Fig. 67.3). 5-FU is also phosphorylated by phosphoribosyl transferase to 5-FUTP which is then incorporated into RNA (fraudulent RNA).

Concurrent administration of leucovorin, rather enhances 5-FU action by facilitating TS inhibition. Leucovorin, occupies an allosteric site on TS to augment its covalent bonding with 5-FdUMP. In absence of leucovorin, an inhibition of TS by 5-FdUMP is not possible.

Capecitabine

It is a fluoropyrimidine carbamate. It is a prodrug which must undergo bioactivation to 5-FU intracellularly, by a series of enzymatic reactions. Its mechanism of action and cytotoxicity resembles 5-FU (see above).

Gemcitabine

It is 2,2'-difluorodeoxycytidine (dFdC) which is an analogue of nucleoside deoxycytidine. It serves as a substrate for an enzyme deoxycytidine kinase which phosphorylates it to dFdCTP (2,2'-difluoro-deoxycytidine triphosphate). The latter then inhibits DNA synthesis and repair by incorporating into DNA fraudulently.

Purine Analogues

6-Mercaptopurine (6-MP)

It is a thiopurine (thiol analogue of hypoxanthine). After penetrating the target cells, it gets converted to a false nucleotide 6-MP ribosephosphate (or 6-thioinosinic acid, Thio-IMP) by an enzyme hypoxanthine guanine phosphoribosyl transferase (HGPRT). Thio-IMP then provides feedback inhibition of the first step of *de novo* purine synthesis. Thio-IMP is also dehydrogenated to thio-GMP, which after phosphorylation gets falsely incorporated into RNA (making it nonfunctional). Similarly, false deoxyribonucleotides are also formed which are incorporated into DNA (Fig. 67.4).

Drug interactions: Allopurinol, being xanthine oxidase inhibitor, prevents metabolism of 6-MP to 6-methyl MP (by xanthine oxidase) leading to an increase in plasma concentration of 6-MP and its toxicity.

Thioguanine (6-TG)

It is another purine analogue like 6-MP. However, it is not metabolised by xanthine oxidase (allopurinol does not potentiate its toxicity). Like 6-MP, it is also converted to 6-thioguanosine-5'-mono-phosphate (6-TGMP) by the enzyme HGPRT, which eventually gets converted to deoxy-6-thioguanosine triphosphate (dTGTP). This thionucleotide analogue then gets falsely incorporated into DNA/RNA and interferes in their function. 6-TGMP, as with 6-MP, also provides feedback inhibition of purine biosynthesis (Fig. 67.4). 6-TG also inhibits purine nucleotide interconversion.

Fludarabine

It is a fluorinated purine analogue of antiviral drug vidarabine. It is converted intracellularly by deoxycytidine kinase to its active metabolite—a triphosphate derivative. The latter interferes with DNA synthesis by inhibiting various enzymes (such as DNA polymerase-α and ribonucleotide reductase) leading to apoptosis.

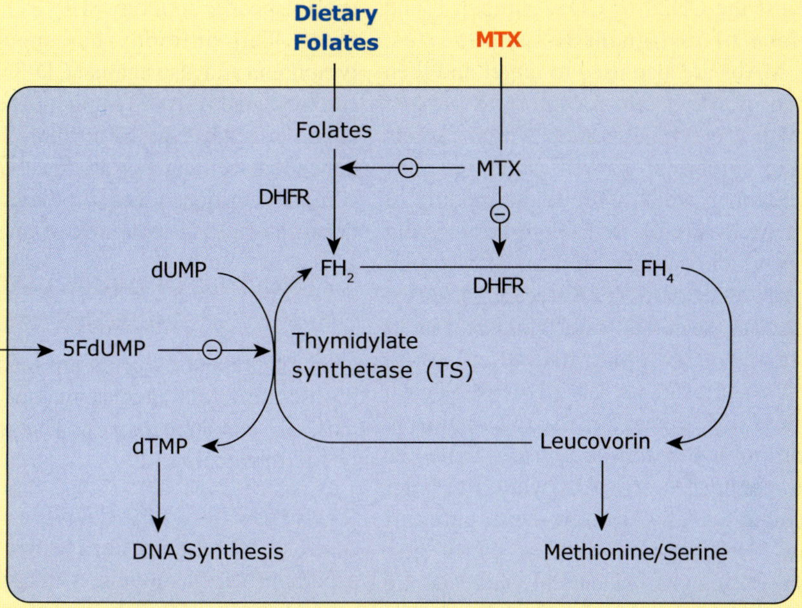

Key: FH_2—Dihydrofolic acid; FH_4—Tetrahydrofolic acid; DHFR—Dihydrofolate reductase; dUMP—Deoxyuridine monophosphate; dTMP—Deoxythymidine monophosphate

Fig 67.3 Mechanism of Action of Methotrexate (MTX) and 5-Fluorouracil (5FU).

Cladribine

It is a synthetic purine nucleoside that is phosphorylated by deoxycytidine kinase to an active metabolite. The latter exhibits its cytotoxic action by fraudulent incorporation into DNA.

Pentostatin

It is a purine analogue isolated from *Streptomyces antibioticus*. It inhibits the enzyme adenosine deaminase which plays a critical role in purine utilisation and DNA synthesis. Adenosine deaminase also converts adenosine to inosine and this inhibition leads to an inhibition of methylation and other reactions.

Monoclonal Antibodies (MAbs)

Malignant cells often have unique antigens expressed on their surface, known as *tumour associated antigens*. Monoclonal antibodies (MAbs) are single species of antibody that recognise and react with a specific antigen only. These are produced by cloning of hybrid cells created by fusing an immortal cell from mouse myeloma with a B-cell producing an antibody against a desired antigen. The resulting hybridomas now have an ability of the B-lymphocytes to secrete a single species of antibody and the capability of the cancer cells to proliferate endlessly. These hybridomas can be cloned and each clone will produce antibodies directed against a single antigen type. Murine (rodents) MAbs, usually, are not preferred as they have a shorter half-life and induce a human antimouse-antibody allergic response. Hence, generally chimerised (part human-part mouse) or humanised forms of MAbs are commonly used therapeutically. The names of chimeric MAbs usually end up with "*ximab*" (e.g., rituximab and cetuximab) while those of humanised MAbs end up with "*umab*" (e.g., trastuzumab and alemtuzumab). For more details refer Ch. 3.

MAbs, such as rituximab and alemtuzumab, are directed against the CD20 or CD52 antigen found on the surface of malignant B-lymphocytes, respectively. MAbs are also used to target and then block selected growth factor receptors to prevent cellular growth (e.g., trastuzumab which targets against human epidermal growth factor receptor protein-2; cetuximab which inhibits the binding of epidermal growth factor to EGF-receptor and bevacizumab which inhibits binding of vascular endothelial growth factor to VEGF-receptor). MAbs may also be used as the missile with "biological smart bombs" carrying a radiopharmaceutical (e.g., ibritumomab-^{90}Y and tostitumomab-^{131}I) or a biological toxin as warhead (e.g., gemtuzumab ozogamicin and denileukin diftitox). The former type are called as radioimmuno-conjugates of MAbs while the latter type are designated as cytotoxic-conjugates of MAbs. The MAbs which do not carry any immunotoxin or radiopharmaceutical warheads are called as "naked monoclonal antibodies". For details refer Table 67.1. Some "bispecific antibodies" have also been engineered. These not only target a specific tumour cell antigen but simultaneously activate neighbouring effector cells, inducing toxicity. One such bispecific antibody 8H9 (Fv) PE38 is in clinical trials. This antibody has specificity to B-cell lymphoma and also against CD-3 which enhances T-cell mediated lysis of lymphoma cells. The cytotoxic action of MAbs may be attributed to their antibody-dependent cellular cytotoxicity (ADCC) or due to complement-dependent cytotoxicity (CDC) and also because of direct induction of apoptosis.

TOXICITIES OF DRUGS USED IN CANCER CHEMOTHERAPY

Chemotherapeutic agents are most toxic to rapidly proliferating cells such as mucous membranes, skin, hair, GIT and bone marrow. The latter toxicity could be life-threatening.

Bone Marrow Suppression

Almost all chemotherapeutic agents, except asparaginase, bleomycin, vincristine, gefitinib and some hormones and hormone antagonists, cause myelosuppression. Drugs that can cause severe myelosuppression include carmustine, cytarabine, daunorubicin, doxorubicin, paclitaxel, alkylating agents and antimetabolites. White blood cells are

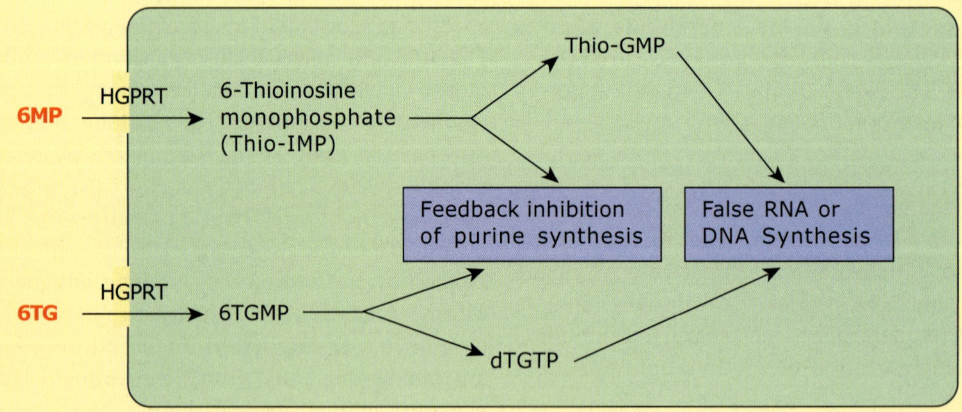

Key: HGPRT—Hypoxanthine guanine phosphoribosyl transferase; 6TGMP—6-Thioguanosine monophosphate; dTGTP—Deoxy-6-thioguanosine triphosphate

Fig 67.4 Mechanism of Action of 6-Mercaptopurine (6MP) and 6-Thioguanine (6TG).

Table 67.1 Classification, Mechanism of Action, Clinical Uses and Adverse Effects of Anticancer Drugs

Drug and Category	Mechanism of Action	Clinical Use	Adverse Effects
I. Alkylating Agents 1. Busulfan	Alkylating agents (1–13) introduce alkyl groups by forming covalent bonds with nucleophilic moieties such as phosphate, sulfhydryl, hydroxyl, carboxyl, amino and imidazole groups present in DNA or RNA. By cross-linking in-between the strands of DNA, they prevent the cell division and protein synthesis. The cytotoxicity of these drugs correlates with the degree of DNA alkylation (or cross-linking). **These are cell cycle-nonspecific agents.**	Chronic myelocytic leukaemia, polycythaemic vera	Myelosuppression, pulmonary and dermatologic toxicity, cataract formation, gynaecomastia
2. Carmustine (Nitrosoureas)		Hodgkin's disease, lymphoma, melanoma, multiple myeloma, CNS tumours, colo-rectal cancer	Myelosuppression, GIT toxicity, hepatotoxicity nephrotoxicity, pulmonary fibrosis
3. Lomustine		– do –	– do –
4. Bendamustine		Chronic lymphocytic leukaemia; Non-Hodgkin's lymphoma	– do –
5. Chlorambucil		Chronic lymphocytic leukaemia, myeloma, lymphoma, Hodgkin's disease, lympho-sarcoma, ovarian cancer	Myelosuppression, nausea, vomiting, pulmonary fibrosis, hepatotoxicity, dermatotoxicity
6. Cyclophospha-mide		Lymphoma, Hodgkin's disease; testicular, lung, breast, prostate and ovarian carcinoma, multiple myeloma	Immuno- and myelo-suppression, hepatotoxicity, alopecia, SIADH, nausea, haemorrhagic cystitis, stomatitis
7. Melphalan		Multiple myeloma, ovarian carcinoma, breast cancer	Myelosuppression, GIT distress, pulmonary fibrosis, SIADH, dermatotoxicity, teratogenicity
8. Dacarbazine		Melanoma, sarcoma, Hodgkin's disease	Myelosuppression, fever, nausea, alopecia, hepato-toxicity, dermatotoxicity
9. Mechlorethamine		Hodgkin's disease, lymphoma	Myelosuppression, neuro-toxicity, alopecia, nausea, tissue necrosis
10. Ifosfamide		Testicular and ovarian carcinoma, sarcoma, multiple myeloma	Myelosuppression, nausea, vomiting, haemorrhagic cystitis, confusion, lethargy
11. Thiotepa		Breast, ovarian cancer; lymphomas, rhabdo-myosarcoma	Myelosuppression, infertility, nausea, vomiting, dermato-toxicity

contd.

Drug and Category	Mechanism of Action	Clinical Use	Adverse Effects
12. Temozolomide		Brain tumour, melanoma	myelosuppression, upper abdominal distress
13. Streptozocin		Islet cell carcinoma of pancreas	Hypoglycaemia, nausea, fever, hepatotoxicity, myelosuppression
14. Estramustine	Though a hybrid structure, it neither acts as alkylating agent nor requires estrogen receptors for its action. Binds to β-tubulin; causes microtubule disassembly; antimitotic actions.	Prostate cancer	Gynaecomastia, thrombophlebitis, nausea, cardiotoxicity (MI)
II. Antimetabolites	**(These are S-phase specific agents)**		
A. ***Folic acid analogues***	See Text		
15. Methotrexate 16. Pemetrexed 17. Pralatrexed		Choriocarcinoma; breast, neck, head, cervical, lung carcinoma; acute lymphoblastic leukaemia, psoriasis, rheumatoid arthritis	Myelosuppression, GIT toxicity (ulcerative mucositis and diarrhoea), nephrotoxicity, neuro-toxicity, hepatotoxicity (prolonged use), alopecia
B. ***Purine analogues***	See Text		
18. Thioguanine		Acute and chronic myelogenous leukaemia	Myelosuppression, hepato-toxicity (less common than mercaptopurine), mild nausea
19. Mercaptopurine		- do -	- do -; stomatitis
20. Fludarabine		Chronic lymphocytic leukaemia	Myelosuppression, mild nausea, alopecia, stomatitis
21. Pentostatin		Hairy cell leukaemia	Myelosuppression, nephro-toxicity, skin rashes, nausea
22. Cladribine		- do -	Myelosuppression
23. Nelarabine		Acute lymphocytic leukaemia (ALL)	- do -; peripheral neuropathy.
24. Clofarabine		ALL; T-cell lymphoma	Myelosuppression; Capillary leak syndrome
C. ***Pyrimidine analogues***	See Text		
25. Cytarabine		Acute and chronic myelogenous leukae-mia, lymphoma	Myelosuppression, stomatitis neurotoxicity, nausea, conjunctivitis

contd.

Drug and Category	Mechanism of Action	Clinical Use	Adverse Effects
26. Fluorouracil		Carcinoma of lung, breast, ovary, cervix, prostate, bladder, head and neck; GIT adenocarcinoma, superficial basal cell skin carcinoma	Myelosuppression, stomatitis, alopecia, photosensitivity, neurotoxicity (cerebellar ataxia)
27. Floxuridine		– do –; preferred in hepatic metastases from GIT adeno-carcinoma	– do – (but mild)
28. Gemcitabine		Adenocarcinoma of the pancreas	Myelosuppression, flu-like symptoms
29. Capecitabine		Colorectal cancer, metastatic breast cancer	Myelosuppression, nausea, vomiting, skin rash, hepatotoxicity
III. Antibiotics			
30. Bleomycin	These drugs bind to DNA through intercalation between specific base pairs. Consequently, they block the synthesis of new DNA and of DNA-dependent RNA and thus inhibit cell replication. These also break DNA strands. **All of them are cell cycle non-specific drugs** except for bleomycin which blocks at G_2 phase of cell cycle. For minor differences in mode of action refer individual drugs. Doxorubicin and daunorubicin, besides binding to DNA, also exert their cytotoxic action by inhibiting topoisomerase II, the activity of which is markedly increased in proliferating cells.	Testicular carcinoma, Hodgkin's and non-Hodgkin's lymphomas, squamous cell carcinoma of head, neck, cervix and skin	Pulmonary toxicity, nausea, vomiting, alopecia, skin rash, fever
31. Dactinomycin (actino-mycin-D)		Wilms tumour, Ewing's sarcoma, rhabdomyo-sarcoma, testicular sarcoma, chorio-carcinoma, neuroblastoma	Myelosuppression, nausea, vomiting, mucositis, tissue necrosis, stomatitis
32. Mitomycin C		Stomach, pancreatic, colon, breast, head, neck and lung carcinoma	Myelosuppression, tissue necrosis, stomatitis, pulmonary toxicity, alopecia, hepatotoxicity (rare)
33. Daunorubicin		Acute myelocytic leukaemia	Myelosuppression, alopecia, cardiotoxicity, stomatitis, tissue necrosis
34. Idarubicin		– do –	– do –

contd.

Drug and Category	Mechanism of Action	Clinical Use	Adverse Effects
35. Doxorubicin		Acute leukaemia, breast, ovarian, endometrial, bladder, thyroid cancer; Hodgkin's disease, Wilms tumour, multiple myeloma	– do –; radiation recall reaction
36. Epirubicin		Breast cancer	Stomatitis, myelosuppression, cardiotoxicity, skin rash, GIT distress
37. Mitoxantrone	Though a synthetic anthraquinone, its structure and mode of action is similar to anthracyclines such as doxorubicin and daunorubicin	Breast cancer, ovarian cancer, non-lymphocytic leukaemias, lymphoma, secondary progressive multiple sclerosis	– do –; hepatotoxicity (rare)
IV. Natural Products			
A. *Vinca alkaloids*			
38. Vincristine sulphate	Obtained from the shrub *Vinca rosea*. Vinorelbine is semisynthetic derivative of vinblastine. These drugs arrest the cell division in the metaphase by binding to microtubular protein tubulin that forms the mitotic spindle. **Thus these are cell cycle specific drugs, arresting mitosis in M-phase** through inhibition of tubulin polymerisation (see also Taxanes below).	Acute lymphocytic leukaemia, Wilms tumour, Hodgkin's disease, non-Hodgkin's lymphoma, rhabdomyosarcoma, cancer of breast, cervix, ovary and lungs.	Neurotoxicity, SIADH, tissue necrosis, alopecia, colicky abdominal pain
39. Vinblastine		Testicular carcinoma, Hodgkin's disease, non-Hodgkin's lymphoma, Kaposi's sarcoma, cancer of breast, lung and bladder	Myelosuppression, tissue necrosis, stomatitis, SIADH, anorexia, diarrhoea, dermatitis, alopecia
40. Vinorelbine tartrate	– do –	– do –; also non-small cell lung carcinoma	– do –; lesser neurotoxicity
B. *Epipodophyllotoxins*			
41. Etoposide	These are semisynthetic derivatives of podophyllotoxins obtained from the roots of American mandrake. They form a complex with topoisomerase II and thus prevent resealing of DNA strands after break, leading to an accumulation of DNA breaks and cell death. **They cause mitotic arrest of cells in S- and G_2 phase of cell cycle.**	Cancer of breast, lung and testis, small cell lung cancer, Hodgkin's disease, non-Hodgkin's lymphoma, Kaposi's sarcoma, acute myelogenous leukaemia	Myelosuppression, nausea, alopecia, hypersensitivity reactions

contd.

Drug and Category	Mechanism of Action	Clinical Use	Adverse Effects
42. Teniposide		– do –; also acute lymphoblastic leukaemia in children	– do –; also neuropathy
C. *Camptothecins*			
43. Topotecan	These are semisynthetic derivatives of camptothecins isolated from an ornamental Chinese tree. They inhibit topoisomerase-I. This allows single strand breaks in the DNA to occur and to accumulate but not its resealing once DNA strands are untwisted. The ultimate cell death, however, occurs due to collision of a DNA replication fork with this cleaved strand of DNA that finally leads to an irreversible double strand DNA break. **These are, therefore, S-phase specific** as ongoing DNA synthesis is necessary for ultimate cytotoxicity and cell death.	Ovarian cancer, colon and lung cancer, small cell lung cancer	Myelosuppression, flu-like symptoms, nausea, vomiting
44. Irinotecan		– do –	– do –
D. *Taxanes*			
45. Paclitaxel	These are derived from the bark of Pacific yew tree. At steady state, microtubules are in a state of assembly and disassembly as tubulin dimers are continually being polymerised at one end and depolymerised at the other end of microtubules. Taxanes stabilise polymerisation of tubulins and thus inhibit disassembly of microtubules even in absence of essential co-factors. Stabilisation of microtubules prevents reorganisation of microtubular filaments essential during mitosis in **G_2 and M-phases of cell cycle** (compare with vincristine which rather blocks microtubule polymerisation and thus disrupts mitotic spindle formation during mitosis).	Breast, ovarian, lung, head and neck cancer,	Myelosuppression, alopecia, hypersensitivity reactions, neuropathy, bradycardia
46. Docetaxel		– do –	– do –
47. Cabazetaxel		Hormone-resistant prostate cancer (best results when given with androgen deprivation therapy	– do –

contd.

Drug and Category	Mechanism of Action	Clinical Use	Adverse Effects
48. Ixabepilone	Semisynthetic analogue. Inhibits normal microtubule dynamics like docetaxel.	Metastatic breast cancer	- do -
E. *Enzymes*			
49. L-Asparaginase (L-Aspg)	Normal tissues are able to synthesise L-asparagine (L-asp) from asparagine synthetase, in amounts sufficient for protein synthesis; but lymphoid malignant cells lack asparagine synthetase enzyme and therefore utilise circulating L-asp from plasma. L-Aspg, an enzyme derived from *E coli*, catalyses the hydrolysis of circulating L-asp to aspartic acid and ammonia. L-Glutamine is also hydrolysed by L-Aspg during therapy. Thus malignant cells get deprived of L-asp and glutamine, necessary for protein synthesis, leading to cell death in the **G_1-phase of cell cycle**.	Acute lymphocytic leukaemia, lymphoma	Nausea, fever, allergic reactions, hepatotoxicity, pancreatitis, mental depression; but insignificant toxicity to bone marrow, GIT and hair follicles
V. Miscellaneous Agents			
50. Hydroxyurea (HU)	HU inhibits ribonucleotide reductase enzyme and prevents conversion of ribonucleotides to deoxyribonucleotides and hence impairs DNA synthesis. It causes arrest of cell growth at **S-phase or near the G_1-S interface**.	Chronic myelogenous leukaemia, polycythaemia vera, sickle cell anaemia	Myelosuppression, alopecia, hyperpigmentation, skin reactions
51. Cisplatin	These drugs are *platinum coordination complexes* and act analogously to alkylating agents. They bind to DNA at nucleophilic sites of guanine producing alterations in DNA structure and inhibit DNA synthesis. Cross-linking of platinum between adjacent guanines on the same DNA strand is primarily responsible for the cytotoxicity. **These are cell cycle non-specific agents**. *Oxaliplatin*, in addition, blocks DNA replication and transcription.	Testicular, ovarian, bladder, lung, prostate head and neck cancer	Nephrotoxicity, nausea, vomiting, hearing loss, anaemia, allergic reactions
52. Carboplatin		- do -	Myelosuppression, other toxicities less than cisplatin
53. Oxaliplatin		- do -; colorectal cancer	Pharyngo-laryngeal dysaesthesia, paraesthesias, diarrhoea, myelosuppression (less)

contd.

Drug and Category	Mechanism of Action	Clinical Use	Adverse Effects
54. Procarbazine	Its active alkylating metabolite methylates DNA and inhibits RNA, DNA and protein synthesis. **A cell cycle non-specific agent**.	Hodgkin's disease, lymphoma, multiple myeloma, brain tumours	Myelosuppression, nausea, vomiting, skin rash, chromosomal damage, disulfiram type reaction with ethanol
55. Hexamethyl-melamine (HMM) or Altretamine	It selectively inhibits the incorporation of thymidine and uridine into DNA and RNA inhibiting their synthesis. **A cell cycle non-specific agent**.	Ovarian cancer	Nausea, vomiting, myelosuppression, neurotoxicity (rare)
56. Arsenic trioxide	Mechanism is uncertain. They promote differentiation of APL cells and promote apoptosis by upregulating the genes involved in apoptosis. Retinoids, however, displace the repressor gene of differentiation in APL cells and activate differentiation program.	Acute promyelocytic leukaemia (APL)	Nausea, vomiting, dermatotoxicity, cardiotoxicity, retinoic acid syndrome
57. Tretinoin (Retinoids)	See above	- do -	Headache, dry skin, cheilitis, teratogenicity, bone tenderness, retinoic acid syndrome
58. Bexarotene (Retinoids)	*Bexarotene* is a retinoid that selectively activates retinoid x receptors which control genes of differentiation. It also increases the level of CD25, low affinity IL-2 receptors on malignant lymphocytes of T-cell origin. *Denileukin diftitox* acts on CD122 and CD132, high affinity IL-2 receptors that are upregulated and expressed on malignant lymphocytes of T-cells. C25, low affinity IL-2 receptors, present on resting T-cells are much less sensitive to denileukin. Hence, to modulate C25 expression and to increase the response rates a combination of denileukin diftitox with bexarotene is being preferred.	Cutaneous T-cell lymphoma	Hyperlipidaemia, skin rash, hypothyroidism, photosensitivity
59. Denileukin diftitox* (Immuno-toxin obtained from genetic recombination of IL-2 and the active fragment of diphtheria toxin)		- do -	Hypersensitivity reactions, vascular leak syndrome

contd.

Drug and Category	Mechanism of Action	Clinical Use	Adverse Effects
60. Thalidomide 61. Lenolidomide	Act by multiple mechanisms. They inhibit angiogenesis to prevent tumour growth and formation of metastases. They also inhibit tumour necrosis factor-α production, stimulate T-cell proliferation and increase interferon as well as IL-2 release.	Multiple myeloma, melanoma. *Other uses:* Leprosy (erythema nodosum leprosum), AIDS-related cachexia, rheumatoid arthritis, graft-versus-host disease.	Teratogenic effects, neurotoxicity, dermatotoxicity, taste alteration, tongue discolouration, GIT distress.
VI. Protein Tyrosine Kinase Inhibitors			
62. Imatinib 63. Dasatinib 64. Nilotinib (Selective Bar-Abl kinase inhibitor)	These drugs are selective inhibitors of tyrosine kinase that causes apoptosis or arrest of growth in cells expressing the Bcr-Abl oncoprotein. This oncoprotein is the product of a specific chromosomal abnormality (Philadelphia chromosome), which is present in the patients of CML. In addition, *imatinib* also inhibits the proliferation of GIT stromal tumour cells dependent on *c-kit* oncogene which increases tyrosine kinase activity.	Chronic myelogenous leukaemia (CML), GIT stromal cell tumour *Dasatinib* and *Nilotinib* overcome imatinib resistance resulting from mutations in Bcr-Abl kinase. Hence preferred in CML with resistance or intolerance to imatinib therapy.	Nausea, vomiting, oedema, muscle cramps, elevation of transaminases, neutropenia, thrombocytopenia
65. Lapatinib	Inhibits tyrosine kinase associated with HER2/neu receptor in breast cancer cells (see trastuzumab monoclonal antibody)	Breast cancer	Diarrhoea, exacerbation of gastro-esophageal reflux skin rash,
66. Sorafenib	Inhibits RAF kinase	Medullary thyroid carcinoma	Nausea, diarrhoea, rash, Hypertension, headache, anorexia, acne, prolongation of QTc, bleeding
67. Pazopanib 68. Vandetanib	Inhibits VEGF receptor tyrosine kinase	- do - - do -	
VII. Epidermal Growth Factor Receptor (EGFR) Inhibitors			
69. Gefitinib (Iressa)	The overexpression of epidermal growth factor receptor tyrosine kinase (EGFR-TK) has been linked to induction, growth and metastatic potential of non-small cell lung cancer as well as head and neck cancer. Upon stimulation by ligands the EGFR dimerises and the intracellularly linked tyrosine kinase (TK) is	Metastatic non-small cell lung cancer and other solid tumours	Diarrhoea, acneiform skin rash, anorexia

contd.

Drug and Category	Mechanism of Action	Clinical Use	Adverse Effects
	activated to transmit pro-growth signals to malignant cells. These drugs inhibit this EGFR linked TK signaling by binding to tyrosine kinase-ATP binding site		
70. Sorafenib	These are smaller molecule inhibitors of vascular endothelial growth factors (VEGF)-receptor associated tyrosine kinase activity. They also inhibit *c-kit* oncogene (a tyrosine kinase stem cell receptor; see above)	Renal cell cancer (both drugs). Hepatocellular cancer	Hypertension, bleeding complications and fatigue (both drugs); skin rash (sorafenib),
71. Sunitinib	– do –	GIT stromal tumours Medullary thyroid cancer	– do – Cardiac dysfunction
72. Carbozatinib	– do –	Medullary thyroid cancer	
73. Erlotinib	– do –	Non-small cell lung cancer (NSCLC)	– do –; interstitial lung disease
VIII. Proteosome Inhibitors			
74. Bortezomib 75. Carfilzomib	It is a proteosome inhibitor. Proteosomes are enzyme complexes which are responsible for degrading proteins that control the cell cycle. Precisely, it prevents the break-up of nuclear factor-κβ (NF-κβ) from its inhibitory partner protein. If NF-κβ is not released, the process of transcription of genes, that promotes cancer growth, is prevented.	Refractory and relapsed multiple myeloma	Diarrhoea, peripheral neuropathy, bone marrow suppression, fatigue
IX. Hormones and Antagonists			
A. *Gonadotrophin release hormone (Gn-RH) agonists* (Ch. 41)			
76. Goserelin 77. Buserelin 78. Leuprolide	These are more potent and longer acting analogues of Gn-RH. They inhibit gonadotrophin (FSH/LH) release and suppress gonadal functions due to down-regulation and desensitisation of Gn-RH receptors. They virtually induce reversible	To treat prostatic carcinoma and estrogen receptor positive (premeno-pausal) breast cancer. Initially, being Gn-RH agonist, they activate testicular/ovarian functions and flare up the symptoms	Hot flushes, headache, nausea, osteoporosis, oedema, loss of libido and allergic manifestations (bronchospasm)

contd.

Drug and Category	Mechanism of Action	Clinical Use	Adverse Effects
	pharmacological oophorectomy or orchiectomy because they decline estradiol or testosterone levels drastically.	of prostatic/breast carcinoma. Hence concurrent use of an antiandrogen (flutamide) prevents this flare up (Ch. 41)	
B. *Gn-RH antagonists* (Ch. 41)			
79. Cetrorelix 80. Ganirelix 81. Abarelix	These are competitive antagonists at pituitary Gn-RH receptors. Like agonists, they do not cause an initial increase in gonadotrophin secretion, and do not exacerbate cancer symptoms.	Prostatic carcinoma	Less toxic than Gn-RH agonists; pain and swelling at the injection site
C. *Corticosteroids* (Ch. 42)			
82. Dexamethasone 83. Prednisolone	Glucocorticoids decrease the release of cytokines (IL-1–IL-6) from lymphocytes which reduces tissue damage. They also decrease the number of lymphocytes (T and B cells). Though the normal lymphoid tissue is not affected, glucocorticoids show marked lympholytic effects on malignant lymphatic cells to reduce cell proliferation, promote cell cycle arrest and induce cell death by apoptosis.	Lymphocytic leukaemia, Hodgkin's disease, multiple myeloma, breast cancer and management of cancer-related hypercalcaemia	Peptic ulcer, hypokalaemia, fluid retention, osteoporosis, diabetes, cataract, Cushingoid appearance, muscle wasting, susceptibility to infections (Ch. 42)
D. *Adrenocortical suppressants*			
84. Aminoglutethimide 85. Trilostane	*Aminoglutethimide* blocks the conversion of cholesterol to pregnelonone (Fig. 42.1) and causes a type of pharmacological adrenalectomy which diminishes the levels of circulating sex hormones. It is also an aromatase enzyme inhibitor and thus reduces estrogen production in the periphery and in the estrogen targeted tissues. *Trilostane* is a 3-β-hydroxy steroid dehydrogenase	Carcinoma of breast, prostate and adrenal cortex. Also for treating Cushing's syndrome associated with adrenal carcinoma	Ataxia, lethargy, rashes, dizziness, hypotension, myelosuppression

contd.

Drug and Category	Mechanism of Action	Clinical Use	Adverse Effects
	inhibitor and therefore retards the synthesis of adrenal and gonadal hormones (Fig. 42.1). Concomitant hydrocortisone supplementation is necessary to avoid unwanted adrenal suppression (with both the drugs).		
E. *Aromatase inhibitors*			
86. Anastrozole 87. Letrozole 88. Exemestane	*Anastrazole* and *Letrozole* are nonsteroidal new generation selective inhibitors of aromatase, an enzyme responsible for converting testosterone to estradiol (Ch. 42, 43). *Exemestane* is an irreversible steroidal aromatase inhibitor (inactivator). Unlike amino-glutethimide, these drugs have no inhibitory effects on adrenal glucocorticoid or mineralocorticoid synthesis.	ER-positive metastatic breast cancer in postmenopausal women, that are resistant to tamoxifen therapy	Mild nausea, headache, fatigue, hot flushes and arthralgias; contra-indicated in premenopausal women (letrozole has been withdrawn)
F. *Estrogen receptor (ER) antagonists*			
89. Tamoxifen 90. Toremifen 91. Fulvestrant (Ch. 43)	*Tamoxifen* and *toremifen* bind to ERs of estrogen sensitive tumours. In addition, they also suppress serum levels of insulin-like growth factor-1 and upregulate local production of transforming growth factor-β. *Fulvestrant* is a steroidal selective ER down-regulator and is termed as "pure antiestrogen."	Breast carcinoma, male breast carcinoma postoperatively. *Fulvestrant* is used for ER-positive metastatic breast cancer that has progressed despite tamoxifen therapy	Transient flare of tumour activity initially (except fulvestrant), oedema, hot flushes, deep vein thrombosis and endome-trial hyperplasia (due to partial ER-agonist effects of tamoxifen on blood vessels and uterus)
G. *Androgen receptor (AR) blockers* (Ch. 44)			
92. Flutamide 93. Bicalutamide 94. Nilutamide	These are nonsteroidal AR antagonists that inhibit testosterone binding to the ARs (Ch. 44). For maximal clinical efficacy, these are not indicated as monotherapy as routine but used in combination with leuprolide to reduce tumour flare-up symptoms (see above).	Prostate carcinoma. *Bicalutamide* and *nilutamide* have longer plasma half-lives that allows once daily oral dosing as compared to flutamide which needs thrice daily dose schedule	Nausea, hot flushes, mild gynaecomastia and transient elevation of liver enzymes

contd.

Drug and Category	Mechanism of Action	Clinical Use	Adverse Effects
H. ***Progestins* (Ch. 43)**			
95. Hydroxyprogesterone 96. Medroxyprogesterone 97. Megestrol acetate	These drugs regress metastatic endometrial mass in high doses only. These are used only as second line hormone therapy and have been superceded by aromatase inhibitors (see above).	Metastatic endometrial and breast carcinomas	Oedema, acne, hirsutism, decreased libido, neurotoxicity
I. ***Estrogens* (Ch. 43)**			
98. Diethylstilbestrol 99. Ethinyl estradiol	They suppress pituitary LH secretion via negative feedback effects and thus inhibit testosterone production in testis. Surprisingly, high-dose estrogen therapy controls the growth of metastatic breast cancer. Estrogens have also been superceded by Gn-RH agonists and antagonists or by anti-estrogen therapy (see above).	Breast and prostate carcinoma	Gynaecomastia (males), breast tenderness (females), oedema, migraine headache, thrombosis
J. ***Androgens* (Ch. 44)**			
100. Testosterone propionate 101. Fluoxymesterone	In premenopausal state they act by modifying the hormonal environment in estrogen/progesterone dependent carcinoma.	ER dependent breast cancer	Masculinisation, oedema, alopecia, acne, cholestatic jaundice, hypercalcaemia
X. Monoclonal Antibodies (MAbs)**			
A. *Naked MAbs*			
102. Rituximab (chimeric)	Targets CD20 B-cell antigen which activates cell cycle initiation and differentiation. Acts through ADCC, CDC and apoptosis.	B-cell lymphoma, chronic lymphocytic leukaemia	Infusion related hypersensitivity (fever, rash, dyspnoea); late onset neutropenia
103. Epratuzumab (humanised)	Binds to CD22 B-cell antigen.	Non-Hodgkin's lymphoma and SLE (Phase III trials)	Not serious
104. Alemtuzumab (humanised)	Targets CD52 antigen present on B- and T-cell lymphomas. Induces cell death through ADCC, CDC and apoptosis.	B-cell chronic lymphoid leukaemia and T-cell lymphoma	Infusion related reaction; immunosuppression, T-cell depletion with risk of infections

contd.

Drug and Category	Mechanism of Action	Clinical Use	Adverse Effects
105. Trastuzumab (Herceptin; humanised)	Targets against human epidermal growth factor receptor protein-2 (HER-2). HER-2/neu receptor is over-expressed in breast cancer. Trastuzumab down-regulates HER-2/neu proliferation by inhibiting HER-2 signaling with G_1 arrest. It induces cytotoxicity through ADCC and apoptosis.	Breast cancer	Infusion related toxicity, GIT enterotoxicity, cardiomyopathy
106. Cetuximab (chimeric) 107. Panitumumab (fully human IgG2 Mab against EGFR)	Block epidermal growth factor receptor (EGFR). Over-expression of EGFR is linked to tumour progression in colorectal cancer and in multiple epithelial cancers of lung, breast, prostate and pancreas. Cytotoxicity involves inhibition of EGF binding to EGFR & its signaling through tyrosine kinase domain leading to apoptosis. Role of ADCC is uncertain with panitumumab but is significant with *cetuximab*.	Colorectal cancer, non-small cell lung carcinoma, breast and pancreatic carcinoma. *Panitumumab* is approved for colorectal cancer.	Infusion related toxicity, skin rash (70–75%). *Panitumumab* is safer but like cetuximab may produce acneiform-type rashes
108. Bevacizumab (humanised)	Targets against vascular endothelial growth factor (VEGF) and inhibits its interaction with VEGF receptors. VEGF is an angiogenic growth factor and its expression is increased in a variety of cancers. Its over-expression correlates with neovascularisation and an increase in micro-vessel density within tumour masses. Bevacizumab inhibits angiogenesis and neovascularisation.	Metastatic colorectal cancer (used with 5-FU), renal cell carcinoma and breast cancer (used with chemotherapy). It is also used to restore hearing in patients suffering deafness due to neurofibromatosis type-2 related tumours.	Hypertension, mild neutropenia, risk of congestive heart failure, pulmonary haemorrhage, proteinuria.
109. Edrecolomab (murine)	Binds to glycoprotein 17-IA.	Colorectal cancer	Infusion related toxicity, skin rash.
110. Ipilimumab	Binds cytotoxic T-lymphocyte associated antigen-4 (CTLA-4) expressed on activated T-cell and causes tumour regression	Metastatic melanoma	Immune mediated entro-colitis, hepatitis and dermatitis
B. *MAbs-Cytotoxic conjugates*			
111. Gemtuzumab ozogamicin (It is a conjugate of MAb against CD33 antigen with a	Directed against CD33 antigen found on most of the acute myeloid leukaemia cells and myelodysplasias. Once bound to CD33, it undergoes endocytosis with discharge	Acute myeloid leukaemia	Infusion related toxicity, myelosuppression, hepatotoxicity

contd.

Drug and Category	Mechanism of Action	Clinical Use	Adverse Effects
potent anticancer-antibiotic calicheamicin)	of calicheamicin within the lysosome which then enters the nucleus to cause double stranded DNA breaks & apoptosis		
112. Brentuximab, Vedotin [It is a conjugate of Mab against CD30 antigen with cytotoxic drug monomethyl auristatin E (MMAE)]	The drug conjugate is directed against CD30 which is a membrane gp in the TNF receptor family. CD30 is express on activative CD4 and CD8 T-cells and B-cells. It is also highly expressed on Reed-Sternberg cells in Hodgkin's lymphoma and on anaplastic large cell lymphoma cells. The drug-Mab conjugate after endocytosis through CD30 binding release MMAE and disrupt microtubule polymerezation during cell cycle G2 to M phase and subsequent apoptosis of CD30 expressing cells.	Relapsed/refractory classic Hodgkin's lymphoma	Peripheral sensory neuropathy, fatigue nausea, vomiting, diarrhoea, neutropenia
C. *Radioisotope based MAbs*			
113. Ibritumomab-^{90}Y (Yttrium-90 radio-nucleotide conjugated to ibritumomab) 114. Tostitumomab-^{131}I (Iodine-131 radio-nucleotide conjugated to tostitumomab)	These are anti-CD20 murine MAbs that are similar to rituximab (see above), but they have additional mechanism of inducing cytotoxicity. The associated radiation source also provides targeted delivery of radioactive particles to nearby tumour clusters in which the blood circulation is unable to deliver MAbS. ^{90}Y is only a β-emitter (no γ-emission as in ^{131}I) and hence is easier and safer to use even in outpatient settings. It also has better radiation penetration in lymphomas of larger diameter.	Follicular low grade non-Hodgkin's lymphoma (NHL), also refractory indolent NHL	Neutropenia, thrombocytopenia, infusion related toxicity, hypothyroidism (with ^{131}I)
XI. Histone Deacetylase (HDAC) Inhibitors			
115. Vorinostat	HDAC are the enzymes which prevent acetylation of lysine residues on histones. Acetylation increases the distance between the DNA	Cutaneous T-cell lymphoma	Nausea, vomiting, anaemia, thrombocytopenia, hyperglycaemia, fatigue and deep vein thrombosis (though rare)

contd.

Drug and Category	Mechanism of Action	Clinical Use	Adverse Effects
	strands and the histone proteins in the nucleosome (a structure that has DNA strands wrapped around histone proteins). This increased distance allows entry of transcription factors which promote transcription of proapoptotic genes and other genes that were selectively repressed in tumour cells. *Vorinostat* being HDAC inhibitor increases histone.		
XII. Hedgehog (Hh) signalling pathway Inhibitor			
116. Vismodegib	Hh family secretes proteins that govern a wide variety of processes during embryonic development and adult tissue homeostasis.	Basal cell carcinoma	Alopecia, dysgeusia, ageusia, weight loss, fatigue, nausea, diarrhoea, decreased appatite, arthralgias
XIII. Protectants* **			
A. *Colony stimulating factors (CSF)*			
117. Filgrastim 118. Sargramostim	Filgrastim is a human recombinant granulocyte colony stimulating factor (rG-CSF), while sargramostim (GM-CSF) is a human recombinant granulocyte and macrophages colony stimulating factor. They enhance neutrophil functions, including phagocytosis and antibody dependent killing, accelerate bone marrow repopulation after high-dose chemotherapy, radiotherapy and bone marrow transplant (Ch. 69)	To prevent chemotherapy induced neutropenia, to increase neutrophil counts, and to prevent infection	Fever, myalgia, bone pain, pericardial effusions
B. *Thiophosphate cytoprotectants*			
119. Amifostine	Amifostine is metabolised by membrane-bound alkaline phosphatase into an active free thiol. Compared to neoplastic tissues, normal tissues rapidly accumulate this free thiol by facilitated	Administered before cisplatin to reduce incidence of nephrotoxicity; and before radiation therapy for head and neck cancer to	Hypotension, nausea, vomiting

contd.

Drug and Category	Mechanism of Action	Clinical Use	Adverse Effects
	diffusion. This active thiol covalently binds to cisplatin, taxanes and anthracycline group of anticancer drugs in normal tissues and inactivates them to minimise the risk of renal toxicity and other cytotoxicities.	reduce xerostomia (where radiation affects a substantial portion of parotid gland)	
C. ***Acrolein conjugator***			
120. Mesna	Acrolein is a nephrotoxic metabolite of cyclophosphamide and ifosfamide causing haemorrhagic cystitis. Mesna conjugates with acrolein in urine reducing the incidence of renal toxicity due to cyclophosphamide and ifosfamide.	Coadministered with cyclophosphamide or ifosfamide to prevent haemorrhagic cystitis	Nausea, vomiting
D. ***Iron chelator***			
121. Dexrazoxane	Anthracycline group of antibiotics, by virtue of their quinone group, generate free radicals which attack DNA and oxidise DNA bases in normal tissues. This production of free radicals is catalysed by their interaction with iron. Dexrazoxane helps natural defense mechanisms, such as action of superoxide dismutase (against free radicals) by chelating the iron and thus protects against cardiotoxicity.	Coadministered with doxorubicin in patients of breast carcinoma to reduce the incidence of cardiomyopathy	Myelosuppression, alterations in liver and renal function test results
E. ***Thrombopoietic growth factors***			
122. Oprelvekin (interleukin-11, IL-11)	IL-11 is a cytokine which stimulates megakaryocytes and their precursors in the bone marrow. Oprelvekin, therefore, prevents severe thrombocytopenia and decreases the need for platelet transfusions in cancer patients receiving highly myelosuppressive	To prevent chemotherapy-induced thrombocytopenia	Peripheral oedema, palpitations, dyspnoea, myalgia, arthralgia, fatigue
123. Thrombopoietin		- do -	Immunogenicity (formation of antirecombinant thrombopoietin antibodies) which subsequently negates the benefits

contd.

Drug and Category	Mechanism of Action	Clinical Use	Adverse Effects
	chemotherapy. *Oprelvekin* is a recombinant human IL-11. **Thrombopoietin** is a high molecular weight glycoprotein and is also a primary regulator of platelet production. Recombinant human thrombopoietin also reduces the duration of thrombocytopenia and the need for platelet transfusion in cancer patients receiving carboplatin or cyclophosphamide.		
124. Levamisole	It is an anthelmintic drug (Ch. 63) that has been found to enhance T-cell functions and cellular immunity	Combined with 5-fluorouracil to improve survival of colorectal cancer patients	Flu-like symptoms, nausea, vomiting
Other New Drugs			
125. Enfortumab vedotin	Binds to Nectin-4, an extracellular adhesion protein and inhibits replication of cells	Refractory bladder cancer	Peripheral neuropathy, fatigue, alopecia, anaemia, rash
126. Darolutamide	Competitively inhibits androgens from binding to their receptors. Decreases prostate cancer cell proliferation	Non-metastatic prostate cancer	Neutropenia, fatigue, increased bilirubin, weight gain, haemorrhage, hypertension
127. Selinexor	Binds and inhibits exportin-1 (XPO1), a nuclear protein which reactivates tumour suppressing proteins and induces apoptosis	Relapsed or refractory multiple myeloma (RRMM)	Leukopenia, thrombocytopenia, fatigue, hyperglycaemia, upper respiratory tract infection
128. Polatuzumab vedotin	It binds to CD79 conjugated to the antineoplastic agent monomethyl auristatin E (MMAE), which inhibits cell proliferation	Refractory large B-cell lymphoma	Increased creatinine, neutropenia, anaemia, hypocalcaemia, infusion reactions
129. Erdafitinib	Selective fibroblast growth factor receptor (FGFR) kinase inhibitor	Advanced or metastatic bladder cancer	Fatigue, dry mouth, increased creatinine, decreased appetite, hyponatraemia
130. Relugolix	Gonadotropin-releasing hormone (GnRH) receptor antagonist	Advanced prostate cancer	Hyperglycaemia, anaemia, fatigue, weight gain, myalgia, hot flush

contd.

Drug and Category	Mechanism of Action	Clinical Use	Adverse Effects
131. Margetuximab	It is an Fc-engineered, monoclonal antibody that targets the HER2 oncoprotein cells	Breast cancer	Nausea, increased ALT, AST, lymphopenia, alopecia, cough
132. Lurbinectedin	It is an alkylating drug that binds to guanine residues in the minor groove of DNA and forms DNA adducts	Metastatic small cell lung cancer	Leukopenia, fatigue, dyspnoea, hyponatraemia, cough
133. Selpercatinib	Potent and selective RET kinase inhibitor	Lung and thyroid cancer	Dry mouth, increase ALT, AST, hyperglycaemia, leukopenia
134. Pemigatinib	Blocks phosphorylation and signalling of FGFR1-3 and reduces cell viability	Cholangiocarcinoma	Alopecia, arthralgia, dry mouth, hyperglycaemia, dysgeusia
135. Tazemetostat	Selective EZH2 inhibitor, which induces cell cycle arrest and apoptosis of lymphoma cells	Epithelioid sarcoma	Injection site pain, hyperglycaemia, hyponatraemia, vomiting, increased triglyceride
136. Tisotumab vedotin	Tissue factor (TF) directed antibody drug conjugate (ADC) having cytotoxic effects	Recurrent or metastatic cervical cancer	Alopecia, epistaxis, myalgia, peripheral neuropathy
137. Sotorasib	Selective inhibitor of KRAS G12C, which inhibits cell proliferation	Non-small cell lung cancer	Myalgia, anaemia, hepatotoxicity, cough, edema
138. Loncastuximab tesirine	Binds to CD19, internalized into the cell, releases SG3199 which forms highly cytotoxic DNA	B-cell lymphoma	Edema, anaemia, thyombocytopenia, dyspnoea, pruritus
139. Umbralisib	Dual inhibitor of phosphoinositide 3 kinase (PI3K) delta and casein kinase 1 (CK1) epsilon	Marginal zone lymphoma	Increased creatinine, neutropenia, upper respiratory tract infection, rash
140. Futibatinib	It is a selective FGFR1-4 inhibitor. It inhibits FGFR phosphorylation and downstream signalling	Intrahepatic cholangiocarcinoma	Alopecia, neutropenia, myalgia, hyponatraemia, dry mouth
141. Sonidegib	An antagonist to Hedgehog (Hh) pathway and inhibits further signalling	Breast cell carcinoma	Muscle spasm, alopecia, decreased appetite, fatigue

contd.

Drug and Category	Mechanism of Action	Clinical Use	Adverse Effects
142. Trifluridine/ Tipiracil	Trifluridine is incorporated in DNA and inhibits DNA synthesis. Tipiracil inhibits thymidine phosphorylase, which degrades trifluridine. Thus, tipiracil boosts the level of trifluridine	Fixed dose combination is used for colorectal cancer	Neutropenia, leukopenia, anaemia, thrombocytopenia, respiratory tract infection
143. Ribociclib	It inhibits cyclin dependent kinases (CDK) 4 and 6; blocks cellular proliferation of G1 to S phase of the cell cycle	Hormone receptor (HR)-positive; human epidermal growth factor receptor 2 (HER2)-negative, metastatic breast cancer	Neutropenia, leukopenia, diarrhoea, rash, back pain
144. Palbociclib	Cyclin-dependent kinases (CDK) 4, 6 inhibitor	Advanced or metastatic breast cancer	Neutropenia, leukopenia, anaemia, alopecia, stomatitis
145. Cobimetinib	Reversible inhibitor of mitogen-activated protein kinase (MAPK)/extracellular signal regulated kinase 1, MEK1 and MEK2	Metastatic melanoma in combination with vemurafenib	Increased alkaline phosphatase, lymphopenia, anaemia, hyponatraemia
146. Olaparib	Inhibitor of poly-ADP-ribose polymerase (PARP) enzyme	Ovarian cancer	Nausea, anaemia, leukopenia, neutropenia
147. Talimogene laherparepvec	It is an oncolytic immuno-therapy for melanoma. Consists of genetically modified herpes simplex virus 1 causes lysis of tumour cells	Melanoma	Fatigue, chills, fever, injection site reactions, myalgia
148. Pralatrexate	Inhibits the enzyme dihydrofolate reductase. Disrupts DNA synthesis	T cell lymphoma	Mucositis, altered liver functions, fever, anaemia, neutropenia
149. Apalutamide	It is an oral anti-androgen. Acts as an androgen receptor inhibitor	Non-metastatic prostate cancer	Hypertension, weight loss, hypothyroidism, QT interval prolongation
150. Tisagenl-ecleucel	This drug is available by using patient's own T cells, then a transgene is introduced encoding a chimeric antigen receptor (CAR). It identifies and eliminate CD19-expressing malignant cells	B-cell precursor acute lymphoblastic leukaemia (ALL)	Cytokine release syndrome, hypotension, coagulopathy, febrile neutropenia, confusion, delirium
151. Abemaciclib	Inhibits cyclin-dependent kinases (CDKs) 4 and 6	Hormone receptor (HR)-positive and HER2 -negative, metastatic breast cancer	Diarrhoea, neutropenia, nausea, increased infections

contd.

Drug and Category	Mechanism of Action	Clinical Use	Adverse Effects
152. Dinutuximab	Binds to the glycolipid disialoganglioside (GD2). Induces lysis of GD2-expressing neuroblastoma cells	Neuroblastoma	Thrombocytopenia, lymphopenia, anaemia, infusion reactions, hypotension, capillary leak syndrome
153. Trabectedin	Alkylating drug, binds to and damages DNA, having cytotoxic and anti-proliferative effects	Soft tissue sarcoma	Neutropenia, thrombocytopenia, increased liver enzymes
154. Axicabtagene ciloleucel	Binds to CD19 has cytolytic activity and stimulates T cell proliferation	Large B-cell lymphoma	Cytokine release syndrome, fever, tachycardia, hypotension, anaemia, thrombocytopenia
155. Carfilzomib	Proteasome inhibitor that irreversibly binds to the 20S proteasome, has anti-proliferative and proapoptotic activities	Multiple myeloma in combination with dexamethasone	Nausea, thrombocytopenia, dyspnoea, diarrhoea, fever, upper respiratory tract infection and hepatic dysfunction
Tyrosine Kinase Inhibitors			
156. Zanubrutinib	It is a Bruton's tyrosine kinase (BTK) inhibitor. Inhibits proliferation and survival of malignant B cells	Mantle cell lymphoma	Upper respiratory tract infection, neutropenia, anaemia, increased uric acid, rash
157. Entrectinib	Inhibits tropomyosin receptor tyrosine kinase (TRK) and anaplastic lymphoma kinase (ALK)	Metastatic non-small cell lung cancer	Increase creatinine, anemia, hyperuricemia, edema, lymphopenia
158. Pexidartinib	Tyrosine kinase inhibitor	Tenosynovial giant cell tumour	Increase cholesterol, LDH, anemia, neutropenia, edema
159. Pralsetinib	Inhibition of the rearranged during Transfection Tyrosine Kinase	To treat non-small lung cancer	Fatigue, myalgia, increase creatinine, fever, edema
160. Ripretinib	Inhibits proto-oncogene receptor Tyrosine Kinase (KIT) and platelet derived growth factor receptor A kinase	Advanced GIT - stromal tumor	Alopecia, fatigue, nausea, myalgia, increased aPTT, arthralgia, edema
161. Tucatinib	An inhibitor of HER2 tyrosine kinase	To treat advanced or metastatic HER2-positive breast cancer	Diarrhoea, anaemia, stomatitis, hepatotoxicity, increased creatinine
162. Avapritinib	Tyrosine Kinase Inhibitor	Gastrointestinal stromal tumour (GIST)	Anaemia, edema, leukopenia, increase bilirubin
163. Asciminib	Allosteric inhibitor of the BCR-ABL1 tyrosine kinase	Chronic myeloid leukaemia	Increased uric acid, thrombocytopenia, rash, fatigue

contd.

Drug and Category	Mechanism of Action	Clinical Use	Adverse Effects
164. Mobocertinib	A potent epidermal growth factor receptor tyrosine kinase inhibitor (TKI)	Advanced or metastatic non-small cell lung cancer	Stomatitis, QTc prolongation, cough, dry skin
165. Infigratinib	Fibroblast growth factor receptor (FGFR)-specific tyrosine kinase inhibitor	To treat cholangio-carcinoma	Fatigue, arthralgia, decreased phosphate, alopecia
166. Tepotinib	It is a MET tyrosine kinase inhibitor. Blocks MET phosphorylation and subsequent downstream signalling	Non-small cell lung cancer	Edema, hypoalbuminaemia, fatigue, myalgia, dyspnoea, leukopenia
167. Cabozantinib	Tyrosine kinase inhibitor that targets RET, MET, VEGFR-1, -2, and -3 and TIE-2 pathways	Renal cell carcinoma	Diarrhoea, hypertension, lymphopenia, stomatitis, weight loss
168. Midostaurin	Inhibits multiple receptor tyrosine kinases including related to FLT3 and KIT, induces apoptosis of leukaemic cells	For adults with acute myeloid leukaemia (AML)	Headache, neutropenia, hypocalcaemia, increased ALT, mucositis
169. Lenvatinib	Receptor tyrosine kinase (RTK) inhibitor that inhibits vascular endothelial growth factor (VEGF) receptors	Thyroid cancer, renal cell cancer	Hypertension, diarrhoea, fatigue, arthralgia, myalgia
170. Alectinib	Tyrosine kinase inhibitor that targets ALK and RET and further signalling	Non-small cell lung cancer	Anaemia, Fatigue, Hyperglycaemia, Edema, Hypokalaemia, Myalgia
171. Ceritinib	Tyrosine kinase inhibitor	Non-small cell lung cancer	Elevated liver enzymes, QT interval prolongation, fatal pneumonitis, hyperglycaemia
172. Neratinib	Irreversible tyrosine kinase inhibitor (TKI), inhibits EGFR, HER2 and HER4 activities	Early-stage HER2-breast cancer, following adjuvant trastuzumab-based therapy	Fatigue, nausea, diarrhoea, stomatitis, muscle spasm
173. Acalabrutinib	Inhibits Bruton Tyrosine Kinase (BTK), inhibits B cell signalling and proliferation	Mantle cell lymphoma, chronic lymphocytic leukaemia	Headache, neutropenia, anemia, thrombocytopenia, bleeding
174. Brigatinib	Tyrosine kinase inhibitor	Anaplastic lymphoma kinase (ALK)–positive, metastatic non-small cell lung cancer	Cough, lymphopenia, anaemia, dyspnoea, anorexia

contd.

Drug and Category	Mechanism of Action	Clinical Use	Adverse Effects
175. Lorlatinib	Inhibitor of C-ros oncogene (ROS1) and anaplastic lymphoma kinase (ALK) tyrosine kinase	Metastatic non-small cell lung cancer (NSCLC)	Hyperlipidaemia, edema, peripheral neuropathy, arthralgia, anaemia
Monoclonal Antibodies			
176. Naxitamab	Humanized anti-GD2 mAb with high receptor affinity. It has antibody-dependent cell-mediated cytotoxicity	Refractory neuroblastoma	Infusion related reaction, tachycardia, lymphopenia, hyperglycaemia, electrolyte abnormalities
177. Tafasitamab	It reduces circulating B-cell counts by binding to a surface antigen, CD19, important for their survival	To treat relapsed or refractory B-cell lymphoma	Hyperglycaemia, neutropenia, diarrhoea, fatigue, cough, hypoalbuminaemia
178. Sacituzumab govitecan	It is a conjugate of the anti-Trop-2 monoclonal antibody linked with SN-38, a metabolite of irinotecan which delivers a drug into tumours.	Metastatic breast cancer	Severe neutropenia, anaemia, fatigue, respiratory tract infection, rash
179. Amivantamab	Bispecific epidermal growth factor (EGF) receptor-directed and mesenchymal-epithelial transition (MET) receptor-directed antibody	Non-small cell lung cancer	Increased AST, ALT, paronychia, hyperglycaemia, stomatitis
180. Dostarlimab	It is a programmed death receptor-1 (PD-1)-blocking antibody	Endometrial cancer	Fatigue, anaemia, hyponatraemia, cough
181. Tremelimumab	Anti-CTLA4 monoclonal antibody that blocks the inhibitory signal resulting from CTLA-4 binding to CD80/86 leads to T-cell activation	Hepatocellular carcinoma	Hyperglycaemia, decreased appetite, fatigue, fever, increased bilirubin, pruritus
182. Atezolizumab	Monoclonal antibody to programmed cell death ligand-1 (PDL1); it inhibits the suppression of immune response against tumour cells	Non-small cell lung cancer	Fatigue, nausea, vomiting, diarrhoea, musculoskeletal pain
183. Inotuzumab	CD22-directed antibody-drug conjugate (ADC) recognizes human CD22. It induces double-strand DNA break and apoptotic death of cells	Acute lymphoblastic leukaemia (ALL)	Febrile neutropenia, fever, sepsis, septic shock, respiratory failure
184. Daratumumab	Monoclonal antibody that binds with high affinity to the CD38 molecule	Multiple myeloma	Neutropenia, anaemia, cough, fatigue

contd.

Drug and Category	Mechanism of Action	Clinical Use	Adverse Effects
185. Avelumab	This immune check point inhibitor binds to the programmed cell death ligand 1, leads to reactivation of immune response to cancer cells	Markel cell carcinoma	Infusion reactions, fatigue, peripheral edema, anaemia
186. Durvalumab	Human IgG1 monoclonal antibody, which blocks PD-L1 binding to PD-1 and CD80 and activates T cells to recognise tumour cells	Non-small cell lung cancer, urothelial carcinoma	Fatigue, nausea, diarrhoea, decreased appetite, fever

* Some texts prefer to classify denileukin diftitox as toxin-based monoclonal antibody.
**For details refer, text and Ch. 3; ADCC—Antibody-dependent cellular cytotoxicity; CDC—Complement-dependent cytotoxicity.
***Also known as *"Biological response modifiers"* or as the *"Fourth modality of cancer therapy."*

most affected because of their shorter life span (6–12 hrs). A significant decrease is observed in neutrophil counts (*neutropenia*) which predisposes the patients to various infections. ***Colony stimulating factors*** (Table 67.1) can be used to increase neutrophil production and to reduce the degree and duration of neutropenia.

Platelets have an intermediate life span (5–10 days) and are affected next. Decreased platelets (*thrombocytopenia*) can lead to bleeding and may require platelet transfusion or the use of thrombopoietic growth factors, e.g., ***oprelvekin*** or ***thrombopoietin*** (Table 67.1).

Anaemia and *fatigue* can also occur but at a later stage because of longer life span of RBCs (120 days). Human recombinant **erythropoietin** may be used to increase haemoglobin and to decrease transfusion requirements. In general, onset of myelosuppression takes about 7–10 days from the start of chemotherapy. Lowest counts are reached in 10–14 days. Recovery occurs after 2–3 weeks of stopping the chemotherapy. Hence the patient's counts must be sufficiently recovered before receiving next chemotherapy.

Dermatological Toxicity

Many anticancer drugs (cyclophosphamide, ifosfamide, doxorubicin, vincristine, methotrexate, mechlorethamine and paclitaxel) damage hair follicles and produce partial or complete alopecia. Hair usually reappear after completion of chemotherapy.

Cancer chemotherapy may cause hyperpigmentation of skin (bleomycin, hydroxyurea, 5-fluorouracil and methotrexate). Local necrosis may result from extravasation of some chemotherapeutic agents like dactinomycin, daunorubicin, doxorubicin, idarubicin, mitomycin, vinca alkaloids and monoclonal antibodies.

GIT Toxicity

Carmustine, cisplatin, cyclophosphamide, dacarbazine, mechlorethamine, cytarabine, doxorubicin, lomustine, procarbazine, temozolomide and thiotepa are highly emetogenic. They stimulate both CTZ as well as vomiting center. ***Ondansetron*** and antihistamines can prevent such type of emesis (Ch. 28). Stomatitis is a common toxicity of many chemotherapeutic agents (e.g., capecitabine, 5-fluorouracil, methotrexate, mercaptopurine, thioguanine, fludarabine, cytarabine and doxorubicin). However, it resolves in 10–14 days of stopping the therapy. Other GI toxicities include *diarrhoea* (e.g., irinotecan, 5-fluorouracil), *constipation* (e.g., vincristine), *anorexia*, *taste changes* and *xerostomia* (e.g., with radiotherapy). ***Amifostine***, a cytoprotective agent (Table 67.1), can reduce the incidence of xerostomia.

Neurotoxicity

Neurotoxicity can occur not only by intrathecal chemotherapy but also by systemic chemotherapy. Vincristine is associated with peripheral neuropathies. Its intrathecal administration results in fatal neurotoxicity. Capecitabine, oxaliplatin, and paclitaxel cause sensory neuropathy (tingling and numbing of hands and feet). Peripheral neuropathy with ototoxicity is a dose limiting toxicity of cisplatin. Cytarabine and 5-fluorouracil cause cerebellar toxicity manifested by ataxia, and loss of coordination between eyes and hands. Arachnoiditis may result with intrathecal administration of cytarabine and methotrexate.

Renal Toxicity

Nephrotoxicity is associated with cisplatin, ifosfamide and methotrexate. ***Amifostine*** may be used to protect the kidneys from the nephrotoxic effects of cisplatin (Table 67.1).

Haemorrhagic Cystitis

This bladder toxicity is most commonly seen with cyclophosphamide and ifosfamide. Acrolein, a toxic metabolite of these agents, causes bladder irritation and damage, resulting in bleeding episodes. ***Mesna*** binds to this active metabolite—acrolein—and provides protection against chemotherapy-induced haemorrhagic cystitis (Table 67.1).

Hepatotoxicity

Asparaginase, cytarabine, mercaptopurine, thioguanine and methotrexate are known to cause hepatotoxicity that is manifested as jaundice, hepatitis and elevation in liver transaminase enzymes.

Cardiotoxicity

Anticancer drugs that are associated with chronic cardiotoxicity (such as precipitation of congestive heart failure) are daunorubicin, doxorubicin, epirubicin, idarubicin and mitoxantrone, trastuzumab and bevacizumab. ***Dexrazoxane*** is a cardioprotectant that can be used with daunorubicin or doxorubicin to minimise their cardiotoxicity (Table 67.1).

Pulmonary Toxicity

Chemotherapeutic agents associated with pulmonary toxicity (pulmonary fibrosis, shortness of breath, cough and low-grade fever) include bleomycin, melphalan, chlorambucil, busulfan, carmustine and mitomycin. Erlotinib produces interstitial lung disease; oxaliplatin causes pharyngo-laryngeal dysaesthesia while bevacizumab leads to pulmonary haemorrhage.

Infertility

Most of the alkylating agents such as cylophosphamide, chlorambucil, thiotepa, mechlorethamine, melphalan, as well as procarbazine are associated with significant incidence of infertility in males as well as females, which may be temporary or even permanent.

Hypersensitivity Reactions

Life-threatening hypersensitivity reactions, including anaphylaxis, appear to be more common with asparaginase, carboplatin, cisplatin, etoposide, teniposide and paclitaxel. Skin rash is more common with procarbazine, retinoids, cetuximab and denileukin diftitox. Chills and fever (temporal site) are commonly associated with bleomycin, cytarabine, monoclonal antibodies and oprelvekin (IL-11).

Tumour Lysis Syndrome (TLS)

This usually occurs in leukaemias and lymphomas, where there is a high tumour cell burden or in rapidly proliferating tumours. During treatment with chemotherapy, there is spontaneous lysis of cells which causes release of intracellular contents such as potassium, phosphate and uric acid. TLS may be prevented by adequate hydration, alkalinisation of urine and by giving allopurinol (to decrease uric acid).

Miscellaneous Side Effects

Conjunctivitis—*Cytarabine*; Inappropriate ADH secretion (SIADH)—*Ifosfamide*, *melphalan*, *cyclophosphamide* and *vinblastine*; Hypocalcaemia and hypokalaemia—*Pilcamycin*; Teratogenesis—*Ifosfamide*, *melphalan*, *retinoids*; Hypothyroidism—*Tostitumomab*-^{131}I and *bexarotene* (*a retinoid*); Haemorrhagic pancreatitis—*Asparaginase*; Disulfiram like effects with alcohol—*Procarbazine*.

RESISTANCE TO CYTOTOXIC DRUGS

Cancers can be regarded as population of cells undergoing spontaneous mutations and as the tumour grows, increasing number of mutations occur. Some tumour types, e.g., malignant melanoma, brain cancer and renal cell cancer, exhibit *primary resistance* (absence of response to standard drug from the very first exposure). *Acquired resistance* develops during continuation of therapy. Primary resistance is associated with the inherent genomic instability linked with the development of cancer, while acquired resistance may result from either adaptation of the tumour cells or due to mutation with amplification or increased expression of one or more specific genes. Tumours that are resistant to drugs at the outset will always have a largely drug-resistant population from the beginning and will be refractory to treatment. The mechanisms of resistance in cancer cells, though imperfectly understood, appear to include:

1) During the course of therapy the tumour cells exhibit either decreased accumulation (uptake) or decreased retention of the cytotoxic drugs. This type of resistance is called *multidrug resistance* and is the major form of resistance to anthracycline group of antibiotics, vinca alkaloids, etoposide, paclitaxel and dactinomycin. The gene that confers **m**ulti**d**rug **r**esistance is termed as MDR-1 gene. In cancer cells, there is an over-expression of this gene which encodes a high molecular weight membrane protein called *P-glycoprotein*. The physiological role of P-glycoprotein is to protect cells against foreign toxins. It picks up drugs as they enter the cell membrane and throws them out. This transport protein

requires ATP to expel a variety of foreign molecules, i.e., its action is not limited to anticancer drugs alone. This protein is present constitutively in normal tissues, e.g., epithelial cells of kidney, intestines, adrenal gland, bile canaliculi and astrocytes in brain. It is generally expressed over a wide range of tumour cells also. Calcium channel blockers such as verapamil, diltiazem, nicardipine, and some other non-cytotoxic drugs like quinidine, cyclosporine and valspodar (immunosuppressive analogue of cyclosporine) may reverse this type of resistance and their use in this situation is being explored.

2) Multidrug resistance also occurs due to an over-expression of a **m**ulti-**d**rug **r**esistant **p**rotein-**1** (MDRP-1). Its over-expression also increases resistance to anthracyclins, vinca alkaloids, taxanes and epipodophyllotoxin by acting as a "drug efflux pump".
3) Three major pathways have been noted for the development of resistance to methotrexate: (i) decreased uptake of the drug into the tumour cell, (ii) alteration in the structure of dihydrofolate reductase (DHFR) enzyme, resulting in a reduced drug affinity and (iii) an increase in DHFR content in tumour cell as a result of its gene amplification.
4) Possible mechanisms of resistance to *alkylating agents* include (i) rapid repair of drug-induced DNA damage, (ii) an increase in cell thiol contents, which in turn can serve as an alternative target of alkylation. Tumour cell resistance to cisplatin is associated with an increase in metallothionein content.
5) Antimetabolites may be ineffective because of insufficient activation of the drug. For example, 5-fluorouracil may not be converted to FdUMP; cytarabine may not undergo phosphorylation and 6-mercaptopurine may not be converted into "fraudulent" nucleotide (see text above).
6) A drug may be inactivated by resistant tumour by enzymatic metabolism, e.g., cytarabine (pyrimidine nucleoside deaminase) and bleomycin (bleomycin hydrolase). On the contrary, leukaemias have been shown to develop resistance to L-asparaginase due to drug related induction of the enzyme asparaginase synthetase (Table 67.1):
7) There may be drug-induced alteration in the activity of target enzyme, e.g., modified topoisomerase-II in case of resistance to doxorubicin.

PREFERRED COMBINATION CHEMOTHERAPY FOR CERTAIN MALIGNANCIES

The combined use of two or more drugs is often superior to a single drug therapy in most of the cancers. The following principles have been used in designing such treatment:

1) Each drug used in combination therapy should have individual therapeutic activity against the tumour being treated.
2) The combined regimens should include drugs that act by different mechanisms. Such a combination provides additive or synergistic therapeutic effects. Furthermore, such a drug combination increases log cell kill and diminishes the probability of emergence of resistance.
3) For the combination, drugs having different dose limiting toxicities should be selected so as to avoid cumulative damage to a single organ.
4) To allow time for recovery from the acute toxic effects of cytotoxic drugs (e.g., bone marrow depression), intermittent schedules of drug treatment should be opted.
5) One or two cycles of chemotherapy are hardly sufficient to eradicate a tumour. Hence, several (4 to 6) cycles of treatment should be given.
6) If the primary tumour has been eradicated with surgery or radiation therapy, adjuvant chemotherapy should be given to decrease the chances of relapse due to micrometastases. Adjuvant chemotherapy has provided good results in breast cancer, colorectal cancer, prostate cancer and osteosarcoma in adults.

The following drug combination regimens have provided encouraging results in some selected malignancies:

1) ***Acute Lymphocytic Leukaemia*** **(ALL)**
   For induction: Vincristine (Oncovin) + Prednisolone + Asparaginase ± Doxorubicin **or** Vincristine + Prednisolone

For maintenance: Mercaptopurine + Methotrexate ± Cyclophosphamide

2) ***Acute Myeloid Leukaemia* (AML)**
For induction: Cytarabine + Daunorubicin (or Mitoxantrone or Idarubicin)
For maintenance: Same as above or etoposide

3) ***Chronic Lymphocytic Leukaemia* (CLL)**
Fludarabine + Prednisone **or** Fludarabine + Cyclophosphamide + Mitoxantrone + Dexamethasone **or** Chlorambucil + Prednisone **or** Alemtuzumab

4) ***Chronic Myeloid Leukaemia* (CML)**
Imatinib; Nilotinib; Hydroxyurea; Busulfan; Interferon alfa.

5) ***Hairy Cell Leukaemia* (HCL)**
Pentostatin **or** Cladribine **or** Interferon alfa.

6) ***Hodgkin's Disease***
Doxorubicin (Adriamycin) + Bleomycin + Vinblastine + Dacarbazine (ABVD regimen) **or** Mechlorethamine + Vincristine (Oncovin) + Procarbazine + Prednisone (MOPP regimen).

7) ***Non-Hodgkin's Lymphoma***
Cyclophosphamide + Doxorubicin + Vincristine (Oncovin) + Prednisone (CDOP or CHOP regimen; because earlier doxorubicin was named as hydroxydoxorubicin) + Rituximab (for better results).

8) ***Multiple Myeloma***
Vincristine + Doxorubicin + Dexamethasone **or** Melphalan + Prednisone (MP protocol) ± Cyclophosphamide; Bortezumab **or** Thalidomide + Dexamethasone for refractory and relapsed cases.

9) ***Polycythaemia Vera***
Busulfan **or** Chlorambucil **or** Hydroxyurea.

10) ***Breast Cancer***
Stage I: Breast surgery followed by Tamoxifen
Stage II: Postoperatively, Cyclophosphamide + Methotrexate + 5-Fluorouracil (CMF protocol)
Stage III and IV: Cyclophosphamide + Doxorubicin (Adriamycin) + 5-Fluorouracil (CAF protocol) **or** Paclitaxel + Trastuzumab (Herceptin) for HER-2 over-expressing breast cancer **or** aromatase inhibitors like Anastrozole, Letrozole or Exemestane with adjuvant chemotherapy (for hormone receptor positive cancers).

11) ***Cancer Head and Neck***
Cisplatin + Fluorouracil (or Paclitaxel or Cetuximab with radiation)

12) ***Cancer Lung***
Small Cell (*oat cell*): Cisplatin + Etoposide **or** Cisplatin + Irinotecan.
Non-small cell: Cisplatin + Gemcitabine **or** Vinorelbine **or** Paclitaxel **or** Gefitinib **or** Erlotinib.

13) ***Endometrium Carcinoma***
Progestins or Tamoxifen

14) ***Carcinoma of Ovary***
Carboplatin or Cisplatin + Paclitaxel **or** Topotecan (in patients with recurrence)

15) ***Carcinoma of Cervix***
Cisplatin + Methotrexate + Doxorubicin + Vinblastine

16) ***Choriocarcinoma***
Methotrexate + Leucovorin **or** Methotrexate + Dactinomycin **or** Etoposide + Cisplatin **or** Dactinomycin + Chlorambucil

17) ***Cancer Testis***
Cisplatin + Bleomycin + Etoposide

18) ***Cancer Prostate***
GnRH agonist (Leuprolide) + Flutamide (or Nilutamide)

19) ***Carcinoma Bladder***
Methotrexate + Vinblastine + Doxorubicin (Adriamycin) + Cisplatin (MVAC protocol)

20) ***Cancer Stomach***
Cisplatin + Fluorouracil **or** Etoposide + Leucovorin + Fluorouracil (ELF protocol) **or** Cisplatin + Irinotecan (or Paclitaxel)

21) ***Cancer Pancreas***
Gemcitabine **or** Docetaxel **or** ELF protocol **or** Erlotinib + Gemcitabine

22) ***Cancer Colon/Rectum***
Fluorouracil + Leucovorin + Irinotecan **or** Oxaliplatin + Leucovorin + 5 Fluorouracil

23) ***Cancer Thyroid***
^{131}I; Cisplatin **or** Doxorubicin

24) ***Melanoma***
Dacarbazine **or** Interferon alfa **or** Cisplatin **or** Interleukin-2

25) ***Insulinoma***
Streptozocin **or** Interferon alfa

26) ***Osteogenic Sarcoma***
Methotrexate + Leucovorin **or** Doxorubicin **or** Vincristine (but after surgery)

27) ***Wilms Tumour***
Vincristine + Dactinomycin (Actinomycin-D) (after surgery and radiotherapy) ± Doxorubicin

28) ***Ewing's Sarcoma***
Cyclophosphamide (or Ifosfamide) + Doxorubicin (Adriamycin) + Vincristine (CAV protocol)

29) ***Kaposi's Sarcoma*** (A multifocal malignant neoplasm of reticuloendothelial cells involving skin—often associated with AIDS): Doxorubicin (Adriamycin) + Bleomycin + Vincristine (ABV protocol)

30) ***Cutaneous T-cell Lymphoma***
Electron beam radiotherapy, Carmustine (topical); Denileukin diftitox ± Bexarotene (a retinoid); Vorinostat.

CURABILITY OF CANCERS WITH CHEMOTHERAPY

a) Advanced cancers with possible cure

Acute lymphoid and Acute myeloid leukaemia (adult or paediatric); Hodgkin's disease (adult or paediatric); Choriocarcinoma; Seminoma and Teratocarcinoma; Small-cell lung carcinoma; Ovarian carcinoma; Burkitt's sarcoma (adult or paediatric, it involves massive jaw lession with extranodal abdominal involvement caused by Epstein-Barr virus); Wilms tumour (paediatric; a nephroblastoma presenting as enormous sized kidney losing shape and looking soft in consistency); Ewing's sarcoma (paediatric; a cancerous bone tumour); Retinoblastoma (paediatric; malignant tumour of retina); Rhabdomyosarcoma (paediatric; tumour of skeletal muscle).

b) Advanced cancers which may be cured by chemotherapy and radiation

Squamous carcinoma (head and neck); Breast cancer; Carcinoma cervix; Small-cell and Non-small cell lung carcinoma.

c) Cancers possibly cured by surgery followed by chemotherapy

Breast cancer; Colorectal carcinoma, Soft tissue sarcoma; Osteogenic sarcoma (malignant bone tumour).

d) Advanced-stage tumours poorly responsive to chemotherapy

Pancreatic carcinoma; Thyroid carcinoma; Prostate carcinoma; Melanoma (tumour of melanin producing cells); Hepatocellular carcinoma; Non-small cell lung carcinoma.

CHAPTER 68

SECTION 13—SPECIAL TOPICS

Heavy Metal Poisoning, Chelating Drugs and Toxicology

COMPETENCY PH1.53

Toxicology deals with the toxicity of drugs and poisonous effects of various chemicals in use (household, environmental or industrial). It is also concerned with the symptoms and management of poisoning. Some of these chemical groups, which may be important health hazards, are listed below:

- ***Air Pollutants*** such as Carbon monoxide (CO), Sulfur dioxide (SO_2), Nitrogen dioxide (NO_2) and Ozone (O_3).
- ***Industrial Solvents*** such as aliphatic alcohols (methyl alcohol), aliphatic hydrocarbons (chloroform, carbon tetrachloride, trichloroethylene) and aromatic hydrocarbons (gasoline, benzene, toluene, xylene).
- ***Agriculture Pollutants*** such as *insecticides* (organophosphorous compounds, carbamates and DDT) and *herbicides* (poisons used to destroy unwanted vegetation), collectively called *pesticides*.
- ***Environmental Pollutants*** such as polychlorinated biphenyls (PCB), cyanide fumes from burning plastics and asbestos.
- ***Heavy Metal Poisons*** such as *inorganic forms* of lead, mercury, copper, iron and arsenic, and *organic forms,* e.g., tetraethyl or tetramethyl lead (a gasoline additive) and alkyl or aryl mercury salts produced by bacteria in seawater from mercury (pollution from a nearby plastic manufacturing plant).

Poisoning from these chemicals can occur due to intentional (suicidal), homicidal, accidental or occupational reasons. Except for poisoning due to heavy metals, organophosphorous compounds, methyl alcohol and cyanides, there is no specific treatment for toxicity due to other pollutants cited above except for providing support for vital functions, oxygen and symptomatic therapy. For other poisons, treatment is done by using a specific antidote and symptomatic therapy with supportive measures. Chemical poisoning due to any reason/hazard or drug poisoning due to overdose and its management has already been dealt in appropriate chapters, e.g., treatment of atropine poisoning (Ch. 11), anticholinesterases (organophosphorous com-pounds; Ch. 11), acetaminophen (paracetamol; Ch. 26), aspirin (Ch. 6 & 26), barbiturates (Ch. 6 & 32), benzodiazepines (Ch. 32), cyanides (Ch. 20), digoxin (Ch. 22), methyl alcohol (Ch. 36), opioids (Ch. 37) and psychotomimetics (Ch. 35).

GENERAL MEASURES IN THE TREATMENT OF POISONING

For all poisoning cases, systemic absorption of poison has to be prevented. *This is done by decontaminating the skin, eyes* and *GIT*. The affected parts (particularly behind the ears, under the nails and in skin folds) should be thoroughly washed with lukewarm water or saline. For oily poisons (e.g., insecticides), skin should be washed twice with soap and hair should be shampooed. Both the eyes should be flushed with copious amount of saline or water under the effects of local anaesthetic drops. Irrigation should be done until the pH of the tears is between 6.5–7.5. GIT decontamination is done either by inducing emesis, or by performing gastric lavage, or whole bowel irrigation or by using cathartics.

Emesis, using a syrup of ipecac, is a convenient and effective way to evacuate gastric poisonous contents if given in an early stage (within 30 min of ingestion). However, it should be avoided in unconscious or convulsing patients and in those cases who have ingested petroleum products (danger of aspiration lipoid pneumonia), corrosive poisons (acid or alkali) or convulsant drug (strychnine). Usual adult dose for syrup of ipecac is 30 ml in 250 ml of water. ***Gastric lavage*** is very effective for liquid or powder form of poison than for tablet or capsule and is very useful when started within 60 min of ingestion. It is useful if results of emesis are unsuccessful or when emesis is contraindicated or when gastric contents are needed for identification of poison. The procedure takes less time (5–10 min) when lavage is done by double lumen tube designed to deliver lavage fluid as well as to aspirate it out, simultaneously. ***Cathartics*** (e.g., 10% magnesium sulfate or 70% sorbitol) are also used to stimulate peristalsis. This hastens the elimination of unabsorbed poison and the activated charcoal slurry (if it has been used, see below). ***Whole bowel irrigation*** utilises large volumes of balanced polyethylene glycol-electrolyte solution, to mechanically cleanse the entire intestinal tract. The balanced electrolyte formula does not disturb the electrolyte balance of the body. It is preferred in massive iron tablets ingestion, for sustained-release tablets and enteric-coated tablets.

In the management of drug poisoning (cited above) and in certain heavy metal poisoning (cited below), *the use of activated charcoal for gastrointestinal decontamination of poison* is quite common. The activated charcoal effectively adsorbs almost all drugs and poisons. However, it should not be used in cyanide, corrosives (acid/alkali), iron, lithium and alcohol poisoning. It should not be used in comatosed or convulsing patients unless it is given by a gastric tube and the airway is protected by an endotracheal intubation. It is also contraindicated in patients with intestinal obstruction or for whom the endoscopic examination is needed.

0.5–2 g/kg of activated charcoal (max. 100 g) is administered orally (or via a gastric tube) mixed in water slurry. Repeat doses may also be given (20–30 g every 4 hr) to accelerate elimination of certain drugs, e.g., digoxin, theophylline and barbiturates ("gut-dialysis"). Emetics or purgatives should not be used concomitantly with activated charcoal mainly because it would also adsorb the emetic or purgative and also because the combination will aggravate dehydration.

Some texts refer to a formulation of activated charcoal + tannic acid + magnesium oxide as ***"Universal antidote"*** for poisoning. Lately it was found that the utility of this mixture was over-rated and the use of last 2 ingredients was redundant.

Drug/poison removal can also be facilitated by urinary manipulations, haemodialysis, haemoperfusion and peritoneal dialysis. Forced diuresis should be avoided as the risk of electrolyte balance and pulmonary oedema outweighs its benefits. Acidic drugs (salicylates, barbiturates) are more rapidly excreted with an alkaline urine; while basic drugs (amphetamine, morphine) are rapidly excreted if urine is made acidic (Ch. 6). But acidification of urine should not be attempted in presence of myoglobinuria and rhabdomyolysis. Haemodialysis or haemoperfusion are very effective but peritoneal dialysis may be employed only when haemodialysis is not available, as it is very inefficient.

TREATMENT OF HEAVY METAL POISONING

Poisoning due to heavy metals such as mercury, lead, nickel, copper, arsenic and iron usually occurs due to occupational reasons, e.g., in persons working in mines, paint industry, glass industry, pesticide industry and petroleum industry. These are also used as salts in some medicines of alternative therapy and used as ashes in many Ayurvedic medicines. Heavy metals exert their toxic effects by combining with and inactivating the functional groups (-SH, -S-S-, -NH_2, -OH, -PO_3) of vital enzymes. By doing so they interfere with the normal physiological functions of these enzymes in the body leading to toxic effects. These groups are called "Ligands". Metal poisoning is treated by using ***chelating agents*** (Greek word, *chele = claw*). A chelating agent usually contains polar groups such as -SH, -OH, -NH_2, or -COOH which can bind a metal ion in a similar fashion as endogenous ligands bind to metal ions. The chelating agents, therefore, compete with body ligands (for heavy metal binding) to form stable, nontoxic, water-soluble complexes, which are then easily excreted from the body. Selectivity of chelators for specific heavy metals and their therapeutic use is discussed below.

Prior to this we discuss the toxicology of heavy metals.

TOXICOLOGY OF HEAVY METALS

Mercury

Mercury exists in 3 chemical forms: ***elemental mercury,*** which is liquid at room temperature and is used as a primary component in making dental amalgam or used to prepare its ash ("Bhasm") in Ayurvedic medicine; ***inorganic mercury salts,*** which are either mercurous (Hg^{+}) or mercuric salts (Hg^{2+}). These are rarely used but mercuric salts are more toxic; ***organic mercury salts,*** of which methylmercury is the most important toxicologically.

Interestingly, all the 3 forms of this single element provide strikingly different toxic effects. For example ***elemental mercury*** is virtually non-toxic as it is not absorbed from GIT. But, if it is vapourised and inhaled, it is absorbed in the blood to produce chest pain, shortness of breath, gastroenteritis, nausea, vomiting, tremors, kidney and CNS damage.

Inorganic mercury salts ($HgCl_2$) on acute poisoning leads to severe haemorrhagic gastroenteritis and acute tubular necrosis. Chronic toxicity with $HgCl_2$ is presented with gingivo-stomatitis and gastroenteritis followed, much later, with renal toxicity; CNS toxicity is rare. Poisoning with ***organic mercury salts*** usually results by eating fish containing high contents of methyl mercury (produced by sea bacteria from mercury waste delivered by nearby plastic manufacturing units). The disease was first noted in 1940 among the inhabitants of local fishing community around Minamata Bay in Japan and was labeled as *Minamata disease.* Organic mercury toxicity also results from eating flour grounded from food-grain preserved with methyl mercury. Its consumption leads to chronic toxicity characterised by birth defects and CNS toxicity with behavioural changes called *erethism* (irritability, memory loss, depression and personality derangement).

Pharmacokinetics: Elemental mercury is adquately absorbed from lungs but not from GIT. Only 10% of the ingested inorganic mercury salts are absorbed from GIT, but being corrosive it can do significant damage. Organic alkylmercury compounds can be absorbed from lungs as well as from GIT. Though, all the 3 types are highly distributed to various tissues, these have highest accumulation in kidney. A small fraction may always be retained in the kidney and brain even after their excretion. Inorganic mercury is excreted by kidney (major) but also through faeces (minor). Same is true for elemental mercury. However, methylmercury undergoes biliary excretion followed by enterohepatic circulation with eventual excretion though faeces. Traces of mercury can always be found in hair and nails as it binds to -SH- groups of keratinised tissues.

Lead

The most common chronic exposure to lead is through diet. In most Asian and Middle East countries utensils used for cooking or for storage of food contain lead. It is also used in plumbing, contaminating drinking water. Lead-based paints contain high concentration of lead and because these paints have a sweet taste, young children frequently consume the chips of this paint (a condition called pica, which means eating of non-food substances). *Organic lead* (tetraethyl- or tetramethyl lead) are used as antiknock agents added to gasoline (in almost all underdeveloped countries) and are readily absorbed through skin and lungs. Occupational exposure to lead also occurs in mine workers, smelters and lead acid battery workers.

Acute inorganic lead poisoning is less common, except from industrial exposure or in children who have eaten large quantities of chips from the wall surfaces of lead-based paint. One early effect of lead exposure (in acute as well as chronic toxicity) is inhibition of haeme biosynthesis with consequent excretion of porphyrins in urine (porphyrins are intermediary products in haeme synthesis). Hence anaemia and urinary porphyrins are characteristic features indicative of lead poisoning. Other features include abdominal colic, reversible or irreversible tubular damage, neuropathies and encephalopathy (particularly in children). As many as 25% of those who develop lead encephalopathy, do not survive and up to 40–50% of those who survive develop severe neurological deficits. ***Chronic lead poisoning*** (plumbism) is much more common than the acute form. Symptoms include microcytic hypochromic anaemia with lethargy and weakness; peripheral neuropathy (wrist-drop or foot-drop), tremors, anorexia, weight loss and GIT disturbances. In children, there is growth retardation, neurocognitive deficits and loss in IQ. ***Organic lead poisoning*** (due to tetraethyl lead in gasoline) is characterised primarily by CNS toxicity which includes hallucinations, convulsions and coma.

Pharmacokinetics: In general, adults absorb about 10% of the ingested amount of lead while children absorb up to about 50%. Once absorbed, these are widely distributed to soft tissues (bone marrow, brain, kidney and liver etc.) and later to the bone matrix. In soft tissues its half-life is 1–2 months; but in skeleton, its half-life may be prolonged to years and even decades. Its route of excretion is primarily renal (70%), then faecal (20%) and rest through bile, skin, hair, nail, sweat and breast milk.

Arsenic

Arsenic exists as trivalent and pentavalent salt forms and also as hydride gas (AsH_3). Commercial applications of arsenic include its use in the manufacture of semiconductors, glass, nonferrous alloys and in veterinary pharmaceuticals. It is also released during burning of hard coke. It has also been found in subsoil water in many regions of West Bengal and Bangladesh. Arsine gas (AsH_3) is generated during the refinement and processing of certain metals. Hence, arsenic is an environmental as well as occupational hazard. Arsenic is also an established carcinogen which can cause cancer of lungs and skin. ***Acute arsenic poisoning*** causes gastroenteritis, laryngitis, dehydration and shock. A sweet garlicky odour in breath and of stool is indicative of arsenic poisoning. ***Chronic arsenic poisoning*** is characterised by skin irritation and colour change, hair loss, nausea, GIT disturbances, bone marrow depression and anaemia. *Arsine causes* massive haemoglobinuria and acute renal failure.

Pharmacokinetics: Inorganic arsenic is absorbed from GIT and skin. Arsine gas is absorbed from lungs. Arsenic crosses placental barrier. It is distributed predominantly in liver, kidney, bone marrow, skin and RBCs; also accumulates in hair and nail where it may lie for years. Its methylated metabolites are excreted in urine (major %) but also through faeces and sweat.

Iron

The pharmacology of iron preparations is discussed in Chapter 50. Haematinics are available as OTC preparations. However, an excessive exposure can lead to significant iron toxicity. Iron toxicity can be either chronic or acute. ***Chronic toxicity*** seems to be more common in people having genetic predisposition to absorb excessive amounts of iron taken orally. It is characterised by haemosiderin accumulation in liver and spleen with haemochromatosis. ***Acute toxicity*** occurs usually in children when they accidentally ingest several iron salts-containing pills. The symptoms start with vomiting and diarrhoea. The vomitus looks brown and the stool bloody. Acidosis and shock occur a few hours later. In a later phase (24–48 hrs), convulsions, cardiovascular collapse and coma ensue. For pharmacokinetics refer Chapter 50.

CHELATING AGENTS IN THE MANAGEMENT OF HEAVY METAL POISONING

Chelators spare endogenous ligands (vital enzymes and proteins) and facilitate excretion of toxic metal as chelator-metal complex (see earlier text). Selectivity for metal ions varies with individual chelator. Hence, for better therapeutic results, the chelator should be matched for the heavy metal responsible for toxicity. Clinically useful chelating agents are discussed below:

Dimercaprol (BAL)

Dimercaprol (2,3-dimercapto-1-propanol) was discovered during World War II, originally as an antidote for poisonous arsenical gas "Lewisite". Hence it is also known as British Anti-Lewisite (BAL). It is used intramuscularly in a peanut oil vehicle, for the treatment of mercury and arsenic poisoning. Two dimercaprol molecules make a complex with single mercury atom and this complex is then excreted in urine. However, the urine must be kept alkaline to avoid dissociation of the complex and subsequent reabsorption of metal. The recommended dose schedule is 5 mg/kg I.M. stat followed by

2–3 mg/kg, 8 hrly for 2 days and then once a day for 10 days. It is contraindicated in iron poisoning as BAL-Fe complex that is formed is itself toxic. In a prescribed protocol with edetate calcium disodium, BAL is also used for the treatment of lead poisoning.

Adverse effects include pain at the site of injection, tachycardia, mild increase in BP, vomiting, tingling and burning sensation in extremities, sweating, cramps and headache.

Succimer

It is 2,3-dimercapto succinic acid, a structural analogue of dimercaprol. Unlike dimercaprol it is orally effective, less toxic and more water soluble. It is more specific for lead chelation and needs no combination with edetate calcium disodium (like dimercaprol, see above). The dose for lead chelation is 10 mg/kg every 8 hrs for 5 days followed by 10 mg/kg every 12 hrs for 14 days. Succimer is equally effective in alleviating acute toxicity and preventing distribution of orally administered mercury (from mercuric chloride) into brain. It also reduces mercury contents of kidney—a key target organ for accumulation of mercury salts. It is more suitable for treating lead posioning in children.

Adverse effects include anorexia, vomiting and diarrhoea (10% incidence); occasionally rashes and elevation of liver aminotransferase enzymes (5% cases).

Disodium Calcium Salt of Ethylene Diamine Tetra-acetic Acid (EDTA)

Edetate calcium disodium complex is a chelator for many divalent (Pb, Zn, Cd, Mn and Hg) as well as trivalent (Fe) metals. In this exchange process, its own calcium is displaced from the molecule. The parent compound ethylene diamine tetra-acetic acid (EDTA) is a stronger chelator for Ca^{2+} and produces life-threatening hypocalcaemia as a side effect. This limitation has been circumvented by using disodium calcium salt of EDTA.

It is a highly polar compound, not absorbed from GIT, poorly crosses cell membranes and does not cross BBB. Hence it is given parenterally. However, I.M. injection is very painful; hence, usually given by slow I.V. route. It is rapidly excreted through glomerular filtration.

Its primary use is in lead poisoning. Edetate-lead complex is water soluble and stable. However, in severe lead poisoning, Ca^{2+} edetate is used in combination with dimercaprol (see above). The treatment protocol includes: 50–75 mg/kg/day of edetate calcium disodium by slow intravenous injection 6 hrly and dimercaprol 4 mg/kg I.M. every 4 hrs for 3–5 days.

Adverse effects include nephrotoxicity (can be prevented by maintaining adequate urine flow), myalgia, lacrimation, hypotension and nasal congestion but these are not serious.

Its related analogue ***diethylenetriamine penta acetic acid*** **(DTPA)** ***calcium disodium*** has been found useful in removing radioactive uranium and plutonium. It is less toxic and more effective but has a very poor tissue distribution. It is still under investigational stage.

Sodium Zirconium Cyclosilicate (ZS-9), Patiromer and Sodium Polystyrene Sulfonate (SPS) as Potassium (K+) Chelating Agents

Sodium Ziroconium Cyclosilicate (ZS-9) is a recently approved inorganic Na+-K+ cation exchange agent administered orally in the dose of 5–10 g dissolved in 240 mL of water alongwith a full meal. It reaches K+ equilibrium in GIT in 20 minutes and show K+-lowering effect within one hr after a 10 g oral dose. No serious AEs are associated with the use of ZS-9 in clinical trials, except GI disturbances (diarrhoea, constipation) and oedema. However, hypokalaemia was another AE (K+=3.0–3.4 mEq/L) but can be resolved after dose adjustments or K+ repletion.

Patiromer is an orally-effective powder form K+ binding polymer for the treatment of hyperkalaemia (dose 8–25 g; maximum 60 g/day). The drug shows an *in vitro* binding capacity of 8.5–8.8 mEq of K+/g of polymer.

Sodium Polystyrene Sulfonate (SPS) is a resin which possesses weakest K+-binding capacity (0.4–0.8 mEq K+/g of resin). It is administered orally in the dose of 5–15 g with 70% of sorbitol four times daily [in patients with oliguric-hyperkalaemia in chronic kidney disease (CKD)]. Sorbitol is intended to prevent SPS-associated constipation. Administration of other cathartics can also enhance the K+-excretion by SPS in the faeces.

All three Potassium Chelating agents are indicated in hyperkalaemic patients of CKD, chronic heart disease, with a history of RAAS Inhibitor drug(s) therapy.

D-Penicillamine

D-Penicillamine (dimethylcysteine or 3-mercapto-D-valine) is a water-soluble degradation product of penicillin. Its D-isomer (instead of L-isomer) is less toxic and is a highly effective chelator of copper. It is also a drug of choice in the management of Wilson's disease (a hepatolenticular degeneration due to accumulation of copper in brain, kidney, liver and cornea). It results due to genetic deficiency of ceruloplasmin whose physiological role is to eliminate excess copper if absorbed from food. For details regarding use of D-penicillamine in the management of Wilson's disease refer Chapter 40. The main use of D-penicillamine, therefore, is in the treatment of copper poisoning. Its recommended dose schedule in the treatment of Cu poisoning is 500 mg orally twice a day, 2 hrs after meal (to avoid chelation of other dietary metals).

It is also used to treat cystinuria (cystine stones) as it complexes with cystine and prevents its precipitation in the urinary tract. It is also occasionally used for the treatment of rheumatoid arthritis but its use has declined (see Ch. 26). Scleroderma patients are also benefited because it increases the solubility of collagen.

Adverse effects include hypersensitivity (not alarming) and proteinuria (rare), leukopenia and aplastic anaemia (careful monitoring is beneficial) and vit. B_6 deficiency.

Trientine (triethylene tetramine dihydrochloride) is another less toxic alternative to penicillamine. It is also effective orally (1 g BD on empty stomach). *Adverse effects* include iron deficiency. Hence, short courses of iron therapy during and after therapy can overcome this problem.

Deferoxamine (Desferrioxamine)

Desferrioxamine means such a ***ferrioxamine*** derivative which is devoid of iron (des = devoid of). Ferrioxamine, an iron chelate, is isolated from *Streptomyces pilosus* and degraded chemically to obtain iron-free ligand *deferoxamine*. It has a very high affinity for Fe^{3+}. On w/w basis 1 g chelates 85 mg of elemental iron. Its unique property is that it can remove iron from ferritin, haemosiderin and to some extent from transferrin, but not from haemoglobin.

It is not absorbed if given orally. For serious iron toxicity, it is given by I.V. route (10–15 mg/kg/hr infusion). In moderately toxic cases, it can be administered intramuscularly (50 mg/kg). For chronic iron intoxication (e.g., thalassemia) an I.M. dose of 0.5–1.0 g/day (or 500 mg B.D.) is recommended. Deferoxamine along with haemodialysis is also useful in the treatment of aluminium toxicity in renal failure. When blood is transfused to the patients of thalassaemia, usually 2 g of deferoxamine is also infused simultaneously at a rate of 15 mg/kg/hr but by a separate I.V. line (to decrease iron overload: transfusion siderosis). *Adverse effects* include diarrhoea, hypotension (if I.V. infusion is rapid), flushing and acute respiratory distress syndrome (rare and with high dose).

Two other orally-effective iron chelators: ***Deferiprone*** and ***Deferasirox*** are also available for the treatment of chronic iron overload due to frequent blood transfusions in patients with beta-thalassaemia where deferoxamine therapy is not tolerated, contraindicated or inadequate. Prolonged use of deferiprone use may lead to Zn depletion. Side effects associated are anorexia, altered taste, joint pain and reversible neutropenia. Due above reasons, it is not widely used in clinical practice.

Deferasirox has very high affinity for iron and least affinity for zinc or copper. It is better tolerated. Iron-Deferasirox chelated complex is secreted through bile and excreted in faeces. GIT upset is the major side effect (25% of the patients).

Prussian Blue (Ferric Hexacyanoferrate)

Oral Prussian Blue has been approved for the treatment of contamination with radioactive cesium (^{137}Cs) and non-radioactive thallium. Prussian Blue traps these metals in intestine and prevents their reabsorption from GIT. The metal complexes are then excreted in faeces. Prussian Blue also reduces the biological half-life of ^{137}Cs from 110 days to 30 days and of thallium from about 9 days to 3 days and therefore reduces time of body exposure to radiation. Usual adult dose is 3 g orally TDS. Monitoring of faecal radioactivity (for ^{137}Cs) and thallium concentration in urine can serve as a guideline for the duration of therapy. Constipation is the side effect of Prussian Blue.

CHAPTER 69 Immunomodulation & Immunotherapy

COMPETENCY PH1.50

Immunology deals with the physiology of "self - non-self discrimination". The immune system must not react with the "self components", otherwise **autoimmune disease** would result. The "non-self components" could be an infectious organism, a transplanted organ or an endogenous cell that can be mistaken as foreign. The immune responses of human body against any non-self are of two types, **(a) innate** (natural or non-specific) **response** and **(b) adaptive** (acquired or specific) **response**. In **immunopharmacology** we study how drugs alter or modify the immune responses of the body, while **immunotherapy** is the clinical application of the knowledge gained from the study of immunopharmacology.

Innate immunity lacks specificity ***as there is no involvement of memory cells.*** It is present since birth and uses only pre-existing but a limited set of components and receptors to recognise and destroy the invading pathogen (see below). **Adaptive** (or acquried) **immunity,** on the other hand, is specifically adapted against the invading pathogen and this response is hightened with subsequent exposure to the same pathogen ***due to the creation of memory cell line.*** In other words, **innate immune system** ***activates*** the response against offending agent (e.g., by activating phagocytosis or complement system to lyse or to kill the pathogen), while **adaptive immune system** ***creates*** a response to kill the invading agents by creating antibodies (and memory cells). The ***adaptive immunity*** is further divided into ***cellular immunity*** and ***humoral immunity.*** The primary cells that mediate the ***cellular immunity*** are ***T-lymphocytes*** while ***humoral immunity*** involves the role of ***B-lymphocytes*** and the production of antigen-specific antibodies by plasma cells (differentiated B-lymphocytes).

To have a clear understanding of the mode of action of various immunomodulatory drugs, it seems logical to provide at least a bird's- eye view of some basic aspects of immune function.

LINEAGE AND DEVELOPMENT OF CELLS INVOLVED IN IMMUNE RESPONSES (Fig. 69.1)

The cellular elements in the blood are *erythrocytes (RBC), leukocytes (WBC)* and *thrombocytes (platelets).* The leukocytes are of 2 types: *granulocytes (neutrophils, eosinophils* and *basophils)* and *agranulocytes* (*T-lymphocytes, B-lymphocytes* and *monocytes*). The process by which blood cells are formed is called *haematopoiesis.* All such cells that are involved in exerting immune response (innate or adaptive) develop from pluripotent haematopoietic stem cells which reside in bone marrow (also in liver). These stem cells give rise to the *lymphoid stem cell, trilineage myeloid stem cell, megakaryocytes* (which form platelets) and *erythroblasts* (which form erythrocytes).

The lymphoid stem cells, through their progenitors, give rise to mature lymphocytes (T-lymphocytes and B-lymphocytes) and natural killer cells (NK cells). T- and B-lymphocytes are involved in mediating adaptive immune responses, while NK cells exert innate immune response. When exposed to specific antigens, B-lymphocytes differentiate into antibody-producing plasma cells in the bone marrow. Simultaneously, T-cells, under the influence of thymic hormones, migrate to the thymus and on appropriate stimulus by antigen presenting cells (APC) acquire T-cell receptor (TCR) and get differentiated to helper T-cells (TH-cells with specific protein *cluster of differentiation*—CD4+) and cytotoxic T-cells (CTL with specific protein *cluster of differentiation*—CD8+). Helper T-cells differentiate further outside the thymus into several phenotypes: TH1, TH2 and TH3, which are distinguished by the different cytokines they synthesise. TH1-cells produce interleukins (IL-2) and interferons (IFN-γ) that stimulate the proliferation and differentiation of T-lymphocytes and NK cells. These cytokines play an important role in *cell mediated immunity* (CMI). TH2-cells release cytokines (IL-4, IL-5, IL-10 and IL-13) that stimulate B-lymphocytes production for *humoral immunity* (see below). TH3- cells play an important role in resting phases of immune response and in the production of anti-inflammatory immunoglobin-A (IgA) antibodies.

Trilineage myeloid stem cells proliferate and differentiate into mature ***granulocyte cells*** (neutrophil, eosinophil and basophil cells), ***mast cell precursor cells*** and ***monocyte-macrophage cells.*** In the tissues, mast cell precursors give rise to *mast cells* and monocytes transform into *macrophages*. All descendent cells of trilineage myeloid stem cells are involved in mediating innate immune response. The development of mature cells from the pluripotent stem cells via their precursor/ progenitor cells is governed by multilineage- or lineage specific growth factors like interleukins (IL-3, IL-5, IL-6, IL-7, IL-9 and IL-11), colony stimulating factors (GM-CSF, G-CSF, M-CSF), erythropoietin and thrombopoietin (refer Ch. 50 and Fig. 69.1).

INNATE IMMUNE RESPONSE (IIR)

When exposed to an invading organism, the nonspecific innate immunity is immediately called into action as it is the first line of defense. However, the antigen-specific responses also start developing side by side for more effective removal of the invading organism (see adaptive immune responses) by creating the antigen - specific memory cells. This

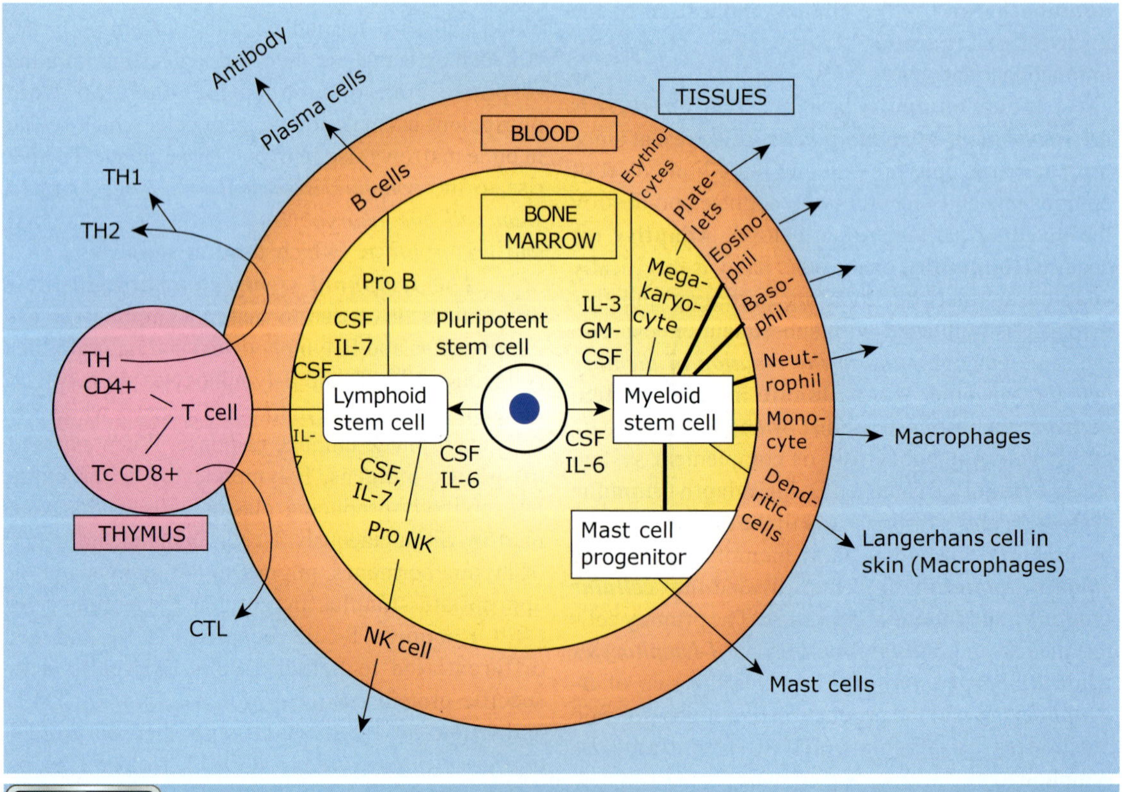

Fig 69.1 Development, Lineage and Location of Blood Cells Involved in Immune Response. Note: Details of growth factors and interleukins involvement have been avoided (see. Ch. 50). Bold lines depict trilineage myeloid stem cell differentiation.

memory and the ability to recognise specific antigen differentiates adaptive from IIR.

The characteristic features of IIRs are: **(a)** immediate onset of action, which remains unchanged howsoever often a pathogen is encountered, **(b)** antigen recognition by a limited set of receptors that can identify only common molecules on the cell surface of microbes, and **(c)** involvement of only macrophages, dendritic cells, neutrophils (also basophils and eosinophils), mast cells, alternative pathway of complement system, interferons and NK cells (but not antigen specific B-cells or T-cells) in killing and neutralising the microbes. Macrophages and dendritic cells usually work as *antigen-presenting cells* (*APCs*) in IIRs.

The innate immune cells perform three important functions: **(1)** Phagocytosis, to kill the offending organism, **(2)** Proteolytic digestion and presentation of the processed pathogen fragments, together with **M**ajor **H**istocompatibility **C**omplex (MHC) class II proteins, on the surface of APCs to activate the T-cells of adaptive immune system and (3) to secrete proper soluble mediators and cytokines to make first two functions more efficient.

Phagocytosis of the offending organism is performed by using ***opsonin-dependent*** or ***opsonin-independent*** mechanisms. ***Opsonisation*** (coating) is a process in which an antibody (IgG/IgE) or complement (e.g., C3b—a fragment of complement-C3) or lectin (e.g., C-reactive protein) coats the invading pathogen and makes it recognisable by the phagocyte cells. Such molecular adapters which coat the foreign agent and signal the phagocytes to recognise and process them are called ***opsonins.*** For opsonin-independent phagocytosis, the innate immune cells utilise "pattern recognition receptors" collectively called PAMP (**P**athogen **A**ssociated **M**olecular **P**attern), which are the members of ***toll-like receptor family.***

Toll-like receptors (TLRs) are pattern recognition receptors as they recognise the generic molecular pattern (related to bacteria or virus) which is different than that of mammalian cells (e.g., bacterial cell wall components, bacterial/viral DNA, viral double stranded RNA, lipopolysaccharide [LPS] of Gram - ive bacteria and teichoic acid of Gram + ive bacteria). They received their name from their similarity to the protein coded by the "Toll gene" identified in a fruit fly called *Drosophila.* This gene on mutation made Drosophila fly look unusual. The researchers were so surprised that they spontaneously shouted out in German "Das ist ja toll" which is translated as "Oh God that is wild".

TLRs are encoded in the host DNA and are expressed on the surface of APCs (dendritic cells and macrophages). There are at least 10 TLRs, each specific for different biologic components of bacteria and virus. For example, even nanoamounts of LPS of *E.coli* are easily detected by CD14 (LPS binding protein associated with TLR4). Interaction of LPS with these components prompts macrophages to produce cytokines (that lead to inflammation) and various enzymes (that digest the microbes). The resultant pathogen fragments are then presented on the surface of APCs to activate T-cells of adaptive immune system. Hence, TLRs mediated phagocytosis and subsequent events are the converging points of interaction between the innate and adaptive immune response.

Role of Different Components in IIR

1) ***The Complement System*** comprises about 20 normally inactive proteins in plasma and on cell membranes that react in a fixed sequence (cascade) on stimulation. When activated, these proteins enhance (or *complement*) certain immune/allergic/inflammatory reactions. There are 11 complement proteins marked C1 through C9 with three subgroups of C1 (totalling 11). The key member of the complement system is C3 which can be activated commonly by either ***classical pathway*** or by an ***alternative pathway.*** The activation of C3 by the *classical pathway* is triggered by antigen-antibody complex formation. In the *alternative pathway* certain polysaccharides or endotoxins on the bacterial cell surface activate C3 directly. Once C3 is activated, by any of the pathways, it activates the cascade of other complement proteins which then attack and destroy (lyse) the invading pathogen by one or more of the following processes:

(a) CHEMOTAXIS: C3a, C4a and C5a cause increased vascular permeability by inducing the release of histamine from mast cells. Among them C5a is also a potent chemotactic factor. Since

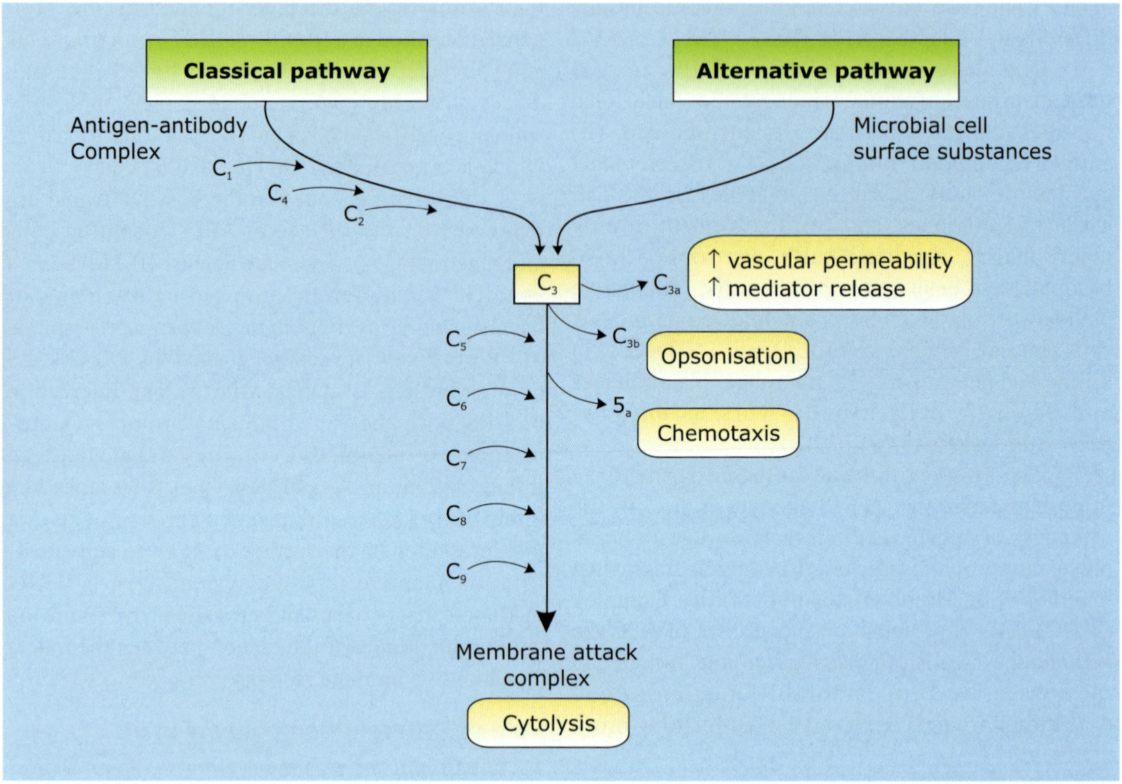

Fig 69.2 The Complement Cascade

histamine increases the permeability of blood capillaries, granulocytes now can easily penetrate tissues to combat the pathogen. Chemotactic action of C5a also attracts phagocytes to the site of microbe invasion, **(b)** OPSONISATION: after coating with an opsonin 3b (see above), and **(c)** CYTOLYSIS: Several complement proteins (C5b, C6, C7, C8 and C9), at the end of cascade reaction, come together to form a ***Membrane attack complex (MAC)*** that punches holes in the plasma membrane of the microbe, which finally ruptures due to cytolysis (Fig. 69.2).

2) ***Neutrophils*** engulf the invading bacteria and after its endocytosis destroy it within the vesicle with the help of endogenous myeloperoxidase enzymes and *defensins*.
3) ***Eosinophils*** are used as defense against parasites which are too large to be engulfed. They attach and secrete the cytotoxic substances onto the parasitic cell wall. Eosinophils also contribute to the pathogenesis of allergic responses (rashes and bronchial asthma).
4) ***Basophils*** and ***Mast Cells*** bind to IgE antibodies and display it onto their cell surface. Like eosinophils, IgE-mediated anaphylaxis is also caused by the stimulation of basophil and mast cell degranulation which releases histamine, 5-HT and also leukotrienes.
5) ***Monocytes*** get differentiated into ***macrophages*** in various tissues including reticulo-endothelial system. Like neutrophils, macrophages have high affinity receptors for antibodies and the complement proteins so that opsonisation of invading microbes occurs to facilitate recognition and phagocytosis of the invading pathogen. Also act as APCs to T-cells.

6) ***Dendritic Cells*** (including Langerhans cells in skin) like macrophages also act as APCs, which normally remain in resting stage. Immature or inactive dendritic cells reside in non-lymphoid tissue but on activation these begin to migrate to lymphoid organs (lymph nodes and spleen) to behave as APCs which present the antigen (through MHC class II protein) to T-lymphocytes for further processing by the adaptive immune mechanisms.

7) ***Natural Killer Cells (NK cells)*** are a special type of lymphocyte which have an intrinsic ability to kill the invading microbes/malignant cells. They recognise and kill the target cells by two mechanisms: (i) NK cells are equipped with IgG-Fc receptor that allows recognition of IgG-coated target cells. The latter are finally killed by antibody-dependent cytotoxicity and (ii) the NK cells also possess *killer activating receptors* (KARs) which recognise virus infected or tumour cells. On activation, KARs are engaged and a kill instruction is issued by NK cells.

There are also *killer-inhibition receptors* (KIRs) expressed on NK cells, which are inhibitory in nature. Their function is to recognise "the self" MHC class I proteins, normally present on all nucleated cells. The killing activity of KARs can be checked by KIRs on recognition of self MHC class I proteins. Malignant cells and virus infected cells are abnormal in the sense that they down-regulate this self MHC class I expression. KIRs, therefore (due to down regulation of the self MHC-I), become ineffectual and cannot inhibit the killer action of KARs. Consequently the malignant cells receive a "kiss of death" from NK cells. The latter then release *perforin* (a pore forming chemical) followed by *granzymes* that cause cytolysis of microbe/malignant cells.

ADAPTIVE (ACQUIRED) IMMUNE RESPONSES (AIRs)

When the IIRs are inadequate, the adaptive immune response system (AIRs) is mobilised because AIR is able **(1)** to respond to a variety of antigens with specificity, **(2)** to discriminate between the "non-self" antigens and the "self" antigens of the host and **(3)** to respond to the previously encountered antigen in a more organised manner by employing memory cells. AIRs comprise two kinds of closely allied immune responses: **(1) cell-mediated (cellular) immune (CMI) responses**, where CD8 cytotoxic T-cells (Tc) directly attack the invading organism and **(2) antibody-mediated (humoral) immune (AMI) responses**, wherein B-lymphocytes transform into plasma cells which synthesise *antibodies* (Abs) that, in turn bind to and inactivate particular antigens. CD4 T-helper cells then aid in processing both CMI (TH1 cells) as well as AMI (TH2 cells). **CMI** is particularly useful against: **(1)** *intracellular* pathogens (like fungi, parasite and viruses), **(2)** cancer cells (excluding leukaemias) and **(3)** tissue transplants. Humoral immunity **(AMI)** works mainly against: **(1)** *antigens dissolved in body fluids* and **(2)** *extracellular pathogens,* such as bacteria which multiply in body fluids but rarely enter the host cells. AIR is endowed with two important characteristics: **(1)** Specificity to foreign antigen which binds to and displayed by **M**ajor **H**istocompatibility **C**omplex **(MHC)** proteins, and **(2) Tolerance** to self antigen, which is provided by regulated immune cell development and by an active role of **costimulator molecules** (see below).

Major Histocompatibility Complex (MHC)

Located in the plasma membrane of most body cells are "self-antigens" called Major Histocompatibility Complex (MHC) antigens (or proteins). These are also called Human Leukocyte Antigens (HLA), because these were first identified on human leukocyes. Several hundred thousand MHC molecules mark the surface of our body cells (except red blood cells). Their normal function is to help T-cells to recognise the foreign antigen, not self, which is an important first step in mediating any immune response. There are 2 types of MHCs: MHC-I are expressed by all nucleated human cells (serving as antigen presenting cells), while MHC-II are expressed by professional APCs like B-cells, macrophages and dendritic cells.

Foreign antigens (bacteria, viruses, pollens) that are present in the fluid *outside* the body cells (i.e., *exogenous antigens*) but have not infected the cell as yet, are first ingested by phagocytosis or endocytosis. These are then digested and broken down to peptide fragments, which then fuse with MHC-II molecules. The antigen + MHC-II complex then undergoes exocytosis and presented on the concerned APC (see above). These are then presented to CD-4 T-helper cells for further processing to mediate either cellular (TH1) or humoral (TH2) immune response (Fig. 69.3 and 69.5A, B). *That means, MHC-II identifies and displays the peptide fragments of an exogenous infectious agent.*

The fragments of the degraded cytoplasmic or secretory proteins of any cell make a complex with MHC class I. This complex is then transported to the surface of human nucleated cells (serving as APCs) where it serves as a fingerprint for the diversity of proteins expressed within that cell. If a cell is expressing a self protein, it will not be attacked by the immune system. However, if a foreign antigen is inside the body cells (endogenous antigen) which is generating a foreign protein within the cytosol of the cell (e.g., viral infected cell or cancer cell itself), then the proteolytic fragments of such foreign proteins (present inside the cell) will complex with MHC-I and presented on the surface of the cell. The CD-8 T-cells (cytotoxic T-lymphocytes) will then recognise the viral or cancerous peptide to trigger cellular immunity (Fig. 69.4). *That means, MHC-I identify and display self proteins (to be ignored by immune system) as well as endogenous protein fragments of an infected cell (not of phagocytosed infectious agent).* MHC-I bound to cytosolic antigen, signals that the cell has been infected and needs help of immune system.

Tolerance

The diversity in the immunoglobulins and T-cell receptors creates the risk that some of these molecules could recognise and attack native proteins. In a process referred to as *tolerance*, cells of the immune system undergo a careful sequence of development to make it sure that mature immune cells ignore the native proteins. In addition, ***costimulation***—a requirement of multiple signals to initiate an immune response—ensures that a faulty stimulation of a single immune receptor (e.g., T-cell receptor) does not initiate a damaging sequence of immune reaction (see below). Defects in the process of tolerance can lead to autoimmune diseases.

Cell-mediated (Cellular) Immunity (CMI)

AIR operates via two major arms: *Humoral immunity* and *cellular* (cell-mediated) *immunity* (CMI). The primary cells that mediate the humoral immunity are B-lymphocytes and plasma cells, which secrete antibodies specific for an antigen (to be discussed later). The CMI is mediated by T-lymphocytes—mainly cytotoxic T-lymphocytes (Tc cells) bearing a cell surface marker CD8 (CD8+ T-cell).

In lymphocytes, the prefix "T" denotes that these cells mature in thymus, whereas "B" denotes that these cells grow and mature in bone marrow; and because both cells require the lymphoid tissue for their operations, both are labelled as *lymphocytes*. Unlike cells of innate immunity (macrophages, dendritic cells and neutrophils etc., i.e., APCs) which kill the pathogen by phagocytosis or complement activation, T-lymphocytes recognise rather processed antigen fragments presented to them by APCs, displayed on their surface via MHC class I or MHC class II proteins.

The Tc cells recognise a specific MHC class I antigen-complex on the *infected cells* and lyse these cells by secreting membrane-perforating *perforins* and apoptosis-inducing *granzymes*. Such cellular immune responses are involved in apoptosis of tumour cells/grafted cells or in an eradication of intracellular pathogens such as virus. The Tc cells may be generated with or without the support of TH (TH1) cells because TH cells also play a pivotal role in regulating the cellular as well as humoral immunity (see below).

All T-cells (Tc or TH) express an *MHC: antigen complex specific T-receptor* designated as *TCR*. The TCR for TH cells differs from TCR of Tc cells in terms of coreceptors and costimulators involved in their function. The TCR of Tc cells identifies the "nonself" antigen bound to MHC protein, while CD8 ensures that the TCR interacts only with APC expressing MHC class I antigen; likewise, CD4 on TH cells ensures that TCR on TH cells interacts only with APC expressing MHC class

II antigens. Each TCR is linked to CD3 complex of molecule that transmit activating signals to the nucleus of T-cells (see below and Fig. 69.3).

Cluster of differention (CD) classification of human leukocyte antigens (only important ones are mentioned):
CD3 (on all T cells; T-cell activation and signal transduction).
CD4 (on TH1 or TH2 cells; T-cell selection and activation).
CD14 (LPS receptor; TLR4, with LPS, mediates activation of innate immune activity)
CD8 (on Tc lymphocytes; T-cell selection and activation).
CD20 (on B-lymphocytes; B-cell activation and cell signaling).
CD28 (on T-cells and plasma cells; costimulator for T-cell activation).
CD40 (on B-cells; B-cell activation, proliferation and differentiation)
CD80 (B 7.1) (on activated T and B-cells; costimulator of T-cell)
CD86 (B 7.2) (on subset of B and activated T cell; costimulator of T-cell)
CD152 (CTLA-4) (on activated T-cell; inhibits T-cell proliferation).
CD154 (CD40L) (on activated T-cells; function as costimulator. Ligand for CD40).

CMI Involving TH1 Mediated Activation of T-Lymphocytes (Fig. 69.3)

At any given time, most T-cells are inactive (naive T-cells—with no prior exposure to an antigen). As discussed above, the peptide fragments of foreign antigen, bound to MHC class II antigens on APC, are first presented to CD4 marker TH cells. The TH cells possess a T-cells receptor (TCR) for the specific peptide:MHC class II complex. The naive TH cell (with CD4) would not set into motion until it receives two activating signals. The "*first signal*" is provided by the binding of TCR with peptide bound MHC class II molecule. But, for T cell to become responsive, a "*second signal*" is also needed, in absence of which the T-cells become "anergic" (unresponsive) and undergo apoptosis. In other words, "signal one" in absence of "signal two" leads to tolerance (see above) or a "functional silencing" of T-cells (anergy). This second signal is provided by the interaction of CD28 on TH cells with the protein of B7 family (B7.1 or CD 80 and B7.2 or CD86) on APC cells. CD28 and B7 are the main costimulatory molecules of second signal. However, the second signal also involves a ligation (attachment) of CD40 present on APC with its respective ligand CD40L (CD154) on T-cells. The presence of one costimulator protein on the surface of T-cells and the second on the surface of APC causes two cells to adhere for sometime for an effective TH cell activation. However, not all signals are stimulatory (some are dampening signals also). For example, binding of CTLA-4 (CD152) on activated TH cell with B7.1 (CD80) on APC, provides negative signals (or negative feedback loop) for self-limiting the immune responses.

The whole situation is similar to starting of your car. When you insert a key (an antigen) in the ignition switch (a TCR) and turn it on (first signal), the engine starts (recognition of specific antigen). But the car would not move unless you shift the gear (costimulator) in drive state (second signal). It is the need to shift the gear (second signal) that had prevented your car to move accidentally after receiving the very first signal. Similarly, the costimulation (i.e., the second signal) ensures that your immune responses may not occur unexpectedly. Just as a reverse gear is also important in functioning of a car, both positive as well as negative signals regulate the immune response on time-to-time requirement basis. It has also been said that "signal one" in absence of "signal two" leads to functional silence (anergy) of T cells or to their apoptosis; similarly, you can imagine your car with its engine running, but in neutral gear, and its becoming functionally silent when it goes out of fuel.

Following the interaction between APC and TH cells, and subsequent two signals, a message is sent through TCR to the CD3 complex into the cell which leads to phosphorylation of tyrosine and the transduction of downstream signals to the nucleus of TH cells. This leads to transcription of various gene sequences for soluble cytokines. The IFN-γ and IL-12 stimulate the formation and profileration of effector TH cell (TH1 cells in this case). Some of these TH1 cells are stored as memory cells. Other

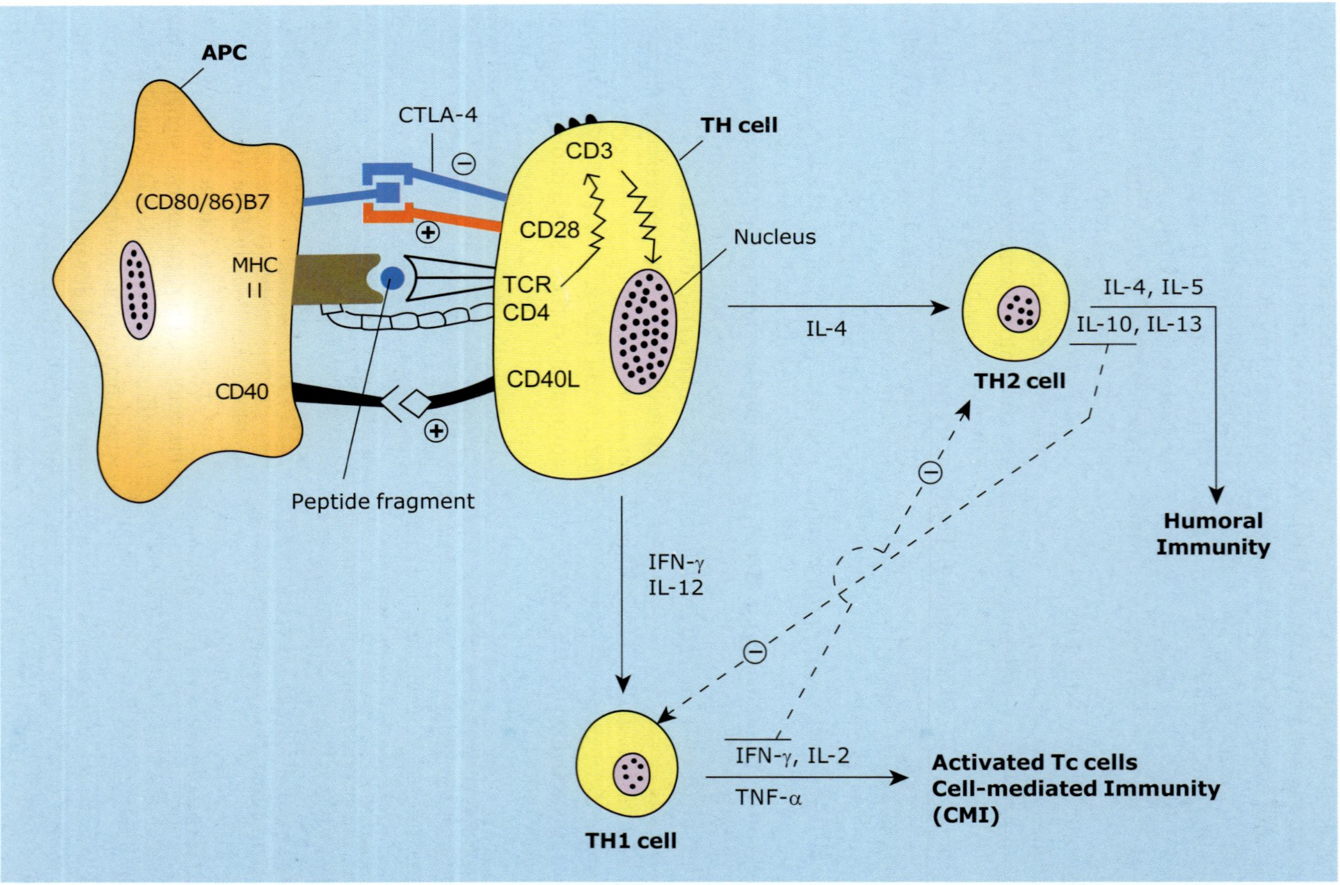

Fig 69.3 Molecular Interactions Between APC and TH Cell and Generation of Cellular and Humoral Immunity (For humoral immunity, see following text).

TH1 cells secrete IL-2, IFN-γ and TNF-α, which result in the activation of macrophages and generation of Tc lymphocytes. Activated Tc cells further secrete IL-2 and stimulate their own proliferation and differentiation of effector Tc cells to perform cell-mediated immune response (lysis by secreting perforins and granzymes, see above). The TH1 and TH2 cells also regulate each other's activity, e.g., secretion of IFN-γ by TH1 cells inhibit activity of TH2 cells, while secretion of IL-10 by TH2 reciprocally inhibits TH1 cells (Fig. 69.3). Such regulatory interactions can be exploited clinically (see following text).

CMI Involving Direct Role of CD8+ T-Lymphocytes (Fig. 69.4)

The cytotoxic T-lymphocytes (CTLs or Tc) can be generated with or without the support of TH1 cells. The CTLs mediate antigen-specific lysis of tumour cells, virus infected cell and graft/transplant cells by a similar mechanism. Naive CTLs also require activation by two signals as described for TH cells. As usual the first signal is delivered by binding of peptide antigen (displayed by APC or by virally infected/tumour cell on their surface in association with MHC class I proteins) to TCR on CD8+ of naive Tc-lymphocyte. The second signal is provided by receptor ligand interactions of costimulatory molecules (CD28 and B7). The activated CD8+ Tc cells kill them by using perforins and granzymes as discussed above. Alternatively, CD8+ Tc cells can express a *Fas* ligand, which can trigger apoptosis in the infected cell by stimulating its *Fas* death receptor.

In addition to killing the target infected cell directly, the CD8+ Tc cells also produce a number of cytokines such as IFN-γ, TNF-α and lymphotoxins. Among these IFN-γ reinforces antiviral defence of CD8+ cells by rendering adjacent cells resistant to viral infection. When CTLs are generated with the support of TH1 cell, then the activated TH1 cell induces an upregulation of costimulatory (B7) molecules on APC and provides a second signal to CTL for its activation. Activated CTLs produce IL-2 which stimulates their proliferation and differentiation. Further steps are same as discussed above.

Humoral Immunity (Fig. 69.5A, B)

Humoral or antibody-mediated immunity (AMI), as discussed, works mainly against antigens dissolved in body fluids and extracellular pathogens such as bacteria which multiplies in body fluids but rarely enters the host cells. The humoral immunity is so named because the factors which mediate this immunity are found in humor, blood or serum. There are millions of different B-cells, each capable of responding to a specific antigen. Whereas CTLs (Tc cells) leave lymphoid tissue to confront the processed foreign antigen, B-cells remain where

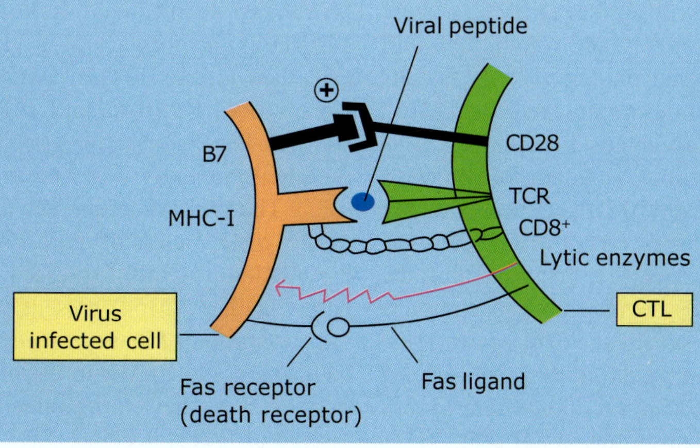

Fig 69.4 Cytotoxic T-Lymphocyte (CTL) Action on Virus Infected Cell (see text)

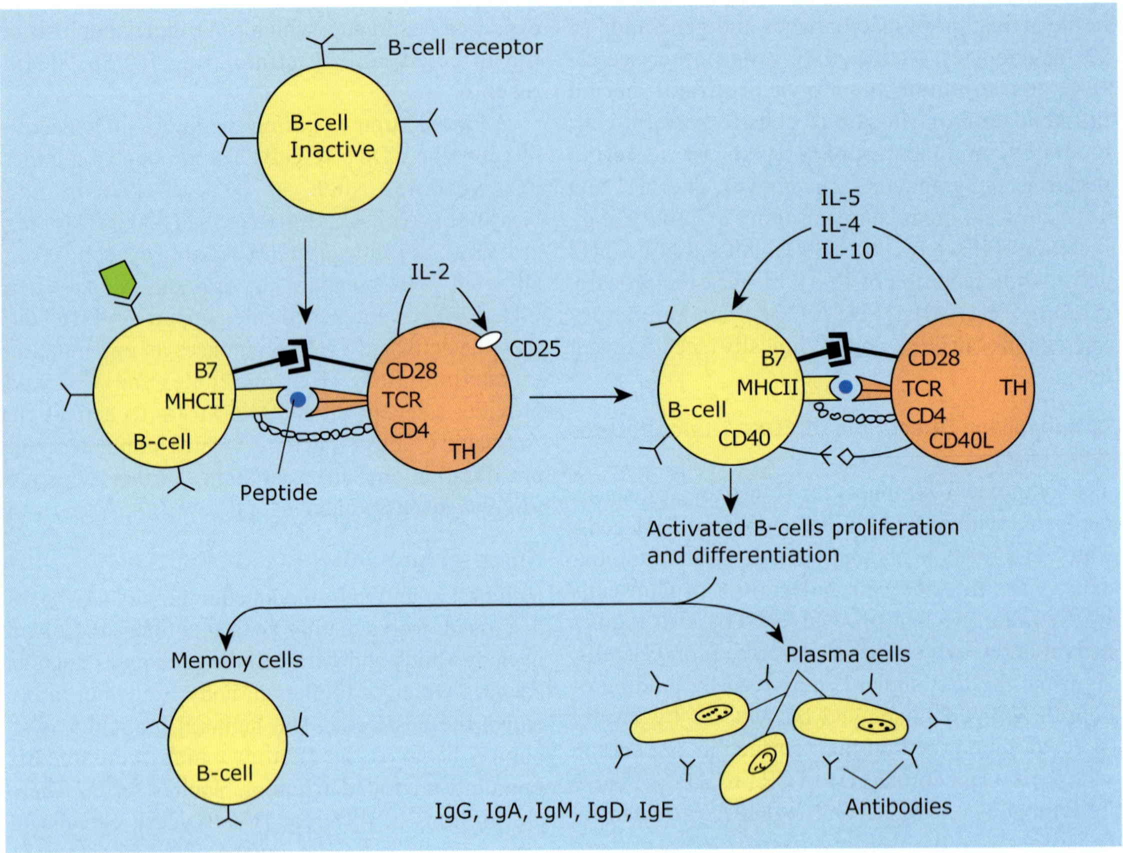

Fig 69.5A Activation, Proliferation and Differentiation of B-Cell During Humoral Immunity

placed. The foreign antigen initially binds to an antigen receptor on the cell surface of B-cell present in lymph nodes, the spleen and other lymphoid tissues. The antigen is then processed by the B-cells and the resulting peptides complexed with MHC class II proteins are presented to the naive CD4+ TH cell. As discussed above, an interaction between the specific TCR:peptide-MHC II pair and the costimulatory molecules (B7 and CD 28) are necessary for activation of TH. For sustaining the activation, the TH cells develop IL-2 receptors as well as generate IL-2—a cytokine that has *autocrine* (acting on the cell that produces it) action, giving rise to a clone of activated TH cells which in turn give rise to two different subsets of TH cells—TH1 and TH2. IL-2 actually causes an upregulation of CD25 which is an active component of IL-2 receptor. Moreover, secretion of IL-4 also, by TH cells, stimulates the formation of TH2 cells. The TH2 cells then secrete IL-4, IL-5 and IL-10 to stimulate B-cell proliferation and differentiation into memory-B cells or antibody secreting plasma cells (humoral immunity; Fig 69.3 and 69.5A).

The primary antibodies formed initially, are mostly of IgM class of immunoglobulin. However, the ligation of CD40 expressed on B-lymphocytes, with CD40L (CD154) present on activated T-cells, induces protein kinase cascade in B-cells, which mediates a switchover in antibody class produced by them, i.e., they start producing IgG, IgA or IgE instead of IgM if need be.

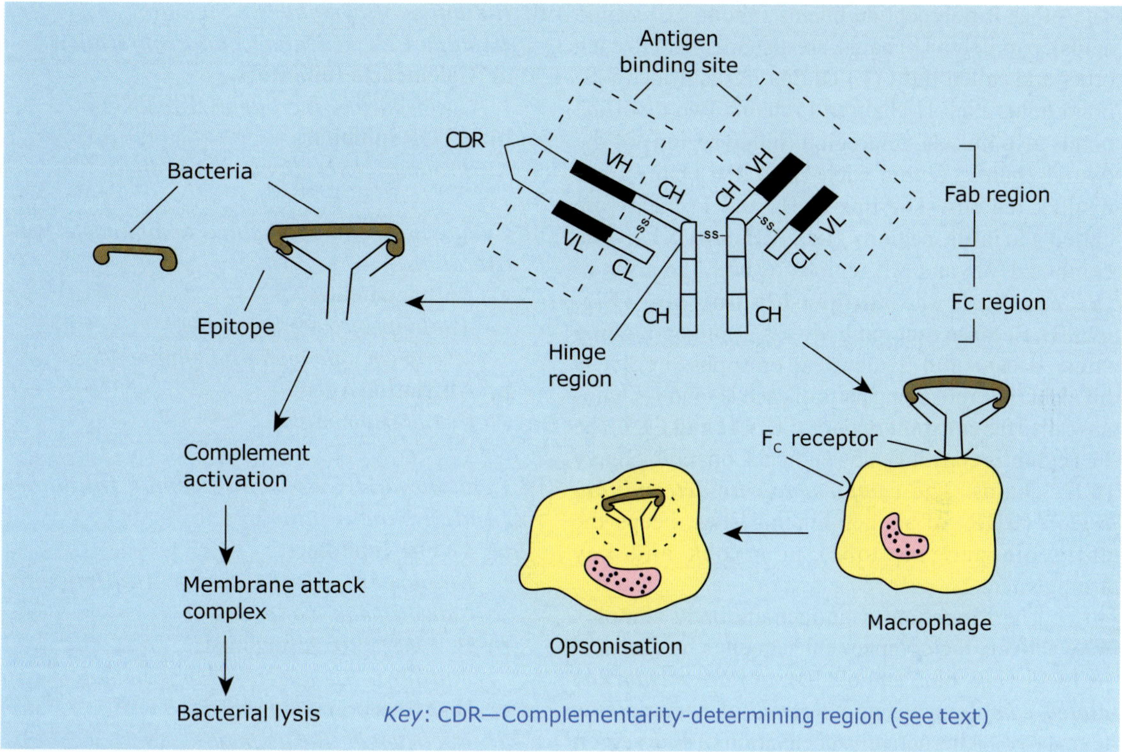

Fig 69.5B Fate of Antigen-Antibody Complex

Different antigens stimulate different B-cells to develop into respective plasma cells and their accompanying memory B-cells. The B-cells of a particular clone are capable of secreting only one kind of antibody, which is identical in its specificity to the antigen receptor displayed by the progenitor B cell that responded to the antigen in the first place. *Memory B cells* remain in the body for a longer time and are always ready to respond more rapidly and vigorously, should the same antigen be encountered in future.

Antibodies belong to a group of immunoglobulins (Igs), and are designated into 5 types:

1) **IgG** – Most abundant (80%) of all antibodies in the blood. Protect against bacteria/virus by enhancing phagocytosis or activating complement system. Only IgG antibodies cross placenta to confer some immune protection to foetus.
2) **IgA** – 15% of all antibodies in the blood. Provide localised protection on mucous membranes (found in tears, sweat, saliva, breast milk, etc).
3) **IgM** – 5–10% of all antibodies in the blood. First antibodies to be secreted by plasma cells (see above). Cause agglutination and lysis of microbes. Also present on surface of B-cells to serve as antigen receptors.
4) **IgD** – Hardly 0.2% of all antibodies in the blood. Involved in the activation of B-cells and also serve as antigen receptors on them.
5) **IgE** – About 0.1% of all antibodies in the blood. Located on mast cells and involved in allergic reactions. Provide protection against parasitic worms.

An antibody is a Y-shaped immunoglobulin in which two arms of the Y (called ***Fab region***) serve as the recognition sites for specific antigens; while the stem of the Y (called the **Fc portion**) is responsible to activate host defence. The arms of Y are made up of 4 polypeptide chains. Two of the chains (on either side) are identical to each other and are called **heavy (H) chains** (about 450 amino acids).

The other 2 polypeptide chains (about 220 amino acids), parallel to H-chains, are also identical to each other and called **light (L) chains.** A disulfide (S-S) bond holds each H-chain to L-chain. Two disulfide bonds also link the midregion (hinge region) of the two H-chains. Within each H- and L-chain are 2 distinct regions. The tips of H- and L-chains are called **variable regions (i.e., VH and VL)**. The combined VH and VL regions of both the arms of 'Y' constitute the **antigen-binding site** (Fig. 69.5B). Because each antibody has 2 antigen-binding sites, it can bind 2 identical epitopes, i.e., it is bivalent. The remaining parts of each H- and L-chains are called the **constant regions (i.e., CH and CL).** The **Fc region** is constituted by vertical **Constant-Heavy (CH) chains.** The ***complementarity-determining region*** (**CDR**) of antigen-binding sites, keeps the antigenic part (epitope) in a lock and key arrangement.

The formation of antigen-antibody complex may activate the complement sequence by classical pathway (Fig. 69.2 and 69.5B), to form ***membrane attack complex*** causing cytolysis of bacteria (see text above). Alternatively, occupation of ***Fab region*** by an antigen can expose the ***Fc domain***. Macrophages or neutrophils possess Fc-receptors on their membranes. The Fc domain of antigen-antibody complex then binds to these Fc-receptors to process opsonin-dependent phagocytosis (Fig. 69.5B).

DRUGS USED FOR IMMUNOMODULATION

All drugs which modify immune responses are generally categorised as immunomodulators. These can either function as *immunosuppressants* or *immunostimulants*. There is also an upcoming generation of immunosuppressants called *tolerogens* (see text).

IMMUNOSUPPRESSANT DRUGS

Depending on their mode of action, these drugs are classified as under:

I. ***Inhibitors of Lymphocyte Gene Expression to Reduce Inflammatory Response***
   Glucocorticoids

II. ***Inhibitors of Lymphocyte Signaling to Prevent Immune Cell Activation and Proliferation***
   a) **Calcineurin Inhibitors**
      Cyclosporine, Tacrolimus, ISATX-247
   b) **mTOR Inhibitors**
      Sirolimus, Everolimus, Zotarolimus

III. ***Cytotoxic Agents to Reduce Lymphocyte Proliferation***
   a) **Antimetabolites**
      Azathioprine, Methotrexate, Mycophenolate mofetil, Leflunomide
   b) **Alkylating Agents**
      Cylophosphamide

IV. ***Cytokine and Cytokine Receptor Inhibitors (Anticytokine-Antibodies)***
   a) **TNF-α Inhibitors**
      Etanercept, Infliximab, Adalimumab, Cetrolizumab, Golimumab
   b) **IL-1 Receptor Antagonists**
      Anakinra, Rilonacept, Canakinumab
   c) **IL-2 Receptor Antagonists**
      Daclizumab, Basiliximab
   d) **IL-6 Receptor Inhibitors**
      Tocilizumab
   e) **IL-12/IL-23 p40 Cytokine Inhibitors**
      Ustekinumab
   f) **IL-17 Cytokine/IL-17 Receptor Inhibitors**
      Ixekizumab, Secukinumab, Brodalumab

V. ***Antibodies Against Specific Immune Cells Molecules***
   a) **Polyclonal Antibodies**
      Antithymocyte Globulin (ATG)
   b) **Monoclonal Antibodies**
      1. **Anti-CD52 Mab**: *Alemtuzumab*
      2. **Anti CD-3 Antibody (OKT-3)**: *Muromonab*
      3. ***Anti-IgE Antibody:*** *Omalizumab*
      4. **Anti-CD20 Mab**: *Rituximab*
      5. **Anti-CD25 Mab**: *Basiliximab*
      6. **B-Lymphocyte Stimulator (BLyS) Cytokine Inhibitor**: *Belimumab*
      7. **Antibody-Drug Conjugate**: *Brentuximab vedotin*
      8. **LFA-3 (CD58) Inhibitor**: *Alefacept*

VI. ***Inhibitors of Immune Cell Adhesion and Activation***
   a) **Anti-LFA-1/LFA-3 Mabs**
      Efaluzumab, Alefacept
   b) **Alpha-4 Integrins Inhibitor/Blocker**
      Natalizumab

VII. ***Inhibitors of Immune Cell Costimulation to Induce Anergy (Tolerogens)***
   a) **Anti-CD80 and Anti-CD86 Mabs**
      Abatacept, Belatacept
   b) **CTLA-4 Inhibitor/Blocker**
      Ipilimumab
   c) **PD-1 Inhibitor/Blocker**
      Nivolumab, Pembrolizumab

VIII. ***Miscellaneous***
      Rho (D) Immune Globulins

I. Inhibitors of Lymphocyte Gene Expression to Reduce Inflammatory Response

Glucocorticoids

When used to prevent graft rejection, glucocorticoids precisely suppress the initiation and generation of a "fresh" immune response more effectively than a response that has already occurred and in which the clonal proliferation of T-cells has already taken place (see following text). Recall that local regulation of cytokine release, from T-cells, stimulates leukocyte recruitment and activation. Glucocorticoids inhibit cytokine synthesis and release (e.g., of IL-1, IL-2, IL-6 and TNF-α), which effectively suppress bizarre immune responses, by inhibiting the activation of cytotoxic T-lymphocyte (Tc) function and proliferation. Glucocorticoids also decrease neutrophils and monocytes chemotaxis and the lysosomal enzyme release. Glucocorticoids induce the transcription of gene for the Inhibitor Factor IFkB. This in turn binds to Nuclear Factor kB (NFkB) transcription factor in the cytosol preventing its translocation to the Tc cell nucleus. Subsequently, the transcription of genes for a variety of inflammatory and immune mediators is inhibited. Glucocorticoids have little effect on humoral immunity and mainly suppress cellular immune responses.

Immunosuppressant Uses: High doses of methyl prednisolone sodium succinate, in pulses, by I.V. route are used to reverse acute transplant rejection and acute exacerbations of certain autoimmune diseases. In combination with other immuno-suppressants, they are also effective in controlling graft *versus* host disease in case of bone marrow transplantation. These are the mainstay of treatment for autoimmune disorders like rheumatoid arthritis, systemic lupus erythematosus (SLE), psoriasis, systemic dermatomyositis and other skin diseases, bronchial asthma, inflammatory bowel and ocular diseases as well as exacerbations of multiple sclerosis. In transplant patients, glucocorticoids are additionally used to block first dose cytokine storm (see text) observed during treatment with muromonab-CD3 (OKT3) and with antithymocyte globulin (though to a lesser extent). These are also used to limit allergic reactions that occur during the use of other immunosuppressive drugs.

For mechanism of their action and adverse effects refer Chapter 42.

II. Inhibitors of Lymphocyte Signalling

a) Calcineurin Inhibitors

Example: Cyclosporine, Tacrolimus

Cyclosporine

Mechanism of Action: Normally when a TH-cell is activated, its cytoplasmic *Ca^{2+}-complexed with calmodulin* stimulates a phosphatase enzyme called *calcineurin*. This Ca^{2+}-calmodulin activated calcineurin phosphatase causes dephosphorylation of **n**uclear **f**actor for **a**ctivated **T** cells (NFAT). Dephosphorylated NFAT is active and enters into the nucleus to enhance the IL-2 gene transcription and in turn IL-2 mRNA formation for IL-2 synthesis. *Cyclosporine* binds to a cytosolic protein of TH cells called cyclophilin (an immunophilin). The drug-cyclophilin complex binds to and inhibits calcineurin activity and thus blocks the activation of TH cells and the production of IL-2 which is necessary for T-cell growth and differentiation (Fig. 69.6). Cyclosporine also increases the expression of transforming growth factor-β (TGF-β) which inhibits IL-2 mediated T-cell proliferation.

Pharmacokinetics: Cyclosporine can be given orally or I.V. Its oral bioavailability is low (about 30%). Food decreases its absorption. It is metabolised by CYP3A which may result in drug-drug interactions. Inactive metabolites are excreted

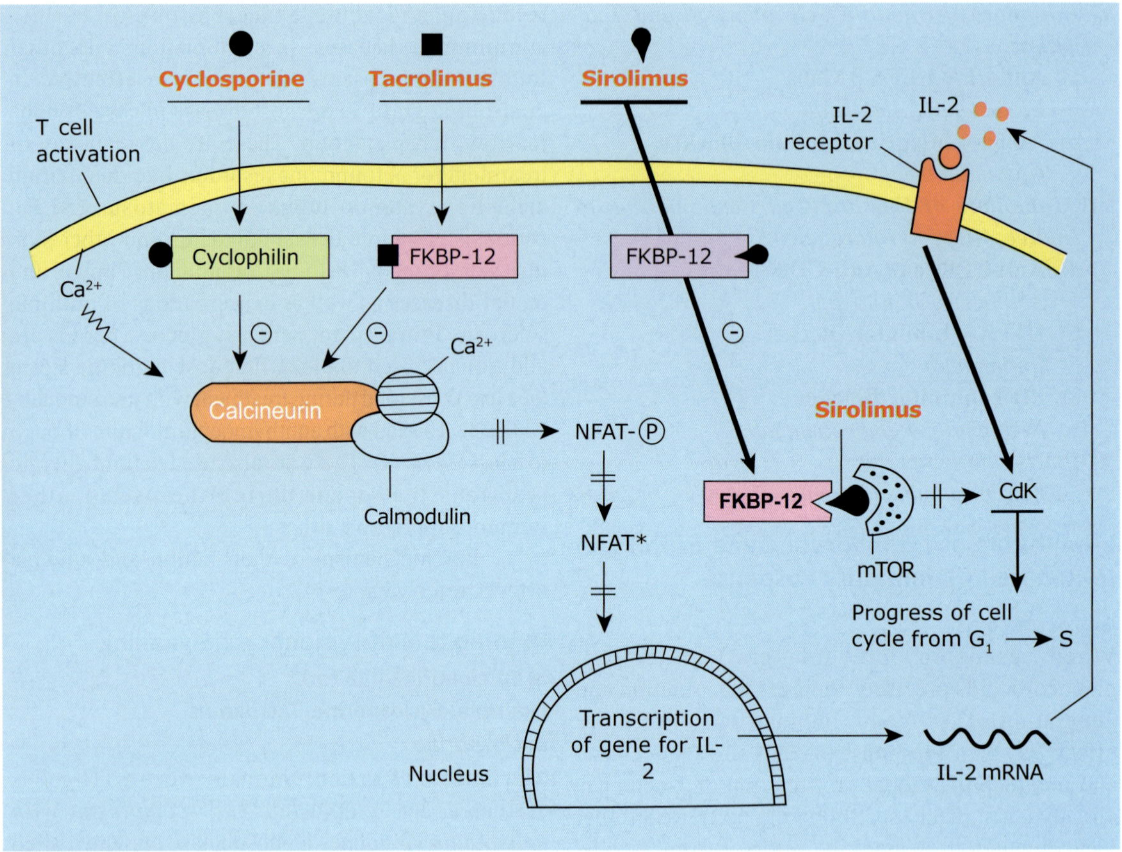

Fig 69.6 Mechanism of Action of Cyclosporine, Tacrolimus and Sirolimus

mainly in bile and then in faeces but minimally in urine. Plasma half-life is about 24 hrs. **Therapeutic Uses**: (1) To prevent graft rejection in solid organ transplant, e.g., heart, kidney and liver, (2) To prevent/control certain autoimmune disorders such as rheumatoid arthritis and psoriasis, and (3) for other T-cell mediated diseases such as atopic dermatitis, endogenous uveitis, inflammatory bowel disease and nephrotic syndrome. **Toxicity**: The drug is nephrotoxic, neurotoxic and hepatotoxic. It can cause hypertension, hyperuricaemia and an increase in LDL. It can also cause tremors, hirsutism and gingival hyperplasia (increase in TGF-β causes growth of extracellular matrix resulting in interstitial fibrosis). Despite these shortcomings, cyclosporine is considered a major step towards the search of specific and selective immunosuppressants.

Its combination with newer agents (see text) has shown considerable efficacy with reduced toxicity.

ISATX-247 is an upcoming semisynthetic analogue of cyclosporine undergoing clinical trials with promising results (more potent and less nephrotoxic compared to cyclosporine with less frequent glucose intolerance compared to tacrolimus treated patients).

Tacrolimus

Tacrolimus is a much more potent immunosuppressant than cyclosporine, with a mechanism of action very much similar to cyclosporine. The main difference is that internal immunophilin-receptor for it is not cyclophilin but the **FK-B**inding **P**rotein (FKBP-12; because tacrolimus was originally called FK-506) The drug-FKBP complex then binds to calcineurin. Subsequent events are same as described above (Fig. 69.6). Tacrolimus can be given orally or I.V. It is 99% metabolised in liver by CYP3A and has a plasma half- life of 7–8 hrs. Its ***therapeutic uses*** are similar to cyclosporine but is quite effective in reversing liver transplant rejection resistant to cyclosporine. Topical tacrolimus ointment is also used in the therapy of atopic dermatitis and psoriasis. Its ***toxicity profile*** is also similar to cyclosporine except that incidence of hirsutism, hyperuricaemia and hyperlipidaemia are significantly less but the risk for post-transplant insulin-dependent diabetes mellitus is more.

b) Mammalian Target of Rapamycin (mTOR) Inhibitors

Example: Sirolimus, Everolimus, Zotarolimus

Sirolimus

Sirolimus, like tacrolimus, is a macrocyclic lactone (a macrolide). It is also known as *rapamycin*. **Mechanism of Action**: Like tacrolimus, sirolimus also binds to the immunophilin FKBP 12 to inhibit T-lymphocyte activation and proliferation, but the sirolimus + FKBP-12 complex does not block calcineurin. Rather, it inhibits the activation of **m**ammalian **t**arget **o**f **r**apamycin (mTOR). The latter is a protein kinase enzyme which plays a key role in the progression of cell cycle by activating *Cdks* (see Ch. 67). Hence, inhibition of mTOR by sirolimus bound FKBP complex blocks the progression of cell cycle from $G_1 \rightarrow$ S phase (Fig. 69.6), i.e., T-cells are arrested in G_1 phase. **Pharmacokinetics**: Oral bioavailability is 15%. Fatty meal decreases its bioavailability. Protein binding is 40–45% mainly with albumin. Extensively metabolised in liver by CYP3A4. Excretion 91% in faeces and only 2.5% in urine. Plasma half-life 62 hrs.

Therapeutic Uses: (1) To prevent acute rejection of solid organ transplant (as of heart, and kidney) in combination with cyclosporine and glucocorticoid (or with mycophenolate mofetil and glucocorticoids). (2) Sirolimus eluted stents are also available for use in coronary angioplasty. This inhibits local cell proliferation and reduces the risk of "in-stent" coronary restenosis. **Toxicity**: Hyperlipidaemia, anaemia, thrombocytopenia, and leukopenia are dose dependent and reversible. Nephrotoxocity is less than cyclosporine and tacrolimus. But, paradoxically, tacrolimus + sirolimus is more nephrotoxic than cyclosporine plus sirolimus. Delayed wound healing has been observed with sirolimus.

Everolimus

It is a hydroxyethyl analogue of sirolimus. The mechanism of action, toxicity and drug-interactions (because of metabolism by CYP3A4) are same as of sirolimus. However, it has a shorter half-life and hence lesser time is needed to achieve steady state plasma concentration, compared to sirolimus.

It has been approoved for provention of kidney transplant rejection and treatment of venous as carcinoma, hormone receptor positive, HER2-negative blood cancer, progressive neuroendocrine tumour originating from pancreas and renal angio-myolipoma.

It has been observed that combined therapy with mTOR inhibitors and calcineurin inhibitors enhances nephrotoxicity and chances of acute rejections.

Zotarolimus

This mTOR inhibitor is approved for loading on the drug-eluting stents.

III. Cytotoxic Agents to Reduce Lymphocyte Proliferation

a) Antimetabolites

Example: Azathioprine (AZA), Methotrexate (MTX), Mycophenolate mofetil, Leflunomide

These drugs compete with essential components of cell metabolism and have been covered in detail in Chapter 26 and 67. Hence, only immuno-suppressant aspects are discussed below.

Azathioprine (AZA)

AZA is prodrug for 6-mercaptopurine (6-MP). The slow conversion of AZA to 6-MP and its final conversion to 6-thioGTP provides a counterfeit product which gets falsely incorporated into DNA of lymphocyte, making it nonfunctional. Even constimulators on the surface of T-cells are not synthesised. Hence, T-cell activation and proliferation is prevented. AZA is used in organ transplant rejection, rheumatoid arthritis and inflammatory bowel disease. **Major side effects** include bone marrow depression, leukopenia, thrombocytopenia, alopecia, increased risk of herpes simplex and varicella infection, neoplasia, hepatotoxicity and GIT toxicity.

Methotrexate (MTX)

MTX, a cytotoxic antimetabolite used in cancer chemotherapy, has immunosuppressant action also due to its action on lymphocytes and other cells of the immune system. The mechanism of these effects is although unknown, but MTX is known to increase adenosine levels. Adenosine has potent endogenous anti-inflammatory effects and also inhibits superoxide anion generation in neutrophils. Recently, MTX has also been reported to enhance apoptosis of activated but not of resting CD4+ and CD8+ T-cells. MTX is used to treat graft *versus* host disease, rheumatoid arthritis and psoriasis.

Mycophenolate Mofetil (MPM)

Mechanism of Action: Its active metabolite *mycophenolic acid* (MPA) inhibits proliferation and activation of T- and B-lymphocytes by inhibiting inosine monophosphate dehydrogenase type II (IMPDH-II) which is highly expressed on lymphocytes and is crucial for *de novo* (afresh) purine biosynthesis (essential for DNA) by T- and B-lymphocytes. MPM also interferes with leukocyte adhesion to endothelial cells. IMPDH inhibition also decreases the levels of guanosine, a precursor of tetrahydrobiopterin (BH4), which regulates the synthesis of inducible nitric oxide synthase (iNOS). Hence, decreased levels of NO also lead to decreased cytotoxicity by T-cells and neutrophils. **Therapeutic Uses**: (1) As prophylaxis of transplant rejection, both acute and chronic. It is generally used with glucocorticoids and calcineurin inhibitors. (2) In rheumatoid arthritis, myasthenia gravis, autoimmune haemolytic anaemia and inflammatory bowel disease and (3) MPM also reduces the replication of HIV virus that infects T-lymphocytes and Epstein-Barr Virus (EBV) which infects B-lymphocytes (because of reduced guanosine-nucleotide levels which inhibits transcription in the infected cell). Moreover, cells infected by EBV shift from type I to type II IMPDH, which makes EBV infected cells easy targets for MPM.

For pharmacokinetics and adverse effects, see Chapter 26.

Leflunomide

Currently leflunomide is being used in rheumatoid arthritis, but has been used successfully in systemic lupus erythematosus, myasthenia gravis, Wegener's granulomatosis and polyoma virus nephropathy seen in immunosuppressed kidney transplant patients.

b) Alkylating Agents

Cyclophosphamide

Cyclophosphamide is a unique immunosuppressant as it suppresses B-lymphocyte proliferation but can enhance T-cell responses. As a result, the use of cyclophosphamide is restricted to diseases of humoral immunity, particularly systemic lupus erythematosus. Other use is in xenotransplant (between animals of different species). For toxicity, mechanism of action refer Chapter 67. Cyclophosphamide causes serious haemorrhagic cystitis due to generation of acrolein, a nephrotoxic metabolite. *Mesna* is usually coadministered with cyclophosphamide to prevent haemorrhagic cystitis. Mesna conjugates with acrolein in urine, reducing the incidence of renal toxicity.

IV. Cytokine and Cytokine Receptor Inhibitors (Anticytokine-Antibodies)

TNF-α, IL-1, IL-2, IL-6, IL-12, IL-17, IL-23 are some proinflammatory cytokines that activate T-lymphocytes and promote their proliferation and are implicated in the pathogenesis of rheumatoid arthritis (Ch. 25, 26) and Crohn's disease (Ch. 29).

a) Tumor Necrosis Factor-α (TNF-α) Inhibitors

These have been discussed in Chapter 26. Activated cytotoxic TH1 cells, macrophages and mast cells secrete TNF-α that binds to TNF receptor ($TNFR_1$ or $TNFR_2$) present on fibroblasts, neutrophils, and vascular endothelial cells. Besides these, there are "*soluble form of TNF-α receptor*" present in serum and synovial fluid. Activation of TNF-α results in the release of cytokines IL-1, IL-6 and adhesion molecules that promote leukocyte activation and migration.

Example: Etanercept, Infliximab, Adalimumab, Cetrolizumab, Golimumab

Etanercept (Ch. 26) is not used that frequently because of the following factors: (1) The drug does not discriminate between TNF-α and TNF-β. Binding to the latter would rather promote IL-2 mediated T-cell proliferation; (2) It has a long serum half-life of 115 hrs which requires weeks to achieve steady state plasma levels and (3) Upon discontinuation of the drug the symptoms of arthritis appear within a month.

Infliximab (Ch. 26) is a chimeric (25% mouse and 75% human) monoclonal antibody. The drug cross-links with membrane bound TNF-α receptors on cell surface to inhibit T-cell and macrophage function and to prevent the release of other proinflammatory cytokines (IL-1, 6 and 8 along with collagenase and metalloproteinases). Though it also has a longer half-life (200 hrs, onset of action 3 weeks), it does not bind TNF-β. It is currently used in Crohn's disease and rheumatoid arthritis. Better clinical benefits are obtained when used with methotrexate as the latter prevents antibody formation against infliximab.

Adalimumab (Ch. 26) is a human recombinant monoclonal antibody to TNF-α (it also does not bind to TNF-β). It is less antigenic than infliximab as it does not contain any foreign component. Its serum half-life is 2 weeks. Patients of rheumatoid arthritis may therefore need to administer single dose of 40 mg/0.8 ml subcutaneously every 14 days.

Cetrolizumab Pegol is a pegylated anti-TNF-α Mab fragment that is devoid of Fc portion of antibody. As a result like other Mabs of its class, it does not cause antibody-dependent cell mediated cytotoxicity. It has been approved for use in rheumatoid arthritis, Crohn's disease, psoriatic arthritis and ankylosing spondylitis.

Golimumab is a fully human IgG1 Mab directed against TNF-alpha that has a long half life as compared to other anti-TNF-α agents. The drug has been approved for the treatment of adult rheumatoid arthritis (in combination with methotrexate), psoriatic arthritis and ankylosing spondylitis.

b) Interleukin-1 (IL-1) Receptor Antagonists

All activated mononuclear cells generate IL-1, which in turn enhances the production of IL-6, of adhesion molecules and the release of metalloproteinase. IL-1 also stimulates cell proliferation. The role of metalloproteinase is to degrade the cellular matrix in preparation for their proliferation. The naturally occurring endogenous antagonist of IL-1 receptor is IL-1RA.

Anakinra is a recombinant form of IL-1RA which inhibits IL-1 interactions with the immune cells and is used for the treatment of rheumatoid arthritis. It is given subcutaneously (100–150 mg daily). Injection site pain and reaction is the most common side effect. Flu-like symptoms with headache may also occur.

Rilonacept is a new fusion protein that binds to IL-1. It is being evaluated (phase III trials) for treating gout.

Canakinumab is a human IgG1 Mab which targetes IL-1 β and shows a prolong action (therefore is administered once in a month). It has been approved for use in cryopyrin-associated periodic syndrome (CAPS) and systemic juvenile idiopathic arthritis.

c) Interleukin-2 (IL-2) Receptor Antagonists

IL-2 mediates early but crucial steps in T-cell activation. CD25 is the high affinity IL-2 receptor expressed on activated T-cells (Fig. 69.5A). Thus, anti-CD25 antibodies can specifically act on those T-cells which have been activated by MHC-antigen complex stimulus. There are two currently available, well tolerated, monoclonal antibodies directed against IL-2α receptor.

Daclizumab is a chimeric humanized monoclonal antibody produced by fusion of murine anti-CD25 antibodies with human IgG_1.

Basiliximab is a murine:human (10% murine, 90% human) chimeric monoclonal anti-CD50 antibody produced by recombinant DNA technology. Both the drugs block the α-chain of IL-2 receptor (CD25) located on the surface of activated T-cells (not of resting cells). Both antibodies are used for the prophylaxis of acute organ transplant rejection. Daclizumab possesses lower affinity to CD25 compared to basiliximab. Both can be used in combination with glucocorticoids, cyclosporine or azathioprine.

d) IL-6 Receptor Inhibitor

IL-6 is an important mediator produced by lymphocytes, monocytes, keratinocytes, fibroblasts, mesangial cells, endothelial cells, and adipocytes. As a result this cytokine is involved in several physiological and pathological processes which include accute phase inflammatory response, neutrophil migration, differentiation and proliferation of TH-cells, metabolism of bone and cartilage, angiogenesis, metabolism of lipids and carcinogenesis. Increased IL-6 levels have been observed in many autoimmune and inflammatory conditions.

Tocilizumab is a Mab directed against the IL-6 receptor and is approved for the treatment of polyarticular juvenile idiopathic arthritis, systemic juvenile idiopathic arthritis and for patients with rheumatoid arthritis who had shown inadequate response to anti-TNF drugs. This drug is administered by I.V. infusion every 4 weeks.

e) IL-12/IL-23 p40 Cytokine Inhibitors

Ustekinumab: is a high effinity human IgG1 Mab that binds to p 40 subunit shared by IL-12 and IL-23 and thereby inhibits the activation of NK cells and CD4 cells. On activation NK cells and CD4 cells secrete inflammatory mediators like IL-2, IL-23, TNF-α and IFN-γ, which are involved in a number of pathophysiological processes like psoriasis, Crohn's disease, multiple sclerosis and sarcoidosis. Thus Ustekinumab has been approved for the treatment of these conditions. The drug is known to increase the risk of infections.

f) IL-17 Cytokine/IL-17 Receptor Inhibitors

Examples: Ixekizumab, Secukinumab, Brodalumab

IL-17 is a proimflammatory cytokine and exerts its effect through two receptor subtypes, IL-17RA and IL-17RC. ***Ixekizumab*** and ***secukinumab*** are two human Mabs which target IL-17, whereas ***brodalumab*** is a human Mab which is directed against IL-17 RA. All these drugs are undergoing investigation for the treatment of rheumotoid arthritis, Crohn's disease and psoriasis.

V. Antibodies Against Specific Immune Cell Molecules

The acquired immune system on recognising the foreign antigens generates an immune response by way of activation and clonal expansion of various immune cell molecules such as CD2, CD3, CD8, etc. Treatment with exogenous antibodies targeted against several such molecules will deplete the immune system of these reactive cells which participate in lymphocyte activation and proliferation.

a) Polyclonal Antibodies

Antithymocyte Globulin (ATG) is a highly purified solution of γ-globulins with antithymocyte activity. It is obtained by immunizing large animals (horses/sheep) with human lymphocytes. It is available as freeze dried sterile powder for I.V. administration. ATGs, being polyclonal cytotoxic antibodies, target several epitopes such as CD2, CD3, CD8, CD11a, CD18, CD25, CD44 and MHC I and II molecules expressed on the cell surface of APCs or T-cells. Administration of ATG , thus results in a depletion of T-lymphocytes as a consequence of complement-dependent lysis followed by opsonisation by macrophage-monocyte system. There is hardly any effect on B-lymphocytes or monocytes. Hence, humoral antibody formation remains relatively intact despite inactivation and depletion of T-cells. The latter event results in an impairment of delayed hypersensitivity and cellular immunity.

ATG is used to prevent allograft (donated by genetically distinct individual but of the same species) rejection, *viz,* kidney transplant. The **adverse effects** of ATG include local pain and erythema at injection site. *Cytokine release syndrome* is the common characteristic side effect of antibodies which target T-lymphocytes. This results due to an initial activation of T-cell and cytokine release before T-cell clearance by macrophages and monocytes. The symptoms include fever, chills, dyspnoea, nausea and vomiting, hypotension and rashes. The symptoms, however, dissipate as T-cells are eliminated. ATG infusion

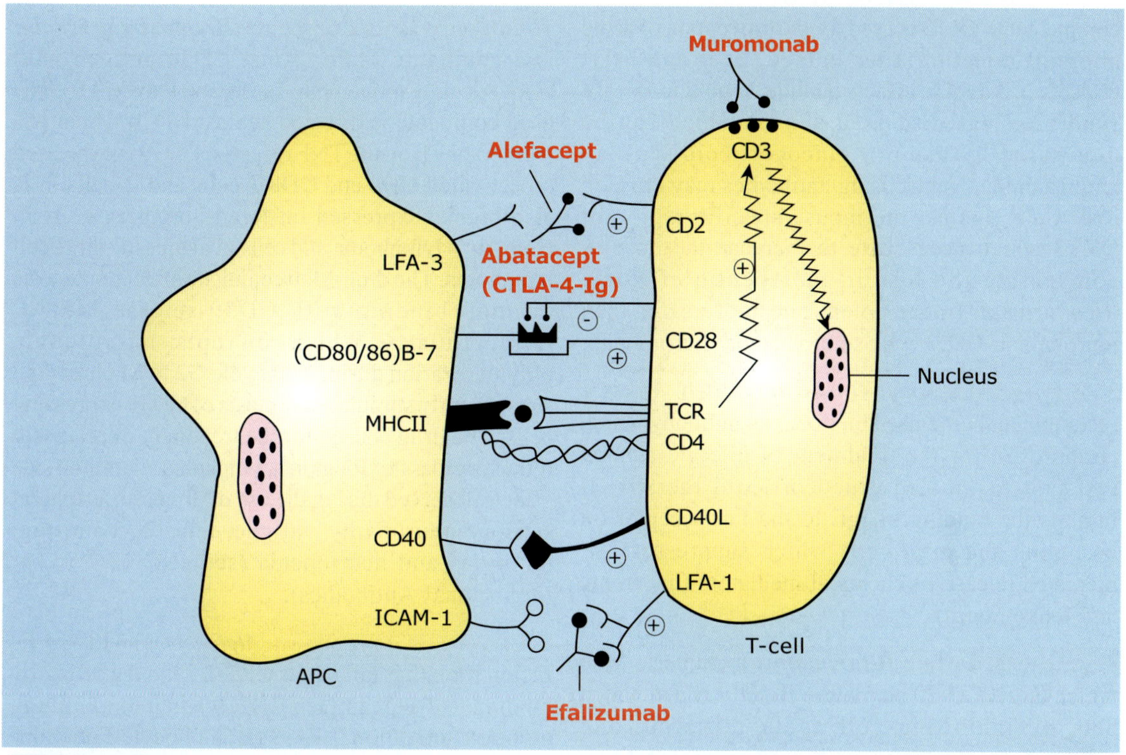

Fig 69.7 Mechanism of Action of Some Monoclonal Antibodies. ***Ipilimumab*** (Table 67.1) binds to CTLA-4 and prevents its association with CD 80/86 to inhibit its cosuppressive signaling to TCR. This MAb is used to treat metastatic melanoma.

under the cover of corticosteroids, an antihistamine and paracetamol reduces the risk of such reactions. The polyclonal antilymphocyte globulins (ALG) are also used to prevent kidney transplant rejection.

b) Monoclonal Antibodies

1. ***Alemtuzumab (Anti-CD52 MAb or Campath-1H)***: CD52 (also called Campath-1) is a glycoprotein expressed on normal and malignant T- and B-lymphocytes, monocytes, NK cells and macrophages. *Alemtuzumab* is a humanised anti-CD52 monoclonal antibody that binds to CD52 and causes prolonged lymphopenia. Hence, recently alemtuzumab has been recommended and used to treat B-cell chronic lymphocytic leukaemia where prolonged and sustained suppression of lymphocytes is desirable. Alemtuzumab induces cell death through antibody-dependent cellular cytotoxicity, complement-dependent cytotoxicity and apoptosis (Ch. 67). **Adverse effects** include infusion-related toxicity, lymphopenia, neutropenia, thrombocytopenia and anaemia, which increases risk for opportunistic infections and bleeding. It can also cause hypertension and kidney failure. It is undergoing phase II trials for use in renal transplantation because it produces long-term B- and T-cell depletion and also allows lowering of drug doses.

2. ***Muromonab-CD3 (anti-CD3 or OKT3)*** is a murine monoclonal antibody against human CD3, one of an important signaling molecules for activation of T-cell receptor (TCR). CD3 is expressed both on CD4+ and CD8+ T-cells (Fig. 69.3). As a result, treatment with muromonab depletes the total circulating T-cells from the blood.

This depletion of T-cell after OKT3 injection results due to cell death (anergy in absence of signal, see earlier text) and antibody mediated activation of complement. OKT3 is used for the prevention of acute allograft rejection after kidney, liver and heart transplant. **Adverse effects** include "cytokine-release syndrome" (as discussed above) which can be minimised by using a glucocorticoid with an antihistamine. Neutralising antibodies may develop over time, against the mouse specific region of OKT3 which necessitate to increase the dose to compensate the loss in therapeutic efficacy. *Alemtuzumab* (more potent and more safer than muromonab-CD3) will soon replace muromonab.

3. ***Anti-IgE Antibody:*** ***Omalizumab*** (Ch. 48) is a recombinant humanised monoclonal antibody which is approved for the treatment of allergic asthma resistant to inhaled glucocorticoid therapy. It inhibits the binding of IgE to the Fcε receptor on basophils and mast cells which suppresses IgE mediated release of chemical mediators (histamine and leukotrienes).

4. **Anti-CD20 Mab**: ***Rituximab*** is a chimeric Mab which target CD-20 on mature B-cell antigen which acts by inhibiting cell cycle initiation and differentiation in these cells, leading to depelition of ciruculating T-cells. It is used for the treatment of B-cell lymphoma ($CD20^+$ non-Hodgkin's lymphoma) and chronic lymphocytic leukaemia. Due to its B-cell depeliting action, rituximab has also been approved for the treatment of rheumatoid arthritis refractory to TNF-α inhibitors.

5. **Anti-CD25 Mab**: ***Basiliximab*** is a Mab directed against CD-25 which is a high affinity IL-2 receptor located on T-cells. IL-2 cytokine mediates T-cell activation. The drug is used for prevention of organ transplant rejection (see above in IL-2 Receptor antagonists).

6. **B-Lymphocyte Stimulator (BLyS) Cytokine Inhibitor**: ***Belimumab*** is a human Mab which targets B-lymphocyte stimulator (BLyS) cytokine. BLyS binding to normal B-lymphocyte activates a chain of events that stimulate cell survival and differentiation to become antibody producing cells. Belimumab acts by blocking normal function of BLyS and thereby inhibits antibody production by B-cells. The drug has potential for the treatment of a number of autoimmune diseases.

7. **Antibody-Drug Conjugate:** ***Brentuximab vedotin*** is a conjugate Mab against CD30 antigen with cytotoxic drug monomethyl auristatin E (MMAE). The drug conjugate is directed against CD30 which is a membrane gp on the TNF receptor. CD30 is expressed on activated CD4 and CD8 T-cells and B-cells. It is also highly expressed on Reed-Sternberg cells in Hodgkin's lymphoma and cells of anaplastic large cell lymphoma. The drug-Mab conjugate after endocytosis through binding with CD30 release MMAE intracellularly which disrupts microtubule polymerezation during cell cycle G2 to M phase and subsequently stimulate apoptosis of CD30 expressing cells. The drug is used for the treatment of relapsed/ refractory classic Hodgkin's lymphoma. Common side effects observed during the use of drug are peripheral sensory neuropathy, fatigue, nausea, vomiting, diarrhoea and neutropenia (see also Table 67.1, Monoclonal Antibodies).

8. **LFA-3 (CD58) Inhibitor**: ***Alefacept*** is an LFA-3/Fc fusion Mab that interrupts CD2-LFA-3 signaling by binding to T-cell antigen CD2, leading to inhibition of T-cell activation. LFA-3 (**L**ymphocyte **F**unction-associated **A**ntigen-3) is a counter receptor for CD2 an antigen expressed on T-cells. Interaction of CD2 on T-cells with LFA-3 on effector T-cells stimulate T-cell proliferation and T-cell cytotoxicity. Alefacept thus blocks the T-cell induced cytotoxicity and is used in the treatment of chronic plaque psoriasis.

VI. Inhibitors of Immune Cell Adhesion and Activation

a) **Anti-LFA-1/LFA-3 Mabs**

Example: Efalizumab, Alefacept

Efalizumab is a humanised IgG_1 monoclonal antibody which targets CD11, a chain of LFA-1 (**L**ymphocyte **F**unction-associated **A**ntigen-**1**) and blocks its activity. Interaction of LFA-1 (expressed on activated T-cells) with ICAM-1, i.e., **I**nter**c**ellular **A**dhesion **M**olecule-1 (expressed on endothelial cells) facilitate T-cell activation, adhesion and diapedesis (migration of cells through pores of blood vessels) to the site of inflammation. Efalizumab binds to LFA-1 and prevents LFF-1 + ICAM interaction.

Efalizumab is used for the treatment of psoriasis but has been reported to decrease the incidence of acute kidney transplant rejection. Its efficacy is increased when used along with glucocorticoids, cyclosporine and MPM. Because of immuno-suppression the drug increases the susceptibility to infections. Phase III trials are being conducted with efalizumab in liver and islet cell transplantation.

Alefacept is an engineered human LFA-3 + IgG_1 fusion protein. The LFA-3 moiety of alefacept binds to CD-2 present on T-lymphocytes blocking the interaction between LFA-3 present on dendiritic cells and CD2 present on T-cells. Hence, alefacept prevents T-cells activation. It is used to treat psoriasis. Clinical trials with alefacept in kidney transplant recipients are underway.

b) **Alpha-4 Integrins Inhibitor/Blocker**

Natalizumab is a Mab directed against alpha-4 integrin. Alpha-4 integrin consists of two units: Alpha-4 β1 and Alpha-4 β7. The Alpha-4 β1 integrin mediates immune cell interaction with cells expressing VCAM-1, while Alpha-4 β7 integrin mediates immune cell binding to cells expressing mucosal addressin cell adhesion molecule (MadCAM-1). ***Natalizumab*** when binds with Alpha-4 integrin inhibits immune cell interaction with cells expressing VCAM-1 and MadCAM-1. ***Natalizumab*** has been approved for the treatment of relapsing-remitting multiple sclerosis (RRMS) (See ch. 40, page 548) and Crohn's disease (See ch. 29, page 419). However, since the use of the drug for the treatment of these conditions was found to be associated with a rare demyelinating disorder similar to the infection by JC virus, one should be watchful of development of progressive multifocal leukoencephalopathy (PML) while using the drug.

VII. Inhibitors of Immune Cell Costimulation (Tolerogens; Fig. 69.7)

a) **Anti-CD80 and Anti-CD86 MAbs**

Example: Abatacept, Belatacept

The focus of research these days is to induce T-cell tolerance in order to have immunosuppression without concomitant risk of developing opportunistic infections and secondary tumours which frequently occur during the use of immunosuppressant drugs. Although there is no drug available for clinical use which can produce T-cell "anergy or tolerance", a term **tolerogens** has been coined for future drugs which by blockade of certain costimulatory mechanisms produce induction of T-cell anergy or tolerance (see earlier text).

As discussed earlier and shown in Fig 69.3, two signals are required for T-cell activation. Signal-1 is an antigen-specific signal mediated *via* TCR. Signal-2 is a permissive signal *via* interaction of molecules such as CD28 on T-lymphocytes with CD80 (B7.1) and CD86 (B7.2) on the antigen-presenting cells (APCs). Another costimulatory pair is CD40 (on APC) with CD40L (CD-154) on T-cell. Both ***costimulatory*** pairs are permissive for T-cell activation. However, for physiological self control of immune responses, a ***cosuppressive pair*** of molecules is also operative. Thus CTLA4 (CD-152) expressed on T-cell surface can also interact with CD80 (B7.1) and CD86 (B7.2) on APC to dampen (downregulate) an immune response (Fig. 69.3). Recently, humanised anti-CD80 MAb (h1F1) and humanised anti-CD86 MAb (h3D1) have been developed and are being evaluated as potential *tolerogens* in renal transplant recipients. Similarly, CTLA4-Ig fusion protein (a homologue of CTLA4, i.e., a part of immunoglobulin molecule and a part of CTLA-4), is also undergoing clinical trials with promising results.

Abatacept is the first generation CTLA4-Ig fusion protein that binds to CD 80/86 on APC and inhibits T-cell costimulation (as done by CTLA-4). It has recently been approved for resistant cases of rheumatoid arthritis and polyarticular juvenile idiopathic arthritis.

Belatacept is a newer CTLA4-Ig fusion protein with much higher affinity for CD80/86 and has been approved for the prevention of organ transplant rejection in patients undergoing kidney transplantation.

Because induction of signal-1, in absence of signal-2, results in "anergy", use of such drugs could be an effective method for down-regulating specific cell (TH1 or TH2) population. Such induction of anergy (or non-responsiveness to antigen specific signal) could lead to long-term acceptance of an organ transplant and would minimise the risk of associated adverse effects as discussed above.

b) **CTLA-4 Inhibitor/Blocker**

Ipilimumab is a recombinant fully human IgG1 Mab which binds to CTLA-4 and blocks the interaction of this receptor with its ligands B7-1 and B7-2 (Fig 69.7). Based on this mechanism, the drug has been shown to provide overall survivial benefit in patient with unresectable or metastatic melanoma who had been previously treated with one or more anticancer drugs. Ipilimumab has been approved for the treatment of advance melanoma. The drug has been shown to produce immune-related hepatotoxicity, immune diarrhoea (enterocolitis, which responds to glucocorticoid therapy) and endocrine problems.

c) **PD-1 Inhibitor/Blocker**

Like Cytotoxic T-Lymphocyte Antigen-4 (CTLA-4), Programmed (cell) Death Protein-1 (PD-1) is another immune check-point signal molecule that regulates antigen specific immune responses. Ligation of both signal molecules (CTLA-4 and PD-1) to T-cells blocks the immune response by inhibiting the T-cell proliferation and activation to produce cytotoxic cytokines. It has been reported that some tumours express and upregulate PD-1 ligands (PDL-1 and PDL-2) and thereby inhibit T-Cell mediated immune surveillance of tumours.

Nivolumab (fully human) and ***Pembrolizumab*** (humanized) are recombinant IgG4 Mabs that bind to PD-1 and thereby inhibit the ligation or binding of PD-1 to tumours that overexpress its ligands PDL-1 and PDL-2. Thus these two anti PD-1 Mabs leads to a downregulation of PD-1 pathway-mediated inhibitation of the immune response. This process results in the enhancement of immunogenic antitumour (tumour-killing) response to T-cells. Both *nivolumab* and *pembrolizumab* are *indicated for the treatment of metastatic or unresectable melanoma* [with disease progression even after the treatment with ipilimumab, and a B-RAF (V600 E) inhibitor (*dabrafenib* or *vemurafenib*) when the tumour is positive for B-RAF V600 E mutation]. These two Mabs are also approved for the treatment of metastatic non-small cell lung cancers (NSCLCs) that express PDL-1 and demonstrate disease progression on or after platinum compound-based chemotherapy.

VIII. Miscellaneous Group

Rho (D) Immune Globulin

The **Rh** system of blood classification is so named because it was first worked out in the blood of *Rhesus monkey*. It is based on the type of antigen present on the surface of erythrocytes. People whose RBCs have Rh (D) antigen are designated as Rh^+ and those who lack are designated as Rh^-. Normally plasma does not have anti-Rh antibodies. But, if a Rh^- person receives Rh^+ blood the body starts to make anti-Rh^+ antibodies which then remain in circulation. Now, if a second transfusion of Rh^+ blood is given later, these antibodies will react and will cause haemolysis of the donated blood with severe reactions.

Such kind of Rh incompatibility may occur during pregnancy. Normally there is no direct contact between the maternal and foetal blood during pregnancy. However, if a small amount of Rh^+ blood leaks from the foetus, through the placenta, into the blood stream of the Rh^- mother (as during delivery or abortion), the mother will start making anti-Rh^+ antibodies. The newborn baby would not be affected (as it is not a second exposure). But, in subsequent pregnancy, the mother's anti-Rh^+ antibodies can cross placenta and enter into foetal circulation. If the foetus is Rh^-, there is no problem because Rh^- blood does not possess Rh^+ antigens. However, if the foetus is Rh^+, haemolysis of foetal blood can occur (**H**aemolytic **D**isease of the **N**ewborn, HDN) resulting in abortion.

HDN can be prevented by giving Rh^- mother, an injection of an anti-Rh gamma globulin RhoGAM) preparation soon after delivery or abortion. These antibodies will bind to foetal Rh^+ antigens (if they had escaped). The mother's own immune system is, thus, spared from generating antibodies against these Rh^+ antigens. Moreover, the foetus of next pregnancy is also protected and is not at risk because the mother has no memory B-cells that can be activated with Rh^+ foetus of second pregnancy. The usual dose of Rho (D) immune globulin is 2 ml I.M. containing about 300 mg of anti-RhoD-IgG. Adverse effects are rare.

IMMUNOSTIMULANTS AND IMMUNOMODULATORS

A number of disorders such as immunodeficiency states (e.g., AIDS), autoimmune disease, cancer and viral infections can be treated with immunostimulant drugs. These agents are nonspecific and may affect innate as well as adaptive immunity. These may work on cellular or humoral immune system or both. Because of their variable effects in different conditions and on different components of immune system, these are more popularly known as *biological response modifiers* or *immunomodulators*.

a) Bacillus Calmette-Guerin (BCG)

BCG is an attenuated live culture of Calmette-Guerin strain of bacillus *Mycobacterium bovis*. Its active constituent is muramyl dipeptide. Its action is nonspecific and stimulates T-cells and NK cells. It is also used for the treatment of urinary bladder cancer where it is instilled and held for 2 hrs before urination.

Common adverse effects include chills, fever, malaise, hypersensitivity reactions and shock.

b) Levamisole

It is an anthelmintic drug discussed in Chapter 63. It stimulates T-cell functions primarily, but also B-cells, monocyte and macrophage activity. It is combined with 5-fluorouracil to improve survival of patients suffering from colorectal cancer. There are reports that patients with slow spreading vitiligo respond to levamisole (150 mg OD orally for 2 consecutive days in a week for 3–4 months). Flu-like symptoms, allergic manifestation, nausea and muscle pain are its usual side effects.

c) Thalidomide and Lenalidomide

Thalidomide is available for restricted use, i.e., to treat erythema nodosum leprosum and multiple myeloma because of its immunomodulatory and anti-inflammatory effects. It decreases TNF-α levels in blood and produces anti-angiogenic effects and therefore is indicated in refractory rheumatoid arthritis and in certain malignancies. Being teratogenic it is contraindicated in pregnancy.

Lenalidomide is a thalidomide analogue with immunomodulatory and anti-angiogenic properties. It has been approved for the treatment of transfusion-dependent anaemia due to myelodysplastic syndrome. *Adverse effects* include neutropenia, thrombocytopenia, risk of deep vein thrombosis and teratogenicity (contraindicated in pregnancy).

d) Recombinant Cytokines

Cytokines are gaining popularity as immunomodulators. With the advent of genetic engineering, cytokines can be produced in bulk and in purified form.

Aldesleukin

These are recombinant IL-2 obtained from cultures of *E. coli*. *Aldesleukin* stimulates TH cells and Tc cells and thus enhances cellular immunity. It is used in the treatment of metastatic renal cell carcinoma and melanoma. *Side effects* include capillary leak syndrome (extravasation of water and plasma proteins), hypotension, reduced tissue perfusion and concomitant infection due to decrease in neutrophil function.

Other Recombinant Interleukins (rIL)

rIL-1 is produced by macrophages and is essential for activation and proliferation of various immune cells. It is given I.V. for general augmentation of immune responses. ***Oprelvekin*** (rIL-11) stimulates megakaryocytes and their precursors in the bone marrow. It is used to prevent thrombocytopenia in the patient of cancer receiving highly myelosuppressive chemotherapy (Ch. 50 and 67).

Colony-Stimulating Factors

Recombinant GM-CSF (***Sargramostim***; Ch. 50 and 67), G-CSF (***Filgrastim***; Ch. 50 and 67) and pegylated recombinant G-CSF (***Pegfilgrastim***; Ch. 50) are some important cytokines that support the survival, proliferation and differentation of haematopoietic cells. ***Sargramostim*** is virtually a multipotent haematopoietic growth factor (granulocytes, erythroids, megakaryocytes and macrophages). ***Filgrastim*** stimulates proliferation and differention of neutrophil progenitor cells, activates the phagocytic activity of mature neutrophils and prolongs their survival in circulation. ***Pegfilgrastim*** is a longer acting analogue of filgrastim which can be given once (I.V.) per chemotherapy cycle. All of them are used to reduce the severity and duration of neutropenia induced by cytotoxic drugs during chemotherapy or following bone marrow transplant. For more details and see Ch. 50.

e) Recombinant Interferons

Interferon-α (IFN-α): Human recombinant IFN-α acts as a immunostimulant as it activates T-lymphocytes, natural killer cells and macrophages. Both IFN-α and IFN-α2b are indicated for a variety of cancers: chronic myeloid leukaemia, hairy cell leukaemia, malignant melanoma, non-Hodgkin's lymphomas and AIDS-related Kaposi's sarcoma (Ch. 67). IFN-α is additionally used in the treatment of hepatitis-B and C virus infections. *Side effects* include flu-like syndrome, blood dyscrasias, nephrotoxicity and neurological symptoms like nervousness and confusion.

Interferon-β1a and β1b are used for the treatment of relapsing type multiple sclerosis. *Side effects* include flu-like symptoms and injection site local reactions.

Interferon-γ, mainly IFN-γ1b, restores macrophages cytotoxicity by generating free radicals and is used for the treatment of chronic granulomatous diseases. *Side effects* include flu-like symptoms, GIT distress, anorexia and skin rashes.

CHAPTER 70 Management of Stroke

Stroke is one of the leading causes of death worldwide these days. It is estimated that death due to stroke will increase drastically in next two decades due to aging of population and our inability to control the risk factors. Atherosclerosis of coronary arteries leads to *ischaemic heart disease (IHD)* and *myocardial infarction (MI)*; while occlusive disease of the arteries in the lower leg and foot leads to *claudication*. On the other hand, atherosclerosis or stenosis of carotid or cerebral arteries results in ***stroke***. A temporary deficit of neurological or monocular functions of acute onset, which lasts for less than 24 hr is called ***transient ischaemic attack (TIA).*** About 30% of the patients of stroke have a history of TIAs and proper treatment of such attacks prevents the possibility of forthcoming stroke. The highest risk of stroke is within a month after the TIA but declines thereafter.

TRANSIENT ISCHAEMIC ATTACK (TIA)

It is an episode of temporary cerebral ischaemia or dysfunction caused by a brief interruption in the blood supply to the brain. ***Symptoms include*** nausea and vomiting, dizziness, weakness, numbness, headache, double vision, partial loss of vision, atypical neurological or extrapyramidal symptoms (e.g., tremors), slurred speech and seldom, however, paralysis in a limb (or on one side of the body) and drooping of face on one side. These symptoms have an abrupt-onset, may last for 15 min to 24 hr, may occur singly or in combination but leave no permanent neurological deficits. An important ***cause of TIA*** is cerebral ischaemia due to embolisation (see below). An ulcerated atherosclerotic plaque in a major artery to the brain may serve as a source of emboli. TIAs can also occur due to atherosclerotic changes in carotid artery (carotid ischaemia) or in subclavian artery proximal to vertebral artery (vertebrobasilar ischaemia).

Management

1) *Use of antiplatelet aggregating drugs*, e.g., *aspirin* in low doses (325 mg orally daily) or *clopidogrel* (75 mg orally daily) or a combination of *aspirin* 25 mg + extended-release preparation of *dipyridamole* 200 mg orally twice daily. For details refer Ch. 51.
2) *Correction of adverse lipid profile by statins*, e.g., Tab. *atorvastatin* 10 mg daily in the evening or a combination of *atorvastatin* 10 mg + *ezetimibe* 10 mg orally daily in the evening. Statins not only ↓ LDL and ↑ HDL, but also normalise vascular endothelial function, prevent plaque rupture and the ensuing thrombosis. For details refer Ch. 23.
3) *Control of blood pressure* preferably by use of an ACE inhibitor (e.g., *perindopril*) with or without a diuretic (e.g., *indapamide*). For details refer Ch.16, 18 and 19.
4) *Cessation of smoking.*

STROKE

Stroke is a state of focal neurological deficit of an abrupt-onset, presumably of vascular origin, which lasts at least for 24 hr. Stroke can be either ***ischaemic*** (85%) or ***haemorrhagic*** (15%). In haemorrhagic strokes, the mortality rates are high (50%); while in ischaemic strokes, mortality is less (20%). ***Risk factors for stroke*** include: **(1)** smoking, **(2)** excessive alcohol intake, **(3)** obesity, **(4)** diabetes, **(5)** hypertension, **(6)** adverse lipid profile (↓ HDL, ↑ LDL), **(7)** stenosis of carotid arteries, **(8)** valvular or rheumatic heart disease and **(9)** atrial fibrillation or arrhythmias.

Ischaemic Stroke

Ischaemic strokes are due to either (1) local thrombus formation (i.e., a ***thrombotic stroke***) or

(2) because of embolism (i.e., an ***embolic stroke***). Both result in an occlusion of cerebral artery. About 60% of cerebral infarcts are thrombotic, while embolic infarcts are 20%. Embolic infarcts have better chances of survival than thrombotic infarcts. If the occlusion is of a major vessel, e.g., of the carotid artery or of a branch vessel, e.g., of the middle cerebral artery or of the posterior cerebral artery, this will lead to ischaemic damage of large areas of brain leading to large ***cerebral infarcts***. If there are multiple smaller infarcts (< 5 mm diameter) due to occlusion/blockage of fine perforating vessels or of fine arterioles in the basal ganglia, pons and cerebellum, these are called ***lacunar infarcts***. In **cerebral infarction**, the resulting neurological deficits depend on the particular vessel involved and the extent of obstruction to cerebral circulation. Yet, there may be headache, hemiplegia, paraplegia, hemianopia (partial blindness) and other motor and sensory deficits (e.g., slurred speech). Cerebral ischaemia leads to the release of excitatory neurotransmitters (Ch. 30) that may augment Ca^{2+} influx into neurons, thereby leading to cell death and an increase in neurological deficits. Infarction in either the carotid or vertebrobasillary region may lead to coma. An infarct involving one cerebral hemisphere may lead to such swelling that the functions of the other hemisphere or the rostral brainstem or of reticular formation is disturbed which leads to loss of consciousness. In **lacunar infarcts** the neurologic deficits are mild, e.g., tremors, nausea, vomiting, clumsiness of hands and slurred speech. These deficits may progress maximum up to 48 hr but later get stabilised and subside within 4–6 weeks in many instances. Early mortality and risk for stroke recurrences is more in patients with *non-lacunar* than *lacunar* infarcts.

Diagnostic Tests

CT scan of head (with contrast for infarcts but without contrast for haemorrhagic stroke) are quite informative and preferable in stroke, compared to MRI. However, with higher resolution, MRI of head can reveal areas of ischaemia earlier than the CT scan. Carotid doppler study can reveal the degree of stenosis (occlusion) in the carotid arteries supplying blood to the brain (extracranial cause of stroke). ECG will determine whether the patient suffers from atrial fibrillation or arrhythmias, a potent aetiologic factor for stroke. A 2-D Echo can reveal valvular heart disease, a probable source of emboli to the brain. Adverse lipid profile and elevated serum homocysteine levels are indicative of increased risk of thrombotic stroke.

Pathophysiology

If there is carotid atherosclerosis, shear stress may result in plaque rupture, collagen exposure, platelet aggregation and clot formation. This clot may remain in the vessel to cause local occlusion or can travel distally as an embolus to eventually lodge downstream in a cerebral vessel. The net result of both thrombotic or embolic stroke is an arterial occlusion, decreasing cerebral blood flow and causing ischaemia distal to the site of occlusion. Normal cerebral blood flow averages 50 ml/100 g/min and this is maintained over a wide range of blood pressures by a process called *cerebral autoregulation* (in the same way as a voltage stabiliser provides a predetermined voltage over a wide range of voltage fluctuations). As a result, cerebral blood vessels keep on dilating or constricting in response to changes in blood pressure if any. This process of cerebral autoregulation gets impaired by atherosclerosis or embolism as happens in stroke. If local cerebral blood flow decreases below 20 ml/100 g/ min, *ischaemia* occurs; and if it decreases below 10 ml/100 g/min and persists too, irreversible damage to brain cells would occur leading to *infarction*.

Drug Treatment of Ischaemic Stroke

1) The only proved effective therapy for acute ischaemic stroke requires intravenous administration of thrombolytic agents preferably ***tissue plasminogen activator (tPA)*** (0.9 mg/kg to a maximum of 90 mg, over one hour) *within 3 hr of the onset of the stroke*. Other thrombolytic agents that can be used are *urokinase*, *alteplase* (a recombinant tPA; rt-PA) and *reteplase* (a modified rt-PA). These are fibrinolytic drugs which dissolve the clot and open up the blocked blood vessel (Ch. 20 and 51). Patients receiving such treatment show a 50% decrease in permanent disability associated with stroke.

Haemorrhagic stroke and *systolic pressure above 185 mm of Hg or diastolic pressure above 110 mm of Hg, are strong contra-indications to this therapy.*

2) Early aspirin therapy also reduces long-term disability and improves the chances of survival *but it should never be given within 24 hr of the administration of tPA because it would increase the risk of bleeding.* However, aspirin (325 mg orally daily) may be started after 24 hr but within 48 hr of the onset.
3) Elevated blood pressure is very common in patients of ischaemic stroke but blood pressure lowering efforts during acute stroke period (first 7 days) may result in decreased cerebral blood flow which may worsen the symptoms (as cerebral autoregulation fails during stroke; see above). If blood pressure is to be lowered, it should be lowered gradually by using short-acting parenteral drugs like *labetalol* or *nicardipine*. Later, during follow-up, the preferred antihypertensive therapy is an ACE inhibitor (e.g., *perindopril*) with or without a thiazide diuretic (e.g., *indapamide*).
4) Statin therapy is an effective way to reduce stroke risk because usually these patients have an adverse lipid profile (↑ LDL, ↓ HDL). It can be corrected by giving *atorvastatin* 10 mg/day or a combination *atorvastatin* 10 mg/day + *ezetimibe* 10 mg/day orally.
5) For follow-up and secondary prevention of non-cardioembolic ishaemic stroke, antiplatelet drugs are normally used, e.g., *aspirin* (325 mg/day orally) or *clopidogrel* (75 mg/day, orally) or a combination of *aspirin* 25 mg + *dipyridamole* 200 mg orally twice daily.
6) Anticoagulant therapy with low molecular weight heparin (LMWH) or with oral anticoagulant like warfarin, has no role in the management of patient with completed stroke EXCEPT when there is a cardiac source of embolism due to atrial fibrillation or valvular disease or MI (i.e., cardioembolic ischaemic stroke). *However, there should be no evidence of any haemo-rrhagic stroke and the CSF fluid should be clear.*
7) ***Other measures*** include (a) cessation of smoking, (b) avoiding the use of any thrombo-genic drug, e.g., oral contraceptives or selective COX-2 inhibitors and (c) use of some adjuvant drugs which lower blood viscosity (e.g., *pentoxifylline*) or which increase cerebral perfusion and protect cerebral cortex from hypoxia (e.g., *piracetam*).
8) Recently, it has been shown that hypothermia provides neuroprotection in patients of acute ischaemic stroke. The "cold therapy" seems to limit the amount of residual damage from the ischaemic stroke by triggering a survival response in which the body requires lesser oxygen. In USA and in some European countries "stroke survival kits" are available which include cooling blankets. Current clinical trials have shown that rewarming the patient after hypothermia provides better results.
9) For ***lacunar infarcts,*** therapy with antiplatelet aggregating drugs and long-term control of risk factors (adverse lipid profile, hypertension, diabetes, and smoking) is usually sufficient.

Haemorrhagic Stroke

Haemorrhagic stroke includes *subarachnoid haemorrhage* (blood entering the subarachnoid space) or *intracerebral haemorrhage* (rupture of blood vessel within the brain parenchyma), *subdural haemorrhage/haematoma* (blood below the dura) and *haemorrhage due to arteriovenous congenital malformation with or without associated aneurysm.* Haemorrhagic stroke, although less common (15%), is significantly more lethal (mortality rates 3–6 times higher) than the ischaemic stroke.

Pathophysiology of haemorrhagic stroke is not well understood. However, presence of blood in brain parenchyma inflicts damage to the surrounding brain tissue (by mass effect). The degradation products of blood components further lead to neurotoxicity. There is an abrupt increase in intracranial pressure which leads to coma, herniation and death.

Management of haemorrhagic stroke usually requires:

1) Surgical intervention to remove haematoma. However, calcium channel blocker *nimodipine* (Ch. 19 and 20) at a dose of 60 mg orally every 4 hr can be used in cases of subarachnoid haemorrhage, and continued for 21 days in such patients. It reduces the incidence and severity of neurologic deficits owing to delayed cerebral ischaemia. Use of nimodipine is sometimes associated with a fairly high incidence of hypotension. This can be managed by reducing the dose to 30 mg every 4 hr.
2) ***Fosphenytoin*** slow I.V./***Phenytoin/Carbamazepine*** can be used to prevent seizures.
3) To decrease cerebral oedema, *prednisolone* (*up to 100 mg per day*) or *dexamethasone* (*up to 16 mg per day*) can be used but benefits are doubtful. Alternatively, hyperosmolar agents such as *glycerine* (oral) or *mannitol* (i.v. infusion) can be used but with poor results because the ensuing oedema is of mixed origin (vasogenic + cytotoxic).
4) Any physical activity or strain should be avoided. Once the patient's condition becomes stable, the drug treatment is accompanied with physiotherapy and occupational therapy (for improving morale, motor skills, muscular strength and speech difficulties).

CHAPTER 71

Management of Shock

COMPETENCY PH1.27

Shock (circulatory failure) occurs when the oxygen perfusion fails to meet the metabolic demands of the tissues. Shock in routine terms is often considered to be synonymus to hypotension (to define the state of circulatory failure). While hypotension is an unfortunate development which is manifested at a later stage of shock, it is the cardiac output and oxygen delivery that is critically low even when the blood pressure remains normal. Shock results in regional hypoxia and subsequent lactic acidosis (from anaerobic metabolism in peripheral tissues) eventually leading to end organ damage and failure.

CLASSIFICATION OF SHOCK

Major types of shocks are classified as under:

1) **Hypovolaemic Shock**: Any condition resulting in a major reduction in blood volume, e.g., due to internal or external haemorrhage; loss of plasma due to burns and loss of fluids and electrolytes due to excessive vomiting and diarrhoea.
2) **Cardiogenic Shock**: A condition resulting due to severe pump failure (due to myocardial infarction or cardiomyopathy), cardiac arrhythmias or valvular dysfunction.
3) **Septic Shock**: A condition secondary to Gram -ive bacteraemia (less often due to Gram +ive cocci or Gram -ive anaerobes). Risk factors include extremes of age, diabetes, immunosuppression or recent invasive procedure. Septic shock is usually associated with massive vasodilatation secondary to the production of endotoxins from pathogenic bacteria. Hence, it is also called "warm shock" to distinguish it from hypovolaemic and cardiogenic shock in which the patient's extremities are usually cold due to inadequate blood flow.
4) **Anaphylactic Shock**: It results due to severe immediate hypersensitivity reaction and is manifested as excessive vasodilatation (warm extremities), increased capillary permeability, exudation of fluid in the tissues, angioneurotic oedema and bronchoconstriction (difficulty in breathing).
5) **Neurogenic Shock**: It is caused by traumatic spinal cord injury or as adverse event during epidural/spinal anaesthesia. This results in a loss in sympathetic tone and reflex vagal parasympathetic stimulation producing vasodilation (warmth of extremities), hypotension, bradycardia and syncope.

The *central venous pressure* (CVP; juglar pressure) *is typically reduced in hypovolaemic and anaphylactic shock,* but *elevated in cardiogenic shock* and *unpredictable (+,- or ±)* in *neurogenic* or *septic shock.* This is an important distinction which may be quite helpful if the physical signs are confusing. All forms of shock require early diagnosis and management because regional hypoxia and deranged tissue perfusion can preciptitate multiple organ failure.

MANAGEMENT OF SHOCK

Volume replacement is critical in the initial management of shock. Hypovolaemia should be corrected by I.V. fluid administration before the use of vasopressors because vasopressors would not be effective if hypovolaemia persists.

1) **Hypovolaemic Shock**: Blood loss is treated with immediate infusions of blood substitues, such as group specific or type O-negative packed red blood cells (PRBC) or whole blood which also provides extra volume and clotting factors. If there is severe dehydration, volume replacement is initiated with the rapid infusion of isotonic saline or by Ringer lactate through large-bore intravenous lines. No distinct benefit from the use of colloid (plasma expanders) over crystalloid solutions were found in hypovolaemic shock due to trauma. Particularly in traumatic brain injury patients, use

of colloids increased mortality while use of hypertonic saline plus dextran increased the survival rate.

Following fluid replacement, the inotropic support with dopamine may be needed to maintain adequate ventricular performance. Use of vasopressor agent like norepinephrine is not recommended because in such patients the circulating catecholamine levels are already high and the fluid loss is accompanied by reflex vasoconstriction. Use of an α_1 blocker, e.g., ***phenoxybenzamine*** (I.V.) can help to (a) counteract vasoconstriction and (b) shift blood from pulmonary to systemic circuit and from extravascular to vascular compartment so as to improve cardiac output.

Dopamine infusion (2–3 mcg/kg/min) stimulates renal dopaminergic (D_1) as well as cardiac β_1-adrenoceptors and is useful as it increases heart rate, contractility as well as glomerular filtration. Supplemental O_2 should also be provided to support respiratory functions. ***Phenylephrine*** may be an useful alternative in patients who are at risk of having tachyarrhythmias with dopamine or norepinephrine.

2) **Cardiogenic Shock**: Vasoactive drug therapy with dobutamine/dopamine can be instituted only after adequate fluid replacement. However, cardiogenic shock requires smaller amounts of fluid replacement. Inotropic drug support can be provided with ***dobutamine*** (β_1-adrenoceptor agonist). Usual dose range is 2.5 mcg/kg/min as I.V. infusion. It increases contractility and decreases afterload, due to reflex reduction in sympathetic tone. Alternatively ***dopamine*** (2–3 mcg/kg/min) by I.V. infusion can also be used. ***Norepinephrine*** is reserved for patients with refractory hypotension particulary those who do not have increased systemic resistance. Usual dose is 2–4 mcg/min. If systolic BP cannot be maintained with a dose of 15 mcg/min, it is unlikely that increasing the dose would be beneficial.

3) **Septic Shock**: Successful management requires urgent measures to treat infection and to provide haemodynamic and respiratory support. Septic shock usually requires large volumes of fluid for resuscitation because the associated capillary leak releases fluid to extravascular space. Empirical antimicrobial therapy with ***meropenem*** (I.V.) or ***ticarcillin*** with ***clavulanic acid*** may be started soon, pending blood-culture reports. Treatment of the known pathogen may start later, after the culture results.

A preparation of recombinant activated protein-C, **drotrecogin alpha (*activated;*** Ch. 51) when given as a continuous infusion of 24 mcg/kg/hr for 96 hr, improves mortality in severe septic shock with multiple organ failure. It has recently been licensed for this indication, by FDA. **Vasopressin (ADH)** is gaining widespread acceptance in the treatment of septic shock. It causes peripheral vasoconstriction via V_1 receptors (located on vascular smooth muscle) and reduces NO synthesis. It also potentiates the effects of catecholamines on vasculature and stimulates cortisol production, and can increase blood pressure even when there is resistance to adrenaline. **Corticosteroids** like hydrocortisone (50 mg QID) with 9-α-fludrocortisone (50 mcg OD) for 7 days suppress the formation of NO and of prostaglandins, as well as shorten the duration of use of vasopessors besides reducing mortality. They also prevent adrenal insufficiency during septic shock. Positive inotropes including **adrenaline, dopamine** and **dobutamine** may also help in certain patients. ***Other measures include*: (a)** maintenance of pulmonary capillary wedge pressure between 12–16 mm Hg or central venous pressure at 8–12 cm H_2O (to avoid pulmonary oedema), **(b)** maintenance of proper urine output (furosemide may be used if needed), **(c)** maintenance of blood glucose levels in a normal range and **(d)** by providing essential respiratory, haemodynamic and metabolic support.

4) **Anaphylactic Shock**: It can be managed by using ***adrenaline*** (I.M. or S.C.) along with other supportive measures. By causing broncho-dilatation and increasing blood pressure, adrenaline counteracts the effects of histamine and other mediators that are released, from mast cells and basophils, during immediate hypersensitivity reaction. A ***antihistamine*** (H_1 antagonist) and a ***glucocorticoid*** are generally used as adjuvants along with adrenaline.

5) **Neurogenic Shock**: Treatment is given on the same lines as with hypovolaemic shock. Once haemorrhage has been ruled out, ***norepinephrine*** or a pure α-adrenoceptor agonist ***phenylephrine*** can be given to augment vascular resistance and maintain mean arterial pressure.

PLASMA EXPANDERS

Ideally, human plasma/whole blood or reconstituted human albumin are preferred to correct hypovolaemia due to haemorrhage. Nevertheless, blood transfusion carries the risk of transmitting hepatitis and AIDS while transfusion of albumin is quite expensive. Hence, high molecular weight synthetic colloids are often used as plasma expanders. When infused I.V., they retain fluid in vascular compartment by exerting osmotic pressure comparable to plasma. Being inert colloids they remain in circulation, do not leak out and are not readily metabolised. Moreover, these are easily sterilised and are cheap. Commonly used plasma expanders are discussed below:

1) **Dextran**: It is a polysaccharide and is available as ***dextran-70*** (mol. wt. 70,000) 6% solution in dextrose or normal saline or as ***dextran-40*** (mol. wt. 40,000) 10% solution in dextrose/normal saline. The most commonly used preparation is ***dextran-70***. It keeps plasma volume expanded for 24 hrs but may interfere with blood grouping and cross matching. It can interfere with coagulation and platelet function (can prolong bleeding time). Allergic reactions may occur but only occasionally. ***Dextran-40*** acts more rapidly, reduces blood viscosity and prevents RBC sludging (as occurs in shock). However, it has a shorter duration of action (rapid glomerular filtration) and may cause tubular obstruction (gets concentrated in tubule if oliguria develops). Dextrans can be stored for several years and are cheap.
2) **Degraded Gelatin Polymer (Polygeline)**: It is a polypeptide (mol. wt. around 30,000). It is not antigenic; hypersensitivity reactions are rare and does not interfere with grouping and cross matching of blood. Expansion of plasma volume lasts for 12 hrs. It remains unmetabolised and is excreted slowly by the kidney. It has a shelf life of 3 yrs and is expensive than dextran.
3) **Hydroxyethyl Starch (Hetastarch)**: Lesser in use because of side effects though it improves haemodynamic status for more than 24 hrs. It contains ethoxylated amylopectin of different molecular sizes. Smaller molecules (40% of the infused dose) is excreted from the kidney within 24 hrs. Remaining larger molecules are degraded first to smaller ones and are excreted very slowly (2 weeks). Its 6% solution has colloidal properties similar to human albumin. *Side effects:* Swelling of salivary glands, periorbital oedema, bronchospasm, vomiting, chills, rigors, flu-like symptoms and urticaria.
4) **Polyvinylpyrrolidone (PVP)**: Obsolete, rarely used because of drug interactions (binds to insulin and penicillins), side effects, antigenicity and histamine releasing property.
5) **Human albumin**: It can be used irrespective of the patient`s blood group. Being heat treated preparation it carries no risk of transmitting hepatitis or AIDS. It does not affect coagulation nor carries any risk of sensitisation with repeated infusion. 100 ml of 20% human albumin solution is equivalent (in osmolarity) to 400 ml of fresh frozen plasma or to 800 ml of the whole blood. However, it is expensive and crystalloid solutions (GNS or normal saline) should also be infused concurrently for optimum results. It can also be use in hypoproteinaemia.

Therapeutic Uses: Plasma expanders can be used as substitutes for plasma in conditions of burns, hypovolaemic and septic shock. These are also used as temporary measure to substitute for blood loss till the same can be arranged.

Contraindications and drawbacks: Plasma expanders do not have O_2 carrying capacity. These are contraindicated in anaemia, cardiac failure, renal insufficiency and pulmonary oedema.

CHAPTER 72 Drug Treatment of Obesity

Our hunger-haunted ancestors survived because any excess calories latent in their food were stored as triglycerides, in adipose tissue, which were then mobilised when food was not available to them. Later, because of economic growth, sedentary lifestyle, cultural influences and availability of a variety of calorie-rich tasty food resulted in an epidemic of "globesity" which in medical terminology is called "obesity". In simple terms, obesity is an illness where the quality as well as the life expectancy is adversely affected by an excess of body fat. According to WHO Expert Committee, calculation of Body Mass Index (BMI; weight in kg divided by the square of height in meters) is a benchmark for assessing obesity. Accordingly, a subject with a BMI of 20–25 kg/m^2 is considered as having normal weight; one with a BMI of 25–30 kg/m^2 as overweight and one with a BMI of more than 30 kg/m^2 as obese. Since BMI depends on an overall energy balance, obesity can be defined as a multifactorial disorder of energy balance in which long-term calorie intake exceeds energy output which results in higher BMI.

HOMEOSTATIC CONTROL OF ENERGY BALANCE AND FAT STORES

Leptin is a peptide secreted by adipose cells and acts through the hypothalamus. Arcuate nucleus of the hypothalamus has two sets of neurons with opposing actions. Both groups express leptin as well as insulin receptors.

One set of neurons contains neuropeptide-Y (NPY) and agouti-related protein (AGRP). The leptin receptors on these neurons sense leptin levels. A fall in leptin levels (due to starvation, weight loss or decreased fat stores) activates these neurons to release NPY and AGRP, resulting in increased food intake (orexigenic effects), decrease in energy expenditure and increase in storage of fat (anabolic effect). Insulin works in concert with leptin but it is not a fat-sensor.

The other set contains neurons of prepro-opiomelanocortin (POMC) which release alfa-melanocyte-stimulating hormone (α-MSH). An increase in leptin levels (due to overeating, weight gain or increased fat stores) activates these neurons to release α-MSH resulting in decreased food intake (anorexigenic effect), increase in energy expenditure and decrease in storage of fat (catabolic effects). The word *leptin* is derived from the Greek word *leptos,* meaning a thinning hormone. As both the sets of neurons have opposing actions, it is implied that if an increase in leptin levels increases α-MSH release, it would simultaneously decrease NPY/AGRP release and *vice versa* (Fig. 72.1).

From the clinical, as well as anecdotal, observation that marijuana and cannabis (Δ^9 tetrahydrocannabinol) stimulate appetite, it appears that CB_1 receptors (in brain) are also involved in the control of food intake and energy balance (see below).

From the leptin story discussed above, it appears that an alteration in leptin kinetics might provide a simple answer to the problem of obesity. Paradoxically, plasma leptin levels are already higher in obese persons (even then their food intake is not affected). It is the resistance to leptin, rather than insufficient hormone, that is the main problem in obesity (for which there is no solution as yet). Hence, such interventions are unlikely to be useful. Attempts are, however, underway to alter CNS levels of NPY and POMC (Fig. 72.1) which transduce changes in leptin signals. Search for Y_5 receptor antagonists, as antiobesity agents, is under process (see Ch. 17).

Currently available drugs target various factors, other than those included in the Figure 72.1, that are involved in regulating food intake and energy expenditure.

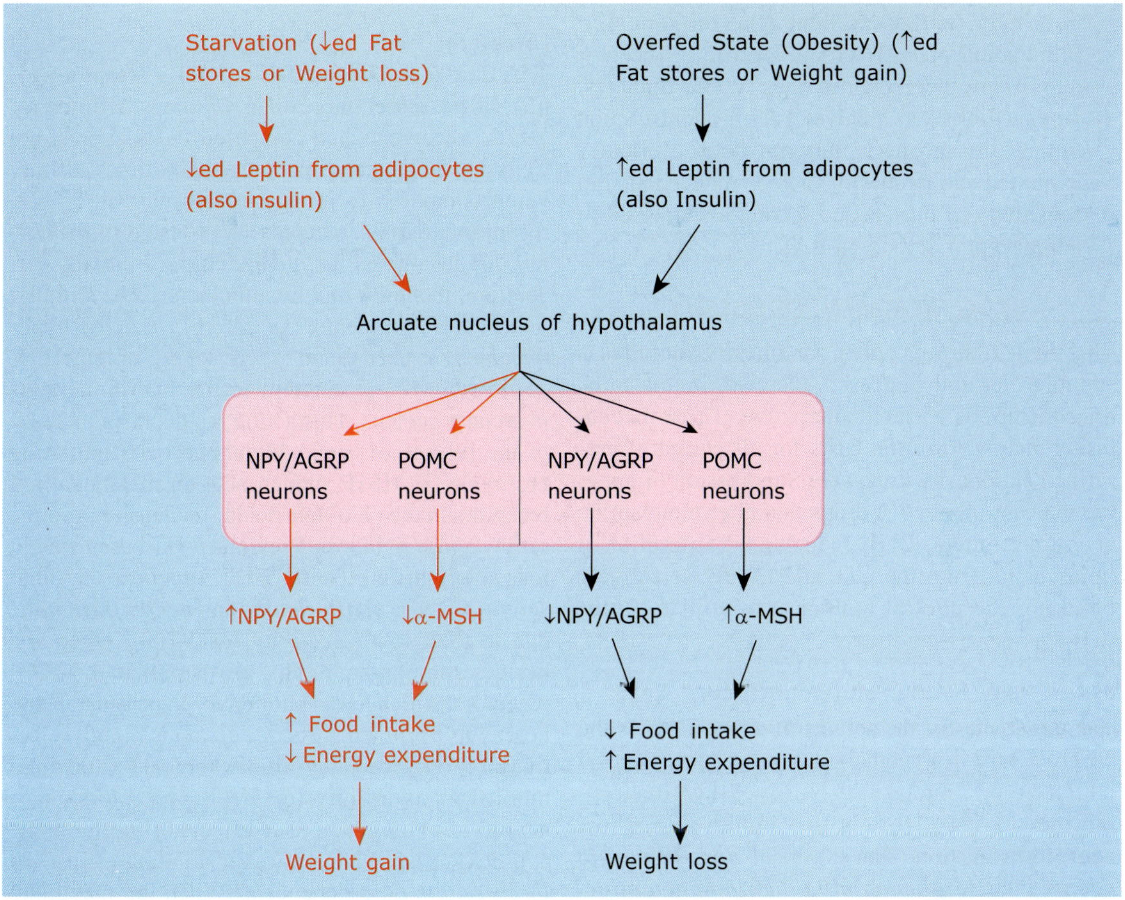

Fig 72.1 The Homeostatic Control of Food Intake and Energy Expenditure Regulated by Leptin

- Common orexigenic factors (which stimulate feeding behaviour) are: melanin – concentrating hormone, GABA, growth-hormone releasing hormone and ghrelin (an endogenous hormone secreted by gastric fundal cells during the fasting state). Ghrelin not only stimulates feeding behaviour but also promotes growth hormone release from the somatotrophs. Orally active ghrelin antagonists are under investigation for appetite control.
- Common anorexigenic factors (which inhibit feeding behaviour) are: corticotrophin-releasing hormone, tumour necrosis factor-α (TNF-α), 5-HT, glucagon like peptide (GLP) and cholecystokinin (CCK; a peptide secreted by the duodenum in respones to eating and digestion of fatty meal). CCK acts on CCK-B receptors in the brain to suppress satiety center.
- The food intake is normally balanced with the energy expenditure required to maintain metabolism, physical activity and thermogenesis (heat production which occurs in brown adipose tissue-BAT). In contrast to white adipose tissue, which stores energy in the form of lipids, BAT expends stored energy as heat. A mitochondrial uncoupling protein-1 (UCP-1) uncouples oxidative phosphorylation while the mitochondria continue oxidative metabolism. Because of absolute uncoupling, the liberated energy (after O_2 consumption) cannot be utilised to couple inorganic phosphates to energy rich organic phosphates (ATP). This unutilised energy

gets manifested as heat (thermogenesis). Stimulation of BAT with a specific β_3 receptor agonist protects against obesity and diabetes. Among β-blockers, **nebivolol** has β_3 agonist action but its this property has not been clinically exploited yet. In obesity, there is reduced insulin sensitivity of muscle and fat and a decreased β_3 adrenoceptor activity in BAT.

DRUG TREATMENT OF OBESITY

The main treatment plan for obesity includes a suitable diet and increased exercise. If this fails, drug therapy is a viable alternative. Three mechanisms mainly form the basis for all currently prescribed antiobesity drugs: **(1)** Suppression of appetite via centrally active drugs that alter monoamine neurotransmitters, **(2)** By reducing the absorption of lipids or fat from the GIT and **(3)** By selectively blocking the central endocannabinoid receptor (CB_1) as discussed above.

a) Centrally Acting Anorexiant Drugs

The target site for the actions of anorexiants is the satiety centre in hypothalamus. All of them act by inhibiting the reuptake of NE or 5-hydroxytryptamine (5-HT) (or both) enhancing their neurotransmission. The classical ***noradrenergic agents*** include ***phentermine***, ***benzamphetamine***, ***diethylpropion*** and ***mazindol***. All of them are amphetamine analogues and are no longer used because of the side effects (CNS stimulation, insomnia, tremors, addiction liability and hypertension). However, tolerance also develops soon to their anorectic action and thus they are unsafe for long-term use. ***Serotonergic agents*** include ***fenfluramine***, ***dexfenfluramine*** and ***lorcaserin***. Of these, the first two agents are no longer used because of their effects such as cardiotoxicity (valvular heart defects/heart valve damage) and pulmonary hypertension as well as sudden deaths particularly with combined formulation of *fenfluramine + phentermine (Fen-Phen)*. However, a combination of ***phentermine*** + ***topiramate*** (an antiseizure drug) by the name ***Qsymia*** has recently been approved as an antiobesity fixed dose combination (FDC) pill.

Lorcaserin

This drug is a selective 5-HT, 5-HT_{2C} receptor agonist (it possesses more than 17 times affinity for 5-HT_{2C} receptor when compared to its agonist activity on 5-HT_{2A} and more than 100 times affinity when compared to its agonist activity on 5-HT_{2B} receptors). 5-HT_{2C} receptors are located in the cortex, hippocampus, amygdala, choroid plexus, cerebellum, thalamus and hypothalamus. The stimulation of 5-HT_{2C} receptors by *lorcaserin* in the hypothalamus has been found to activate pro-opiomelanocortin (POMC) production in the POMC neurons in arcuate nucleus. This action results in an increase in the release of *alpha*-**M**elanocortin-**S**timulating **H**ormone (α-**MSH**), which acts on melanocotin-4 receptors in the para-ventricular nucleus to promote satiety and weight loss. Previous 5-HT based weight loss medications (with 5-HT receptors agonist activity) such as ***fenfluramine*** and ***dexfenfluramine***, due to their low selectivity for 5-HT_{2C} receptors, besides stimulating 5-HT_{2C} also stimulated 5-HT_{2B} receptors, which led to pulmonary hypertension and heart valve problems. As *lorcaserin* is highly selective for 5-HT_{2C} receptors (affinity for 5-HT_{2C} 100 times more than its affinity for 5-HT_{2B} receptors), it is devoid of on-target adverse effects of fenfluramine and dexfenfluramine. However, binding affinity of *lorcaserin* is dose-dependent. When the maximum dose of 20 mg/day is exceeded, it may bind to other 5-HT receptors such as 5-HT_{2A}. When these receptors are stimulated hallucinations, euphoria and altered mood may occur. *Lorcaserin* is thus approved as antiobesity drug (to be given in the dose of 10 mg BD with or without food) as an adjunct to a reduced calorie diet and increased physical activity for chronic weight management in obese adults (with a BMI equal to or more than 30 kg/m^2) or in overweight patients (with a BMI of >27 kg/m^2) with at least one weight-related co-morbidity such as hypertension, type-2 diabetes or dyslipidaemia. It is advised that if patients do not achieve 50% reduction in weight by week 12 of taking the drug, they should stop taking *lorcaserin* because it is unlikely that they will be benefitted by this agent. Further increase in the dose is not advisable due to development of non-specificity of 5-HT receptors (5-

HT_{2A} and $5HT_{2B}$) agonist activity if higher doses than the 20 mg/day are administered.

If administered orally, *lorcaserin* is well absorbed, metabolized by CYP enzymes in the liver and excreted more in urine and less in faeces. Its $t_{1/2}$ is 11 hrs. As a result the dose adjustments are not required in patient with mild-to-moderate hepatic or mild renal impairment. However, in patients with severe hepatic and moderate-to-severe renal impairment or end-stage renal failure, the drug is not recommended. The safety and efficacy of this drug for paediatric patients (<18 yrs) has not been established. *Lorcaserin* is contraindicated in pregnancy.

Qsymia

The drug is an extended release (ER) or controlled release (CR) combination of two older drugs, ***phentermine*** *and* ***topiramate (PHEN/TPM -ER, -CR)****. Phentermine* is a noradrenergic sympathomitic amine, amphetamine derivative approved earlier as an anorexic agent for short-term weight loss (with restrictions on use due to its cardiotoxicity). Compared to amphetamine, phentermine is not a habit forming drug and produces its anorexic effect by increasing the release of noradrenaline (NA) dopamine (DA) from central nerve terminals as well as by blocking the reuptake of these monoamines, thereby increasing the concentration of these neuro-transmitters in the brain. An increase in NA in hypothalamus decreases appetite. However, since phentermine acts indirectly by increasing the release of NA and DA, tolerance to the anorexic effect occurs within weeks and weight loss effect plateaus. An increase in doses does not result in further weight loss and therefore there is a need of combining this event with other drug(s) having different weight loss mechanism of action. *Topiramate* is a sulphamate-substituted monosaccharide derivative of the natural sugar monosaccharide D-fructose approved as an antiseizure (see Ch. 39) and antimigraine drug, which has shown weight loss as an adverse reaction when it was used for its approved antiseizure indication. An ER or CR fixed dose combination (FDC) of PHEN/TPM is available as an immediate-release phentermine and CR-release topiramate for long-term use in the treatment of obesity. This FDC is available in four dosage formulations. For initial treatment: **(1)** PHEN/TPM in the ratio of 3.75 mg/23 mg to be taken once orally in the morning for 14 days, and for maintenance treatment; **(2)** In the ratio of 7.5 mg/46 mg to be taken once orally in the morning from day 15 for 12 weeks (including the first 14 days). Weight loss should be evaluated after 12 weeks of taking the formulation (2) and if the patient does not loose 3% of baseline body weight, treatment is discontinued or escalation of doses should be considered, as it is unlikely that the patient will achieve and sustain clinically useful weight loss at this dose [formulation (2)]. If escalation in doses is considered formulation (3) and (4) have to be used: **(3)** PHEN/TPM in the ratio of 11.25 mg/69 mg to be taken once orally in the morning for 14 days, followed by maintenance dose treatment; **(4)** In the ratio of 15 mg/92 mg to be taken once orally in the morning from day 15 for 12 weeks (including the first 14 days). Weight loss should be evaluated after 12 weeks of taking the formulation (4) and if the patient does not loose atleast 5% of baseline body weight, after the subsequent 12 weeks of taking the formulation (4), the treatment should be discontinued **gradually**, as it is unlikely that the patient will achieve and sustain a clinically meaningful weight loss with continued treatment.

It is important to remember that the formulations (1) 3.75 mg/23 mg and (3) 11.25 mg/69 mg dosage strengths are for titration purposes only, whereas formulations (2) 7.5 mg/46 mg and (4) 15 mg/92 mg dosage strengths are for maintenance purposes only. Besides when the treatment is decided to be discontinued, it should be done **gradually** with both the maintenance formulations (2) and (4) by taking a dose every other day (after 12 weeks of continuous therapy in each case) for at least 1 week before stopping the treatment altogether due to the possibility of precipitating a seizure (even if the patient is not an epileptic). *This instruction has particularly been advised to be followed strictly when formulation (4) of highest dosage ratio has been used.*

The antiobesity treatment with *Qsymia* should be started with the lowest dose ER FDC ratio formulation pill administered for 12 weeks as an adjunct to a reduced calorie diet and increased physical activity for chronic weight management in obese adults (with a BMI >30 kg/m^2) or in overweight patients (with a BMI > 27 kg/m^2) with at least one weight-related co-morbidity such as hypertension, type-2 diabetes or increased LDL cholesterol and dysplipidaemia.

The adverse effects of individual drugs used in the FDC combination in *Qsymia* should be kept in mind and informed to the patient. *Phentermine* is an adrenergic drug having both central and peripheral actions and thus may cause hypertension, tachycardia (which warrant caution in patients with history of cardiac and cerebrovascular disease), insomnia, anxiety, dizziness, impaired coordination, etc. Adverse effects associated with topiramate are glaucoma (acute myopia with secondary angle-closure glaucoma has been reported with topiramate), urolethiasis (urinary stone formation, metabolic acidosis and non-anion gap may occur as *topiramate* is known to posses carbonic anhydrase inhibitory activity), sedation, somnolence, amnesia, impairment of concentration/attention, speech or language problems (particularly word finding difficulties due to disturbed memory; more reported when rapid titration or high initial doses are used to start weight loss therapy with *Qsymia*).

Besides weight loss achieved by the drugs in combination with *Qsymia*, these may increase the risk of hypoglycaemia in type-2 diabetes treated with insulin or insulin secretogogues. In patients with hypertension, weight loss may increase the risk of hypotension. Therefore, strict monitoring and dose adjustments are required when *Qsymia* is used for weight loss in patients with type-2 diabetes mellitus and essential hypertension. Co-administration with alcohol and CNS depressant drugs with PHEN/TPM combination may potentiate CNS depression or other centrally mediated effects of these agents, e.g., dizziness, drowsiness, somnolence and cognitive impairment.

Qsymia is contraindicated in pregnancy and its safety and efficacy is not known in paediatric patients younger than 18 years. *Qsymia* has been approved for **R**isk **E**valuation and **M**itigation **S**trategy **(REMS)** programme to insure that benefits of treatment outway the risks because of the teratogenic risk (oral cleft in offspring of women treated with topiramate for migraine prophylaxis) associated with the PHEN/TPM CR therapy.

Naltrexone and Bupropion Combination

US-FDA has approved a combination of ***naltrexone and bupropion (NB)*** as weight loss drug therapy. It was shown in clinical trials that administration of a sustained release fixed-dose combination (FDC) tablet of *naltrexone HCl* (8 mg) *plus bupropion HCl* (90 mg) administered in the following dose escalating schedule: **Week 1**: *1 tablet once in the morning*; **Week 2**: *1 tablet twice in the morning and evening*; **Week 3**: *2 tablets in the morning and 1 tablet in the evening*; **Week 4**: *2 tablets in the morning and evening*. When a total daily dose of two tablets twice daily (i.e., 32 mg/360 mg) is reached at the start of the week 4, the dosage schedule is continued further until desired weight loss goal is met. Clinical response should be evaluated after 4 months of treatment. Therapy is discontinued, if clinically meaningful weight loss (>5%) is not observed after this period. Clinical trials with *naltrexone-bupropion* combination therapy have demonstrated 2–4% weight loss compared to placebo after 1 year.

Bupropion component may increase the risk of seizures, suicidal ideation and anxiety behaviours, other neuropsychiatric events and elevation of blood pressure and heart rate. Other adverse effects that can be seen are headache, nausea and vomiting, diarrhoea and constipation and dry mouth. When drugs which inhibit CYP2B6 enzyme (e.g., ticlopidine or clopidogrel), are co-administered with this combination, the dose should not exceed one tablet b.i.d. Other condition which need dose reduction to this level are mild-to-moderate hepatic and renal impairment.

The exact mechanism of neurochemical effect of *naltrexone/bupropion* leading to weight loss is not fully understood. However, it has been suggested that the effect may be mediated through an action in areas of brain involved in the regulation of food intake: the hypothalamic appetite regulatory centre, where *naltrexone* produces an aversion to food intake right from the beginning by blocking *mu*-opioid receptors (see Ch. 37) and bupropion (see

Ch. 34) in the long term may reduce activity of dopamine-mediated reward system in the mesolimbic dopaminergic neurocircuitry.

Liraglutide

Liraglutide is an injectable modified incretin, i.e., an acylated GLP-1 analogue [where a soluble fatty acid (palmitic acid) is attached to the side chain of lysine], which acts as **GLP-1 R**eceptor **A**gonist (GLP-1 RA). This chemical modification in the native GLP-1 molecule causes it to bind to serum and tissue albumin (much like *insulin detemir,* which also possesses fatty acid acylated amino acid lysine like *liraglutide*). This increases the half-life of *liraglutide* to approximately 12 hrs from 1–2 min of the native GLP-1, permitting once daily injection dosing. As such it has been approved by the US-FDA (in 2010) and DCGI (in 2014) for patients with type-2 diabetes who achieve inadequate control with diet and exercise and even after concurrent therapy with metformin, a sulfonyl urea or a glitazone with which it can be combined (but not with DPP-4 inhibitors; in the latter combination the risk of pancreatitis is increased). Treatment is started with 0.6 mg s.c. daily and increased after 1 week to 1.2 mg daily. If needed the doses can be increased to a maximum of 1.8 mg daily as the most common adverse effect noted are nausea (28%) and vomiting (10%).

Recently *liraglutide* was approved by the FDA (in 2014) for the weight loss therapy in obese people based on the observation that GLP-1 analogues are known to produce an enhanced satiety effect mediated in the hypothalamus leading to loss of appetite. Clinical trials have demonstrated a 3.7–4.5% weight loss compared to placebo after 1 year of therapy in the doses of 0.6–1.8 mg/day administered by s.c. route [pre-filled, multi-dose pen that delivers doses of 0.6 mg, 1.2 mg or 1.8 mg (6 mg/mL; total 3 mL) are available]. Concerns include thyroid-C-cell tumour observed in animal studies (obese patients are specially advised to watch for any change in the thyroid gland size), pancreatitis, gall bladder disease, renal impairment, increased heart rate and suicidal thoughts. Frequently observed adverse effects include nausea, vomiting, diarrhoea, constipation and hypoglycaemia (as the obese patient are already regulating their dietary requirements).

Albiglutide, Dulaglutide, Semaglutide

Three other long-acting GLP-1 analogues, ***albiglutide*** [GLP-1 dimer is genetically fused to human albumin, has a half-life of 4–5 days, thereby permitting a weekly S.C. dose (30 mg)]; ***dulaglutide*** [in which two native GLP-1 analogue are covalently linked to an Fc fragment of human IgG4, enabling it to withstand degradation by DPP-4, as a result of which it has a half-life of approximately 5 days and thus can be injected S.C. (in the dose of 0.75–1.5 mg) at weekly intervals] have been approved for the patients with type-2 diabetes (t-2 DM); ***semaglutide*** is a once-daily glucagon-like peptide-1 analog that differs by the presence of an acyl group with a steric diacid at *Lys26* and a large synthetic spacer and modified by the presence of a α-aminobutyric acid in position 8 which gives stability against the DPP-4. The stability of semaglutide by the acylation permits a high-affinity albumin binding and gives it a long plasma half-life which allows the once-daily dosage. Although weight loss is much less with these three drugs but they do cause weight loss in obese (t-2 DM) patients, albeit less than that seen with *liraglutide*.

Sibutramine

It functions as a 5-HT and NE reuptake inhibitor at hypothalamic site that regulates food intake. It is not related to amphetamine and carries no addiction liability. It reduces food intake and causes dose dependent weight loss with reduction in visceral fat. In addition, it decreases plasma triglycerides, LDL, VLDL but increases HDL. It also stimulates thermogenesis by activating β_3 receptors in adipose tissue. Usual dose is 10–15 mg once daily orally.

Adverse effects: Increase in heart rate and blood pressure, dry mouth, constipation and insomnia (contraindicated in patients of hypertension, CHF, stroke and cardiac arrhythmia).

Drug interactions: It should not be used concomitantly with SSRIs like *fluoxetine* and 5-HT agonist used for migraine like *sumatriptan* (risk of serotonin syndrome). Because of its cardiotoxicity it has been withdrawn by FDA in October 2010, and immediately after by the DCGI in the Indian market.

b) GI Lipase Inhibitor

Orlistat

Orlistat is a synthetic ester that inhibits gastric and pancreatic lipases which are required for the hydrolysis of dietary fat into fatty acids (a step prior to their absorption). Orlistat is also suitable for obese persons with additional risk factors like diabetes and hypertension.

Taken at a therapeutic dose of 120 mg TDS orally it blocks the digestion and absorption of fats by 30 percent.

Adverse effects include flatulence, oily spotting and faecal urgency. It causes deficiency of fat-soluble vitamins A, D, E and K. Vitamin supplements are needed but should not be given within 2 hrs of orlistat administration. Orlistat is contraindicated in patients with malabsorption of fats or cholestasis. It has been approved as OTC drug by FDA.

If the drug treatment of obesity does not give desired reduction in the weight loss, ***bariatric surgery*** is an increasingly prevalent treatment option for the patients with severe obesity. Currently three types of surgeries are recommended: (1) Most popular is the ***Roux-en-Y Gastric Bypass (RYGB)*** surgery. RYGB typically results in substantial amount of weight loss over 30% of initial body weight in some studies. However, some complications occur in 40% of persons undergoing RYGB which include peritonitis due to anastomotic leak; abdominal hernias; gall stones; neuropathy; stomal stenosis; thromboembolic disease; gastrointestinal symptoms and nutrition deficiencies, including iron, B_{12}, folate, calcium and vitamin D. (2) ***Gastric banding*** procedure results in less dramatic weight loss than RYGB. (3) ***Sleeve gastrectomy***, which is gaining in popularity; with this procedure approximately three-quarters of the stomach is resected, but the intestinal tract is otherwise left intact. Weight loss results are some what less than RYGB but greater than gastric banding.

Setmelanotide

Setmelanotide is recently approved by US-FDA for the management of obesity. It is an agonist to melanocortin-4 receptors to induce a feeling of satiety for chronic weight management. It is used to treat obesity and the control of hunger associated with pro-opiomelanocortin deficiency, a rare disorder that causes severe obesity in early age. It is administered subcutaneously. *Adverse effects*: Nausea, injection site reaction, disturbances in sexual arousal, depression, suicidal ideation and skin pigmentation.

CHAPTER 73

Prescription Writing and Common Latin Abbreviations

COMPETENCY PH1.10

After examining the patient and making a diagnosis, a clinician may have various therapeutic options such as medication or surgery or physiotherapy and even no therapy at all. If he opts for drug therapy, he has to write a ***prescription*** which ***is a written directive by a clinician to the pharmacist/chemist to prepare and/or dispense a specific medicine for a particular patient.*** Medicine is a drug that is used clinically in therapeutic practice. That means, all medicines are drugs but all drugs are not medicines. ***A prescription is a medicolegal document*** and hence it should be written in ink. It should not only be accurate and precise but should be written with particular care, with clarity and legibility, to avoid possibilities of error or misinterpretation on the part of pharmacist/ chemist/ patient.

In 1999, the Institution of Safe Medication Practices, USA, and the Institute of Medicine, Washington DC, USA, published a report which documented an increasing frequency of medical errors. Later, a detailed list of such possible errors was made available at the websites of the Institute of Safe Medication Practices (ISMP) and of Joint Commission for the Accreditation of Healthcare Organisation (JCAHO) USA. The following are a few examples of safe writing rules suggested on these websites:

1) There should be a space between a number and its units to make it easier to read. There should not be any periods (full stop/dot) after the abbreviations:

Incorrect	Correct
10mg or 10mg.	10 mg
10ml or 10ml.	10 ml

2) Trailing zeros should be avoided because if decimal point is misinterpreted or missed, a ten-fold overdose can occur.

Incorrect	Correct
2.0 mg	2 mg

3) On the contrary, leading zeros should be preferred for numbers less than one. That means a zero should always be placed before a decimal.

Incorrect	Correct
.5 mg	0.5 mg

4) There is no safe abbreviation for "once daily dosing". It must be written out in full. O.D. can be confused for right eye (o.d.). Hence, if there is a liquid medicament (e.g., Lugol's iodine), it can harm the patient due to incorrect administration. On the contrary, Q.D. can be misinterpreted as QID (sloppy dot in between Q and D can give an impression of I). If this happens, there would be a four-fold overdose of the drug
5) Never abbreviate Units as U, because handwritten U may look like 0 (zero) and may lead to 10-fold overdose error.
6) Similarly, never abbreviate International Units as IU, because hand written IU can be misread as IV which may create a havoc. Write in full as International Units or Int. Units, instead.
7) Never abbreviate micrograms as µg, as µg can be misinterpreted as mg. Instead use mcg or microgram.
8) Never abbreviate drug names, e.g., MTX (for methotrexate) and INH (for isoniazid), because different people can interpret them differently.
9) Blank space between the body of prescription and the signature of the doctor should not be left. If blank space is present, it should be striked off to avoid misuse of this space for obtaining some drugs illegally.

PARTS OF A PRESCRIPTION

A correct and a complete prescription can prevent the clinician, the pharmacist and the patient from making a mistake and can eliminate the need for further clarification. A good prescription should contain:

1) Name, address and qualification of the prescribing doctor. Usually it is printed at the top of the prescriber's letter pad.
2) Date of writing the prescription.
3) Name, age, sex and the address of the patient.
4) ***Superscription*** (to be written on outside-left at the top of the body of prescription): It consists of the symbol (R_x) meaning "take thou". R_x is also considered as a prayer to the Greek Gods of healing—Jupiter and Horus. Hence, in short, R_x means "Take thou in the name of God".
5) ***Inscription****:* Earlier it was known as the main body of prescription. Through this part of prescription, the physician used to direct the pharmacist to compound the preparation. Hence, the physician used to write the main drug responsible for the desired effect (***Basis*** part of inscription). Next, he used to write what was to be added to promote the effect of the main drug (***Adjuvant***). Then, what to be added to minimise the undesirable effects of the main and/or adjuvant drug (***corrective***) and finally, what should be used as a ***solvent/vehicle/excipient*** for preparing the drug in requisite amount. Such preparations used to be either syrups/mixtures/powders/ointments. Since these were compounded formulations delivered to the patient by the pharmacist, such prescriptions (written by the physician) were called "***compounded prescriptions***". With the rapid advancement of dosage forms of the drugs, the pharmacist now is no longer required to prepare and dispense the drugs written in compounded prescription because this is done for him by the pharmaceutical manufacturers.

   Nowadays, the prescriptions are the "***precompounded prescriptions***" as these are written for a drug with its ***brand/proprietary name***. It directs for the dosage form (Cap/Tab/Inj/Mix/Syrup) to be used, its strength, the dose interval and the duration for which the drug is to be taken. Since a number of drugs are available in the market by their generic names, the precompounded prescription can also be written for a generic drug. During the past two decades, there has been a gradual change in the method of prescribing a drug. More emphasis is now laid on the directives written on prescription for the correct use of medicine. These directions should be clear, simple and understandable to the patient. These should also be explained to the patient by the physician and pharmacist/chemist. To avoid errors or misinterpretation, safe writing practices for prescription writing should be followed (see above). *Latin abbreviations, very popular earlier, are usually avoided nowadays. Rather, the instructions such as "at bed-time", "once a day" or "before/after meals" are now written clearly on the prescription itself.*
6) ***Subscription (Mft)****:* This part of prescription was used to provide directions to the pharmacist regarding dispensing of the preparation written in prescription. However, with the advent of branded formulations, this part is rarely described in modern prescriptions.
7) ***Signa or Signatura****:* This part of prescription includes instruction to the patient regarding the intake of the prescribed drug(s). These instructions, in modern prescriptions, can also be written in the local language for the benefit of the patient.
8) ***Physician's Signature with Registration Number****:* The prescription ends with the signature of the doctor with his registration number. No blank space should be left between the body of the prescription and the signatures (see above).

A sample of traditional (compounded) prescription and of a modern (precompounded) prescription is given below:

TRADITIONAL (COMPOUNDED) PRESCRIPTION (NOW OBSOLETE)

1) Doctor's Name and Qualifications — Address: Clinic/Residence, Tel. No.:
2) Date
3) Patient's name, age, sex and address
4) R_x
5) *Inscription*:

Basis:	Bismuth carbonate	1 g
Adjuvant:	Sodium bicarbonate	1 g
	Light Kaolin	4 g

Corrective:	Tinct. Catechu	2.5 g
Vehicle:	Pulv. Tragacanth	0.15 g
	Chloroform water	q.s. 30 ml

6) *Subscription* (Mft): Prepare the mixture. Send such 3 doses
7) *Signa/Signatura*: One dose (30 ml) to be taken every 4 hr
8) Doctor's signature and registration number.

CURRENT MODEL OF PRESCRIPTION

1) Doctor's Name and Qualifications — Address: Clinic/Residence Tel. No.:
2) Date
3) Patient's name, age, sex and address
4) ℞
5) Tab. Ciplox* 500 mg • - • 1 tab 12 hrly x 5 days
   Tab. Alerid* 10 mg • - x 1 tab once a day x 5 days
   Cap. Becosule • - x 1 cap once a day x 5 days
6) Doctor's signature and registration number.

**Ciplox and Alerid are brand names and can also be prescribed by their generic names as Ciprofloxacin and Cetirizine, respectively.*

THE COMPLIANCE OF A PRESCRIPTION

The compliance is the extent to which the patient follows and adheres the directives given to him, in his prescription, by the doctor. The patient's compliance, or more accurately the noncompliance, is a subject of current interest regarding the directions provided in the prescription. Usually, 30–60% of the patients fail to take medications as intended by the doctor due to various reasons: **(1)** One such reason could be the financial constraints. Little is accomplished by prescribing a drug that the patient cannot buy. One way to solve this problem is to substitute the branded drug by a generic one because generic drugs are much cheaper. Secondly, only bare minimum drugs should be prescribed to reduce the cost, and lastly the physician can make use of some cheaper brands (if generic drug cannot be prescribed) marketed by some good manufacturer, **(2)** Another reason could be the patient's lack of knowledge about the purpose for which the drug(s) have been prescribed. In such cases, compliance can be improved if the doctor explains the condition for which the patient is being treated and the anticipated benefits from the drug(s) that have been prescribed. However, the therapeutic purpose should be explained to him in layman's terms so that the patient is able to comprehend and recognise the importance of each drug prescribed, **(3)** Another reason for non-compliance or discontinuation of drug could be because of delayed response or experience of side effects. Hence, the patient should be instructed clearly about the use of the drug, i.e., how and when to take the medicine, what dose to be taken, what should be the interval between the doses, what type of food should be avoided, what type of side effects he may experience which do not require discontinuation of the drug and what type of adverse effects (e.g., allergy) require immediate reporting so that the drug can be discountinued. In short, for better compliance the doctor should have better interaction with the patient. Writing the instructions, about taking the drug, in the native language and then explaining it may, in addition to enhancing the compliance, enable the patient to detect any error or to clear the doubts that may occur during prescribing and to recall oral instructions thereafter, **(4)** For better compliance, the patient should also be informed what to do if one dose is missed (e.g., in case of oral contraceptives) on some day, or when the dose has been missed for 2–3 days in succession. The patient should always be encouraged to ask questions and to clarify the confusion about the instructions, **(5)** Patient compliance can also be improved by selecting drugs that are given on once daily or at 12 hrly interval basis; as administration of drugs at 6 hrly or 8 hrly basis is not suitable for geriatric patients or to business executives, **(6)** If multidrug therapy is essential, generic drug prescribing should be avoided because "pill profusion creates more confusion" and a poor compliance. Prescribing branded formulations of combination drugs is helpful in improving the compliance in such situations, and **(7)** The compliance problem in illiterate patients can be minimised by prescribing drugs with distinctive physical characteristics, e.g., one red tab, one white tab, one yellow tab and one capsule instead of 4 white tablets.

Though the use of Latin abbreviations, that once was very popular, is on the decline nowadays. Some common abbreviations still being used by many practitioners are given below.

ABBREVIATIONS USED IN PRESCRIPTION

Abbreviation	Latin Equivalent	English Meaning
ac	ante cibum	before meals
ad lib	ad libitum	as desired
b.i.d or b.d.	bis in die	twice a day
h.s.	hora somni	at bed time
mft	misc fiat	prepare and send (instructions to the pharmacist)
o.d.	omni die	once a day
p.c.	post cibum	after meals
p.o.	per os	by mouth
PRN	Prorata need	Taken as required
q.d.	—	once a day (see o.d.)
q.i.d.	quarter in die	four times a day
q.s.	quantum sufficit	in sufficient amount
signa	signatura	let it be labelled (instructions to the patient)
s.o.s.	si opus sit	when necessary
stat	statim	immediately
t.i.d.	ter in die	three times a day
t.d.s	ter die sumendrum	to be taken three times a day

CHAPTER 74 Drugs Used in Paediatrics and Geriatrics

COMPETENCY PH1.56

DRUGS USED IN PAEDIATRICS

Paediatric pharmacology is a challenge for prescribers as there is pharmacokinetic and pharmacodynamic variations of drugs, which makes them vulnerable for adverse effects.

Pharmacokinetics in paediatrics

Absorption

Gastrointestinal tract: In paediatric age group, oral route of drug administration is preferred. In neonates, there is more gastric pH (>4), which affects degree of ionization of drugs. Hence, absorption of weak acidic drugs like phenytoin and phenobarbital is variable; dose adjustment of these antiepileptic drugs is needed. In neonates, there is low basal acid output. So, oral administration of acid labile drugs like penicillin G, ampicillin and nafcillin have more bioavailability.

In neonates and young infants: a) Gastric emptying is delayed; b) Slow rate of absorption of drugs. Neonates also have low concentrations of bile acids and lipase, which may decrease the absorption of lipid soluble drugs.

Skin: In children, there is thinner stratum corneum of skin than adults. Hence, more absorption of topically applied drugs like corticosteroids, antiseptics and antihistaminics. Methylphenidate transdermal patch is available for attention deficit hyperactive disorder (ADHD).

Intramuscular: In infants, low blood flow to skeletal muscles which may affect drug absorption. Example: Low rate of absorption of diazepam. In conditions like cardiovascular shock and heart failure there is less peripheral perfusion. If perfusion suddenly improves, increase in absorption and the higher amount of drug in circulation can cause toxicities e.g., cardiac glycosides, aminoglycosides and anti-convulsants.

Rectal: The rectal route of administration can be useful for infants or children who are unable to take oral medications. The bioavailability of rectal route (suppository) is 30 to <100%. About 50% of a rectal dose can be assumed to bypass the liver, e.g., bisacodyl, glycerin.

Distribution

During development of child, body composition changes which affect volume of distribution (Vd) of drugs. Preterm infants have much less fat than full-term infants.

Infants have higher percentage of its body weight in the form of water (70–75%) than adults (50–60%). Examples: Vd of gentamicin in neonates is 0.48 L/kg, while 0.20 L/kg in adults. In premature infants, Vd of tobramycin is more. Further, there is less amount of total plasma proteins binding like albumin and acid glycoprotein in neonates. It leads to more availability of unbound free drug and more displacement interactions like bilirubin and free fatty acids, which displace drug from albumin binding sites, e.g., Kernicterus in premature newborn: Sulphonamides displace bilirubin from its plasma protein binding sites which cross BBB and cause kernicterus.

Drugs excreted through breast milk: Toxicities of drugs are likely, if taken during lactation. Examples: Lithium, cyclophosphamide, bromocriptine, ergotamine, amphetamine , alcohol, aspirin, atenolol, phenobarbitone, sulfasalazine, etc. Hence, lactating mother should avoid these drugs.

Metabolism

In infant (<1 year), metabolizing enzymes in liver are less mature than adults. *In children (1–6 years)*, more level of metabolizing enzymes than adults. *In children (>6 years)*, similar level of metabolizing enzymes as adults. *Examples*: Dose of phenytoin, diazepam, phenobarbital should be less.

There is large variation in level of CYP3A4 enzymes during first 3 years. Conjugation reactions in phase II metabolism are less mature than adults. Glucuronidation pathway is less developed in infants. Examples: Less glucuronidation of chloramphenicol to its inactive metabolites causes Grey baby syndrome in infants. Premature infants cannot metabolize morphine to its more potent metabolite. Hence, higher dose of morphine is required.

In children, due to high level of CYP3A4 enzymes, plasma clearance of carbamazepine and midazolam is faster than adults, i.e. higher dose of drug in mg/kg is required.

Excretion

The glomerular filtration rate (GFR) is much lower in newborn than in older infants, children or adults. Glomerular filtration rate increases rapidly during first 2 weeks of life. Subsequently, it exceeds adult values, often necessitating larger doses per kilogram than in adults. At 8–12 months of age, adult value of GFR is achieved. There is less tubular secretion in newborn and at 1-year than adults. Examples: Dosing regimen of some drugs like famotidine and ceftazidime should be less in newborn. A decreased rate of renal elimination in the neonate has also been observed with aminoglycoside antibiotics (kanamycin, gentamicin, neomycin and streptomycin).

Pharmacodynamics of Drugs in Paediatrics

In infants, there is variation in receptor binding ability of drugs. Examples: There is low binding ability of digoxin to Na^+-K^+-ATPase. Hence, high maintenance dose should be given. In premature infants, prokinetic effect of erythromycin is variable due to age dependent expression of motilin receptors. At birth, the function of drug transporters may be very low, e.g., P-glycoprotein.

Dosing Regimen

Many formulae are available for calculating the dose for a child who, obviously, requires a lesser dose than an adult. These formulae are based on age, weight or body surface area of a child.

i) Young's Formula

This is applicable for children up to 12 years of age, and makes the assumption that a 12yr-old-should receive one-half of the adult dose.

$$\text{Child's Dose} = \frac{\text{Age in years}}{\text{Age} + 12} \times \text{Adult Dose}$$

ii) Dilling's Formula

It makes an assumption that a 20-year-old should receive an adult dose.

$$\text{Child's Dose} = \frac{\text{Age in years}}{20} \times \text{Adult Dose}$$

iii) Clark's Formula

This is based simply on proportional body weight as related to an average adult weighing about 70 kg (150 lb).

$$\text{Child's Dose} = \frac{\text{Wt. of child (lb)}}{150} \times \text{Adult Dose}$$

However, for children, ***body surface area (BSA)***, which is based on both height and weight, is a more precise index than body weight alone for adjustment of drug doses. Hence, a more accurate method for calculating a dose for a child should be on the basis of his body surface area. On obtaining the BSA, the child's dose can be calculated by the following formula:

$$\text{Child's Dose} = \frac{\text{BSA (m}^2\text{)}}{1.8} \times \text{Adult Dose}$$

The surface area rule is based on the assumption that the average adult weighing about 70 kg has a corresponding surface area of about 1.8 (approximately).

Nomograms are available which are generally used for finding out BSA from height and weight. In case, nomograms are not readily available with the physician, the following formula can also be used for a simplified approximation:

$(1.5 \times \text{wt in kg}) + 10 =$ Percentage of adult dose to be given to the child

OR

$(0.7 \times \text{wt in lb}) + 10 =$ Percentage of adult dose to be given to the child

Paediatric Dosage Forms and Adherence

Drugs prepared for children are in the form of liquid formulation like elixirs or suspensions. ***Elixirs*** are solutions in which the drug molecules are dissolved and evenly distributed. ***Suspensions*** contain undissolved particles of drug that must be distributed throughout the vehicle by shaking. Common challenge in paediatric age group is adherence. For example, one teaspoon can accommodate the volume from 2.5 to 7.8 mL of drug. Parents should obtain a calibrated medicine spoon or syringe to improve the accuracy of dose measurements and simplify administration of drugs to children.

Therapeutic Drug Monitoring (TDM)

In selected cases, when drug is administered to children, TDM should be essential to achieve and maintain therapeutic drug concentration within therapeutic range. It is important for drugs having narrow therapeutic window. TDM is required for carbamazepine, valproate, phenytoin, theophylline, aminoglycosides, sirolimus, 5-Fluorouracil, tacrolimus, cyclosporin and digoxin.

DRUGS USED IN GERIATRICS

The problems found more commonly in older people are of multiple diseases which are referred to "13 Is" of geriatrics. These include: (1) Immobility, (2) Isolation, (3) Incontinence, (4) Infection, (5) Inanition (marked weight loss with weakness), (6) Immuno-deficiency, (7) Insomnia, (8) Impotence, (9) Impaired visual and auditory senses, (10) Impaction, (11) Intellectual loss, (12) Instability and (13) Iatrogenic responses. The treating physician, therefore has to be aware of the alterations in drug response that may occur in elderly due to physiological and pharmacological changes associated with ageing. This chapter enlists the drugs to be avoided in elderly (with reasons) and outlines the preferable alternatives to the therapeutic management of various disease entities prevalent in elderly.

Altered Drug Response in Elderly

Geriatric patients seem to be "more sensitive" to the action of several drugs because of altered pharmacodynamic interactions with their receptors or due to a diminished homeostatic response. For example, reflex tachycardia, seen commonly with vasodilator therapy, is often blunted in the elderly, perhaps owing to dampened baroreceptor function. Elderly suffer from postural hypotension in response to many drugs for this reason (e.g., neuroleptics, tricyclic antidepressants, antiparkinsonism drugs and with many antihypertensive agents). Many drugs, particularly sedative-hypnotics-antianxiety agents significantly impair the normal postural control mechanism, which leads to sudden falls and injuries in elderly people.

Some age-related decline in central neurotransmitter function also occurs in elderly. Thus, due to degeneration of dopaminergic neurons in basal ganglia, these patients suffer from Parkinson's disease. Similarly, there is a marked decrease in choline acetyltransferase and other markers of cholinergic neuron activity, which eventually leads to cognition deficits and Alzheimer's disease in elderly. For similar reasons, drug-induced confusion is a common adverse effect in elderly by a diverse group of drugs, which include hypnotics, sedatives, theophylline, anticholinergics and even β-blockers. Average blood pressure goes up with age after 50 while the average 2 hr post-meal blood sugar increases by about 1 mg/dL for each year of age after 50. Temperature regulation is also impaired in old age and hence a classical neuroleptic-induced hypothermia is poorly tolerated by an elderly. In addition, the elderly demonstrate an enhanced responsiveness to anticoagulants such as warfarin and heparin as well as to thrombolytic therapy. In contrast, the elderly exhibit decreased responsiveness to β_2- agonists and β_1-antagonists. Thus, higher doses of salbutamol and atenolol are needed to treat bronchial asthma and hypertension, respectively. Elderly are more sensitive to some antianxiety agents like diazepam, to narcotic analgesics like pethidine, to general anaesthetics like halothane and to sedative hypnotics such as phenobarbitone.

Hence, pharmacotherapy in elderly has a considerable potential for both "useful" and "harmful" effects of the drugs. This balance may be tilted in the desired direction by considering some safer alternatives provided in Table 74.1.

ADVERSE DRUG REACTIONS IN ELDERLY

The overall incidence of adverse drug reactions in the elderly is 2 to 3 times that found in young adults. Commonly used drugs which produce unwanted effects in elderly are listed below:

1) ***Postural hypotension***
   Isosorbide dinitrate, tricyclic antidepressants, levodopa, bromocriptine, antipsychotics, debrisoquine, guanethidine, β-blockers, diuretics, antihistamines (with anticholinergic effects).
2) ***Constipation***
   Anticholinergics,antidepressants, antipsycho tics, opioids, disopyramide, nifedipine.
3) ***Urinary incontinence***
   β-Blockers, antipsychotics, diuretics, prazosin, lithium, labetalol.
4) ***Parkinsonism***
   Antipsychotics, metoclopramide, reserpine, drugs for vertigo, methyldopa.
5) ***Depression***
   Antipsychotics, anxiolytics, β-blockers, methyldopa, sedatives.
6) ***Confusional state***
   Anticholinergics, antihistamines, β-blockers, theophylline, sedative-hypnotics, anticonvulsants, antidepressants.
7) ***Loss of postural reflexes (Fall)***
   Benzodiazepines, neuroleptics, antidepressants, carbamazepine, phenobarbital, antihistamines.

• Chronic use of certain drugs can cause vitamin/mineral deficiency. It would probably be useful to advise all elderly individuals to take vitamin supplements (except for megadoses of vitamin A and D, as overdoses of these vitamins are toxic). Such drugs include:

Alcohol:	Causes deficiency of vitamin B_1, B_2, B_6, C, folic acid and also of vitamin A, D and K.
Antacids:	Reduce absorption of iron. Aluminium hydroxide containing antacids cause hypophosphataemia.
Phenytoin:	Causes deficiency of vitamin D and folic acid as well as of vit. K.
Corticosteroids:	Cause deficiency of vitamin D and of calcium.
Cholestyramine and liquid paraffin:	Cause deficiency of vitamin A, D, E and K.
Methotrexate, trimethoprim + pyrimethamine:	Cause deficiency of folic acid.
Isoniazid:	Causes deficiency of vitamin B_6.
Oral anticoagulants:	Cause deficiency of vitamin K.
Vitamin E:	Interferes with oral absorption of iron.

(refer Table 74.1)

Table 74.1 Drugs to be Avoided in Elderly and their Safer Alternatives

Drugs to be Avoided	Reasons	Safer Alternatives
1. CNS drugs		
a) **Sedative-Hypnotics-Antianxiety drugs** - Chlordiazepoxide - Diazepam - Barbiturates - Clorazepate - Flurazepam	Prolongation of half-life due to age-related decline of renal and hepatic functions. Elderly are highly sensitive, leading to ataxia, loss of postural reflex and fall causing fractures and injuries	Oxazepam, lorazepam, alprazolam and temazepam. These do not form active metabolites, have shorter half-life and are less sedating
b) **Analgesics** i) Opioids	Elderly are very sensitive to their respiratory depressant effects. However, in chronic painful condition such as cancer, their use is justified. Pentazocine and dextropropoxyphene should be avoided (Ch. 37). Risk is more, efficacy is less.	Prefer codeine, meperidine, morphine and buprenorphine. Titrate optimum dose and frequency of administration
ii) NSAIDs	These should be used very carefully as they may cause GIT bleeding and renal damage (renal functions are already compromised in old age). Indomethacin should be avoided due to its CNS side effects while phenylbutazone has haematological toxicity. Long-term use of naproxen or piroxicam should be avoided (cumulative toxicity).	Ibuprofen, nimesulide, Cox-2 inhibitors may be preferred but should be carefully watched as Cox-2 inhibitors carry cardiovascular risk particularly in elderly. Corticosteroids may be used along with calcium and vitamin-D supplements (to avoid osteoporosis) and with H_2 antagonist (to prevent gastric acidity). NSAIDs, as a rule, should be started at a low dose to the elderly and the dose be increased only if the therapeutic effect is insufficient.
c) **Antipsychotics** - Phenothiazine analogues and - Haloperidol analogues	To be avoided because of greater risk of extrapyramidal side effects and postural hypotension. Elderly are very sensitive to their anticholinergic side effects	Thioridazine, olanzapine, risperidone, ziprasidone or aripiprazole are safe in this regard. Pimozide is also safe but QT interval in the ECG should be watched. Atypical neuroleptics in elderly demented patients, sometimes ↑ the mortality rate.

contd.

Drugs to be Avoided	Reasons	Safer Alternatives
d) **Antidepressants** - Tricyclic antidepressants	Avoid due to postural hypotension and anticholinergic side effects. Combinations of tricyclic antidepressant + antipsychotic should be avoided	Prefer SSRIs (e.g., sertraline). Its elimination is not affected with ageing. If tricyclics are to be used, prefer nortriptyline or desipramine
e) **Antimania** - Lithium	Renal toxicity. Thiazide diuretics further reduce Li^+ clearance and ↑ its toxicity in elderly	Prefer carbamazepine or valproic acid
f) **General anaesthetics** - Halothane - Enflurane - Thiopental - Pancuronium	Elderly are more sensitive to halothane and are more prone to its hepatotoxicity. Enflurane precipitates epilepsy. Elderly are very sensitive to thiopental as well	Prefer isoflurane, albeit expensive. For minor surgical procedure prefer midazolam or propofol. Thiopental and pancuronium should be used in low doses
g) **Drugs for Alzheimer's disease** - Tacrine	Patients with Alzheimer's disease are very sensitive to CNS toxicity of drugs having anticholinergic effects. Tacrine has hepatotoxicity	Donepezil, rivastigmine, galantamine and memantine are preferred, being safer
2. CVS drugs a) **Antihypertensive drugs** - Propranolol - Methyldopa - Thiazide diuretics in high doses	Frequent use of thiazides in high doses causes hypokalaemia, hyperglycaemia & hyperuricaemia which in elderly increase the risk of precipitating arrhythmias, type-2 diabetes and gout. Methyldopa produces deep sedation & postural hypotension in elderly. Propranolol is not safe in elderly suffering from asthma, peripheral vascular disease and congestive heart failure. Its bioavailability and half-life also increase with age	Prefer thiazides in minimum effective dose or along with potassium-sparing diuretic. Prefer selective β_1-receptor blocker or an ACE inhibitor or angiotensin receptor antagonist or a Ca^{2+} channel blocker

contd.

Drugs to be Avoided	Reasons	Safer Alternatives
b) **Cardiac glycosides** - Digoxin	There is an increase in the sensitivity to the toxic arrhythmogenic actions of digoxin. Hypokalaemia hypomagnesaemia, hypoxaemia (due to associated pulmonary disease) and coronary artery disease further aggravate this toxicity in elderly. Clearance of digoxin is usually decreased and its half-life is prolonged	Loading dose should be reduced. Maintenance dose should also be reduced and properly titrated
c) **Antiarrhythmic drugs** - Disopyramide - Quinidine - Xylocaine	The clearance of quinidine is decreased and its half-life is prolonged in elderly. It also has antimuscarinic effects. Disopyramide should also be avoided because of its anti-muscarinic effects and negative inotropic cardiac effects. Half-life of xylocaine is also increased in elderly, besides old patients are quite sensitive to its toxic effects	Disopyramide should be avoided. However, if quinidine or xylocaine are to be used, their doses must be reduced
d) **Platelet inhibitors** - Dipyridamole	Causes postural hypotension and coronary steal phenomenon in elderly	Prefer clopidogrel or aspirin (if tolerated)
e) **Antianginal drugs** - Isosorbide dinitrate - Verapamil	Elderly are more sensitive to hypotensive action and tachycardia caused by isosorbide dinitrate. They are also very sensitive to verapamil causing conduction abnormalities	Prefer diltiazem
3. Drugs for respiratory diseases - Ephedrine - Isoproterenol - Theophylline	Ephedrine is no longer used. It causes rise in BP, tachycardia and urinary hesitancy. Isoprenaline causes tremors, tachycardia and even arrhythmias. Theophylline half-life is prolonged in old age causing tremors, CNS stimulation, diuresis and arrhythmia (in high dose)	Prefer salbutamol and its congeners or budesonide or beclomethasone. Terbutaline may also be used

contd.

Drugs to be Avoided	Reasons	Safer Alternatives
4. Antibiotics - Penicillins - Cephalosporins - Fluoroquinolones - Nitrofurantoin	Because of the decline in renal functions in elderly, half-life of these antibiotics is prolonged. Elderly are very sensitive to peripheral neuritis and pulmonary reaction caused by nitrofurantoin. Gatifloxacin may cause episodes of hypo- as well as hyperglycaemia (caution! diabetes).	Some trials indicate that half-life of tobramycin is not prolonged in elderly. This could be one alternative. Use of ceftriaxone or cefoperazone, which are excreted through bile, could be other alternatives. Otherwise dose adjustment of these drugs is needed.
5. Antihistamines - Chlorpheniramine - Cyproheptadine - Hydroxyzine	Avoid due to anticholinergic and sedative side effects	Prefer second generation drugs, e.g., levocetrizine
6. Antispasmodics - Atropine - Scopolamine - Dicyclomine - Clidinium bromide	Avoid due to anticholinergic side effects	Prefer oxybutynine, tolterodine (lesser side effects)
7. Drugs for BPH - Tamsulosin - Finasteride	Tamsulosin causes intraoperative floppy iris syndrome (problematic during cataract surgery). Finasteride, on long-term use, surprisingly ↑es the risk for prostate cancer	Prefer dutasteride with or without doxazosin
8. Laxatives-Purgatives - Castor oil - Magnesium sulfate - Liquid paraffin - Phenolphthalein	Castor oil causes pelvic congestion, damage to intestinal mucosa and other complications if there is fecal impaction. Magnesium sulfate may cause hypermagnesaemia (if renal functions are compromised - as in elderly). Liq. paraffin, in elderly, may pass into intestinal mucosa to produce foreign body granulomas in intestinal submucosa. It also causes deficiency of fat-soluble vitamins. Phenolphthalein, because of its cardiotoxicity, has been withdrawn from market in several countries	Prefer bran preparations, senna preparations, bisacodyl, milk of magnesia (Mg-hydroxide) and enema if there is faecal impaction

contd.

Drugs to be Avoided	Reasons	Safer Alternatives
9. IBS with predominant diarrhoea in women		
- Tegaserod	Unpredictable cardiotoxicity	Prefer alosetron (Ch. 28)
10. Antiemetics and Gastrokinetics		
- Antihistamine group - Metoclopramide - Cisapride	Antihistamine group (promethazine) should be avoided due to their anticholinergic side effects. Metoclopramide may be avoided due to its extrapyramidal side effects. Cisapride causes QT prolongation	Prefer domperidone or ondansetron. Mosapride, however, is weaker antiemetic but safer gastrokinetic
11. Antidiabetic drugs		
- Chlorpropamide - Glibenclamide - Rosiglitazone	Half-lives of these drugs get increased in elderly. Moreover, these are known to cause serious hypoglycaemic episodes. Rosiglitazone causes fluid retention (may ppt CHF)	Glipizide, gliclazide or a combination of nateglinide + metformin may be used

Key: IBS—Irritable bowel syndrome; BPH—Benign prostatic hyperplasia

CHAPTER 75 Management of Micronutrients Deficiency Disorders

COMPETENCY PH1.61

Micronutrients are vitamins, antioxidant phytochemicals/bioflavonoids and minerals, which are needed in small amounts (in micro- or milligram quantities) for maintaining optimal health. That is all are vital for improving physical and mental performance, enhancing immunity, preventing cancer and adding healthy years to life. *Micronutrients are not produced by the body and mostly must be derived from the diet.* Phytochemicals play a key role in scavenging the oxidative free radicals. If these free radicals attain an excessive dimension (due to exhaustion of the endogenous antioxidant system), it may lead to eventual tissue damage and injury resulting in a disease or worsening of an already existing disease. Micronutrients deficiency, until one is critically needed for a particular function, as such do not cause specific diseases, but they act as exacerbating factors in infections and chronic diseases greatly impacting morbidity, mortality and quality of life. An adequate intake therefore is necessary, but provision of excess supplements to people who do not need them may be harmful. Single micronutrient deficiency states are comparatively easily recognized and treated. Subclinical deficiency, often of multiple micronutrients, is more difficult to recognize. Clinical benefit is most likely to occur in those people who are severely depleted and at risk of complications and is unlikely to be seen, if this is not the case.

Most micronutrients were discovered as a result of specific diseases occurring in particular geographical areas or groups with atypical diets resulting into a severe depletion of a particular micronutrient (Table 75.1).

Micronutrient deficiency is often called '***hidden hunger***.' It is given less importance than the obvious starvation of people who are unable to get enough food to survive. Instead, it refers to sickness that affects people who can afford only low-cost filling food that is deficient in essential vitamins and mineral trace elements. ***Micronutrient malnutrition*** is a term used to refer to diseases caused by a dietary deficiency of vitamins and minerals. More than 2 billion of people in the world today may be affected by micronutrient malnutrition, including both vitamin and mineral deficiencies. Hence, discussions in this chapter will focus only on the generally accepted essential inorganic micronutrient trace elements and wherever necessary organic micronutrient (fat soluble and water soluble vitamins) for which deficiency states with biochemical, physiological and structural changes have been clearly demonstrated. Such states occur after prolonged consumption of a diet lacking the single nutrient or result due to the selective loss of the micronutrient under consideration and are uniquely corrected by addition of the nutrient back into the diet or through supplementation, with special reference to the role of zinc in childhood diarrhoea.

TYPES OF MICRONUTRIENTS

Atleast 28–30 chemical entities constitute micronutrients that are classified into three categories: (i) *essential organic micronutrient vitamins*, (ii) *phytochemicals* and (iii) *essential inorganic micronutrient minerals*. All these three classes of micronutrients play an important role in the metabolism of carbohydrate, fat and protein for timely formation of structures of the body and development of different physiological and biochemical activities.

(i) Essential Organic Micronutrient: Fat Soluble and Water Soluble Vitamins

These include *fat soluble vitamins*: A, D, E and K; *water soluble vitamins*: B-complex group of vitamins – B_1 (*thiamine*), B_2 (*riboflavin*), B_3 (*niacin*), B_5 (*pentothenic acid*), B_6 (*pyridoxine*), B_7 (*biotin*), folic acid and B_{12} (*cyanocobalamin and hydroxocobalamin*) and non-B-complex group of vitamin (*vit C*). Details of all these vitamins have been covered in Ch. 50.

Table 75.1 Typical diseases or health disorders that characteristically indicate the severe or sub-clinical micronutrients deficiency

Typical diseases/Health disorders	Implicated micronutrients severe depletion or sub-clinical deficiency
Goitre and cretinism	Iodine
Microcytic anaemia	Iron
Macrocytic anaemia	Folic acid and Vitamin B_{12}
Beri beri	Thiamine
Pellagra	Niacin
Peripheral neuritis	Pyridoxine
Scurvy	Vitamin C
Bleeding tendencies	Vitamin K
Osteomalacia and ricket	Vitamin D and Calcium
Xerophthalmia and vision problems (night blindness)	Vitamin A
Disturbed protein synthesis, low immune function, enteropathies in children (childhood diarrhoea) and acrodermatitis	Zinc
Myopathy	Selenium
Hyper-homocysteinaemia	Folic acid (subclinical deficiency)
Low immune and cognitive function	Institutionalized elderly (on monotonous low-cost diet)

(ii) Phytochemicals

An increased body of evidence indicates that nutrients called phytochemicals that include a number of bioflavonoids act as exogenous antioxidants. In general, populations eating greater amounts of phytochemical-containing foods (e.g., fruits, vegetables and whole grains) have a significantly lower risk of certain diseases; such as heart disease, hypertension, diabetes, arthritis and cancer. Some of these phytochemicals have been briefly discussed in Ch.50.

(iii) Essential Inorganic Micronutrients: Mineral Trace Elements

These include ***calcium, phosphorus, iron, copper, chromium, magnesium, manganese, zinc, selenium, molybdenum, sodium, potassium, iodine, chloride and fluoride***.

Table 75.2 depicts the role of each one of these mineral trace elements in the regulation of physiological and metabolic functions and their recommended daily dietary requirements. However, salient feature of physiological functions are described below.

Physiological and Metabolic Functions of Inorganic Micronutrients

1. **Coenzymes in metabolism**: Many vitamins or metabolites of vitamins are required to play an active part within complex biochemical reactions, e.g., *riboflavin* and *niacin* in the electron transport chain or *folic acid* as part of methyl group transfer. These reactions are critical to intermediary metabolism and ensure utilization of the major nutrients to provide energy, proteins and nucleic acids. Two examples as given below will

Table 75.2 Essential inorganic micronutrients: Mineral trace elements

Minerals(Trace elements)	Functions/Roles in metabolism/adverse effects	Recommended daily dietary requirement
Calcium	Component of teeth and bones; essential for blood vessel, muscle and nerve function	Adults (19–70 yrs) Male: 1000 mg; Female: 1200 mg Aged 70+: 1200 mg
Phosphorus	Component of most cell membranes & DNA molecules;maintains normal pH	Adults (19+ yrs): 700 mg
Iron	Component of enzymes and haemoglobin in red blood cells; poor brain development	Adults: Men (19+ yrs), Women (51+): 8 mg; Women (19–50): 18 mg; Pregnancy: 27 mg (total 1000 mg started from the 4th month of pregnancy)
Copper	Part of enzymes;anaemia;less growth	Adults (19+ yrs): 900 μg
Chromium	Helps in insulin action	Adults (19–50 yrs): 30–35 μg
Magnesium	Required as cofactor for over 300 enzymes; DNA and RNA synthesis; myopathy	Adults (19–30 yrs): Men: 400 mg; (31+): 420 mg; Women: (19–30): 310 mg; (31+): 320 mg
Manganese	Component of certain enzymes	Adults (19+ yrs): Men: 2.3 mg; Women: 1.8 mg
Zinc	Component of about 100 enzymes; antioxidant function as part of zinc-copper/zinc-manganese superoxide dismutase; integral to healthy pregnancy outcome; decreases childhood diarrhoea & respiratory infections; lowers all cause mortality	Adults (19+ yrs): Men: 11 mg; Women: 8 mg; Infants/children: Boys/Girls: (0–6 months): 2 mg; (7 months - 3 yrs): 3 mg; (4–8 yrs): 5 mg; (9–13 yrs): 8 mg; (14–18 yrs): 11 mg; Girls (14–18 yrs): 9 mg
Selenium	Antioxidant; regulation of thyroid hormone action; myopathy	Adults (19+ yrs) 55 μg
Molybdenum	Component of certain enzymes	Adults (19+ yrs) 45 μg
Sodium	Maintenance of blood volume and electrochemical gradient across the cell/neuronal membranes	Adults (19–50 yrs): 1500 mg; (51–70 yrs): 1300 mg; (70+ yrs): 1200 mg
Potassium	Nerve function; muscle contraction; blood vessel tone	Adults & children (>14 yrs of age): 4700 mg
Iodine	Part of thyroid hormones; cretinism	Adults (19+ yrs): 150 μg
Chloride (Cl^-) (anion of chlorine)	Important component of gastric acid	Adults (19–50 yrs): 2300 mg; (51–70 yrs): 2000 mg; (>70 yrs): 1800 mg
Fluoride (F^-) (anion of fluorine)	Helps in formation of bone matrix by forming fluoroapatite, used for protection from dental caries by strengthening the damaged dental enamel (does not prevent but repairs caries)	Not determined

further explain the role of *zinc* in protein metabolism and of *chromium* in glucose tolerance.

- A positive zinc balance was associated with improved nitrogen retention and a better nitrogen balance. Interestingly, plasma insulin was also found to increase when a negative zinc balance was converted to a positive one. Adequate zinc provision is therefore necessary not only to stimulate protein synthesis, probably as a result of increasing the activity of the many zinc-dependent enzymes in the protein synthetic pathway, but also to stimulate an adequate insulin response and utilization of glucose as well as amino acids.
- An interesting interaction between a trace element and substrate utilization is the *role of chromium in improving insulin action*. A low molecular weight intracellular octapeptide, known as *chromomodulin*, binds trivalent chromium and increases the response of the insulin receptors. This has been seen in nondiabetic obese subjects with a family history of type-2 diabetes, during long-term total parenteral nutrition (TPN) and especially in type-1 diabetic patients. There is growing evidence for the value of added chromium in maintaining glucose tolerance, reducing body fat and increasing lean tissue mass.

2. **Cofactors in metabolism**: Trace elements are frequently involved in modulating enzyme activity or are an integral part of enzyme prosthetic groups; e.g., *zinc* is a cofactor for over 100 enzymes, whereas *selenium* is required in the form of selenocysteine within the enzyme glutathione peroxidase.
3. **Genetic control**: Zinc "fingers" are transcription control factors that bind to DNA and regulate transcription of receptors for steroid hormones and other factors.
4. **Antioxidant action**: Much of the popular interest in the micronutrients stems from the recognition that many of the micronutrients have antioxidant properties. Oxidative metabolism inevitably leads to generation of reactive oxygen species (ROS) or "free radicals," which have the potential to cause further oxidative reactions, especially in those parts of the cell that remain in a relatively reduced state such as cell membranes or nucleic acids. The potential to cause damage is limited by mechanisms that include direct quenching of oxidant activity by tocopherols (vit E) or carotenoids (vit A), or enzyme systems to dispose the products of oxidation-superoxide dismutase (either zinc–copper- or manganese-dependent) and glutathione peroxidase (selenium-dependent).

People at Risk of Micronutrient Deficiency

Certain people including children are more likely to have micronutrient deficiencies and may require dietary changes or supplementation.

Alcohol Abuse

Low blood levels of vit B, vit C, vit E, carotenoids and selenium have been found in alcohol-dependent patients. Folic acid intake may be especially important for alcohol consumers. For example, individuals who consume alcohol appear to be at twice the risk for breast cancer when folic acid intakes are below recommendations, compared with those with higher intakes.

Smokers

Smokers often have poorer diets in general than nonsmoking individuals, and generally consume fewer fruits and vegetables and more saturated fat. Also, smokers have significantly lower blood levels of carotenoids and vit C.

Inappropriately Restricted Diets

Nutritional deficiency can result from overly strict dietary restrictions, particularly those that eliminate the most nutrient-rich foods (e.g., vegetables, fruits and whole grains). Individuals who consume low-carbohydrate, high-meat diets may have vit C intakes that are nearly 50% lower than those of persons eating more plant-based diets.

The Elderly

Particularly those in hospitals or long-term-care facilities, and vegetarians are at risk of deficiency of vitamins D and B_{12}. Poor protein intake more commonly is accompanied by the B_{12}. Poor intakes in these and other groups have led to the suggestion that all adults take a dose of multiple vitamins daily.

Drug Therapy

Medication may interact with nutrients to cause deficiencies. Folic acid deficiency may occur due to treatment with many seizure mediations (e.g., phenytoin, carbamazepine, phenobarbital and valproic acid).

- Vit B_{12} absorption decreases as a result of long-term acid reflux therapy (e.g., proton-pump blockers) and treatment with the anti-diabetic drug, metformin.
- Low potassium commonly occurs due to diuretics, amphotericin B, corticosteroids and insulin. Excessively high potassium can occur due to use of heparin and certain diuretics (e.g., spironolactone).
- Thiamine deficiency may occur due to diuretic therapy.
- Magnesium deficiency frequently results from diuretics, amphotericin B, certain antibiotics and cyclosporine.

Socioeconomic Conditions

Many groups in the population have a poor intake of nutrients as a result of a complex interaction between social and economic circumstances. Thus, people from a poorer background may well take less fresh fruit and vegetables. Such groups may benefit from some form of micronutrient supplement. Certain groups within the population are known to have a poor or inadequate intake. For example, adolescents and teenagers may have an inadequate intake of milk and other sources of calcium and elderly people in nursing homes and residential care have an inadequate vit D intake.

Reduced Intake States

Anorexia is common as a result of disease, e.g., because of chronic inflammation, acute infection or neoplastic disease. This is especially likely in the institutionalized elderly population. As mentioned above, the lower the protein energy intake, the lower the micronutrient intake.

Increased Requirements for Metabolism

The catabolism associated with acute infection, surgery or trauma leads to increased energy expenditure and net protein breakdown. Requirements for water soluble vitamins, as coenzymes for these metabolic pathways, will be increased, as will the requirements for various trace elements. Some intracellular elements such as zinc will be released during cell breakdown, so that increased amounts may not be required at this time.

Anabolism increases the requirement for all nutrients; hence, increased micronutrients should be supplied when patients are gaining weight. Trace element deficiencies are more likely when patients become anabolic, after a prolonged period of catabolism.

Certain groups have increased requirements – expectant mothers require increased folate both before conception and specially in the first trimester and also thereafter, and people who are recovering from an acute illness or after surgery probably have multiple nutrient requirements.

Infections in Children

As discussed above zinc deficiency is prevalent in children in developing countries where diarrhoea is also an important problem. In a number of clinical trials, zinc supplementation was observed not only to significantly reduce the incidence of diarrhoea, but also there was a lower incidence of pneumonia. Moreover, in acute diarrhoea trials, zinc supplemented children had a 15% lower probability of continuing diarrhoea on a given day, and in persistent diarrhoea trials, there was a 24% lower probability of continuing diarrhoea.

Vit A supplements in populations with poor vit A status, have been shown to reduce mortality from diarrhoea and pneumonia in community studies.

Role and Mechanism of Action of Zinc Supplementation in Childhood Diarrhoea

Diarrhoea has multiple aetiologies varying from infections by enteric organisms (*E. coli, Shigella, Salmonella, Staph. aureus, Vibrio cholerae, Clostridium difficile, Giardia lamblia, Entamoeba histolytica, Rota virus,* etc.), which may stimulate secretion or disrupt absorption in the gut lumen, to nutrient malabsorption due to a variety of intestinal diseases.

Intra-enterocytic nucleotides – cAMP and cGMP – are important regulators of both absorption and secretion in the intestine (where latter exerts a weaker effect than the former). Both nucleotides' formation is enhanced by toxins of the diarrhoea-causing bacteria like *E. coli, Shigella, Salmonella, Staph. aureus and Vibrio cholerae* that upregulate adenylate cyclase activity and *Clostridium difficile, Giardia lamblia and Entamoeba histolytica* that primarily upregulate guanylate cyclase activity. The resulting increased intestinal intracellular concentration of cAMP and cGMP produced net loss of salt and water by inhibiting Na/H-exchanger 3, which blocks NaCl absorption in the villous cells and promotes Cl^- and HCO_3^- secretion (with accompanying Na^+ and water) through the crypt cells. The diarrhoea-producing effect of bacterial toxins via cAMP and cGMP peaks after 3–4 hrs and continues for 24–36 hrs until the stimulated enteric cells are shed down in normal turnover. Both second messenger nucleotides also contribute to inflammation in the intestine by enhancing synthesis of prostaglandins, leukotrienes and increased intracellular Ca^{2+}, all of which further stimulate secretory process of salt and water leading to full-fledged secretory diarrhoea.

Through data obtained in a number of studies, it has been demonstrated that supplementation of elemental zinc in the dose of 10 mg/day to children of 0–6 months and 20 mg/day to children of more than 6 months age for 10–14 days of occurrence of diarrhoea show remarkable anticharrhoeal effect. Such zinc supplementation alongwith low molar oral rehydration salt solution (ORS) not only reduced the duration and severity of diarrhoea episodes, but also reduced the recurrence of diarrhoea for up to next 3 months.

Although the mechanism of antidiarrhoeal action of zinc is not clearly understood, it has been suggested that zinc inhibits second messenger (cAMP and cGMP)-activated chloride and fluid secretion by blocking basolateral K^+ channels (similar to its effects in *in vitro* studies in rat ileum). Furthermore, the long-term beneficial effects of zinc are related to its effect on: (i) improved absorption of electrolyte (NaCl) and water by stimulating Na/H$^-$ exchanger 3, which as such is known to be inhibited by increased concentration of cAMP in the enterocyte, (ii) enhanced regeneration of intestinal epithelium through its effects on brush-border enzymes, (iii) the antioxidant enzyme zinc-copper superoxide dismutase activity and (iv) an increased immune response. All these effects lead to a better clearance of pathogens and reduction in pathogen induced inflammation.

A possible interaction between zinc and vit A has been explored and it was shown that combined administration of zinc and vit A for 2 weeks and followed up for 6 months synergistically reduced the prevalence of persistent diarrhoea. Furthermore, it was observed that zinc alone was associated with a significant increase in acute lower respiratory infection, but this adverse effect was reduced by the interaction of zinc and vit A. Similarly in other studies, it was demonstrated that supplementation of zinc with vit A led to much earlier resolution of radiological changes and time to sputum negativity in patients of tuberculosis and multi-micronutrient supplementation containing zinc and vit A in children with biochemical evidence of micronutrient deficiency although did not reduce the incidence of common childhood infections, but did reduce the duration of such illnesses.

These studies show that zinc supplementation may work better, if combined with vit A and may be other micronutrients, especially when multiple micronutrient deficiency is suspected in the patient.

Zinc supplementation is a relatively easily implemented and inexpensive intervention that could help address zinc deficiency. Zinc supplements come in various physical forms, including liquid solutions, syrups, pills tablets, capsules, powders and pastes. Supplements also come in various chemical forms, such as *zinc sulphate* and *zinc acetate*, with water soluble compounds often preferred because they may be more efficiently absorbed. In addition, zinc is sometimes administered with other micronutrients such as vit A or iron. Zinc supplements have been provided at various doses, daily and weekly, for a few weeks to over a year.

However, preventive zinc supplementation is not a sufficient or long-term solution to the nutrition and health challenges facing children in resource-scarce settings. Children ultimately need well-balanced diets, and poverty is often a risk factor for undernutrition and pathogen exposure. The evidence suggests that preventive zinc supplementation offers a short-term intervention to help alleviate these problems in resource-scarce settings. It may also be pragmatic and effective to deliver zinc supplementation along with other public health interventions such as growth monitoring. Furthermore, fortification may be beneficial in areas where food production and processing systems could enrich foods with zinc. Therefore, deficiency of micronutrients in some group of people including the children at severe risk, require supplementation but the most effective way to meet the community health needs safely is by population-based approaches involving food fortification. These complementary methods along with food security, education and monitoring are challenges for public health medicine.

CHAPTER 76 Drug Regulations, Acts and Other Legal Aspects

COMPETENCY PH1.63

Drug regulations play a key role across the world in ensuring safety and efficacy of drugs. Every country has its own drug regulations. Aim is to maintain the standards of drug quality. Poor quality drugs can lead to adverse effects, treatment failure and prolonged illness. Hence, drug regulation must be strengthened.

Drug regulation includes:
1. Drug regulatory bodies
2. Drug laws
3. Quality control

DRUG REGULATORY BODIES

In India, main regulatory bodies for the approval of product, manufacturing quality drugs at reasonable prices are Central Drug Standard and Control Organization (CDSCO), Drug Controller General of India (DCGI) and National Pharmaceutical Pricing Authority. Ministry of Health and Family Welfare is responsible for ensuring quality manufacturing, sales and distribution of drugs.

Central Drug Standard and Control Organization (CDSCO)

The Drug and Cosmetic Act, 1940 and rules 1945 had given various responsibilities to Central and State regulators for drug regulations. Head quarter of CDSCO is located at Delhi.

CDSCO is responsible for the approval of drugs and clinical trials, quality standard of drugs, quality control of imported drugs, import registration and licensing, licence approval of blood banks, vaccines, r-DNA products and medical devices. It is also involved in Amendment in Drug and Cosmetic Act and rules, banning of drugs and cosmetics, testing of new drugs and approval for export.

CDSCO receives application from applicants requesting for approval to carry BA/BE study with various dosage formulations. The DCGI ensures safety and tolerability of generics against innovator drugs. It is also responsible for regulation of biologics, approval of clinical trials for human vaccines, stem cells, cell based products and veterinary vaccines.

Functions of State Licencing Authorities are approval of drug formulation for manufacture, licencing of drug testing laboratories and monitoring of quality of Drugs and Cosmetics.

CDSCO is also involved in application of new Ethics Committee, registration and re-registration. The application shall be made to the licencing Authority in accordance with Schedule Y. After fulfil criteria, it may grant registration of Ethics Committee. Ethics committee ensures right, safety and wellbeing of Human subjects involved in clinical trials. It is a Committee for reviewing and approving various protocols of clinical trials. Schedule Y of Drugs and Cosmetic Act explains the ethical guidelines for conducting clinical trial. CDSCO is also involved in evaluation of dosage form, indication additional dose or route of Fixed Dose Combination for manufacture and marketing. It regulates processing of application for *Investigational New Drug (IND)* review and approval and handling of all processed documents. '***Sugam***' is an online portal for application, submission, processing & grant permission for quick services.

Schedules in India

In India, the legislative laws related to drugs have a wider coverage. According to the Drugs and Cosmetic Act 1940 with amendments, various Schedules of drugs are explained.

Schedule Y

Schedule Y is a guideline required for approval of Clinical Trials and/or to import or manufacture of new drug for marketing in India. It explains guidelines for the following:

- To import new drugs.

- To manufacture new drugs.
- To import or manufacture fixed dose combinations.
- To conduct Clinical Trials for new drug.
- Definition of Clinical Trial.
- Registration of Ethics Committee.
- Report Serious Adverse Events (SAEs) including death.

Schedule Y also explains the process of informed consent, role of Ethics Committee, undertaking by investigator, contents of protocol, documents to report SAE, special situation like geriatric, paediatrics, pregnancy along with post-marketing surveillance. It also explains guidelines for bioavailability/ bioequivalence studies.

Other schedules of drugs and Controlled Substance Act (CSA) in United States are explained in Chapter 1 (Page 5).

Good Clinical Practice (GCP)

Good Clinical Practice (GCP) is an international ethical and scientific quality standard for designing, conducting, recording and reporting clinical trials that involve the participation of human subjects. It ensures to protect the rights, safety and wellbeing of human subjects along with integrity and confidentiality of research subjects. It provides assurance that the data and results are credible and accurate with Global Acceptance. The International Conference on Harmonization (ICH) of Technical Requirements of Pharmaceuticals for Human Use is an initiative with principle that clinical trials should be conducted in accordance with the ethical principles consistent with GCP and other regulatory requirements.

Indian Council of Medical Research (ICMR)

The *Indian Council of Medical Research (ICMR)* is the apex body in India for the formulation, coordination and promotion of biomedical research. ICMR is involved in planning, formulation, co-ordination, implementation and conduct of biomedical research in India. The council promotes research in the country through intramural research (through institutes totally funded by ICMR) and extramural research (at college or university). The policies of ICMR coincide with national health policies such as control and management of communicable disease, fertility control, maternity and child health, control of nutritional disorders, non-communicable diseases like cancer, cardiovascular diseases, metabolic and haematological disorders and drug research including traditional remedies. All efforts are undertaken with aim to reduce total burden of disease and to promote health and well-being of the population.

Drug Testing Advisory Board (DTAB)

Drugs Technical Advisory Board (DTAB) and Drugs *Consultative Committee (DCC)* discuss recommendations on the matters raised for Drugs and Cosmetics Act and Rules.

Functions of DTAB

- Advise the Central and the State Governments on technical matters arising out of the administration of the Drugs and Cosmetics Act, 1940.
- Initiate the amendments in the Drugs and Cosmetics Rules, 1945 as per the recommendations and co-ordinate with Ministry of Health & Family Welfare.
- Examination, compilation and consideration of comments/suggestions/objections.
- Processing of representations, *Right to Information (RTIs)* queries, Public Grievances with respect to Drugs and Cosmetics Act.

Narcotic Drugs and Psychotropic Substances (NDPS) Act, 1985

Main objective of *Narcotic Drugs and Psychotropic Substances (NDPS)* Act is to consolidate and amend the law relating to narcotic drugs. The NDPS Act launched in 1985 and then been amended four times in 1988, 2001, 2014 and 2021. It includes substances like Ampheta-mine, Cannabis, Charas, Ganja, Cocaine, Heroin, Methadone, Opium and LSD. Anyone who contravenes the NDPS Act, will face punishment based on the quantity of the banned substance. There may be imprisonment for up to10 years, with fine also. There is prohibition to produce, manufacture, possess, sale, purchase, transport, ware-house, use, consume, import inter-state, export inter-state, import into India, export from India any narcotic drug or psychotropic substance except for medical and scientific purpose. It is aimed that no person can consume, import and export these narcotic agents.

New Drug and Clinical Trial Rules, 2019

New Drug and Clinical Trial Rules apply to Clinical Trials, Bioavailability and Bioequivalence Studies of New Drugs and *Investigational New Drugs (INDs)*. As per this rule, if a new drug discovered in India, application shall be processed within 30 working days. It explains post-trial access of New Drug or Investigational New Drug. The rule explains that after completion of clinical trial, the post-trial access shall be provided free of cost.

In case of an injury, the sponsor shall provide free medical management. If the death or the injury is related to clinical trials, the compensation is payable as per the formula specified in the Schedule and Rules. Permission to manufacture unapproved new drug in special circumstances explains that any new drug for a patient suffering from serious or life-threatening disease for which no satisfactory therapy is available, new drug may be approved for manufacturing in limited quantity subject to provisions of these rules.

DRUG LAWS

1. The Drugs and Cosmetics Act, 1940
2. Pharmacy Act, 1948
3. Drugs and Magic Remedies Act, 1954
4. Drugs Pricing Control Order, 1995

The Drugs and Cosmetics Act, 1940

Objectives of The Drug and Cosmetic Act are to regulate the import, manufacturing, distribution and sale of drug and cosmetics by qualified persons. Other objectives are to maintain standard quality of drugs, to regulate the manufacture and sale of Ayurvedic, Siddha and Unani drugs and to establish *Drugs Technical Advisory Board (DTAB)* and Drug *Consultative Committees (DCC)* for allopathic drugs and cosmetics. It also explains role of drug inspector, adherence to manufacture guidelines and regulation on sale of drugs. It deals with import of biological drugs and related penalties, prohibition of misbranded and substandard drugs.

Pharmacy Act, 1948

Objectives of Pharmacy Act are regulation and raising the status of the profession of Pharmacy, providing uniform education, training and control of persons entering in profession of pharmacy. Pharmacy Council of India is formed to fulfil these objectives along with State Pharmacy Council.

Drugs and Magic Remedies Act, 1954

Objectives of this act are to control certain types of advertisements related to drugs, to control over magic remedies for the treatment of certain diseases, marketing with false claims and misleading public, prohibition of import and export of drugs without permission and related advertisement. Offences and penalties must be applied, if any provisions like fine and imprisonment.

Trade and Merchandise Marks Act (TMMA), 1958

The Brand or Trade mark is regulated by the Trade and *Merchandise Marks Act (TMMA)*. It provides better protection of trade marks and prevents the use of fraudulent logo or mark by any firm or company. It provides registration of trademark for 7 years at a time. At specific time interval it should be revised. Registered trademark should not be used elsewhere in India. But a foreign trademark can be used in India without any restriction.

Drugs Pricing Control Order (DPCO), 1995

Objectives of DPCO are to ensure the availability of essential and life-saving good quality drugs at reasonable prices and promoting rational usage of drugs for cost-effective production and marketing. It involves guideline to regulate the price of drugs by Government, list of controlled drugs and provision of penalties for overpriced drugs.

QUALITY CONTROL

Good Manufacturing Practice (GMP)

Good Manufacturing Practice (GMP) is a set of regulations, codes and guidelines for the manufacture of drugs, medical device, diagnostic products and food. Objective is to supply standard quality products to target population.

GMP includes WHO Guidelines

a) ***Pharmaceutical Quality System***: It ensures safety and efficacy of drugs.
b) ***GMP for pharmaceutical products***: It is a part of production and quality control measures. It ensures that drugs are constantly produced under strict guidelines.
c) ***Sanitation and Hygiene***: Potential source of contamination must be eliminated in every step of production, complains and product recall strategies must be specified and documented.
d) ***Qualification and Validation***: Every pharmaceutical industry should document various aspect of qualification of work like premises, utilities and equipments.
e) ***Training and Infrastructure***: Training of staff should be given regularly. Premises should be designed properly. Materials and documentation should be comprehensive. In production premise, smoking, drinking and eating should not be allowed.
f) ***Quality Audits and Approval***: Self-inspection should be implemented regularly. All recommendations for corrective measures should be done. Various procedures, handling of product, cleaning, sampling, storage, labelling, distribution must be predefined and strictly followed.

CHAPTER 77 Rational Use of Antimicrobials and Antibiotic Stewardship Programme

COMPETENCY PH1.43

RATIONAL USE OF ANTIMICROBIALS

Rational use of medicines include appropriate drug in right dose, duration and frequency. Irrational use of antimicrobials is common Worldwide. It can cause antibiotic resistance, adverse effects and high cost. Hence, rational use of antibiotics must be strengthened. Choice of antimicrobials for infections should be based on patient factors, organism-related factors and drug factors.

Factors for Rational Drug Usage

A. Patient Factors

1. **Age**:
   Examples: Chloramphenicol causes '***Gray baby syndrome***' because of immature metabolism and excretion in newborns. Sulfonamides cause kernicterus because they displace bilirubin from its plasma protein binding sites. In elderly, aminoglycoside causes ototoxicity and nephro toxicity. Tetracyclines cause teeth and bone malformation in children.
2. **Local factors**:
   a) *Pus*: In the presence of pus, efficacy of sulfonamide and aminoglycoside activity is reduced. Abscess creates anaerobic environment. So, aminoglycosides cannot be concentrated inside abscess. Drainage of abscess suppresses anaerobic bacteria due to exposure of oxygen.
   b) *pH*: Acidic pH decreases effects of aminoglycosides and macrolides.
   c) *Necrotic tissue*: Presence of necrotic tissue, implant or catheter favours bacterial colonization. Adhesion of bacteria creates biofilm and multiplies around surfaces. Hence efficacy of antimicrobials is reduced.
   d) *Haematoma* favours bacterial growth. Penicillins and cephalosporins are effective in haematoma.
3. **Host defense**: In immunocompromised patients, potent and high dose of antibiotic is required. Bactericidal drugs are preferred over bacteriostatic drugs. Complete eradication of organism may not occur in immunocompromised patients which can cause relapse.
4. **Allergy**: Antibiotic should not be given to the patients with history of allergy. If syphilitic patient is allergic to penicillin, erythromycin should be given.
5. **Pregnancy**: Penicillin, cephalosporins and erythromycin are safe in pregnancy. All others are contraindicated due to risk of teratogenicity. Tetracyclines may affect fetal teeth and bone. Drugs avoided during pregnancy: Sulfonamides, cotrimoxazole, chloramphenicol, fluoroquinolones and nitrofurantoin.
6. **Liver and renal function**: Impairment of kidney and liver functions causes toxicity.
   - *Antimicrobials avoided in liver dysfunctions*: Nalidixic acid, nitrofurantoin, tetracyclines (except doxycycline), pyrazinamide, erythromycin estolate and pefloxacin.
   - *Antimicrobials dose has to be reduced in renal failure*: Nalidixic acid, tetracyclines, pyrazinamide, nitrofurantoin, aminoglycosides, cephalosporins, flucytosine, vancomycin, ethambutol, imipenem and meropenem
   - *Drugs not eliminated by kidney*: Doxycycline, rifampicin, erythromycin, ceftriaxone, chloramphenicol and cefoperazone.
7. **Genetic**: Drugs can cause haemolytic anaemia in G6-PD deficient patients. Examples: Sulfonamides, nitrofurantoin and fluoroquinolones.

B. Drug Factors

1. **Spectrum of action**: For definitive therapy, specific drug is used. For empirical therapy, broad spectrum antibiotic is given.

2. **Efficacy**: On the basis of results of clinical trials, efficacy of antibiotic should be evaluated with dose, duration and frequency. With bacteriostatic drugs, bacteria can start dividing after MIC level falls. Bactericidal drugs are more efficacious than bacteriostatic drugs.
   Minimum inhibitory concentration (MIC): It is the lowest concentration of antibiotic which prevents visible growth of bacteria after 24 hrs incubation.
3. **Pharmaco-kinetic profile**: Ciprofloxacin has better tissue penetration. Ceftriaxone has good CSF penetration.
   Concentration-dependent killing: Aminoglycosides, fluoroquinolones and metronidazole have concentration-dependent killing, i.e., they kill bacteria more rapidly, if their serum concentrations are kept above MIC, e.g., Gentamicin produces better effect, if given as a single dose rather than 8 hourly.
   Time-dependent killing: β-Lactam antibiotics, clindamycin and macrolides have time-dependent killing. Maintain the serum concentration of drug above MIC for as long as possible. e.g., β-lactams are given 6–8 hourly.
4. **Route of drug**: For mild infections, oral antibiotics are preferred while in serious infections like meningitis, parenteral antimicrobials are used. Aminoglycosides, vancomycin, penicillin and some cephalosporins are given only by parenteral route.
5. **Type of infection**: Severe acute bacterial infections are better cured with bactericidal drugs. In immunocompromised patients also, bactericidal drugs are preferred.
6. **Cost**: Cheap antimicrobials should be prescribed routinely to reduce cost burden.

C. Organism-related Factors

The infecting microorganism should be sensitive to antibiotic to be used.

- **If drug sensitivity pattern is known**: When physician knows drug sensitivity pattern, selection of antimicrobial is easy. Examples: Syphilis, tetanus, diphtheria, TB, leprosy, herpes simples, cholera, plague.
- **Guess bacterial infection** by experience and knowledge about type of organism and its sensitivity. Examples: Tonsilitis, boil, vaginitis, urethritis, etc.
- **Based on identification of bacteria**: It includes empirical and specific therapy.
  1) ***Empirical therapy***: Before specific bacteria are identified by culture and sensitivity, broad spectrum antibiotics are used. It covers Gram positive and Gram-negative bacteria. Called as 'Empirical therapy', e.g., tetracycline, chloramphenicol, fluoroquinolone or combination of cephalosporin and gentamicin. If anaerobes are suspected, metronidazole or clindamycin can be administered.
  2) ***Definitive therapy***: After culture and sensitivity testing; specific drug is prescribed as per identification of bacteria.

Other aspects of antimicrobial usage are discussed in Chapter 52.

ANTIBIOTIC STEWARDSHIP PROGRAMME

Antimicrobial resistance (AMR) is an emerging global issue for concern. AMR increases medication cost, length of hospitalization and the total burden on healthcare system.

WHO AWaRe Classification of Antibiotics

Rational use of antibiotics is one of the key interventions to prevent emergence and spread of antimicrobial resistance (AMR). **A**ccess, **Wa**tch, **Re**serve (AWaRe) classification of antibiotics is a tool for antibiotic stewardship at local, national and global levels with the aim of reducing AMR.

Access Group Antibiotics

This group includes antibiotics that have activity against a wide range of susceptible pathogens while also showing lower resistance than other groups. It includes 48 antibiotics, 19 of which are included in WHO Model List of Essential Medicines. Examples: Amikacin, amoxicillin, cefadroxil, cefazolin, doxycycline, gentamicin, metronidazole, sulfamethoxazole, etc.

Watch Group Antibiotics

This group includes antibiotics that have higher resistance potential. It includes most of the highest priority agents among the Critically Important Antimicrobials. It includes 110 antibiotics, 11 of which are included in WHO Model List of Essential Medicines. Examples: Azithromycin, carbenicillin, cefepime, ceftriaxone, clarithromycin, levofloxacin, rifampicin, Tobramycin, etc.

Reserve Group Antibiotics

This group includes antibiotics reserved for treatment of infections due to multi-drug-resistant organisms. Antibiotics in reserve group should be treated as "last resort" options, when other alternatives have failed. 22 antibiotics have been classified as reserve group. Examples: Tigecycline, daptomycin, polymyxin-B, linezolid, colistin, telavancin, etc.

Usage of Antibiotics

- **Overuse**: Antimicrobials are prescribed regularly for variety of diseases, but use of too many medicines 'Polypharmacy' cause irrational usage. Examples: Administration of i.v. drugs instead of oral tablets. Self-administration of antibiotics for fever of non-infectious conditions. Antibiotics are usually prescribed for viral cough and cold which is not required.
- **Misuse**: Antibiotics are commonly misused when broad-spectrum antibiotics are prescribed for drug sensitive micro-organisms.
- **Underuse**: Unavailability, inadequate dosing and premature discontinuation of antibiotics lead to ineffective treatment and antibiotic resistance.

Definition of Antibiotic Stewardship

It is a coordinated intervention designed to improve and measure the appropriate use of antimicrobial agents, by promoting the selection of optimal antimicrobial drug regimen including dosing, duration of therapy and route of administration.

Objectives

The primary objective of Stewardship Programme is usage of safe and appropriate antibiotics to improve outcome of patient and to reduce associated adverse effects. The secondary objectives are to reduce cost burden due to antibiotics and to reduce the incidence of AMR or any other adverse antimicrobial event.

The balance between safe appropriate antibiotic and broad-spectrum antibiotic is essential (Fig 77.1).

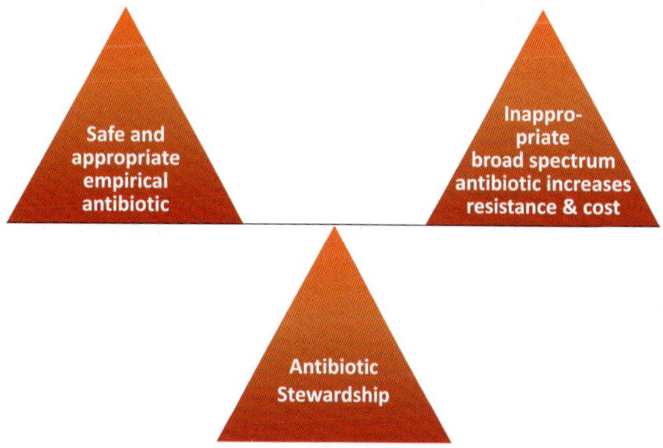

Fig 77.1 Balance of Antibiotic Stewardship in healthcare system

Various strategies implemented in Antimicrobial Stewardship:

- Appropriate antimicrobial therapy.
- Rational antimicrobial prophylaxis for surgical procedures (to prevent Surgical Site Infection).
- To form standard treatment guidelines and implementation of antibiotic policies.
- To conduct audit, evaluation, feedback, intervention for rational usage of antibiotics.
- To implement formulary restriction or pre-authorization.
- Various educational and administrative activities to improve antimicrobial prescription.

Components of Antimicrobial Stewardship

There are four components of Antimicrobial Stewardship: 4**D**s, Right drug, Right dose, Dosing interval and Right duration. Other components are switching from parental to oral antimicrobial therapy, streamlining strategies, infection control and appropriate use of microbiology laboratory.

Antibiotic Cycling

"Antimicrobial cycling" refers to the scheduled withdrawal of antimicrobial and substitution with a specific antimicrobial aiming to prevent or reverse risk of antimicrobial resistance.

Antibiotic Use Strategies

Antibiotic use can be measured mainly by two strategies: *Days of Therapy (DOT)* or *Defined Daily Dose (DDD)*. Rational usage of DOT and DDD improves patient outcome with less adverse effects.

Combination Therapy

In certain conditions, antimicrobial combinations are unnecessary. It increases cost burden, risk of resistance and adverse effects. Some beneficial combinations are sulfamethoxazole + trimethoprim, penicillin + gentamicin or streptomycin for SABE, rifampicin + isoniazid for TB and carbenicillin + gentamicin for Pseudomonas infection.

Dose Optimization

Several factors influence optimization of antimicrobial dose like pharmacokinetic and pharmacodynamic characteristics of drug, causative micro-organism, site of infection, patient characteristics like age, comorbidities, etc.

Duration Optimization

Recommended duration of antibiotics in various diseases is given in Table 77.1.

Table 77.1 Recommended duration of antibiotics

Disease	Duration*
Uncomplicated UTI**	5 days
Community acquired pneumonia	7 days
Ventilator associated pneumonia	8 days
Meningococcal meningitis	7 days
Uncomplicated secondary peritonitis	7 days
Uncomplicated SSTI***	5 days

*Some physician extends duration to 10–14 days as per patient's condition.
**UTI: Urinary Tract Infection.
***SSTI: Skin and Soft tissue infection.

Switch from Parenteral to Oral Therapy

For patients admitted in hospital suffering from serious infections, parenteral antimicrobial is preferred. But, many factors are responsible before switching to oral therapy. Appropriate culture and sensitivity test should be done, start drug accordingly and review the effects after 48–72 hrs.

Following criteria are important for switching:

a) Oral absorption is good.
b) Adequate oral antibiotic is available.
c) Normal body temperature since last 24–48 hrs.
d) No signs of sepsis.

Monitoring of Process

To find out impact of Antimicrobial Stewardship on antimicrobial use and resistance patterns, several programmes are conducted. These programmes evaluate challenges and other unintended consequences of antimicrobial use. Clinical outcomes should also be correlated with usage of antimicrobials.

Antimicrobial Stewardship Team

Antimicrobial Stewardship Team includes infectious disease clinicians, medical directors, pharmacist and microbiologist.

Standard Treatment Guidelines (STG)

Standard Treatment Guidelines (STG) should be published and revised. It improves patient's care in accordance with current AMR data.

Disposal of Antibiotics

Inappropriate disposal of unused or expiry dated antibiotics can cause hazardous effects to humans and environment. These medicines can be returned to the pharmacy for safe collection and disposal by incineration and other methods. Liquid anti-infective drugs should be diluted in water and after 2 weeks disposed in sewage.

CHAPTER 78 Pharmacogenomics and Pharmacoeconomics

COMPETENCY PH1.60

PHARMACOGENOMICS

Pharmacogenetics involves the study of genetic basis for variation in drug response and deals with how gene can modify the drug response. **Pharmacogenomics** is the study how an individual's genomic profile influences the response to drugs. It is an emerging tool to optimize drug therapy. Pharmacogenetics mainly focuses on single drug gene interactions while pharmacogenomics deals with multiple genes affecting drug response. Knowledge of pharmacogenomics into clinical practise helps prescribers for drug selection with optimal dosage to improve outcome of treatment and reduce adverse effects. It is a rapidly growing field in the area of personalized medicine. Over the past few decades, due to advancement in genetic testing, pharmacogenomics becomes stronger in clinical practice for betterment of patients.

Various examples of pharmacogenetic variations are discussed in Chapter 7.

PHARMACOECONOMICS

Pharmacoeconomics is the science which compares the cost of various treatment alternatives along with its outcome. It involves the research which identifies and compares the costs of diseases and/or drug treatments. It focuses on the costs and benefits of various drug treatments. It also involves impact on psychosocial wellbeing, known also as "**Health-related Quality Of Life**" (**HRQOL**). Pharmacoeconomics is a division of outcomes research which can be used to quantify and compare the value of drug treatments.

Components of Pharmacoeconomics

Economic

- Cost minimization analysis
- Cost-effective analysis
- Cost–benefit analysis
- Cost utility analysis

Humanistic

- Quality of life
- Patient satisfaction
- Patient preferences

Types of Cost

To evaluate the economics of drug therapy, cost is categorized into direct, indirect and intangible cost. ***Direct*** cost means costs from the perspective of the healthcare personnel including staff costs, capital costs and drug acquisition costs. Also includes physician's consultation fees, cost of administering the drugs and cost to treat any adverse drug reaction. ***Indirect cost*** means costs from the perspective of personal and society. For example, cost of travel to hospital, due to illness, loss of earnings, loss of productivity, etc. ***Intangible cost*** involves illness related pain, anxiety, apprehension or other distress from which person and whole family might suffer. In monetary terms, it may not be possible to measure, but sometimes evaluated in terms of health-related quality of life.

Steps in Economic Evaluation

- **Step 1**: Quantify the costs of the intervention/drug (input)
- **Step 2**: Quantify the outcomes/consequences (output)
- **Step 3**: Compare magnitude of differences in costs and evaluate "value money" (e.g., by cost-effectiveness ratio)
- **Step 4**: Evaluate the precision of these comparison.

Methods of Economic Evaluation

Cost Minimization Analysis (CMA)

Cost minimization analysis (CMA) compares the costs of treatment which provides the same outcome. Aim is to identify the cheapest option and when two or more treatments are evaluated, costs associated with each treatment may be evaluated and compared, e.g., prescribing drugs with generic names instead of brand names. Prescribing with generic names is always cheaper than brand names. Even different brands have different costs. Hence, CMA compares various treatment alternatives and their therapeutic equivalence of the alternatives. Hence, CMA indicates a cost savings management over another options.

Cost-Effective Analysis (CEA)

In cost-effective analysis, there is comparison of costs and effects (outcomes) of two or more treatments. The effects of drug treatment are evaluated as duration of treatment, length of hospital stay and mortality rate. However, the result of CEA is expressed as a ratio, either as an average cost-effectiveness ratio (ACER) or as an incremental cost-effectiveness ratio (ICER). An ACER represents the total cost of treatment divided by its clinical outcome.

$$\text{Average cost-effectiveness ratio (ACER)} = \frac{\text{Heath care cost}}{\text{Clinical outcome}}$$

Incremental CEA can be used to determine the additional cost and effectiveness gained when one treatment alternative is compared with the next best treatment alternative. Here, additional cost of treatment alternative imposes over another treatment is compared along with benefit or outcome.

$$\text{Incremental cost-effectiveness ratio (ICER)} = \frac{\text{Cost of drug A - Cost of drug B}}{\text{Benefits of drug A - Benefits of drug B}}$$

The cost effectiveness can be expressed in terms of Life Years Gained (LYG) or infection prevented, i.e., COST/LYG. Cost-effective analysis is helpful in balancing cost with other measures like outcome of patient. The four possible results arising in a CEA when costs and effects of the one drug is analysed with its alternative are shown in Fig. 78.1.

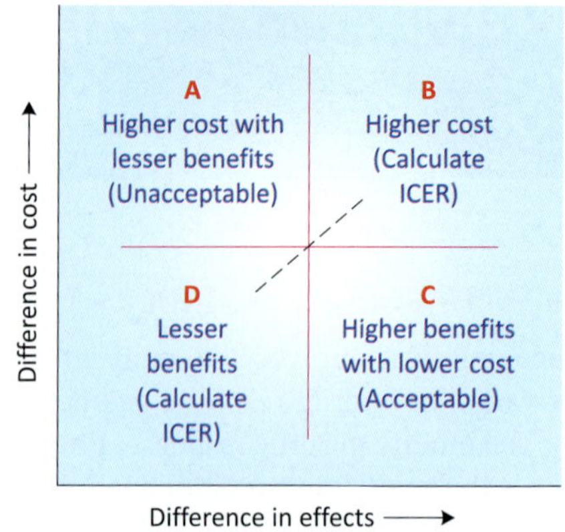

Fig 78.1 Cost-effective diagram

Cost–Benefit Analysis (CBA)

Cost-benefit analysis is a systematic process for calculating and comparing benefits and costs of treatment. Aim is to identify, measure and compare the costs and benefits of various treatment alternatives. The benefits and costs are compared as a ratio 'benefit to cost ratio', i.e., either net benefit or net cost. Physician can select treatment with highest net benefit or greater benefit to cost (B/C) ratio.

Example:

- If B/C ratio > 1, the treatment is of value, i.e., the benefits are higher and outweigh the cost providing it.
- If B/C ratio = 1, the benefits equal the cost. The benefits of treatment alternative are equivalent to the cost.
- If B/C ratio < 1, the treatment is not economically beneficial. The cost of treatment alternative outweighs the benefits.

CBA is also used to evaluate a single or multiple treatment alternatives. However, exact calculation of health benefits in monetary terms is subjective and difficult to measure.

Cost Utility Analysis (CUA)

Cost utility analysis is a type of pharmacoeconomics in which the denominator is measured typically using a metric called the *quality-adjusted life year* (**QALY**).

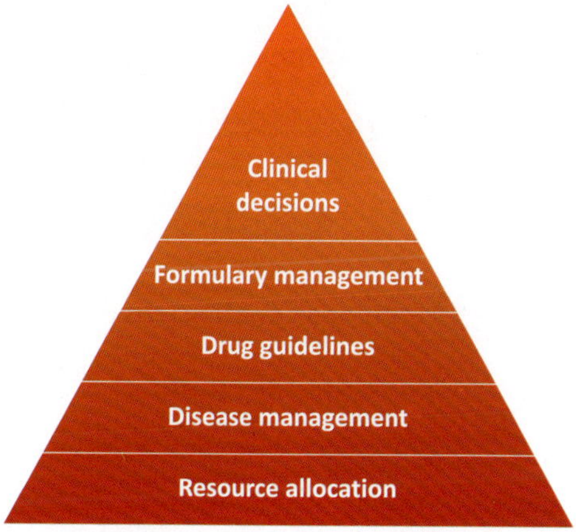

Fig 78.2 Application of PE data

Aim of cost-utility analysis is to compare the cost per quality adjusted life-year for two or more interventions that provide varying outcomes. It involves integration with patient preferences and **Health Related Quality of Life (HRQOL)**. In general, CUA can compare different parameters including cost, quality of life and QALY. Example: In a disease-free patient, it would be 1.0 QALY (in a year) but with a specific disease it would be significantly lower, about 0.5 QALY (varies depending on disease). This method evaluates HRQOL, the most important outcome of health. It measures reductions in morbidity rather than mortality. The outcome is measured as a unit of utility (e.g., QALY depending on disease).

Pharmacoeconomic data is important for various formulary management, resource allocation, clinical decisions, drug guidelines and disease management (Fig. 78.2).

Various Challenges during Pharmacoeconomic Evaluation

- To establish guidelines or standards of practice.
- To train personnel for quality pharmacoeconomic evaluation.
- To increase awareness and education on the relevant features of pharmacoeconomics.
- To provide fund for pharmacoeconomic research.

Pharmacoeconomics is primarily used to inform decision making at different levels like drug therapy evaluations. Nowadays, pharmacoeconomics evolves as an important area of interest to explore the optimal therapy for patients at the lowest price as healthcare facilities are not easily affordable and accessible to some patients. Numerous drug alternatives and empowered consumers also fuel the need for economic evaluations of pharmaceutical products. In a developing country like India, the pharmacoeconomics helps the patients to obtain better healthcare services.

CHAPTER 79

National Health Programmes

COMPETENCY PH1.55

National health programmes are an integral part of our health care system to improve the health status of Indian population. Objective of major National Health Programmes is to provide health care facilities to society especially to vulnerable population like children, pregnant females and elderly.

In India, the three main health services are:

a) National Health Policy 2017
b) National Nutrition Policy 1998
c) National Population Policy 2000.

Under *National Health Mission (NHM)*, National Rural Health Mission (NRHM) was launched in 2005. Various health programmes under NHM are listed in Table 79.1. Various activities are community-based approach through training of ASHA workers, health action plan, strengthening Primary Health Centre (PHC) and Community Health Centre (CHC). Implementation of programmes with help of ASHA workers, district administration, Anganwadi workers, NGOs and State Government. *National Urban Health Mission (NUHM)* is implemented with aiming to improve health status of the urban population.

UNIVERSAL IMMUNIZATION PROGRAMME

Universal Immunization Programme in India was launched in 1989 by Ministry of Health and Family Welfare. Under this programme, several vaccines are administered to infants, children and pregnant women (Table 79.2).

Other activities of Universal Immunization Programme are training of health care workers for routine immunization, planning and implementation, monitoring adverse effects and vaccine cold storage. Programme Implementation Plan (PIP) includes support for alternative vaccine delivery from primary health centre to sub-centre.

Table 79.2 National immunization schedule

Age	Vaccine schedule
Birth	BCG, OPV, Hepatitis B birth dose
6 weeks	OPV-1, Pentavalent-1, RVV-1, fIPV-1, PCV-1
10 weeks	OPV-2, Pentavalent-2, RVV-2
14 weeks	OPV-, Pentavalent -3, fIPV -2, RVV-3, PCV-2
9-12 months	MR-1, JE-1, PCV-booster
16-24 months	MR-2, JE-2, DPT-Booster-1, OPV-Booster
5-6 years	DPT-Booster-2
10 years	Td
16 years	Td
Pregnant mother	Td-1, Td-2 or Td-booster

BCG—Bacillus Calmette Guerin; OPV—Oral Polio Vaccine; RVV—Rotavirus Vaccine; fIPV—Fractional dose of inactivate polio vaccine-1; PCV—Pneumococcal conjugate vaccine; MR—Measles rubella vaccine; JE—Japanese Encepha-litis; DPT—Diphtheria, Pertussis & Tetanus; Td—tetanus and adult diphtheria toxoid.

Cold chain is a system of storing and transporting vaccine at the recommended range of temperature. It requires to maintain temperature between 2°C and 8°C (36°F and 46°F) from the point of manufacturer till it reaches to the beneficiaries. Monitoring of temperature should be done at specific intervals.

POSHAN ABHIYAAN

POSHAN Abhiyaan earlier called the 'National Nutrition Mission' is a systematic approach in

Table 79.1 Classification of health programmes under National Health Mission (NHM)

Category	Programmes
National nutrition programmes	Mid-day Meal Program National Vitamin A Prophylaxis Program National program for Prevention and Control of Fluorosis Mothers Absolute Affection (MAA) National Iodine Deficiency Disorder Control Program Infant and Young Child Feeding Anemia Mukht Bharat
Communicable diseases	National TB Elimination Program (NTEP) National Leprosy Elimination Program National AIDS Control Program National Vector Borne Disease Control Integrated Disease Surveillance Program National Program on Containment of anti-microbial Resistance
Non-communicable diseases	National Mental Health Program National Tobacco Control Program National Program for healthcare of elderly National Program for Prevention and Control of Deafness National Oral Health Program National Program for Control of Blindness and Visual Impairment National Program for Prevention of Cancer, Diabetes, Cardiovascular Diseases and Stroke
Reproductive, Maternal, Newborn, Child plus Adolescent Health (RMNCH + A)	Universal Immunization Program Janani Suraksha Yojana Janani Shishu Suraksha Karyakram (JSSK) Rashtriya Kishor Swasthya Karyakram (RKSK) Rashtriya Bal Swasthya Karyakram (RBSK) Mission Indradhanush Navjaat Shishu Suraksha Karyakram (NSSK) Pradhan Mantri Surakshit Matritva Abhiyan
Health system strengthening	LaQshya Pradhan Mantri Swasthya Suraksha Yojana (PMSSY) Ayushman Bharat PM Jay

addressing the life cycle issues of malnutrition. Efforts are underway to improve the integration of various nutritional interventions in India.

Key Nutrition Strategies

1. Infant and Young child feeding (IYCF)
2. Poshan (Overall nutrition)
3. Food fortification
4. Dietary diversification
5. Early childhood development (ECD) /Early Childhood care and education (ECCE)
6. ORS-Zinc supplementation for diarrhoea
7. Maternal health and nutrition
8. Hygiene, sanitation and safe water drinking
9. Monitoring of growth of child and Promotion
10. Prevention of anaemia in children adolescents girls and women: diet and deworming

11. Girl's education, diet and age of marriage
12. Immunization for every child and Vitamin A supplementation

MID-DAY MEAL PROGRAMME

It is a nutritional programme launched in 1995, also called as 'School Lunch Programme.' Objectives are to provide healthy food, give nutritional education and to attract children for school admission. This programme combines nutrition and formal education for children. Principle is to supply 1/3rd energy and ½ total protein requirement per day. But meal should be supplement not in replace of home diet. (Table 79.3)

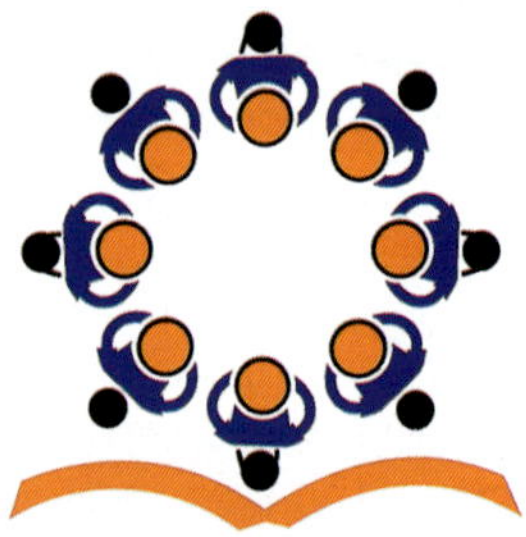

Mid Day Meal Scheme

Table 79.3 Food items in Mid-day Meal Programme

Food items	Primary level (Class I-V)	Secondary level (Class VI-VIII)
Food grains	100 g	150 g
Pulses	20 g	30 g
Vegetables	50 g	75 g
Oil and fat	5 g	7.5 g
Salt	2 g	4 g
Calory intake	450 calories	700 calories
Protein	12 g	20 g

NATIONAL PROPHYLAXIS PROGRAMME AGAINST NUTRITION BLINDNESS (NPPNB)

Objective of this programme is to reduce incidence of blindness due to vitamin A deficiency. Programme is implemented by primary health centres and subcentres. *For prophylaxis*: Give Vitamin A tablet 1 lac IU (1 mL) for 6–12 months of age and then 2 lac IU (2 mL) at every 6 months interval till 5 years of age. *For treatment*: Give 2 lac IU (2 mL) followed by same dose after 4 weeks.

NATIONAL IRON PLUS INITIATIVE (NIPI)

National Iron Plus Initiative (NIPI) is an initiative to prevent iron deficiency anaemia in adolescents and women of reproductive age group also. Aim is to supplement iron and folic acid to prevent deficiency (Table 79.4).

NATIONAL IODINE DEFICIENCY DISORDER CONTROL PROGRAMME (NIDDCP)

Aims of this programme are to decrease magnitude of iodine deficiency disorders in India and consumption of iodized salt at the household level. The standards of salt iodisation must be followed like fixed iodine content in salt (30 ppm of iodine at manufacturer level and 15 ppm at consumer level), moisture and transport. Regular surveys should be conducted to assess magnitude of iodine deficiency (goitre) and health educational activities to prevent iodine deficiency.

MOTHER'S ABSOLUTE AFFECTION (MAA) PROGRAMME

Objectives are to encourage early breastfeeding via awareness activities, educating pregnant and lactating mothers and their family members. Breastfeeding should be started within one hour of child birth including colostrum feeding.

NATIONAL PROGRAMME FOR PREVENTION AND CONTROL OF FLUOROSIS (NPPCF)

Fluorosis is caused by excessive intake of fluoride through food or drinking water. Dental *Fluorosis* affects children leading to discoloured and disfigured teeth. *Skeletal Fluorosis* affects bones and major joints like shoulder, hip and knee. Aims of NPPCF are to prevent and treat fluorosis in India. Various activities are to evaluate the burden of fluorosis, prevention, diagnosis and management of cases including supplementation of vitamin C, D, calcium and antioxidants for treatment.

Table 79.4 Iron regimen and its dose in children

Age group	Dose	Regimen
6–60 months	1 mL iron syrup (20 mg elemental iron) and 100 μg folic acid	Given biweekly and deworming for children 12 months and above.
5–10 years	Iron tablet 45 mg elemental iron and 400 μg folic acid	Given weekly and deworming biannual.
10–19 years	Iron tablet 100 mg elemental iron and 500 μg folic acid	Given weekly and deworming biannual
Pregnant and lactating females	Iron tablet 100 mg elemental iron and 500 μg folic acid	Daily iron tablet for 100 days starting after first trimester.
Women in reproductive age group	Iron tablet 100 mg elemental iron and 500 μg folic acid	Weekly throughout reproductive period.

DIARRHOEA CONTROL PROGRAMME

Objective of this programme is to reduce morbidity and mortality due to diarrhoeal diseases. The mainstay treatment is administration of oral rehydration salt (ORS). Administration of zinc with ORS can reduce severity and duration of diarrheal episodes. Dose of zinc: For 2–6 months of age - 10 mg dispersible tablets. > 6 months of age: 20 mg tablets for 2 weeks.

NATIONAL PROGRAMME FOR PREVENTION & CONTROL OF CANCER, DIABETES, CARDIO-VASCULAR DISEASE AND STROKE (NPCDCS)

In India, non-communicable diseases like cardio-vascular diseases, cancer, diabetes and respiratory diseases are major causes of morbidity and mortality. Objectives of NPCDCS are to screen these diseases and to provide cost effective treatment. Newer initiatives are inclusion respiratory diseases like Chronic Obstructive Pulmonary Disease (COPD), chronic kidney disease and Rheumatic Heart Disease (RHD).

NATIONAL MENTAL HEALTH PROGRAMME (NMHP)

Objectives of this programme are treatment of mental disorders, rehabilitation of patient, prevention and promotion of positive mental health. Various components are to ensure the availability of mental health care, promote participation of community and to eradicate stigma associated with mentally ill patients. It also involves early detection of psychiatric illness and counselling.

NATIONAL TOBACCO CONTROL PROGRAMME

Objectives of National Tobacco Control Programme are to increase awareness regarding hazards of tobacco and to facilitate effective implementation of tobacco control laws. It also involves prohibition for advertisement, production, distribution and supply. Implementation of programme by educational activities, treat tobacco dependent persons and establishment of tobacco cessation centres in dental institutions.

NATIONAL TB ELIMINATION PROGRAMME (NTEP)

Tuberculosis is a leading cause of morbidity and mortality in India. Large numbers of multidrug resistant TB (MDR-TB) cases reported every year. Revised National TB Control Programme (RNTCP) is revised to NTEP. Aim is to eliminate TB by 2025 from

India. There are four strategic pillars, a) Detect b) Treat c) Prevent and d) Built.

- **Detect**
  Objective is to find drug sensitive TB (DS-TB), drug resistant TB (DR-TB) and undiagnosed TB cases. Various activities are providing affordable and quality diagnostic tests and distribution of drug free of cost. NIKSHAY portal (http://niskshay.gov.in) is case based surveillance system for Government and private health care facilities.
- **Treat**
  Directly Observed Treatment (DOT) is a specific strategy to improve adherence when a patient takes drugs in his/her presence.

  For drug sensitive cases, there is only one category, a) Intensive phase: 2 months 4 drugs are given, Isoniazid, Rifampicin; Pyrazinamide and Ethambutol. b) Continuation phase: 4 months 3 drugs are given; Isoniazid, Rifampicin and Ethambutol.

  'Nikshya Poshak Yojana' gives free nutritional supplement to patients.
- **Prevent**
  It includes BCG vaccination and isoniazid chemoprophylaxis for 6 months. Contact tracing to all close contacts must be evaluated. Social and other barriers should be addressed like malnutrition, poverty and pollution.
- **Build**
  It includes building and strengthening policies, empowering institutions and human resources to strengthen health system to fight against TB.

NATIONAL ANTI-MALARIA PROGRAMME

Malaria is one of the most common diseases in India caused by female anopheles mosquito. Objective of this programme is to reduce transmission of malaria, active case detection, early diagnosis and treatment. Various activities include environmental control, chemical control, residual sprays and space sprays.

KALA-AZAR CONTROL PROGRAMME

Kala-Azar is a disease caused by protozoa leishmania species and transmitted to humans by bite of sand fly. Aim of this programme is to interrupt transmission through indoor residual insecticides, early diagnosis and treatment of cases and health education for awareness.

NATIONAL FILARIA CONTROL PROGRAMME

Filariasis has been a major public concern in India caused by *W. Bancrofti*. It is transmitted to humans by biting of mosquito. Aim is to eliminate filariasis from India. Various activities are to identify cases, treat with drugs and prevent complications. The activities are mainly confined to areas with high incidence of filariasis.

DENGUE AND DENGUE HAEMORRHAGIC FEVER (DHF)

Dengue is a mosquito borne disease caused by dengue virus. It is prevalent in India and outbreaks are reported in tropical and subtropical areas. The guidelines are explained in Integrated Vector Control and Management. Various activities are increase awareness, prevent dengue by larvae spray, prompt diagnosis and management.

NATIONAL AIDS CONTROL PROGRAMME (NACP)

Objective of NACP is to prevent and slow down the spread of HIV transmission. Various activities under this programme are diagnosis and prevention strategies, comprehensive care, support and management. HIV surveillance should be conducted to determine level of HIV infection among general population and to identify causes of spread.

'Counselling and HIV Testing Centres' are working for early detection of HIV and providing basic information on transmission. Patients receive free

National AIDS Control Organisation
India's Voice against AIDS
Ministry of Health & Family Welfare, Government of India

Anti-Retroviral Therapy (ART). Various activities are regular health check-up, rehabilitation, psychological and social support prevention and treatment of opportunistic infections. HIV screening of pregnant females should be done to prevent transmission from mother to child. HIV and TB collaborative activities are conducted by combined work of NACP and NTEP. Preventive measures include awareness for usage of barrier contraceptive (condom) and implementation of regulations for blood transfusion.

NATIONAL LEPROSY ERADICATION PROGRAMME (NLEP)

Objectives of this programme are to reduce incidence and prevalence of leprosy, to reduce disability cases, to neutralize stigma and discrimination of leprosy patients.

Strategies are integrated anti-leprosy services, detection and management, Information, Education and Communication (IEC) including behaviour change communication (BCC). Others are Disability prevention and Medical Rehabilitation (DPMR) and collaboration with NGO services. To reduce stigma and discrimination, 'Sparsh leprosy awareness campaign' was launched.

NATIONAL PROGRAMME ON CONTAINMENT OF ANTI-MICROBIAL RESISTANCE

Due to widespread usage of antibiotics, antimicrobial resistance (AMR) is a growing public health concern. Objectives are to establish a laboratory-based AMR surveillance system and usage of antimicrobial among population and promote rational use of antibiotics. For anti-microbial resistance, seven common bacterial pathogens are E. coli, Pseudomonas, salmonella, Acinetobacter, klebsiella and staphylococcus aureus.

NATIONAL PROGRAMME FOR PALLIATIVE CARE

Palliative care is also known as supportive care for patients suffering from terminal illness like AIDS, cancer etc. Objectives of this programme are to improve the capacity to provide palliative care services in various government health programs like cardiovascular diseases, diabetes, stroke and cancer.

NATIONAL PROGRAMME FOR PREVENTION AND CONTROL OF DEAFNESS (NPPCD)

This programme was initiated with objectives to prevent avoidable hearing loss due to disease or injury, early identification, diagnosis and treatment of ear problems. It also includes how to prevent and control major causes of hearing impairment and deafness.

NATIONAL PROGRAMME ON HEALTH CARE FOR ELDERLY

This programme provides dedicated health care facilities for elderly (>60 years of age). Objectives are to provide high quality affordable care services to elderly in collaboration with National Rural Health Mission and AYUSH. Various activities are geriatric health assessment for elderly geriatric clinic, rehabilitation of bed ridden patients and dedicated geriatric OPD services.

CHAPTER 80 Evidence-Based Medicine (EBM) & Therapeutic Drug Monitoring (TDM)

COMPETENCY PH1.2

EVIDENCE-BASED MEDICINE (EBM)

Definition

Evidence-based medicine (EBM) is the integration of best research evidence with clinical expertise and patient values. Due to interest in research by medical and other professionals, the quantity of clinical research is escalated and further publishing the research, evidence-based journals have emerged. The search of any scientific article for physician, the rational practice of EBM should be employed to find the best and updated reliable information and it application for the benefit of the patient. Hence, EBM focuses to develop decision making for benefit of patient by emphasizing the use of evidence from well-designed conducted medical research. It is an integration of evidence, clinical knowledge and patient values.

Various types of study are randomized controlled trials (RCTs), non-randomized intervention studies, systematic reviews, meta-analyses, observational studies, non-experimental studies and expert opinion.

The Process of EBM

The process of EBM comprises five basic steps to be followed by an individual or physician.

Step 1: Clinical Question Development

To find and evaluate accurate clinical question according to the objective, **PICO** format is used:

- **P**: *Patient or population* – It includes age, gender, demographic data of patient, etc.
- **I**: *Intervention* – By drug, procedure, surgery, diagnostic test or vaccine.
- **C**: *Comparison* – It includes comparison of new with standard drug therapy or placebo.
- **O**: *Outcome* – It describes the result like reduced mortality or morbidity, less risk of infection improvement in quality of life, etc.

Step 2: Searching the Best Evidence from Literature

To find research of interest, several options are available but aim is to acquire ideal research from various available sources, which will provide the best answer to our question. Appropriate sources for search are PubMed, Medscape and Medline. Various standard journals are also available. Others like Evidence summaries, Clinical Evidence, Clinical guidelines, etc. Out of these, ideal source of information must be selected on basis of relevance and validity (Table 80.1).

Table 80.1 Various types of study design

Descriptive studies	Case series Case reports Ecological studies
Analytical studies	Case-control study Cross-sectional study Cohort study
Experimental studies	Randomized control trials Non-randomized control trial Community trial Pre- and post-test study design

Ideal Type of Study:

- *For therapy*: Randomized Controlled Trial (RCT)
- *For prevention*: RCT > Cohort > Case control
- *For prognosis*: Cohort > Case-control > Case series/Case report
- *For cost analysis*: Economical analysis study
- *Aetiology/Harm*: RCT > Cohort > Case-control

Step 3: Critical Appraisal of the Evidence

Once information is available, a physician further evaluates its importance, reliability, quality, validity and relevance. Validity should be checked by objectives of the study, time of study, sample population, study group, appropriate test or control group and methodology. Evaluate the following parameters: Content is accurately presented or not, result should be checked with tables, charts, statistical tests, any conflict of interest and any evidence of bias.

Evidence-based Medicine Pyramid

To understand the importance of different types of study designs, Evidence-based medicine pyramid is created (Fig. 80.1).

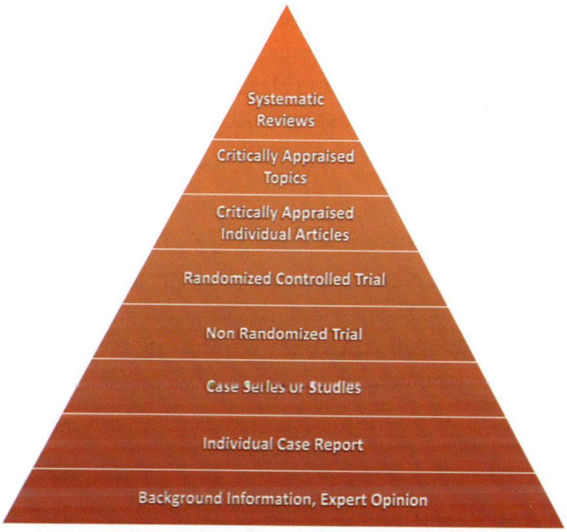
Systematic Reviews
Critically Appraised Topics
Critically Appraised Individual Articles
Randomized Controlled Trial
Non Randomized Trial
Case Series or Studies
Individual Case Report
Background Information, Expert Opinion

Fig 80.1 Evidence-based Medicine Pyramid

Step 4: Applying Evidence to the Patient

Once knowledge of EBM is obtained, the physician has to take decision whether apply it to patient or not. For decision making, information is correlated with patient's value, preferences, requirements and physician's own expertise.

Step 5: Efficacy Evaluation in Terms of Benefits

After applying knowledge of EBM, efficacy should be evaluated in terms of *benefit to patient* that up to which extent.

Advantages of EBM

EBM keeps physician with upgraded knowledge, improves data search skills, critically evaluate information available from different sources which helps them for better management decision.

Disadvantages of EBM

It is time consuming, confusion among various information and improper application of EBM can harm the patient.

Real-World Data (RWD) and Real-World Evidence (RWE)

The Food and Drug Administration (FDA) had created a framework for evaluating potential use of RWD and RWE to monitor post-marketing safety and adverse events and to make regulatory decisions.

Real-World Data (RWD)

It includes data of drugs collected from a variety of sources like Electronic Health Records (EHRs), claims and billing activities, product and disease registries, etc.

Real-World Evidence (RWE)

It includes clinical evidence regarding usage, potential benefits and risks of drugs for new indication. This framework is also intended for biological products. RWE can be generated by different study designs or analyses including Randomized Controlled Trials, observational studies, etc.

Challenges in Implementing Evidence-based Medicine

Many quality research articles are expensive and not universally available. There is lack of free access to all available information. Physicians currently have no free or reasonably priced services to access a comprehensive database of full text research articles and journals. It affects the search of valid and reliable research resource. Further, during busy schedule in routine daily working hours, physician has time constraints and for EBM additional time is required for search and evaluation.

THERAPEUTIC DRUG MONITORING

Therapeutic drug monitoring (TDM) is defined as measurement of concentration in biological fluid and interpretation of its concentration. TDM is the clinical assessment of a drug's pharmacokinetic properties. Many drugs have direct relationship between their plasma level and clinical effects. TDM refers to the individualization of drug dosage by maintaining plasma or blood drug concentrations within a targeted therapeutic range or window.

Indications of TDM

1. Drugs with low safety margin, narrow therapeutic index, to avoid their toxicities. Examples: Lithium, digitoxin, digoxin, etc.
2. Drugs having saturable kinetic, e.g., Phenytoin.
3. When renal disease alter relationship between dose and plasma concentration and to reduce toxicities, e.g., aminoglycosides in the presence of renal failure.
4. When failure to respond to therapy without any known reason – to check patient compliance.
5. Poisoning of drugs.
6. To measure bioavailability.
7. Monitoring and detecting drug–drug interactions, e.g., Plasma concentration of lithium is increased by thiazide.
8. To evaluate compliance of patient.

TDM is required for the following drugs

- Cardiovascular drugs: Amiodarone, Digoxin, Digitoxin, Procainamide, Quinidine.
- Antibiotics: Gentamycin, Tobramycin.
- Antidepressants and mood stabilizers: Tricyclic antidepressants, Lithium.
- Antiepileptic drugs: Phenytoin, Phenobarbitone, Carbamazepine, Valproic acid.
- Bronchodilator: Theophylline.
- Cancer chemotherapy: Methotrexate.
- Immunosuppressants: Cyclosporin, Tacrolimus

TDM is not required for the following drugs

1. For hit and run drugs (omeprazole).
2. Drugs causes tolerance (morphine).
3. Drugs with high therapeutic index, safer drugs (paracetamol).
4. When effects can be measured easily (blood pressure measurement for antihypertensives).
5. Effects can be measured using available laboratory tests (anticoagulants).
6. Effects of drug continues for a long time even after the drug is eliminated.
7. Effects of the relationship remains undefined (selective serotonin reuptake inhibitors).

Principles of TDM

Drug concentration should be measured at an appropriate time after administration. Knowledge of pharmacokinetic and pharmacological profiles of drug is essential. TDM can be a part of individualized drug therapy as per patient's demographic data, clinical condition and laboratory tests.

Samples

Plasma or serum is commonly taken for measuring drug concentration. Whole blood is taken for drugs like cyclosporin, tacrolimus as there is large shift of drug between red cells and plasma. Saliva can be taken for drugs like phenytoin and lithium as an alternative to blood samples.

Timing

The importance of proper timing of a sample collection should be given sufficient attention. The best sampling time is when drug reaches steady state level, i.e., after 4–5 half-life. Before collecting the sample, confirm that drug achieves steady state level and sufficient time after administration to ensure drug is absorbed and distributed in the body.

Blood sample can be taken at two times, during highest therapeutic concentration ('peak' level) and lowest ('trough' level). Peak level shows risk of toxicities and trough level indicates sufficient lower level for the effect. For i.v. administration, sample should be taken according to half-life. Poisoning or toxicity can be identified by one sample only when the symptoms of poisoning or toxicity are prominent.

Examples

1. ***Cyclosporin***: After oral administration, sample should be taken every 2–3 days for first 4 weeks then monthly for three months. Aim is to prevent nephrotoxicity and excessive immunosuppression. Therapeutic range: 0.6–0.8 μg/mL.
2. ***Phenytoin***
   a) After administration of oral tablet, blood sample is taken 24 hrs after last dose.
   b) Following dose adjustment: Within 6–7 days, sample is taken 8 hrs after last dose.
   c) For toxicity: Sample to be taken immediately. Therapeutic range: 10–20 μg/mL.

3. ***Digoxin***: The blood sample should be taken 6 hrs after dose. Many drug–drug interactions also increase risk of toxicities. Plasma concentrations between 0.5 and 0.8 ng/mL are associated with beneficial effects, and concentration 1.2 ng/mL and greater are associated with increased mortality.
4. ***Theophylline*** has narrow therapeutic index. Drug concentration is measured:
   a) For oral solution, 1–2 hrs after administration.
   b) For extended-release tablets, 4–12 hrs after administration.
   c) For injection, ½ hr after administration.

   Therapeutic range: 5–20 μg/mL.

Analytical Methods

Several analytical techniques are available to measure drug concentration in sample like High Pressure Liquid Chromatography (HPLC), Liquid Chromatography Mass Spectrometry (LC/MS), Gas Chromatography (GC), Enzyme Immuno-assay (EIA), Radio Immunoassay (RIA) and Fluorescence Polarization Immunoassay (FPIA).

Interpretation of Sample Concentration

In collected sample, if lower concentration is measured, may be due to missed dosing regimen, non-compliance of patient, error in timing of sample collection, poor bioavailability and rapid elimination. If higher concentration is measured, may be due to higher dose administration, slow elimination, renal or hepatic dysfunction.

Factors which Affect TDM

- Pharmacokinetic parameters like bioavailability, half-life, clearance, volume of distribution and plasma protein binding can affect TDM. Other conditions like age (neonates, elderly), diseases (hepatic, renal, cardiovascular), pregnancy and drug–drug interactions lead to variations in TDM.
- Other factors like pharmacodynamics of drug, dose of drug and sampling time affect TDM.

Free Drug Monitoring

The active concentration of drug is a 'free drug' level which gives better idea about TDM. Recently, to detect the level of free unbound drug, various new filtration devices like dialysis, ultrafiltration and ultracentrifugation are developed.

CHAPTER 81

Drugs Used in Skin Disorders

COMPETENCY PH1.57

Skin disorders are common among population globally. Topical route of drugs is appropriate, i.e., drug is applied directly on skin or mucus membrane. Certain properties of drugs are responsible for them to be effective topically. Factors which determine drug response are:

1. Highly lipid soluble and low molecular weight drugs are more effective topically.
2. Thickness of skin affects drug penetration. Example: application on palm, scrotum, lips or scalp.
3. Concentration gradient: Increasing the concentration gradient increases delivery of drug.
4. Age: In children, absorption is faster than adults.
5. Vehicle: An appropriate vehicle maximizes the ability of the drug to penetrate the outer layers of the skin.

DRUGS FOR PSORIASIS

Psoriasis is an autoimmune disorder characterized by localized or widespread erythematous scaling lesions or plaques. Size and shape of erythematous plaques may vary with silvery scales. Plaques are localized or involve many areas like skin, scalp, fingers and nails.

A. Topical Drugs

Glucocorticoids are highly effective in mild, moderate and severe cases of psoriasis. The usefulness of topical corticosteroids is due to anti-inflammatory activity. The antimitotic effects of corticosteroids may account for an additional mechanism of action. Gradual response is seen over 3 weeks. ***Keratolytics***: Salicylic acid, urea, formalin and lactic acid can be used in combination with other drugs.

Tazarotene is a topical synthetic retinoid used in psoriasis. It is a prodrug, converted to tazarotene acid which has anti-inflammatory and anti-proliferative properties. After applying, skin irritation, burning and photosensitivity is common. Hence, minimize exposure sunlight and use sunscreens. It can be combined with topical steroids.

Emollients hydrate the skin and soft paraffin softens the skin.

Calcipotriol is a synthetic vitamin D_3 analogue effective in the treatment of plaque-type psoriasis. It inhibits proliferation of keratinocytes and can be combined with topical steroids. *Adverse effects*: Burning, itching, mild irritation with dryness, erythema and ocular irritation. ***Coaltar*** acts via different mechanism. It has phototoxic actions leading to decreased epithelial proliferation and resolution of plaques. First apply ointment of coaltar on psoriatic plaques followed by direct exposure to sunlight. Side effects are bad odour, irritation, allergy of skin and carcinogenicity.

B. Systemic Drugs (Oral)

i) **Antimetabolites**: ***Methotrexate*** *and* ***azathioprine*** are antiproliferative drugs which inhibit replication and function of T cells. These are effective in moderate to severe psoriasis. *Side effects*: Myelosuppression and increase liver enzymes.
ii) **Immunosuppressants**: ***Tacrolimus*** is an orally effective drug in severe psoriasis. Cyclosporine inhibits IL-2 production. ***Mycophenolate Mofetil*** is used (1–2 g/day) in severe psoriasis.
iii) **Biological agents** are useful for moderate to severe chronic plaque psoriasis. It includes the TNF-α inhibitors adalimumab, etanercept and infliximab, and the cytokine inhibitors secukinumab and ustekinumab. They inhibit TNF-α and T cell activation and migration lead to inhibition of antibody synthesis.

    Alefacept: It blocks the interaction between the leukocyte-function-associated antigen (LFA)-3 and CD2 and inhibits activation and proliferation of T cells. It can be used for moderate to severe chronic plaque psoriasis in adult patients.

    Efalizumab: It is a humanized IgG1 Mab inhibits LFA-1, prevents interaction of the LFA-1 and intercellular adhesion molecule-1 (ICAM) which blocks T-cell adhesion and activation. It is approved for moderate to severe chronic plaque psoriasis.

iv) **Others**:

Acitretin is a synthetic retinoid used orally for severe and pustular psoriasis. *Side effects*: Gingivitis, dry skin, myalgia and liver damage. It is a teratogenic drug, not given during pregnancy and at least 3 years after treatment is discontinued.

Psoralen (phototherapy): Oral methoxasalen is given followed by exposure to UV radiation after 1–2 hrs. It inhibits DNA synthesis and DNA turnover. Side effects are burns, insomnia, skin cancer and cataract. Glucocorticoids are used orally in severe cases.

Risankizumab is a monoclonal antibody recently approved drug by US-FDA for moderate to severe psoriasis. It inhibits interleukin-23 involved in inflammation.

Deucravacitinib is a newly approved drug by US-FDA to treat moderate-to-severe plaque psoriasis. It has a novel mechanism of action via inhibiting *Janus Kinase (JAK)* pathway. It binds to a unique pocket in the regulatory domain of TYK2 catalytic site.

Spesolimab acts by inhibiting the inflammatory signalling pathway of IL-6 which is overexpressed in psoriasis. It is US-FDA approved drug for the treatment of generalized pustular psoriasis flares in adults.

Ixekizumab is a monoclonal antibody at targets interleukin 17A. It inhibits proliferation of keratinocytes. It is indicated for moderate to severe psoriasis.

Tildrakizumab is a humanized IgG1 monoclonal antibody which selectively binds to interleukin-23 (IL-23) and inhibits the release of proinflammatory cytokines and chemokines. It is used in moderate-to-severe plaque psoriasis in adults. *Adverse effects*: Upper respiratory infections, injection site reactions and diarrhoea.

Guselkumab is a monoclonal antibody (IgG1) that inhibits IL-23 by selectively binding to p19 subunit of IL-23 and inhibits cytokine and chemokine release. It is approved for chronic plaque psoriasis. *Adverse effects*: Injection site reaction, increase risk of infections and hypersensitivity reactions.

Tapinarof binds with therapeutic *Aryl hydrocarbon receptor Modulating Agent (TAMA)* and stimulates it. Tapinarof has anti-inflammatory effects and approved for treatment of chronic plaque psoriasis in adults.

DRUGS USED IN ACNE VULGARIS

Acne vulgaris is a common skin problem in adolescents. High androgenic activity leads to more sebum production and blockade of the follicular opening. Growth of bacteria in the hair follicles (*P. acne*) produces lipase, which cause lipid breakdown. It produces free fatty acids which irritate the follicular ducts leads to formation of black heads (Comedones).

A. Topical Therapy

Benzoyl peroxide releases oxygen and kills the anaerobic bacteria (*Propionibacterium acne*). It has antibacterial, comedolytic and keratolytic properties. Production of irritant fatty acids is also reduced. *Adverse effects*: Local burning and stinging sensation initially but tolerance develops gradually. Avoid direct contact with mucus membrane, eyes and lips. It can cause swelling, edema and erythema. It is available as 5–10% cream, gel and lotion.

Retinoic acid (Tretinoin) prevents the formation of comedones; has comedolytic and keratinolytic properties. Response is slow, may take 6–10 weeks. *Advantages*: It decreases pigmentation on skin, photoaging, wrinkles, mottling and sagging of loose skin. *Adverse effects*: Stinging, redness, edema and crusting may develop. Avoid tretinoin during pregnancy due to risk of teratogenicity. Available as 0.05% cream or gel. It causes erythema with mild peeling. If too much irritation occurs, reduce concentration or discontinue the drug.

Adapalene is a synthetic drug resembles retinoic acid in structure and effects. It is available for daily application as a 0.1% gel, lotion and cream. It is effective in patients with mild to moderate acne vulgaris.

Tazarotene is a retinoid derivative available as a 0.1% gel and cream for the treatment of mild to moderate facial acne.

Azelaic acid inhibits bacterial density of *P. acne*, free fatty acids and keratinocytes. It is available as 10–20% cream.

Antibiotics: ***Clindamycin*** is effective against *P. acne*. About 10% of an applied dose is absorbed. It may cause drying, irritation of the skin, burning and stinging. *Erythromycin* has inhibitory effects on *P acne*. But, antibiotic resistance may develop. So topical erythromycin should be discontinued and appropriate systemic antibiotic therapy started. *Adverse reactions* include burning sensation, drying and irritation of the skin. *Sodium Sulfacetamide* is available as single (10% lotion) or in combination for the treatment of acne vulgaris.

B. Systemic Therapy

Oral antibiotics like erythromycin, doxycycline or minocycline are effective for acne. ***Isotretinoin*** is a synthetic retinoid for oral treatment of severe cystic acne. It acts by inhibiting the function of sebaceous gland and decreases sebum production. *Adverse effects*: Dryness and itching of the skin and mucous membranes. Teratogenicity is a significant risk, so the FDA mandates the childbearing women must use contraception for at least 1 month before, throughout therapy, and for 1 or more months after discontinuation.

Trifarotene is a recently US-FDA approved drug for acne vulgaris. It is an agonist to retinoic acid receptor and used as cream.

Clascoterone is a newly approved drug by US-FDA to treat acne. It is an androgen receptor antagonist. It competes with the androgen dihydrotestosterone for binding to androgen receptors in the sebaceous gland and hair follicles. It is used topically in patients 12 years of age or older.

DRUGS FOR SCABIES AND PEDICULOSIS

In scabies, mite enters the body from finger web which spreads to forearm, lower limbs and genital. It forms papules with redness and itchy skin. Pediculosis is due to entry of lice on head and body. It causes intense itching.

Treatment

Permethrin is a broad spectrum, most effective and most convenient drug for scabies and pediculosis. It causes paralysis in insects. Single application achieves up to 100% cure rate. Some patients have itching, burning, redness and rash after application. *For scabies*: Apply 5% cream over the body except face and head and wash after 12 hrs. *For pediculosis*: 1% cream/lotion to be applied on the scalp and wash after 10 min.

Lindane (gamma benzene hexachloride: BHC) kills mite and lice by affecting its nervous system. It is effective but less potent than permethrin for scabies and pediculosis. *For scabies*: Lotion or cream to be applied from neck to toes and take scrub bath after 12–24 hrs to washout the drug. *For pediculosis*: Apply on the scalp and head without touching the eyes and then wash off. Repeat after 1 week. *Adverse effects*: Skin rash, headache, vertigo, convulsions and arrhythmias.

Benzyl benzoate: After scrub bath, emulsion of benzyl benzoate is applied on skin of whole body except face and neck. Next day, second application and wash after 24 hrs. ***Crotamiton*** is a scabicide, pediculocide and antipruritic. It is safer in children. After scrub bath, apply drug over the skin below face two times at 24-hrs interval.

Ivermectin is an anthelmintic drug. Orally effective against scabies and pediculosis. Single dose (12 mg) causes almost complete cure. Contraindicated in children, pregnancy and lactation.

Sulfur is a weak scabicidal and pediculocidal. It has bad odour and requires repeated application.

ANTISEBORRHOEIC AGENTS

For the treatment of seborrhoeic dermatitis or dandruff, several topical drugs are available. The efficacy of these drugs is variable and can be combined with topical corticosteroids in severe cases. Various antiseborrhoeic agents are Ketoconazole shampoo, Chloroxine, Zinc pyrithione, Selenium sulfide shampoo and Betamethasone valerate foam.

DRUGS FOR ECZEMA

- As a moisturizing agent, petroleum jelly can be used.
- Hydrocortisone cream and antihistaminic like levocetirizine orally used.
- Calamine lotion or coal tar application.

- Phototherapy (using ultraviolet light).
- Injectable dupilumab can be used in severe eczema.
- Topical immunosuppressants like pimecrolimus and tacrolimus can be used.

TOPICAL ANTIFUNGALS

- ***Topical azoles***: Clotrimazole is used in ring worm, otomycosis, athlete's foot and vaginal candidiasis. Miconazole and econazole are used in otomycosis and dermatophytosis.
- ***Nystatin*** is effective against Candida infection.
- ***Terbinafine*** cream is used in tinea cruris, corporis and pedis.
- ***Tolnaftate*** is used in tinea cruris and corporis.
- ***Butenafine*** is used in dermatophytosis, tinea cruris, corporis and pedis.
- ***Ciclopirox olamine*** has high cure rate in tinea infections, candidiasis and *P. versicolor*.
- ***Benzoic acid*** is used along with salicylic acid as a Whitfield ointment: benzoic acid + salicylic acid. It helps to remove infected tissue.
- ***Haloprogin*** is fungicidal and principal use is against tinea infection.
- ***Naftifine*** is used in tinea cruris and tinea corporis.

TOPICAL ANTIVIRALS

Acyclovir, valacyclovir, penciclovir and famciclovir have inhibitory activity against members of the Herpes virus family, including Herpes simplex type 1 and 2. Topical penciclovir (1% cream) is used for the treatment of recurrent orolabial herpes simplex virus infection. *Adverse effects*: Pruritus, mild pain with transient stinging or burning sensation.

TOPICAL NSAIDs

Many topical preparations are available containing NSAIDs. Usually, NSAID is combined with counterirritants like menthol, methyl salicylate, camphor, etc. *Drugs*: Diclofenac 1% gel, Ibuprofen 10% gel, Flurbiprofen 5% gel, Naproxen 10% gel. Used in minor injury, osteoarthritis, sprain, spasm, backache, spondylitis, etc.

CHEMICAL AND PHYSICAL SUNSCREENS

Sunscreens are drugs which protect the skin from the harmful effects of the UV rays (sunlight).

a) ***Chemical sunscreens*** are agents which reduce the effects of UV rays on skin. *Drugs*: Para-aminobenzoic acid (PABA), benzophenones and cinnamates. Efficacy of sunscreens is measured by '*Sun Protection Factor (SPF)*.'

$$\text{SPF} = \frac{\text{Dose of UV-B radiation that produce minimal erythema on protected skin}}{\text{Same to unprotected skin}}$$

Most of the sunscreens have SPF 15 (more SPF is better). They are used to prevent and treat sunburn.

b) ***Physical sunscreens*** block or reflect the UV rays. Also called as '*Sun Shades*.' *Drugs*: Calamine, petroleum jelly and titanium oxide.

KERATOLYTIC DRUGS

These drugs dissolve the intercellular substance in the layer of skin. They cause peeling of superficial layer of skin. *Drugs*: Salicylic acid, urea, lactic acid, sulfur, propylene glycol and benzyl peroxide. *Uses*: Corns, psoriasis, warts, ringworm, chronic dermatitis, ringworm and athlete's foot.

MELANIZING AND DEMELANIZING AGENTS

- ***Melanizing agents***: Psoralen, Methoxsalen and Trioxsalen. Topical or oral application sensitizes the skin to sunlight and causes pigmentation. These can be used in vitiligo.
- ***Demelanizing agents***: Hydroquinone, Monobenzone and Azelaic acid. They lighten the hyperpigmented skin. These agents are used in melasma, chloasma of pregnancy and in sunscreens.

DRUGS FOR VITILIGO

- ***Vitiligo*** is a progressive autoimmune depigmentation disorder of the skin due to loss of epidermal melanocytes. The characteristic lesions are white patches of various sizes on skin.

- ***Topical corticosteroid*** is the first line treatment for localized vitiligo. On chronic usage, it may cause skin atrophy. Depending on the area treated, topical steroids can be applied daily for a period of months and then tapering of dose is required.
- ***Calcineurin inhibitors***: Tacrolimus ointment (0.03–0.1%) or pimecrolimus cream is effective for vitiligo.
- ***Vitamin D analogues***: Calcipotriol is used topically for vitiligo.
- ***Phototherapy***: Psoralen is combined with ultraviolet radiation (UV-A) also known as **PUVA**. Psoralen can be used topically, followed by exposure to UV-A radiation or natural sunlight. Repigmentation slowly begins in perifollicular area and periphery of lesion.
- ***Ruxolitinib is*** a Janus Kinase inhibitor (JAK1 and JAK2) and recently US-FDA approved drug for the treatment of nonsegmental vitiligo in adults and children more than 12 years of age.

IRRITANTS AND COUNTER-IRRITANTS

Drugs: Turpentine oil, clove oil, eucalyptus oil, camphor, menthol, capsicum, cantharidin and methyl salicylates. *Mechanism of action*: When counter-irritant is applied on skin, produces vasodilatation and redness of the skin. It irritates the nerve endings. Nerves supplying skin and deeper parts (muscles, joints) are same, so impulses from skin or deeper parts are not clear to the brain and underlying pain is relieved. It is used to reduce deeper pain and inflammation. Counter-irritants should be applied for headache, joint pain, muscular pain, etc.

TOPICAL CORTICOSTEROIDS

Beclomethasone, Betamethasone, Dexamethasone, Clobetasone, Hydrocortisone and Triamcinolone. Topical steroids are used in allergic dermatitis, eczema, psoriasis, cystic acne, lichen planus, lichen simplex and alopecia. Side effects are local dermal thinning, easy bruising and fungal infection, HPA axis suppression and Cushing's syndrome.

IMMUNOMODULATORS

- ***Imiquimod*** is used for the treatment of external genital and perianal warts in adults. It stimulates mononuclear cells to release interferon alpha.
- ***Tacrolimus*** *and* ***pimecrolimus*** are immunosuppressants can be used in atopic dermatitis. Both agents inhibit T-lymphocyte activation and prevent the release of inflammatory cytokines.

TRICHOGENIC AND ANTI-TRICHOGENIC AGENTS

- ***Minoxidil*** is available as topical formulation which is effective in androgenic alopecia. It is more effective in Vertex balding than frontal balding.
- ***Finasteride*** is a 5α-reductase inhibitor that blocks the conversion of testosterone to dihydrotestosterone. It promotes hair growth in males having androgenic alopecia.
- ***Bimatoprost*** is a prostaglandin analogue available as a 0.03% ophthalmic solution and used for hypotrichosis of the eyelashes.

ANTI-NEOPLASTIC AGENTS

- ***Alitretinoin*** is an anti-neoplastic agent used topically for the treatment of cutaneous lesions in patients with AIDS-related Kaposi's sarcoma.
- ***Bexarotene*** binds and activates retinoid X receptors. It is used topically for the treatment of cutaneous T-cell lymphoma.

CHAPTER 82 Drugs Used in Ocular Disorders

COMPETENCY PH1.58

Ocular structures are divided into anterior and posterior segments. Anterior segment includes the cornea, limbus, trabecular meshwork, Schlemm's canal, iris, lens and ciliary body. The posterior segment includes the retina, vitreous, choroid, sclera and optic nerve.

PHARMACOKINETICS

It determines the time course of drug action in the eye. *Absorption*: After topical application of drug, rate and extent of absorption is determined by the dwell time of the drug in the cul-de-sac, precorneal tear film and elimination by nasolacrimal drainage. Nasolacrimal drainage contributes to systemic absorption of topically administered ophthalmic medications. Absorption from the nasal mucosa avoids first-pass metabolism by the liver; thus, topical ophthalmic medications can cause significant systemic side effects. *Distribution*: Topically administered drugs may undergo systemic distribution primarily by nasal mucosal absorption and possibly via local ocular distribution by transcorneal/transconjunctival absorption. Transcorneal drug penetration has a differential solubility process; the cornea resembles a trilaminar "fat-water-fat" structure corresponding to the epithelial, stromal and endothelial layers, respectively. Following absorption, the aqueous humour accumulates the drug, then drug is distributed into intraocular structures. *Metabolism*: Biotransformation of ocular drugs may be significant due to variety of enzymes, including esterases, oxidoreductases, lysosomal enzymes, peptidases, COMT, MAO, etc.

DRUG DELIVERY STRATEGIES

Several drug formulations prolong the time a drug remains on the surface of the eye. These include gels, ointments, solid inserts and soft contact lens. Ophthalmic gels (e.g., pilocarpine 4% gel) release drugs by diffusion. Ointments usually contain mineral oil and a petrolatum base, e.g. antibiotics, cycloplegics and miotics (Table 82.1).

GENERAL PRINCIPLES FOR EYE DISORDERS

Non-pharmacological treatment includes protection of eyes from strong light, trauma and infection, advice for eye exercise and hot or cold compression.

Pharmacological Treatment

1. Consider strict aseptic precautions while instilling eye drops.
2. Only one drop to be inserted into eye, the capacity of conjunctival sac. Then, eyes should be kept close for at least 5 min.
3. Ointment has longer duration of action but may cause blurred vision.
4. In severe ocular conditions, oral therapy should be started.

MYDRIATICS AND MIOTICS

Mydriatics cause dilatation of pupil and used in fundoscopic examination of eyes. Also used to identify refractive error, to break adhesions between lens and ciliary body, along with miotics and in iridocyclitis. Salient features of some mydriatics are given in Table 82.2.

The actions of Cholinergic and Anti-cholinergic drugs on eye are discussed in Chapter 11.

Miotics cause constriction of pupil. They are used in glaucoma, to break adhesions between lens and ciliary body and along with mydriatics. Pilocarpine 0.5% drops and Ocusert, physostigmine 1% can be used. *Adverse effects*: Headache, browache, burning and blurred vision.

Table 82.1 Characteristics of ocular routes of drug administration

Route	Absorption	Indication	Precaution
Topical	Depending on concentration, fast absorption	Most commonly used, safe, economical and convenient	Corneal and conjunctival irritation can occur. Nasal mucosal toxicity and systemic side effects
Intraocular (intracameral) injections	Fast absorption, short duration of action	Anterior segment surgery, infections	Corneal and intraocular toxicity
Subconjunctival, sub-tenon, and retrobulbar injections	Prompt or sustained, depending on formulation	Anterior segment infections, posterior uveitis, macular edema	Local toxicity, tissue injury, globe perforation, optic nerve trauma, retinal artery occlusion
Intravitreal injection or device	Immediate local effect, sustained effect	Endophthalmitis, retinitis, age related macular degeneration	Retinal toxicity

Table 82.2 Characteristics of Mydriatics

Mydriatics	Peculiarities
Atropine (0.5–2%)	Mydriasis is seen within 30–40 min, while cycloplegia occurs within 1–3 hrs. Actions last for very long duration; about 7 days.
Homatropine (2–5%)	Less potent than atropine. Onset of action is within 45–60 min. Duration of action is about 1–3 days.
Cyclopentolate (0.5–2%)	Onset of action is within 30–60 min. Duration of action is about 24 hrs.
Tropicamide (0.5–2%)	Onset of action within 20–40 min. Duration of action about 3–6 hrs. It has quickest onset of action and shortest duration of action. It is used commonly for refraction testing and fundoscopy.
Phenylephrine (2.5%)	It stimulates α_1 receptors, causes contraction of radial muscles of iris. So, mydriasis (active mydriasis) occurs without cycloplegia (no blurred vision).

Effects of Adrenergic agonists and antagonists on eye are explained in Chapter 12.

For drugs used in Glaucoma, refer Chapter 11.

TOPICAL ANTIBACTERIAL AGENTS

Micro-organisms like bacteria, virus, fungi and protozoa can infect eyes. *Blepharitis,* a common inflammatory condition of the eyelids characterized by ocular irritation and burning.

Conjunctivitis (inflammation of conjunctiva) characterized by mild hyperaemia to severe purulent discharge. The common causes include bacteria, viruses, allergies, irritants, contact lenses and chemicals. *Keratitis* (inflammation of cornea) is due to bacteria, viruses, fungi, spirochetes and parasites. Severe infections may cause corneal ulcers which should be treated more aggressively. *Endophthalmitis* is a severe inflammatory and usually infectious disease involving the intraocular tissues. When there is inflammation of the entire globe, it is called *panophthalmitis*. Various topical antibacterial agents for ophthalmic use is given in Table 82.3.

ANTIVIRAL AGENTS

Viral keratitis is an infection of the cornea which involves epithelium. It is caused by Herpes simplex virus, Epstein-Barr virus and cytomegalovirus. Topical trifluridine (1% solution) is used in Herpes simplex keratitis and keratoconjunctivitis. Topical ganciclovir (0.15% gel) is effective in Herpes simplex keratitis and cytomegalovirus retinitis. Acyclovir is used in herpes zoster ophthalmicus and herpes simplex iridocyclitis. Valacyclovir and famciclovir are effective in herpes simplex keratitis. Herpes zoster ophthalmicus is a reactivation of a varicella zoster virus in the trigeminal cranial nerve. Acyclovir, valacyclovir and famciclovir can be used in herpes zoster ophthalmicus.

ANTIFUNGALS AGENTS

Fungal infections of eye involve cornea, conjunctiva, sclera and intraocular structures. Fungal infections are common in ocular trauma, chronic ocular disease, contact lens and chronic usage of topical steroids. Amphotericin-B (0.1–0.5%) topical solution is used in fungal keratitis and endophthalmitis. Natamycin (5% topical suspension) is used in fungal blepharitis, conjunctivitis and keratitis. Fluconazole is used in keratitis and endophthalmitis. Itraconazole and ketoconazole are used topically in fungal keratitis and endophthalmitis. Miconazole and voriconazole can be used as topical solution and intravitreal injection.

Uveitis

Uveitis is an inflammation of the uvea. Topical

Table 82.3 Topical antibacterial agents for ophthalmic use

Antibacterial agent	Formulation	Indications
Azithromycin	1% solution	Conjunctivitis
Bacitracin	500 units/g ointment	Conjunctivitis, blepharitis, keratitis, corneal ulcers
Chloramphenicol	1% ointment	Conjunctivitis, keratitis
Ciprofloxacin	0.3% solution, ointment	Conjunctivitis, keratitis, corneal ulcers, blepharitis
Erythromycin	0.5% ointment	Superficial ocular infections involving the conjunctiva or cornea
Gatifloxacin	0.3% and 0.5% solutions	Conjunctivitis
Gentamicin	0.3% solution, 0.3% ointment	Conjunctivitis
Levofloxacin	0.5% solution	Conjunctivitis, blepharitis, keratitis, corneal ulcers
Moxifloxacin	0.5% solution	Conjunctivitis
Sulfacetamide	10% solution	Conjunctivitis

cyclopentolate, tropicamide, atropine, scopolamine and homatropine are frequently used to prevent posterior synechia between lens and iris. It relieves ciliary muscle spasm and associated painful eye.

PROTOZOAL INFECTIONS

Parasitic infections involving the eye are *Acanthamoeba* and *Toxoplasma gondii*. Polyhexamethylene is an antiseptic used in Acanthamoeba keratitis. Topical chlorhexidine can be used. Oral imidazoles (e.g., itraconazole, fluconazole, ketoconazole, voriconazole) are also effective. For toxoplasmosis involving eyes, systemic corticosteroids, sulfadiazine and clindamycin can be used.

GLUCOCORTICOIDS

Glucocorticoids have an important role in treating many ocular inflammatory conditions. They are used in anterior and posterior uveitis and postoperative inflammation of eye. Dexamethasone 0.1% eye drops are used in many inflammatory conditions of conjunctiva and cornea. It can be used in infective conjunctivitis to reduce edema. Also effective in treating corneal injury from chemical, radiation or thermal burns and post-operative inflammation. Fluorometholone is used in allergic conjunctivitis, keratitis, ocular burns and postoperative ocular inflammation. Prednisolone is effective in allergic conjunctivitis, corneal ulcer and endophthalmitis. Fluocinolone acetonide is used as ophthalmic implant intravitreally for Diabetic macular edema. Loteprednol etabonate ointment is used for allergic conjunctivitis. Difluprednat emulsion is used for ocular pain and postoperative ocular inflammation.

Adverse effects of topical glucocorticoids: Open angle glaucoma, posterior subcapsular cataract and risk of infection. In herpes simplex eye infection, usage of glucocorticoids may cause blindness.

Systemic corticosteroids like triamcinolone, betamethasone and dexamethasone can be used in ocular inflammation, uveitis and other conditions.

ANTIHISTAMINICS

Topical solution of levocabastine and antazoline are available for allergic conjunctivitis. Mast cell stabilizer like cromolyn sodium and nedocromil can be used. Pheniramine in combination with naphazoline (vasoconstrictor) is effective in allergic conjunctivitis. Olopatadine ophthalmic eye drops is used for allergic conjunctivitis. It relieves itching, redness, burning and watering from eyes. Side effects are headache, irritation, blurred vision and eye discomfort.

NONSTEROIDAL ANTI-INFLAMMATORY DRUGS (NSAIDS)

NSAIDs are used as solution and suspension for topical use to reduce inflammation, pain and edema. Diclofenac is used topically to reduce postoperative inflammation and pain. A combination ketorolac/ phenylephrine intraocular solution is available. Flurbiprofen can also be used.

LOCAL ANAESTHETICS

Lignocaine, tetracaine and bupivacaine are used before before operation to induce anaesthesia. They are also used to remove foreign body from eye, prior to tonometry and for infiltration anaesthesia.

IMMUNOSUPPRESSIVES AND ANTIMITOTIC DRUGS

Topical cyclosporine is approved for the treatment of chronic dry eye associated with inflammation. It increases tear production, improve vision and comfort. Lifitegrast is used topically for dry eye. 5-Fluorouracil is used to prevent subconjunctival scarring. Mitomycin is used topically in glaucoma surgery, pterygium surgery and surface ablation surgery.

Treatment of Retinal Neovascularization, Macular Degeneration

For retinal neovascularization and macular degeneration, current treatment employs agents that inhibit the actions of Vascular Endothelial Growth Factor (VEGF). Anti-VEGF agents are described in Table 82.5.

Diagnostic Dyes

Fluorescein is used to detect epithelial damage due to foreign body in the cornea. Also used to detect leakage of aqueous humour due to eye surgery or trauma. Can detect nasolacrimal duct patency. Rose

Bengal can stain devitalized tissue of the conjunctiva and cornea. Indocyanine green is used for retinal angiography.

Treatment of Dry Eye

Artificial tears or lubricants can be used, e.g., Carboxymethyl cellulose is an artificial substitute for tears.

Ophthalmic Effects of Vitamin Deficiencies

- **Vitamin A or retinal deficiency causes**:
  In anterior segment: Conjunctiva (Bitot spots, xerosis), Cornea (keratomalacia, punctate keratopathy).
  In posterior segment: Retina (night blindness), retinal pigment epithelium (hypopigmentation).
- **Vitamin B6 (pyridoxine) deficiency** causes neovascularization of cornea and atrophy of retina.
- **Vitamin B12 (cyanocobalamin) deficiency** causes visual field defects as it affects optic nerve.
- **Vitamin K deficiency** causes haemorrhage in conjunctiva and retina.

Table 82.4 Drugs causing ocular side effects

Drug	Ocular side effect
Chloroquine	Retinopathy
Ethambutol	Optic neuritis
Digoxin	Scotoma
Sildenafil	Blue colour vision defect
Glucocorticoids	Cataract
Chlorpromazine	Pigmentation of retina
Alendronate	Iritis, conjunctivitis

Table 82.5 Anti-VEGF agents for ocular use

Drug	Formulation	Use
Verteporfin	2 mg/mL reconstituted solution for intravenous infusion	Retinal neovascularization with macular degeneration
Pegaptanib	0.3 mg intravitreal injection	0.3 mg intravitreal injection
Aflibercept	2 mg/0.5 mL intravitreal injection	Same as verteporfin plus diabetic macular edema (DME), diabetic retinopathy
Bevacizumab	Intravitreal injection	Same as above
Brolucizumab	Intravitreal injection	Macular degeneration

CHAPTER 83

Treatment of Urinary Tract Infection and Sexually Transmitted Diseases (STDs)

COMPETENCY PH1.48

Urinary tract infection (UTI) is a common health problem in community and nosocomial settings. It affects bladder, urethra, kidney and ureter. UTI is one of the most common infections in females.

CLASSIFICATION OF UTI

- **Acute and chronic UTI**
  Acute urinary infection: Infection of kidney termed as upper UTI or pyelonephritis. Infection of bladder and urethra, termed as lower UTI or cysto-urethritis. *Chronic urinary infection* is characterized by weight loss, anaemia and hypertension with renal dysfunction.
- **Uncomplicated, complicated UTI and Asymptomatic bacteriuria**
  In uncomplicated UTI, infection in normal urinary tract without prior surgery or instrumentation. *In complicated UTI*, there are functional or structural abnormalities, history of urinary surgery or instrumentation with increased risk of complications. *Asymptomatic bacteriuria* is the presence of bacteria in urine culture in absence of signs and symptoms of UTI. It is common during pregnancy.

Symptoms

Burning in urination, increased frequency of urination, urgency, blood in urine, cloudy urine, pelvic pain, fever, chills, nausea and vomiting.

Pathogens

Escherichia coli, Klebsiella pneumoniae, Proteus mirabilis, Enterococcus faecalis, Staphylococcus species, etc.

Predisposing or Risk Factors of UTI

Age (older adults), obstruction due to kidney stone, enlarged prostate, cancer, prolonged urinary catheter, diabetes, pregnancy and developmental anomalies in urinary structures. UTI is common in females due to: (a) short urethra; (b) use of spermicide; (c) after menopause.

CLASSIFICATION OF DRUGS USED IN UTI

1. ***Bacteriostatic drugs***: Doxycycline, Sulfonamides, Nitrofurantoin
2. ***Bactericidal drugs***: Cotrimoxazole, Penicillin, Fluoroquinolones, Aminoglycosides, Cephalosporins, Azithromycin
3. ***Urinary antiseptics***: Nalidixic acid, Nitrofurantoin, Methenamine

Goals of Therapy

- To provide symptomatic relief.
- To eradicate infective bacteria.
- To prevent recurrence.
- To prevent predisposing factors.

Principles of Treatment

1. In acute UTI: Start single drug as early as possible to prevent complications.
2. In chronic UTI: Mixed infection is suspected with renal dysfunction.
3. Drugs to be given with adequate dose, frequency and duration.
4. Alkalization of urine (pH > 7.5) by 2 g sodium bicarbonate
5. Pregnant females may suffer from asymptomatic bacteriuria.
6. High fluid intake reduces bacterial growth in urine.

MANAGEMENT OF ACUTE LOWER UTI (CYSTO-URETHRITIS)

For acute lower UTI, tablet co-trimoxazole (2 tablets BD) and nitrofurantoin (100 mg BD) are prescribed. Alternatively, ampicillin or trimethoprim can be given for 3 days. Ciprofloxacin or norfloxacin is also effective. Longer duration (1–2 weeks) therapy is required in: (a) failure of previous treatment; (b) associated with DM, renal disease; (c) symptomatic elderly patients; (d) children.

MANAGEMENT OF CHRONIC UTI

Chronic UTI may be due to indwelling catheter or kidney stone. Chronic UTI is common in children; growth of child may be delayed and often complicated by renal failure. It is treated by norfloxacin or ofloxacin for up to 12 weeks.

RECURRENT INFECTION

Within 2 weeks of treatment, recurrence of UTI is very common. It is treated by co-trimoxazole or ciprofloxacin or amoxicillin + clavulanic acid or cefixime for 4–6 weeks.

For Prophylaxis of Recurrent Cystitis

Tab. Cotrimoxazole is used at bed time. During pregnancy, cephalexin is safer.

Nalidixic Acid

It is a first quinolone effective against Gram-negative bacteria like *E. coli, Proteus, Klebsiella* and *Shigella.* Nalidixic acid is concentrated in the urine and gut lumen, hence useful as a urinary antiseptic. It is given in uncomplicated UTI and diarrhoea due to Gram negative organism. *Adverse effects:* Neurological symptoms like drowsiness, visual problems, seizures, rash and haemolysis.

Other Measures

- Follow up for acute UTI should be up to 6 months.
- For chronic UTI, follow up may be required for up to 2 years.
- Urine culture should be repeated at 1–2-month interval, if required.
- For severe pyelonephritis, parenteral nitrofurantoin can be administered for longer period as '*Chronic suppressive therapy.*'
- In infants, cephalexin is safer.

TREATMENT OF UPPER UTI

Acute Pyelonephritis

- ***In mild upper UTI***, give ciprofloxacin 500 mg BD or co-trimoxazole or cephalosporin for10–21 days. As an alternative, amoxicillin + clavulanic acid with gentamicin can be used.
- ***In severe upper UTI*** due to Pseudomonas infection or chronic urinary obstruction, give ciprofloxacin or piperacillin or ticarcillin + tazobactam or ceftriaxone for 21 days.
- Urine and blood culture should be done before therapy.

Chronic Pyelonephritis

Chronic pyelonephritis is a severe infection often complicated by secondary hypertension or chronic renal failure. According to culture and sensitivity, drug should be started for longer period of time. If one drug is not effective, it should be replaced by more effective drug.

Urinary pH

Nitrofurantoin, tetracyclines, methicillin and cloxacillin work better in acidic urinary pH. Urinary alkalisers should not be used with them. On the other hand, cotrimoxazole, gentamicin, cephalosporins and fluoroquinolones work effectively at alkaline urinary pH. Use of urinary alkalisers with them either enhances efficacy or reduces toxicity. For nalidixic acid, chloramphenicol and ampicillin, urinary pH is immaterial.

Urinary Analgesic: Phenazopyridine

It is a dye having analgesic effects in UTI and provides symptomatic relief from burning sensation, dysuria and urgency. *Adverse effects:* Nausea, epigastric pain. Urine colour turns orange red due to its metabolites. It is used as urinary tract analgesic.

Prophylaxis of UTI

It is required in following:

- Long time catheter in bladder
- Recurrent UTI > 3 attacks
- Developmental abnormalities in urinary tract.

Give cotrimoxazole, nitrofurantoin, cephalexin and ampicillin for prophylaxis of UTI. Aseptic precautions are required before catheterization.

Antibiotic Resistance in Treatment of UTI

Urinary tract infection is often treated by broad spectrum antibiotics and the treatment is started empirically without culture and sensitivity test. The inappropriate usage of antibiotics has emerged as antibiotic resistance Worldwide. Development of multidrug resistant (MDR) bacterial strains can cause treatment failure, high morbidity and mortality. Hence, it is necessary to prescribe most appropriate antibiotics for first choice empirical treatment. For selection of antibiotic therapy, UTI treatment guidelines should be followed. Individual patient characteristics should be kept in mind to minimise antibiotic resistance by supporting antibiotic stewardship initiatives for rational prescription.

TREATMENT OF SEXUALLY TRANSMITTED DISEASES (STDS)

Sexually transmitted diseases (STDs) also known as '**Venereal diseases**' are caused by a wide range of bacteria, virus and other pathogens, transmitted via sexual contact. Major pathogens are HIV (AIDS), *Chlamydia trachomatis* (cervicitis, urethritis), *Neisseria gonorrhoeae* (gonorrhoea), *Treponema pallidum* (syphilis) and Herpes simplex virus (genital herpes). Common symptoms of STDs are unusual discharge from genitals, unusual vaginal bleeding, itching around genitals, sore on genitals, rectal or anal area, enlarged lymph nodes, rash, pain or discomfort during sexual activity, etc *(Treatment of various STDs are given in Table 83.1)*.

Drugs for HIV (Antiretroviral drugs) are described in Chapter 62.

Table 83.1 Treatment of various Sexually Transmitted Diseases

Disease	Treatment	Alternatives
Gonorrhoea		
- Uncomplicated	Ceftriaxone 250 mg single dose i.m. or Ciprofloxacin 500 mg single dose orally or cefixime 400 mg single dose orally	Levofloxacin 250 mg single dose orally or Cotrimoxazole 2 tablets BD for 5 days or Spectinomycin 2 g single dose i.m.
- Complicated	Ofloxacin 400 mg BD for 14 days with Clindamycin 450 mg QID for 14 days 100 mg BD for 14 days	Procaine penicillin 2 MU i.m. for 10 days with doxycycline
Syphilis	Procaine penicillin 6 L units daily i.m. for 10 days or Benzathine penicillin 2.4 MU single dose i.m.	Erythromycin 500 mg QID for 15 days or Doxycycline 100 mg BD for 15 days
Chancroid	Azithromycin 1 g single dose orally or Erythromycin 500 mg QID for 7–10 days or Ceftriaxone 250 mg i.m. single dose	Cotrimoxazole 2 tablets BD for 7 days or Ciprofloxacin 500 mg BD for 3 days
Granuloma inguinale	Azithromycin 1 g once a week for 4 wks or Doxycycline 100 mg BD for 3–4 wks	Cotrimoxazole 2 tablets BD for 3–4 weeks
Lymphogranu-loma venereum	Azithromycin 1 g single dose orally or Doxycycline 100mg BD orally for 21 days	Tetracycline 500 mg QID for 21 days
Chlamydial urethritis/ Cervicitis	Doxycycline 100 mg BD or a single dose of azithromycin 500 mg for 7 days	Ofloxacin 400 mg BD or Levofloxacin 500 mg OD for 7 days
Acute epididymitis	A single injection of ceftriaxone (250 mg) plus doxycycline 100 mg BD for 10 days.	Cotrimoxazole 2 tablets BD or Ciprofloxacin can be used
Trichomoniasis	Metronidazole 2 g single dose orally	Secnidazole 2 g single dose orally

CHAPTER 84

Dietary Supplements & Nutraceuticals

COMPETENCY PH1.61

Changes in lifestyle since last few decades influenced paradigm due to high stress level, eating habits and work pattern. It leads to many lifestyle diseases like obesity, hypertension, diabetes mellitus and ischaemic heart disease (IHD). The demand for dietary supplements and nutraceuticals has increased and they are being used by people for various therapeutic outcomes.

DIETARY SUPPLEMENTS

Dietary supplements are usually used to improve and maintain overall health of patient. They are marketed as tablet, capsule, powder and liquid. Various dietary supplements are vitamins, minerals, amino acids and enzymes, components of multivitamin tablets. Regulation of dietary supplements is under the Dietary Supplement Health and Education Act of 1994 (DSHEA) and Food and Drug Administration (FDA). It deals with prohibition of misbranded or adulterated product manufacturing and marketing. DSHEA and FDA have authority to take strict action against manufacturer of these products.

NUTRACEUTICALS

The term '**Nutraceutical**' was coined by Stephen DeFelice in 1989, Founder and Chairman of the 'Foundation for Innovation in Medicine.' He described nutraceutical as a food (or part of a food) that provides medical or health benefits including the prevention and/or treatment of a disease. Nutraceuticals also termed as '**superfood**' or '**bioceuticals**.' Differences between Pharmaceutical and Nutraceutical are given in Table 84.1.

Various Nutraceuticals

Various substances used as nutraceuticals are natural and can be categorized like Dietary fibres, Probiotics, Polyunsaturated fatty acids, Antioxidant vitamin, minerals and polyphenols. Various sources and beneficial effects of nutraceuticals are given in Table 84.2.

Dietary Fibres

Dietary fibres are composed of lignins and non-digestible carbohydrates present in intrinsic and intact plants. They are used to relieve constipation and soluble dietary fibres delay gastric emptying. Dietary fibres prevent breast cancer and also inhibit reabsorption of bile acid.

Probiotics

Probiotics are ingestion of live helpful bacteria like *Lactobacillus*, the most common probiotic. *Bifidobacterium* is helpful to relieve diarrhoea and reduces symptoms of Inflammatory Bowel Disease (IBD), Irritable Bowel Syndrome (IBS), etc.

Table 84.1 Differences between Pharmaceutical and Nutraceutical

Pharmaceutical	Nutraceutical
Pharmaceutical is referred as a drug	Nutraceutical is a health product
Used as prophylaxis and treatment of diseases	Nutraceutical is used for prophylaxis of diseases
Prescription is mandatory for pharmaceutical (except OTC drugs)	Prescription is not mandatory for nutraceuticals
Requires licence for regulatory authorities	For marketing, licence is not mandatory

Table 84.2 Various sources and beneficial effects of nutraceuticals

Nutraceutical	Sources	Beneficial effects
Carotenoids		
Lycopene	Guava, papaya, watermelon, tomato	Reduces cholesterol levels, antioxidant, protects against cancer
β-Carotene	Vegetables, fruits, oats, carrots	Antioxidant
Lutein	Spinach, corn, avocado, egg yolk	Anticancer, protects eyes against muscular degenerations, cataracts
Tocotrienol	Palm oil, different grains	Improves cardiovascular health, prevents, breast cancer
Saponins	Beans like soya beans, chickpeas	Effective in colon cancer, reduces cholesterol level
Phytoestrogens		
Isoflavones	Legumes, beans like soya beans	Antioxidant, lowers LDL cholesterol
Lignans	Vegetables, rye	Prevents colon and breast cancer
Dietary fibre		
Soluble fibre	Beans like legumes, cereals like oats, barley	Maintain healthy digestive tract and have anticancer activity
Insoluble fibre	Whole grain foods wheat and corn	Maintains healthy digestive tract and have anticancer activity
Fatty acids		
Omega 3 fatty acids	Present in salmon and flax seed	Anti-inflammatory, maintains brain function
Monosaturated fatty acids	Present in tree nuts	Reduces the risk of coronary heart disease
Probiotics	Lactobacilli, bifidobacteriae present in yogurt	Production of bacteriocins and organic acids, modulation of immune response, inhibits colonization of pathogens

Polyunsaturated Fatty Acids (PUFAs)

They are divided into two groups: omega-3 (ω-3) and omega-6 (ω-6) polyunsaturated fatty acids (PUFAs). The major ω-3 fatty acids (FA) are α-linoleic acid (ALA), eicosapentaenoic acid (EPA) and docosahexaenoic acid (DHA). The sources of these FA are various fatty fishes or fish oil like herring, salmon, mackerel and tuna.

Various clinical trials show benefits of fish oil and PUFA. They can reduce lipid level (LDL-Ch), reduce risk of sudden cardiac death and coronary artery disease (CAD). They also have antiarrhythmic and antithrombotic properties.

Dietary Antioxidants

Dietary antioxidants are available as nutraceutical. Examples: Beta carotene, carotenoids, lycopene, lutein, flavones, flavonoids and polyphenols. Other antioxidants are vitamin C (ascorbic acid), vitamin E, tocopherols, lipoic acid and glutathione.

Coenzyme Q10

Coenzyme Q10 (CoQ10) is an antioxidant, which inhibits generation of free radicals and prevents damage to lipids, proteins and DNA. It is commonly used as a purified dietary supplement. It is prescribed in various diseases like heart failure, hypertension and statin induced myopathy. CoQ10 can be used to boost immunity, increase energy level and to relieve fatigue. Some studies found that it delays progression of degenerative diseases like Alzheimer's disease and Parkinson's disease. It is also beneficial in muscle pains, myopathies, ischaemic heart disease, hypertension, heart failure and radiation injury. The oral tablet is well tolerated and can cause side effects like nausea, diarrhoea, anorexia and heart burn.

Several Antioxidant Enzymes

Several antioxidant enzymes are also used and a component of multivitamin tablets. Examples: Glutathione peroxidase, glutathione reductase and superoxide dismutase which are scavengers for many oxidants or free radicals.

Metal Binding Proteins

Metal binding proteins are albumin, ceruloplasmin and ferritin which sequester free form of metals like iron and copper which can participate in oxidative reactions.

Glucosamine Sulfate and Chondroitin Sulfate

Glucosamine and chondroitin are natural compounds found in healthy cartilage. Supplements are available as glucosamine sulfate and glucosamine hydrochloride. In osteoarthritis, they have anti-inflammatory and cartilage protecting effects.

Prebiotics

Prebiotics are non-digestible substances which stimulates the growth of intestinal flora and thereby prevent growth of pathogenic micro-organism. Examples are raw oats, wheat, soyabeans, barley, lactulose and unrefined sugars. These prebiotics facilitate the growth and survival of probiotic flora. These are non-digestible substances. Combination of prebiotics and probiotics are called as ***Synbiotics***.

Flavones (Polyphenols)

Flavones (Polyphenols) are a large family of naturally occurring organic compounds characterized by multiples of phenol units. They are structurally diverse and abundant in fruits, vegetables, cereals and plant beverages. Various beneficial effects of phenols are studied. They protect cells from photosynthetic stress and reactive oxygen species (ROS). The most important polyphenols are flavones, flavonoids and phenolic acids.

Dietary polyphenols have various beneficial properties like antioxidant, anti-inflammatory, antiatherogenic and anticarcinogenic. These are used for protection in various CVS diseases like hypertension, coronary artery diseases, etc. They are also beneficial in diabetes mellitus, Parkinson's disease, Alzheimer's disease and cancer.

Curcumin, a polyphenol found in turmeric. It is commonly used in Indian cooking. It has beneficial properties like antioxidant, anti-inflammatory and anticarcinogenic. It inhibits lipid peroxidation and has free radial scavenging effects. It also suppresses various pro-inflammatory ILs, cytokines, PGs and TNFα.

Red wine also has polyphenol compounds and can reduce the incidence of coronary artery disease. The proposed mechanism is that red wine reduces the synthesis of endothelin-1 (ET-1) which is responsible for atherogenesis in artery.

Tea, an aromatic beverage is a rich source of polyphenols and amino acids. Polyphenols include flavonoids, epigallocatechin gallate (EGCG) and other catechins. It has beneficial effects when consumed as black tea or green tea. It can prevent various cancers of skin, esophagus, pancreas, stomach, colon, breast and lungs.

Diacerein also known as diacetylrhein, is a slow-acting medicine of the class anthraquinone. It has chondroprotective effect due to inhibition of synthesis of cytokines IL-1. It decreases breakdown of collagen and stimulates proliferation of chondrocyte. It also inhibits generation of superoxide, phagocytic action of neutrophils and chemotaxis. It prevents development of degenerative joint diseases such as osteoarthritis. It is well tolerated orally and can cause side effects like diarrhoea, allergic reaction, rash and hepatobiliary dysfunction.

Micronutrients like vitamins and minerals are discussed in Chapter 50 and Chapter 75, respectively.

Alzheimer's Disease

Alzheimer is a neurodegenerative disease which affects millions of patients all over the World. β-Carotene, lycopene, curcumin and lutein are useful in the management of Alzheimer's disease. They have anti-oxidant property, reduce oxidative stress and mitochondrial dysfunction.

Cancer

Lycopene and *carotenoids* prevent different cancers including prostate cancer. Plant extracts rich in isoflavones, tannins, biochanin and derivatives like curcumin have remarkable potency against many cancers. *Flax seeds* have beneficial role in reducing risk of colon and rectal cancer.

Currently, a wide range of nutraceutical products are marketed successfully. The regulatory authority for the manufacturing, distribution, storage, import of nutraceuticals is '***Food Safety and Security Act***' *and* '***Food Safety and Standards Authority of India (FSSAI)***.' Future research and development of nutraceutical products are essential for better health outcome and to fight against deadly diseases.

CHAPTER 85 Herbal Medicines

COMPETENCY PH1.59

Herbal medicines are medicinal plant preparations which include '***traditional medicines***', explained in classical Indian literature like Rigveda, Charak Samhita and Sushruta. Herbal medicine contains active ingredients made from whole plant or leaves, roots or flowers. Herbal medicines have effects on body systems and should be taken with same caution like conventional medicines.

The clinical trial and safety data of herbal medicines are of great concern as:

1. During manufacturing process of herbal medicines, there is no well-defined purification steps.
2. Variation in quality among different brands.
3. Herb–drug interaction is common, if modern medicines are taken with self-medication of herbal drugs.
4. Some of them add lead, arsenic or mercury like harmful substances can cause renal and hepatic dysfunction.
5. When medicinal plants are not properly stored, fungus like *Aspergillus flavus* can grow and it produces a mycotoxin (aflatoxin).

Herbal medicines are available in various routes and dosage forms. Various oral dosage forms are tablets, capsules, syrups, drops and elixirs. Topical preparations are also available as creams, gels and ointments. They can be combined with allopathic drugs in topical dosage forms.

St. John's Wort or *Hypericum perforatum*

St. John wort is a flowering plant contains flavonoids, phenolic acid, etc. Mechanism of action is inhibition of reuptake of serotonin, noradrenaline and dopamine in presynaptic membrane. It can be used in depression, anxiety and premenstrual disorders. *Adverse effects*: Sedation, headache, fatigue and dry mouth.

Ginseng

It is derived from *Panax ginseng* having various effects like immunomodulatory, anti-inflammatory, antioxidant, analgesic, improves physical and mental health. It can be used in common cold, prophylaxis of cancer and diabetes mellitus. *Adverse effects*: Vaginal bleeding, insomnia and hypertension.

Ginko

Ginko biloba is obtained from Ginko tree. It causes vasodilation and increases blood flow. It has antioxidant and radical scavenging property. It can be used in dementia.

Garlic (*Allium sativum*)

Allicin is a content in raw garlic while *organosulfur* compound is present in aged garlic. Various properties of garlic are lipid lowering effect via inhibition of HMG-CoA reductase, antiplatelet, anticancer and antioxidant.

Amalaki

Amalaki powder is made from the dried fruits of Amalaki. It is used in hyperacidity, gastritis, non-ulcer dyspepsia and duodenal ulcer. Clinical evidence suggests that it is safe without adverse effect.

Trikatu

Trikatu powder consists of three commonly used herbal drugs in equal quantity namely dry ginger (Shunthi), black pepper (Maricha) and long pepper (Pippali). It has anti-inflammatory, analgesic and expectorant properties. *Uses*: Cough, cold, rhinitis and bronchial asthma.

Haritaki

Haritaki powder is a simple formulation made of dried ripe fruits. It has laxative, digestive and antispasmodic properties. Haritaki is useful in constipation, haemorrhoids and hyperacidity.

Daruharidra (*Berberis aristate*)

Daruharidra has anti-inflammatory, antimicrobial, antidiarrhoeal properties. It is used in conjunctivitis, trachoma and chronic eye inflammation.

Pippali

Pippali powder has properties like anti-inflammatory, decongestant, expectorant and anti-allergic. *Uses*:

Common cold, cough, pharyngitis, laryngitis and bronchitis. It is considered safe in recommended doses.

Shirisha

Shirisha bark has anti-histaminic, anti-allergic, antifungal and anti-bacterial properties. The bark is useful in allergic and chronic skin diseases like eczema.

Triphala Decoction

Triphala decoction is mainly used for washing inflamed eyes in conjunctivitis. It has decongestant, anti-inflammatory and soothing effects on eyes.

Karanja

Karanja has anthelmintic, insecticidal, anti-bacterial and anti-fungal properties. It is indicated for skin diseases such as ringworm, scabies, eczema, urticaria, leucoderma, herpes and impetigo.

Pippali Moola

The roots of Pippali have thermogenic, tonic, expectorant, anti-bacterial, anti-inflammatory properties. It is used in headache, insomnia, cough, cold and chronic bronchitis.

Katuka

Katuka is a bitter tonic with carminative, digestive, hepato-protective and anti-spasmodic properties. It is useful in flatulence, jaundice and liver dysfunctions.

Ashwagandha Powder

Ashwagandha is one of the most commonly used medicinal plants in Indian medicine for a varied range of physical and psychological ailments. It acts as tonic, anti-stress, simulant, aphrodisiac, immuno-modulatory and antioxidant. It is used to relieve weakness, malaise, impotence and mental stress.

Shatpushpa

It has anti-spasmodic, carminative and anti-flatulent properties. Various reports are published regarding its efficacy in painful menstruation.

Surana

Surana has carminative, appetizing, digestive and analgesic properties. It can be used in abdominal pain, constipation, piles and liver disorders.

Gandhaka Ointment

Gandhaka ointment is an effective preparation made from Gandhaka (sulphur) and Tila oil (sesame oil). It has bactericidal and fungicidal properties. It can be used in infections of skin, scabies and eczema.

Kapikacchu

It has aphrodisiac and anti-inflammatory properties. It can be used in sexual disorders like oligospermia, loss of libido, erectile dysfunctions and premature ejaculation.

Lavanga

Lavanga is the dried flower bud of *Syzygium aromaticum*. Clove oil has analgesic, anaesthetic, antiseptic, digestive and carminative properties. *Uses*: Toothache, dental caries and painful condition after tooth extraction.

Gokshura (*Tribulus terrestris*)

Gokshura has anti-urolithiatic, muscle relaxant and anti-inflammatory properties. *Uses*: Burning urination, difficulty in urination and urinary stones.

Ela

Ela (Cardamom) is one of the common spices used in almost every Indian kitchen. Therapeutic properties are anti-emetic, carminative, digestive and as appetizer.

Haridra (*Curcuma longa*)

Haridra is a widely used as medicinal plant in India. It is known for its wound healing effects. It has anti-inflammatory, anti-allergic and antiseptic properties. Commonly used externally in acute and chronic wounds.

Oscimum sanctum (Tulsi)

Oscimum sanctum is recommended for the treatment of cough, bronchitis, bronchial asthma, diarrhoea, skin diseases, arthritis, painful eye diseases etc. Tulsi has various properties like antioxidant, anti-inflammatory, antimicrobial, anticancer, cardio-protective and analgesic effect. Eugenol is the active constituent in *Ocimum sanctum*.

Azadirachta indica (Neem)

Neem plant is extensively used in Ayurvedic System of Medicine for various disorders. Neem is a herb having properties like anti-fungal, anti-bacterial, anti-diabetic, antiviral and anti-helminthic. It can be used in skin disorders, wounds, ulcer, loss of appetite and diabetes mellitus.

Aloe Vera

Aloe is a plant that usually grows in hot and dry climates. It has anti-inflammatory activity due to polyphenols, a group of antioxidant-rich compounds. It can be used for various skin conditions including psoriasis, minor burns, skin abrasions and acne. It reduces wrinkles on skin. Aloe vera helps to lower blood glucose and cholesterol level.

Most of the herbal medicines are manufactured in combination preparations. Multi-ingredient of Ayurveda, Unani and Siddha including herbal medicines form a compounded medicament. *Chyawanprash* is an ayurvedic product which contains ashwagandha, pipli, cardamom, Cinnamon, vasaka etc. with honey, sugar , ghee or butter oil and added flavour for good taste compatibility. It is marketed to boost immunity, decrease fatigue, to maintain vitality, functions of lungs, and overall health of body.

REGULATORY BODIES FOR HERBAL DRUGS

In India, Herbal Medicines are regulated by the *Ministry of Ayurveda, Yoga and Naturopathy, Unani, Siddha and Homoeopathy (AYUSH)*. Regulatory provisions are laid down in Drugs and Cosmetics (D & C) Act 1940 and Rules 1945.The D&C Act extends the control over licensing, formulation composition, manufacture, labelling, packing, quality and export. Schedule T described good manufacturing practices for Ayurvedic, Siddha and Yunani which include herbal medications. The ***National Medicinal Plant Board of India (NMPB)*** and the ***Quality Council of Indla (QCI)*** are important which regulate the quality, safety and efficacy of the herbal medicine.

Good Manufacturing Practices (GMPs) should be employed to ensure that raw material used in drugs are of good quality and free from contamination. Adequate quality control measures are adopted.

CHAPTER 86

Enzymes in Therapy

Enzymes are chemical catalysts of biological systems. Enzymes are involved to accelerate the targeted biochemical modifications. They catalyse many stepwise metabolic reactions and generating macromolecules from their precursors. The active enzymatic activity depends on their specific protein structure or confirmation. Hence the activity of one or more enzymes is impaired due to mutation in structural components. The enzyme-based drugs should have following criteria: Half-life of drug should be long, actions of the enzymes should be targeted and accurate and lack of immune response.

CLASSIFICATION OF ENZYMES USED AS THERAPY

1. ***Mammalian enzymes***: Hyaluronidase, chymotrypsin, alpha chymotrypsin, trypsin, dornase.
2. ***Bacterial enzymes***: Streptokinase, streptodornase, collagenase, serratopeptidase, L-asparaginase.
3. ***Plant enzyme***: Papain.

Collagenase

Collagenase is a matrix metalloproteinase enzyme which breaks peptide bonds in collagen. Collagenase is obtained from *Clostridium histolyticum* and approved by US-FDA, as a novel nonsurgical treatment for *Dupuytren's contracture*. It provides a safer and effective alternative to surgery with quick recovery. It can be used in debridement of dermal ulcers and burns. It also promotes growth of granulation tissue.

Pancreatic Enzymes

Trypsin

It is obtained from bovine pancreas. It is a proteolytic enzyme, which hydrolyses proteins. It is given in various routes like oral, sublingual and topical.

Uses:

1. Topically used for debridement of necrotic tissues, as it digests bacteria and dead tissue.
2. To irrigate nasal cavity.
3. For deep contusions, thrombophlebitis.
4. Topically effective to liquify coagulated blood and exudates.

Chymotrypsin

It is obtained from bovine pancreas. It can be used in abscess, ulcers to reduce postoperative edema and inflammation. Chymotrypsin is also used for tooth impaction and after tooth extraction. *Adverse effects*: Rare but can cause diarrhoea, itching, shortness of breath and allergic reactions like rash.

Alpha chymotrypsin

It is like chymotrypsin having proteolytic property. It is used during cataract surgery to dissolve the suspensory ligament of lens which helps to remove the lens.

Insufficiency of ***pancreatic enzymes*** leads to indigestion and inadequate absorption of fat leading to steatorrhoea. Pancreatic dysfunction due to pancreatitis, pancreatic cancer can be treated by pancreatic enzyme replacement. Currently used pancreatic enzyme supplements are combination of lipase, protease and amylase, known as **pancreatin**.

Lipases

They are enzymes which catalyse the hydrolysis of lipids like phospholipids and triacylglycerol. Lipases are a part of oral pancreatic enzyme preparations.

Hyaluronidase

Hyaluronidase causes hydrolysis of hyaluronic acid, lowers the viscosity and increases tissue permeability. Given subcutaneously.

Uses:

1. For retrobulbar and peribulbar block along with local anaesthetic.
2. To facilitate penetration of anticancer agents to reach malignant cells.

Asparaginase

Asparaginase is an anticancer drug. In the presence of asparaginase, neoplastic cells are unable to produce sufficient asparagine for protein synthesis leads to cell death during G1 phase of cell cycle. It is used for the treatment of acute lymphoblastic leukaemia (ALL).

L-Glutaminase

L-Glutaminase is an amidohydrolase enzyme, which hydrolyses L-glutamine into glutamate and ammonia. Various cancer cells like lymphatic tumour cells, require high amount of L-glutamine for rapid growth. So, use of L-glutaminase deprives the tumour cells from L-glutamine and causes selective death of lymphatic tumour cells.

DNA and RNA Enzymes

DNA and RNA enzymes can be used to block the expression of specific genes in cells. These enzymes can cleave DNA or RNA, which inactivate abnormal gene expression.

Dornase-alfa: It is a recombinant human deoxyribonuclease (DNAase). It is an enzyme which breaks accumulated DNA of sputum and reduces the viscosity. It is used in cystic fibrosis. RNA-based therapeutics are investigated for diseases like HIV, hepatitis B and cancer.

Fibrinolytics

Streptokinase is obtained from culture of β-haemolytic streptococci having fibrinolytic action by indirectly activating the circulatory plasminogen. *Urokinase* is an enzyme obtained from human urine. *Alteplase* is tissue type plasminogen activator (tPA). It is non-antigenic, non-pyrogenic, rapid acting and more potent.

Fibrinolytics are used in ST elevation myocardial infarction (STEMI), deep vein thrombosis, pulmonary embolism and acute thrombotic or ischaemic stroke. *Adverse effects*: Bleeding, allergic reactions like fever, chills, skin rash, hypotension, anaphylactoid reaction, etc. Alteplase causes less bleeding and allergic reactions.

Serratiopeptidase

It is a proteolytic enzyme obtained from the *Serratia* species. It is effective orally and prescribed widely to relieve inflammatory edema of soft tissue. It has anti-inflammatory and analgesic effects. The proposed mechanism is digestion of the necrotic tissue, exudates and clots which are cleared faster from the site of injury or inflammation. Serratiopeptidase can be tried in different conditions like osteoarthritis, rheumatoid arthritis, ankylosing spondylitis and fracture. Other conditions are bronchitis, pulmonary tuberculosis, traumatic injury, following dental surgery, etc.

Lysosomal Hydrolases

Deficiency of lysosomal hydrolases enzyme causes lysosomal storage diseases (LSDs). It leads to dysfunction of intracellular turnover, degradation of a variety of substrates present in lysosomes. Enzyme replacement therapy is approved for various lysosomal storage diseases (LSDs).

Papain

Papain, also known as **papaya proteinase I** found in species of papaya, *Carica papaya*. The enzyme is found on the skin of papaya. It is known for its anti-inflammatory properties. It also acts as a digestive enzyme. It can be used as a digestive aid and for inflammation of throat, pharynx and running nose. It can be directly applied on skin to treat infected wounds and ulcers.

CHAPTER 87 Vaccines and Antisera

COMPETENCY PH1.54

VACCINES

Vaccines are biological agents that elicit an immune response against a disease-producing specific pathogen. Edward Jenner developed first vaccine against smallpox in 1796. Vaccines prevent the spread of several diseases like polio. The administration of vaccine is termed as **vaccination**; it is one of the most effective methods for the prevention of infectious diseases.

ANTISERA

Antisera is a blood serum containing monoclonal or polyclonal antibodies and provides passive immunity against specified micro organism. Source of antibody is mainly sera of actively immunised horse against micro organism. The most common use of antiserum in human is as antitoxin or antivenom also termed as '**serotherapy**.' When preformed antibodies are given, they trigger immune system against specific antigen. Examples: Tetanus antitoxin, diphtheria antitoxin. *Adverse effects*: Immediate type of allergic reactions, Serum sickness, urticaria, rash, fever, joint pain and anaphylaxis.

IMMUNOGLOBULINS

Immunoglobulins obtained from human plasma were first used in 1952 to treat primary immune deficiency. Intravenous immunoglobulin (IVIG) contains the pooled immunoglobulin G (IgG) immunoglobulins from the plasma of approximately a thousand or more blood donors. Nonspecific (normal) and specific (hyperimmune) immunoglobulins against specific antigen are obtained. These are more efficacious than antisera and less or no risk of allergic reactions. Examples: Normal human gamma globulin (viral hepatitis A and B, measles, mumps), tetanus Ig, rabies Ig, hepatitis B Ig and anti-diphtheria Ig. *Adverse effects:* Allergic reactions, nausea, vomiting, chills, fever, flushing, muscle pain and joint pain (Table 87.1).

HERD IMMUNITY

Herd immunity describes a state of immunity when a significant number of population become immune to an infectious agent. The percentage of immune population may differ and it is not always possible. Once herd immunity is reached, disease incidence or virulence is gradually reduced. Herd immunity develops either with mass vaccination or mass infection. Hence, it takes longer time to develop herd immunity.

Table 87.1 Differences between active and passive immunity

Active immunity	Passive immunity
Active immunity refers to immunity due to production of antibodies by person's own immune system	Passive immunity refers due to direct administration of antibodies.
Pathogen in direct contact with body cells	Pathogen does not have direct contact
Immunity lasts for long time	Immunity does not last for long time
Less adverse effects like allergy	More risk of allergy
Not given in immunocompromised people	Can be given to immunocompromised people

IMMUNISATION

Primary immunisation gives primary immunity to children like first dose of DPT is administered to infant. Secondary immunisation includes administration of booster dose to induce immunity.

CLASSIFICATION OF VACCINES (Table 87.2)

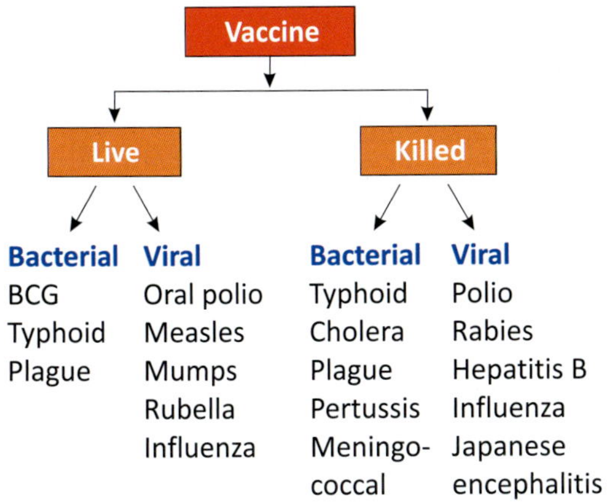

Fig 87.1 Classification of vaccines

TYPES OF VACCINES

Live attenuated vaccine	Killed vaccine
Consist of live bacteria or viruses.	Microorganisms are killed by heat or chemicals.
More efficacious	Less efficacious
Long lasting immunity	Short lasting immunity

Toxoid Vaccines

Bacteria produce toxins or harmful chemicals. Toxoid vaccines are used when a bacterial toxin is main cause of disease. Bacterial exotoxins are modified to reduce toxicity but retain it antigenic property as toxin. To neutralize these toxins, various toxoid vaccines are available like against diphtheria and tetanus (Table 87.3).

Subunit, Recombinant Vaccines

Subunit vaccines are manufactured by the isolation of specific antigens from virus or bacteria to strengthen immune response. Recombinant vaccines are made through genetic engineering. The gene carries protein for virus or bacteria is identified, isolated and placed inside another cell. When that cell multiplies, it produces vaccine proteins to induce immune response.

Site of Vaccine

Intramuscular vaccine is given at anterolateral side of thigh or deltoid. Subcutaneous or intradermal vaccine is given in left upper arm or anterolateral aspect of thigh.

Other Vaccines

Fractional dose inactivated polio vaccination (fIPV): Intradermal (ID) administration of a fractional dose of IPV (fIPV) is safe, effective and immunogenic. fIPV can benefit children previously vaccinated for polio and zero-dose children. For children who have previously received oral polio vaccine (OPV), fIPV will help to "boost" their immunity. fIPV may be used for VDPV2 outbreak or event response in settings where immunity is already high. It is administered via intradermal injection 0.1 mL.

JAPANESE ENCEPHALITIS VACCINES AVAILABLE IN INDIA

a) Live-attenuated, cell culture-derived SA 14-14-2
b) Inactivated SA 14-14-2 vaccine
c) Inactivated Vero cell culture-derived Kolar strain, 821564XY, JE vaccine (JENVAC® by Bharat Biotech).

a) **Live-Attenuated Cell Culture-Derived SA 14-14-2 Vaccine**: *Japanese encephalitis virus (JEV)* is a mosquito borne disease. The most commonly used vaccine used to prevent JE is the live-attenuated strain SA14-14-2, which was generated by serial passage of the wild-type (WT) JEV strain SA14. It is a live, attenuated vaccine. In India, JE prevalent areas can receive this vaccine. Usually, two dose administered s.c. at 9–12 months and 16–24 months of age. Common adverse effects are transient fever, rash, local pain and irritability.
b) **Inactivated SA 14-14-2 vaccine**: This is an inactivated vaccine (JE-VC) derived from the attenu-

ated SA 14-14-2 JEV strain propagated in Vero cell. It can be used in travellers with an increased risk for JE on the basis of planned travel duration, season and location. Two doses 4 weeks apart will be given for all age groups (2 months to 65 years). *Dose*: <3 years – 0.25 mL, >3 years – 0.5 mL.

c) **Kolar 821564XY strain inactivated JE vaccine (JENVAC)**: JENVAC is a Vero cell culture derived, inactivated, Kolar strain, vaccine developed by Bharat Biotech International Ltd. JENVAC (5 μg/0.5 mL/dose) was administered intramuscularly on day 0 and day 28. Efficacy is up to 90%.

d) **Live-Attenuated Recombinant SA 14-14-2 Chimeric Vaccine**: A promising new genetic approach is adopted; this novel, live, recombinant vaccine, is a safe, highly immunogenic and capable of inducing long-lasting immunity. The clinical development of this vaccine is under clinical trial.

VACCINE FOR CERVICAL CANCER

Human Papillomavirus (HPV) is a virus which can cause cancers later in life. HPV infections can cause cancers of the cervix, vagina and vulva in women and penis in men. The US-FDA has approved vaccine for Human Papillomavirus (HPV). A first dose of HPV vaccination is recommended for 11- and 12-year-old girls. It can be given to 13–26 years of girls and women who have not yet vaccinated. Routine vaccination is also effective for males 9–26 years of age. Two doses are recommended, given 0.5 mL intramuscularly. *Adverse effects*: Fever, dizziness, nausea, fainting and allergy.

VACCINES FOR COVID-19

Coronaviruses are a large group of viruses which can infect animals as well as humans. Recently faced global pandemic of novel **coronavirus disease 2019 (COVID-19)** is caused by **severe acute respiratory syndrome coronavirus 2 (SARS-CoV-2)**. Vaccination probably the best option for the prevention of COVID-19 infection. Vaccine-induced humoral immune responses, especially involving the production of neutralizing antibodies are crucial to prevent infection and reinfection. Current COVID-19 vaccines continue to provide strong protection against severe disease and death. Booster dose of vaccines is essential to sustain immunity against COVID-19. Some COVID-19 vaccines are in *WHO emergency use listing* (Table 87.4).

iNCOVACC (SARS-CoV-S COVID-19 Vaccine)

iNCOVACC (recombinant) is a recently approved nasal vaccine developed by Bharat Biotech International Limited (BBIL) indicated for active immunization against SARS-CoV-2 virus infection in adults. iNCOVACC is an Adenoviral vector-based (expressing a stabilized spike protein) SARS-CoV-2 vaccine for nasal administration only. Phase 1, 2 and 3 clinical studies for safety and immunogenicity found that the vaccine is safe and immunogenic. The vaccine shown satisfactory immune response against several variants of SARS-CoV-2. Cell mediated immune response, both T and B cell phenotype distribution is evaluated against SARS-CoV-2 variants and found that the response is persistent across these variants. iNCOVACC vaccination course consists of two separate doses of 0.5 mL (8 drops, 4 drops in each nostril). The second dose should be administered after 28 days (4 weeks from the first dose). Once opened, Multi-dose vial should be used within 6 hrs and stored at 2–8°C between administrations. Post 6 hrs after opening, the vial should be discarded. *Contraindication*: Hypersensitivity to any constituents of the vaccine. Administration of iNCOVACC should be postponed in individuals suffering from an acute severe febrile illness/acute infection. Some *side effects* include headache, fever, running nose, sneezing and sore throat. Currently, data are not available for the use of iNCOVACC in paediatric population.

Table 87.2 Vaccine, types and recommended schedules

Vaccines	Type	Dose and route	Primary immunisation	Booster	Indication
BCG	Live-attenuated	0.1 mL (0.05 mL until 1 mo of age) SC, ID	At birth	7 and 14 yrs	Childhood tuberculosis
Diphtheria	Toxoid	0.5 mL IM	6, 10, 14 weeks of age	18 months and 4–6 yrs	Diphtheria
Pertussis	Inactivated	0.5 mL IM	6, 10, 14 weeks of age	18 months & 4–6 yrs	Pertussis
Tetanus	Toxoid	0.5 mL IM	6, 10, 14 weeks of age	18 months & 4–6 yrs	Tetanus
Typhoid & paratyphoid	Inactivated	0.5 mL SC	>3 yrs at any age, 2 doses 4 weeks apart	Every 3 yrs	Childhood typhoid and paratyphoid fever
Typhoid conjugated vaccine	Conjugate	0.5 mL IM	Single dose	–	Childhood typhoid fever
Typhoral	Live-attenuated	Oral capsules	>6 yrs at any age, 1 capsules alternate day (total 3) 1 hr before food	Every 3 yrs	Childhood typhoid fever
Plague	Inactivated	IM	Single dose	–	In Plague epidemic and persons at risk
Pneumo-coccal	Bacterial polysaccha ride	IM	Single dose	-	Pneumococcal infections
Haemo-philus influenza (type B)	Bacterial polysaccha-ride	SC	Single dose	–	*H. influenza* infections
Meningo-coccal	Bacterial polysaccha-ride	SC	Single dose	–	Prevents outbreak, among travellers in epidemic
Oral polio vaccine	Live (Salk type)	Oral 2 drops	6, 10, 14 weeks	18 months, 4–6 yrs	Poliomyelitis
Injectable polio vaccine	Killed (Salk type)	0.5 mL IM	14 weeks	–	Poliomyelitis

contd.

Vaccines	Type	Dose and route	Primary immunisation	Booster	Indication
Hepatitis A	Inactivated	IM	2–4 weeks before travelling, 2 doses	After 6–12 months	To prevent Hepatitis A in occupational risk, homosexual
Hepatitis B	Inactivated	0.5 mL IM	At birth, 6, 10, 14 weeks	After 5 yrs	To all children, post-exposure prophylaxis
Measles	Live	0.5 mL SC	9 months	16–24 mo	Measles
Rubella	Live	0.5 mL SC	9 months	16–24 mo	Rubella
Rabies	Inactivated	1 mL IM or ID	Pre-exposure: 3 doses, 0, 7, 21 days. Post-exposure: 6 doses, 0, 3, 7, 4, 30, 90	After 1 yr then 2–5 yrs	Pre- and post-exposure prophylaxis of rabies
Influenza (Type A, B, H1N1)	Inactivated	0.5 mL IM	Single dose	Yearly	To prevent meningitis in high-risk persons like pregnancy, asthma, elderly
Yellow fever	Live	0.5 mL SC	Single dose	Every 10 yrs	Travelling to yellow fever prevalent regions
Varicella	Live	0.5 mL SC	2 doses, 4–8 weeks apart at 18 months	–	All children above 18 months to prevent Varicella infection
Rotavirus	Live	5 drops oral	3 doses, 6, 10, 14 weeks	–	Protection against rotavirus diarrhoea
Japanese encephalitis	Live	0.5 mL SC	9 months	16–24 months	High-risk persons
Herpes zoster	Live	0.5 mL SC	1 dose	–	Herpes zoster
Human papilloma virus	Capsid protein	0.5 mL IM	3 doses, 0, 2, 6 months	–	Females 9–26 yrs
Pentavalent vaccine (DPT, Hepatitis B, HiB)	–	0.5 mL IM	6, 10, 14 weeks	–	All children

Table 87.3 Passive immunisation

	Indications	Source	Dose	Route
Immunoglobulins				
Tetanus immunoglobulin	Tetanus and post-exposure prophylaxis in persons not immunised previously	Human	Prophylaxis: 2500 IU; Treatment: 3000–6000 IU	IM
Rabies immunoglobulin	Combined with rabies vaccine for post exposure prophylaxis	Human	20 IU/kg	Half dose given around wound and other half IM
Hepatitis B immunoglobulin	Along with hepatitis B vaccine, post exposure prophylaxis	Immuno-globulin	0.06 mL/kg	IM
Anti-RhD immunoglobulin	To Rh +ve newborn of Rh -ve mother, administer within 72 hrs of delivery		300 μg	IM
Antisera antitoxins				
Tetanus antitoxin	Tetanus	Horse	Prophylaxis: 1500–3000 IU; Treatment: 50,000–1,00,000 IU	SC/IM
Gas gangrene antitoxin	Gas gangrene	Horse	Prophylaxis: 10,000 IU' Treatment: 30,000–75,000 IU	IV, IM, SC
Diphtheria antitoxin	Diphtheria	Horse	20,000–1,20,000 IU	IV, IM
Botulinum antitoxin	Post-exposure prophylaxis and treatment of botulism		10,000 IU	IV, IM
Anti-rabies serum	Can be used, if rabies Ig is not available	Horse	40 IU/kg	IM
Anti-snake venom polyvalent	Snake bite	Horse	20–30 mL as early as possible, repeat dose, if required	IV

Table 87.4 Vaccines for COVID-19

Vaccine Platforms	Manufacturer and Brand Name	Description
Messenger Ribonucleic acid (mRNA)	Comirnaty (Pfizer/BioNtech), Spikevax (Moderna)	mRNA vaccines induce human cells to produce spike protein of SARS-CoV-2. The spike protein triggers the immune system to develop a protective response, which protects against SARS-CoV-2 infection.
DNA vaccine	Zydus Cadila (ZyCoV-D)	ZyCoV-D is a DNA vaccine which comprises a plasmid DNA carrying spike-S gene of SARS-CoV-2 virus along with gene coding for signal peptide. This DNA vaccine induces antibody response including neutralizing antibodies against SARS-CoV-2.
Recombinant viral vector	Vaxzevria (Astra Zeneca) Covishield (Serum Institute of India) Janssen (Johnson & Johnson)	A modified virus (the viral vector), other than the virus causing COVID-19, is used to induce human cells to synthesize a part of the SARS-CoV-2 spike protein. The spike protein triggers the immune system to develop a protective response against SARS-CoV-2.
	Sputnik V (Dr Reddy's Laboratories Limited)	A combined vector vaccine, a heterologous recombinant adenovirus approach using Adenovirus 26 (Ad26) and Adenovirus 5 (Ad5) as vectors both of which carry the gene for SARS-CoV-2 spike protein. The reduction in the severity of COVID-19 and less hospitalization.
Inactivated virus	Coronavac (Sinovac) Sinopharm (Vero cell) Beijing Institute of Biological Products Covaxin (Bharat Biotech)	An inactivated vaccine consists of killed virus or particles that are recognized by the immune system to elicit an immune response.
Recombinant spike protein nanoparticle	Covovax (Novavax)	Subunit vaccines contain specific fragments of the SARS-CoV-2 spike protein, which have been carefully selected to produce combinations of these molecules likely to produce a strong and effective immune response.
	Convidecia (CanSino Biologic)	A genetically engineered vaccine with the replication-defective Adenovirus type 5 vector expressing the SARS-CoV-2 coronavirus spike protein.

CHAPTER 88 Common Stings & Bites

COMPETENCY PH1.52

DOG BITE

According to WHO, India is an endemic for rabies responsible for about 36% of the World's rabies death. About 30–60% rabies cases in India are children under 15 years of age. The rabies is caused by virus transmitted to humans via saliva, bite, lick on broken skin and scratch. Several symptoms of rabies are muscle pain, dizziness, fatigue, excessive salivation, high grade fever, muscle spasm, paralysis, aggression, irritability, dilated pupil, seizure, coma and death. Person at risk of rabies must be treated immediately if bitten by dog. *National Rabies Control Programme* was launched for implementation and focus on human health component after animal bite management. For uniformity of management, a guideline is published based on WHO recommendations.

After dog bite suturing of wound should be avoided initially. If required, it should be delayed. To prevent sepsis in wound, suitable antibiotic course is recommended.

POST-EXPOSURE PROPHYLAXIS

Type of exposure and management of dog bite is given in Table 88.1.

Rabies Immunoglobulin (RIG)

The anti-rabies serum of rabies immunoglobulin (RIG) provides passive immunity in the form of preformed antibodies. RIG binds to the rabies virus, which causes neutralization of virus and loss of infectivity. Two types of RIG are available:

1. ***Equine rabies immunoglobulin (ERIG)***: It is produced by hyperimmunization of horse. Currently produced and highly purified Fab fragment is used which has less risk of adverse effects like allergic reactions. Dose: 40 IU/kg body weight.
2. ***Human rabies immunoglobulins (HRIG)***: It is relatively free from allergic reactions. It has longer half-life and costly. Dose: 20 IU/kg body weight.

Table 88.1 Type of exposure and management of dog bite

Category	Type of exposure	Management
Category I exposure	Contact of intact skin with secretions of rabid animal	Immediately wash the exposed area with soap and apply antiseptic
Category II exposure	Mild abrasion without scratches or bleeding at site	Examine wound, immediately wash area with soap and water for 15 min thoroughly to remove local viral invasion. Let dry wound area and apply antiseptic like povidone iodine or alcohol to kill virus. Rabies vaccine is given.
Category III exposure	Contamination of mucus membrane with bites, saliva, scratches with bleeding, licks on scratched skin	Rabies vaccine, Treat wound as above. Rabies immunoglobulin to neutralize virus

Indication

Category III exposure. In immunocompromised patient, RIG is given to category I and II also.

Adverse Effects

Pain at injection site, anaphylaxis, serum sickness. Patient should be observed atleast 15 min after injection. RIG is administered only once as single dose, within 24 hrs after the exposure on day 0 along with anti-rabies vaccine. Other supportive therapy should be given. RIG is directly infiltered or injected into or around wound.

Anti-rabies Vaccine (Table 88.2)

Active immunization is achieved by administration of safe and effective cell culture vaccine (CCV) or purified duck embryo vaccine (PDEV).

Indication

Category II and III exposure irrespective of age and body weight same number of injections are required. RIG is administered to category I and category II immunocompromised individuals along with vaccine as discussed earlier.

Storage and Transport

In freeze-dried form, vaccine should be kept and transported. Temperature to be maintained 2–8°C and protected from sunlight. The lyophilised vaccine should be kept with diluent and to be used immediately prior to use.

Duration of Immunity

Protection ranges from 5 to 21 years after vaccination.

Pre-exposure Prophylaxis

In high-risk group like staff handling virus in laboratory, veterinarians, animal handlers, etc., should receive 0.1 mL intradermal vaccine on 0, 7, 21 days. *Adverse effects*: Pain at injection site, redness, itching, swelling, headache, nausea and dizziness.

BEE STING

Honey bee and wasps sting is common in India. Bee stings differ from other insect bite as toxin of sting is quite different.

Symptoms

- ***Mild local reaction***: Pain, tenderness, burning, itching, redness and swelling.
- ***Moderate local reaction***: Massive swelling at the sting site, severe redness, tenderness which lasts up to week without treatment.
- ***Severe allergic reaction***: Anaphylaxis, hypotension, respiratory distress, swelling of throat and tongues fainting and unconscious.

Management

- ***For minor reaction***: Wash the area with soap and water and cold compression.
- ***For moderate reaction***: Remove the sting quickly by scraping with fingernails, if it is still in the skin. Sting can release remaining venom in blood which can worsen symptoms. Wash thoroughly the affected part with soap and water. Apply a cold compression for 20 min to reduce swelling.

Table 88.2 Dosing schedule of Anti-rabies vaccine*

Route	Dosing schedule	Cost
Intradermal*	0, 3, 7, 28 days. Vaccine to be administered at two sites: 0.1 mL per site over 1 inch above insertion of deltoid at both sites.	Cheap, covers wide range of PEP available and available in large quantity.
Intramuscular	0, 3, 7, 14 and 28 days. 0.5–1 mL is administered into the deltoid in adults and anterolateral aspect of thigh in infants and children.	Costly

*According to National Rabies Control Programme 2021

- ***NSAID like ibuprofen or acetaminophen*** is used to relieve pain and inflammation. If sting is on arm or leg, elevate to reduce edema. Apply corticosteroid cream (e.g., hydrocortisone) 3 times a day or calamine lotion to reduce redness & itching.
- ***For severe reaction***: In emergency treatment of anaphylactic reaction, epinephrine (adrenaline) is administered i.v. along with antihistaminics, salbutamol and hydrocortisone.

SCORPION STING

Scorpion sting is common in tropical and subtropical regions like India. The mortality is high in rural areas due to nonavailability of medical facilities, delay in hospital admission and faith in village local healers. In farmers, scorpion sting is common. Various species of scorpion are red scorpion (*M. tamulus*) and black scorpion (*P. swammerdami*). Toxins like neurotoxin is most important, which interferes with neurotransmission and causes massive release of endogenous catecholamines. Other toxins are alpha toxin, beta toxins, iberiotoxin, charybdotoxin and others.

Symptoms

- ***Early***: Mild pain, burning, tingling, cold extremities, sweating.
- ***Local manifestations***: Severe pain, edema, redness, urticaria, fasciculation and spasm of muscles.
- ***Systemic***: Tachycardia or bradycardia, hyper- or hypotension, chest discomfort, anxiety, coma and convulsion in severe cases.

The venom of *M. tamulus* scorpion is neurotoxic. It delays recovery of Na^+ channel and causes autonomic Storm i.e., massive release of catecholamines into circulation leads to severe sympathetic stimulation. Cardiogenic shock, organ failure and death can occur.

Management

- Wash the site with soap and water thoroughly. For mild pain, application of ice packs over the site of sting. NSAID is given to relieve pain and inflammation. Opioid analgesic can be given to relieve pain, anxiety and apprehension.
- *Scorpion antivenom (SAV)*: It is infused i.v. after dilution in normal saline. Early use of scorpion antivenom and prazosin improves recovery. It blocks various effects of toxins circulating in blood. Allergic reactions are common after administration of SAV. Adrenaline is administered for anaphylactic shock. *Dose of SAV*: 30 mL (3 vials) of reconstituted SAV infused I.V. slowly over 30 min after dilution in 100 mL saline. Supplemental dose can be administered after 6 hrs.
- Oxygen inhalation should be started to prevent hypoxia.
- Prazosin (selective α_1-blocker) prevents risk of pulmonary edema via reducing effects of excessive catecholamines. It reduces mortality significantly if given early. *Dose*: 5 mg in adults, 0.25 mg in children every 3 hrs.
- Convulsion can be controlled by i.v. diazepam. It relieves muscle spasm also.
- For vomiting, ondansetron or metoclopramide is given.
  To prevent secondary infection, antibiotics can be given in combination. If required. Tetanus toxoid injection is given i.m.
- Intravenous fluid should be administered to correct dehydration. Blood pressure should be measured regularly.
- Inotropic drug like dobutamine is effective to correct hypotension due to cardiogenic shock.

SNAKE BITE

Vipers, Kraits and Cobras are common poisonous snakes in India. According to WHO, it is estimated that about 5 million snake bite occurs every year. Out of which 81,000–1,38,000 deaths occur. Snake bite envenoming causes many amputations and other permanent disabilities. Snake venoms are a complex mixture of enzymes, various proteins, lipids, amines and nucleosides. *Composition*: Venom contains enzymes like phosphodiesterase, heparinase, metalloproteinase, hyaluronidase, paraoxonases, etc. Other toxins are three finger toxins, C-type lectins, disintegrins, myotoxins, etc. The Krait venom contains β-bungarotoxin which attacks the presynaptic terminal at the neuromuscular junction leads to release of ACh followed by flaccid paralysis.

Signs and Symptoms

- ***Viper bite (haematotoxic)***: Local swelling, bleeding, blister formation, discolouration, bleeding from gums, haematuria, disseminated intravascular coagulant on.
- ***Elapid bite (neurotoxic; Krait, Cobra)***: Local pain, burning, swelling, bleeding, blisters, local necrosis. Other symptoms are headache, vomiting, unconsciousness, fixed eyes in central position, convulsion and paralysis.
- ***Sea snakes (myotoxic)***: Pain, swelling, muscle pain, liver and kidney dysfunction.

First Aid Management

- Reassure the patient who is very anxious that most snake bites are nonvenomous.
- Immobilize the affected limb using splint or sling which should be not too tight.
- Avoid any procedure or application on the bitten wound, as it may increase absorption of venom.
- *Pressure immobilization method*: Elastic, crape bandage is bound firmly around entire bitten limb starting distally to proximally. Compression bandage should not be released until the patient gets admission in hospital and anti-snake venom is administered.
- *Treatment of elevated part*: Elevate the bitten limb to hasten reabsorption of fluid, prophylactic antibiotics should be started.
  Debridement of necrotic tissues should be done.

Anti-snake Venom (ASV)

Anti-snake Venom is immunoglobulin (Fab fragment of IgG) purified from the serum or plasma. Polyvalent ASV can neutralize the venom of several species of snakes.

Dose of Antivenom

1 cc of ASC can neutralize 0.60 mg of Russel Viper and Cobra venom and 0.45 mg of Saw scaled viper and Krait venom. For mild envenomation: 3–5 vials, moderate: 5–10 vials and severe: 10–20 vials are administered.

Indications of ASV

Excessive bleeding, neurotoxic signs, cardiovascular abnormalities like hypotension, shock, acute renal failure and severe local edema.

Administration of ASV

Liquid ASV is diluted in 5–10 mL of isotonic fluid per kg body weight (200–500 mL). It should be infused at a constant rate over 1 hr. Children and pregnant females should receive the same dosage as adults.

Observation of Response to ASV

Hypersensitivity reactions like anaphylactic shock can occur. Adrenaline should be kept ready before injection of ASV. Symptoms of snake bite like bleeding, nausea, pain and hypotension disappear gradually.

Other Measures

- Investigations like whole blood clotting test, platelet count, WBC count, biochemical abnormalities, urine examination, ECG should be done after hospital admission.
- To relieve pain, paracetamol or tramadol can be given.
- Area of bite should be cleaned with antiseptic like povidone iodine.
- To relieve neuromuscular blockade, neostigmine is administered with atropine.
- 'Do not': Do not apply ice or heat on wound. Do not apply bandage and tourniquet. Do not cut the wound. Do not inject ASV intramuscularly (slow absorption) or locally on the wound directly (painful).
- Give normal saline 0.5% and then infuse dopamine 0.2–0.5 mg/min if BP is reduced.
- To prevent wound infection, ceftriaxone or cefpodoxime + gentamicin should be infused.
- Treatment of coagulopathy: Fresh blood or fresh frozen plasma can be infused.
- *Neostigmine and atropine for Cobra bite*: The cobra venom is a neurotoxic. Neostigmine (anticholinesterase) is administered with atropine (to prevent muscarinic actions). *Dose*: Initially, give atropine 0.6 mg (10 μg/kg) then neostigmine 1.5 mg (30–50 μg/mL). The dose can be given every 30 mins till ptosis is reversed i.e., weakness of muscles is reduced.

  For Krait venom, paralysis can be reduced by slow I.V. administration of 5–10 mL (10%) calcium gluconate.

CHAPTER 89 Pesticides, Food Adulterants, Pollutants and Insect Repellents

COMPETENCY PH1.51

PESTICIDES

Pesticides are compounds which inhibit growth or kill any pest. The pest can be insects, rodents, plant pathogens, weeds, etc. Pesticides, the term includes various insecticides, herbicides, fungicides and rodenticides. Pesticides are toxic to living organisms, including humans and animals. Hence, it is necessary to use it cautiously, keep out of reach from children and dispose safely.

INSECTICIDES

Insecticide is any toxic substance that is used to kill insects. Such substances are used primarily to control pests that infest cultivated plants or to eliminate disease-carrying insects in specific areas.

Classification of Insecticides

1. **Organophosphates**: Malathion, Diazinon (TIK-20), Chlorpyriphos, Dimethoate, Dichlorvos.
2. **Carbamates**: Propoxur, Carbaryl, Aldicarb.
3. **Pyrethroids**: Cyhalothrin, Allethrin, Deltamethrin, Cypermethrin.
4. **Chlorinated hydrocarbons**: Lindane, DDT (Dichlorodiphenyl trichloroethane). (Table 89.1)

Organophosphates

Organophosphate pesticides are widely used and are one of the broad-spectrum pesticides, which control a wide range of pests. Organophosphates are irreversible inhibitor of acetylcholinesterase enzyme, so excess acetylcholine in synapse causes rapid twitching of muscles, paralysis and death. Organophosphate compounds include parathion, malathion and diazinon.

Carbamates

Carbamates are reversible inhibitor of acetylcholinesterase enzyme. Examples: Carbaryl, aldicarb, propoxur and aminocarb.

Organochlorine

Organochlorine insecticides can disrupt nervous system of the insects leading to convulsions and paralysis followed by death. Most commonly used organochlorines are DDT and lindane.

DDT is a colourless, tasteless and odourless crystalline chemical compound. In insects, DDT opens voltage-sensitive sodium ion channels in neurons.

Table 89.1 WHO classifications of pesticides

WHO class	Toxicity level	LD50 for the rat (mg/kg) oral	Examples
Class Ia	Extremely hazardous	<5	Parathion
Class Ib	Highly hazardous	5–50	Eldrin
Class II	Moderately hazardous	50–200	DDT
Class III	Slightly hazardous	>2000	Malathion
Class IV	Unlikely to present acute hazards	≥5000	Carbetamide

Spontaneous depolarization of neurons may lead to spasms and eventual death. It also binds to picrotoxin binding site of $GABA_A$ receptors.

DDT is a persistent organic pollutant that is readily adsorbed to soils and sediments, which can act both as sinks and as long-term sources of exposure affecting organisms. DDT is toxic to a wide range of living organisms, including marine animals such as crayfish, daphnids, sea shrimp and many species of fish. In humans, DDT can cause nausea, vomiting, irritation, burning and watering from eyes and redness in mucous membranes, tremors and seizures. Resistant to DDT is common, insects with certain mutations in the sodium channel gene are resistant to DDT and similar insecticides.

Synthetic-Pyrethroid

Synthetic pyrethroid insecticides were introduced into widespread use for the control of insect pests and disease vectors. The insecticidal actions of pyrethroids depend on their ability to bind to and disrupt the voltage-gated sodium channels of insect nerves. Human sodium channels are less sensitive to synthetic pyrethroids. At higher concentrations, disruption of neurological activity is thought to contribute to their irreversible effects on insects. Various studies show that pyrethroid also affects voltage-gated calcium channels. Exposure to pyrethroids is usually harmless. Higher amount of contact may irritate the skin, watering and burning from eyes, nose. It also causes cough, dyspnoea and wheezing if inhaled. There is no specific antidote of pyrethroid. Treatment is usually symptomatic. Pyrethroids are harmful to marine lives like various fishes and lobsters. However, studies showed that they are non-carcinogenic.

Cypermethrin is one of the most used synthetic pyrethroid pesticides. Synthetic-pyrethroid pesticides are highly toxic to insects. They are used as insect repellents in household as mosquito coil, mats and spray. Acute exposure to this pesticide causes irritation of eyes, skin and respiratory mucosa. Chronic exposure may cause paraesthesia in industry workers.

Botanical Pesticides

Botanical pesticides include nicotine, rotenone and pyrethrum. Rotenone is derived from *Derris elliptica*. Exposure to rotenone can cause nausea, vomiting, dermatitis, conjunctivitis, pharyngitis and rhinitis.

- ***Pyrethrum***: It is derived from *Chrysanthamum* having esters of insecticides. CNS toxicity is common, causes convulsion and tetanic paralysis in insects.
- ***Nicotine*** analogues like neonicotinoids can be used to collapse bee colonies.

Health and Environmental Hazards

Pesticides enter the human body through skin via direct exposure, inhalation, dust, vapour containing pesticide or consumption of contaminated food and water. Further, pesticides are directly sprayed on fruits and vegetables and consumption of such contaminated food causes various health hazards.

Environmental Hazards

Pesticides can cause environmental hazards because pesticides in soil enters through water sediment from ground water into surface water. Drinking of such contaminated water causes various health hazards.

Acute Effects of Pesticides

Common routes are topical (skin), inhalation (lungs) and oral (mouth). After exposure to pesticide, acute harmful effects are seen. Symptoms are according to dose of pesticide exposure include irritation of the nose, eyes and skin, nausea, vomiting, inability to breathe, headache, excessive salivation, sweating, weakness, cough, thirst, abdominal cramps, rapid pulse, unconsciousness and death.

Chronic Effects

Exposure to pesticide over long period of time can cause various chronic complications like brain, renal and blood cancer, neurodegenerative diseases including Parkinson disease, Alzheimer disease, cardio-vascular disease including coronary artery disease, type-2 diabetes mellitus, reproductive disorders and birth defects.

HERBICIDES

Herbicides are mainly used to control undesired plants like destruction of weeds.

Types of Herbicides

- ***Selective herbicide (Diclofop-methyl, Atrazine)***: This chemical is formulated to be extremely potent to specific types of plants only, such as grass and broadleaf weeds. However, it is not harmful to other plant species.
- ***Nonselective herbicide (Glyphosate, Paraquat)*** also called *knockdown herbicides*. This variant is designed to eliminate a broad range of weeds and plants. It works either by contact or systemic mode of action.
- ***Systemic herbicides (Glyphosate)*** are absorbed and transported through the plant's vascular system, killing the entire plant.
- ***Contact herbicides (Paraquat, oxyfluorfen, diquat and bromoxynil)*** kill the part of the plant in contact with the chemical but the roots may survive and the plant may regrow.
- ***Residual herbicides*** remain active in the soil for an extended period of time till months.
- ***Non-residual herbicides***, such as paraquat and glyphosate have little or no soil activity and are quickly deactivated in the soil.

Amino-acid Inhibitors

Glyphosate is one of the most commonly used herbicide. It is absorbed in the leaves and roots of plants. It is commonly used for resistant variety of soya beans, corn and cotton. Exposure to these compounds causes skin and eye irritation, burning, esophageal erosions, aspiration pneumonia and kidney failure. *Imazethapyr* is usually applied to control weeds in soya beans, wheat and alfalfa. *Thifensulfuron* is commonly used to control weeds in small grains, corn and soya beans.

Photosynthesis Inhibitors

Atrazine and *cyanazine* can be applied to crops of corn, sorghum and *soya beans*.

Cell Division Inhibitors

Trifluralin is used to control weeds in crops of beans, cotton and peanuts.

Paraquat

It is a nonselective herbicide. It kills all types of plants and used to clear waste grounds. It can be sprayed on emerging weeds to kill grasses and weeds. Paraquat is toxic to humans (Category I) by the oral route and moderately toxic (Category II) through the skin. It is toxic to human beings and lethal to animals due to its redox activity, which produces superoxide anions.

It can cause bloody stool, lung edema, alveolitis, fibrosis and haematemesis. Some studies suggested that it can cause degenerative disease like Parkinson's disease. *Treatment*: There is no antidote of paraquat, but antioxidants, activated charcoal and cyclophosphamide can be administered. The treatment is usually symptomatic. Herbicide resistant weeds are grown and identified in fields after regular application.

Glyphosate

It is a broad-spectrum systemic herbicide and crop desiccant. It is an organophosphorus compound. Glyphosate is absorbed minimally through roots, and transported to growing parts. It inhibits a plant enzyme involved in the synthesis of three aromatic amino acids: tyrosine, tryptophan and phenylalanine. It is effective only on actively growing plants. Glyphosate can be applied in agricultural, residential and commercial settings using a wide range of application methods, including aerial sprays, ground broadcast sprayers of various types, shielded and hooded sprayers, wiper applicators. Agricultural uses include corn, cotton, canola, soybean, sugar beet, alfalfa, berry crops, brassica vegetables, leafy vegetables, legumes, etc. Non-agricultural uses include conservation land, pastures, rangeland, aquatic areas, forests, turf grass, etc.

Oral ingestion of the 40% formulation is toxic to humans, can cause dyspnoea, arrhythmia and shock. It is corrosive to throat, larynx, pharynx and esophagus leads to dysphagia and stricture.

Genetically modified crops: Genetic modification (GM) is a technology that involves inserting DNA into the genome of an organism. To produce a GM plant, new DNA is transferred into cells of a plant. They are resisitant to insects, pests and herbicides, e.g., genetically modified corn that are resistant to larval pests. They can grow in the prescence of glyphosate.

Chlorophenoxy Herbicides

Chlorophenoxy herbicides are used to control lean weed. Large dose can cause generalized hypotonia. It produces a human carcinogen dimethyl nitrosamine.

RODENTICIDES (RAT POISON)

Rodenticides are pesticides which kill rodents, commonly referred as '**rat poison**'. It kills rat, mice, woodchucks, beavers and voles. Examples: Warfarin, chlorphacinone, diphacinone, bromadiolone, zinc phosphide, difethialone, bromethalin, brodifacoum and strychnine. Warfarin is an anticoagulant which causes uncontrolled bleeding in rodents. It acts slowly; causes bleeding due to blockade of vitamin K dependent clotting factors. Death of rodent occurs after about 1 week or more due to excessive bleeding. For bait, it is lethal after single administration. Baits, nowadays are resistant to warfarin and termed as '***Superwarfarins***'. Rodenticide like *Bromethalin* causes muscle tremors, seizures and hyperexcitability in animals. *Strychnine* can cause involuntary muscle spasms in animals. Severe spasm can cause extreme extension of limbs and death. These are highly toxic for humans and must be out of reach from children and pets. *Treatment*: Vitamin K supplement if warfarin ingestion. Symptomatic management include mechanical ventilation, oxygen, infusion of dextrose or normal saline.

FUNGICIDES

Fungicides are one of the major groups of agricultural pesticides but quantities used are smaller than insecticides and herbicides.

a) *Organic sulfur fungicides* (Propineb, Thiram)
b) *Inorganic fungicides* (Copper sulfate)
c) *Natural fungicides* are α-Cadinol (present in essential oils of different plants), Citronella

Fungicide resistance is common after chronic application. Several mechanisms of resistance have been identified. The evolution of fungicide resistance can be gradual or sudden.

LARVICIDES

A larvicide is an insecticide that is specifically targeted against the larval life stage of an insect. Their most common use is against mosquitoes. *Methoprene* is an insect growth regulator agent which inhibits growth cycle of insect larvae. Larvicides are usually applied to larger bodies of water in the form of time-release formulations that can last from 1 to 5 months. *Temephos*, marketed as Abate which prevents mosquito larvae and used to treat water infested with insects including mosquito.

FOOD ADULTERANTS

Food is our basic need for life but sometimes nutritional value of food is affected by the addition of different adulterants. Food adulteration has been a concern since long. The Food Safety and Standards Act (2006) of India defines *food adulterant* as "Any material which is or could be employed for making food unsafe or substandard or misbranded or containing extraneous matter." Adulterant food consumption in our daily life without our knowledge is unsafe and unhygienic. Adulteration in food items can reduce its nutritional value and can cause various health hazards. (Table 89.2)

Types of Food Adulteration

a) ***Intended Adulterants***: Intentional adulteration of food is common in India. *Example*: Addition of various chemicals and urea. To increase volume of food, starch, cane sugar, flour, water, skim milk, vegetable oil, sand, chalk powder, stone and molasses are added. Inclusion of these substances is difficult to detect. Consumption of contaminated food is harmful to the human body.
b) ***Metallic Contamination***: Addition of metals in food like arsenic in pesticides and lead in water are responsible for health hazards. These metals can cause cancer, liver or kidney dysfunction.
c) ***Accidental Adulterants***: Various causes of accidental adulterants are unhygienic practice, contamination with pesticide residues, presence of larvae of parasite in foods, etc. Accidental metallic contamination can occur by arsenic, lead and mercury.

Human health is highly sensitive to these food adulterants either consumed acutely or chronically. Generalized hazardous effects on body include diarrhoea, abdominal pain, nausea, vomiting, burning of eyes, headache, anaemia and serious diseases like cancer.

Table 89.2 Adulterant and their harmful effects

Food	Adulterant	Harmful effects
Milk	Water, starch powder, skim milk	Abdominal disorders like diarrhoea
Ice cream	Starch, rice powder	Abdominal disorders
Butter, ghee	Vegetable oil, starch powder, banana	Diarrhoea
Sugar	Chalk powder, washing soda, urea	Abdominal disorders
Tea	Black/Bengal gram dal husk with artificial colouring agent	Liver disorders
Coffee powder	Roasted barley powder, tamarind seeds	Diarrhoea
Jaggery	Chalk powder, washing soda	Vomiting, diarrhoea
Honey	Molasses, cane sugar	Abdominal disorders
Common salt	White powdered stone, chalk	Abdominal disorders like diarrhoea
Turmeric powder	Pesticide residues, sawdust, dyes, chalk dust, lead, arsenic	Cancer and GIT disorders
Edible oil	Mineral oil, castor oil, artificial colours	Allergy, gall bladder cancer, stroke, high LDL level, cardiac arrest
Pepper	Dry papaya seeds, blackberries	Allergy
Pulses	Dyes, lead compound	Abdominal disorders
Grains	Weed seeds, dust, stones, mixing with old or damaged grain	Abdominal and liver disorders
Cumin seeds	Sawdust, charcoal dust, coloured grass seeds	Abdominal disorders
Vegetables	Malachite green, dyes, copper sulphate, wax	Carcinogenic

Other methods of food adulteration are artificial ripening of fruits, misbranding and using decomposed food.

Reasons for Adulteration

- Better selling
- Financial gain
- Lack in proper hygienic in processing, storage, transportation and ignorance.
- To increase food volume or weight.
- To add bulk and to darken the colour of food like yellow for turmeric.

Other specific food adulterations are the addition of chemicals and colours in fruits and vegetables. These are highly poisonous for health, e.g., calcium carbide is used in mangoes, bananas, copper sulphate is added to ripen some fruits faster, oxytocin (a hormone) is used for faster growth of watermelon. In children and elderly, these chemicals cause nausea, vomiting, diarrhoea and kidney failure.

Epidemic Dropsy (Argemone Poisoning)

Epidemic dropsy is a form of edema of extremities due to poisoning by *Argemone mexicana.*

Use of edible oils adulterated with *Argemone mexicana* seed oil leads to argemone poisoning. Sanguinarine and dihydrosanguinarine are two major toxic alkaloids of argemone oil, which cause widespread capillary dilatation, proliferation and increased capillary permeability. *Treatment*: Withdrawal of the contaminated cooking oil. Supplements of antioxidants, vitamins like B, C and E and calcium can be given. Protein-rich diet and bed rest is recommended. Oral corticosteroids and antihistamines can be used.

Lathyrism

Consumption of *Lathyrus sativus* can cause lathyrism. A pulse 'Khesari Dal or grass pea' can cause lathyrism. If Khesari Dal mixed with Arhar dal or other pulses and consumed for 3–6 months or more can cause lathyrism.

a) *Neurolathyrism*: The responsible neurotoxin is β-N-oxalylamino-l-alanine (BOAA), an AMPA glutamate receptor agonist. Increased levels of reactive oxygen species (ROS) and impairment of the mitochondrial phosphorylation chain. It causes degeneration of spinal motor tracts followed by sclerosis causing paralysis of both legs.
b) *Osteolathyrism* affects the bones and connecting tissues, instead of the nervous system.
c) *Angiolathyrism* affects the collagen in blood capillaries. High dose of vitamin C may have some beneficial effects against lathyrism in early stages.

Ergotism

It occurs due to the ingestion of the alkaloids produced by the *Claviceps purpurea* fungus which grows on rye, pearl millet (Bajra) and other grains. It is also known as *ergot poisoning* and *Saint Anthony's fire*. It is common in animals like cattles. *Symptoms of egotism*: Convulsive symptoms are painful seizures and spasms, diarrhoea, paraesthesia, itching, mental effects including mania or psychosis. Other vascular complications are dry gangrene due to severe vasoconstriction induced by the ergotamine. The ergotism can be prevented by discarding the infested grains.

Aflatoxicosis

It is caused by the fungus *Aspergillus favus* which grows in soil, decaying vegetation and on food like hay, sweetcorn, wheat, millet and cassava. The fungus grows on these seeds during storage under dirty and humid conditions like rainy season and in coastal areas. *Signs and symptoms* are nausea, vomiting, jaundice, anorexia, edema and liver enlargement.

Prevention

1. Grains, pulses and other food products should be cleaned and stored.
2. Before use, wash vegetables and fruits thoroughly in running water.
3. Avoid dark coloured and junk foods.
4. Check seal before buying the food products like milk, butter, oil, etc.
5. Seal on product should contain licence number, list of ingredients, manufacturer details and expiry date.

Safety Measures at Level of Producers and Manufacturers

Farmers should avoid food contamination in crops before and after harvest and they should follow Good Agricultural Practices (GAP) including pest management and reducing chemical usage. Other measures are regular follow up by health authorities for acceptable quality food standards, labelling and strict action against sources of food contamination.

Role of Government Agencies

- ***Food Safety and Standards Authority of India (FSSAI)***: Food Safety and Standards Authority of India (FSSAI) is an autonomous body established under the Food Safety and Standards Act, 2006 (FSS Act).

  FSS Act, 2006 consolidates various acts and orders in various Ministries and Departments:
  - Prevention of Food Adulteration Act, 1954

- Fruit Products Order, 1955
- Meat Food Products Order, 1973
- Vegetable Oil Products (Control) Order, 1947
- Edible Oils Packaging (Regulation) Order 1988
- Milk and Milk Products Order, 1992

The FSSAI has under the Food Safety and Standards Act (2006) is responsible for regulating manufacture, storage, import and marketing of food. It is responsible for regulations to lay down the standards and guidelines of food safety.

- ***Indian Standards Institution (ISI) standards***: A producer who wants to adopt a quality standard for his product, has to obtain a license from the ISI under its marking scheme. Companies can obtain 'ISI' logo on their product. If any producer is found to be using the ISI mark fraudulently, he will be liable for punishment. Its main objective is to lay down quality standards for consumer and industrial goods.
- Market surveys should be conducted about presence of toxins in food which help to prevent intentional adulteration. The health authorities should be vigilant on such illegal activities. At the level of retail shops, regular food sampling and testing should be done.
- Recently, cold chain is being introduced in the food transport and supply system. National Food *Quality Control Board* is formed and *Ministry of Health and Family Welfare* in collaboration with *National Codex Committee* are working on all aspects of food adulteration.

ENVIRONMENTAL POLLUTION

The Environmental Protection Agency (EPA) defines pollution as "Any substances in water, air or soil that deranges the natural quantity of the environment can cause health hazards or impairs the usefulness of natural resources." Air pollution, water pollution and soil pollution are three major forms of environmental pollution.

Air Pollution (Table 89.2)

Air pollutant is explained as "any substance either chemical, biological or physical agent, which can affect the atmosphere." Several air pollutants are from natural and human activities (incineration, vehicles, fumes, emissions from power plant or emissions from industries). Major air pollutants are sulphur dioxide (SO_2), Particulate matter (PM10, PM2.5), Ozone (O_3), Carbon monoxide (CO) and Volatile organic compounds (VOCs).

Carbon Monoxide (CO)

Carbon monoxide (CO) binds to oxygen carrying site on haemoglobin, which reduces oxygen supply to the tissues and leads to hypoxia. ***Signs and symptoms***: Nausea, headache, confusion, loss of vision, tachycardia, tachypnea, vertigo and syncope. Further severe intoxication causes convulsion, coma, respiratory failure and death. In pregnancy, CO can cause birth defects and fetal death. Environmental hazard occurs when CO is oxidised to form CO_2 in the atmosphere, a greenhouse effect gas.

Treatment of intoxication: Patient must be detached from the source of CO exposure. Admit the patient, high flow oxygen should be started to treat hypoxia. If required, do mechanical ventilation. Further, treatment is given according to symptoms.

Sulfur Dioxide (SO_2)

Sulfur dioxide pollution is due to emission of sulphur containing fossil fuels mainly fuel oil and coal. Other sources of SO_2 are petroleum refining industry, electricity production and various heating systems. Diesel motor vehicles are also responsible for such emissions. It is a respiratory irritant gas. Sulfuric acid is generated when SO_2 in contact with moist membrane.

Signs and symptoms: Nonspecific symptoms like headache, cough, difficulty in breathing, irritation of eyes, skin, nose and throat. It may worsen respiratory diseases; it precipitates acute attack of bronchial asthma. Pulmonary edema can occur on chronic exposure.

Nitrogen Oxides (NO_2)

Sources: Automobile sector including heavy road traffic is mainly responsible for emission of NO_2. Others are fires, mining, agriculture, forestry and manufacturing industries.

Table 89.3 Health and environmental hazards of various air pollutants

Air pollutant	Source	Health hazards	Environmental hazards
Lead	Emissions from metal industry or other manufacturing industry	Lead is accumulated in body causes CNS and renal dysfunction especially in children (lead poisoning)	
Particulate matter (PM)	Particulate matter or particle pollution is a complex mixture of solid particles and liquid droplets found in the air. PM is made of particles that vary in size, composition and concentration. Examples: Emission from vehicles, industry, burning wood and incineration of waste. The particle diameter <10 µm (PM10; big particles) can stay in the air for minutes or hours, PM2.5 (fine particles) are lighter and stay in the air for days or weeks	PM10 causes nose and throat irritation, cough, bronchitis	Smoke and dust cause dirty or dark coloured surfaces and structures
Volatile organic compounds	Due to petroleum, chemical industries and transportation	Cancer, CNS dysfunction and developmental defects	Can combine with NO_2 to form O_3
Ozone (O_3)	From vehicular traffic, industrial boiler, refineries, chemical plants	Eye and respiratory tract irritation, severe coughing, shortness of breath, bronchitis, pneumonia, asthma	Damages plants and trees

Signs and symptoms: Irritation of eyes, nose, throat, cough with sputum and difficulty in breathing. It can cause pulmonary edema within 1–2 hrs and it precipitates Acute Respiratory Distress Syndrome (ARDS). Some patients develop chronic nonallergic asthma and bronchiolitis obliterans. Environmental hazards are common when NO_2 is oxidised in the atmosphere to nitric acid which is a major reason of acid rain.

Air Quality Index (AQI)

The National Air Quality Index (AQI) was launched in India in 2014 under the Swachh Bharat Abhiyan. It is composed of 8 pollutants: Carbon monoxide (CO), Ozone (O_3), Sulphur dioxide (SO_2), Nitric dioxide (NO_2), Ammonia (NH_3), Lead, PM 10 and PM 2.5. It measures the quality of air by transforming weighted values of individual pollution parameters into a single number, and graded into six categories namely Good, Satisfactory, Moderate, Poor, Severe and Hazardous.

WATER POLLUTION

Water pollution is caused by the emission of domestic or urban sewage, agricultural waste and industrial effluents into waterbodies. Nowadays, one of the main sources of water pollution is the waste material discharged by industrial units. The *major organic pollutants* are malathion, lindane, DDT and hexachlorocyclohexane (HCH). Various other pollutants are petroleum hydrocarbons, detergents, industrial effluent, organic content, suspended solids, ammonium-nitrogen, microbacteria, heavy metals, lead, cuprum, cadmium and pesticides. Water pollution causes several water borne diseases like amoebiasis, giardiasis, hookworm, ascariasis and typhoid. It can cause food poisoning and skin allergy. Contaminated water causes epigastric pain, diarrhoea, vomiting and hepatitis. Various tests are available to check water quality like *total suspended solids* (TSS) and *total dissolved solids* (TDS). Water pollution can be prevented by measures like affordable and easy treatment of industrial effluent and sewage, some persistent pesticides should be discontinued and special water storage should be created for waste water effluent.

Soil Pollution

Soil pollution is commonly due to dumping of large quantity of solid wastes, unused and rejected chemicals like calcium carbonate, magnesium sulphate, fly ashes, bottles, etc. Exposure to these hazardous substances cause irritation of the skin and eyes, difficulty in breathing, headache, nausea and behavioural abnormalities. Soil and water pollution cause death of fish and other marine lives.

Pharmaceutical Pollution

Sources: Discarded medication, unused drugs, medical containers and devices. Many pharmaceutical industries produce toxic effluent generated from machines and dump in river or soil can lead to many human and environmental hazards. The waste water generated from industries are solids, toxic biodegradable and non-degradable organic compounds. Traces of drugs are found in ground water and affects aquatic life.

INSECT REPELLENTS

Insect repellent (also termed as '**bug spray**') is a substance used to repel insects like mosquitoes, flies, ticks and other biting insects or arthropods. Insect repellents help to prevent and control outbreak like malaria, dengue fever, plague and other insect borne diseases.

Synthetic repellents are more effective and longer acting than 'natural' repellents. Various insect repellents include active ingredients like DEET (N,N-Diethyl-meta-toluamide), picaridin (icaridin), oil of lemon eucalyptus and ethyl butylacetylamino-propionate. Essential oil containing repellents have short duration of action, so less used.

Biopesticides

Biopesticides are biological substances that kill or damage microorganisms (microbial pesticides). They are obtained from organisms including bacteria, fungi and nematodes. It includes insect pheromones, IR535, chitosan and BT toxin from bacteria like *B. thuringiensis*.

Permethrin

Permethrin is an insecticide and also used to treat scabies and lice. It is applied topically as a cream or lotion. It can be applied directly on human skin (not mucosa) as spray or wipe.

As insecticide, it is used in agriculture to protect crops like wheat, cotton and alfalfa, to kill live parasites and to prevent insect attack of woollen products. It can be applied on cloths or impregnated cloth or mosquito nets.

The available or allowable concentration for DEET 5–40%, picaridin 5–20%, IR355 7.5–15% and permethrin 4–70%.

Protection time for DEET (5–12 hrs), Picaridin (2–8 hrs), IR55 (2–4 hrs) and permethrin (at least 2 weeks).

Side Effects

Mild topical side effects are rash and burning sensation. Excessive exposure can cause muscle weakness, salivation, nausea and shortness of breath. DEET can cause eye, skin and respiratory irritation, neurological dysfunction and seizures. Picaridin and oil of lemon eucalyptus can cause eye irritation. Specific instructions should be followed and used cautiously. Children are at higher risk for accidental exposure. So lowest concentration should be used for children. To prevent accidental eye contact or ingestion, they must be kept out of reach from children. Pregnant females should also take care to avoid exposure. DEET can damage plastic surfaces, eyeglass frames, rayon and varnished surfaces.

APPENDIX I Drugs to be Avoided During Pregnancy

Most clinicians would like to avoid use of drugs during pregnancy, if it is possible. Pre-existing and other medical problems occurring during pregnancy sometimes require continuation of the old drug or intiation of the new drug therapy. The FDA, in 1979, developed a classification system which groups drugs under **category A,B,C, D** and **X,** according to the degree of their potential risk of foetal teratogenicity during pregnancy. It has not been revised since then, despite introduction of a huge number of new drugs. With many drugs there is a paucity of human data that makes categorization difficult. Therefore, the drugs enlisted in Table A1.1 are those drugs which belong to **category D** or **X**.

Category D includes those drugs where studies, well controlled or observational, in pregnant women have demonstrated a risk to the foetus. *However, the benefits of therapy may outweigh the potential risks.*

Category X includes those drugs where studies, well controlled or observational, in animals or pregnant women, have demonstrated a positive evidence of foetal abnormalities. *The use of such drugs is contraindicated in women who are or may become pregnant.*

Table A1.1 Drugs to be Avoided During Pregnancy

A) Drugs Affecting Renal and Cardiovascular System	
• **Renin inhibitor** like Aliskiren	To be avoided in 2nd and 3rd trimesters
• **Diuretics** like amiloride, chlorothiazide, chlorthalidone, ethacrynic acid, furosemide, hydrochlorothiazide, indapamide, metolazone, polythiazide, spironolactone and triamterene.	All to be avoided in gestational hypertension
• **ACE inhibitors** like benazepril, captopril, cilazepril, enalapril, fosinopril, lisinopril, perindopril, quinapril, ramipril and trandolapril.	All to be avoided in 2nd and 3rd trimesters
• **Angiotensin receptor antagonists** like candesartan, eprosartan, irbesartan, losartan, olmesartan, telmisartan and valsartan.	All to be avoided during in 2nd and 3rd trimesters
• **β-Blockers (cardioselective and non-selective)** like atenolol, betaxolol, bisoprolol, carteolol, carvedilol, celiprolol, metoprolol, nadolol, oxprenolol, pindolol, propranolol, sotalo and timolol.	Atenolol should be avoided in all trimesters Others to be avoided during 2nd & 3rd trimesters

contd.

• **Antihyperlipidaemic agents** like atorvastatin, cerivastatin, fluvastatin, lovastatin, pitavastatin, pravastatin, rosuvastatin and simvastatin	To be avoided in all trimesters. All are Category-X drugs.
• **Fixed dose formulations of**:	
a) amlodipine + above cited ACE inhibitors.	To be avoided during 2nd and 3rd trimesters
b) amlodipine + above cited angiotensin receptor antagonists.	To be avoided during 2nd and 3rd trimesters
c) ezetimibe + above cited statins.	To be avoided in all trimesters
d) amlodipine + atorvastatin or lovastatin + nicotinic acid.	To be avoided in all trimesters
e) atenolol + chlorthalidone or bisoprolol + hydrochlorothiazide or metoprolol + hydrochlorothiazide.	To be avoided in 2nd and 3rd trimesters
f) hydrochlorothiazide in combination with ACE inhibitors like benazepril, captopril, enalapril, lisinopril or quinapril.	To be avoided in 2nd and 3rd trimesters
g) hydrochlorothiazide in combination with angiotensin receptor antagonists like candesartan, eprosartan, irbesartan, losartan, olmesartan, telmisartan or valsartan.	To be avoided in 2nd and 3rd trimesters
• **Antiarrhythmics** like amiodarone	To be avoided in all trimesters
• **Antiplatelet-aggregatory drugs** Aspirin + dipyridamole	To be avoided in all trimesters
• **Anticoagulants** like coumarin and warfarin	To be avoided in all trimesters. Both are Category-X drugs.
B) Drugs Affecting Central Nervous System	
• Alcohol	To be avoided in all trimesters (Fetal alcohol syndrome and spontaneous abortions).
• **Benzodiazepines** like alprazolam, chlordiazepoxide, clonazepam, chlorazepate, diazepam, estazolam, flunitrazepam, flurazepam, midazolam, oxazepam, temazepam and triazolam.	To be avoided in all trimesters. Estazolam, flurazepam, triazolam and temazepam belong to Category-X
• **Anticonvulsants** like carbamazepine, phenytoin, phenobarbitone, primidone and valproic acid.	To be avoided in all trimesters
• **Barbiturates and other sedative hypnotics** like amobarbital, meprobamate and pentobarbital.	To be avoided in all trimesters

contd.

• **Opioid analgesics** like alfentanil, butorphanol, codeine, fentanyl, hydrocodone, morphine, nalorphine, pentazocine, pethidine and sufentanil.	Avoid prolonged use or higher doses at term (respiratory depression or withdrawal syndrome)
• **Antidepressants and antimanic drugs** like lithium	To be avoided in all trimesters
• **Others**: Caffeine + ergotamine and ergotamine alone.	To be avoided in all trimesters. Category-X combination.
C) NSAIDs, Related Autacoids, Drugs for Gout and Rheumatoid arthritis	
Aspirin, celecoxib, diclofenac, diflunisal, etodolac, fenoprofen, flurbiprofen, ibuprofen, indomethacin, ketoprofen, ketorolac, leflunomide, mefenamic acid, meloxicam, methotrexate, mycophenolic acid, nabumetone, naproxen, nimesulide, oxaprozine, piroxicam, sulindac, tolmetin.	NSAIDs to be avoided in 3rd trimester or at term (premature closure of ductus). Leflunomide and methotrexate belong to Category-X, while mycophenolic acid to Category-D. These should be avoided in all trimesters.
• Colchicine	To be avoided in all trimesters
• Alprostadil, misoprostol, diclofenac + misoprostol.	To be avoided in all trimesters. All Category-X drugs.
• Sulfasalazine (for ulcerative colitis).	To be avoided near term.
D) Drugs Affecting Endocrine System	
• **Glucocorticoids** like betamethasone, cortisone, dexamethasone, hydrocortisone, prednisone, prednisolone and triamcinolone.	To be avoided during first trimester
• **Androgens** like nandrolone, oxandrolone, oxymetholone, stanozolol, methyltestosterone and testosterone. **Antiandrogen** like danazol.	To be avoided in all trimesters. All Category-X drugs
• **Estrogens** like dienestrol, diethylstilbesterol, estradiol, estriol, estrone, ethinyl estradiol and mestranol. **Selective estrogen receptor modulator** like clomiphene and raloxifene	To be avoided in all trimesters. All Category-X drugs.
• **Progestins** like hydroxy-progesterone, levonorgestrel, lynestrenol, medroxy-progesterone, megestrol, norethisterone, norgestrel and progesterone. **Antiprogestin** like mifepristone.	To be avoided in all trimesters. All Category-X drugs.
• **Combinations** of estrogens + methyltestosterone, ethinyl estradiol + levonorgestrel and ethinyl estradiol + norgesterol, etc.	To be avoided in all trimesters. All Category-X drugs

contd.

• **Gonadotrophins** like human chorionic gonadotrophin, follitropin alfa/beta, human menopausal gonadotrophin or menotrophin and urofollitropin (uFSH).	To be avoided in all trimesters. All Category-X drugs.
• **Antithyroid drugs** like carbimazole, methimazole and propylthiouracil. Also potassium iodide.	To be avoided in all trimesters
• **Drugs for osteoporosis** like pamidronic acid, raloxifene and zolendronic acid.	To be avoided in all trimesters. Raloxifen is a Category-X drug.
• **Uterine stimulants** like ergometrine, dihydroergotamine, ergotamine, and oxytocin.	To be avoided in all trimesters. All Category-X drugs.
E) Antibiotics and Antifungals	
Amikacin, chlortetracycline, clarithromycin, demeclocycline, doxycycline, erythromycin estolate, kanamycin, minocycline, netilmicin, oxytetracycline, streptomycin, tetracycline and tobramycin.	To be avoided in all trimesters.
• Sulfadiazine and cotrimoxazole.	To be avoided near term.
• Levofloxacin, lomefloxacin, norfloxacin, ofloxacin and sparfloxacin.	Contraindicated in first trimester.
• **Antifungals** like econazole and voriconazole	Econazole to be avoided in 1st trimester. Voriconazole to be avoided in all trimesters (Category-D drug)
F) Antiviral Drugs and Anti-HIV Drugs	
• Efavirenz and ribavirin.	To be avoided in all trimesters. Ribavirin is Category-X drug
• Combined formulations of efavirenz + emtricitabine + tenofovir.	To be avoided in all trimesters
G) Antiamoebic Drugs	
Metronidazole	Mutagenic from animal studies only. Best to be avoided in 1st trimester.
H) Immunosuppressants	
Azathioprine and temsirolimus.	To be avoided in all trimesters.
I) Vitamins	
• **Retinoids (Vit. A analogues)** like acitretin, bexarotene, etretinate, isotretinoin and tretinoin.	To be avoided in all trimesters. Except for tretinoin (Cat.D) all are Category-X drugs.
• **Vit. D derivatives** like calcifediol, calcitriol, cholecalciferol, ergocalciferol.	Category-D drugs in high doses

contd.

J) Anticancer Drugs (see also under section-C) Abarelix*, altretamine, anastrozol, azacitidine, bilcalutamide*, bleomycin, bortezomib, capecitabine, carboplatin, carmustine, cetrorelix*, chlorambucil, cisplatin, cladribine, cyclophosphamide, cytarabine, dasatinib, daunorubicin, docetaxel, doxorubicin, dutasteride*, erlotinib, estramustine*, etoposide, exemestane, finasteride*, floxuridine, fludarabine, 5-fluorouracil*, flutamide, fulvestrant, ganirelix*, gefitinib, gemcitabine, gemtuzumab, ozogamicin, goserelin*, histrelin*, hydroxurea, ibritumomab, idarubicin, ifosfamide, imatinib, irinotecan, ixabepilone, lenalidomide*, lapatinib, letrozole, leuprorelin*, lomustine, melphalan, mercaptopurine, mitoxantorne, nafarelin*, pemetrexed, paclitaxel, procarbazine, sunitinib, tamoxifen, teniposide, thalidomide*, thioguanine, thiotepa, topotecan, toremifene, triptorelin*, vinblastine, vincristine, vinorelbine, and vorinostat.	Ideally to be avoided in pregnancy, but can be used if benefits from use are acceptable despite the risk. Drugs marked '*' belong to Category-X; Others belong to Category-D.
K) Miscellaneous	
• Cigarette smoking, nicotine chewing or transdermal patch.	Intrauterine growth retardation, spontaneous abortions and perinatal complications.
• D-Penicillamine (for Cu poisoning and rheumatoid arthritis).	Category-D drug; to be avoided.
• Terpin hydrate in cough mixtures.	Category-D drug; avoid frequent or prolonged use.

APPENDIX II
Bioassay of Drugs

The quantitative estimation of drugs or of their active constituents can be done by:

- *Biological methods (bioassay)*
- Physico-chemical methods (e.g., by chromatographic, spectrophotometric, fluorimetric and mass spectrometric techniques)
- Radio-immunological methods, and by
- Microbiological methods.

BIOLOGICAL METHODS (BIOASSAY)

BIOASSAY means the measurement of the concentration or potency of a drug from the magnitude of its main biological effect. In this method, one of the main pharmacological effects of the drug under test is compared with that of the standard drug (or preparation) and their potency ratios are then compared quantitatively. For example:

a) The unknown preparation having acetylcholine like action is compared with standard solution of acetylcholine by measuring contractile responses on frog rectus abdominus muscle.

b) Analogously, histamine-like preparations are compared with histamine for their contractile responses on isolated guinea pig ileum.

The bioassay methods are usually applied:

a) To measure the pharmacological activity of new or chemically undefined substances;

b) To measure the concentration of known substance (e.g., acetylcholine, histamine, serotonin or catecholamine) in a tissue extract or body fluids;

c) To measure ED_{50} or LD_{50} of a drug (see Ch. 7 also);

d) For biological standardisation of drugs from natural sources which cannot be obtained in a chemically pure form, e.g., vasopressin, oxytocin, insulin and heparin.

PRINCIPLES OF BIOASSAY

a) The bioassay usually involves the comparison of the main pharmacological response of the unknown preparation with that of the standard. The best kind of standard, of course, is the pure substance; but at times it is often necessary to utilise the standardised preparations of hormones or natural products against which the unknown sample can be calibrated, even though the standard preparation used is not chemically pure.

b) The reference standard and the test sample should have similar pharmacological effects and should have the same mode of action, so that their log dose-response (LDR) curves run parallel and their potency ratios can be conveniently compared.

c) The test solution and the reference standard should be compared for their established pharmacological effect using a specified pharmacological technique, e.g., acetylcholine and histamine can be compared with their respective test samples for their contractile responses on frog rectus abdominus muscle or isolated guinea pig ileum (or tracheal ring chain preparation), respectively; adrenaline and its related test sample for the rise in blood pressure in dogs or cats, and so on. However, some exceptions can be made, e.g., insulin preparations should ideally be assayed by estimating blood sugar levels, but, for the sake of convenience, the most commonly used method is the comparison of hypoglycaemic convulsions in mice.

d) The methods selected should be reliable, sensitive, reproducible, and should minimise errors due to biological variations and methodology. Hence, the animals used should always be of the same species, sex and weight and if an isolated preparation is used, it should be sensitive. The number of animals should be large enough to permit statistical analysis and the experimental conditions should always be kept constant.

TYPES OF BIOASSAYS

Quantal Assays (direct end-point assay)

In this type of bioassay, the dose of the standard and that of the unknown which provides a predetermined "all or none" response is measured and then their potency ratios are compared. For example, digitalis induced "cardiac arrest" in guinea pigs or cats; insulin induced "hypoglycaemic convulsions" in mice; "head drop" assay for d-tubocurarine in rabbits and calculation of "LD_{50}" of drugs in mice or rats.

A simplified and arbitrary example can be given for the bioassay of digitalis by this method. The extract containing digitalis (standard or unknown) is infused into the vein of the anaesthetised cats at the rate of 1 ml/min till the heart stops and the blood pressure falls to zero level. The volume of the fluid passed into the vein (to produce this end-point) is noted for each animal. This is called as the *threshold dose*. Two series of experiments are done: one with the standard preparation and the other with test solution, using at least 10 cats in each series. The LDR curves for both the test drug and the standard are plotted between the cumulative percentage of the subjects showing cardiac arrest and the respective threshold doses (on log scale).

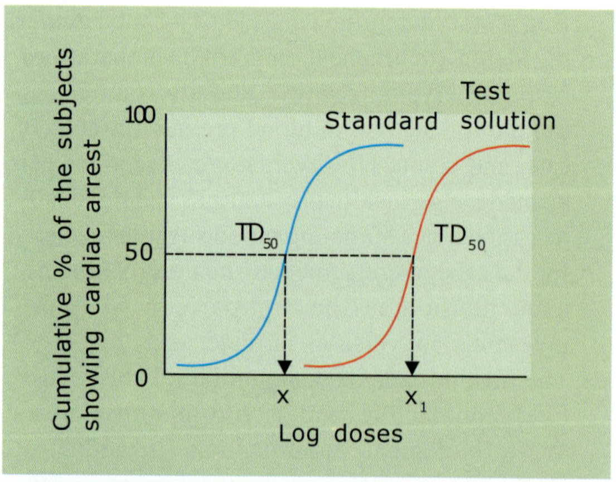

Fig AII.1 Calculation of Threshold Toxic Dose

TD_{50} (threshold dose producing cardiac arrest in 50% of the subjects) is then calculated for the standard (log x) and for the unknown (log x_1). The toxicity/potency ratios are then compared and strength of unknown calculated (Fig. AII.1) (for details, refer Ch.7).

Graded Response Assays

These are called as graded response assays because the responses to varying doses of a drug are graded and measured.

Here, the effect of the standard drug and of the unknown are measured repeatedly on the same tissue, e.g., bioassay of histamine on guinea pig ileum and bioassay of acetylcholine on frog rectus abdominus muscle. Any of the following methods can be employed:

i) **Matching Assay**
It is used when the test sample is too small. In this method, a concentration of the unknown which matches in its response with the known dose of the standard, is found by trial and error. From this, the potency ratio of the two can be approximately found and the strength of the unknown test solution can be calculated.

ii) **Bracketing Assay**
It is also used when the test sample is too small. The observed response with the test drug is bracketed between the one higher and one lower response of the standard. The strength of the unknown can be found by simple interpolation of this bracketed response on the dose axis.

iii) **Interpolation Method**
It is based on the principles of LDR curves discussed earlier (Ch. 7). In this method, the LDR curve of the standard drug is obtained first. Later two or three such responses of the unknown, which fall in between the linear portion of the LDR curve, are obtained by trial and error. Then, by interpolation of these responses at the dose axis, and taking the antilog (of x and x_1), the concentration of the unknown test solution can be found (Fig. AII.2).

All the three methods described above are not reliable because they do not take into account (a) changes in the sensitivity of the tissue

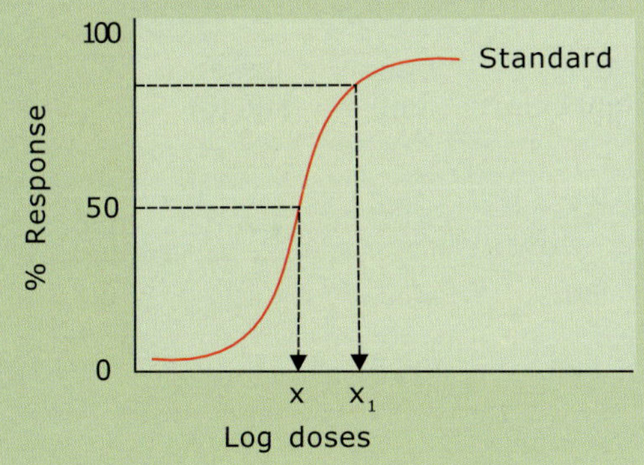

Fig AII.2 Graded Response Assay

with respect to time, (b) the timing of the doses, (c) variations in the mode of application of drugs, and are based on the application of a single dose (or few doses) and hence cannot be subjected to statistical evaluation.

iv) **Multiple Point Assays**

1. ***Three-point Assay (2 + 1 dose assay)***

This is a faster bioassay procedure having general utility. The steps are discussed by taking an example of bioassay of acetylcholine (ACh) in some tissue homogenate.

- First of all, a LDR curve is plotted with varying concentrations (doses) of the standard ACh solution. The doses are plotted in log scale (on X-axis).
- Two such doses (s_1 and s_2) are then selected whose responses (S_1 and S_2) lie in between the linear part of this LDR curve. Care should be observed in selecting these doses so that their concentrations are in simple ratio (e.g., 2, as in 1:2 or 2:4 ratio), since its log value has to be used in the calculations.
- Subsequently, a dose (t) of the test sample, which produces a response (T), in between S_1 and S_2, is found. Bioassay is then performed in four sets using three doses (s_1, s_2 and t), in a randomised fashion, in each set, e.g., using s_1, s_2, t; t, s_1, s_2; s_2, s_1, t and t, s_2, s_1 (one can observe from the latin square design shown in Fig. App. II.3, that none of the sequences is repeated, i.e., the doses have been randomised to reduce error).

s_1	s_2	t
t	s_1	s_2
s_2	s_1	t
t	s_2	s_1

Fig AII.3 Latin-Square Design for Three-Point Assay

- The respective mean responses (of these four sets) are then plotted on the graph paper (Fig. AII.4). The results have been arbitrarily tabulated as under (Table AII.1) and mathematically computed to find out the strength of the test solution.

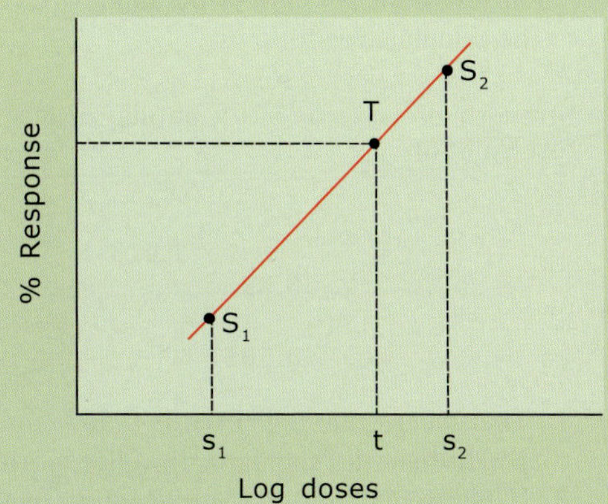

Fig AII.4 Plotting of LDR in Three-Point Assay

Table AII.1 Tabulation of Arbitrary Data for 3-Point Bioassay

Response	Height of contractions (mm) I	II	III	IV	Mean height (mm)	Dose (ml)	Dose ratio (d)
S_1	35	40	40	45	40	0.1	$\frac{s_2}{s_1} = \frac{0.2}{0.1}$
S_2	75	80	80	85	80	0.2	
T	55	60	60	65	60	0.25	= 2

From these data, log potency ratio (M) is calculated from the formula:

$$M = \frac{T - S_1}{S_2 - S_1} \times \log d$$

Where 'd' is the dose ratio.

Hence,

$$M = \frac{60 - 40}{80 - 40} \times \log 2$$

OR

$$M = \frac{20}{40} \times 0.301 = 0.150$$

From M, the strength of the unknown can be calculated as follows:

$$\text{Strength of test solution} = \frac{s_1}{t} \times \text{antilog of } M$$

$$= \frac{0.1}{0.25} \times 1.413$$

$$= 0.5652$$

That means, the unknown is 0.565 times potent than the standard. In other words, if the strength of the standard solution is 1 mg/ml, the test solution strength would be 0.565 mg/ml. The significance (P value) of the results or the fiducial limits of this estimate can, however, be evaluated statistically.

2. ***Four-point Assay (2+2 dose assay)***
This type of bioassay, though cumbersome, provides fairly accurate results. The steps with mathematical computation of results are discussed below, using a hypothetical example of bioassay of ACh obtained from a tissue homogenate.
   - First of all, the log dose-response curves for both the standard and the test solution are constructed as described above.
   - Then, two such doses of the standard (s_1 and s_2) and two such doses of the test solution (t_1 and t_2) are selected whose respective responses (S_1, S_2 and T_1, T_2) fall within the linear portion of their LDR curves, respectively. In selecting these doses care should be taken so that the responses due to the lower doses of the standard (S_1) and the test solution (T_1) and due to the higher doses of the standard (S_2) and the test solution (T_2) should be similar amongst themselves. Furthermore, the ratio between the higher and the lower doses of the standard (i.e., s_2/s_1) and of the test solution (i.e., t_2/t_1) should not only be the same but simpler too (e.g., $s_2/s_1 = t_2/t_1 = 2$, as in 1:2 or 2:4) because their log values are to be used in calculations.
   - Four sets of bioassay are then performed using 4 doses (s_1, s_2, t_1 and t_2), in a randomised fashion, in each set (i.e., 4 x 4= 16 doses). Each set could use doses in a sequence, like s_1, s_2, t_1, t_2; s_2, t_1, t_2, s_1; t_1, t_2, s_1, s_2; and t_2, s_1, s_2, t_1.

s_1	s_2	t_1	t_2
s_2	t_1	t_2	s_1
t_1	t_2	s_1	s_2
t_2	s_1	s_2	t_1

Fig AII.5 Latin Square Design for Four-Point Assay

From the latin square design (Fig. AII.5) it is obvious that none of these sequences is repeated, i.e., the doses have been properly randomised to reduce error. The respective mean responses (S_1, S_2, T_1 and T_2) are then plotted on the graph (Fig. AII.6 a,b). The results have been arbitrarily tabulated and computed as under (Table AII.2).

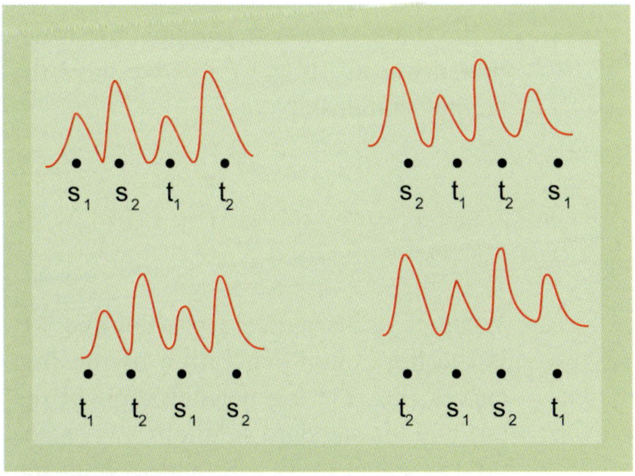

Fig AII.6a Dose Responses in Four-Point Assay

- Note that the log dose ratio (d) of t_1 and t_2 and of s_1 and s_2 are same.
- Lower doses, s_1 and t_1, are providing similar response. The same is true for higher doses s_2 and t_2.

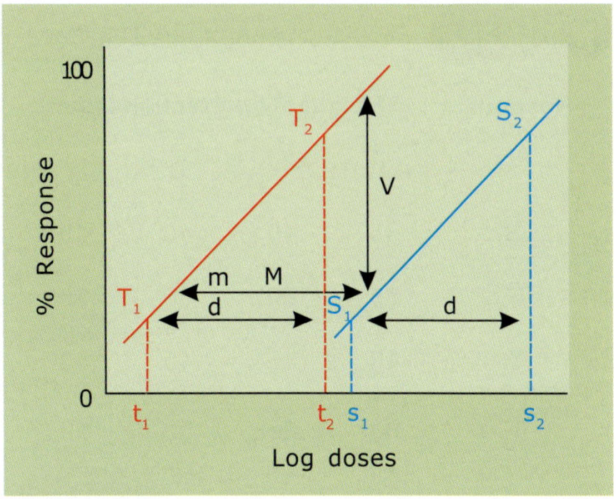

Fig AII.6b Plotting of Graphic Data in Four-Point Assay

- The horizontal separation M of the two curves represents the log potency ratio of the concentration of the test material and of the standard.

From these data (see Table AII.2), the log potency ratio (M) is calculated from the formula (for derivation of the formula, see below):

$$M = \frac{T_1 - S_1 + T_2 - S_2}{S_2 - S_1 + T_2 - T_1} \times \log d$$

Where 'd' is the dose ratio.
Hence,

$$M = \frac{45 - 40 + 85 - 80}{80 - 40 + 85 - 45} \times \log 2$$

$$= \frac{10}{80} \times 0.\ 301$$

$$= 0.037 \text{ (log potency ratio).}$$

From M, the strength of the unknown can be calculated as follows:

Table AII.2 Tabulation of Arbitrary Data for 4-Point Bioassay

Response	Height of contractions (mm)				Mean height (mm)	Dose (ml)	Dose ratio (d)
	I	II	III	IV			
S_1	35	40	40	45	40	0.1	$\frac{s_2}{s_1} = \frac{t_2}{t_1}$
S_2	75	80	80	85	80	0.2	
T_1	40	45	45	50	45	0.15	$\frac{0.2}{0.1} = \frac{0.3}{0.15}$
T_2	80	85	85	90	85	0.3	$= 2$

$$\text{Strength of test solution} = \frac{s_1}{t_1} \times \text{antilog of } M$$

$$= \frac{0.1}{0.15} \times 1.089$$

$$= 0.726 \text{ times the standard}$$

In other words, if the strength of the standard is 1 mg/ml, the strength of the test solution would be 0.726 mg/ml. The significance (P value) or the fiducial limits of the results can further be calculated using statistical analysis.

The figure (Fig. AII.6b) representing the graphic data of the 4-point assay is only a simplified presentation because in the situation illustrated therein, the test solution is clearly more active than the standard. Hence the question arises as to why a cumbersome mathematical procedure should be adopted when the horizontal separation 'M' (the log potency ratio) can be measured directly from the two curves. Certainly it can be done, but practically it is not; because the experimentally determined points S_1, S_2 and T_1, T_2 of the 4-point assay rarely make two perfectly parallel lines (because of biological variations). Hence for strict statistical analysis, it is necessary to show that the difference in the parallelism of the lines is not significant.

This is, therefore, done by calculating M, as follows:

If the slope of the two parallel lines is depicted by 'm' (Fig. AII.6b) we have the simple relationship

$$m = \frac{v}{M} \quad \text{or} \quad M = \frac{v}{m} \qquad \textbf{(1)}$$

Where 'v' is the vertical separation and 'M' is the horizontal separation of the two curves (i.e., the log potency ratio of the test and the standard solution). "v" is obviously equal to $T_1 - S_1$ and as both the lines are parallel it should be the same as $T_2 - S_2$. However, the better estimates of "v" can be obtained by taking the average of these two values.

$$\text{Hence } v = \frac{T_1 - S_1 + T_2 - S_2}{2}$$

"m" is the slope which is equal to

$$\frac{S_2 - S_1}{\log s_2 - s_1} \quad \text{or} \quad \frac{S_2 - S_1}{\log d}$$

where "d' is the dose ratio ($s_2:s_1$) in log scale.

"m" is also equal to:

$$\frac{T_2 - T_1}{\log t_2 - t_1} \quad \text{or} \quad \frac{T_2 - T_1}{\log d}$$

For more accuracy, the better estimate of 'm' can be obtained by taking the mean of these two values.

$$\text{Hence } m = \frac{S_2 - S_1 + T_2 - T_1}{2 \times \log d}$$

Substituting the values of 'v' and 'm' in equation (1) we get

$$M = \frac{T_1 - S_1 + T_2 - S_2}{2} \times \frac{\log d \times 2}{S_2 - S_1 + T_2 - T_1}$$

$$M = \frac{T_1 - S_1 + T_2 - S_2}{S_2 - S_1 + T_2 - T_1} \times \log d$$

Taking the antilog of the value of M, thus obtained, would provide the potency ratio of the unknown and the standard.

Again, the volume of the test and the standard solution, used in the 4-point assay, need not in fact be the same although it is ideally supposed that the ratio of the larger to the smaller dose of test solution should be the same as that of the standard solution. In case, if the volumes of the test and of the standard solution are not the same, the calculation of M given above must be modified by multiplying the term on the right by the factor s_1/t_1 (or by s_2/t_2, which is the same). Hence precisely speaking 'M' which is calculated by the following modified formula, provides the potency ratio directly:

$$M = \frac{s_1}{t_1} \times \text{antilog} \frac{T_1 - S_1 + T_2 - S_2}{S_2 - S_1 + T_2 - T_1} \times \log d$$

3. ***Six-point Assay (3 + 3 dose assay)***

The reliability of this bioassay is excellent but it is too time consuming, and hence lesser in use. It differs from the 4-point assay (2+2 dose assay) in the sense that here three concentrations of the standard and 3 concentrations of the test substance are used in six sets of experiments using six doses in each set (i.e., 6 x 6 = 36 doses) in the randomised fashion as discussed above.

BIBLIOGRAPHY

1. Brunton LL, Chabner BA, Knollmann BC, Eds. *Goodman and Gilman's: The Pharmacological Basis of Therapeutics*, 14th ed. NY, USA: McGraw Hill; 2022.
2. Papadakis MA, McPhee SJ, Rabow MW, Eds. *Current Medical Diagnosis and Treatment*, 55th ed. NY, USA: Lange Medical Books, McGraw Hill Education; 2016.
3. Whalen K, Finkel R, Panavelil TA, Eds. *Lippincott Illustrated Reviews: Pharmacology*, 7th ed. Philadelphia, USA: Wolter Kluwer; 2018.
4. Male D, Brostoff J, Roth DB, Roitt I. *Immunology*, 7th ed. Philadelphia, USA: Elsevier Mosby; 2007.
5. Kasper DL, Braunwald E, Fauci AS, Eds., et al. *Harrison's Principles of Internal Medicine, Vols. I and II*, 19th ed. NY, USA: McGraw Hill; 2015.
6. Golan DE, Armstrong EJ, Armstrong AW, Eds. *Principles of Pharmacology: The Pathophysiologic Basis of Drug Therapy*, 4th ed. Philadelphia, USA: Wolter Kluwer; 2017 (Indian Reprint).
7. Satoskar RS, Bhandarker SD, Nirmala NR. *Pharmacology and Pharmacotherapeutics*, 26th ed. Mumbai, India: Popular Prakashan; 2020.
8. Katzung BG, Trevor AJ, Eds. *Basic and Clinical Pharmacology*, 15th ed. NY, USA: McGraw Hill Education; 2020 (Indian Reprint).
9. Shargel L, Mutnik AH, Souney PF, Swanson LN, Eds. *Comprehensive Pharmacy Review*, 7th ed. Philadelphia, USA: Lippincott Williams & Wilkins; 2010.
10. Rang HP, Ritter JM, Flower RJ, Henders G. *Rang and Dale's Pharmacology*, 9th ed. Philadelphia, USA: Elsevier Churchill Livingston; 2019.
11. Bennet PN, Brown MJ. *Clinical Pharmacology*, 11th ed. Philadelphia, USA: Churchill Livingston; 2012.
12. Tripathi KD. *Essentials of Medical Pharmacology*, 8th ed. New Delhi, India: Jaypee Brothers Medical Publishers; 2018.
13. Sweetman SC, Ed. *Martindale: The Complete Drug Reference*, 40th ed. London, UK: Pharmaceutical Press; 2020.
14. Satyanarayana U, Chakrapani U. *Biochemistry*, 6th ed. Kolkata, India: Books and Allied(P) Ltd; 2021.
15. Page C, Curtis M, Walker M, Hoffman B. Integrated Pharmacology, 3rd ed. Philadelphia, USA: Elsevier Mosby; 2006 (Indian reprint 2009).
16. Gerbino PP. *Remington: The Science and Practice of Pharmacy, Vol. I & II*, 21st ed. Philadelphia, USA: Lippincott Williams & Wilkins; 2006.
17. Tortora GJ, Derrickson B. *Principles of Anatomy and Physiology*, 15th ed. NY, USA: John Wiley & Sons, Inc.; 2016.
18. Brenner GM, Stevens CW. *Pharmacology*, 6th ed. NY, USA: Saunders Elsevier; 2022.
19. Walker BR, Colledge NR, Ralston SH, Penman ID, Eds. *Davidson's Principles and Practice of Medicine*, 24th ed. NY, USA: Churchill Livingstone; 2022.
20. Briggs GG, Freeman RK, Yaffe SJ. *Drugs in Pregnancy and Lactation*, 12th ed. Philadelphia, USA: Lippincott Williams; 2021.
21. *Drugs Facts and Comparisons*, 65th ed. St. Louis, USA: Published by Facts and Comparisons, Wolter Kluwer Health; 2017.
22. Minneman KP, Wecker J, Eds. *Brody's Human Pharmacology: Molecular to Clinical*, 6th Ed. Philadelphia, USA: Elsevier Mosby; 2018.
23. Dipiro JT, Talbert RL, Yee GC, Matzke GR, Wells BG, Posey LM, Eds. *Pharmacotherapy: A Pathophysiologic Approach*, 12th ed. NY, USA: McGraw Hill; 2022.
24. Craig CR, Stitzel RE, Eds. *Modern Pharmacology with Clinical Applications*, 6th ed. Philadelphia, USA: Lippincott Williams & Wilkins; 2004.
25. Walker R, Edward C. *Clinical Pharmacy and Therapeutics*, 4th ed. Philadelphia, USA: Churchill Livingston; 2008.
26. Wynn RL, Miller TF, Crossley HL, Eds. *Drug Information Hand Book for Dentistry*, 27th ed. OH, USA: Lexi Comp.; 2021.
27. van Boxtel CJ, Santoso B, Edwards IR, Eds. *Drug Benefits and Risks. International Text-Book of Pharmacology*, 2nd revised ed. NJ, USA: John Wiley Sons Inc.; 2008.
28. Campbell PN, Smith AD. Philadelphia, USA: *Biochemistry Illustrated*, 5th ed. Churchill Livingston; 2005.
29. Levinson WE, *Review of Microbiology and Immunology*, 16th ed. NY, USA: McGraw Hill Education; 2020.
30. A number of scientific medical journals and official sites of Drug Regulatory Bodies and health authorities constituted the consulting material, all of which cannot be enumerated; however, important once are mentioned: *Pharmacological Review*; *British Journal of Pharmacology/Clinical Pharmacology*; *European Journal of Pharmacology/Clinical Pharmacology; JPEP*; *TIPS*; *TIBS*; *TIIS*; *Brain Research*; *Psychopharmacology*; *Diabetes Research/Care*; *Epilepsy*; *Endocrinology*; *Australian Prescriber*; *NEJM*; *BMJ*; *Lancet*; A number of *Nature Review* in selected specialities; Official sites of *US-FDA*; *EMEA*; *Indian-FDA (DCGI)*; Several notifications of *Ministry of Health & Family Welfare, Govt. of India, New Delhi*.

INDEX

B

PRINCIPLES OF PHARMACOLOGY

PRINCIPLES OF PHARMACOLOGY

PRINCIPLES OF PHARMACOLOGY

PRINCIPLES OF PHARMACOLOGY

F

G

H

J

K

L

M

N

PRINCIPLES OF PHARMACOLOGY